EMERGENCY
EMERGENCY
EMERGENCY
EMERGENCY
EMERGENCY

FLINT'S EMERGENCY TREATMENT AND MANAGEMENT

SEVENTH EDITION

HARVEY D. CAIN, M.D., J.D.

Chief of Occupational Medicine and Rehabilitation
Permanente Medical Group and Kaiser Foundation Hospital
Sacramento, California

1985 W.B. SAUNDERS COMPANY
Philadelphia London Toronto Mexico City Rio de Janeiro
Sydney Tokyo Hong Kong

W. B. Saunders Company: West Washington Square
Philadelphia, PA 19105

Library of Congress Cataloging in Publication Data

Flint, Thomas, 1903–1977

Flint's Emergency treatment and management.

Includes index.

1. Emergency medicine. I. Cain, Harvey D., 1930–
II. Title. III. Title: Emergency treatment and management. [DNLM:
1. Emergencies. 2. Emergency medicine. WB 105 F625e]

RC86.7.F63 1985 616'.025 83–20393

ISBN 0–7216–2313–1

Listed here is the latest translated edition of this book together with the language of the translation and the publisher.

Greek (*3rd Edition*)—Asklepios, Athens, Greece

Spanish (*3rd Edition*)—Editorial Jims, Barcelona, Spain

Italian (*4th Edition*)—Piccin Editore, Padova, Italy

Flint's Emergency Treatment and Management ISBN 0-7216-2313-1

Last digit is the print number: 9 8 7 6 5 4 3 2 1

To
All stalwarts who in the time of another's urgent medical need come forth to offer the best of their time, talent and teaching

and

In Fondest Memory of
My Mother, Ruth D. Cain,

and

My Son, Norman J. Cain

Preface to the Seventh Edition

Coming into stride with the great interest in personal physical fitness are further benefits to the overall level of health throughout the nation being achieved by the ever-enlarging individual and community involvement in CPR training and preparedness for emergencies, including mass disasters. A correlation may exist between the former and the latter, since people are better able to appreciate the health needs of others when they understand their own. There is an increasing recognition both by the public and by public officials that emergency medical care is not an isolated component of medical care restricted to the hospital emergency ward but, rather, comprises a continuum of care that begins with the patient and extends to family members, friends and bystanders; progresses to contact with Emergency Medical Services (EMS)—governmental agencies that include fire, police and rescue units; incorporates the assistance, as needed, of organized volunteer groups; and finally, concludes with the provision of further care at qualified treatment centers.

Objectives and Use of this Handbook

The principal objective of this handbook remains to assist the emergency professional in providing a form of adequate "portal to portal" care (i.e., from scene, field or office to hospital), in order to stabilize the patient's condition and initiate early definitive care whenever feasible. Lengthy dissertations on all possible theories and solutions to problems are not feasible here; rather, the aim of this book has been to put into clear, concise and readily locatable form at least one current and workable solution to a wide variety of emergency situations.

The second objective and special challenge of this edition has been to present new valuable information that the increasingly widespread interest in emergency medicine is bringing forth while at the same time retaining the text's compact handbook dimensions.

Efforts to achieve the first objective have included the following: addition of 22 new experienced contributors, who joined the prior assembly of 50 contributors in providing input from their various specialized fields of knowledge; vigorous updating and revision of all sections; introduction of the five "ABC's" sections at the beginning of the book, to abet early management; addition of approximately 70 new figures and tables; and further incorporation of critically important ACLS data, including more details on IV cannulation for lifeline establishment.

In order to fulfill the second objective, the size of the book has been kept within desirable handbook dimensions while presenting an even greater breadth and depth of information by incorporating the following: new, more legible, space-saving print; format redesign with less empty space; reduction of illustration size to only that required for clear presentation of concepts; new high-quality paper which itself reduced the thickness of the book by about one-half inch; elimination of older, less important data (it can be just as noble to erase as to write!); and increased use of standard medical abbreviations throughout the text.

Regarding the last of these points, it is common knowledge that medical personnel writing in urgent situations must make copious use of abbreviations. A standardized list (in accordance with JCAH guidelines) of the most commonly used medical abbreviations is now presented in the Appendix. While an attempt has been made to write out the abbreviation each time it is first used in the text, the reader can always rapidly refer to this extensive list of Commonly Used Abbreviations and Symbols, which begins on page 759. Many concepts are more rapidly conveyed by means of abbreviations and symbols, in addition to which they are time-saving in everyday writing, are just as accurate when standardized and are space-saving in the text.

To aid in making certain data readily accessible, three sections of page tabs have been introduced. The first of these comprises the five ABC's chapters, which provide the initial data most frequently needed in emergency care situations; for easy location, an outline of the most commonly used emergency medications is found on the last four pages of this section. The second tabbed section contains the comprehensive Acute Poisoning chapter, and the third concerns medicolegal data.

A Note on DMSO

Although an estimated 20 million people use DMSO sporadically (and sometimes improperly) for relief of sequelae of acute soft tissue injuries (I have included DMSO in my personal first-aid kit for over 20 years, but rarely use it in chronic conditions), the medicolegal status of the product remains nearly unchanged since the last edition. DMSO is an FDA-approved medication for instillation into the bladder for treatment of interstitial cystitis; prescription by a physician of DMSO for any other use, although legal, constitutes unapproved use of an approved drug and carries with it a greater professional and medicolegal burden. Research and investigation continues.

Acknowledgments

I am indebted to experts in many disciplines and to many other people—too numerous to mention in all—for their excellent assistance with this seventh edition; some are listed in the list of reviewers and contributors. Again I wish to especially thank Larry Broadbridge, M.D., Diplomate of the American Board of Emergency Medicine and member of the Emergency Department at the Sacramento Kaiser-Permanente Medical Center, for his careful review and suggestions concerning many sections of the manuscript. The work done on manuscript preparation by Ruth Burkholder, Nora Hoffman, Bess Flint, and particularly Janet Peyton and Joan Caron, my principal assistants, is most appreciated. The new illustrations were provided through the fine capabilities of artist Hal Pullum of the University of California Medical School at Davis. All members of my department have been most supportive during the book's revision, and their assistance is appreciated. Finally, I wish to thank the entire publishing staff who worked on this edition at W. B. Saunders Company, and foremost Carroll Cann, Senior Medical Editor; Erika Shapiro, Copy Editor; and Bill Donnelly, Designer, who created the new format for the book and designed the book cover. As always, my children—Tom, Phillip, Lori and Harvey—have served as a source of inspiration.

HARVEY D. CAIN

Preface to the First Edition

Many excellent texts are available covering first aid procedures and surgical and medical care in acute conditions. The following pages, however, have a much more limited objective—the presentation of the treatment and management of the patient by the Emergency Physician from first examination until disposition for definitive treatment can be arranged. To borrow a phrase from current labor relations, I have endeavored to outline *in a rapidly available form* "portal-to-portal" care in emergency situations.

The term "Emergency Physician" has been used throughout this book to designate the physician in charge of the patient in the emergency room, department, or private office. In large hospitals this physician may be on a full-time basis; in smaller units he may have numerous other duties, or be on part-time emergency call. Too often he is an intern, resident, or general practitioner of very limited experience in the management and treatment of acute conditions. To all these physicians whose contribution to the welfare of the patient is often overshadowed by a spectacular surgical procedure or a brilliant medical diagnosis, I am dedicating this book with the hope that the information herein contained may be of some assistance to them in fulfilling their very great, and often unrecognized, responsibilities.

"Emergency Care" is used in this book in the sense of the examination, treatment, and disposition of a person who has developed or sustained an unforeseen condition which is believed to call for prompt action. Examination may disclose no urgent or pressing need for treatment, and reassurance of the patient or his family may be all that is necessary. On the other hand, prompt and proper handling of the case may result in saving a life, preventing a long illness, or preserving maximum function.

In the first section are grouped some important generally applicable miscellaneous medical procedures. Administrative medicolegal and clerical principles and procedures which I have found to be of value in the operation of an efficient emergency service are covered in the third section. Since, by the nature of the cases which he is called upon to handle, the physician treating emergencies is especially vulnerable to legal action, the medicolegal aspects have been outlined in considerable detail. The underlying legal principles used as the basis for the medicolegal points involved are widely accepted, although minor variations may occur in some localities.

In order to facilitate rapid reference all conditions covered in the second section are listed alphabetically, and cross references are indicated. Although in some instances the most important diagnostic points have been given, I have made no attempt to cover this aspect fully. The methods of treatment suggested are *not necessarily the only proper therapeutic methods,* but they are based upon several years of experience in the handling of a large volume of emergency cases as well as upon accepted methods of emergency care. The drugs mentioned are those available in any well equipped emergency room or office. The dosages given are for adults unless otherwise specified and should, of course, be modified for infants, children, or elderly persons. Whenever the use of Plazmoid is recommended, dextran, PVP (polyvinylpyrrolidone), serum albumin, or any of the other accepted plasma volume expanders can be substituted. If facilities for typing and cross matching are available the use of whole blood transfusions is even more desirable.

No attempt has been made to specify or suggest therapeutic measures after immediate emergency care with the exception of supportive therapy during ambulance transportation and occasional instructions to be carried out at home before receiving hospital or office treatment.

It will be noted that repetition and duplication occur rather frequently, particularly in the section covering *Poisoning, Acute* [Topic 49]. I believe that *for the purpose of quick reference* this repetition will be found to be of value.

The political and social unrest so prevalent throughout the world suggest the possibility that many physicians not familiar with emergency measures may be called upon to treat large numbers of serious civilian casualties. This possibility—remote though it may be—in my opinion justifies the presentation of this summary at this time.

I should like to express my thanks to Dr. E. M. MacKay for his encouragement, constructive criticism and guidance in the preparation of this book. I am also grateful to Dr. Glenn Lubeck for his suggestions on *Cardiac Emergencies* and to Dr. Arthur Michels for the section on *Shock*. The interpretation and clarification of the medicolegal problems by Mr. James French and Mr. C. H. Brandon have been invaluable. Finally, I wish to thank Miss Dernice Turkovich for her very great assistance in the preparation of the manuscript.

THOS. FLINT, JR.

Appreciative Acknowledgments To Reviewers and Contributors*

Timothy E. Albertson, M.D., Ph.D.
Medical Director, University of California Davis Regional Poison Center
Sacramento, California

Leslie A. Bard, M.D.
Chief, Ophthalmology Department

Douglas A. Benner, M.D.
Coordinator, Occupational Medicine
Northern California Kaiser Foundation Hospitals and Permanente Medical Group
Oakland, California

E. Richard Bollinger, E.M.T. (II)
Supervisor, Metropolitan Ambulance Co.
Sacramento, California

Jean A. Bollinger, R.N.
Supervisor, Emergency Services

Louis K. Boswell, M.D.
Medical Hypnosis and Pain Management, Private Practice
Walnut Creek, California

Lawrence W. Broadbridge, M.D., F.A.C.E.P.
Emergency Department

David W. Chipman, M.D.
Division Chief, Gastroenterology

Louise L. Chiu, M.D., Pharm.D., J.D.
Assistant Physician-in-Chief, Obstetrics and Gynecology Department

Macey Dennis, M.D.
Department of Allergy and Pulmonary Medicine

Sgt. James Duckworth, E.M.T.(I)
E.M.T. Staff Coordinator
California Highway Patrol Academy
Bryte, California

William E. Durston, M.D.
Chief, Emergency Department
South Sacramento Kaiser-Permanente Medical Center

Thomas O. Evans, M.D.
Division Chief, Cardiology

Judith A. Fairchild, M.D.
Emergency Department

Jean-Guy Fecteau, M.D.
Surgery Department

Nihal N. Fernando, M.D.
Division Chief, Endocrinology

Douglas W. Freeman, M.D.
Chief, Department of Otolaryngology

Jose A. Ganel, M.D., F.A.C.P.
Division Chief, Nephrology

Gail L. Gilbert, R.N.
Assistant Supervisor, Emergency Services

Jack W. Graffin, M.D.
Dermatology Department

Stanley E. Hanna, E.M.T.(I)
Chief, Station 8,
Sacramento Fire Department

Edward W. Hearn, M.D.
Division Chief, Hematology

Charles C. Henriques, M.D.
Chief, Allergy Department

*Unless indicated otherwise, the specialists listed are in practice at the Kaiser-Permanente Medical Center, Sacramento, California.

Donald M. Hopkins, M.D.
Thoracic Surgery, Private Practice
Sacramento, California

Jacob Igra, M.D.
Neurology Department

James R. Johnson, M.D.
Psychiatry Department

Gregory A. Joy, M.D.
Orthopedic and Hand Surgery
Placerville, California

Albert J. Kahane, M.D.
Physician-in-Chief, Obstetrics
and Gynecology

Penny J. Karr, M.S.W., L.C.S.W.
Medical Social Worker,
Private Practice
Sacramento, California

Earl F. King, M.D.
General and Hand Surgery

Jit Seng Khoo, M.D.
Plastic Surgery, Private Practice
Carmichael, California

Peter B. Lau, M.D.
Emergency Department

Chinh T. Le, M.D.
Pediatrics Department

Alvin Lee, Pharm.D.
Pharmacy Department

Kenneth K. Lee, M.D.
Internal Medicine, Communicable
Diseases

Gregory M. Leo, M.D., F.A.C.E.P.
Emergency and Family Practice
Departments

Linda Leong, Pharm.D.
Pharmacy Department

Howard B. Liebgold, M.D.
Medical Director, Kaiser Foundation
Rehabilitation Center
Vallejo, California

Howard Maccabee, M.D., Ph.D.
Nuclear Medicine and Nuclear
Physicist
President, Doctors for Disaster
Preparedness
Walnut Creek, California

Gerard L. MacDonald, M.D.
Chief, Orthopedics Department

Robert C. Midgley, Jr., M.D.
Chief, Internal Medicine/
Gastroenterology
South Sacramento Kaiser
Permanente Medical Center

Carter G. Mosher, M.D.
Chief, Neurology Department

Gopal R. Nemana, M.D.
Cardiology Department

Donald C. Oliver, M.D.
Chief, Emergency Department

William M. Pelander, M.D.
Department of Surgery
Denver Kaiser-Permanente
Medical Center
Denver, Colorado

Glenn W. Pett, M.D.
Radiology Department

Susan H. Pieper
Director of Public Affairs

Jack Rozance, M.D.
Neurology Department

Findlay E. Russell, M.D., Ph.D.
Research Professor, Department of
Pharmacology/Toxicology
University of Arizona
Tucson, Arizona

Michael A. Russo, M.D.
Chief, Urology Department

Hartzell D. Schlecter
Medical Coordinator, Office of
Emergency Services, State of
California
Sacramento, California

Lawrence E. Sheridan, D.P.M.
Chief, Podiatry Department

Michael P. Sherman, M.D.
Assistant Professor,
Pediatric Department
Division of Neonatology
University of California School of Medicine
Los Angeles, California

Kirkham Smith, R.P.T.
Chief Physical Therapist

Roderick L. Smith, M.D.
Chief, Neurosurgery Department

Kenneth E. Stinson, R.R.T.
Chief Respiratory Therapist

Sajio Sumida, M.D.
Chief, Division of Cardiovascular and Medical Low Temperature Unit
The National Fukuoka Central Hospital
Fukuoka, Japan

Gerald R. Swafford, M.D.
Surgery Department

Robert L. Tilly, D.D.S.
Dentistry, Private Practice
Carmichael, California

Bill L. Vandermeer, M.D.
Chief, Anesthesiology Department
South Sacramento Kaiser Permanente Medical Center

George H. Williamson, J.D.
Deputy District Attorney
Sacramento County, California

Stuart C. Zeman, M.D.
Team Physician,
Oakland Invaders, U.S.F.L.
Chairman, Medical Advisory Board, U.S.F.L.
Orthopedic Surgery and Sports Medicine
Private Practice, Berkeley, California

TABLE OF CONTENTS

Find immediately inside front cover for convenience and quick reference.

EMERGENCY TELEPHONE NUMBERS

Find immediately inside back cover for convenience and quick reference.

ABBREVIATIONS

See first section of APPENDIX for Table of Abbreviations used in this book.

MEDICATION NOTICE

Every effort has been made to prevent errata in dosage recommendations and to keep the dosages found in this text in agreement with official standards at the time of publication.

However, dosage recommendations do sometimes change. I therefore urge you to check the manufacturer's brochure, particularly before using any drug with which you are not familiar or have not used for some time.

Unless otherwise specified, doses and recommendations are for an average 75-kg adult without other severe complicating factors. Initial doses and loading doses recommended presume no immediate prior administration of the same, similar or complicating medications.

HARVEY D. CAIN

General Medical Principles and Procedures

1. ABC's of Emergency Problem Analysis

A systematic inventory plan is of great benefit in analyzing the scope and magnitude of complex emergency problems. This is particularly true for multiple trauma cases, in which less obvious problems may be life-threatening and go undetected if there is not a methodical method for discovering them. While circumstances will quickly modify what is done, the following outline, rapidly performed, should aid in appraising complicated injury and illness situations and establishing appropriate therapeutic interventions.

1–1. EMERGENCY SCENE ANALYSIS ("AN IDEA")

The health care or emergency medical service (EMS) personnel who come to the scene of an emergency should try to obtain, while in transit, general information regarding the overall status at the scene, in order to evaluate current and potential problems, as well as assets. The acronym "AN IDEA" is a useful aid for remembering the six major areas of concern, as outlined below.

Area Quarantine
Are there hazards of the environment (e.g., chemicals, gases, explosives, fire, radiation) that may require area quarantine, evacuation or crowd control?* If so, make sure that fire, police and any necessary rescue department are notified.

Numbers
How many ill people or victims are involved, and to what degree? If there are large numbers of seriously involved people, initiate or direct appropriate action and call for adequate help. (See also 2, *Triage*, and 3–1).

Identification
Give your name and training (MD, RN, EMT, BLS, Paramedic, ACLS, ALS, etc.) to any earlier arrivers on the scene (or control officer if established) and indicate your willingness to participate. Establish through quick direct constructive discussion how your talents may be utilized.

Detection
Determine as much as possible from the surrounding circumstances the most probable cause or causes (pathogenesis) of the victim's illness or injury. Note the people and materials surrounding the victim—Do they have any significance to the victim's status?

---

*See Appendix for tables on identification of hazardous materials in vehicles and cargo carriers.

Examination

Keep an eye out for any evidence—unusual as well as routine—that may be relevant to the situation (e.g., bottles, containers, weapons, body position, notes). If criminal activity appears likely, attempt to preserve such evidence for future reference.

Aid

Ensure that adequate personnel and equipment are brought to the scene of the emergency, including someone who can establish a two-way report transmission.

1–2. PATIENT HISTORY ANALYSIS

(*Note:* If patient is in great distress, go to *1–3, Patient Physical Analysis,* and return to this section when feasible.)

- The health care professional should always first identify himself/herself to the patient and indicate that the purpose is to help—give a few words of assurance first, even if it is not evident that the patient can hear you.
- If the condition appears life-threatening, history taking is minimal (or may be unobtainable); in such cases, proceed rapidly to *1–3, Patient Physical Analysis.*
- Get input also from family/friends/witnesses to supplement or corroborate data (another person may assist in this area).

Illness

- *Chief Complaint (CC)*
  Onset: When did onset occur, and how rapidly did symptoms progress? Any preceding events or circumstances of possible significance?
  Magnitude: What are the characteristics and severity of the problem?
  Variance: If pain is present, is it radiating or local? Any other signs or symptoms? Is it constant or intermittent, or is it varying in intensity? If variant, what relieves or aggravates it?
- *Prior Health Status.* Good health previously? Any similar problems in the past in self, family members or close contacts?
- *Drugs.* Has patient recently taken any prescription or non-prescription medications, alcohol, (illicit) drugs?
- *Allergies?*

Injury

- *Predisposing Medical Problems.* Any preceding medical difficulties such as alcohol, drugs, seizures, TIA's, illness, emotional problems?
- *Dynamics of Event.* What are mechanisms and forces involved (e.g., speed(s), weight, impact, angles)? Any known contributing causes? Any observed changes in surrounding materials to indicate magnitude of force (bent or broken objects)? Note presence or absence of safety equipment; was it in use when the injury occurred?
- *Consequence of Injury.* Get inventory of complaints or symptoms as for illness above (plus additional data outlined in *1–3*).

1–3. PATIENT PHYSICAL ANALYSIS

I. QUICK INITIAL EXAM (15–30 second ABBCS exam in the field, office, or ED. In mass casualty the initial field triage stops with ABB.)

	Procedures	Further Data
Airway	Check for obstruction	If problems exist, see 5, *Resuscitation* Clear or bypass any obstruction (see also Table 5–3; *39–5* and *39–6* [for foreign bodies in the airway]; Fig. 5–3 [abdominal/chest thrust])
Breathing	Check thoracic and abdominal (diaphragmatic) excursion and gross rate Evaluate for ventilatory effort, distress and fatigue	Cover any sucking wounds (see also *31–13* for traumatic pneumothorax) and *31–11* (penetrating/perforating wounds)
Bleeding	Check for any major hemorrhage that is peripherally controllable	*45–1, Control of Bleeding;* arterial spurting establishes circulation presence
Circulation	Check for presence of pulse and approximate rate, rhythm and quality or amplitude Check skin color, moistness and gross temperature	If no pulse, start EHC; see 5, *Resuscitation* If in circulatory collapse, see also 57, *Shock.*
Sensorium	Check quality and quantity of responsiveness to questions or, if necessary, to painful stimuli	Briefly reassure patient If still not clearing after completion of examination, consider approaches outlined in 32, *Coma;* 44, *Head Injuries;* 53, *Poisoning*

Comments

- If the patient is unconscious from unknown circumstances that suggest trauma or has any evidence of head injury *(44), immobilize the neck immediately* (see Fig. 4–3).
- If the patient has cessation or severe impairment of ABC functions, reestablishment of these functions takes precedence over any other measures.
- If breathing and circulation are mechanically adequate and the patient is still in respiratory distress, see Table 5–2.
- If body temperature is severely abnormal, see 62.

II. SYSTEMATIC PHYSICAL EXAMINATION (Few minutes exam *with later return to any positive findings. Immobilize neck first* if any signs or symptoms of head/neck trauma; include back if paralysis/trauma (see Fig. 4–3). Perform in the field or office; repeat in the ED.)

	Procedures (Inspect/Palpate/Listen)	Further Data
Head/Face	Observe for gross deformity and blood Palpate face (see Fig. 61–2) Inspect oropharynx: Check for foreign matter, dentures, broken teeth, occlusion Check eyes for wounds, foreign bodies, contact lens, gross EOM. PERL? Ask if can see all right	44, Head Injuries 61, Teeth and Orofacial Conditions 38, Eye Conditions 35, Ear Conditions 48, Nasal Conditions 49, Neurologic Conditions 59, Soft Tissue Injuries
Neck/Chest	If neck immobilized, do not check further at this time Check for neck tenderness, movement, wounds, venous distention, medical alert tags	47, Musculoskeletal Disorders 31, Chest 56, Respiratory Tract Conditions 29, Cardiac Emergencies 55, Pulmonary Edema

Table continued on following page

	Procedures (Inspect/Palpate/Listen)	Further Data
	Listen for gross wheezing, altered voice, sucking wounds, crepitus Look for accessory muscles of respiration activity, symmetrical vertical and lateral chest excursion, deformity, wounds Compress chest gently to check for stability, pain response, fractures, crepitant feeling	
Abdomen	Look for distention, wounds, diaphragm movement Check for rigidity, tenderness, femoral pulses Listen to bowel sounds if there is pain or tenderness, or if poisoning is suspected	22, Abdominal Pain 40, Gastrointestinal Emergencies 53, Poisoning (Table 53–2) 47, Musculoskeletal Disorders 42, Gynecologic Conditions 41, Genitourinary Tract Emergencies
Pelvis	Pubic symphysis and lateral bimanual palpation and compression for stability/tenderness Look for gross trauma to perineum and genitalia	
Upper and Lower Extremities	Look for deformities, swelling, asymmetry, wounds, skin color, medical alert tag Feel for pulses, skin temperature, tenderness, instability of structure Check for gross sensation, strength and, if no evident contraindication, active ROM.	43, Hand Injuries 47, Musculoskeletal Disorders 59, Soft Tissue Injuries
Back	Observe for wounds, deformity, asymmetry. Check for focal tenderness, vertebral dislocation, spinous process "step off" (suspect if motor/sensory deficit)	47, Musculoskeletal Disorders 41, Genitourinary Tract Emergencies 22, Abdominal Pain (referred)
Neurologic	See 49, *Neurologic Conditions*, for survey as appropriate	44, Head Injuries 49, Neurologic Conditions

III. EXAMINATION COMPLETION

- Measure pulse, respiratory rate, blood pressure (and temperature if at extremes).
- Establish periodicity for recheck of vital signs according to patient condition.
- Return for second look, as needed, at any positive findings detected.

1–4. LIFE SUPPORT AND SPECIFIC INITIAL TREATMENT

- If in the field or office, proceed with support and specific initial treatment (e.g., splints, IV's, pneumatic trousers (MAST suit), thermal protection, airway and ventilation maintenance, analgesics) as appropriate and available pending and during any necessary transportation for definitive care.
- If in the ED, recheck that measures initiated are appropriate and functioning properly at this time (e.g., IV solution and rate correct; circulation under splints satisfactory) before proceeding to more definitive care.

2. ABC's of Urgency Evaluation (Triage)

Rapid classification of emergency cases by the urgency with which treatment is required (triage) is one of the most important functions and responsibilities of those called upon to treat such cases. Accurate urgency evaluation, often complicated by the presence of multiple serious conditions in the same individual and almost always in an unstable, excited environment, calls not only for extensive basic knowledge of surgery, medicine, toxicology, psychology (especially crowd psychology) and psychiatry, but also for the ability to translate this knowledge into immediate effective action under stressful circumstances. In mass casualty situations, the individual in charge of triage should be the best trained and most experienced person available.

2–1. PRIORITY CLASSIFICATION (INDIVIDUAL TREATMENT)

The usual order of initial treatment measures for emergency problems in an individual (or a small group of patients) is as follows (with as many measures being performed simultaneously as feasible):

1. Cessation of bleeding of major proportions that is peripherally controllable (*see 45–1*).
2. Airway and breathing or ventilation management (5–*1*), including occlusion of any sucking chest wound (*31*).
3. Restoration of circulation (5–*1*).
4. Splinting of fractures of major bones (47–6, *Fractures*).
5. Treatment of shock (57), including correction of severe endocrine (*36*) and metabolic (*46*) problems.
6. Restoration of normal body temperature, if severely altered (62).
7. Treatment of sepsis of profound degree (33, *Contagious and Communicable Diseases*).
8. Management of massive soft tissue injuries (59).
9. Other measures pertinent to treatment of the specific illness or injury.

2–2. PRIORITY CLASSIFICATION IN MASS CASUALTY INCIDENTS*

In the mass casualty situation, the early responders must first treat the greatest number who have serious injury who can survive with care immediately available who would not survive otherwise.

- All victims must be helped with peripheral control of major bleeding (45–*1*) and rapid airway control (5–*1*) and occlusion of any sucking chest wound before anything else is done. Patients with catastrophic events, such as cardiac arrest, cannot be tended to in this type of situation.
- Table 2–1 provides a guide for determining the severity of injuries.
- Victims should be tagged to indicate that they have been assessed and their priority for transportation has been determined. A skin marking pen can be used to mark the patient's status on the forehead. The simplest division is transport *Now* and transport *Later*. Color coding and numbering of treat-

---

*The term Mass Casualty Incident (MCI) refers to disasters that occur in one location in the absence of similar or related occurrences in neighboring towns or counties. Some use the term *multiple* to refer to from 10 to 100 cases and *mass* to refer to incidents involving hundreds and thousands of cases.

Table 2–1. CLASSIFICATION OF MULTIPLE INJURIES*

Injury Severity	General	Head and Neck	Chest	Abdominal	Extremities
No injury	None; possible emotional reaction	None	None	None	None
Minor	Minor lacerations, contusions and abrasions All 1°, small 2° and 3° burns	Cerebral injury without loss of consciousness "Whip-lash" without vertebral damage Ocular abrasions and contusions	Minor chest wall contusions, abrasions	Muscle contusions; seat belt abrasion	Minor sprains and fractures, and/or dislocation of digits
Moderate	Extensive contusions, abrasions; large lacerations; avulsions (<3" diameter). 10–20% 2° or 3° burns	Cerebral injury with <15 minutes unconsciousness; no amnesia Undisplaced skull or facial bone fractures Eye lacerations, retinal detachment "Whiplash" with vertebral injury	Simple rib or sternal fractures Major contusions of chest wall without hemo- or pneumothorax, or respiratory embarrassment	Major contusion of abdominal wall without intra-abdominal injury	Compound fractures of digits or nose Undisplaced long bone or pelvic fractures Major joint sprains
Severe (Not life-threatening)	Extensive contusions or abrasions; large lacerations or avulsions (>3" diameter). 20–30% 2° or 3° burns	Cerebral injury with unconsciousness >15 minutes without severe neurologic signs; <3 hours post-traumatic amnesia Displaced closed skull fractures without signs of intracranial injury Loss of eye or avulsion of optic nerve Facial bone fractures, displaced or without antral or orbital involvement Cervical spine fractures without cord damage	Multiple rib fracture without respiratory embarrassment Simple hemo- or pneumothorax Rupture of diaphragm Moderate pulmonary contusion	Contusion of abdominal organs Extraperitoneal bladder rupture Retroperitoneal hemorrhage Avulsion of ureter Laceration of urethra Thoracic or lumbar spine fractures without neurologic involvement	Displaced simple long bone fractures, and/or multiple hand and foot fractures Single open long bone fractures Pelvic fractures with displacement Dislocation of major joints Lacerations of major nerves or vessels of extremities

Most Severe (Life-threatening, survival probable)	Severe lacerations and/or avulsions with dangerous hemorrhage 30–50% 2° or 3° burns	Cerebral injury with or without skull fracture, with unconsciousness of >15 minutes with definite abnormal neurologic signs; post-traumatic amnesia 3–12 hours Compound skull fracture	Open chest wounds; flail chest; pneumomediastinum; myocardial contusion and pericardial injuries without circulatory embarrassment	Minor lacerations of intra-abdominal viscera, including kidney, spleen and tail of pancreas Intraperitoneal bladder rupture Avulsion of genitals Dorsal and/or lumbar spine fractures with paraplegia	Multiple closed long bone fractures Amputation of limbs
Critical (Survival relatively improbable or uncertain)	Over 50% 2° or 3° burns	Cerebral injury with unconsciousness of >24 hours; post-traumatic amnesia >12 hours; intracranial hemorrhage; signs of increased intracranial pressure Cervical spine injury with quadriplegia Major airway obstruction	Chest injuries with major respiratory embarrassment (laceration of trachea, hemomediastinum, etc.) Aortic laceration Myocardial rupture or contusion with circulatory embarrassment	Rupture, avulsion, or severe laceration of abdominal vessels or organs, except kidney, spleen or ureter	Multiple open limb fractures
Dead Tag: Black or Mark: D or Dead					
Contaminated Case Tag: Blue					

*Modified from the abbreviated outline of the AMA Committee on the Medical Aspects of Automotive Safety as it appears in Ballinger, W. F., Rutherford, R. B., and Zuidema, G. D.: *The Management of Trauma*, 2nd ed. Philadelphia, W. B. Saunders Co., 1973.

NOTE: Other nontraumatic conditions that can *rapidly* change from lesser severity to greater severity include the following: cessation or acute embarrassment of ventilation and respiration (*5*); massive bleeding from any cause (*45*); cardiac arrest (*29–8*); severe heat stroke with rapidly rising temperature (*62–7*); profound shock from any cause (*57*); near drowning (*25–3*); rapidly acting poisons (*53*); anaphylactic reactions (*24–1*); acute overwhelming bacteremia and toxemia (*33, Contagious and Communicable Diseases*); acute endocrine (*36*) and metabolic (*46*) emergencies; acute maniacal states (*54, Psychiatric Emergencies*); rupture of a viscus (*40–4*).

Smoke and toxic inhalation (*25–4*) can be a serious compounding problem in accident cases complicated by fire.

ment and transportation priorities at the scene can aid management. One color tag coding system (from Journal of Civil Defense, Starke, Florida) is as follows:
Red: First priority (1) (most urgent)
Yellow: Second priority (2) (*Note:* a designation of 2′ indicates higher urgency)
Green: Third priority (3)
Black: Dead (D)
Blue: Addition of a blue tag indicates that the victim is contaminated.

- Victims are reassessed at the nearest primary receiving hospital.
- Triage, to be effective, must be efficiently coordinated with transportation under central leadership (e.g., Incident Control Center [ICC] or Scene Manager).

2–3. JUDGMENT EVALUATION

Through experience and confidence in their own knowledge and judgment, plus discipline and training in following a carefully designed team approach to the management of multiple casualties, emergency medical service personnel will develop the ability to determine priorities and respond appropriately. The team includes fire, police, ambulance, military, radiocommunications and other available community resources such as the American Red Cross (ARC). Extensive preplanning and trials help to change management in mass emergencies from innovation to exercise (*see also* 3).

The medical personnel's function has been performed well if the best decisions possible under the circumstances have been made. Guidelines that can be used to reach the best (SMARTEST) decisions and action program are outlined (though not in any particular order of importance) in the following mnemonic:

Support: Will the patient, other reviewers, your peers and superiors and even you yourself later substantially understand and approve or defend this action?

Material: Are more materials needed? If so, have they been ordered? When could they reasonably arrive?

Achievement of goal: Will this action logically lead to fulfillment of the objective that has been decided upon?

Risk: Does the action planned offer the widest therapeutic index of likelihood of benefit: likelihood of harm? Is there a less risky way to achieve nearly the same objective?

Time: Does time permit actions to be taken in this order, especially if the best quality of survival of the greatest number is the objective?

Economy: Considering all the resources available, is this their best utilization?

Staff: Is there sufficient personnel to perform the management required? Can and should more personnel be called? When could they reasonably arrive? How should the present staff function in the interim?

Training: Is the training adequate to technically perform the decided action? Can and should more adequately trained personnel be recruited? When could they reasonably arrive? Who is best qualified to function in the interim?

Another acronym long used by fire departments in instituting action programs is: F—POD—P, which stands for *F*acts, *P*robabilities, *O*wn situation (need help?), *D*ecision (make one), *P*ut plan into action. The plan results are assessed, and if there is still a problem, the acronym is used again.

3. ABC's of Mass Civilian Casualty in "Peace" and Wartime

3–1. GENERAL CONSIDERATIONS *(See also 1, Emergency Problem Analysis, and 2, Urgency Evaluation [Triage])*

Even during the best of modern times, the civilian population is subject to potential mass injury and illness from natural disasters, transportation accidents, widespread toxin exposures, large structural collapses, blasts, terrorist devastation and nuclear reactor accidents. The results of food and water contamination, bombing of various types, blast injuries, bullet wounds, shrapnel injuries, effects of gases, bacterial and viral infections, burns, concussions, contusions, dislocations, fractures, infectious and contagious diseases, lacerations, effects of radioactivity and stress-induced psychiatric symptoms are often compounded by poor communications and transportation, inadequate medical supplies and shortage of personnel. When tremendous numbers of casualties occur,* on-site treatment must of necessity be restricted to the simplest possible effective procedures (*1*, *2*), with removal of the victims to a safe area for definitive care as soon as possible (*4*).

In both wartime emergencies and "peacetime" mass civilian casualty disasters, there are many similarities in the general measures instituted for evaluation and care (with resources and personnel frequently being inadequate to meet the needs of the situation). These measures are summarized in Table 3–1; the mnemonic "TNT SCREAMS STOP" may be helpful for recalling important elements. The items are not in an order of priority, although the first three items, TNT, indicate the individual first response to the disaster. It is essential that civilian defense programs and protocols be developed for such emergencies, and that stockpiling of materials be prearranged. Preplanning and drill are mandatory for successful program activation. *Failing to plan is planning to fail.*

In an era when nuclear bomb production by diverse nations (and potentially by individuals associated with radical groups) is becoming more common,

*Some use the term *multiple* to refer to 10–100 cases and *mass* to refer to hundreds and thousands of cases.

Table 3–1. MASS CASUALTY EMS DISASTER PROGRAM (MAJOR NEEDS)

Item	Comment
Triage team	Advance EMS triage team at incident or disaster scene should quickly perform an initial survey (*1–3*) of all victims, initially providing only for adequate airway/ventilation (5) as quickly as achievable and stoppage of major bleeding (*45–1*); tags are put on victims as priority status is established. Patients in immediate environmental peril (e.g., smoke, fire, toxins, particularly in enclosed areas) are moved first. An Incident Control Center (ICC) and a Patient Collecting Station (PCS) are set up in safe convenient locations. First 3 EMS personnel on scene are Control Officer (Chief of EMS), Triage Officer, Transport Officer until replaced. Call for adequate help ASAP (it is better to overestimate needs). Summon special rescue units as required for extrication of victims. If an open-field casualty event, include wide area survey for victims when help arrives.
News (Communications)	Establish immediate two-way radio contact with hospital(s) and disaster headquarters to communicate supply and personnel needs. Channel F-3 (155.340 MHz) can be used for all ambulance-to-scene, ambulance-to-ambulance, and ground scene communications. Channel F-4 (155.400 MHz) is used for triage officers and ambulances returning to nearby hospitals. F-1 position is used for individual agency communications and F-2 for other interagency/local government use. Sirens and radio are used in special instances to alert citizens (all AM/FM stations refer to local Emergency Broadcast System [EBS]).
Transporters	Transporters entirely immobilize the most seriously injured, preferably on a "long board" (or split litter, backboard, or any firm board); 4 people (if available) carry patient to PCS; (see *4*). Patients are placed in priority rows according to tagging done by triage team; those with red tags (first priority) are placed closest to ambulance arrival area. Stabilization efforts and reassessment continue. Transportation Officer directs transfer by ambulance, bus or truck to nearby hospitals in numbers proportionate to hospital size, if possible, to limit impact on any one facility. Hospitals should accept all such directed patients. Ambulances may need to restock prior to returning to disaster scene. Ambulances should have separate entrance/exit sites at the scene.
Supplies and personnel	Mobilization of necessary supplies and personnel commensurate with magnitude of disaster should be started immediately in accordance with preplanning. Personnel include physicians and surgeons; nurses; paramedics; emergency medical technicians, corpsmen and other technicians; pharmacists; dentists/oral surgeons; and security and support personnel. Reserve supplies should include 50 to 100 long boards (no cots) with 6 to 8 cravat-rolled triangular bandages (Fig. 47–1) to accompany each one (Fig. 4–3).
Contamination abatement	Decontaminators, specially trained, are essential not only to lessen further exposure of the victims to poisonous substances (e.g., gases, chemicals, radiation) but also to protect emergency medical staff from secondary exposure. Showering, washing, clothing change, radiation check and communicable disease control are common measures necessary.

Reports/tags	Tags indicating status are tied on the victim at the scene. This aids in continuity of care and saves time; if tags are unavailable, mark patient's forehead with skin pen or lipstick (see Table 2–1). Records are started during transport or at hospital and may be supplemented by a serially numbered carbon control sheet. Original record stays with patient, one copy goes to public information and one to admitting hospital.
Emergency treatment areas	Victims should be distributed from priority rows of PCS and preferably sent sequentially to different nearby hospital intake areas as feasible. At intake hospital triage area (often located in parking lot near—but not blocking—ED entrance) reassessment is necessary to evaluate for condition change during transportation.
Admitting	The most seriously injured require admission. Hospital admissions department must communicate with disaster operation headquarters as to capacity to handle more victims and is responsible for all aspects of patient tabulations. After stabilization, patients with special needs may be transferred to other hospitals.
Morgue	A morgue area, separate from treatment areas, must be established. Public relations center is notified of identified victims.
Security	Security personnel (police/sheriff/security guards/occasionally national guard) are essential to protect and aid victims and staff, direct traffic flow and maintain law and order. Limiting ingress of unauthorized vehicles to the emergency scene and providing room for rapid movement of emergency vehicles is critical.
Sustenance	Food and fluid needs for both victims and staff must be met. Those minimally injured may receive food and fluids; the moderately injured may receive oral fluids unless surgery pending; the severely injured receive nothing by mouth because of usual nausea, vomiting, gastric retention and, frequently, pending surgery.
Team work	Maximum salvage of life and limb is attained only by the fullest cooperation and discipline of *all* personnel involved in the operation. Police/Fire/Rescue personnel often perform best owing to experience with plan/drill/discipline method of operating. At ICC, Chief Town Executive/Chief of Operations directs chiefs of Fire/Police/Rescue/EMS teams. EMS Chief (Control) directs Triage Officer and Transportation Officer.
Operations (Surgical area)	Surgical areas with all necessary personnel must be established, plus expanded space for postoperative intensive care and recovery.
Public relations and management	A concerned populace, relatives and communications representatives need reasonably rapid dissemination of the best available information, given in a calm, conservative and sincere manner. This is the primary task of the public relations section, which receives information principally from disaster headquarters, the hospital admitting area and the morgue.

citizens may find themselves as hostage pawns in international blackmail schemes. Even though massive destruction of life and property would be inevitable in any such conflict, a nation with the best civilian preparedness may not have to be the first to blink in negotiations.

In mass casualty situations, emergency treatment and management of many conditions will vary in important details from those outlined in other sections of this book. The most important points are summarized in the following paragraphs.

3–2. BACTERIAL OR VIRAL INFECTIONS (Biologic Warfare)

In spite of highly publicized and supposedly sacred covenants between nations, inoculation of the population with lethal microorganisms in a given area is always a possibility. It is difficult to outline in advance comprehensive emergency procedures to cope with such a situation. However, the well-known public health principles applicable to any epidemic should be put into effect as soon as possible. These principles are: identification and confinement of the source, segregation of cases, decontamination and symptomatic treatment, followed by specific therapy and preventive inoculations as soon as available after the causative organisms have been identified and their sensitivities determined. See also 33, *Contagious and Communicable Diseases*.

Decrease in resistance of the body to infection may also be expected to occur following massive injuries, radiation exposure or as a result of protracted stress due to interference with adequate sleep, poor food, extreme fatigue and mental strain.

3–3. BLAST INJURIES

Direct blast effects usually consist of multiple massive contusions of the lungs and are characterized by dyspnea, cyanosis and unconsciousness; in many cases, pulmonary edema may develop. Remarkably, there may be no signs of external trauma.

Preliminary decontamination measures should be taken (if the blast involves a fissionable or other noxious material) and victims transferred from the disaster site for definitive care as soon as possible.

Indirect blast effects are caused by being struck by objects collapsing or propelled by the blast and are similar to injuries encountered in industry, automobile accidents, explosions or in the home.

3–4. EXPLOSIVES AND FIRE BOMBS

These may cause many casualties if employed in saturation or area bombing. The types of injuries to be expected are the same as for blast injuries (3–3). Immediate decontamination from persisting chemicals, such as phosphorus, must be carried out.

3–5. NUCLEAR BOMBS

Nuclear bomb explosions cause mass death, injury and destruction from their blast, light, heat and radiation effects.* If a nuclear bomb is exploded at

---

*The efforts of Physicians for Social Responsibility to republicize and reemphasize the horrors of nuclear war are noteworthy. Likewise, Doctors for Disaster Preparedness has a most important role in urging the populace to be as ready as possible for any natural disaster, mass casualty incident, or other catastrophe, including the regrettably thinkable possibility of nuclear aggression and its aftermath. The address of Doctors for Diaster Preparedness is P.O. Box 1057, Starke, FL 32091.

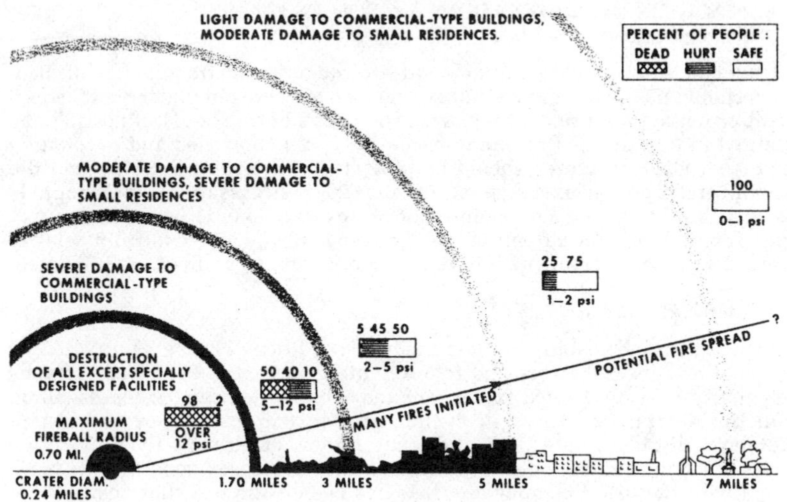

Figure 3–1. Estimated damage area from 1-megaton nuclear weapon blast (most likely military weapon size). A 25-megaton blast would increase the radius of each of these zones about threefold. (From *In Time of Emergency,* Federal Emergency Management Agency, Washington, D. C. 20472.)

a considerable distance above the earth's surface, gamma rays and, under certain circumstances, neutrons may cause serious and fatal injury. Extreme thermal radiation also may cause flash burns (*28–15*) as well as secondary burns. If the fireball comes in contact with the earth's surface, the blast and thermal effects are decreased, but the ground or water is contaminated with fission products. Radioactive fallout, although it may have serious delayed effects, is not an urgent emergency problem in the ordinary sense except for the need for decontamination as soon as possible. Determination of the intensity of radioactive contamination is essential for estimating prognosis if the person survives the other effects (*see 3–12*). Medical resources should be located at a distance suitable for preservation of survivors and medical care personnel (see Fig. 3–1).

Blast injuries, if direct, need no practical consideration following nuclear bombing, since any person injured by blast pressure would undoubtedly be killed immediately.

Ionizing radiation effects are discussed in section *3–12*.

3–6. THERMAL EFFECTS OF NUCLEAR BLASTS AND FIRES *(See 28, Burns)*

3–7. BULLET AND OTHER PENETRATING WOUNDS *(See also 59–9)*

On-site treatment should be limited to insurance of an adequate airway, covering of sucking chest wounds, respiratory assistance (*5–1*) and control of hemorrhage (*45–1*) and shock (*57–5*), with transfer as soon as possible to a hospital equipped for definitive care.

3–8. FRACTURES AND DISLOCATIONS *(See Table 47–1, Initial Immobilization)*

Under mass casualty conditions, on-site reduction of fractures or dislocations should not be attempted unless evidence of acute circulatory embarrassment or nerve pressure is conclusive. The injured part should, if possible, be splinted in a position of minimal discomfort, pain controlled and evacuation arranged. Open fractures should be protected by a sterile dressing and the patient given prophylaxis against tetanus (*20*) if necessary. No sulfonamide powder, antibiotic powder or ointment of any kind should be applied to any open fracture. Oral or parenteral antibiotics should be given only if a delay of more than 6 hours before definitive treatment can be obtained is anticipated.

3–9. MEDICAL EMERGENCIES

In a catastrophe, many chronic medical conditions can be aggravated by physical and mental stress and require emergency care. Poor food, nervous strain, exposure, prolonged excitement and overexertion can trigger disabling, sometimes fatal, increases in symptoms primarily caused by preexistent metabolic disorders, infections and other chronic conditions. Even moderate doses of ionizing radiation can gradually cause decreased general body resistance with the usual complications. It has been estimated that about 2% of all casualties following a major catastrophe would involve known or latent diabetics; those requiring insulin need to be provided for. Anyone dependent on daily medications should be encouraged to preplan for any mass disaster and to put a fresh supply of medication with their emergency gear. If insulin or other refrigerated medicines need to be carried in a mass evacuation, they can be put in a small thermally insulated canister with ice, which will keep it cool for a few days.

3–10. POISONOUS GASES (Chemical Warfare)

If, in violation of worldwide international covenants, chemical warfare is ever used again, it is probable that phosphate ester "nerve gases" will almost completely supplant lacrimators, pulmonary irritants, irritant smokes and vesicants (*53–746, War Gases*). All of the "nerve gases" are strongly cholinesterase-inhibiting and result in profound stimulation of the parasympathetic nervous system. For treatment, including the use of atropine, see *53–497, Organic Phosphates*.

3–11. SPRAINS AND STRAINS *(See also 47–3, Sprains)*

The only valid indication for treatment of damaged ligaments and adjacent structures is for control of pain (by immediate infiltration with a local anesthetic) in order to allow ambulatory evacuation from a life-threatening location, or when there are severe sprains of the lower extremities, which could cause serious permanent disability from laxity of ligamentous structures unless splinting or some means of support is provided.

3–12. RADIATION INJURIES: EVALUATION AND TREATMENT

Nuclear power plant and isotope production facility accidents differ from nuclear bomb attacks in that little or no explosion or blast is involved, and radiation is the primary problem.* Other important sources of radiation to individuals are x-ray units, open radionuclides and radioactive material in transit.

For measures that can be taken to protect against radiation effects, see Table 3–2.

---

*As fossil fuel supplies continue to decrease and the problems of nuclear waste disposal are resolved, the use of nuclear power with its considerable advantages will certainly increase. The relative safety of the peaceful use of fissionable material has been impressive and continues to improve thanks to more rigid construction standards, closer maintenance and increased regulation.

Table 3–2. PROTECTION FROM RADIATION

Note: The three modes of protection from radiation are (1) increasing distance from the radiation source, (2) shielding, and (3) minimizing time of exposure.

Distance

- Nuclear power plants are monitored so closely that there would undoubtedly be time for safe evacuation if an accident occurred (provided that citizens adhered without panic to an adequate preplanned evacuation scheme). An evacuation radius of 3 miles is considered adequate, and 10 miles is considered sufficient even in the event of a core melt down (although preplanning can encompass a 50-mile radius). Radiation exposure decreases by the square of distance from the source.

Shielding

- If time does not permit evacuation from the source area, then deep subterranean shielding is next best alternative.
- If possible, stay away from sites downwind from radiation source. If this is not possible, stay indoors, close all doors and windows, turn off any ventilators and wear a mask over nose and mouth to decrease inhalation of contaminated particles.
- Do not touch metallic objects.

Minimize Time of Exposure (Radiation dose is directly proportional to the time of exposure)

Decontaminate

- Remove contaminated clothing (reduces contamination by 70–90%); wash with soap (or Betadyne if available) and water, and shower as soon as possible. Put contaminated articles and clothing into plastic bags. *Note:* Water used in cleaning contaminated articles should be diked to prevent it from flowing into sewer system.
- Thoroughly cleanse all body canals, crevices and hair.
- Clip all long hair to short length (don't shave) if contamination still detected after cleaning.
- Avoid irritating or abrading the skin, and keep hands and all contaminated substances out of the mouth.
- If radioactive material was ingested, lavage the stomach and follow with alkalinization (Alka Seltzer, oral antacids are fine), but *not* if radioactive chromium was ingested. Magnesium sulfate also helps form insoluble salts and reduces bowel transit time. Sodium alginates are given if radioactive strontium has been ingested.
- Irrigate all wounds well, promote bleeding, and debride as necessary. If Geiger counter monitoring shows 2000 counts per minute or less, wound closure is all right.

Reduce Thyroid Gland Uptake of Radioactive Material

- If thyroid exposure (from radioactive iodine) to more than 25 rads has occurred or is likely to occur (i.e., if within 3 miles of source, or if downwind) immediately start 1 tablet (130 mg) of potassium iodide (½ tablet for those 5 years of age or younger) p.o. daily for 10 days (6 drops of saturated solution of potassium iodine (SSKI) may be used instead of tablet form).

Ionizing Radiation Effects

Alpha rays, emitted by unfissioned bomb residue containing plutonium or uranium are of very low penetrance (i.e., they will not penetrate a piece of paper) but are a problem if they pass through wounds or are ingested. If even small amounts of an alpha-emitting substance are deposited in the bones, under certain circumstances serious damage may occur from long-term bombardment of tissues.

Beta rays are emitted from fission products. Although they are relatively nonpenetrating as compared with gamma rays, the products by which they are emitted may enter the body through inhalation or ingestion or through a break in the skin. Many of these products have the same tendency as alpha rays to localize in the bones and cause severe signs and symptoms, often delayed, through constant bombardment.

Gamma rays are liberated for only a few seconds after a high air burst and are similar in effect to those emitted by a high energy x-ray machine. Their range in air varies directly with the size of the bomb, and they may be lethal for several miles from the point of explosion. These rays have a tremendous penetrating power (even through thick concrete walls) and are the most important causative factor in radiation injuries.

Neutrons are formed in nuclear fission and other fusion reactions. These particles have a relatively short range as compared with gamma rays; their chief importance is that, on being absorbed by the surface of the earth, they may induce radioactive products that emit beta or gamma rays. Persons relatively close to a nuclear blast may be shielded by a barrier from gamma rays but may develop acute symptoms from neutron exposure.

Magnitude of Radiation

The distance from the radiation source and the amount of radiation exposure have been considered possible criteria for determining the need for and extent of treatment. It is important to note the following:

- There should be no delay of any required medical assistance in order to initiate decontamination.
- Exposure and contamination are *not* synonymous.
- The effects of radionuclide contamination rarely, if ever, constitute an emergency.

The possible phases following radiation exposure are:

- *Prodromal phase:* Patient is all right for about 2 days, then vomits for 2 days, then is okay if dose was low.
- *Latent phase:* 2 to 20 days; shorter if dose greater than 1000 rads.
- *Bone marrow depression phase:* 20 to 40 days; the period in which medical treatment is most important. Decrease in Hb/WBC/platelets exhibited.
- *Recovery phase:* 40 to 60 days.
- Table 3–3 gives further details.

Actions of Radiation Exposure Team

- Decontaminate (see Table 3–2, under "Minimize Time of Exposure").
- Administer first aid; do not delay necessary first aid while awaiting decontamination. Wipe or wash away any material around the victim's mouth before performing any mouth-to-mouth resuscitation.
- Administer potassium iodide.
- Administer antacids, except in cases of chromium exposure.
- Determine degree of exposure by dosimetry, evaluation with Geiger counters, and accident reconstruction. *Remember:* Exposure and contamination are not the same.
- Direct relocation of exposed persons; classify by degree of exposure, contamination and injury.
- Local reactor operators and Health Department can give advisory assistance.
- Professionals can call REACTS (615-482-2441, Beeper 241, for 24-hour emergency advice).

Reminder to Citizens

- Remember: Sirens mean TURN ON RADIO to EBS for instructions.

Table 3–3. ACUTE WHOLE BODY RADIATION (X OR GAMMA); DOSE–EFFECT RELATIONSHIP (AFTER WELD)

Whole Body Dose (Rem)	Clinical and Laboratory Findings	Medical Treatment After Decontamination*
5–25	Asymptomatic; CBC/diff. normal; chromosome aberration detectable	None
50–75	Asymptomatic; can be minor decrease in WBC/platelets	Give KI for this and greater exposures
75–125	Minimal prodromal symptoms of fatigue, anorexia, nausea or vomiting in 20% of patients within 2 days; decreased WBC/platelets in some	Control of vomiting; symptoms should clear in 2 days
125–200	Same symptoms as for 75–125 rem, plus transient disability; WBC/platelet decrease in majority of exposed persons	• Hospitalize patients if there is nausea and vomiting; localized erythema; decreasing CBC and lymphocyte count; psychologic problems; seizures • Corticoids not of value • Provide relief to all, but if medications in short supply, restrict administration to those most likely to survive
250–450	Serious disabling illness in most persons, with about 50% mortality if untreated; lymphocyte depression in approximately 75% of patients within 48 hours	• LD_{50} for humans thought to be 400–450 rads
500+	Rapid intense course of above symptoms (250–350 rem), with gastrointestinal slough within 2 weeks; bleeding and death in most exposed persons.	
5000+	Patients die within 24–72 hours from CV/GI/CNS complications	

*Management and treatment of excitement states (37) may be an additional major problem regardless of exposure level.

3–13. EARTHQUAKES, VOLCANIC ERUPTIONS, TORNADOS, HURRICANES AND OTHER MASSIVE FORCE DISASTERS

PRE-EVENT

Modern seismic monitoring and weather forecasting help greatly in predicting the occurrence of these types of natural disasters and aid the timely, orderly institution of prearranged plans and evacuation, but when they occur suddenly or in densely populated areas, there will still be substantial injuries to remaining occupants. See *3–14* and *3–15* for advice to individuals.

DURING EVENT

To reduce the frequency and magnitude of injury, individuals should be advised (in addition to remaining alert, cool and collected) to do the following:

- ***If in a vehicle:*** Stay in the vehicle. In the event of an earthquake, tornado or explosion, stop the vehicle (away from unsturdy structures if possible); lying in the floorboard space below seat level gives further protection. In the event of a volcanic eruption or hurricane, evacuate area directly and drive cautiously at safe speed according to radio directive; if no directions to safety are available by radio, proceed to the nearest safe area. Noxious volcanic ash and fumes may be as lethal as the lava itself; protect respiratory system as much as possible by using a mask or cloth for ash exposure and a self-contained breathing apparatus, if available, for fume exposure.
- ***If indoors:*** Stay indoors, get clear of windows, seek protection of sturdy structure (get under table or bed or get in doorway). An underground area offers the best protection from surface blast forces. This is the best place to stay unless subsequent fire, noxious fumes or inundation forces evacuation.
- ***If outdoors:*** If in a tornado, earthquake or hurricane, get down and away from power lines or structures that may collapse; a ditch or culvert provides the best protection against blast forces from such events.

POST EVENT *(See also 3–14 and 3–15)*

- ***Evaluate injuries*** and institute initial needed care (see 2 [Triage] and Table 3–1).
- ***Evaluate safety of immediate environment.*** Look for fire and act accordingly; do not light match. • Turn off gas and electricity; use outdoor cooking fire until safety is assured. • Look for and avoid broken electric power lines; consider all electric wires energized. If electric wires must be moved out of the way, use a long board to push them aside. • Avoid structurally damaged areas, including chimneys. • Step cautiously; wear shoes. • Stand clear when opening all doors; watch for teetering objects, especially shelves. • Clear away potentially dangerous or combustible materials (gasoline, acids, lye, pesticides, etc.).

3–14. INDIVIDUAL PREPAREDNESS FOR DISASTER

No government agency, civilian defense unit, or other outside group can come close to doing as good a job of meeting the basic needs of individuals (or individual households) in a catastrophe or holocaust as can the individuals themselves through preplanning and preparation.

Following is a list of items that each individual household should be encouraged to arrange or store in a permanent area:

- Potable water *(see 3–16)*.
- Nonperishable food supply. Dried and powdered foods are the lightest, most compact and easiest to transport. For bottled and canned foods, remember to include a can opener. Have enough food available to serve the needs of each person for at least 7 days. Periodically rotate foods to preserve freshness. Use foods from refrigerator and freezer first if electricity is off.
- First-aid kit *(see 10)*, daily medications and an emergency handbook.
- Flashlight and portable radio (for immediate instructions from EBS*) plus several sets of reserve batteries (these preserve best if kept in refrigerator; rotate stock regularly).
- A written plan with which all household members are thoroughly familiar; this should include the following:
  —Prearranged contingency meeting sites.

---

*Emergency Broadcast System

—General safety measures for varying situations.
—Information on an alternative communication system that is not dependent upon public utilities. CB radios with independent energy supply can be invaluable.
—Location and technique (including use of a wrench) for turning off household utilities when applicable: electricity (main switch usually pulled to down position); gas (valve turned from open [vertical] position to closed [horizontal] position); water (usually closed by turning main valve tightly clockwise).
—Instructions on the use of firearms (if any) and other self-defense measures. *Note:* The former should be stored with great caution and used only by those with special safety training. Indiscriminate use can create far more problems than it resolves in the civilian setting.

3–15. INDIVIDUAL RESPONSIBILITY TO THE COMMUNITY IN DISASTERS

Health care professionals and those responsible for maintaining law and order should inform individuals not officially involved to:

- Stay away from disaster areas if not already in the area.
- Leave the area promptly in accordance with official instructions when directed.
- Turn on portable radio to Civil Defense frequency (EBS) for area to obtain information and public directives.
- Keep personal vehicles out of the way of emergency vehicles. Traveling, when necessary, can be quicker and surer by foot or bicycle than on vehicle-congested or mechanically disrupted roadways.
- Stay alert, since follow-up disruptions and explosions can occur.
- Be cautious and considerate of fellow community members who may act foolishly through panic, bewilderment or grief.
- Be individually prepared for mass disasters.

3–16. POTABLE WATER

Availability of plain potable water for drinking is essential. If main sources of public water are disrupted or contaminated (and it is best to initially presume contamination following great disasters such as warfare or earthquakes), the individual must use acceptable alternative sources, as described below:

- Water stockpiled by the individual in sealed inert containers (several gallons for each household member).
- Usual household reservoirs (4 to 5 gallons in each toilet tank; 30 to 50 gallons in hot water tanks; water filled in pots or bathtubs when there has been sufficient warning time).
- Dirty water may be settled, decanted to another container, filtered (e.g., through a clean cloth or handkerchief) and boiled (8 minutes).
- Clear water may be disinfected with 4 drops of *plain* 5.25% sodium hypochlorite (household chlorine bleach without additives) to each gallon of water (use 8 to 12 drops if water is cloudy).
- Iodine solution or tablets are satisfactory for purification but require 30 minutes' exposure time.
- "Purification Straws" containing an iodide-based ion exchange resin column can be used to purify small amounts of drinking water.

4. ABC's of Transportation and Transfer of Care

4–1. GENERAL CONSIDERATIONS

There are multiple objectives in achieving satisfactory transportation from the scene to the treating facility for patients requiring ongoing evaluation and treatment. Among them are:

- **Prompt notification** for need of EMS transport vehicle to reduce waiting time and reduce need for speed in transit. Indicate type and magnitude of medical problem (determine number of vehicles and what emergency medical technicians (EMT-I, EMT-P [Paramedic], etc.) will be sent).
- **Call for special rescue extrication equipment** if more than the light rescue equipment carried on standard EMS vehicle is needed. Power saws, power winches and rigging are carried on EMS vehicles equipped to perform moderate or heavy rescue, as with severe impaction collision and rescue from heights, depths and other perilous positions.
- **Prompt response of transport vehicle,** aided by two-way radio dispatch of closest appropriate vehicle, by public education in not overutilizing system and by establishment of a mutual aid program to provide a back-up when one unit is already engaged.
- **Prompt short-range evacuation** from area of immediate danger. In disasters involving fire, explosion, smoke, toxins, inundation, etc., evacuation takes precedence over patient assessment and immobilization; in other situations rescue workers must quickly assess the risks of such movement vs. the risks of delay. Evacuation of victims unable to move themselves is carried out as follows:
  —*By 1 person:* See Figure 4–1.
  —*By 2 persons:* See Figure 4–2.
  —*By 3 or more persons:* See Figure 4–2, *D* to *G*. As shown in Figure 4–2 *D*, one rescuer's sole task is to lift and stabilize head and neck while others lift on same side of body from shoulders to knees, cradling body in their arms. (*Note:* even with careful handling, actual spine immobilization is minimal.) A 15-foot synthetic rope, ½″ to ¾″ in diameter, can be snaked back and forth under the body 5 to 6 times to provide rope loop handles for an impromptu stretcher.
- **Immobilization of all possible fracture sites** prior to movement (unless prompt evacuation necessary, as described above):
  —*Presume neck/spine fracture* (fx) until proved otherwise in all patients with: unconsciousness due to trauma, unconsciousness for unknown reasons, head/neck injury (especially in diving and motor vehicle accidents [MVA]), paralysis or complaining of burning in the hands or extremities. Immobilize with hard neck collar and boards as shown in Figures 4–3 and 4–4. (See page 24 for measures to be taken while awaiting transportation of head-injured patients. For special measures in the event of head/neck injury involving a helmet, see p. 25.)
  —*Immobilize suspected extremity fractures* as described in *18–25* and *18–30.*
  —*Long board (72″ × 18″) immobilization* using straps or cravat (Figs. 4–3 and 4–4) is best for patients with serious multiple injuries—particularly in an MCI. Scoop stretchers and wheeled ambulance cots can also be used.

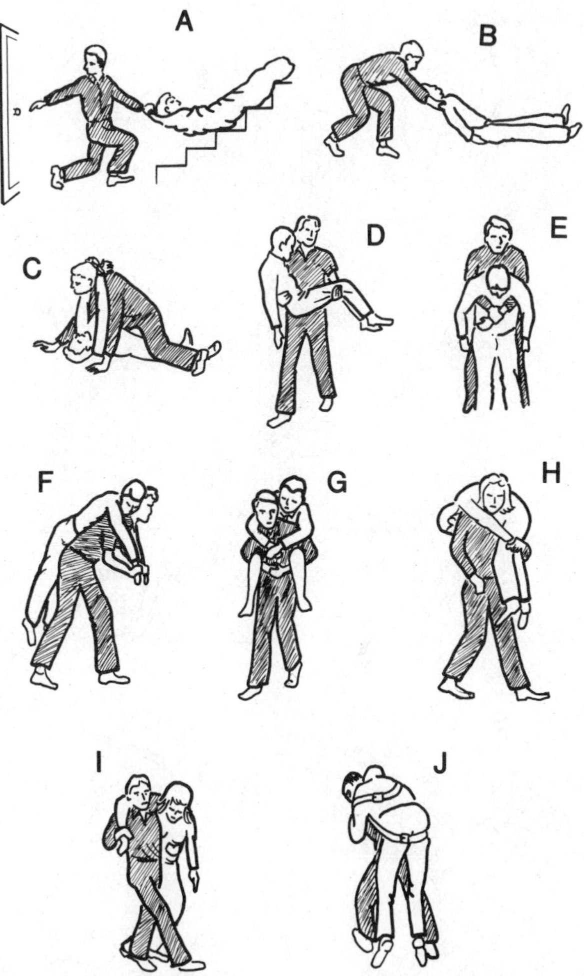

Figure 4–1. Single rescuer expedient transport. *A,* Blanket drag. *B,* Clothes drag. *C,* Firefighter's drag. (Victim's wrists are tied together, preferably with any soft broad material available). *D,* Arm carry. *E,* Chest lift and drag. *F,* Pack strap or back carry. *G,* Saddle or "piggyback" carry. *H,* Firefighter's carry. *I,* Walking assist. *J,* Belt carry. (Two or more belts are buckled together to form a sling positioned on the victim as shown. Initially sling is positioned with victim lying on his back; the single rescuer in a comparable position then slides one arm through each side of sling, turns himself and victim over to kneeling position and stands up.)

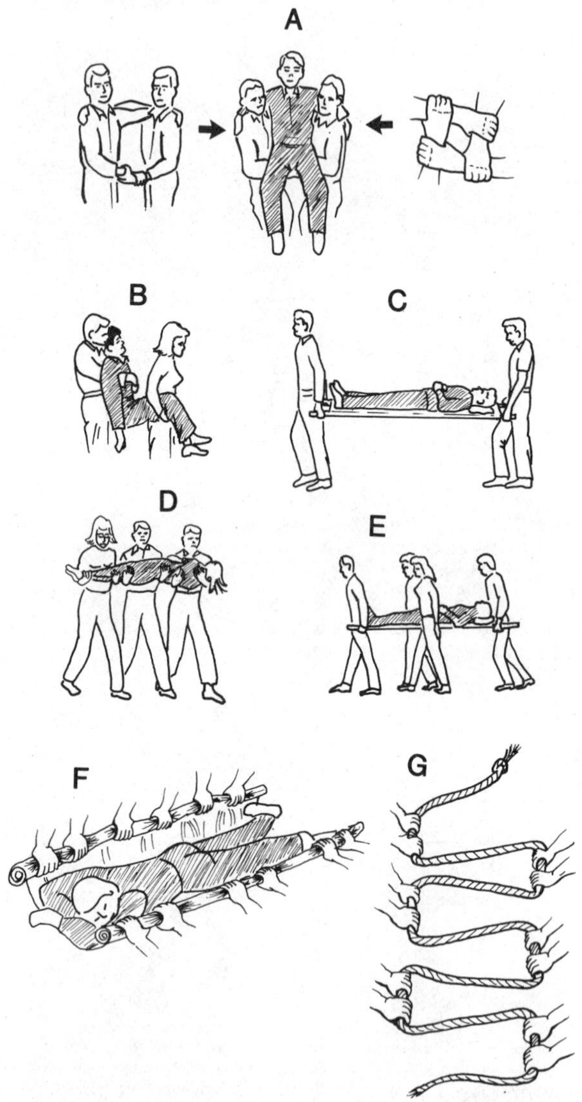

Figure 4–2. *A,* Two-person arm carry. *B,* Chair-position carry. (Victim can also actually be seated in a chair as an alternative.) *C,* Two-person stretcher carry. *D,* Three-person carry. (*Note*: Stability of the spine is only partial in this position and inadequate if a fracture is present.) *E,* Four-person stretcher carry. (Alternatively two people can be positioned at each end.) *F,* Blanket carry. *G,* Rope carry.

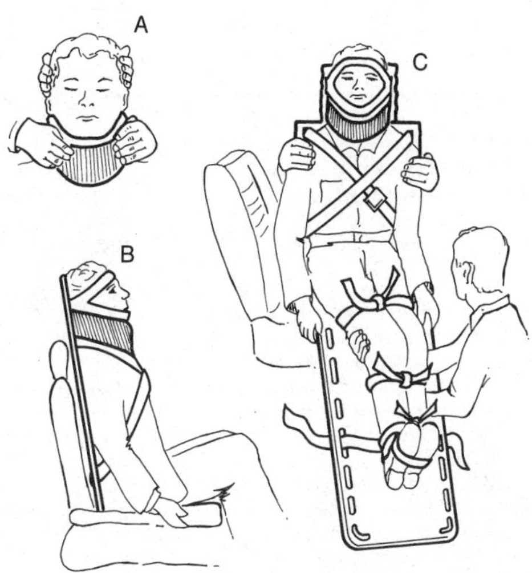

Figure 4–3. *A,* If head or neck injury is evident or suspected or there is general body trauma, stabilize the head and apply a hard cervical collar. *B,* Next apply short board, if long board will not fit in confined area. Note that the chin strap and forehead band are diagonally crossed to add stability when fixed to short board. See comments under Figure 4–4, including alternative use of neck roll in some (infrequent) circumstances. *C,* After patient is moved cautiously from confined area, immobilization on a long board may take place. When the short board is used first, it can then be fixed directly to the long board.

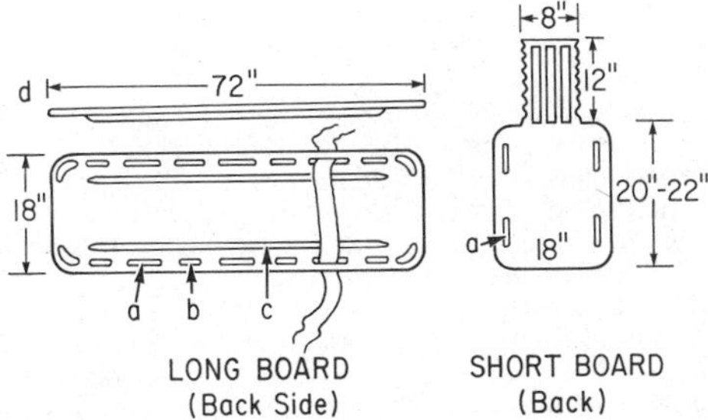

Figure 4–4. Long board and short board. These smoothly finished plywood boards are sturdy (¾" and ½" thick respectively), with notches or slots for insertion of head band and chin straps (both about 42" long with a center padded section and Velcro fastener ends; these straps are placed obliquely to each other to increase head fixation) and for other body fixation straps. If a hard cervical collar is not available, use a 4" diameter foam rubber neck roll between the posterior neck and the board to help stabilize neck position and contour. The neck roll is particularly helpful in maintaining neck position if a helmet is on and should not or could not be removed, making it impossible to put on a hard cervical collar. Adhesive taping of helmet to board is usually preferable to other fixation methods. The long board has hand slots at the corners to aid lifting and carrying. (Redrawn from *Emergency Care and Transportation of the Sick and Injured.* American Academy of Orthopedic Surgeons, 1977.)

MANAGEMENT OF PATIENTS WITH SERIOUS HEAD INJURIES AWAITING TRANSPORT FOR HOSPITAL CARE: ROUTINE THERAPY AND HANDLING

- Initially treat with cervical splinting, back board, and careful handling (see Figs. 4–3 to 4–5), particularly if patient is comatose, has had a concussion with an unconscious episode or paralysis, if a skull fracture is evident or if the patient had a helmet on and it is dented, crushed, cracked or gouged. Treat as if patient had also had a cervical spine fracture until this possibility is ruled out by a cross-table lateral cervical spine x-ray.
- Any helmet should be left on (with a posterior neck roll to keep straight cervical alignment) unless the rescue worker is skilled in removal (see p. 25) and there is a compelling reason for doing it (e.g., to administer CPR, evaluate underlying injury, stop bleeding).
- Ensure an adequate airway by support of the angles of the jaw or oropharyngeal airway, positional drainage and application of suction as needed. Comatose patients should be intubated. Ventilate as needed.
- Administer oxygen as needed for dyspnea and cyanosis.
- Avoid use of oral medications, food and fluids initially, and anything that may induce vomiting.
- If there is evidence of CSF leak (low viscosity/clear/colorless fluid stained with blood giving "halo" appearance [*18–29*] on materials) from the nose or ear, elevate head of the long board or cot approximately 30 degrees. If fluid is from nose, do not put anything in nose; see *44–17*. If fluid is from ear, cover ear with sterile gauze; put nothing in ear; see *44–18*.
- Make frequent checks of patient's state of consciousness, pulse, blood pressure, respiration, temperature and neurologic status. These findings should be recorded on the patient's emergency record. If the patient is being transferred from an initial hospital rather than from the field, send a summary of events together with any x-rays with the patient to the next destination.
- Use of gentle restraint is preferable to any sedation. Forcible physical restraint should be kept to a minimum; intermittent reassurance in a compassionate but firm, distinct voice often has a quieting effect. A skilled, able-bodied attendant should be present at all times.
- Use cooling measures as available (ice bags, cold compresses, blower, etc.) if the patient's temperature is higher than 39° C (102.2° F).
- Treat gross cerebral edema (*44–7*) if present.
- Ensure tactful and sympathetic handling of the patient's family, friends or other interested persons, avoiding specific statements concerning the extent of injuries, condition of patient, type and duration of further treatment, possible complications and prognosis.
- With the airway established and the neck/spine splinted, the comatose patient may be transported in the recumbent position. If the patient is vomiting, turn into the semiprone position after first firmly immobilizing the head, neck and back. If available and necessary, a nasogastric tube can be inserted and the stomach emptied. The semiprone position (Fig. 4–5*A*) is also one of the preferred positions for head injury or comatose patients once the presence of cervical fracture is not of concern.
- Keep patient recumbent and quiet.

HELMET (MOTORCYCLE/FOOTBALL TYPE) MANAGEMENT WITH POSSIBLE HEAD/NECK INJURIES

Leave Helmet on During Transportation to the Emergency Department

- Unskilled removal of or pulling on the helmet can aggravate neck injuries.
- Leave helmet on with known or suspected head/neck injuries unless removal is imperative; this applies particularly to helmets providing entire head protection, such as football and motorcycle helmets. Partial or upper head helmets do not generally present a removal problem after the neck is stabilized.
- Hold the head and helmet in a stable position with two hands while sliding a neck roll (of sufficient diameter to help stabilize and maintain the cervical curvature) behind the neck.
- Secure the helmet to the short or long board with adhesive tape.
- Tie through and around the rigid chin piece of a full face mask with cloth bindings if adhesive tape is not available; then secure bindings to the board. Nonadhesive straps, bandages and cravats tend to slip off the hard, smooth helmet surface.
- If adhesive tape is not available, stabilize neutral position of the head with sandbags or hands, with the patient in a recumbent position, for as long as is necessary during transportation. The hands can also be used to apply gentle traction in a neutral position (however, firm neck fixation is preferable).
- Place the secured patient in a recumbent position.
- The above procedure is a substitute measure for the hard cervical collar, which is usually impossible to apply with helmets that cover the entire head.

If the Helmet Must Be Removed

- Possible problems with the helmet on the head include:
  —Difficulty or impossibility (with full face mask) of giving CPR.
  —Control of any gross bleeding beneath the helmet.
  —Application of hard cervical collar; use procedures outlined above.
  —Obstruction and management problems during vomiting with full face mask on.
- Remove or cut chin strap; take off face shield and glasses (if any) first.
- The easiest manner of removal is to cut the helmet off with a cast saw when available.
- If no cast saw is available, have an assistant stabilize the neck posteriorly with one hand and the jaw anteriorly with the other hand. The assistant also observes and places a finger, if necessary, on each side of the patient's nose under the rigid chin guard, to guide the chin guard over the nose during removal. Spread the helmet apart laterally with one hand placed under the lower helmet edge at each ear level (requires strength to pull helmet sides apart laterally with a tight-fitting helmet). While assistant stabilizes head and neck, tilt or pivot the front of the helmet backward slightly until the greatest length of the helmet is in line with the frontal-occipital length of the head (the forehead will now be mostly uncovered from the brow of the helmet); then pull the helmet off with a gentle sliding motion. The slight pivoting and alignment of the helmet (while keeping the head and neck stable) before pulling is the essential maneuver.

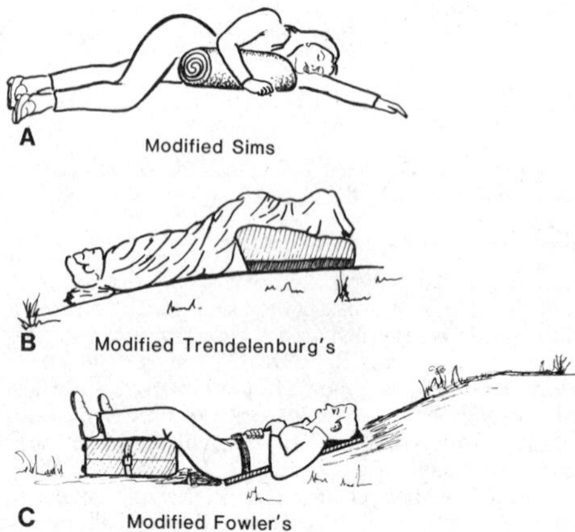

Figure 4–5. Body position placement in emergencies. *A,* Modified Sims position is preferable for lethargic, comatose or nauseated patients. If chest or lung injury also is present, it is usually best to lay patient with uninjured or least injured side up. *B,* Modified Trendelenburg position is used for patients in shock. *C,* Modified Fowler position may be helpful for patients in cardiopulmonary distress. (*Note:* following trauma, awkwardly positioned bodies [or body parts that probably have been fractured] should generally be left as is until they can be appropriately immobilized in the same or a similar position.)

- **Initiation of specific management** according to the problem present (e.g., for burn victims, see 28–3) and the resources available at the scene of injury and during transportation to a care facility.
- **Safety of EMS vehicles in transit.** Stabilization treatment en route reduces need for speed. Multiple blinking lights and siren are essential when moving through traffic (Code 3). Other vehicles (e.g., buses, trucks) may be enlisted in mass casualty events to move less seriously wounded patients.
- **Proper destination of EMS vehicle** should be a facility that can give adequate care. Patients with severe injuries should be taken to a Trauma Center if available. Whenever possible, patients should be sent to an in-hospital facility that meets the Emergency Care Guidelines of the American College of Emergency Physicians. Special problems such as burns, behavioral crises, neonatal emergencies and rape cases may be preferentially referred to hospitals with special care facilities for that problem.

Special Problems

- **Patient reluctance to be transported** to a hospital by ambulance occasionally occurs. Patients needing physician evaluation prior to release should be gently and firmly convinced that proceeding to a hospital is in their best interest.
  —If the patient still refuses and is competent, he or she should sign a release from care. (If the patient refuses to sign the form, this should be noted in writing.)
  —If the patient refuses and is not competent, he or she should be taken under custody by police (or by EMT where state law permits).
- **Transportation from difficult areas** (hazardous, distant, across congested areas, etc.) is often better handled by airborne vehicles (helicopter, air

ambulance). Assistance may be obtained from the military or state highway patrol.

4–2. TRANSFER OF CARE

In the period just *before, during* and *after* patient transfer there is a great risk of poor communication and missed assignments or even of a finding of abandonment and malpractice, regardless of how unintentional. In the emergency situation, this applies to transfer of patient care from one physician to another at the same location as well as patient transfers from one location to another. Prior to transfer, the patient should be stabilized and programmed for care during transportation as much as is feasible. Placement of at least one IV line is advisable for patients requiring emergency interfacility transfer. Communication problems can be avoided by the following measures:

- Personal direct communication by phone or radio between the responsible medical personnel before and during transportation, at intervals as frequent as new information and patient condition require.
- Clear, concise transfer notes, when possible, giving a summary of laboratory work, x-rays and treatment to date and noting areas of special concern and reason for transfer. These notes, which accompany the patient, should be given to the transporting professionals rather than to the patient's family or friends.
- Prearranged protocols whenever possible as to when, where and how responsibility for patient care will be transferred—this is applicable also in hospital staff procedures concerning emergency department–to–hospital physician transfers.
- Adequate availability of equipment for specific needs of the patient during time of transfer. In some instances in which the patient's condition is particularly critical, the attendance of a physician in addition to other adequately trained professional personnel during transportation is advisable when feasible; this is particularly so with long distance aeromedical patient transport (the medical personnel accompanying the patient should not only be capable for the situation medically but also—when light aircraft are used—preferably have demonstrated their ability to perform in the heat, lower oxygenation, noise, close quarters and turbulence that can occur). See also comments concerning patient air travel (26–7, *Barotrauma*).

5. ABC's of Resuscitation (CPR)

5–1. BASIC LIFE SUPPORT (BLS) AND OTHER CPR PHASES

Cardiopulmonary resuscitation (CPR) may be divided into 3 phases:

Phase I: Basic Life Support (BLS)

This phase involves (1) initial airway management; (2) breathing or ventilation assistance; and (3) circulation augmentation with external heart compression (EHC).

These steps are outlined in Figures 5–1 and 5–1A and are taught to medical personnel and interested members of the general public by certified AHA and ARC instructors. The final outcome in any CPR case can be no better than the promptness and efficacy of BLS permits.

Text continues on page 35

PHASE I: BASIC LIFE SUPPORT

IF UNCONSCIOUS

AIRWAY

- Tilt head back*
to open airway
- Do not overextend,
particularly in infants
- If trauma, get cervical
collar, but do not delay CPR

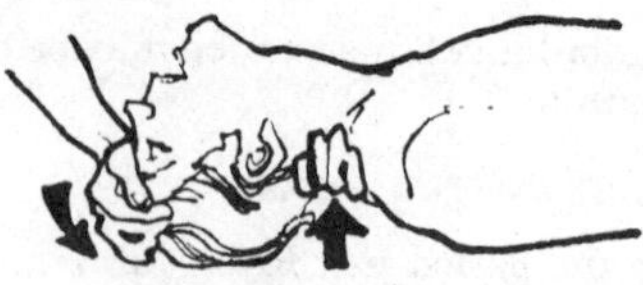

IF NOT BREATHING

BREATHE

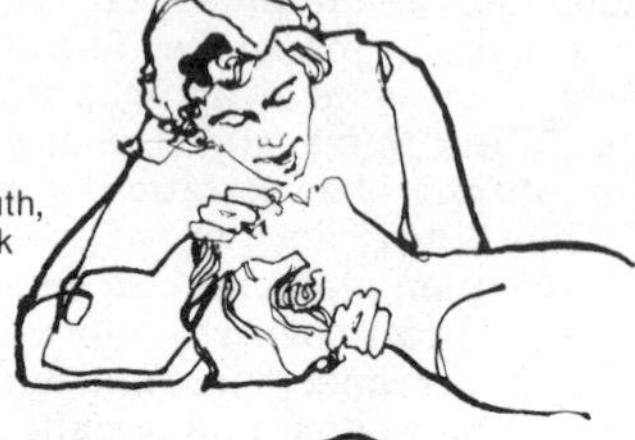

- Inflate lungs rapidly 4 times mouth-to mouth, mouth-to-nose, mouth-to-adjunct, bag-mask
- MAINTAIN HEAD TILT*
  - — Feel carotid pulse
  - — If pulse present, continue lung inflations as follows:
    adult: 12/min; child: 15/min;
    infant: 20/min; neonate: 24/min

IF PULSE ABSENT (with pupils dilated and deathlike appearance)

CIRCULATE (See also 5-23,EHC)

ONE-RESCUER CPR (see Table 5-4):
Adult (80/min):
Alternate 2 quick lung inflations with 15 chest compressions

Child (80/min) or infant (100/min):
Alternate 1 quick lung inflation with 5 chest compressions

TWO-RESCUER CPR:
Interpose 1 lung inflation after every 5th compression (no pause for ventilation), at following rates:
adult: 60/min; child: 80/min;
infant: 100/min; neonate: 124/min

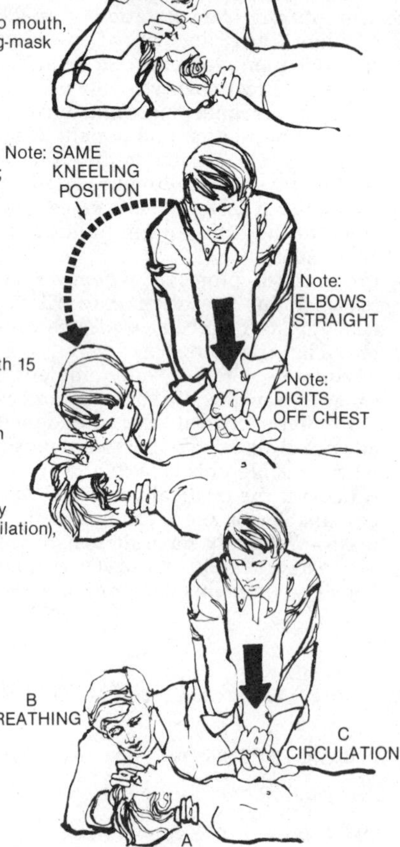

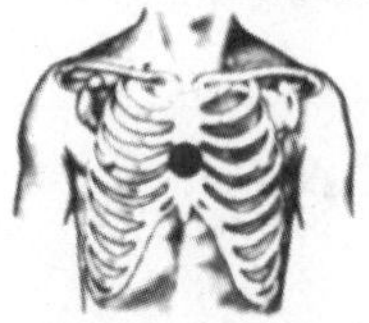

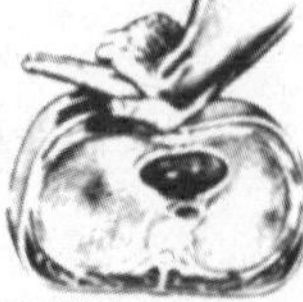

DEPRESS LOWER STERNUM:
Adult: 1½ – 2" (4 – 5 cm) (use 2 hands)
Child: ¾ – 1½" (2 – 4 cm) (use 1 hand)
Infant: ½ – ¾" (1 – 2 cm) (use 2 fingers)
Neonate: See 52 – 1

CONTINUE RESUSCITATION until spontaneous pulse returns
(Check pulse at 1 min and then every few min)

Figure 5–1. Basic life support (BLS) measures. (Figure on left from Schwartz, G. R., et al.: *Principles and Practice of Emergency Medicine,* Vol. I. Philadelphia, W. B. Saunders Co., 1978, p. 178; Figures on right from Committee of the American Medical Association: Standards for cardiopulmonary resuscitation [CPR] and emergency cardiac care [ECC]. JAMA, 227:841, 1974. Reprinted by permission of the American Heart Association, Inc.) **Lift jaw instead if possible neck injury.*

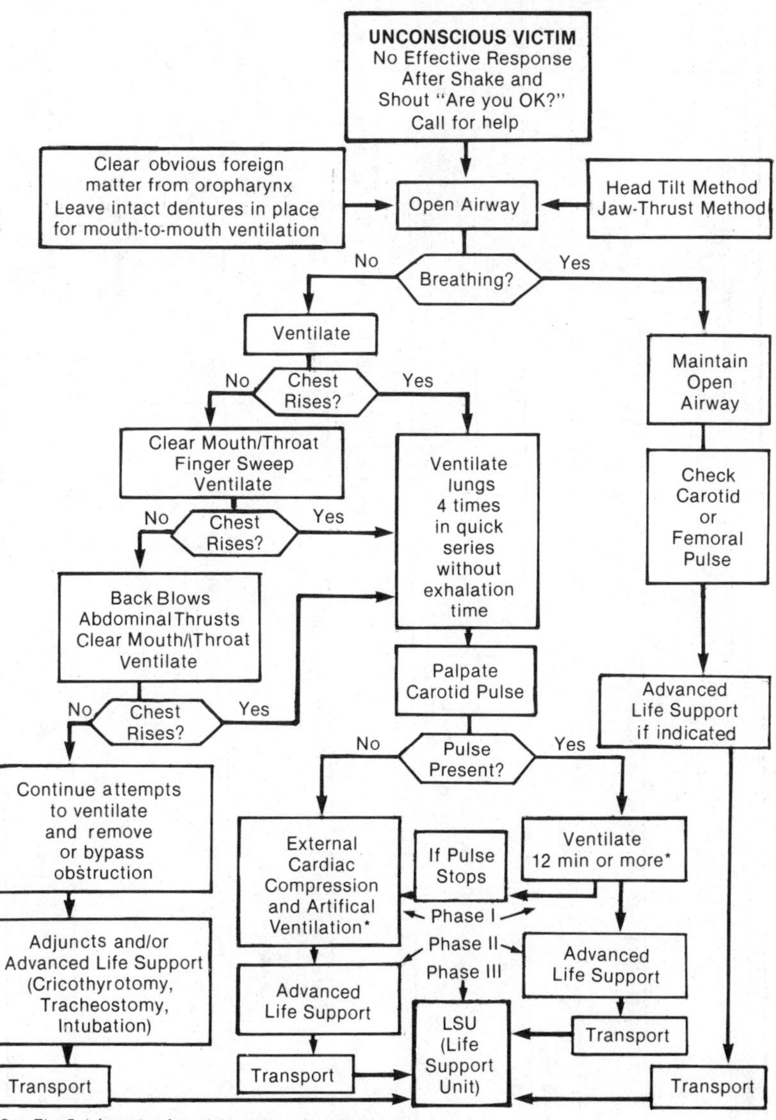

*See Fig. 5-1 for rates for adult, child, infant. Recheck pulse after 1 minute CPR; if present and effective, continue ventilation and supportive measures as needed; if absent, continue CPR and recheck pulse every few minutes.

Figure 5–1A. Life Support Decision Tree (unwitnessed arrest). *Note*: Call for help should activate Emergency Medical Service (EMS) system; dialing 911 activates EMS in many communities. (Modified from JAMA, 227, 1974.)

Table 5–1. PHASE II: ADVANCED CARDIAC LIFE SUPPORT (ACLS—AHA GUIDELINES/FOR USE WITH FIG. 5–2)

ACLS Drugs and Symbols	Conc/Vol Prefilled Syr/Amp	Initial Dose	Infusion Preparation†	Comments/Cautions
ATRO Atropine	0.1 mg/ml in 10-ml syringe	0.1 ml/kg or (0.01–0.03 mg/kg); in children, no single dose over 0.4 mg (4 ml)	—	Avg adult: 0.5 to 1.0 mg/dose Repeat at 5-min intervals to desired ↑ HR, or to total of 2 mg
BRET Bretylium tosylate	50 mg/ml in 10-ml ampule	5 mg/kg loading dose	500 mg in 500 ml or 250 ml D5W = 1 or 2 mg/ml	Avg adult: 1–2 mg/min after loading dose for control of recurrent VT/VF; caution if <12 yr
CA Calcium chloride, 10%	100 mg/ml in 10-ml syringe	0.1 ml/kg or 5–7 mg/kg	—	Don't give in same IV tube with $NaHCO_3$ Use bolus q 10 min prn
DOP Dopamine	200 mg in 5-ml ampule	—	200 mg/250 ml D5W = 800 μg/ml	Infuse at 2–10 μg/kg/min Monitor BP ↑ to adjust rate
EPI * Epinephrine, 1:10,000	0.1 mg/ml in 10-ml syringe	0.1 ml/kg (or 0.01 mg/kg) IV or 10 ml into adult trachea	1 mg/500 ml D5W = 2 μg/ml; Adult: 1 μg/min	Repeat bolus q 5 min prn in cardiac arrest Avoid intracardiac injection Monitor BP ↑/ECG
ISO Isoproterenol	0.2 mg/ml; 5 ml = 1 mg	0.1 μg/kg/min initially; may increase to 0.2–2 μg/kg/min	Adult: 1 mg/500 ml D5W = 2 μg/ml Child: 1 mg/100 ml D5W = 10 μg/ml	Adult: 2 to 20 μg/min; titrate Child: max 6–24 ml/hr Monitor closely; adjust rate or discontinue if tachycardia or PVC's develop
LIDO * Lidocaine, 1%, 2%, 4%	Bolus: Use either 1% (10 mg/ml); 2% (20 mg/ml); or 4% (40 mg/ml)	1 mg/kg; must follow with infusion drip	Adult: 2 g in 500 ml D5W = 4 mg/ml Child: 2 g in 100 ml D5W = 20 mg/ml	For breakthrough ventricular ectopy, may give additional bolus of 0.5 mg/kg q 5 min to suppress, to max 3 mg/kg Adult infusion: 1–4 mg/min Ped infusion: 25–50 μg/kg/min
PRO Procainamide	Bolus: Use 100 mg/ml in 10-ml vial	Adult: 20 mg/min until one of the conditions listed under "Cautions" occurs (see last column) Child: Doses in children not well established	After bolus, 1 g/250 ml D5W = 4 mg/ml; for continuous infusion with precautions	Give bolus until one of the following occurs: suppression of dysrhythmia; BP ↓; QRS width increases by 50%; or until total of 1 g is given Adult infusion: 1–4 mg/min Monitor ECG and BP Use with caution in acute MI
NaBi or $NaHCO_3$ Sodium bicarbonate	1 mEq/ml or usual prefilled 50-ml syringes (44.6 mEq)	Adult: 1 mEq/kg, or by pH Child: 1–2 mEq/kg	—	Repeat according to pH; if pH determination not possible, use ½ initial dose q 10 min during cardiac arrest

*Can be given endotracheally with increased dose.
†Best to use infusion pump for drip administration.

Table 5–2. RESPIRATORY DISTRESS EVALUATION (LIFE SUPPORT: PHASES I, II and III)

Cause of Respiratory Distress	Emergency Correlations
1. Environment abnormality in gas content (e.g., low oxygen, high carbon dioxide); suffocation	Move to normal gas environment; administer oxygen (see 25, *Asphyxiation*); consider use of HBO
2. Partial or complete mechanical ventilatory failure of muscles (diaphragm, intercostals, accessory muscles); impaired anatomic problems of the thorax: post-traumatic flail chest *(31)*; impaired elastic recoil of the lungs; immobile thorax; or CNS/peripheral nerve impairment	Ventilate *(5–21, Artificial Ventilation)* Check for and treat cause of impaired neuromuscular capacity—e.g., drugs/poisons *[53]*, paralytic disease (polio, myasthenia gravis, myelitis, neuritis *[49]*, botulism toxin), trauma (especially cervical spinal cord and head injury)
3. Airway obstruction, partial or complete (see Table 5–3). With COPD (chronic obstructive emphysema, chronic bronchitis, or combinations of the two), *use O_2 with extreme caution* (no more than 1 to 2 liters/min), and monitor ABG's closely	Remove bypass or alleviate obstruction. See 5–1, *Basic Life Support;* 5–13, *Abdominal Thrust and Back Blow;* 18–34, *Tracheostomy;* 18–10, *Endotracheal Intubation;* 18–20, *Nasotracheal Intubation;* 38–6, *Foreign Bodies in the Larynx, Trachea or Bronchi;* 56–4, *Asthma*
4. Impairment of gas exchange between alveolar air and pulmonary capillary blood due to: Structural/functional changes of the alveolar wall	Improve ventilation and partial gas pressures (see also treatment in cause 6) Refer for surgical evaluation of potentially correctable segmental lesions
Abnormal segmental gas distribution and/or abnormal segmental pulmonary capillary blood flow to significant proportions of the alveoli	Treat any specific infections or inflammatory processes See also 55–4, *Noncardiogenic Pulmonary Edema;* 56–20, *Pulmonary Artery Embolism;* 56–2, *ARDS;* and 56–3, *ARF*
5. Mechanical or electrical failure, partial or complete, of the cardiovascular pump function	See treatment in cause 6. Also see 5, *ABC's of Resuscitation;* 29–8, *Cardiac Arrest;* 55–3, *Congestive Heart Failure;* and 59, *Shock.* Surgical evaluation for installation of a temporary pump mechanism may be of value
6. Inadequate blood gas carrying mechanism due to insufficient hemoglobin or to abnormal alteration of hemoglobin (congenital or acquired [poisoning, e.g., carbon monoxide, methemoglobin])	Administration of oxygen by nasal tube to enhance hemoglobin and soluble oxygen content of blood. Transfusion of whole blood or packed blood cells. Removal from exposure to poisoning substance; give specific antidote if available. Consider exchange transfusion; hyperbaric oxygen
7. Impaired cellular metabolism due to enzymatic poisons, shock, metabolic disorders and acid-base or electrolyte disorders	See: *Fluid Replacement (11)* *Metabolic Disorders (46)* *Poisoning (53)* *Shock (57)* *Peritoneal Dialysis (18–24)*

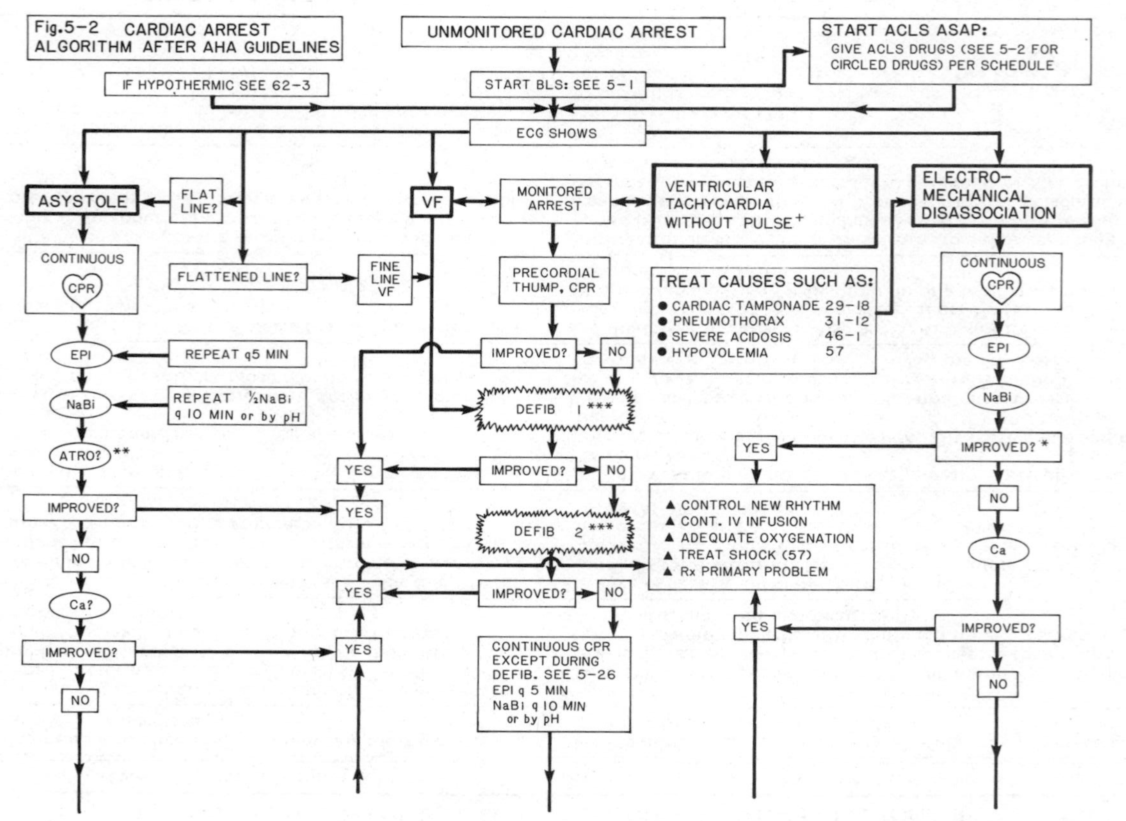

Fig.5-2 CARDIAC ARREST ALGORITHM AFTER AHA GUIDELINES

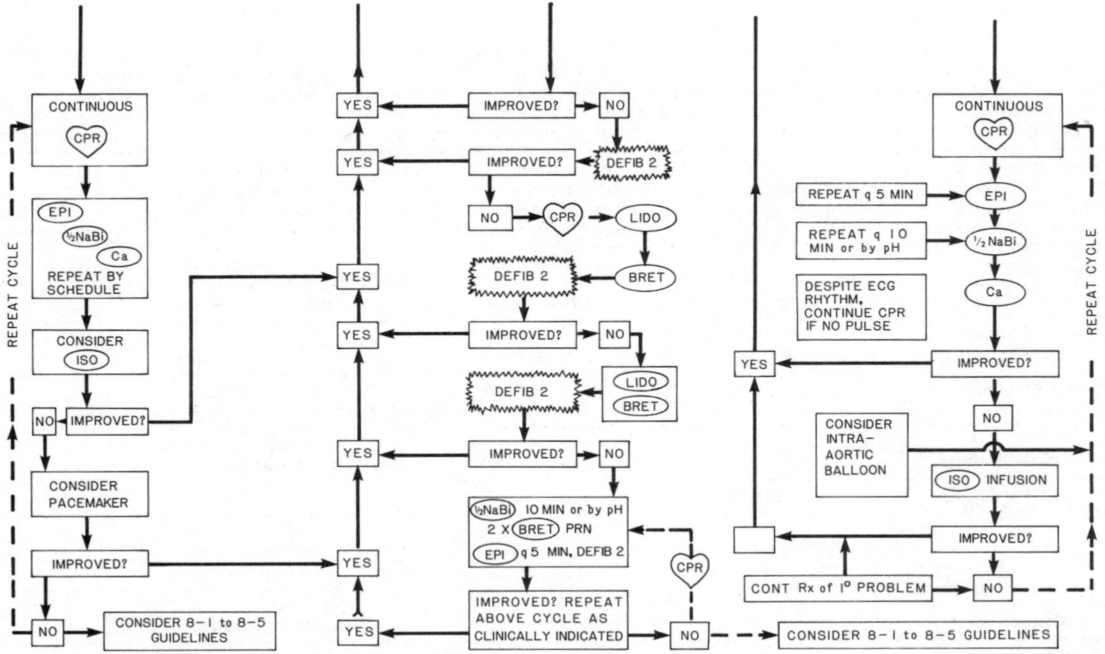

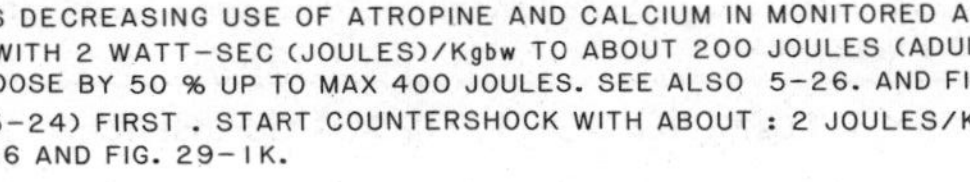

* IMPROVED MEANS PATIENT'S OWN PULSE HAS RETURNED AND ECG SHOWS A SELF-SUSTAINING RHYTHM.

** IF ARREST 2° to ↑K^+, GIVE Ca^{++} FIRST. ATROPINE EFFICACY GENERALLY UNDER REEVALUATION AS IS CALCIUM UNDER OTHER CIRCUMSTANCES. THERE IS DECREASING USE OF ATROPINE AND CALCIUM IN MONITORED ASYSTOLE.

*** DEFIB 1.. DEFIBRILLATION WITH 2 WATT-SEC (JOULES)/Kgbw TO ABOUT 200 JOULES (ADULTS).
DEFIB 2.. INCREASE LAST DOSE BY 50 % UP TO MAX 400 JOULES. SEE ALSO 5-26. AND FIG.29-1 L

+ USE PRECORDIAL THUMP (5-24) FIRST . START COUNTERSHOCK WITH ABOUT : 2 JOULES/Kg, UP TO 200 JOULES (ADULTS). SEE ALSO 29-26 AND FIG. 29-1K.

Figure 5–2.

Table 5–3. GUIDE TO LOCALIZATION OF PARTIAL AIRWAY OBSTRUCTION*

Sign or Symptom	Level of Obstruction			
	Pharynx	*Larynx*	*Trachea*	*Bronchi*
Voice changes	Slurred or thick	Hoarse or absent	Decreased volume	Decreased volume
Cough	Persistent, scratchy	Harsh (stridor), "croupy"	Reflex irritative	Reflex irritative
Swallowing	Difficult; drooling; patient juts head forward and down to aid egress	Difficult; may be drooling	Usually normal but sometimes painful	Normal
Dyspnea	Positional	Inspiratory	Inspiratory	Often present with wheezing
Cyanosis	May be present—relieved by position changes	May be present	May be present	Often present
Intercostal/neck retractions	Usually not present unless severe airway block	Inspiratory	Inspiratory	If a large bronchus is blocked; may be unilateral
Breath sounds	Normal	Roughened—coarse	Loud rales and rhonchi	Rhonchi; may be decreased or absent
Restlessness, excitement, apprehension	Intermittent; acute during episodes of dysphagia and dyspnea	Often acute	Variable; depends on % obstruction	Acute if a large bronchus is blocked
X-ray†: lateral, neck and chest films	"Thumb sign" of swollen epiglottis; retropharyngeal swelling wider than patient's little finger	May be normal; esophageal foreign body indentation	May be normal; esophageal foreign body indentation	Acute ball valve obstruction: bilateral expiration decubitus AP, film-involved side stays expanded; late-collapse

*Note: *Complete obstruction* is indicated by the acute onset of complete loss of voice and inability to cough or breathe in a struggling conscious person whose hand is clutching the throat. The Heimlich hug and/or back slap (*5–13*) should be instituted immediately.

See also *39–5, Foreign Bodies in the Larynx, Trachea or Bronchi; 56–4, Asthma and Severe Bronchospasm;* and *56–8, Epiglottitis.*

†Obtain portable film or have an experienced person with complete airway equipment accompany patient. Radiopaque or air-displacing foreign bodies may also be seen. All of the films listed may be normal.

Phase II: Advanced Cardiac Life Support (ACLS)

This phase is most often begun outside the hospital by specially trained medical personnel under the direction of a physician; measures are continued during transportation and maintained until administration of efforts is assumed by ED and hospital personnel. ACLS includes: (1) continuous lung ventilation and necessary cardiac compression (EHC) as with BLS; (2) intubation of the trachea (or use of EOA/EGTA) ASAP, with hyperventilation before the procedure, which should interrupt CPR for no more than 15 to 30 seconds; and (3) administration of ACLS drugs (Table 5–1) and fluids via IV life lines, performance of ECG monitoring and continuation of cardiac arrest management (Fig. 5–2).

Phase III: Life Support Unit (LSU)

The staff of the hospital or trauma center continues efforts of the prior phases while further tests, procedures and responses may be performed to determine: (1) need for additional efforts or advisability of cessation (see 8); (2) later phases of resuscitation (including cerebral resuscitation) and intensive care unit (ICU) management; (3) definitive management of any continuing/preexisting/predisposing pathology, including any indicated surgery.

5–2. CARDIAC ARREST (*For treatment, see Figs. 5–1, 5–1A and 5–2; Table 5–1*)

Characterized by loss of arterial pulse, pulse pressure and respiration, cardiac arrest may be due to cardiac asystole, ventricular fibrillation, ventricular tachycardia without a pulse, or electromechanical disassociation (see Fig. 5–2). It represents one of the most urgent conditions that may be encountered in the practice of medicine. Rapid recognition of the condition and prompt reestablishment of adequate oxygenation and circulation represent the only possible chance of saving the patient's life. Because severe hypoxemia for more than 3 to 5 minutes will usually result in irreparable damage to the higher centers of the brain, success depends upon carrying out an already planned course of action without delay.

Causes of Cardiac Arrest

- Acute myocardial infarction or severe progressive myocardial ischemia.
- Too rapid or unregulated administration of, or overdosage of, any anesthetic (inhalation, intravenous, spinal or local), with lack of close observation for and recognition of changes in condition.
- Obstruction of the respiratory tract (mucus, vomitus, foreign bodies [39], trauma, angioedema [24–2], bronchospasm [24–3]).
- Preexistent conditions (acute anxiety states [37], anemia, cardiac disease, dehydration, hyperpyrexia, pulmonary edema [55], shock [57] or severe hypothermia [62]).
- Excessive medications or street drugs or poisons.
- Mechanical errors (faulty gauges, mislabeled tanks, poor valves, etc.).
- Position of the patient. The sitting position (sometimes used for throat operations) and the deep Trendelenburg are the most dangerous positions. Rapid shifting on the operating table may precipitate cardiac arrest.
- Electrical shock (32–5; see also 28–12, *Electrical Burns*).
- Air emboli (63–6) (rarely).

Preliminary Warning Signs of Incipient Cardiac Arrest

- Signs and symptoms of respiratory obstruction with hypoxemia (see Tables 5–2 and 5–3).

- Conditions of severe progressive acidosis and shock.
- Electrocardiographic evidence of multifocal or frequent premature ventricular systoles (particularly bigeminy).

Note: Failure to recognize the preliminary warning signs of incipient cardiac arrest when the patient is under immediate medical care (i.e., hospitalized) and to institute prompt and proper treatment has been held to constitute negligence.

Successful Resuscitation After Cardiac Arrest

This requires a combination of the following:

- Prompt institution of corrective measures.
- Adequate pulmonary ventilation.
- Adequate coronary artery flow and adequate perfusion of vital organs with oxygenated blood.
- Adequate correction of acidosis and electrolyte imbalance.
- Adequate defibrillating current for an effective period of time with good skin contact of the electrodes with the chest.
- Restoration of a functional cardiac rate, rhythm and stroke volume, with assistance of an artificial pacemaker if necessary. When functional rhythm, rate and stroke volume have been established, the following measures to facilitate recovery can be started:

—Determination and treatment of the cause of cardiac arrest; further treatment of shock *(57)*.

—Intravenous supportive or replacement therapy *(11, Fluid Replacement in Emergencies; 18–35, Transfusions)* based on frequent arterial pH, blood gas and electrolyte determinations and CVP monitoring.

—Lidocaine loading dose (1 mg/kg) and IV drips 1.5 mg/kg/hr, generally not to exceed 100 mg/hr, helps prevent repeat ventricular fibrillation. Propranolol, 1 mg IV, may also help in repeated ventricular fibrillation, particularly if associated with excess amounts of catecholamines or digitalis. It may be repeated with monitoring 1 to 2 times.

—Vasopressor drugs if indicated for hypotension.

—Continuous electrocardiographic monitoring.

—Cardiac pacemaker (external or intracardiac via intravenous route) on operative or standby basis is indicated with Mobitz II 2nd degree atrioventricular (AV) block, with 3rd degree AV block and with bifascicular block with acute MI.

Note: Early communication with and support of family members is an important concomitant of care.

5–3. VENTRICULAR ASYSTOLE *(See Fig. 5–2)*

Usually caused by severe generalized hypoxemia or focal myocardial lack of oxygen, this condition is rapidly terminal if not corrected.

5–4. VENTRICULAR FIBRILLATION *(See Fig. 29–1L)*

This extremely serious arrhythmia, incompatible with life if not rapidly corrected, may occur with any of the causes listed under cardiac arrest *(5–2)*. It is particularly to be suspected when sudden unconsciousness and asystole follow electrical shock.

Treatment *(See Figs. 5–1 and 5–2)*

- Direct current defibrillation is the immediate treatment of choice.

- Precordial thump (*5–24;* Fig. 5–8) may be immediately administered in cases of monitored cardiac arrest due to VF.

Prophylaxis Against Ventricular Fibrillation *(See 29–27)*

Agonal Arrhythmias

Ventricular fibrillation followed by cardiac standstill is the common agonal arrhythmia seen terminally in persons with serious chronic diseases. Management of ventricular fibrillation under these circumstances when death is anticipated should be approached with discernment (See *8, Guidelines for Death and Dying Cases*).

5–5. VENTRICULAR TACHYCARDIA WITHOUT PULSE *(See Fig. 5–2; see also 29–26, Ventricular Tachycardia)*

- CPR, BLS and ACLS should be started.
- Synchronized cardioversion with 20 to 200 joules is used instead of unsynchronized direct current defibrillation.

5–6. ELECTROMECHANICAL DISASSOCIATION *(See Fig. 5–2)*

5–7. CEREBROCARDIOPULMONARY RESUSCITATION (CCPR)

Treatment with the current common measures for cerebral edema reduction is presented in 44–7. Further improvements and refinements in protection of the brain after hypoxemic insult continue to be vigorously sought, with research focusing on slow-acting calcium channel blockers, thiopental/barbiturate coma therapy, hypothermia, DMSO (a free radical scavenger that reduces cerebral edema by vasodilatation and diuresis) and osmotherapy as means of cerebral resuscitation.

5–8. FURTHER RESEARCH DEVELOPMENTS IN CARDIAC RESUSCITATION TECHNIQUES

Though not as yet considered standard resuscitation techniques, the following have demonstrated value and are under evaluation:

- Intermittent abdominal compression (IAC) with CPR. In this modified CPR technique (so far used only in animal experimentation), CPR would be conducted in the standard way by two rescuers as previously described, and a third rescuer would perform IAC. This involves applying perpendicular, downward mid-abdominal pressure (about 100 mm Hg) with the palms placed side by side in the vertical line just after EHC (external heart compression) pressure is released. The third rescuer would kneel on the opposite side of the second rescuer. Improved tissue oxygenation and circulatory hemodynamics are the objectives accomplished in the animal experimentation. Intra-abdominal tissue trauma is a problem consideration.
- "High-impulse" CPR using rates of 150 EHC/min with pressure of moderate intensity has demonstrated in animal experimentation significant increases in cardiac output and arterial BP.

5–9. TERMINATION OF RESUSCITATIVE EFFORTS

See sections *8–1* to *8–6* for guidelines for determining the point at which resuscitation measures have failed and may be terminated.

RESUSCITATION TECHNIQUES AND PROCEDURES

5–10. AIRWAY MANAGEMENT *(See 5–11 to 5–20)*

5–11. HEAD TILT WITH NECK OR CHIN LIFT *(See Figs. 5–1 and 5–7)*

In unconscious people, the tongue, which is affixed to the lower jaw (mandible), slides back into the oropharynx and completely or partially occludes it in older children and adults. Tilting the head backward gently with one hand under the neck or with 2 fingers under the chin automatically lifts the tongue, which opens the airway and prepares it for ventilation resuscitation via the mouth. The other hand is used to seal off the nose. This technique is not used if there is a cervical injury; in such cases the jaw lift is used instead *(5–12)*. In infants and neonates the head should be brought only to a neutral face-up position or "sniff position", since overextension in these patients will actually close the airway.

5–12. JAW LIFT (OR THRUST)

In patients who have actually or potentially sustained a neck injury, the neck must be stabilized in a neutral position, and therefore head tilt is inappropriate to clear the tongue. Instead, with the head left in a neutral position, one hand is placed under the angle of the jaw and the jaw is manually lifted to open the airway by lifting the affixed tongue; the airway is now patent for the patient's own ventilations or for mouth-to-mouth ventilation resuscitation. This position must be maintained each time for ventilation.

5–13. BACK BLOWS; ABDOMINAL OR CHEST THRUSTS *(See Fig. 5–3)*

These techniques are used in the event of a "café coronary," or choking emergency, in which a conscious person, while eating, suddenly clutches a hand to the throat, becomes unable to cough or make any sound, and in response to questioning becomes frantic, signaling an acute complete obstruction of the trachea or hypopharynx from food.* Abdominal (or chest) thrusts or back blows must be instituted immediately. Which is preferably done first is still a matter of some controversy. Either technique may be effective; if back blows are done first and prove unsuccessful, the rescuer may switch to abdominal (or chest) thrusts, and vice versa. The AHA and ARC recommend four back blows first, whereas Dr. Henry Heimlich and followers advise thrusts first (abdominal preferred over chest thrusts unless the patient is pregnant, is grossly obese, or is an infant or child). The AHA does not recommend abdominal thrusts for infants or children, while Dr. Heimlich advises using the pressure of two fingers of each hand in applying abdominal thrusts to infants and young children.

**Note:* In a conscious person, first very quickly explain technique and purpose, to obtain cooperation and allay apprehension. If obstruction is *not* complete, and adequate ventilation is occurring, it is best not to do anything until emergency bronchoscopy can be performed (see 39–6).

Abdominal Thrusts

The rescuer *should not* compress or squeeze the victim's chest at the same time as the abdomen or turn the victim's head to the side, even when the victim is in the recumbent or supine position. The foreign body will be removed from the mouth by the victim if conscious; if the victim is unconscious, the rescuer should remove it from the oropharynx with the fingers.

Complications are infrequent if the technique is properly performed, with vomiting being the most common. Potential complications include viscous rupture or hemorrhage of the spleen, liver or stomach, or a combination of these conditions. Rupture of the stomach has been reported only once. Rib fractures occurred before the technique was modified.

If the abdominal thrust maneuver fails, back blows with the head dependent, finger probe, hypopharynx forceps removal, cricothyrotomy and tracheotomy are subsequent available procedures to be attempted until one proves effective.

Victim Standing or Sitting (Fig. 5–3*A*)

Actions by Rescuer: Rescuer stands behind victim • Wraps arms around victim's waist • Places fist with thumb side just above victim's navel and

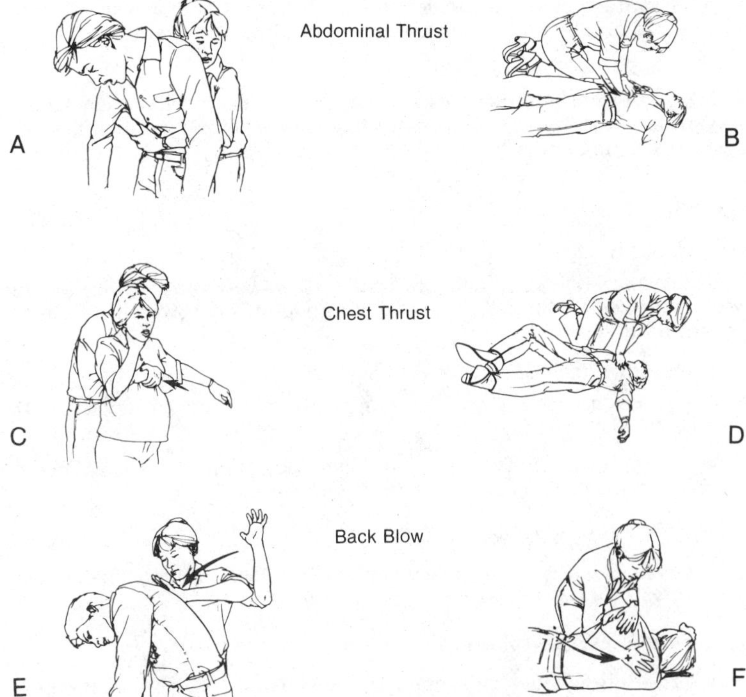

Figure 5–3. Six methods to externally extrude material causing complete airway obstruction. (From American Heart Association: *Student Manual for Basic Life Support: Cardiopulmonary Resuscitation,* 1981, pp. 32, 36, 40.)

below (distal to) the rib cage (and distal sternum) • Places other hand over first and makes 4 quick upward thrusts, pressing into victim's abdomen toward the diaphragm • Repeats prn (rescuer generally gradually becomes more adept in exerting the proper effective pressure; in unusual instances, success may come as late as the seventh attempt).

Victim Lying Face Up (Fig. 5–3*B*; *note:* if victim lying face down, turn victim face up)

Actions by Rescuer: Rescuer faces victim • Kneels so that victim's hips are between rescuer's knees • Places one open hand palm down on victim's abdomen above the navel and below (distal to) the rib cage (and distal sternum) • Places the other open hand (also palm down) over the first hand and makes 4 quick upward thrusts, pressing into victim's abdomen toward the diaphragm • Repeats prn.

Chest Thrusts (Use in pregnancy along with back blows)

Victim Standing or Sitting (Fig. 5–3*C*)

Actions of Rescuer: Rescuer stands behind victim • Places arms under victim's armpits to encircle the chest • Places thumb side of one hand against middle of victim's sternum (breast bone) • Covers the first with other hand and then hands jointly press with 4 quick backward thrusts.

Victim Lying Face Up (Fig. 5–3*D*)

Actions of Rescuer: Rescuer uses same body position and hand placement as for external chest (heart) compressions (EHC) • Exerts 4 quick downward thrusts • Clears foreign body with finger sweep.

Back Blows

Victim Standing (Fig. 5–3*E*)

Actions of Rescuer: Rescuer delivers 4 sharp blows between scapulae (shoulder blades) with heel of hand while supporting victim's chest with second hand on sternum (breast bone).

Victim on Side (Fig. 5–3*F*)

Actions of Rescuer: Same as for victim standing, except supports victim's body with hand on shoulder.

Note: In an unconscious person, the back blows and thrusts are not done first—instead the order is as shown in Figure 5–1*A*.

5–14. OROPHARYNGEAL AIRWAY

This semiovoid device, used only in unconscious patients, helps keep a patent airway between the tongue and pharynx.

5–15. NASOPHARYNGEAL AIRWAY

This thinly lubricated device, approximately 6″ long, is eased along the floor of either nostril into the pharynx and is tolerated by conscious patients. (*Note:* Do not force if one nostril if blocked by a deviated septum; the other side is usually patent.)

5–16. ESOPHAGEAL OBTURATOR AIRWAY (EOA) AND ESOPHAGEAL GASTRIC TUBE AIRWAY (EGTA)

Both these tube devices (each about 15″ long) are eased down the esophagus into the stomach the same way (see Fig. 5–4) and have the same general appearance. One important difference is that in the EGTA there is a hole through the center of the tube (whereas the EOA has a blind end) through which a gastric tube can be passed into the stomach to withdraw contents; the EGTA is therefore more versatile. To check patency and position of the tube before inflating the gastric cuff (which prevents airflow into the stomach), blow a large breath into the air-intake vent once the face mask is sealed; clear expansion of chest and breath sounds in the lung indicates the tube is in proper position—if not, the tube has gone into the trachea and must be repositioned. A few cases of laceration and rupture of the esophagus have been reported with use of these tubes, and on occasion a misplaced tube has been left in the trachea; on balance, however, the devices are useful field instruments, although tracheal intubation gives better oxygenation.

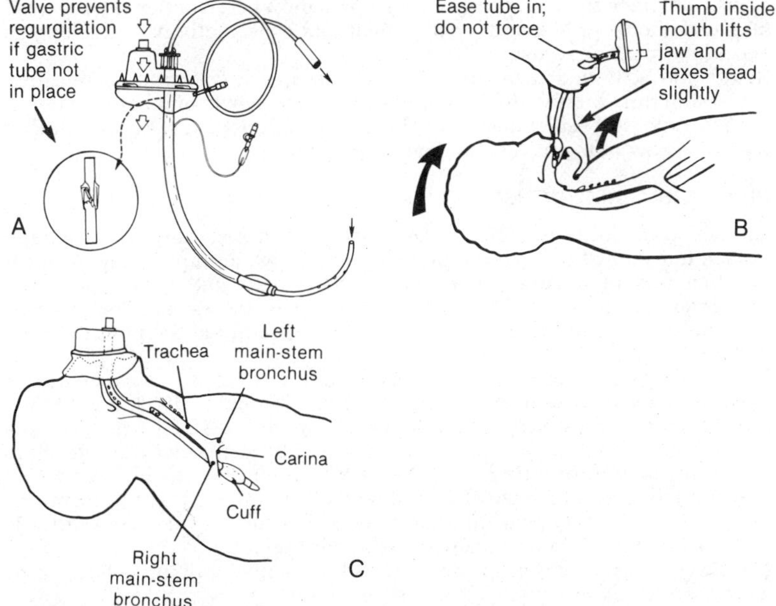

Figure 5–4. *A,* Esophageal gastric tube airway (EGTA), for use only in unconscious patients 16 years of age or greater. Gastric tube can be passed through lumen of airway. Ventilation is carried out by standard mask technique, with mask held securely against face. *B,* Positioning of tube (same as for esophageal obturator airway [EOA]. Check that chest rises/expands with blowing into vent (top arrow) before inflating gastric cuff; if chest expansion does not occur, reposition tube until it does. Then inflate cuff, using no more than 30 ml of air. *C,* Final position of esophageal airway and mask. *Note:* When removing tube, suction stomach first. (From American Heart Association: *Textbook of Advanced Cardiac Life Support,* 1981, pp. IV-2, IV-3.)

5–17. NASOTRACHEAL INTUBATION

Though an endotracheal tube may be inserted in this manner, passage, via the nose into the bronchi, of a *clean* "nasogastric" tube (now a nasotracheal tube), thinly lubricated with a water-soluble jelly also serves a valuable function in suctioning of thickened secretions from the tracheobronchial tree with a minimal procedure. No anesthetic is needed for passage of the nasotracheal (NT) tube. Tell the patient that coughing will occur right after the tube goes into the trachea but nothing more will be done until the patient has "regrouped" and given a "go ahead."

- Place the patient in a semi-sitting position with the neck in a neutral to slightly flexed position (except in neck trauma cases).
- Position the tube so that it is arced in an anterior direction as it passes via the floor of the nose (inferior turbinate) into the hypopharynx. When a swallowing reflex is elicited or loud breath sounds are coming from the tube, stop tube advancement.
- Tickle the hypopharynx with the tube end or rub the trachea externally to initiate a swallowing reflex, *immediately* after which the tube is advanced and slid into the trachea. It also helps to tell patients to take a deep breath immediately after they swallow.
- Gentle advancement of the tube and periodic short suctioning are well tolerated. Constantly monitor the patient and cease activity for as long as necessary to allow recovery.
- Rotate the body and turn the neck the opposite direction to suction into each bronchus. Instill 1 to 2 ml of normal saline slowly and periodically as needed to loosen secretions. Give the patient frequent rest periods during which no suctioning or tube motion is occurring.

5–18. ENDOTRACHEAL INTUBATION *(Fig. 5–5)*

The endotracheal tube offers a rapid, secure and generally nontraumatic approach to establishing and maintaining an airway, administering artificial ventilation and managing posttrauma patients with an unstable chest or tracheobronchial damage. This is best tolerated in the unconscious patient and for not more than several days. Measures that can aid the procedure are as follows.

- If the tube is not going to be passed blindly through the nose or mouth (possibly with the use of two fingers to locate the epiglottis and guide the tube), select a laryngoscope blade that is of appropriate size for the patient's oropharynx in addition to a proper-sized tube. The easiest way to determine this is by the "rule of little finger," i.e., a tube is chosen that has an outside size comparable to the size of the patient's little finger. It is also common in an extreme emergency situation to choose a tube diameter size that is about 1 mm less than that shown on standard tables.
- If a cervical fracture is suspected, instead use a fiberoptic bronchoscope or a cricotracheal approach to establish an airway.
- Make as straight a line as possible from the upper incisors of the teeth to the larynx (Fig. 5–5C). With the patient supine, this is aided by elevating the head to 1 to 2 inches with a towel, then hyperextending the head.
- Open the mouth (unless the nasal route is to be used) and move the jaw upward and forward. Clear any foreign objects.
- Insert the blade of the laryngoscope over the tongue and perform a lifting maneuver with the arm rather than a lever motion with the wrist to get the tongue out of the way. A straight blade (Fig. 5–5*A*) goes gently beyond the epiglottis; a curved blade goes above it. In general, it is easier to pass the

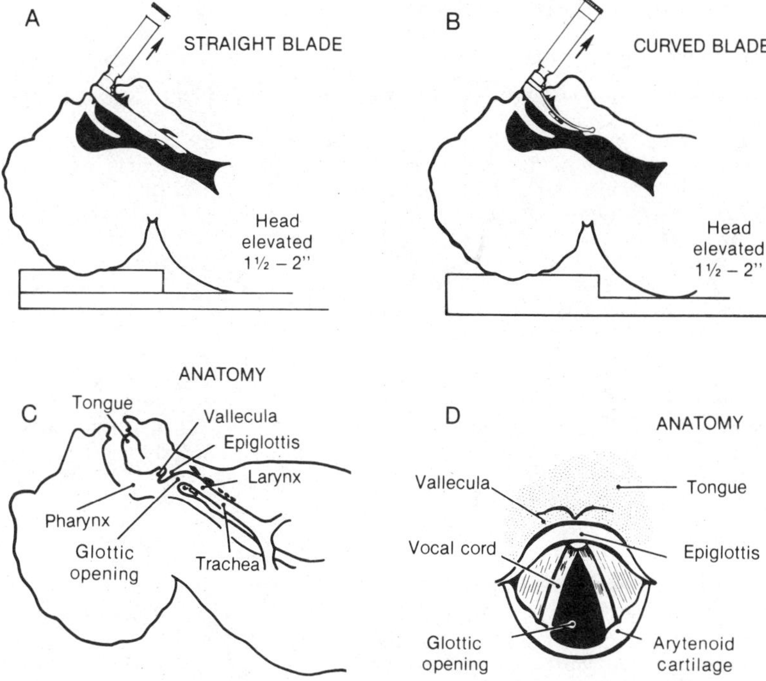

Figure 5–5. Endotracheal intubation. *A,* Laryngoscopic technique with straight blade; epiglottis is elevated anteriorly to expose glottic aperture. Force must be exerted in the direction of the arrow. *B,* When curved blade is used, epiglottis is displaced anteriorly by upward traction, with tip of blade in vallecula, resulting in exposure of the glottis. *C,* Essential landmarks in direct laryngoscopy. *D,* Anatomic structure to be visualized during direct laryngoscopy. (From American Heart Association: *Textbook of Advanced Cardiac Life Support,* 1981, pp. IV-4, IV-5.)

tube with a straight blade, though lifting the tongue out of the way is harder with this method than it is with a curved blade (Fig. 5–5*B*). Do not press against the incisors, as the teeth may break.

- After visualizing the larynx, pass the appropriate-sized tube prepared with a water-soluble lubricant alongside—not through—the blade into the triangular-shaped opening of the larynx (Fig. 5–5*D*). Check that air is coming into and out of the tube.
- Insert the cuff just beyond the vocal cords and stop. The label on the tube should be about 2 cm from the teeth.
- Inflate the cuff with just enough air to stop leakage while ventilation is being given—this is generally a preferable technique to instilling a set volume of air (which is approximately 5 to 8 ml of air).
- Check that both lungs are being ventilated. If not, withdraw the tube 1 to 2 cm and recheck aeration until evident that both sides are being ventilated.
- Connect the airway to any necessary ventilation tubes.
- Tape the endotracheal tube to the side of the mouth.
- Oral position of the tube is protected from biting by also putting in a firm oropharyngeal tube. Obtain chest x-ray after intubation.

5–19. CRICOTHYROTOMY (PUNCTURE) AND TRACHEOSTOMY

Indications

- Emergency bypass or removal of airway obstruction not attainable by other methods.
- These procedures may be necessary because of airway obstruction or ventilation problems due to burns, infection and inflammation, paralysis, coma, laryngeal spasm or foreign bodies that cannot be initially managed with an oropharyngeal airway or endotracheal tube. Cricothyrotomy or puncture is the simpler and faster procedure in dire emergency. In situations necessitating prolonged intubation (i.e., beyond 48 to 72 hours), tracheostomy is usually required. However, that is not an invariable time limit; sometimes that period has been greatly exceeded without difficulty and at other times there have been significant ill effects.
- Anticipation of airway problems is the best policy for minimizing rushed procedures and turning them into safer elective procedures. This is particularly important in treatment of children, in whom emergency tracheostomy is fraught with a high incidence of complications and even death. Whenever possible, convert an emergency tracheostomy to an orderly tracheostomy with good lighting and technique and adequate assistance by first inserting an endotracheal tube or bronchoscope.

Methods

Cricothyroid Membrane Puncture

This procedure may be a lifesaving measure and can be done with any sharp instrument, such as sharp-pointed scissors, knife blade, nail file or one or more large hollow needles (preferably No. 14 or larger); a special instrument designed for cricothyrotomy puncture is most desirable. The commercially available NuTrake, which comes in a variety of sizes, is a readily usable satisfactory device; care must be taken to ensure that the correct size is selected. It must be supplanted by a regular tracheostomy within 2 days.

- Locate the space between the two most prominent cartilages with the neck slightly hyperextended.
- Make a 1-inch transverse incision in the soft space between the cartilages. This incision should go through the skin only (Fig. 5–6*A* and *B*).
- Stabilize the larynx between the left thumb and middle finger; press the index fingernail firmly into the exposed cricothyroid ligament.
- Using the index fingernail as a guide and holding the instrument blade transversely, work the blade through the ligament and into the trachea. Avoid excess pressure with damage to the posterior wall.
- Spread by turning the blade handle through 90 degrees.
- If necessary, substitute a key or pen barrel for the blade. Large-bore hollow needles may be left in place pending elective procedure. DO NOT USE SMALL OBJECTS THAT MIGHT BE ASPIRATED.

5–20. LOW TRACHEOSTOMY *(Tracheostomy location of choice)*

- Place the patient on his or her back with the neck slightly hyperextended by a support under the shoulders.
- With the patient under local anesthesia, make a longitudinal incision (better exposure) or transverse incision (more cosmetic closure) through the skin and subcutaneous tissue from below the cricoid to just above the sternal notch.

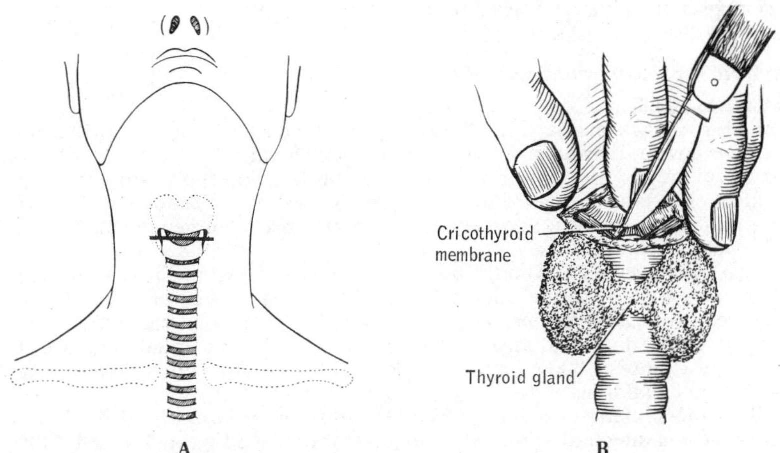

Figure 5–6. *A,* Drawing of cricothyroid membrane. Solid line shows incision. *B,* Cricothyroid membrane puncture. To establish an emergency airway, a 1-inch transverse skin incision is made over the cricothyroid membrane. The larynx is stabilized between the thumb and middle finger of the left hand. A sharp instrument is then passed along the nail of the index finger, which is pressed firmly into the membrane. (*A* from Nicholas, T. H., and Rumer, G. F.: JAMA, *179*:1933, 1960. *B,* Modified from Nicholas, T. H., and Rumer, G. F.: Mod. Med., April 17, 1961.)

- Separate the muscles by blunt dissection.
- Locate the inferior border of cricoid with the finger transversely. Avoid the inferior thyroid veins. If necessary, clamp, suture and retract the thyroid isthmus after cutting between clamps, exposing the 1st through 5th tracheal rings.
- Incise the 3rd or 4th tracheal ring and excise a small "window" of anterior trachea just large enough for the cannula; control the window flap with a clamp during excision to prevent aspiration.
- Insert the cannula followed by the inner tube. Complete hemostasis is important. If ventilatory assistance is required, use an inflatable cuffed tube.
- Suture the upper angles of the wound loosely to allow escape of air and avoid possible extensive subcutaneous emphysema.
- Fasten the tapes snugly around the neck.
- Arrange for tracheostomy care. Specific instructions regarding suction, insertion of saline drops for loosening of secretions, aspiration of the trachea and bronchi and cleansing of the tube should be given. It is important not to keep the suction valve closed while advancing or withdrawing the catheter, since injury to the mucosa can occur. Instead, open the valve while repositioning.
- Check by auscultation and percussion for adequate aeration of both lungs. Recheck tube length if one lung is underventilated; at times the tube may be too long and go down one main-stem bronchus and occlude the other.
- Check the position of the tracheostomy tube and pulmonary findings by x-ray when the patient's condition permits.

5–21. BREATHING–VENTILATION *(See also 52–1 for technique variation in neonates and infants)*

*Expired Air Ventilation Methods**

Mouth-to-Mouth

- In adults, place one hand under the nape of the neck and lift; this will bring the tongue and lower jaw forward and open the airway. (*Note:* If there is cervical injury, use jaw lift instead.) If preferable, apply firm, upward-lifting chin pressure with fingers. If air exchange and filling of the chest with the patient's own efforts do not spontaneously commence, follow with the next steps.
- Place the opposite hand on the patient's forehead, pressing down, compressing the nostrils with the fingers. Take a deep breath; then breathe directly between the patient's lips. The lips must form an airtight seal. Watch the chest for adequate expansion (Fig. 5–1). Give 4 rapid inhalations (each about 1½ pints or 800 ml volume in an adult) initially without waiting for effective exhalation.
- Allow the patient to exhale. Check the ipsilateral carotid pulse; if it is present and adequate, proceed as follows; if not, see Figure 5–1 and Table 5–4 (single rescuer techniques) for timing in coordination of ventilation with external heart compressions (see also 5–23 for EHC techniques).
- See Figure 5–1 for rates of assisted ventilation for various age groups. Regular rhythm is not as important as adequate ventilation volume per minute.

Mouth-to-Nose. Same as mouth-to-mouth, except that the mouth is held closed with the fingers of one hand and air is blown into the nostrils.

Mouth-to-Airway. Proceed as for mouth-to-mouth; make seal of patient's lips around tube as tight as possible. (Not preferred because of air leakage at mouth around tube; generally recommended only for patients who are deeply unconscious.)

Mouth-to-Mask. Success depends upon holding the mask firmly in place and keeping the airway patent; use with oropharyngeal airway in deeply unconscious patients. Use of the "pocket mask" has distinct advantages with regard to portability, good ventilation, hygiene and allowing the rescuer's two hands to be free to combine the jaw thrust maneuver with a secure seal (Fig. 5–7). It is usable in patients with cervical injuries, since neutral alignment is maintained.

Mouth-to-Laryngectomy Site. When resuscitating a patient who has had a laryngectomy, the rescuer forms a seal with his lips over the laryngectomy site and blows as in the mouth-to-mouth technique except that additionally the mouth and nose of the victim must also be sealed. Alternatively, a round infant resuscitation mask (if available) usually will seal the laryngectomy site well, and the rescuer can blow into the mask.

Advantages of Expired Air Methods. These expired air methods have the following major advantages over manual push-pull techniques (Schaefer, Sylvester, Holger-Nielsen, and so forth and the Richard prone tilting visceral shift "teeter board" method in infants):

**Note:* If, despite changes in position of neck, gastric distention becomes so severe that lung filling is compromised, and no endotracheal tube is available, it may be necessary to use abdominal thrusts to achieve gastric decompression.

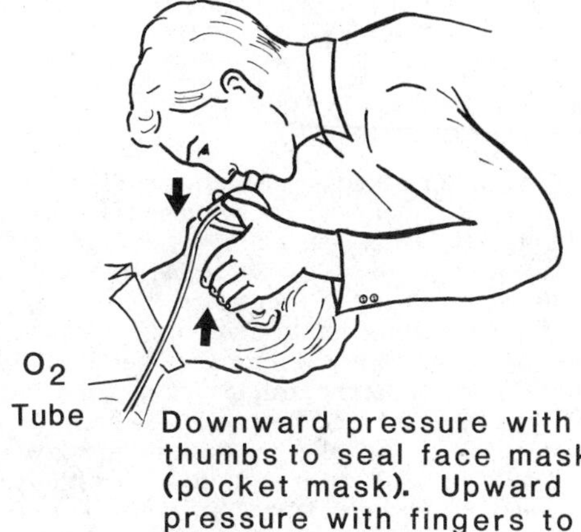
O2
Tube
Downward pressure with thumbs to seal face mask (pocket mask). Upward pressure with fingers to lift mandible.

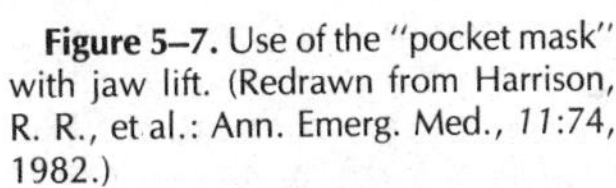
Figure 5–7. Use of the "pocket mask" with jaw lift. (Redrawn from Harrison, R. R., et al.: Ann. Emerg. Med., *11*:74, 1982.)

- Better pulmonary ventilation—enough to sustain life.
- The rescuer's hands are free to extend the head, pinch shut the nostrils, or form a mask seal and perform the jaw thrust maneuver.
- Special positioning is not necessary; therefore, expired air respiration can be performed in cramped or unusual circumstances—for instance, while bringing a drowning victim to shore, or treating a patient in the upright position (e.g., electrical lineman).
- The presence of an obstruction can be recognized. If it is impossible to force air in, an obstruction in the respiratory tract is present.
- Can be used in the presence of fractures of the upper extremities or thorax.

Manual Ventilation Methods

All of the previous well-known manual methods (Schaefer, Sylvester, Holger-Nielsen) are inefficient and unsatisfactory and do not uniformly supply enough ventilation to sustain life.

Mechanical Ventilation Methods

- Bag-valve mask used with oropharyngeal airway or preferably a cuffed endotracheal tube and air or oxygen.
- Intermittent pressure ventilatory apparatus (available from Bennett, Bird, Ohio, Emerson and other companies) with manually triggered (time-cycled) devices can be used when external cardiac compression is being administered, but conventional pressure cycled automatic resuscitators cannot be used in this situation.
- Coordinated time-cycled ventilatory apparatus with external cardiac compression apparatus offers a good method for sustaining prolonged combined mechanical ventilation and cardiac resuscitation when functioning well, but requires constant monitoring for position and mechanical adjustment.

5–22. CIRCULATION ASSISTANCE TECHNIQUES *(See 5–23, 5–24, 5–25)*

5–23. CLOSED CHEST EXTERNAL HEART COMPRESSION (EHC) TECHNIQUES

- The patient should be supine on a hard surface. If the patient must remain in a bed, a bed board or spine board must be slid under the patient for upper thoracic resistance. The individual performing resuscitation must kneel at the patient's side in order to perform with adequate technique and effective pressure. For electric shock victims, if tetany persists, several Holger-Nielsen maneuvers (raising the upper extremities over the head) will help relieve the tetany and produce better ventilation.
- In the adult, start cardiac compression by placing the heel of one palm over the distal (inferior) portion of the body of the sternum, avoiding the xiphoid process (the distal edge of the palm is two fingerbreadths above the xiphoid notch in adults and proportionately the same in children; *in infants and small children, compress at midsternum*). Cover this hand crosswise with the heel of the other hand and exert forcible downward pressure. Keep the even steady down pressure (½ second) and release (quick and non-jerky) in a vertical plane over the sternum. Keep the fingers and elbows straight; let the shoulders and body weight do the work. Pressure (usually amounting to more than 60 pounds for an average-sized adult) should be applied with two hands (see Fig. 5–1), producing a forceful thrust followed by a quick release to give 1½ to 2 inches sternum excursion in an adult. One hand is used to give ¾ to 1½ inches sternal excursion in a child, and two fingers are adequate to give ¾ to ½ inch of movement in an infant. (For neonates, see *52–1*.) Mnemonic for single rescuer management and details for CPR in adults/children/infants is given in Table 5–4.
- With two rescuers, repeat the series of 1 expired air ventilation to each 5 EHC at the rates indicated in Figure 5–1.

5–24. PRECORDIAL THUMP

In cases of ventricular tachycardia (with or without pulse or consciousness) or monitored arrest due to ventricular fibrillation, when this procedure can be done within the first few minutes, strike the precordial (midsternum) area of an adult with the closed medial (ulnar or hypothenar) fleshy part of the fist (see Fig. 5–8). If this results in a sinus mechanism, proceed with lidocaine drip infusion; if VF persists, proceed with defibrillation and ACLS (Fig. 5–2). There is evidence that delayed use of the precordial thump makes the heart more difficult to resuscitate. *Note:* Precordial thump is not recommended in children.

If rhythmic precordial thumps produce a QRS complex and associated myocardial contraction in ventricular asystole due to heart block, continue until a pacemaker can be inserted. Use EHC if cardiac output is not adequate.

Table 5–4. COMPARISON OF SINGLE RESCUER TECHNIQUES AFTER AHA BLS PROGRAM

	Infant	Child	Adult
Compress with . . .	2–3 fingers	Heel of 1 hand	2 hands
to a depth of . . .	½″ to 1″	1″ to 1½″	1½″ to 2″
at this rate . . .	100 per minute	80 per minute	80 per minute
with this ratio . . .	5:1	5:1	15:2
and mnemonic	One, two, three, four, five, BREATHE One, two, three, four, five, BREATHE	1 and 2 and 3 and 4 and 5 and BREATHE 1 and 2 and 3 and 4 and 5 and BREATHE	1 and 2 and 3 and 4 and 5 and 1 and 2 and 3 and 4 and 10 and 1 and 2 and 3 and 4 and 15 and BREATHE BREATHE

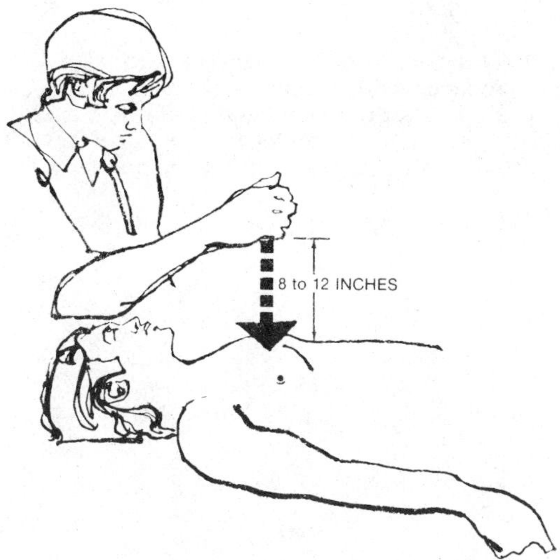

Figure 5–8. Precordial thump. (From Committee of the American Medical Association: Standards for cardiopulmonary resuscitation [CPR] and emergency cardiac care [ECC]. JAMA, *227*:841, 1974. Reprinted by permission of the American Heart Association, Inc.) If witnessed arrest over 2 minutes long, precordial thump considered not helpful. Not recommended for pediatric cases.

5–25. OPEN CHEST INTERNAL HEART COMPRESSION

Since the cardiac output obtained by external cardiac compression is, for practical purposes, as good as that obtained by direct open chest compression, there are few indications for the open chest procedure. However, among these are the following:

- If the chest has already been opened for some operative procedure.
- Presence of chest wall restricting deformities or extensive fractures causing instability and possible perforations.
- Cardiac tamponade or penetrating wounds.
- In rare instances, closed chest external heart compression, even when properly performed, is not effective in producing adequate pulses.

5–26. CARDIOVERSION AND DEFIBRILLATION

Cardioversion is the synchronized electrical shock management technique of choice for treatment of serious cardiac dysrhythmias, except for ventricular fibrillation, for which defibrillation is appropriate.

Cardioversion (Direct current synchronized for delivery usually 10 millisec after peak of first R wave following pressing of discharge buttons)

- If patient is conscious, slowly administer IV diazepam or morphine sulfate to reduce tension and produce amnesia for procedure.
- Uncover patient's chest.
- Turn on the main switch of the defibrillator, select energy level and then turn on the synchronizer circuit switch (not needed for VT without pulse).
- Charge in accordance with condition (from 5 to 50 joules for non-VT conditions, with an average of 25 joules [lowest amounts are used in digitalized patients]; up to 200 joules initially for VT in adults). In infants and children use 0.5 to 1.5 joules/kg up to a maximum of 2 joules/kg initially in VT.
- At locations indicated on Figure 5–9, place paddles coated (not excessively) with conductive jelly.

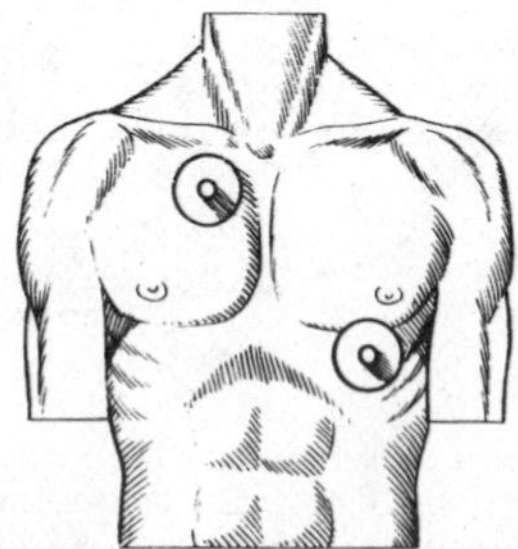

Figure 5–9. Position of paddle electrodes for countershock. Alternatively can put the second paddle on chest wall directly posterior to the precordial paddle if this positioning not adequate. Recommended paddle diameter size: adult (10-13 cm); children (8 cm); small infant (4.5 cm).

- Kneel or stand at patient's side. Stand clear of metal frames of bed; surface underneath rescuer should be dry.
- Place one paddle (either regular or "Quick-Look" [engineered to alternatively be ECG electrodes] paddles) at each location shown in Figure 5–9.
- Grasp paddle handle firmly with each hand and press firmly onto patient's chest (about 10 kg or 25 pounds).
- Call out in loud enough voice for all around to hear: "STAND BACK! CONVERT ON THREE! ONE, TWO, THREE!"
- On count of THREE, depress both paddle buttons.
- Monitor ECG/pulse response and proceed accordingly.

Defibrillation (Direct current delivered at time of depressing paddle buttons; see Fig. 5–2)

- Used for correction of ventricular fibrillation.
- Procedure is the same as for cardioversion, EXCEPT be sure to turn off synchronizer switch and start with 2 watt-seconds (joules)/kg for first and (if necessary) second attempts; usual initial adult dose is 200 joules (300 joules in large, heavy-set adults). For third and subsequent attempts (when necessary), increase dose by 25 to 50%, to a maximum of 400 joules.

Failure of Defibrillation. Attempts at defibrillation may fail as a result of:

- Severity of patient disease.
- Prolonged period of cardiac arrest before starting CPR.
- CPR inadequate (insufficient ventilation and/or EHC with secondary hypoxemia, acidosis, hypercarbia).
- Drug toxicity (digitalis, antiarrhythmic agents, etc.) and electrolyte imbalance—particularly lowered K levels or lowered or raised Ca levels (increase in K usually leads to asystole).
- Insufficient sympathetic tone or inadequate epinephrine.
- Insufficient direct current to heart. (Check paddle position and increase pressure to chest; check for excess conductive jelly, which dissipates current; use maximum current in barrel-chested victims).

5–27. COMMON MEDICATIONS USED IN URGENT CONDITIONS AND FIRST AID

(*Note:* Although only some of the following medications are used in resuscitation, this list is placed on the following pages for easy reference. The reader is also referred to the Appendix for tables giving therapeutic serum levels of some common medications and for a table giving the starting doses of commonly used antibacterial drugs.

COMMON MEDICATIONS USED IN URGENT

Item	Name	How Given	Usual Initial Dose
* 1.	Aminophylline	IV	*Loading dose:* 6 mg/kg given over 20 minutes *Maintenance dose:* 0.5–0.9 mg/kg/hour, continuous IV drip
2.	Amobarbital (Amytal) sodium	IV, IM	65–500 mg, slowly 3–5 mg/kg; use not advised for patients under 6 yr
3.	Ampicillin sodium (injectable)	IM, IV	< 40 kg: 50–100 mg/kg/day in divided doses; > 40 kg: 1–2 g/day in divided doses. Double dosage in more severe cases. (Doses apply to both items 3 & 4)
† 4.	Ampicillin trihydrate (oral)	PO	
†* 5.	Ammonia (pearl)		One crushed pearl
6.	Amyl nitrate		0.3 ml pearl
* 7.	Atropine sulfate	IM, IV	0.01–0.03 mg/kg/dose, up to 0.4 mg dose (usual). Repeat q 5 min prn
8.	Bretylium tosylate	IV	5 mg/kg bolus for VF
* 9.	Calcium chloride (10%) 100 mg/ml 1.36 mEq Ca^{++}/ml	IV	0.1–0.2 ml/kg bolus slowly, up to 250–500 mg (2.5 to 5 ml)
*10.	Calcium gluconate (10%) 100 mg/ml 0.45 mEq Ca^{++}/ml	IV	0.1–0.3 ml/kg, up to 500 mg to 1 g (to 10 ml). Slow push up to 1.0 ml/min
*11.	Codeine sulfate or codeine phosphate	PO, IM	0.25–1.0 mg/kg/dose every 4 hours
12.	Dexamethasone (Decadron)	IV, IM PO	0.5–9 mg/day 0.75–9 mg/day
13.	Dextrose (50%)	IV	2 ml/kg/bolus dose
*14.	Diazepam (Valium)	IV	0.05–0.20 mg/kg/dose, up to 5–10 mg, slowly
15.	Diazepam (Valium)	PO	0.10–0.20 mg/kg/dose
*16.	Digoxin (Lanoxin)	PO	See *29–10*
*17.	Digoxin (Lanoxin)	IM IV	See *29–10*
*18.	Diphenhydramine (Benadryl)	IV PO	Adult: 0.2–0.5 mg/kg Child: 0.5–1.25 mg/kg q 6 h 1 mg/kg; maximum 50 mg
‡*19.	Epinephrine hydrochloride 1:10,000 = 0.1 mg/ml	IM IV	1:1000; 0.01 ml/kg/dose 1:10,000; 0.05–0.1 ml/kg/dose
20.	Flurazepam hydrochloride (Dalmane)	PO	15–30 mg (adult)
21.	Furosemide (Lasix)	IV	0.5 to 1.0 mg/kg to maximum 40 mg; repeat: adults 1 hour, children 2 hours. Give slowly
22.	Heparin, sodium	IV	Adult: 70–140 units/kg Child: 50 USP units/kg bolus, followed by continuous IV infusion of 10–25 units/kg/hr

*This item or its near equivalent is contained in one or more of the commercially prepackaged emergency kits.

†Advisable item for first-aid or travel kit.

‡See also 57–5 for other vasopressors.

CONDITIONS AND FIRST AID

Item	Comments and Considerations	Average Dose for 70-kg Person
1.	Therapeutic serum level: 10–20 μg/ml For patients with cardiac decompensation or impaired liver function, 0.2–0.4 mg/kg/hour; also low for neonates/infants	Loading dose: 420 mg Maintenance dose: 63 mg/hour Check serum level if there has been prior use
2.	Not more than 1 ml/min of 10% solution Deep IM; not more than 5 ml injected at any one site; avoid if liver disease	Varies with purpose: 65–500 mg; maximum dose, 1 g
3.	Dose varies with organism/severity May be penicillin hypersensitivity	250–500 mg every 6 hours; 8 g/day usual maximum
4.	Most severe pediatric cases may require 200–400 mg/kg/day	
5.	Inhale whiffs from crushed pearl	One; repeat prn
6.	Inhale every 30 sec for 2 min until $NaNO_2$ ready	One; repeat prn
7.	Larger doses required in poisoning cases (see *53–10*) and cardiac asystole	0.4 mg common 0.6–1.0 mg in more severe cases
8.	Rapid, undiluted IV bolus for VF only; dilute 1:4 for VT; may repeat in 10 min	350–500 mg; not for use in children
9.	Do not mix with sodium bicarbonate. Do not give if digitalis toxicity present. Dilute 1:1 for intracardiac injection	250–500 mg (2.5–5.0 ml 10% solution) Give slowly: < 1 ml/min
10.	As for Calcium chloride Monitor with ECG as possible May repeat in 8–10 min	(10 ml 10% solution)
11.	IM dose usually half of oral dose	32–65 mg/dose
12.	Dosage individualized by disease Do not use for fungal infection	0.75–3 mg/day; taper to dc (see *44–7*)
13.	Follow with 10% drip infusion or food	30–50 ml
14.	Administer cautiously in presence of any other CNS depressing medication	5 mg
15.	Same as above; wide range of response	2–10 mg
16.	Tablets and pediatric elixir	See *29–10*
17.	Oral route preferred unless urgent	See *29–10*
18.	Administer slowly Warn about drowsiness, use of other sedative drugs	25–50 mg
19.	Maximum 0.5 ml dose usual in asthma; may repeat every 5 min	0.3–0.5 ml (1:1000) 5–10 ml (1:10,000)
20.	Or may use temazepam (Restoril), same dose for sleep	15–30 mg; may repeat
21.	May increase to 2–3 mg/kg/ for hypertensive crisis with pulmonary edema or acute renal failure	40 mg; may repeat in 1 hour
22.	Dose adjusted according to clotting time every 4 hours (keep at 2.5 to 3 times control) For average adult after giving 5000 units IV, use maintenance doses	Initial dose: 5000–10,000 units Maintenance dose: 5000–7500 units every 6 hours (or 1000 units/hr by pump continuous infusion

Table continued on following page

COMMON MEDICATIONS USED IN URGENT

Item	Name	How Given	Usual Initial Dose
*†23.	Ipecac, syrup (See also *53–7*)	PO	Child < 1 yr: 5–10 ml; caution Child (1–12 yr): 15–30 ml Adult: 30 ml
24.	Isoproterenol hydrochloride (Isuprel; 1:5000)	IV	Complete heart block: See discussion in *29–13* *Shock:* 0.5–5.0 μg/min (rare use) *Severe ↓ pulse:* 2–20 μg/min
*25.	Lidocaine hydrochloride (Xylocaine)	IV IM	*Cardiac arrhythmia*: bolus 1 mg/kg 4 mg/kg maximum
*26.	Meperidine hydrochloride (Demerol)	IM IV	1–2 mg/kg/dose 0.2–0.4 mg/kg
*27.	Methoxamine hydrochloride (Vasoxyl)	IV IM	0.08 mg/kg (IV preferred) 0.15 mg/kg
28.	Methylergonovine maleate (Methergine)	IM IV	0.2 mg IM preferred If IV, slowly over 1–3 min
*29.	Methylprednisolone sodium succinate (Solu-Medrol)	IV, IM	0.5–5.0 mg/kg every 6 hours; in severe shock, 30 mg/kg
30.	Morphine sulfate	IM IV	0.1–0.2 mg/kg/dose ⅓–½ IM dose
*31.	Naloxone hydrochloride (Narcan)	IV	Child: 0.01 mg/kg, up to 0.1 mg/kg on repeats Adult: 0.4–2 mg or > if needed
*32.	Nitroglycerin‡	SL	One tablet (0.15–0.6 mg) every 5 min up to 3 doses sublingually
†33.	Pepto-Bismol	PO tablets	Child (5–10 yr): ½–1 tab Adult: 2 tab; every ½–1 hour
*34.	Phenytoin (Dilantin)	IM, IV	*Status seizures*: 150–250 mg IV (adult); 10–15 mg/kg (child)
35.	Procainamide hydrochloride (Pronestyl)	IM IV	0.5–1.0 g (adult) 100 mg over 2–5 min (adult) See Table 5–1 for child doses
*36.	Prochlorperazine (Compazine)	IM IV	0.05–0.1 mg/kg every 3–4 hours to maximum 40 mg/day
37.	Proparacaine hydrochloride (Ophthaine)		1–2 drops topically (eye)
*38.	Propranolol (Inderal)	IV PO	Adult: 1–3 mg slowly Child: 0.01–0.1 mg/kg to maximum 1 mg/dose 10–30 mg (adult)
*39.	Sodium bicarbonate	IV	1 mEq/kg with cardiac arrest: bolus IV
40.	Tetanus immune globulin, human	IM	See *20–2*
*41.	Verapamil (Isoptin)	IV	0.075 to 0.15 mg/kg
42.	Water (sterile normal saline)	IV, IM	Diluent for desired volume

*This item or its near equivalent is contained in one or more of the commercially prepackaged emergency kits.

†Advisable item for first-aid or travel kits.

‡Consider maintenance with transdermal preparation.

CONDITIONS AND FIRST AID (*Continued*)

Item	Comments and Considerations	Average Dose for 70-kg Person
23.	Follow with 16–32 oz water; less for children (see 9). May repeat in 20–30 min; lavage if still no results	30 ml
24.	Dilute 1 mg (5 ml) in 500 ml D/W: equals 2 μg/ml. Titrate by pulse and blood pressure	For shock: 1 μg/min initially and titrate For ↓ pulse: 2–20 μg/min
25.	Second bolus ⅓ to ½ of initial dose if no response. Monitor with ECG if available. Continuous infusion: 20–50 μg/kg/min	70 mg bolus IV; 1–4 mg/min infusion
26.	Avoid use within 15 days of MAO inhibitor. Dilute to 5 mg/ml for slow infusion	75–150 mg 10–30 mg
27.	Administer slowly; monitor BP increase response; repeat q 10 min prn	3–5 mg (↑ if poor BP/P response) 10 mg
28.	0.2 mg after delivery of anterior shoulder or placenta or during puerperium	0.2 mg
29.	IV dose given over 1–4 min. Dose may be increased 4- to 6-fold in severest cases	40–125 mg; largest doses for 48–72 hours only
30.	Maximum 15–20 mg; may repeat every 3–4 hours. Dilute to 10 ml for titrated infusion (5 min)	5–15 mg 2–10 mg
31.	May repeat in 3 min up to 5 times as necessary; if severe known narcotic OD, can give adult up to 2–4 mg stat	0.4–2 mg, to total of 10 mg
32.	If anginal pain persists after 3 tablets, evaluate for myocardial infarction	1 tablet (0.4 mg)
33.	For indigestion or diarrhea; may darken tongue/stool; watch for salicylate OD in pediatric patients	2 tab every ½–1 hour; maximum 8 doses/day
34.	IV, not to exceed 50 mg/min; repeat ⅔ initial dose in 30 min if needed	100 mg q 8h; therapeutic level 10–15 μg/ml
35.	May repeat every 4–6 hours May repeat every 5 min to maximum 1 g; monitor with BP and ECG (QRS widens)	0.5–1.0 g 100-mg increments or 20 mg/min to maximum 1 g
36.	Caution with IV use and acute febrile illnesses (↑ extrapyramidal reaction)	5–10 mg IM
37.	For examination, not home use	1–2 drops
38.	Not more than 1 mg/min; monitor BP, ECG. Avoid in CHF and asthma Repeat every 6–8 hours prn for arrhythmia	1 mg 10 mg
39.	Repeat 0.5 mEq/kg every 5–10 min of arrest or dosage according to arterial blood gases and pH	70 mEq (70 ml 8.4% solution)
40.		250 units
41.	Calcium blocker; used for supraventricular tachycardia; best for adults and older children Caution when used with digitalis or propranolol, in cases of shock or congestive heart failure, and in younger children	5–10 mg; monitor closely; may repeat in 20–30 min
42.	Best to use single-dose vials	Not applicable

6. Achievements in Urgency Care

There is an increasing recognition by the public that emergency medical care is a continuum beginning with the patient, family, friends and bystanders; progressing to Emergency Medical Services (EMS); governmental agencies including fire, police and rescue units; and organized volunteer groups as needed; and concluding with provision of care at qualified treatment centers.

Yearly national recognition of Emergency Medicine Week during September, beginning in 1982, has further increased public awareness of this concept. In addition, in 1980, the field of Emergency Medicine was established as a fully recognized specialty, the culmination of a program fostered by the ACEP when first organized in 1968.

ORGANIZATIONAL ACHIEVEMENTS

- Special award presented to ACEP by FDA in recognition of its role in the establishment and success of the National Medicine Device and Laboratory Product Problem Reporting Program (headquarters at 12601 Twin Brook Parkway, Rockville, MD 20852; phone 1-800-638-6725).
- American Board of Medical Specialty recognition for Certification of Special Competence in Critical Care Medicine (CCM) and Board Examination.
- Establishment by ACEP of standards to be met by centers providing emergency medical care.
- Uniform interstate standardization of training, nomenclature and registry of EMT's under the EMS system.
- Health Evaluation System and Information Service (HESIS) (occupational health consultation service) available free to all California health care providers (phone 1-800-792-0720) during business hours and backed up by regional Poison Centers for 24-hour service, including advice on hazardous substance spills and victim treatment.
- Establishment of identification numbers for hazardous substance carrier vehicles. These are outlined by the Department of Transportation in the *Emergency Response Guidebook* and placed with numbered, colored, diamond-shaped placards and numbered rectangular panels on the vehicle. The color informs of general fire, explosion and health hazards, and the number gives specific substance identification (see Appendix).
- Establishment of Doctors for Disaster Preparedness to promote nationally and better organize professional and civilian resources for management of consequences of all types of disasters, including nuclear war.
- Major improvements in hospital and community preparations for individual and mass disaster management, including better response time in provision of Emergency Medical Services.
- Community and statewide acceptance of policies (e.g., concerning who will be the scene manager or head the Incident Control Center when multiple agencies respond to an emergency) aimed at reducing conflict and promoting effective care and survival activities. Drills greatly aid this process.
- Improvement of EMT services by critical care protocols and radio-communicated medical control; these are increasingly approved by legislation vesting regulatory authority in the appropriate state agency.
- Continued improvement of Advanced Life Support (ALS) programs, including new programs in Trauma (ATLS) and Pediatric (APLS or PALS).

- A new emphasis dealing with mass/multiple trauma has been fostered by the International Society on Disaster Medicine (Switzerland). Simplification of medical assistance and treatment—plus coordinated cooperation among all levels of health personnel—is stressed.

TECHNICAL IMPROVEMENTS

- Rotorcraft (helicopter) transport of severe trauma cases to appropriate trauma centers, allowing more rapid definitive treatment with significantly improved survival. Helicoptor transport is particularly important for evacuation from congested or obstructed sites or urban areas where fixed wing transport is impractical or impossible and where surface transportation is slowed by impassable, congested or circuitous routes.
- Easier telephone accesss to EMS through use of "911" numbers, aided by current conversion of pay phone booths to a system not requiring a coin to call for emergency services or operator.
- Improved emergency medical kits for inflight emergencies aboard commercial airlines.
- Use of "Medic Alert" and "Life Alert" bracelet/necklace data backed by 24-hour collect-call information service from anywhere in the world for people with high-risk medical problems. Other systems that provide valuable medical information include: Alert Along (orange laminated tag generally affixed anywhere to clothing, shoelaces or luggage); SOS Talisman (strip worn in jewelry containing information in 6 languages); Vial of Life (3″ tall vial with medical data—decal on refrigerator door calls attention to vial taped under right side of top shelf); Emerg-Alert (data on jewelry); and various medical data cards for carrying in wallet or purse.
- Reduction of trauma to children in MVA's as result of legislation passed in some states to hold parent drivers liable if their child is not in a car seat. Also, some hospital nurseries allow release of newborn infants only if an infant car seat is present in vehicle.
- Increasing number of major lifesaving measures initiated in the ED when it is obvious the patient will succumb before an OR becomes available. With an adequately trained physician, such operations as thoracotomy (higher level of benefit), craniotomy, cardiorrhaphy and abdominal laparotomy (lower level of benefit) may be performed in the ED, although the orderliness and resources of the OR remain the preferred location whenever feasible.
- Development of calcium antagonists (slow channel blockers) as a prime therapy for PAT, vasospastic (Prinzmetal's) angina and for cerebral resuscitation following cardiac arrest.
- Development of IV and/or intra–coronary artery administration of streptokinase/urokinase under angiographic control for thrombolysis of intra-arterial clots within 90 to 120 minutes of onset of event in acute MI and other conditions.
- Establishment of civil air patrol assistance in a nationwide program to help with organ retrieval and transport (see *8–13*).

EDUCATION

- Established formal residency programs in Emergency Medicine (EM) are approaching 70 in number nationwise, and program content is more comprehensive and standardized.
- Medical school curricula are including EM orientation.
- Education in EM has been promoted by (1) organization of the Society of

Teachers of Emergency Medicine (STEM), (2) awards by ACEP for journalism excellence, (3) emergency care research project support by the Emergency Medical Foundation (P.O. Box 61911, Dallas, TX 75261; phone 1-214-659-0911).

- *Emergindex* has been developed as a microfiche system presentation of current clinical data for emergency care, similar to the Poisondex program for treatment of poisoning.
- Computers are being used increasingly in ED and critical care units to aid therapeutic calculations, retrieve medical literature and present current protocols.

7. Addiction

7–1. GENERAL CONSIDERATIONS

- Physicians treating the emergency problems of patients who are narcotics addicts are often concerned as to what measures they can legally take regarding pain relief and acute withdrawal problems (see 7–4). In general, the physician in the emergency situation should identify the drug being used and order whatever substance (including controlled drugs) is medically reasonably necessary for pain relief now.
- In any jurisdiction, it is required that the physician take a competent history, perform an adequate physical examination and arrive at a diagnosis or clinical impression on which to base any treatment. Recording of this is particularly important when administration of controlled substances to narcotics addicts comes under legal scrutiny. The physician is specifically required to make an effort to detect the presence of narcotics addiction (see 7–2).
- Many states do not require reporting of addicts and do not limit administration of narcotic "controlled" substances except as a breach of "legitimate medical practice." Some states, however, such as California, have laws codifying specific restrictions on narcotics administration, and any physician in compliance with them should meet other broader standards with ease.

7–2. ADDICTION DEFINED

- The word addict comes from the Latin word meaning to surrender. Legally, the word is used to refer to someone who has developed the following characteristics:
  —*Emotional Dependence*: The user has a compulsive need to continue the drug.
  —*Physical Dependence*: Deprivation of the drug causes withdrawal signs and symptoms.
  —*Tolerance*: Larger, more frequent and more potent doses are required as the user develops greater physiologic need and resistance.
- Habituation and drug dependence are somewhat vague terms indicating something less than addiction but a compulsive need to continue use of the substance despite the lack of physical dependence and tolerance. They are thus included in the California Health and Safety Code Section 11156, which states that "No person shall prescribe for or administer or dispense a controlled substance to an addict or habitual user, or to any person

presenting himself as such except as permitted by this division." See 7–5 for permitted exceptions to this rule.

- Common types of substances to which people may become addicted or habituated to or develop dependence on are: alcohol (*53–295*), amphetamines (*53–66*), barbiturates (*53–110*), cannabis (*53–409*), cocaine (*53–218*), opiates (*53–496*), PCP (*53–532*), and volatile solvents and nitrates (*53–481*). All of these are controlled or illegal substances except ethyl alcohol, for which the prohibition years exercised a futile attempt at federal and state control. Even though access to alcohol is only marginally controlled, penalties for driving while under the influence are gradually increasing. Two other addictive substances that are in common everyday use, caffeine (*53–159*) and tobacco (*53–711*), are slowly coming under closer public and government scrutiny.

7–3. NARCOTICS

Narcotics are substances that relieve pain, lead to tolerance, cause withdrawal signs and symptoms after prolonged use, and, finally, if administered to a morphine addict who is having withdrawal signs and symptoms will relieve those signs and symptoms. Some substances that do not fit this definition are also controlled under The Narcotics Act because of their high frequency of abuse; cocaine being one such drug.

Whenever addiction to, or self-administration of, any of the substances covered by the Narcotics Act is known or suspected, certain restrictions (7–5) apply. Most of the substances covered are included in the following list; for further information on any of these, see the individual listing in the chapter on Poisoning (53).

Alphaprodine (Nisentil)
Apomorphine
Cocaine and its salts, preparations, compounds and derivatives
Codeine and its salts, preparations, compounds and derivatives
Hemp and its extracts and compounds
Heroin
Hydromorphone (Dilaudid)
Lophophora (mescal, peyote)
Marihuana
Meperidine (Demerol)
Methadone (Adanon, Dolophine)
Morphine and its salts, preparations, compounds and derivatives
Opium and its salts, preparations, compounds and derivatives
Pantopon (pantopium hydrochloride)
Paregoric (camphorated tincture of opium)

Though not classified as narcotics and quantitatively less prominent in effect, propoxyphene hydrochloride (Darvon) and pentazocine lactate (Talwin) fit the criteria of narcotics and should be prescribed with the same degree of caution appropriate to the prescription of codeine. Naloxone hydrochloride (Narcan) is a specific and effective antagonist for respiratory depression caused by use of the above drugs.

7–4. ADDICTION TO NARCOTIC DRUGS: SIGNS AND SYMPTOMS

- A habitual user of opium derivatives or opiate-like synthetics who is taking regular doses of a pure preparation at accustomed intervals may not show outward evidence of dependence on the drug until use of the drug is interrupted. Denial of use by the addict is common.

- Scars on the extremities—old, recently healed, healing or fresh—are evident from subcutaneous, intramuscular or intravenous injections.
- Conjunctival inflammation may be bothersome, and users often wear sunglasses to protect themselves from light sensitivity and to hide the bloodshot appearance of their eyes.
- Chronic sniffing, nasal congestion and septal ulceration may occur, particularly in cocaine users.
- Piloerection, diaphoresis, rhinorrhea, lacrimation, tremors, yawning, increased respiratory rate and muscle aching are common upon withdrawal.
- Pinpoint nonreactive pupils or small pupils that react sluggishly to light are characteristic of narcotics addicts. Cocaine causes pupillary dilatation (normal range is 3 to 6 mm). Pupillary signs demonstrable by the usual tests may be completely absent in persons accustomed to large doses of narcotic drugs. The naloxone hydrochloride (Narcan) test (*19–5*) is of great diagnostic value in the opiate addict.
- Evidence of narcotic in a urine specimen will confirm suspicions in questionable cases.

7–5. RECOMMENDATIONS ON ACUTE MANAGEMENT AND CONTROLLED SUBSTANCE ADMINISTRATION TO NARCOTICS ADDICTS IN CALIFORNIA

- Identify the narcotics addict and fill out a report (see Fig. 7–1) as required if controlled substances are prescribed or dispensed in treatment. At this time, propoxyphene HCl (Darvon) and napsylate (Darvon N) and pentazocine lactate (Talwin) are not regulated as narcotics, but precautions are advised.
- Physicians may administer (in the office or ED), prescribe, or even dispense (provided treatment beyond 3 days not expected; see *13–1*) for a 72-hour supply any medically reasonable substance—including controlled drugs—in the following situations:

- Acute bona fide emergency conditions. (*Note*: If narcotic is only *administered* for emergency pain, reporting is not required.) It is important to keep in mind that narcotics users may become rather proficient at feigning acute emergency pain

MAIL TO:
BUREAU OF NARCOTIC ENFORCEMENT

NAME OF PATIENT ______ AGE ______

ADDRESS ______
STREET ______ CITY ______

QUANTITY AND KIND OF NARCOTIC ______

DAILY DOSAGE ______

DIAGNOSIS OF INJURY OR AILMENT ______

______

HAS PATIENT PREVIOUSLY USED NARCOTICS? ______ YES OR NO ADDICTED? ______ YES OR NO

PHYSICIAN'S SIGNATURE ______

ADDRESS ______
STREET ______ CITY ______

DATE OF REPORT ______ FED. REG. NO. ______

Figure 7–1. Report form usually required to be sent by registered mail within 5 days of first treatment.

problems (for example, to simulate an acute ureteral stone they may go so far as to put a drop of blood from a finger puncture into their urine sample).

- Complications of incurable disease, serious accident or injury, or infirmities of old age requiring treatment with narcotics. The burden of proof is on the physician to show that administration of the drug was necessary in such cases, since usually even nonaddicted patients generally cope better with these chronic problems when not on narcotics or when taking only minimal amounts.
- Prescription of methadone in accordance with formal provisions of stage-adopted detoxification and maintenance treatments. (*Note*: The emergency physician will ordinarily not become involved in this situation.)
- Acute withdrawal symptoms in an addict. These can be treated without reporting if noncontrolled substances are used. Clonidine, for example, can stop practically all opiate withdrawal symptoms and signs in some cases; in others, combinations of other medications such as prochlorperazine or trimethobenzamide for nausea, pentazocine lactate for pain relief, and methocarbamol or carisoprodol for relief of muscle spasm and tension, may be used.
- Acute withdrawal symptoms that require administration of controlled substances present another situation. Emergency physicians (unless working in a government-certified institution for detoxification or in a jail where there is more prescribing liberty) should administer controlled substances only if a true emergency requiring narcotics exists, and even then only for one or possibly two doses, while arrangements are made for treating the patient in a government-certified institution.

8. Guidelines for Death and Dying Cases

8–1. ABSENCE OF ACCEPTED CRITERIA FOR DETERMINING TIME OF DEATH

Modern methods of resuscitation (5) have been spectacularly successful—so much so that the point at which death ends human existence has become difficult to determine. Although higher nervous system centers have been destroyed by prolonged anoxia, the viability of what has been termed "a human heart-lung preparation" may be continued for lengthy periods by various supportive means. Civil and criminal actions are still in the process of distinguishing acceptable basic medicolegal criteria for establishing "life" and "death" and even when it is proper for the judiciary to approve or order termination of supportive measures.

Medical and institutional facilities are finding it advantageous to hold a formal "ethics committee" hearing, to which *all* professional personnel caring for the patient plus concerned relatives and legal counsel are invited, to discuss any cessation of life support *before* such an event occurs. Legal counsel can be of benefit before "pulling the plug" on any patient on an artificial life support system. Some comparable dilemmas are involved in decisions not to institute cardiopulmonary life support ("no code blue").

The conflict arises in part from the archaic common law definition of death, which was established before the utilization of electricity in medicine, when there was no electrodiagnostic or electromonitoring equipment. The common law, which was still the law in 23 states as of 1982, requires in essence that there be complete cessation of cardiovascular and respiratory functions for death to have occurred. This definition is inadequate for two important reasons:

1. Every day patients are restored to functional alive states after clinically

appearing to have had complete cessation of cardiovascular and respiratory functions before initiation of resuscitation measures.

2. If one extends the definition to mean complete, irreversible cessation of cardiovascular and respiratory functions (approximating "pancytologic death"), the definition is excessive, in that patients and their relatives are often subjected to prolonged, inhumane, futile and costly processes wherein a body with "brain death"—physiologically nearly the equivalent of a decapitated person—is forced to maintain a few vestiges of meaningless organic activity. The philosophies of the major Western religions and the moral, ethical and scientific considerations of modern medicine do not require such measures, and the requisite of neural or "brain death" (*8–4*) is ample to establish cessation of meaningful life.

A succinct and generally workable standard definition of "death" (albeit still not uncontroversial or flawless) is that recommended in the Uniform Determination of Death Act, approved by the AMA in October 1980: "An individual who has sustained either (1) irreversible cessation of circulatory and respiratory functions, or (2) irreversible cessation of all functions of the entire brain, including the brain stem, is dead. A determination of death must be made in accordance with accepted medical standards." States are increasingly utilizing this format in their statutory definitions; no state has rejected it, but, as noted earlier, 23 states as of 1982 still used the common law definition and had no legal authorization for pronouncing death based on brain criteria (*8–4*). When the neural or "brain death" criteria just discussed are used in the absence of irreversible cessation of cardiovascular and respiratory functions, two physicians (at least one a neurologist) should evaluate the patient's terminus, and both should sign the death certificate.

8–2. PRESUMPTIVE SIGNS OF DEATH

- No response to painful stimuli.
- No carotid, femoral or other pulse or heartbeat or blood pressure by palpation or auscultation.
- No breath sounds on auscultation or chest motion for 3 or more minutes; no fogging of a freshly polished mirror held close to the nostrils or mouth.
- Complete absence of corneal and deep tendon reflexes.
- Absence of ocular motion upon passive head motion or ice water flushing of either ear.
- A flat baseline on all electrocardiographic (ECG) leads.
- Doughy resistance to passive motion, suggestive of developing rigor mortis.
- Dependent lividity and cyanosis.
- Decreased body temperature plus severe disparity between body temperature and that of environment (e.g., body temperature of 80° F found in 95° F environment).

These presumptive signs are usually considered to be adequate for determination of death when they occur in the terminal stages of chronic illnesses such as malignancy with metastases or uremia in a patient with whom the attending physician is thoroughly familiar and whose death is not unexpected—particularly if a Natural Death Act form has been signed. They are not adequate for determination of sudden and unexpected death in catastrophic emergency conditions such as trauma; acute poisoning (*53*) (including use of anesthetic and muscle-relaxing or paralyzing drugs); induced hypothermia (*62*); cardiogenic shock; or in instances in which the attending physician is not familiar with the patient's underlying condition, the events leading up to and climaxed by the apparent terminal state or the interval (in minutes) since onset of presumptive signs of death.

8–3. CONCLUSIVE SIGNS OF DEATH

Patients in this category are clinically described as having sustained "pancytologic" death, when presumptive signs of death (8–2) are accompanied by any of the following criteria:

- Complete partition of the body into parts incompatible with life (*example*: decapitation).
- Generalized body putrefaction.
- Fully established rigor mortis.

8–4. SIGNS OF BRAIN DEATH

Immutable, steadfast criteria for "death" in difficult cases (e.g., severe hypothermia or poisoning cases)—particularly in young people—are not established. Each year with improved medical therapies people miraculously recover from situations previously considered impossible for survival, although many others achieve merely a vegetative existence. The guidelines discussed in this section do not indicate conclusive signs of death but rather give criteria for determining, to a reasonable medical certainty, that the patient is in an irreversible permanent coma or chronic vegetative state, and that the likelihood of cognitive brain function returning is nonexistent by known standards. Because of the length of time required for these studies and observations to be made, admission to the hospital directly from the ED is performed.

"Brain dead" patients can maintain a heartbeat, circulate blood, sometimes breathe unassisted, digest food, perform exothermic body metabolism, filter waste products, and grow new tissue—all on a progressively deteriorating basis. However, there is persistently no evidence of cognitive brain function or nonverbal response to the environment. The "brain-dead" person medicolegally can be pronounced "dead."*

Following are guidelines and methods used to establish that a person is brain dead. (*Note:* These guidelines are *not* reliable in patients with hypothermia below the range of 32.2° C (90° F); prior electrical or cardiogenic shock; elevated or toxic levels of any removable or isoelectric-producing drugs such as barbiturates, diazepam, meprobamate, and methaqualone within the past 24 hours, as determined by toxicologic screening; or in very young patients, particularly those under age 5.)

- Flat lines without evidence of rhythm in all leads of an electroencephalographic (EEG) tracing that is taken at maximum gain and is not modified by loud noises. Absence of change over a 2- to 24-hour period is presumptive evidence of "brain death."
- At least 6 hours after onset of coma and apnea, presence of all of the following for at least 30 minutes (and more definitively 24 hours):†
  1. Coma with no cerebral response to stimuli.
  2. Apnea (ventilate with pure oxygen or O_2-CO_2 mixture for 10 minutes before removing ventilator; follow with ordinary passive O_2 flow).
  3. Dilated pupils.

---

*Since less than "pancytologic death" is present and there are vestiges of "life" in a "brain-dead" person, the term "quasi-death," which has the same criteria and medicolegal status as "brain-death," may be a more appropriate term in describing the status of the total body.

†Minimal criteria for "brain death" (all appropriate diagnostic and therapeutic procedures having been done without producing evidence of beneficial response) established following a collaborative study of cerebral death (JAMA, 237:982, 1977). These criteria are not as yet accepted by all as definitively authoritative.

4. Absent cephalic reflexes.
5. Electrocerebral silence (see precautionary *Note* in introduction to guidelines, above).

- A confirmatory test for the absence of cerebral and brainstem bloodflow is done with intracarotid injections of radionuclide or intravenous isotope angiography with a gamma camera or computed axial tomography (CAT) scan; one of these confirmatory tests is done if the most definitive test of brain death is needed or if the other listed criteria are indefinite or untestable (e.g., fixed, anatomically narrowed pupils or in patients undergoing therapeutic procedures that make examination of one or more of the cranial nerves impossible). Four-vessel angiography after IV radioactive sodium pertechnetate and a portable gamma camera also offer simple, specific and rapid determination of status of cerebral-brainstem bloodflow.
- Other guidelines (after Eliastam*) that are less definitive but are sometimes helpful for the clinician in considering cessation of CPR (even if agonal cardiac ECG activity is present) are:
  —Absence of all signs of life and a flat baseline ECG for at least 10 minutes after all appropriate resuscitative measures have been instituted. (See *Note* in introduction to guidelines, above, for circumstances in which these criteria are not applicable.)
  —Absence of response after 30 minutes of adequate combined prehospital care and ACLS.
  —Apnea and pulselessness known to have existed for 5 to 10 minutes before CPR instituted.
  —Pre-existing terminal illness and suffering.
- Two physicians, at least one a neurologist should certify "brain death."

8–5. CERTIFYING DEATH

The physician is justified in certifying a patient as "dead" when any of the following criteria are fulfilled:

- Any of the conclusive signs of death are present *(8–3)*.
- The presumptive signs of death are present *(8–2)* and the problems that led to this state have been corrected to the greatest degree that is reasonably possible (see conditions to be evaluated with special caution in *8–4*); in addition, resuscitative efforts, when indicated, have been instituted to the fullest extent (including resuscitation team exhaustion) and no evidence of improvement has ensued.
- "Brain death" ("quasi-death") in the absence of pancytologic death has been established beyond a reasonable doubt. (See *8–4* for clinical, EEG, ECG, and radiologic criteria for establishing "brain death.")

If the patient is about to be pronounced dead or has just been declared dead, consider any further actions to be taken *before* support measures are ceased (e.g., organ donation [*8–13*] if the patient had previously decided to make an anatomic gift). In situations in which immediate transplant of organs is planned, the two physicians certifying "brain death" should not be part of the transplant team.

8–6. NATURAL DEATH ACT CASES

See form 69–19, which, when in effect, may morally, ethically and legally alter the physician's responsibility and actions in a given case.

---

*Eliastam, M., et al.: Cardiac arrest in the emergency medical services system: Guidelines for resuscitation. JACEP, 6:569, 1977.

8–7. DEAD ON ARRIVAL (DOA) CASES

These should be registered in the usual manner, using *John Doe* or *Jane Doe* if the body is unidentified. Any available information regarding details of the illness or accident, cause of death, and so forth, together with external signs of trauma and other objective findings, should be entered in detail on the emergency record.

Any physician called upon to examine a patient suspected to be DOA has the very great responsibility of determining to the best of his ability if life has, in fact, ceased. If there is any suspicion in the physician's mind that some degree of life might still be present, immediate and vigorous resuscitative and supportive measures *(5)* should be begun, particularly if any of the conditions listed in *8–4*—which make life status determination so difficult—are present. A known period of 5 to 10 minutes of "down-time" (absence of vital signs before effective BLS measures are instituted) is often difficult to specifically determine and is only a *relative* indicator not to institute resuscitative measures. Careful recheck examination should be done again in 3 minutes and repeated as necessary until there is ABSOLUTELY no doubt in the mind of the attending physician that life is no longer present. If it is immediately available, the opinion of another physician should be obtained regarding confirmation.

PATIENTS IN WHOM ANY EVIDENCE OF LIFE IS DETECTED AND WHO RECEIVE FORMAL TREATMENT SHOULD NOT BE CLASSIFIED AS "DOA." However, patients who are considered dead and who show no response to the painful vigors and stimuli of resuscitative efforts may still be classified as "DOA." With the increasing prevalence of resuscitation measures in the field, the presentation of this type of case is more likely to be termed "DAR" (Dead After Resuscitation).

All DOA patients whose cause of death is unknown to a current physician must be reported at once to the coroner's office, and the remains, together with any personal belongings, turned over undisturbed to the coroner or the coroner's representative, avoiding altering of any evidence.

8–8. CORONER'S OR MEDICAL EXAMINER'S CASES

The circumstances under which a death case comes under the jurisdiction of the coroner (in some areas called the medical examiner) vary in minor details in different localities, but, in general, responsibility is transferred from the attending physician to the coroner or medical examiner for the locality or political subdivision in which the death occurs in the instances listed in Table 8–1. When a coroner or medical examiner assumes responsibility, this official's authority is supreme and completely supersedes the usual rights of the surviving spouse or next of kin *(8–9)*.

The attending physician CANNOT sign the death certificate *(65–6)* in coroner's cases unless specifically designated to do so by the coroner or the coroner's representative. The decision regarding the need for an autopsy and its extent is made solely by the coroner, although he or she may delegate the actual performance of the postmortem examination to another person. In this case, the person who authorized the autopsy, not the person who actually performed it, is completely responsible.

8–9. NOTIFICATION AND ASSISTANCE TO RELATIVES

Order of Notification

Although there is no absolute order of priority as to the person to notify, an acceptable guide is the jurisdictional order of intestate succession, which is commonly as follows:

Table 8–1. CORONER'S CASES

Section 10250 (Health and Safety Code, State of California)

A PHYSICIAN, FUNERAL DIRECTOR OR OTHER PERSON SHALL IMMEDIATELY NOTIFY THE CORONER WHEN HE HAS KNOWLEDGE OF A DEATH WHICH OCCURRED OR HAS CHARGE OF A BODY IN WHICH DEATH OCCURRED:

a. Without medical attendance
b. During the continued absence of the attending physician
c. Where the attending physician is unable to state the cause of death
d. Where the deceased person was killed or committed suicide
e. Where the deceased person died as the result of an accident
f. Under such circumstances as to afford a reasonable ground to suspect that the death was caused by the criminal act of another

Section 27491 of the Government Code, State of California—Classification of deaths requiring inquiry; determination of cause; signature on death certificates.

It shall be the duty of the coroner to inquire into and determine the circumstances, manner and cause of all violent, sudden or unusual deaths; unattended deaths; deaths wherein the deceased has not been attended by a physician in the 20 days before death; deaths related to or following known or suspected self-induced or criminal abortion; known or suspected homicide, suicide, or accidental poisoning; deaths known or suspected as resulting in whole or in part from or related to accident or injury either old or recent; deaths due to drowning, fire, hanging, gunshot, stabbing, cutting, exposure, starvation, acute alcoholism, drug addiction, strangulation, or aspiration, or where the suspected cause of death is sudden infant death syndrome; death in whole or in part occasioned by criminal means; deaths associated with a known or alleged rape or crime against nature; deaths in prison or while under sentence; deaths known or suspected as due to contagious disease and constituting a public hazard; deaths from occupational diseases or occupational hazards; deaths under such circumstances as to afford a reasonable ground to suspect that the death was caused by the criminal act of another; or any deaths reported by physicians or other persons having knowledge of death for inquiry by coroner. Inquiry in this section does not include those investigative functions usually performed by other law enforcement agencies.

- The surviving spouse.
- Surviving children who have reached majority age.
- Surviving parents of the deceased.
- Surviving adult siblings of the deceased.
- Other surviving adult kin in order of closest blood relationship.

An acceptable alternative, especially when there is advanced age or infirmity of a relative of prior right, is notification of the relative who is the apparent or specified spokesman for the family or a specified friend.

Manner of Notification

Particularly in emergency cases—in which there has been little or no time for preparatory grief—the role of the physician in notification of the patient's death is quite important. The following guidelines may be of assistance:

- Do not assume the relatives already know of the death; it is preferable to have the relatives taken to a private room where they may sit and be physically comfortable prior to notification.
- If the family is not in the ED and knows nothing of the event, it may be preferable to delay notification until meeting in person, or to send a professional to the home. (With any call from the ED, regardless of circumstances, caution the call recipient to drive carefully to the ED.)

- Be compassionate; assure that all reasonable efforts were made to save the deceased's life. Make every effort to comfort the bereaved, and in particular to assuage any guilt or sense of responsibility they may feel for the patient's death. (*Note:* At times such guilt may be projected onto others, including the physician and other medical personnel.)
- Spend enough time to answer important questions in order to facilitate constructive mourning.
- Aid in follow-up assistance; if necessary, offer a few days' supply of a fast-acting sedative for rest.
- If the body has not been badly disfigured, it is appropriate that members of the family who wish to be permitted to spend a few moments with the body in private in the ED; the grieving process can be aided by letting at least one mature family member make a personal observation of the actuality of the event.
- If necessary, an autopsy (*8–10*) may be requested after the family has had an opportunity to initially adjust to the fact of death. If an autopsy is performed, offer to answer any questions that subsequently occur, and to review the autopsy findings.
- It is of aid to the family to make arrangements for a mortuary service before they leave.
- The assistance of a medical facility chaplain or the family's own spiritual counselor can be of great comfort. Many hospitals and communities have follow-up counseling facilities or support groups available for the bereaved. Provision of written information for such for later consideration may be helpful.

8–10. AUTOPSIES (POSTMORTEM EXAMINATIONS)

Coroner's Cases

All requests for autopsies must be signed by a representative of the coroner's office. The signature of any other person is invalid.

Non–Coroner's Cases

Request and Permit for Autopsy. Any type of postmortem examination, with or without removal of tissue or organs, requires completion of a properly signed and witnessed autopsy permit BEFORE THE EXAMINATION IS BEGUN. Any type of postmortem examination without such permission constitutes actionable assault. There are no universal specifications in regard to the persons who may authorize postmortem examinations but, in general, priority is the same as indicated for notification of death (*8–9*).

Although the signature of only one of several persons of the same degree of blood relationship is required by law if there is no surviving spouse, it is always desirable and advisable to obtain as many as practical.

Purposes of Autopsy in Non–Coroner's Cases. The purposes of autopsy are to determine the cause of death and any contibutory factors, evaluate for transmissible disease—both genetic and infectious—and promote medical science.

Limitations. Any limitations or restrictions on the extent and scope of the postmortem examination or unusual special instructions must be specified on the Autopsy Permit form and must be scrupulously observed by the autopsy surgeon or pathologist. Any examination or removal of tissues or organs in excess of, or in addition to, those specifically authorized is prima facie evidence of law violation even if, in the opinion of the autopsy surgeon, such additional examination is absolutely necessary to determine the cause of death. Example: "no brain examination."

8–11. DISPOSAL OF REMAINS

If the decedent leaves written instructions in a will or other document *(69–17, Uniform Donor Card),* his or her remains should be disposed of in accordance with the instructions even if other provisions of the will are subject to dispute. If the decedent leaves no will or written instructions, the decision regading disposition rests with survivors, following the same priority outlined under *Order of Notification (8–9).*

STILLBIRTHS. (For definition, see *65–4.*) When the parents do not wish custody of a dead fetus, a permit for disposal should be properly signed and witnessed.

8–12. RELIGIOUS RITES NEAR AND AFTER DEATH

Considerable variation exists among religious groups regarding procedural rites before, at and after death. Accepted procedures, in some of which the attending physician may of necessity be forced to participate, are outlined in Tables 8–2 to 8–4.

8–13. ORGAN DONATION AND TRANSPORT

Kidneys for individuals with end-stage renal disease, corneas for the curably blind, middle ears for the deaf, pituitary gland extract for the dwarfed, plus bone, cartilage, dura, liver, heart, lungs, and skin, among other tissues and organs can greatly benefit and in many cases save the lives of recipients. Another valuable factor can be aid to research.

The Uniform Anatomical Gift Act (UAGA) is curently in effect in all 50 states. If the deceased had expressly made *(69–18)* or declined to make an anatomic gift, then further action proceeds accordingly. If, however, no action was made by the deceased one way or another, the next of kin *(8–9)* manage and control the deceased's body and can authorize an anatomic gift from the individual.

If an anatomic gift is donated, certain preparations are necessary to preserve its quality for the recipient. Specific directions from the transplant center concerning qualification and procedure are essential and should be obtained immediately. (In "brain death" cases *[8–4]* these preparations should precede termination of artificial life support measures. Among the 24-hour transplant banks that will give assistance are the following:

- Northern California Transport Bank: (408) 289–8200.
- University of Colorado Medical Center: (303) 394–5252.
- Association of Illinois Transplant Surgeons: (312) 263–3655.
- University of Texas, Houston: (713) 797–4284.
- Delaware Valley Regional Transplant Program (Philadelphia): (215) 543–6391.

In the continental United States, the Air Force Rescue Coordination Center (AFRCC) at Scott Air Force Base, Illinois, helps coordinate the services of the Civil Air Patrol and assists in matters of life or death, including prevention of loss of limb, and in transportation of organs for transplant. AFRCC can be reached by telephoning 800-851-3051. The following information should also be available upon contacting AFRCC: (1) confirmation that investigation has established that there is no local or commercial transportation that can effectively provide this critically needed service; (2) the name, age and residence of the patient; (3) the problem at hand and the objective of the request being made; (4) the location of the starting point and the destination point of the transport, also noting whether there is a helicopter landing pad (helipad) at each location; (5) what specialized equipment, provisions and personnel are required and are they already available.

Table 8–2. RELIGIOUS RITES FOR PERSONS ON CRITICAL LIST FOR ANY REASON

	Roman Catholic	Jewish	Protestant	Buddhist	Hindu	Moslem
Medical personnel's responsibility	Call a priest to administer the required sacraments of Penance, Holy Communion and Anointing of the Sick (Extreme Unction). Arrange complete privacy for confession.	Call a rabbi—preferably of the branch (Conservative, Orthodox, Reformed) to which the patient belongs.	Call a minister—preferably of the patient's own denomination. In certain instances, Holy Communion, Penance and Extreme Unction may be required. Arrange for privacy.	Call a priest of indicated sect (e.g. Jodosh inshu) *only at patient or family request.* There is no specific prayer or rite.	None; no formal religious visits, prayers or rites before death.	None; no formal religious visits, prayers or rites before death.

Table 8–3. RELIGIOUS RITES FOR PREMATURE OR OTHER INFANTS IN CRITICAL CONDITION; STILLBIRTHS; ABORTIONS

	Roman Catholic	Jewish	Protestant	Buddhist	Hindu	Moslem
	Excluding Anglo-Catholic, Eastern Orthodox and Polish National Catholic.	The Conservative, Orthodox and Reform branches specify minor differences in certain rites.	Presbyterian, Episcopalian, Lutheran, Moravian, etc.			
General Instructions						
Notify the closest representative of the parents' church group at parents' request, but if death is imment, do not await his or her arrival to perform last rites.	Call a priest (addressed as *Father*).	Call a rabbi (addressed as *Rabbi*).	Call a minister (addressed generally as *Mister* or *Doctor*, rather than *Reverend;* Lutheran, *Pastor;* high church Episcopal, *Father*).	Call a priest (addressed as *Reverend)* only at family request. No specific rite or prayer.	No religious representative need be contacted.	No religious representative need be contacted.

Baptism or Circumcision "I baptize you in the name of the Father and of the Son and of the Holy Spirit, Amen."	Required for infants in danger of death and for all products of conception, no matter how early. Water must flow on the skin. If born with membranes intact, immerse in water and break membranes. If in utero, hypodermic injection of sterile water through membranes.	No baptism. Jewish males are circumcised on the 8th day after birth—no religious rites of any type for females.	Required for all viable infants and stillbirths (65–4), not for early products of conception. (Exceptions—Baptists and Disciples of Christ not baptized.) Water must touch skin—excess poured off—cloths, cotton, etc., used to wipe skin or head must be burned at once.	No baptism, religious circumcision or specific pre-death rite.	No baptism. No specific religious rite.	No baptism. No specific religious rite.
Name Necessary?	No. Give full details to priest on his arrival.	No.	Yes. If no given name, specify *Baby Boy Doe*. Give full details to minister on his arrival.			

Table 8–4. RELIGIOUS RITES FOR DEATH CASES

	Roman Catholic	Jewish	Protestant	Buddhist	Hindu	Moslem
Last Rites	Call a priest. If last rites have not been given before death, the Sacrament of Anointing of the Sick (Extreme Unction) can be administered conditionally for several hours afterward, provided the body has not been shrouded or covered.	No last rites. Notify a rabbi or a responsible member of the Jewish community so, that arrangements for disposition of remains, burial, etc., can be made.	No last rites after death.	No specific predeath rite. At family request call priest to place of death (or next day at funeral home if family chooses) for Makur Geyo (sutra plus incense).	No last rites.	No last rites. Conservative sects have burial before next sundown.
Permission for Autopsy?	No objection on religious grounds.	Because of religious objections, permission will have to be obtained through a rabbi.	No moral or religious objection to autopsy.	No moral or religious objection to autopsy.	No objection to autopsy.	No autopsy generally.

9. Drug Dosage in Children

Except in those instances in which a specific dose per age, dose per weight or dose per skin surface ratio is given in the text or in the brochure of the manufacturers, the following dosage guidelines are satisfactory for emergency use.

Dosage Guidelines by Mg per Kilogram of Body Weight

The best policy in prescribing drugs is to use the manufacturer's recommended dosage, which is most frequently given in mg per kilogram of body weight and is available in the package insert brochure or in the *Physician's Desk Reference* (PDR); at times, the manufacturer will prefer to give dosage by age and weight range, and that should be used in these instances.

In the text, dosage for many common emergency drugs is given (see also 5–27). In the absence of any of the above information, Table 9–1 may be an aid in an emergency situation. *Note:* Infants and young children are especially susceptible to the action of narcotics; from the age of 6 months to 2 years, doses should be reduced below these schedules by at least one-half, and these drugs should be avoided in infants less than 6 months of age.

Table 9–1. CHILDREN'S DRUG DOSAGES BY SKIN SURFACE FOR AGE, WEIGHT AND HEIGHT

Age	Weight		Height		Surface Area (sq m)	Approximate Percentage of Adult Dose*
	kg	lb	cm	in		
Birth	3.4	7.4	50	20	0.21	11
3 months	5.7	12.5	60	23.5	0.29	16
6 months	7.4	16	66	26	0.36	21
1 year	10.0	22	75	29.4	0.45	26
2 years	12.4	27	87	34	0.54	31
3 years	14.5	31	96	38	0.60	35
4 years	16.5	36	103	40.5	0.68	39
5 years	19.0	41	110	43.5	0.73	42
6 years	21.5	47	116	46	0.82	47
7 years	24.1	53	123	48.5	0.90	53
8 years	26.8	59	129	51	0.97	57
9 years	29.4	65	134	53	1.05	61
10 years	32.3	71	139	55	1.12	65
11 years	35.5	78	144	57	1.20	69
12 years	39.0	86	151	59.5	1.28	74

*Based on average adult skin surface of 1.73 sq m. See nomogram (Fig. 9–1) to determine skin surface for a greater range of heights and weights.

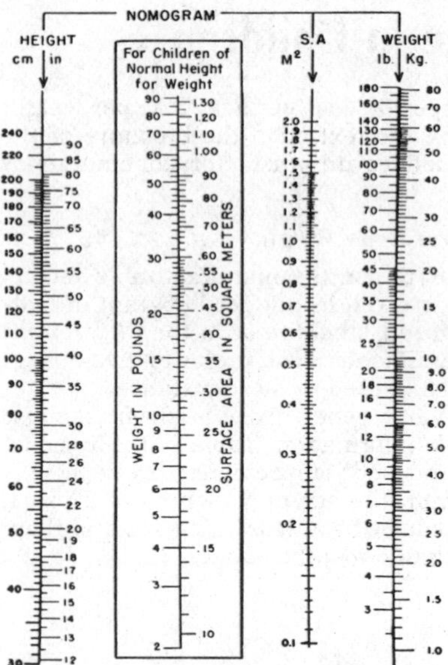

Figure 9–1. West nomogram (for estimation of surface areas). The surface area is indicated where a straight line connecting the height and weight intersects the surface area column, or, if the patient is roughly of average size, from weight alone (enclosed area). Nomogram modified from data of E. Boyd by C. D. West, from Shirkey, H. C.: Drug therapy. *In* Vaughan, V. C., and McKay, R. J. (eds.): *Nelson Textbook of Pediatrics,* 10th ed. Philadelphia, W. B. Saunders Co., 1975.

10. Emergency Medical Supplies and Bag Contents

The contents of an emergency bag will, of course, vary considerably according to the owner's type of practice and individual preferences. Depending on the proximity of a well-equipped emergency room or hospital, and the availability of a well-organized EMS program, some may wish to add to or delete items from the lists given in sections *10–1* to *10–4*. However, these basic items will allow efficient and satisfactory care for most urgent conditions. Compact preassembled emergency kits (e.g., the Banyan or Emergi-Stat bags and the Biotek case) offer many advantages for the physician who is not in a remote area or for whom, as is usually the case, management of cardiopulmonary resuscitations is of foremost concern.

The basic emergency bag and ancillary materials to be kept in the trunk of the car include diagnostic equipment *(10–1)*, medications *(5–27)* and therapeutic supplies *(10–3)* listed alphabetically, not in order of importance. Each article should be packaged separately, labeled clearly for rapid identification and kept in a specific place in the bag. Medications (especially solutions) preferably should be in separate individual doses and not in stock bottles. Parenteral medications should be carried in single-dose sterile vials; preloaded syringes are a convenience and advantage for some medications. Plastic nonbreakable bottles should be used for all liquids.

REPLACEMENT OF EACH ITEM AS SOON AS POSSIBLE AFTER USE IS IMPERATIVE! A list of items on each call facilitates replacement as soon as the physician returns to the office. The expiration date of each item should be checked periodically.

10–1. DIAGNOSTIC EQUIPMENT

Item	Quantity	Description and Use
1	1 set	Batteries and bulb (spare) to fit diagnostic equipment; a battery-containing universal handle to fit flashlight, laryngoscope and otoscope saves space and weight. A nickle-cadmium battery unit, rechargeable in 5 minutes, may obviate the need for carrying spare batteries
2	10	"Dip sticks" for urinary sugar/acetone/protein,and Dextrostix for blood sugar tests
3	4	Finger cots, assorted sizes, for digital examination, finger dressings and use as *flutter valves (31–12)*
†4	1	Flashlight, small (may use item 1, *above*)
5	2	Fluorescein ophthalmic solution (1%); single application packages or strips
6	2 pairs	Gloves: sterile, disposable, plastic or rubber
*7	1	Laryngoscope with 3 blades (infant, medium, large) to fit universal handle (see item 1)
8	1	Neurologic reflex hammer with pinwheel, soft hair tuft and tuning fork incorporated
9	1	Ophthalmoscope-otoscope to fit universal handle (item 1)
*10	3	Oropharyngeal airways, assorted sizes
11	1	Phenylephrine hydrochloride (Neo-Synephrine), 10% ophthalmic solution, 5 ml dropper vial (for funduscopic examination)
12	2	Pontocaine, ½% ophthalmic solution, single application container for eye examinations
13	2	Rectal lubricant, water soluble (K-Y Jelly), single application packages
*14	1	Sphygmomanometer, aneroid, with self-adherent cuff
15	1	Spinal puncture needle with stylet (22 gauge)
*16	1	Stethoscope, folding type with flexible tubes
17	1	Stylet with obturator 12 to 14 gauge for cricothyroid airway
†18	2	Thermometers (oral and rectal) in break-resistant cases
19	1	Thoracentesis needle, 4 inch, 18 gauge short bevel, with stylet
†20	4	Tongue blades, individually packaged (can double for use as small temporary splints)

*This item or its near equivalent is contained in one or more of the commercially prepackaged emergency kits.

†Included in basic first-aid kit; should also include acetaminophen/aspirin, calamine lotion, Dramamine. Consider also inclusion of DMSO.

10–2. MEDICATIONS *(See 5–27)*

10–3. THERAPEUTIC SUPPLIES

Item	Quantity	Description
*†1	1 roll	Adhesive tape—3″
†2	1	Alcohol 70%, 60 ml in plastic bottle with screw top
*3	6	Alcohol-saturated gauze pads, small, individually packaged
†4	4 oz	Antiseptic solution for wounds (Betadine or Hibielens)

Table continued on next page

Item	Quantity	Description
†5	6	Applicators, cotton-tipped, sterile, individually packaged
*6	1	Bag-valve-mask; hand-operated ventilation bag with tubing and adaptors for other respiratory aid equipment
7	1	Bandage/clothes scissors (medium size)
†8	1 box	Bandages, sterile, assorted sizes (Band-Aids)
9	2	Catheters (urinary bladder), plastic No. 12 and No. 16 Foley, 5-ml reservoir, sterile
10	2	Eye patches
11	1	File for opening ampules and vials
†12	4	Gauze roller bandages, sterile, 1″ and 2″
†13	8	Gauze pads, sterile, 2″ × 2″, individually packaged
†14	4	Gauze pads, sterile, 4″ × 4″, individually packaged
15	9	Hypodermic needles, sterile, individually packaged and labeled: 2 #26 gauge, ⅞″ long 2 #24 gauge, 1½″ long *†3 #22 gauge, 2″ long *1 #18 gauge, 3″ long, with stylet *†1 #14 gauge, 3″ long, with stylet (emergency tracheal airway canula also)
16	6	Hypodermic syringes, sterile, individually packaged and labeled: 1 syringe, 1 ml (tuberculin) *1 syringe, 2 ml *1 syringe, 5 ml *1 syringe, 50 ml
17	2	Intravenous catheters
*18	3	Laryngeal intubation tubes (assorted sizes)
*†19	1 dozen	Matches, friction type, in waterproof container
†20	1 tube	Petroleum jelly
21	1	Pocket knife, large pointed blade
22	1 dozen	Safety pins, assorted sizes, in plastic box
†23	3	Sanitary napkins (Kotex), individually wrapped, for use as compression bandages for profuse hemorrhage
24	1 roll	Scotch tape, ¾″ width
25	3 packs	Sterile adhesives, assorted widths (steristrips)
26	1	Suction cup (small), for removal of contact lenses
27	2 oz	Tincture of benzoin
†28	1	Tweezers

10–4. ADDITIONAL EQUIPMENT *(Optional—can be carried in the car trunk)*

Electrocardiograph (portable, with electrolyte jelly).

Intravenous Starter Set

Item	Quantity	Description
1	1	Dextran, 500 ml
2	1	Dextrose, 5% in water, 500-ml flask or 125-ml starter bottle
*3	2	Ringer's lactate, 500 ml
4	2	Needles, short-bevel, 20 gauge, 2″ long
*5	2	Disposable tubing sets

*This item or its near equivalent is contained in one or more of the commercially prepackaged emergency kits.

†Included in basic first-aid kit.

Lavage and Catheterization Setup

Item	Quantity	Description
1	2	Adaptors (plastic or metal, *not* glass) to fit funnel, catheters, gastric lavage tubes and rubber tubing
2	2	Adaptors (plastic or metal), Y-tube
3	4	Catheters (sterile), individually packaged, 3 male (small, medium and large), one female (plastic, nonbreakable); with adaptors to fit plastic funnel, syringe and tubing
4	1	Funnel (plastic) with adaptors to fit lavage tubes, catheters and tubing
5	2	Gastric lavage tubes (Ewald type), small and medium
6	1	Syringe, large, with tubing and adaptor
7	2 pairs	Sterile gloves

Obstetric–Gynecologic Supplies

Item	Quantity	Description
1	1	Clamp (Kocher), large, sterile
2	1	Forceps, thumb, sterile
3	2 ampules	Silver nitrate solution (1%), individual dose package
4	2	Umbilical cord ties (sterile)
5	1	Vaginal speculum, medium size
6	1	Episiotomy set (spring retractor, scissors, needle holder, sutures)
7	1	Bulb syringe (for suctioning infant)
8	2	Infant blankets
9	2 pairs	Sterile gloves

Orthopedic Supplies

Item	Quantity	Description
1	1	Aluminum, sheet, malleable, 6″ × 8″ for small splints
2	1	Mechanics' pliers with side-cutting jaws
3	1	Metal shears, heavy enough to cut sheet aluminum
4	2	Pneumatic splints (upper/lower extremity)
5	6 rolls	Plaster of Paris: (2) 2″ rolls (2) 3″ rolls (2) 4″ rolls
6	2 rolls	Sheet wadding, 3″
†7	1	Sling, muslin (Red Cross type, or clean old triangular bed sheet, 36″ × 36″ × 54″
8	1 roll	Stockinette, bias-cut, 3″

Oxygen Tank.* Small portable, with tubing and adaptors to bag-valve-mask.

Poison Kit. Some physicians like to carry a separate kit for treatment of acute poisoning. This should contain the following items:

Acetic acid, 5%
†Activated charcoal
Ammonia water, 0.2%
Amyl nitrite pearls
†Amobarbital (Amytal) sodium parenteral)
Atropine sulfate (parenteral)
Caffeine and sodiobenzoate (parenteral)
†Calcium gluconate, 10% (parenteral)
‡Cyanide Antidote Kit
Dimercaprol (BAL)
Edathamil calcium disodium (EDTA)
†Ipecac, syrup of
†Magnesium hydroxide (milk of magnesia)
†Metaraminol bitartrate (Aramine)
Methylene blue, 1% aqueous (parenteral)

Table continued on next page

*This item or its near equivalent is contained in one or more of the commercially prepackaged emergency kits.

†Included in basic first-aid kit.

‡Can be kept separately from other supplies; available from Eli Lilly, stock #76.

Poison Kit *(Continued)*

Methylprednisolone sodium succinate (parenteral)
Naloxone (Narcan)
Paraldehyde
Phenylephrine hydrochloride (parenteral)
Potassium chloride (tablets and parenteral)
Potassium permanganate
†Procainamide (parenteral)
Sodium bicarbonate (parenteral)
Sodium formaldehyde sulfoxylate
Sodium nitrite, 3%
Sodium thiosulfate, 25% (parenteral)
Starch
Vitamin K_1 oxide (AquaMEPHYTON)
†Water (distilled, sterile)

Specimen Collection Setup

Item	Quantity	Description
1	2	Bottles, plastic, sterile, large mouth, screw top, 60 ml for specimens of urine, vomitus, stool, etc.
2	2	Culture tubes, 5 ml, plastic, screw top
3	1 box	Labels, gummed, small
4	4	Microscope slides, sterile, in container
5	2	Vials, sterile, 10 ml, screw top, for blood samples
6	6	Small envelopes for containing and labeling specimens and evidence

Surgical Setup

Item	Quantity	Description
*1	4	Clamps (hemostats), sterile, individually packaged: 2 small (mosquito or Kelly) 2 large (Carmalt or Kocher)
2	1	Eye scalpel, bistoury point, sterile
3	1	Eye spud, small, sterile
*4	3	Forceps (sterile), individually packaged and labeled: 1 thumb forceps, plain tip 1 thumb forceps, rat-tooth tip
5	4	Needles, surgical, cutting edge, half curved, assorted sizes, sterile, in individual envelopes
6	1	Probe, flexible wire, ball tip
7	1	Razor, safety, with package of blades
8	2	Small retractors (may supplement with bent paper clips for small areas)
9	1	Scalpel handle (Bard-Parker No. 3) with 3 individually packaged sterile blades, assorted shapes, to fit handle
*†10	1	Scissors, Mayo type (1 sharp, 1 rounded point)
*11	1	Skin hook (may substitute bent safety pin)
12	1	Ring cutter in case
*13	6	Sutures with fixed needles in individual sterile tubes or envelopes: (2) 3-0 Dermalon or Prolene (2) 5-0 Dermalon or Prolene (1) 2-0 Plain catgut (1) 4-0 Plain catgut
*14	1	Tourniquet (may use sphygmomanometer in its place).

Miscellaneous Supplies

Emergency textbook
Prescription pad
Road and street map
Restraint straps (4), 1″ webbing, airplane-type quick release buckles, or 4 slings rolled into cravats
[illegible]ber tubing (2 rolls), ¼″ to ⅜″ bore, 18 to 36 inches long for use as tourniquets, etc.

[illegible] item or its near equivalent is contained in one or more of the commercially [illegible]kaged emergency kits.
[illegible]ded in basic first-aid kit.

Supplemental Equipment for Emergency Transport Vehicles

Additional blankets
Body splint system: head/neck/shoulder, separable extrication splint (Greene)
Hard cervical collar
Cardiac monitor/defibrillator
Extremity traction splint, adult and pediatric sizes (Hare)
Fire extinguisher
K-Bar-T vehicle entry tool
Medical anti-shock trousers (MAST)
Oxygen tank
Suction equipment
Tow chain
Two-way communication system (radio or telephone)

10–5. PRECAUTIONS

The basic emergency bag, as well as optional kits, should be kept out of public view as much as possible, preferably locked in the luggage compartment. If carried on the seat or floor of the car, they should be covered. All equipment will be safer if the car does not carry M.D. identification.

When an emergency night call is received, a spotlight, either transportable or mounted on the car, and a good map of any unfamiliar localities are invaluable. Transportation of the patient to the ED is often preferable.

If calls for emergency treatment are received from persons who are not known or if the circumstances of the call are unusual and the patient cannot be brought to the emergency department, it may be prudent for the physician to request a police escort, particularly if the area to be visited has a high crime rate.

11. Fluid Replacement in Emergencies*

Proper replacement of fluid and electrolytes (prior losses plus ongoing special and normal losses) is an often overlooked and neglected aspect of the care of emergency cases; proper management may be lifesaving. The following principles of replacement therapy may require modification because of limited facilities for laboratory determination, but in many instances, clinical examination will allow institution of therapy that can be continued during transfer to a hospital in which accurate confirmatory laboratory tests can be obtained. In all instances, an *accurate* record of intake, both parenteral and oral, and of output must be sent with the patient. Monitoring with central venous pressures (CVP; see *18–7*) and multiple large IV catheters (*18–36*) is usually required to rapidly and properly administer the numerous liters of solution required in severe adult dehydration and shock.

Calculations for repair of electrolyte imbalance are usually expressed in milliequivalents per liter (abbreviated mEq/L) as in the following formula:

---

*See also *46–1* (Acidosis); *46–3* (Alkalosis); and sections on fluid replacement in special conditions, e.g., burns (28) and shock (57; especially Tables 57–1 to 57–5 for identification, severity evaluation, monitoring and treatment of hypovolemic shock).

$$\text{mEq/L} = \frac{\text{mg/100 ml} \times 10}{\text{atomic weight}} \times \text{valence}$$

Values for the normal range of concentration of the major elements in electrolyte balance are given in Table 11–1.

Table 11–1. MAJOR BASIC ELEMENTS IN ELECTROLYTE BALANCE

Element	Chemical Symbol	Atomic Weight	Valence	Range of Concentration in Extracellular Fluid (mEq/L)
Sodium	Na	23	1	135–148
Potassium	K	39	1	4.4–5.6
Carbon dioxide combining power	CO_2	. .	1	25.0–30.0
Chloride	Cl	35	1	99–108
Calcium	Ca	40	2	4.5–5.5

11–1. BASIC CONSIDERATIONS IN MANAGEMENT AND TREATMENT

*1. **Estimation of volume and type of prior loss*** of water, sodium and other electrolytes and of degrees of acid-base imbalance or blood-plasma loss (see *11–2* and *11–3*).

- Duration, site (e.g., upper/lower GI, urine, drainage tubes) and rate of losses or lack of intake (history and observation). Include sweat losses, especially if there is fever.
- Weight loss: Estimate or compare current and normal weight (1 pint water ≅ 1 pound).
- Urinary specific gravity.
- Skin turgor (look for persistent skin tenting after lifting up).
- Presence of loss into *third compartment* (e.g., pleural cavity and peritoneal cavity).
- Direct measurement of losses (volume and type): urine, GI, drainage tubes.
- Specific determinations of urine and blood electrolytes, pH, ABG's and blood volume, as needed. Electrocardiograms can be of assistance in emergency evaluation of calcium and potassium levels (Fig. 46–1). Do CVP as needed.

*2. **Estimation or determination of rate of current abnormal losses*** by volume and type for the next 24 hours (see *11–2* and *11–3*).

*3. **Estimation of anticipated normal loss of water and electrolytes*** for the next 24 hours.

*4. **Total body losses of water and electrolytes*** estimated by end of next 24 hours (estimated by sum of *1*, 2, and 3).

*5. **Determination of the type and rate of correction*** over the next 24 hours based on the considerations above, plus the patient's age, severity of condition and cardiovascular and renal status. (*Note:* Lactic acidosis must be treated more vigorously than other types of acidosis.) Specific orders should be written covering the first 24 hours of replacement therapy, giving type of fluids (*11–4*), amount of fluids and route and rate of administration. Number all bottles of fluids consecutively. The following summary form can be helpful:

Day 1 Balance Form	Water (ml)	Na (mEq)	K (mEq)	Cl (mEq)	Ca (mEq)	Other*
1. Prior loss						
2. Current abnormal loss						
3. Normal loss in 24 hours						
4. Total loss at end of next 24 hours						
5. Replacement to be ordered for next 24 hours						

*Blood; plasma; trace metals, etc.

11–2. BASIC REQUIREMENTS (FLUIDS AND ELECTROLYTES) PER DAY

The amount of fluids and electrolytes required every 24 hours depends upon the patient's age, weight and skin surface (usually indicated in square meters; abbreviated sq m); see nomogram (Fig. 9–1).

Water (H_2O) Requirements Per Day *(See also 28–3, Burns, Principles of Treatment)*. The following list gives daily water requirements according to physical condition.

Average physical condition	1500 ml/sq m
Moderately dehydrated	2400 ml/sq m
Severely dehydrated	3000 ml/sq m
Hyperventilating	500 ml/sq m
Hyperpyrexic	1500 ml/sq m +4.5% for each Centigrade degree above normal (2.5% for each degree Fahrenheit)

Potassium Ion Requirements Per Day: 40 mEq/sq m.

Sodium Chloride (NaCl) Requirements Per Day.

The following table gives daily NaCl requirements according to age.

Age	NaCl g	NaCl mEq
Newborn	0.25	4
1–3 months	0.35	6
3–6 months	0.5	8
6–12 months	0.75	12
1–2 years	1.0	17
2–4 years	2.0	34
4–7 years	3.0	51
7–12 years	4.0	68
12–18 years	5.0	85
18 years up	6.0–7.0	100–120

Table 11–2. TYPES AND APPROXIMATE AVERAGE AMOUNTS OF OUTPUT

Type	Na	mEq/L K	Cl	HCO_3	Average Output Per Day in ml (70-kg adult)
Bile	140	10	100	30	500
Bowel	120	10	105	25	3000
Gastric	35	12	125	—	2500
Pancreatic	140	10	75	75	700
Saliva	10	25	10	10	1000
Urine	40	30	70	—	1500
Sensible and insensible (skin and lungs)					
At rest	0	0	0		1000
Moderate activity	25	0	25		1500
Extreme activity	50	0	50		2000+

11–3. OUTPUT

Physiologic output of fluids and electrolytes must be given full consideration in estimating replacement therapy (see Table 11–2). Pathologic processes (excessive perspiration, hyperpyrexia, rapid respiration, vomiting, diarrhea, bleeding) must also be considered. In edematous patients, no loss of electrolytes is considered to occur through the skin.

11–4. REPLACEMENT SOLUTIONS (mEq to volume indicated)

	Volume or Amount	Na	K	Cl	Lactate
Normal saline (0.9% NaCl)	Per liter	154	—	154	—
Ringer's lactate	Per liter	131	4	110	28
Sodium bicarbonate (3.75 gm)	Per 50 ml	44.6	—	—	—
Sodium lactate (1/6 molar solution)	Per liter	166	—	—	166
Plasma	Per 250 ml	35	1.2	25	—
Whole blood (approximate*)	Per 500 ml	70	2.5*	52	—
5% DW (dextrose in H_2O)	Per liter	—	—	—	—
5% Saline†	Per liter	855	—	855	—
Ammonium chloride† (0.9% solution)	Per liter	—	—	167	—
Butler's solution†	Per liter	57	25	50	25
Darrow's solution†	Per liter	117	35	99	53
Potassium penicillin	Per million units	—	1.7	—	—
Sodium penicillin	Per million units	1.6	—	—	—

*Potassium increases in hemolyzed blood; calcium is reduced in stored blood.
†Rarely used.

11–5. FLUID REQUIREMENTS FOR BURN PATIENTS IN THE FIRST 24 HOURS *(See 28–3)*

11–6. ORAL SOLUTION FOR MASS CASUALTY USE

Usually, plentiful oral intake of potable water is the most important measure for patients who have no contraindication to ingestion of oral fluids. See 3–*16* for instructions on making contaminated water into potable water.

Periodic oral intake of one to two glasses of a solution containing 1 level teaspoonful of table salt and ½ teaspoonful of baking sodium dissolved in a gallon of water may aid persons who show evidence of water, saline and base depletion. Follow with administration of potable water ad lib.

12. Pain Management: Analgesia and Anesthesia

Control of acute pain may require anesthetic (either general, with obliteration of conscious functioning, or local) measures to eliminate all pain response, such as needed during surgical procedures, or analgesic measures to raise the pain threshold and reduce pain perception without causing serious alterations in consciousness. Details concerning any necessary informed consent and signing are best achieved before giving stronger analgesics.

Measures may be medicinal or nonmedicinal and systemic or focal; usage depends on factors such as the condition under treatment, the measures available and the intensity aand duration of pain control required.

MEDICINAL MEASURES

12–1. SYSTEMIC ANALGESICS

For usage and toxicity of other substances listed under the Narcotics Act 7–3), see *53* (Poisons). See also *13* (Prescription Restrictions; particularly *13–2*, Schedules 2 and 3) and the table on common emergency medications in section 5–27 (pp. 52–55).

EMERGENCY USE OF NARCOTICS

Opium derivatives as well as synthetic narcotics are of great value in emergency treatment, provided indiscriminate use is avoided and the following principles are kept in mind.

Definite indications for use are present. These include the following:

- Control of acute intense pain and associated apprehension.
- Desire to achieve specific effects—e.g., apomorphine to induce vomiting under unusual circumstances (generally best avoided); naloxone hydrochloride (Narcan) to counteract overdoses of opiates and synthetic narcotics; morphine to control acute pain.

Contraindications. The most important contraindications to narcotics use include:

- Head injuries *(44)*. Important changes in vital signs may be masked by even small doses of narcotics.
- Respiratory depression from any cause.
- Chest injuries *(31)*.
- Undiagnosed abdominal pain (22).
- Addiction withdrawal treatment, unless special circumstances *(7)*.
- Abnormal or allergic reactions to previous doses *(24)*.
- Infancy or early childhood *(9)*.
- Pregnancy at or near term—respiratory depression may be dangerous to the child.
- Myxedema *(36–12)*.

- Concomitant administration of other drugs that accentuate or potentiate the action of narcotics; beware of nondisclosed prior administration of such drugs.

Minimal effective dosage should be used, based on age or weight *(9)* and physical condition of the patient.

Proper means of administration is chosen. Oral administration is contraindicated if vomiting is present or may occur. Subcutaneous or intramuscular injections may be temporarily ineffective if the patient is in any stage of circulatory collapse but will result in an overwhelming cumulative toxic effect once the circulation improves. The intravenous route offers the most rapid result. Doses should be diluted to 10 ml for slow administration with monitoring, and the physician should observe for, and be prepared to treat, any respiratory distress.

The appropriate drug must be used. Consideration must be given to possible side effects as well as to intensity and duration of action. Morphine sulfate is a most useful narcotic for general emergency use not only because of its general availability and low cost but also because of its ability to control severe pain and at the same time allay apprehension. If marked contraction of smooth muscle and decreased respiratory rate will be detrimental, atropine sulfate may be given additionally or meperidine hydrochloride (Demerol) may be substituted. Meperidine hydrochloride, however, has relatively less effect on severe pain and does not control acute apprehension; therefore, as a rule it preferably is not used alone in emergencies such as fractures. This deficit may be overcome by using meperidine hydrochloride in combination with an ataraxic medication of comparable short action, e.g., reduced doses of hydroxyzine HCl (Vistaril), for its sedative and anticholinergic effect (promethazine [Phenergan] is longer-acting). Codeine sulfate is satisfactory for control of acute pain of moderate intensity.

In severe pain situations such as experienced by terminal cancer patients, morphine solution (morphine sulfate 45 mg; 90% alcohol, 5.4 ml; simple syrup, 10.5 ml; and water, qs ad 30 ml) has been found effective in oral doses of ½ to 1 tsp. q several hours prn.

Another narcotic that is as effective as morphine sulfate but slightly more toxic is hydromorphone hydrocloride (Dilaudid), 2 mg q 3–4 hr IM, PO or even slowly IV, or 3 mg by rectal suppository.

Minor procedures such as minor fracture reductions, particularly in children, can often be done after an IM dose of meperidine (Demerol), 1 mg/kg, plus 0.5 mg/kg of hydroxyzine HCI (Vistaril). Chlorpromazine (Thorazine), 0.5 mg/kg, is added by some to this combination, but this medication has a different half-life and requires extra caution.

Intravenous analgesia with 2 μg/kg fentanyl (Sublimaze), sometimes used in conjunction with IV diazepam (Valium), can be used in adults in such procedures as fracture reductions of large bones or dislocated joints. It should be used only under the close supervision of professionals trained in airway/ventilation management, with "crash cart" and oxygen available.

USE OF NON-NARCOTICS

Many non-narcotic analgesics require prescriptions because of their greater potency, side effects and/or tendency to cause drug dependence. Use of multiple drugs or drugs in conjunction with ethyl alcohol can be hazardous. The prostaglandin inhibition of many of the new nonsteroidal anti-inflammatory drugs (NSAID) (a class to which aspirin and acetaminophen also belong) makes them also valuable analgesics.

Prescription Analgesics

Some prescription analgesics that are effective for slight to moderate acute pain are given below (adult doses). (*Note*: All of these have the potential for gastrointestinal upset, but symptoms are generally less severe than with aspirin.)

- Pentazocine hydrochloride (Talwin hydrochloride), 50 mg, plain (or with naloxone HCl [Talwin NX], 0.5 mg) or with aspirin (Talwin Compound), 12.5 mg PO q 4–6 hr. (Can be addicting.)
- Pentazocine lactate (Talwin lactate), 30 mg/ml, injected, 30 mg IM or 15 to 30 mg IV q 4–6 hr. Avoid use in acute MI. (Can be addicting.)
- Ibuprofen (Motrin), 400 to 600 mg PO q 4–6 hr (maximum benefit may be delayed several days). Also available in nonprescription strengths.
- Diflunisal (Dolobid), 1000 mg loading dose, PO, followed by 250 to usually a 500 mg dose given generally bid, but not oftener than tid.
- Fenoprofen calcium (Nalfon), 200 mg PO q 4–6 hr.
- Mefenamic acid (Ponstel), 250 mg PO q 6 hr; 500 mg initially.
- Naproxen (Naprosyn), 250 mg PO q 6–8 hr.
- Naproxen sodium (Anaprox), 275 mg PO q 6–8 hr (more rapidly absorbed than Naprosyn; do not give these two drugs together).
- Propoxyphenes (Darvon and Darvon Compounds) have the potential to be highly addictive and are mild analgesics.

Nonprescription Analgesics

Among the nonprescription analgesics that are effective for slight to moderate acute pain and are given about every 4 to 8 hours are the fllowing:

- Aspirin, plain (Bayer); adult (5 or 10 grains or a 325- to 650-mg tablet) or pediatric (1.25 grains, or 81 mg)—1 grain per year of age/dose.
- Aspirin with antacid (Bufferin, Ascriptin).
- Aspirin compound (contains caffeine).
- Acetaminophen (APAP or AAP) (Tylenol, Datril or Tempra) pediatric drops (1 grain or 65 mg per 0.6 ml) or pediatric syrup (2 grains per 5 ml tsp). *Adult acetaminophen dosage*: 0.3 to 0.6 g every 4 to 6 hours. *Pediatric acetaminophen dosage*: See Table 12–1.
- Ibuprofen, 200 mg, available as Advil or Nuprin.

Approach to Usage

An effective approach to use of oral analgesics is to have the patient take one of the nonprescription analgesics just described on a regular or periodic "as necessary" basis and to supplement as necessary with one of the *plain* non-narcotic prescription medications if relief is not achieved. Codeine (15 to 32 mg) is, however, preferably prescribed with aspirin compound or acetaminophen because the tendency to overuse it is lessened when it is in this form (a triplicate prescription blank is not necessary for that reason).

Other Preparations

Other non-narcotic system preparations that may help to reduce acute pain perception are phenothiazines and antidepressants (more rapid acting, such as thioridazine hydrochloride [Mellaril], 25 mg PO tid.). Doxepin, 75–100 mg PO at hs is also effective. These are also particularly valuable adjuncts to other analgesics used in chronic pain management (for which narcotic use is best minimized except in terminal situations).

Other non-narcotic, nonprescription systemic preparations with analgesic effect that are occasionally used are:

Table 12–1. PEDIATRIC DOSAGE OF ACETAMINOPHEN (APAP or AAP)*

Age	Pediatric Drops† (0.8 ml per full dropper = 80 mg)	Pediatric Syrup† (160 mg/5 ml, or 160 mg/tsp)	Pediatric Chewable Tablets (scored) (80 mg/tab)	Regular Adult Tablets‡ (scored) (325 mg/tab)
Birth to 3 mo	0.3–0.4 ml	0	0	0
4–11 mo	0.6–0.8 ml	½ tsp	0	0
12–23 mo	0.9–1.2 ml	¾ tsp	1½	0
2–3 yr	1.6 ml	1 tsp	2	0
4–5 yr	2.4 ml	1½ tsp	3	0
6–8 yr	—	2 tsp	4	1
9–10 yr	—	2½ tsp	5	1
11–12 yr	—	3 tsp	6	1–1½
12 yr (= adult)	—	—	6–8	1–2

**Note:* Single doses shown; start with the lower recommended dose, to a maximum of 5 doses/24 hr.

†Not extra-strength adult liquid pain reliever, which contains 500 mg acetaminophen/tblsp.

‡Not extra-strength tablets or capsules, which contain 500 mg acetaminophen each.

- Ethyl alcohol, several ounces taken orally, is a historically effective analgesic but is preferably not used if other alternatives are available, since it can cause a hazardous compound of side effects when used with other medications, sometimes inducing vomiting and increasing the risks of hypothermia and shock, as well as aggravating many primary problems.
- L-Tryptophan. This amino acid in oral doses of 0.5 to 1.0 g has been reported to reduce pain.

12–2. TOPICAL MEDICATIONS AND PREPARATIONS

Topical preparations can be effective both in controlling pain, by chemically or physically raising the pain threshold and reducing perception, and in alleviating the primary condition, e.g., by reducing inflammation or by diminishing edema and improving local circulatory dynamics and cellular metabolism.

Following are some of the more frequently used topical preparations:

- Topical lidocaine (Xylocaine, 2% viscous solution) for use on irritated mucous membranes.
- Dibucaine NF and other "caine" preparations (Nupercainal, Surfacaine, Xylocaine, Rectal Medicone Suppositories) for relief from skin irritations and hemorrhoids. (*Note:* Allergic reaction to these may occur.)
- Dilute phenol preparations (U.S.P. calamine solution with 0.25% phenol) for skin application prn.
- Topical cryotherapy spray (ethyl chloride—explosive; Fluori-Methane—nonexplosive) for relief of pain prior to injections or rapid incisions or for reflex reduction of muscle spasm and pain prior to stretching.
- Ice packs to reduce acute pain and edema may be devised from ice chips placed in a sandwich bag, a wet wrung-out towel placed in the freezer till "crinkly" or a large ice cube formed in a paper cup for use in ice massage. An ice pack can also be made by putting 3 cups of water and 1 cup of rubbing alcohol into a 1-gallon size zip-lock bag, which is then put in the freezer overnight until slushy, covered with a wet towel and applied to

affected areas for 5 to 10 minutes prn. Ice packs are especially useful during the first 24 to 48 hours after injury.

- Warm moist heat. This is best applied either through total immersion (e.g., getting into a hot tub with jet pressurization or a bathtub with water heated to approximately 105–110° F [*note:* there is a risk of syncope in older people or those using vasodilators, including alcohol]) or by local application of warm towels wrung out after being dipped in hot water, cooled to tolerance and then applied to the skin and covered with plastic wrap (e.g., Saran Wrap); the process is repeated and towels are reapplied after cooling. Heat is most beneficial when used 24 to 48 hours after injury. Watch burning.
- Methyl salicylate preparations (e.g., Banalg Liniment, Ben-Gay, Heet). If wide areas are repeatedly treated, it should be remembered that a tablespoon of methyl salicylate solution contains the equivalent of about 12 aspirin tablets (though this would be more dilute in commercial liniments and solution preparations) and this is absorbed through the skin, so signs of hypersalicylism *(53–614)* can occur.
- Dimethyl sulfoxide (DMSO), 5 ml of 50% to 70% solution applied topically over small areas several times a day for several days, will reduce acute post-traumatic swelling and acute pain and improve function. DMSO has been observed to give gratifying relief and results when applied as soon as possible over minor burns. To date, this drug has received Food and Drug Administration approval only for treatment of bladder wall edema with chronic inflammation and pain (chronic cystitis). DMSO must be used with caution (reduce dosage or do not use) in patients on other medications, such as insulin or digitalis, since their absorption and rate of utilization is enhanced, which could lead to overdosage. A garlic odor of breath and sweat will occur, and skin blistering may develop with concentrations over 60%. Prior application of 50% glycerin solution reduces skin reaction.

12–3. LOCAL AND REGIONAL ANESTHETIC BLOCKS

Surgical procedures of more than a few moments' duration require a greater degree of elimination of pain perception. Many times this can be achieved with injection of various "caine" preparations around the nerves going to and from the affected areas.

Lidocaine (Xylocaine) in 0.25% (2.5 mg/ml) to 1% (10 mg/ml) solution, with or without epinephrine, is most commonly used for short local procedures, such as laceration repair, simple debridement or exploration for foreign bodies. See Step 7 under Suggestions After Preliminary Cleaning for indications for avoidance of use of epinephrine-containing solutions and for comments about bupivacaine HCl (Marcaine). See also Figures 12–1 and 12–2 for a guide to injections for the wrist/hand and ankle/foot respectively.

Suggestions After Preliminary Cleaning *(See also 59–1)*

1. Total dosage of lidocaine should not exceed 2 *mg* per pound of 4.4 *mg* per kilogram or 300 *mg* total dose without epinephrine. Total dose should not exceed 3 *mg* per pound or 6.6 *mg* per kilogram with epinephrine.
2. A small amount of lidocaine solution sprayed on the wound brings relief before injection.
3. A preliminary spraying of the skin for a few seconds with Fluori-Methane reduces even the pain of initial skin puncture or wheal. Lidocaine solution can be injected with the use of a 25-gauge needle. Always aspirate before injecting to assure that the needle is not in an intravenous location.
4. Use of 2% lidocaine reduces the volume of fluid and lessens skin

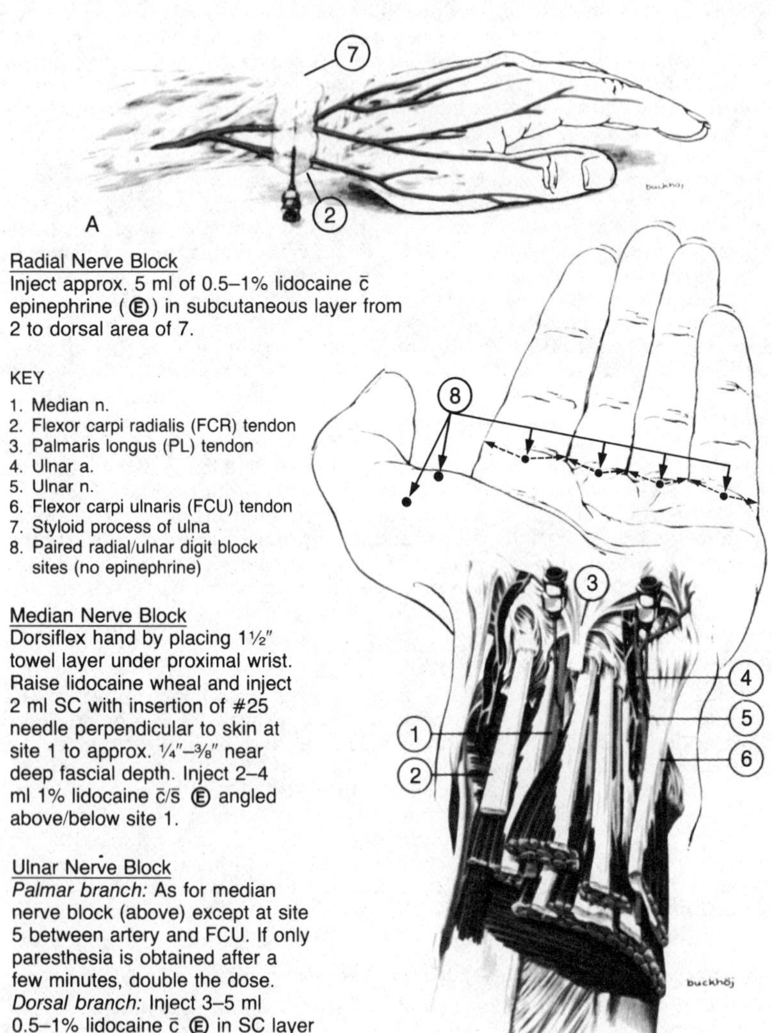

7
2
A
Radial Nerve Block
Inject approx. 5 ml of 0.5–1% lidocaine c̄ epinephrine (Ⓔ) in subcutaneous layer from 2 to dorsal area of 7.
KEY
1. Median n.
2. Flexor carpi radialis (FCR) tendon
3. Palmaris longus (PL) tendon
4. Ulnar a.
5. Ulnar n.
6. Flexor carpi ulnaris (FCU) tendon
7. Styloid process of ulna
8. Paired radial/ulnar digit block sites (no epinephrine)
Median Nerve Block
Dorsiflex hand by placing 1½″ towel layer under proximal wrist. Raise lidocaine wheal and inject 2 ml SC with insertion of #25 needle perpendicular to skin at site 1 to approx. ¼″–⅜″ near deep fascial depth. Inject 2–4 ml 1% lidocaine c̄/s̄ Ⓔ angled above/below site 1.
Ulnar Nerve Block
Palmar branch: As for median nerve block (above) except at site 5 between artery and FCU. If only paresthesia is obtained after a few minutes, double the dose.
Dorsal branch: Inject 3–5 ml 0.5–1% lidocaine c̄ Ⓔ in SC layer from site 6 to site 7.
8
3
4
5
1
6
2
buckhöj
B

Figure 12–1. Nerve blocks for the hand (to be used in conjunction with Fig. 49–2). For assistance in location of upper extremity nerve sites at higher level, see Figures 47–12 and 47–13. (Modified from Ericksson, E.: *Illustrated Handbook in Local Anesthesia,* 2nd ed. Philadelphia, W. B. Saunders Co., 1980, pp. 90, 92.)

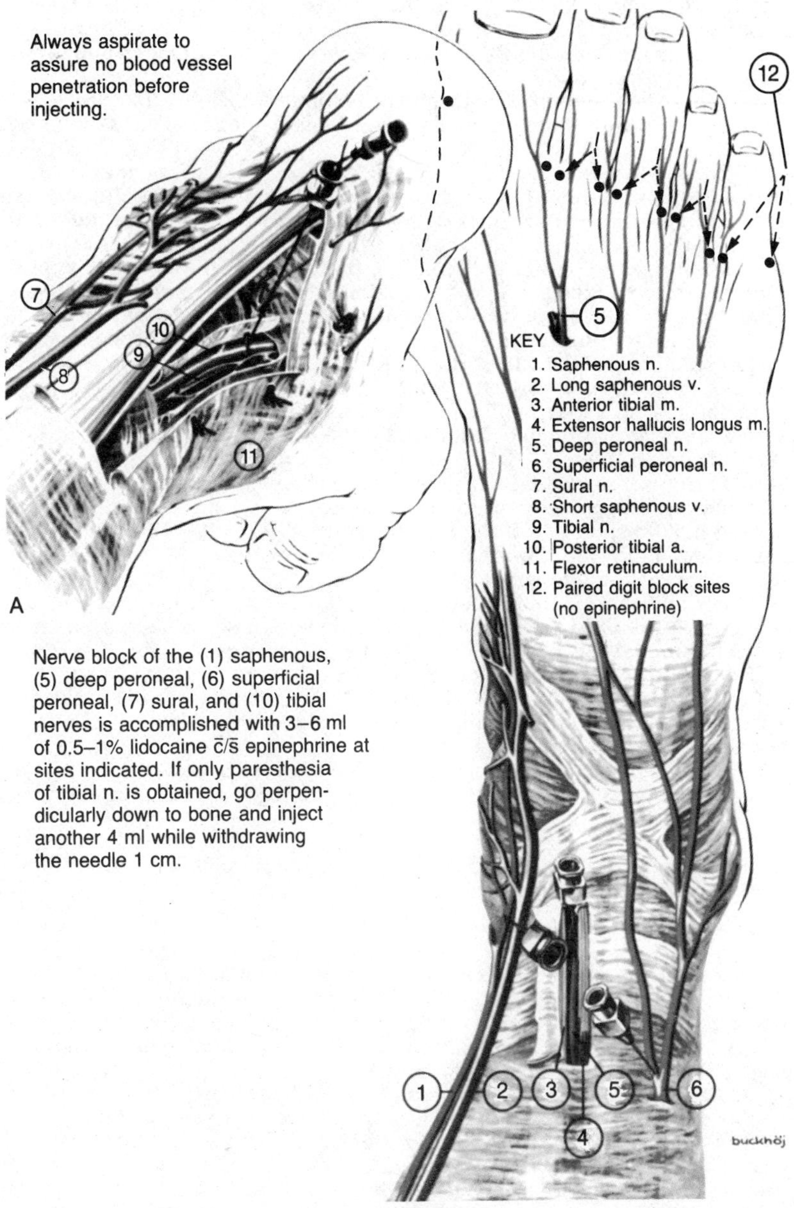
Always aspirate to assure no blood vessel penetration before injecting.
7
8
9
10
11
12
5
A
KEY
1. Saphenous n.
2. Long saphenous v.
3. Anterior tibial m.
4. Extensor hallucis longus m.
5. Deep peroneal n.
6. Superficial peroneal n.
7. Sural n.
8. Short saphenous v.
9. Tibial n.
10. Posterior tibial a.
11. Flexor retinaculum.
12. Paired digit block sites (no epinephrine)
Nerve block of the (1) saphenous, (5) deep peroneal, (6) superficial peroneal, (7) sural, and (10) tibial nerves is accomplished with 3–6 ml of 0.5–1% lidocaine c̄/s̄ epinephrine at sites indicated. If only paresthesia of tibial n. is obtained, go perpendicularly down to bone and inject another 4 ml while withdrawing the needle 1 cm.
1
2
3
4
5
6
buckhöj
B

Figure 12–2. Nerve blocks for the foot (to be used in conjunction with Fig. 49–2). For assistance in location of lower extremity nerve sites at higher level see Figures 47–14 and 47–15. Watch total lidocaine dose *(12–3)*. (Modified from Eriksson, E.: *Illustrated Handbook in Local Anesthesia,* 2nd ed. Philadelphia, W. B. Saunders Co., 1980, pp. 112, 114.)

distortion for repair. Slow injection through the intradermal layer of lacerations is well tolerated.

5. Wait about 3 minutes for anesthetic effect to occur after injection before starting the procedure.

6. Repeat lidocaine injections may be required for longer procedures, but after administration of maximum dosage, it should not be repeated within 90 minutes.

7. Planned longer procedures or work in vascular areas may require lidocaine with epinephrine; total dosage can be increased about 50%. *Do not inject epinephrine-containing solution around tissues with terminal arteries (includes all digits, nose, earlobes, penis, scrotum).* Bupivacaine hydrochloride (Marcaine), 0.25% for local infiltration, or 0.25% to 0.5% without epinephrine for peripheral nerves (maximum total individual dose recommended approx 175 mg) or with epinephrine (maximum total dose approx 225 mg), has a longer anesthetic effect than plain lidocaine, but it should not be used in children less than 12 years of age; dose should not be repeated within 3 hours. Intravascular injection of Marcaine must be avoided and great caution used near very vascular areas such as the paracervical (uterine) area; Marcaine is also contraindicated in epidural blocks, as ventricular fibrillation has occurred.

8. Digital nerve blocks in an adult can be obtained with about 1 ml of 1% lidocaine, without epinephrine, injected through the volar surface of the hand (or foot) next to each side of the metacarpal head (see Figs. 12–1 and 12–2). Never force fluid into the area, as secondary ischemia can occur (47–60); preferably block at a proximal site.

9. For major nerve and regional blocks, use of a simple nerve stimulator-locator, metal-hubbed glass syringe and Teflon-coated needle aids localization and can diminish the amount of anesthetic solution needed for anesthesia; the lowest effective dose is always desirable.

10. Resuscitative equipment and medication for treatment of shock from sensitivity reactions and convulsions should always be at hand. See also 53 for discussion of toxic reactions.

11. Special training should be obtained for use of central neural blocks, such as epidurals or caudals and intravenous regional anesthesia ("Bier block").

12. Hematoma block can be useful in some fracture reductions, such as around the wrist. First aspirate the hematoma, as possible, then inject 3 to 5 ml of 1% lidocaine into the hematoma of the fracture.

12–4. INHALATION ANESTHETICS

General anesthesia for surgery is usually not administered within 6 hours after the patient has eaten and without assurance that the stomach is empty. The urgency of the need for surgery, however, may require that there be no delay; in these cases, persons experienced in crash intubation techniques and anesthesia should be called upon.

Nitrous oxide (N_2O) in 50% concentration (Dolonox/Nitronox) with 50% O_2 has been steadily increasing in field and ED use as a safe analgesic when properly prescribed. The patient self-administers it by mask or mouth airway after instruction. Its benefits are: rapid onset, short duration of effect and freedom from serious side effects; also, it does not seriously interfere with the patient's consciousness or pain evaluation shortly after cessation of use. (*Note:* Increase to 70% N_2O and 30% O_2 has been found necessary to raise effective pN_2O to therapeutic levels at altitudes over 5000 feet.)

Side effects are common but are mild and generally rapidly reversible with return to air or 100% O_2 ventilation. They include drowsiness, lightheadedness and confusion; 2 to 10% of patients experience nausea, with vomiting uncommon. Contraindications to use are: head injury and altered consciousness from poisonings (difficulty in evaluation plus nausea and vomiting); COPD (hazards of $\uparrow O_2$), CHF and shock (possibility of $\downarrow$ CO); possible maxillary fractures (difficulty with airway, nausea and potential vomiting); potential problems from hollow structures in a diseased state into which N_2O can expand (e.g., obstructed bowel or eustachian tube; pneumothorax or decompression).

Nitrous oxide appears to be a safe analgesic for self-administration when properly supervised.

NONMEDICINAL PAIN MANAGEMENT

Frequent emergency problems are relief of pain; relaxation of skeletal or smooth muscle spasm causing ischemia, venous congestion, impairment of microcirculation, edema and more pain; and relief of apprehension—all of which have variable degrees of effect on the function of diverse organs. Unfortunately, the precise physiologic mechanisms of pain and the exact actions of the autonomic nervous system are among the largest and oldest areas of medical ignorance. A medication approach to the treatment of these problems is sometimes not effective for several reasons, including (a) unavailability, (b) contraindications to use and (c) therapeutic failure. Under these circumstances, various forms of reflex therapy may be used as an adjunctive measure for relief. Embryologically, the entire central, peripheral and autonomic nervous systems are derived from ectoderm, and critical functional relationships with the skin persist throughout life. Skin stimulation and the spinal reflex suggest the existence of a dermatomyosplanchnic response, which may result in relief of pain and muscle spasm. Physical therapy (e.g. ice/massage) aids this process.

12–5. ACUPUNCTURE AND ACUPRESSURE

Experimental evidence that this therapeutic modality can augment endorphin release or utilization, or both, has added to the status of this modality, as have practical clinical observations. Sir William Osler in the late 1800s made note of the responsiveness of local soft tissue–muscle tenderness to needling in the area ("dry needling"). In the absence of a needle, firm rubbing pressure for 10 to 15 seconds with the tip of a digit (acupressure), repeated as necessary, can bring relief. Tenderness from focal fibromyositic nodules and smooth/skeletal muscle spasms generally respond well to this modality.

For more diffuse pain, stimulation of a proximal and distal point on a dermatome covering the affected area and some of the major acupuncture points (e.g., Li4, Liv3, S36, Sp7, GB20, CV21) will be associated with improvement. Contrary to traditional Chinese theory, the points have not been proved to have high degrees of specificity for disease processes. Instruction in use of the modality is of value, however.

12–6. HYPNOSIS

Since 1958, the AMA has officially recognized that there are definite and proper uses of hypnosis in medical and dental practice when it is employed by those who are properly trained.

Hypnosis has a place in emergency treatment of acute pain and apprehension, particularly in situations in which other modes of treatment are not yet available. If the patient has had prior exposure to hypnosis or similar experiences, induction is easier, but even without prior experience, dissociation can be achieved if the patient is receptive.

In addition to relief from pain, the physiologic benefits from hypnosis include easier control of hemorrhage, less swelling and edema and more rapid healing. In situations in which narcotics cannot be used, such as brain injury to a still-conscious patient, the relief of pain, thrashing, apprehension and related increased intravascular pressure by a nonmedicinal approach is evident.

Suggestions for induction (to be used, for example, to treat acute post-traumatic pain when in remote areas pending arrival of assistance) are as follows:

1. Proceed with usual triage protocol of priorities (2), performing as many measures simultaneously as feasible.

2. Establish verbal, touch and eye contact with the patient. Tell who you are, that you are able to help and that you will help if the patient desires—get some indication of assent, if feasible. Tell the patient what you are doing (e.g., applying splints or compressions) as you are doing it.

3. After the basic treatment has been accomplished (or while it is being performed) and the patient is physically as comfortably situated as is feasible, tell the patient (a man in this example) you believe the situation could be more comfortable if he were more relaxed and ask if he would like to see what happens. If the answer is affirmative, proceed. It is usually best to start by having the patient slowly take 3 slow, deep breaths and exhalations. Many techniques can be employed to achieve relaxation and disassociation; the following is one that can be used in any emergency situation:

4. Tell the patient to concentrate entirely on the sound of your voice and to focus his eyes on the tip of your finger (which is held by your eye) and that as he focuses all of his mind's attention on the sound of your voice and his eye on the tip of your finger his eyelids will become very, very heavy and that gradually, try as he may, he will no longer be able to keep them open and they will shut. Keep repeating this until the patient's eyelids flutter and close (or if the patient starts to just stare blankly, tell him his eyelids may now be closed). Following this, have the patient perform a few deep breaths and slow exhalations and start feelings of muscle relaxation in the fingers and toes and work proximally, i.e., fingers relaxed like lumps of lead, then hands, wrists, forearms, elbows, shoulders, toes and so forth. Telling the patient to imagine traveling down a series of 100 escalators may produce further deepening. Then take the patient on a verbal adventure (e.g., visualizing scenes seen while floating down a river, riding a train, walking through a forest, etc.) to further aid the process of disassociation from current problems and pain.

When transportation arrives, tell the patient you are going to move him now, that he may open his eyes to assist as needed but as soon as he is moved to the vehicle his eyes may be closed again. Tell all personnel that the patient is under hypnosis.

When it is indicated to have the patient come out of hypnosis, state that he will be clear-headed and wide awake when you count from 3 to 1 as follows: 1, coming up; 2, nearly there; 3, clear-headed, wide awake and refreshed. If need be, the patient can be preprogrammed under hypnosis to come out of the hypnotic trance later when these words are spoken by someone else.

5. If the patient is distracted or involved in the problem at hand—particularly as happens with children—voice control must be more decisive and direct attention away from the situation to some remote situation

that can be pursued, e.g., "Did you hear that fire engine?" then pursue narrative trip.

6. If hypnosis is effective, much has been gained; if not, nothing has been lost. Training and experience help improve assistance.

12–7. BIOFEEDBACK

Electronic biofeedback apparatus (electromyogram, temperature control, galvanic skin resistance), though of help in chronic pain states, is not of much help in acute emergency conditions. Human biofeedback, which is directive (and approximates hypnosis), is of assistance.

12–8. TRANSCUTANEOUS NERVE STIMULATORS (TNS)

TNS, with electrodes applied generally proximally and distally to the area of involvement, can be of relief for acute pain in some circumstances. Back, thorax and extremity pain are particularly amenable to this modality.

12–9. RELIGION AND PRAYER

Spiritual counseling, prayer, laying on of hands and other religious actions consistent with a person's personal belief system can unquestionably aid in the relief of acute pain. There is almost a direct proportional relationship between the strength of the patient's belief system and the response of the patient's body to prayer.

13. Prescription Restrictions

13–1. AMOUNTS

Only small amounts of medications of any kind should be prescribed for patients seen solely on an emergency basis—that is, just enough to obtain the desired effect until the patient can report elsewhere for definitive care. (See also 7, *Addiction*.) Dispensing of controlled substances is also limited, but restrictions may vary from state to state. Dispensing of up to a 72-hour supply for the patient's "immediate needs" may be permissible provided there is adequate prior examination, a triplicate record is sent to the Bureau of Narcotics Enforcement and further medication need is not anticipated.

13–2. CONTROLLED DRUGS OR DEVICES

In many areas, strict restrictions are in effect with regard to prescription not only of narcotics *(13–3)* but also of a large number of drugs of various actions specified as unsafe for self-medication and classified as controlled substances. Certain instruments used in administration of drugs are also included. These classifications usually include the following:

- Any hypnotic drug—defined as "any compounds, mixtures or preparations that may be used for producing hypnotic effect."
- Amphetamines.
- Diethylstilbestrol.
- Ergot, cotton root or their contained or derived active compounds.
- Oils of croton, rue, savin or tansy.

- Phenylhydantoin derivatives.
- Thyroid and its contained or derived active compounds.
- Any drug whose packaging bears the legend: "Caution: Federal law prohibits dispensing without prescription."
- Hypodermic syringes and needles.

For a guide to prescribing controlled substances, see Table 13–1.

CLASSIFICATION OF CONTROLLED DRUGS*

Schedule I—Not applicable to prescription of drugs for emergency care.

Schedule II

A. NARCOTICS—STATE TRIPLICATE PRESCRIPTION BLANK REQUIRED		B. NON-NARCOTICS—REGULAR PRESCRIPTION MAY BE ACCEPTABLE†	
Cocaine	Paregoric	Amphetamine	Methamphetamine
Codeine, plain	Percodan	Amytal	Nembutal
Demerol	Percocet-5	Biphetamine	Parest
Dilaudid	Sublimaze	Desoxyn	Preludin
Innovar	Tylox	Dexedrine	Ritalin
Morphine			Seconal
			Tuinal

Schedule III

A. NARCOTICS		B. NON-NARCOTICS
A.P.C. with codeine	Hycodan	Butisol
Empirin with codeine (Nos. 1, 2, 3, 4)	Hycomine	Doriden
Fiorinal with codeine (Nos. 1, 2, 3)	Paregoric mixtures	Fiorinal
Phenaphen with codeine (Nos. 2, 3, 4)	Percogesic C	Noludar
Tylenol with codeine (nos. 1, 2, 3, 4)		

Schedules IV and V

A. SCHEDULE IV		B. SCHEDULE V
Chloral hydrate	Milpath	Actifed-C
Dalmane	Miltown	Donnagel-PG
Darvon	Phenobarbital	Lomotil
Equagesic	Placidyl	Parepectolin
Equanil	Serax	Phenergan with codeine
Librium	Valium	Robitussin A-C
Meprobamate		Terpin hydrate & codeine elixir

NONCONTROLLED PRESCRIPTION DRUGS

- New prescription or refill authorization may be phoned in by prescriber or authorized employee (written evidence of authorization must be on file with pharmacy or provided within a reasonable time).

---

*The controlled drugs listed here are for example only; the lists are not complete.

†Since January 1, 1981, California physicians have been required to use triplicate prescription forms for these drugs.

Table 13–1. QUICK REFERENCE CHART ON PRESCRIBING CONTROLLED SUBSTANCES (BASED ON FEDERAL AND CALIFORNIA REGULATIONS)

Prescription Item	Schedule (see text)			
	II	III	IV	V
1. Date, patient's name and address; prescriber's BNDD* number, signature and telephone number must be on prescription.	Yes	Yes	Yes	Yes
2. Patient's name, address and drug prescription must be wholly written in PHYSICIAN'S OWN HANDWRITING.	Yes	Yes	No	No
3. State control (triplicate) prescription blank required.	Yes	No	No	No
4. Prescription can be phoned in by prescriber.	No	Yes	Yes	Yes
5. Prescription can be phoned in by authorized employee.	No	No	Yes	Yes
6. Maximum period in which prescription can be filled.	7 days	6 months	6 months	6 months
7. Limit of five refills over a 6-month period.	No refills	Yes	Yes	Yes
8. Federal order form required to obtain drugs for office use.	Yes	No	No	No

*Bureau of Narcotics and Dangerous Drugs.

- Need patient's address.
- Need prescriber's state license number on prescriptions.
- Refill limit discretionary with prescriber.

Examples: Antibiotics, antihistamines, diuretics, oral contraceptives.

13–3. NARCOTICS

Although regulations regarding prescription of narcotics vary in different countries, it is usually required that the prescription be completely in the physician's handwriting and that his or her office address, telephone number and narcotic registration number be given. Only the minimal amount necessary to obtain the desired effect should be used in adjustment of the dose to the age in children *(9)* and in elderly or debilitated persons. Schedule II prescriptions, as a rule, cannot be filled, although Schedule III narcotics can. Some states require the use of triplicate forms.

For restrictions on prescription of narcotics for treatment of addiction, see 7–5.

13–4. SOMNIFACIENTS

Antihistaminics, hypnotics, muscle relaxants, narcotics, sedatives and tranquilizers are among the commonly used drugs that may cause drowsiness and slowing of reflexes. Therefore, persons for whom any of these drugs have been prescribed should be cautioned against operating any type of motor-driven vehicle during the duration of the effect of the drug. The same warning should be given to persons exposed to changes in barometric pressure *(26)*.

14. Rape and Sexual Assault

Definition of Rape

The older legal definition of rape is "the carnal knowledge, to a lesser or greater degree, of a female [most states still add that the female not be the wife of the assailant] without her consent and by compulsion, either through fear, force or fraud, singly or in combination." As long as the penis entered any portion of the female genitalia, the assailant need not have an orgasm or even an erection.

More states now are defining rape as any oral, anal or vaginal act committed by force or threat of force with a person (sex not specified) not the spouse of the offender. Many states have established "the age of consent" (usually 16 to 18 years) below which sexual intercourse, even with the girl's consent, constitutes statutory rape or "unlawful intercourse." Rape is properly considered a crime of violence and aggression.

Examination in Rape Cases

- People offering initial aid should, insofar as possible, avoid destroying evidence that may be needed in criminal prosecution.
- The patient should be instructed not to shower, wash, douche or change clothes prior to examination. Fresh clothes should be brought for the patient to change into after the examination.
- Collection of evidence is aided by having the patient undress over a clean sheet. All items (including sanitary napkins or tampons if menstruating) are then bundled and sent to the police laboratory for examination with other evidence. Areas of clothing with wet secretions should be outlined with a laundry marker.
- Direct referral to or close coordination by emergency personnel with a rape crisis center is desirable because the staff at such a center is familiar with handling such cases, can facilitate proper collection of evidence, and includes trained psychological–social service counselors.
- Examination for possible rape should *never* be done—even when requested by law enforcement officers—without either the properly witnessed written consent (69–7) of the patient (or, if she is a minor, of a parent [both parents if possible] or legal guardian) or a court order (obtainable when necessary in about 20 to 30 minutes from the jurisdictional judge on 24-hour call).
- Examination and treatment should include the measures described in sections *14–1* through *14–5*.

14–1. CARE OF PHYSICAL INJURIES

These may be diffuse and severe (see *59, Soft Tissue Injuries; 20, Tetanus Immunization;* and other specific pertinent sections) or nonexistent (the victim's prudence may have dictated nonresistance for life-preservation) except for emotional distress and terror, which may be medically and legally tantamount to "great bodily harm." Carefully record all medical findings but generally avoid recording historical statements other than the patient stated a sexual attack occurred. A female member of the staff should be present at all examinations.

14–2. PREVENTION AND TREATMENT OF PSYCHOLOGIC DAMAGE

- In all dealings with the patient, maintain a calming and compassionate attitude. Assiduously avoid careless comments that may in any way imply blame or irresponsibility on the part of the patient or close associates. Carefully explain each step in the examination before or while performing it, or at both times.

- No nonmedical personnel should be present during examination without the patient's request or consent; unless the person is a member of the immediate family, such a request or consent should be in writing and signed.
- Prescription of a 1-week supply of a tranquilizer such as diazepam (Valium) 2.0 to 5.0 mg (qid), or a sleeping medication such as flurazepam HCl (Dalmane), 30 mg at bedtime, is often advisable.
- Feelings of revulsion, anger, helplessness, numbness, indignation and guilt, as well as thoughts of suicide are common, and the patient should be encouraged to express her emotions. Carefully selected members of the community or organizations such as rape crisis centers may also render valuable services. If the patient does not have a family to go home to, arrangements for staying with a friend for a few days can be of help. Follow-up psychologic counseling should be arranged.

14–3. PREVENTION AND TREATMENT OF VENEREAL DISEASE

1. Culture and gram-stain a cervical mucus specimen while collecting other samples.

2. Draw a blood sample for the Venereal Disease Research Laboratory (VDRL) and repeat in 4 to 6 weeks.

3. Give 1 g probenecid (Benemid) PO *30 minutes prior* to giving 4.8 million units of procaine penicillin G IM in divided locations for prophylaxis against gonorrhea; additional prophylaxis treatment against syphilis is not recommended. If penicillin allergy is present, use tetracycline, 500 mg qid for 15 days, or spectinomycin, 2 gm intramuscularly.

4. Permit the patient to douche and shower—*but only after examination and collection of specimens*—for hygienic and psychologic reasons.

14–4. PREVENTION OR TREATMENT OF PREGNANCY

1. Unless the patient is unequivocally sterile, perform a pregnancy test (urine or serum) to determine status prior to the rape.

2. Consider and discuss use of IV conjugated estrogens (25 mg Premarin repeated in 12 hours) or diethylstilbestrol (DES) for prophylaxis or, alternatively, early therapeutic abortion, if needed.

The absolute contraindications to use of DES are the presence of a wanted pregnancy prior to the rape and the presence of malignancy. Relative contraindications to use of DES are pre-existent gastrointestinal disorders (because of the high incidence of moderate to severe nausea and vomiting from DES), menstruation at time of the attack, fear of malignancy and, possibly, prior administration of DES to the rape victim or her mother during gestation, because of indications of some increased incidence of malignancy in these individuals. An additional consideration is that conception from a rape attack is infrequent, occurring in about 5% of cases. A stronger indication for DES use is in the woman who is probably ovulating at the time of the rape and who prefers this to an indicated therapeutic abortion if conception did occur. However, in such cases there must be a signed pre-existent agreement that if DES is used and fails, an elective abortion will follow; otherwise, avoidance of DES is advisable.

3. DES dosage is 25 mg twice daily (bid) PO for 5 days if that course is decided upon; order anticholinergic suppositories, e.g., trimethobenzamide hydrochloride (Tigan), to relieve vomiting, as needed.

4. Usually a simple vacuum curettage therapeutic abortion is the preferable approach should pregnancy occur.

5. Permit the patient to douche (after examination and taking of specimens) for hygienic and psychologic reasons—though this procedure is of limited anticonception value.

6. Arrange follow-up evaluation.

14–5. MEDICOLEGAL DOCUMENTATION

1. Initial Instructions. First instruct the patient-victim not to shower, douche or change clothes prior to coming for examination. A change of clothes should be brought for use afterwards.

2. Questioning and Examination. Questioning and examination should always be done in the presence of a third person (certainly a woman if the physician is male and the victim is female) and should cover the points listed below. Pertinent negative as well as positive findings should be noted in detail in the Emergency Department record.

- Note the date and time of the alleged act.
- Record the patient's statement that the alleged act occurred and the time elapsed since any previous recent sexual relations. Since the patient is generally initially very upset and the physician has principally many medical responsibilities that attenuate his or her attention for legal recording, it is preferable not to embark on any precise documentation in the medical record of circumstances of the alleged act unless time and conditions permit.
- Physical examination is performed as soon as possible after the alleged act. In a small child, the assistance of an anesthetist may be necessary.
- Make notations regarding condition of the clothing, development of the genitalia, all external signs of bodily injury (abrasions, lacerations, contusions, edema, bleeding and so forth), presence or absence of excessive secretion (type?), abrasions or lacerations of the vaginal canal or anus and condition of the hymen. The diagnosis should state the medical conditions found, plus "History of Sexual Assault" rather than "Rape," which is properly a legal term.

3. Collection of Specimens/Evidence. Particular care must be taken to assure *accurate immediate labeling and continuous control* of all items that may be used as legal evidence. Put items in individual, clean, empty containers. The hand-carrying of items for transfer, the written signature of each person receiving evidence and the use of a taped or locked box for collection of material being taken to the police laboratory (give the key to the officer and get a receipt for itemized contents) help reduce any confusion and the need for appearance of medical personnel in court.

- Using sterile pipets, collect specimens of secretions from the labia, introitus and cervix and from the rectum and perianal area if anal intercourse may have occurred. Sperm may still be found in the cervical os mucus even if the patient has just douched.
- Examine these secretions IMMEDIATELY as wet-mount preparations for the presence or absence of motile or nonmotile sperm and record findings immediately. Sperm may be absent because of vasectomy.
- Test these secretions and any dried secretions from the vulva, upper thighs or perineal area for the presence of seminal fluid (acid phosphatase test (*19–8*) and the blood group antigen of semen and perform precipitin tests against human blood and sperm.

- Send smears of these secretions to a qualified laboratory also for staining for spermatozoa and gonococci.
- Obtain material for cultures, particularly gonococci.
- Comb the pubic hair with a *clean* comb, take scrapings from under the patient's fingernails for portions of the assailant's skin, collect any other particulars that may be attributable to the assailant (smeared blood, threads and so forth); place each of these, as well as the patient's clothing worn at time of the attack, in appropriate individual, labeled, clean, empty containers to turn over to the police. Place sample of the patient's *clipped* pubic hairs separately in an envelope for comparison.

4. Photographs. Photographs are usually taken by the police investigators after the medical examination, but if they are taken by a hospital employee, obtain special consent (*69–14*). Evidence of rape (attempted or accomplished) must be reported at once to the proper law enforcement authorities. Even if there is no evidence of penetration or seminal emission, findings indicative of trauma may help to substantiate the occurrence of criminal assault.

Due to the complexities of treatment and investigation, many communities in conjunction with law enforcement agencies have selected specific medical centers to treat rape victims.

FORCED SODOMY

The preceding comments are applicable to male victims of criminal or forced sodomy, with the exception, of course, of references to pregnancy and female anatomy.

LABORATORY AND EVIDENCE KIT

The following items are prepared as a kit and are being used and tested in 25 metropolitan Chicago hospitals in conjunction with local law enforcement agencies:

- 3 cotton-tipped swabs in test tubes for use in obtaining smears and swabs
- 2 microscopic slide mailers, each with 2 frosted-end slides
- 5 prelabeled pill boxes: 1 each for head hair, pubic hair, right and left hand fingernails or scrapings and 1 for other material, such as foreign fibers, hairs, dirt
- 1 small comb and 1 nail clipper in plastic bag
- 2 strips of white pre-gummed lables (6 labels per strip)
- 2 small paper bags for small undergarments only
- 1 roll cellophane tape for sealing outside of kit to preserve evidence
- 1 victim information card
- 1 authorization for release of information/evidence to law enforcement agency form
- 1 medical report form

After the kit is sealed with the evidence collection tape, it is signed over to the local Police Department evidence technician, the legal chain of evidence thereby being preserved.

If the patient undresses while standing on a clean sheet, all the clothing can be dropped on the sheet, then everything is bundled in the sheet, which is secured and identified for evidence.

15. Reportable Diseases and Conditions

Public health regulations regarding certain diseases require that special forms be completed and signed by the physician who established the diagnosis.

15–1. REPORTABLE DISEASES

The list of diseases reportable to the local health department usually includes the following:

Acquired Immune Deficiency Syndrome (AIDS) *(33–2)*
Amebiasis *(33–3)*
Anthrax *(33–5)*
Aseptic meningitis *(33–20)*
Botulism *(33–8)*
Brucellosis (undulant fever) *(33–75)*
Chancroid *(33–10)*
Chickenpox (varicella) *(33–11)*
Cholera (Table 40–5)
Coccidioidomycosis *(33–12)*
Conjunctivitis, acute infections of the newborn (gonorrheal ophthalmia, ophthalmia neonatorum and babies' sore eyes in the first 21 days of life)
Dengue *(33–17)*
Diarrhea of the newborn
Diphtheria *(33–18)*
Dysentery, bacillary *(33–19, 33–63)*
Encephalitis, acute *(33–20)*
Epilepsy *(32–7)*
Food poisoning *(53–314)*
Gonococcus infection *(33–25)*
Granuloma inguinale *(33–26)*
Hepatitis (B, A, unspecified) *(33–28)*
Legionnaire's disease *(33–35)*
Leprosy (Hansen's disease *(33–36)*
Leptospirosis, including Weil's disease
Lymphogranuloma venereum (lymphogranuloma inguinale)
Malaria *(33–38)*
Measles (rubeola) *(33–39)*
Meningitis, meningococcal or meningococcemia *(33–40, 33–41)*
Mumps *(33–43)*
Paratyphoid fever, A, B and C (see *53–314, Food Poisoning)*
Pertussis (whooping cough) *(33–48, 33–80)*
Plague *(33–49)*
Pneumonia, primary infectious *(33–51)*
Poliomyelitis, acute anterior *(33–52)*
Psittacosis *(33–53)*
Q fever (see *33–56, Rickettsial Infections)*
Rabies, human or animal *(33–54)*
Relapsing fever
Reye's syndrome
Rheumatic fever, acute
Rocky Mountain spotted fever *(33–57)*
Salmonella infections (exclusive of typhoid fever) *(33–60;* see also *53–314, Food Poisoning)*
Scarlet fever *(33–62)*
Shigella infections *(33–63)*
Smallpox (variola) *(33–64)*
Streptococcal infections (including scarlet fever and streptococcal sore throat) *(33–62)*
Syphilis *(33–66)*
Tetanus *(33–68)*
Trachoma *(33–71)*
Trichinosis
Tuberculosis *(33–72)*
Tularemia
Typhoid fever, cases and carriers *(33–73)*
Typhus fever, tick- or flea-borne *(33–74)*
Venereal diseases *(33–78)*
Yellow Fever *(33–81)*

Official cards (Fig. 15–1) for reporting these cases should be completed as soon as the diagnosis is made and mailed to the local health officer. Botulism, cholera, dengue, relapsing fever, plague, smallpox, typhus (louse-borne epidemic type), diarrhea of the newborn, diphtheria, food poisoning, rabies, syphilis, yellow fever and unusual outbreaks of any disease must be reported immediately to the director of the state department of public health, preferably by telephone or telegraph.

Physicians should be especially mindful in reporting communicable diseases in food handlers. Failure to perform obligatory reporting exposes the physician

CONFIDENTIAL MORBIDITY REPORT
(SEND TO LOCAL HEALTH OFFICER) STATE OF

CONFIDENTIAL

PATIENT'S LAST NAME | FIRST NAME AND MIDDLE INITIAL | RACE OR COLOR | SEX | AGE | DATE OF BIRTH

PRESENT ADDRESS: NUMBER | STREET | CITY | COUNTY

USUAL RESIDENCE IF DIFFERENT FROM ABOVE: STREET OR RURAL ADDRESS | CITY OR TOWN | COUNTY | ☐ OUTSIDE CORPORATE LIMITS ☐ INSIDE CORPORATE LIMITS

DISEASE—TUBERCULOSIS: SEE BELOW—SYPHILIS: SEE OVER | DATE OF ONSET

ATTENDING PHYSICIAN (NAME AND ADDRESS) | DATE OF DIAGNOSIS

HOSPITAL, INSTITUTION OR OTHER AGENCY REPORTING

TUBERCULOSIS ONLY

PRIMARY
☐ POS. TUBERCULIN TEST
☐ CONVERTER ONLY
☐ X-RAY EVIDENCE
☐ HISTOLOGIC EVIDENCE
☐ BACTERIOLOGIC EVID.

PULMONARY
☐ MINIMAL
☐ MODERATELY ADV.
☐ FAR ADVANCED

REACTIVATION
☐ YES ☐ NO

TUBERCLE BACCILLI DEMONSTRATED (COMPLETE FOR PRIMARY, PULMONARY AND OTHER FORMS)
☐ YES ☐ SMEAR
☐ NO ☐ CULTURE
☐ NOT DONE ☐ OTHER, SPECIFY

IF REPORTED AFTER DEATH
DATE OF DEATH

SYPHILIS Diagnostic Information

INFECTIOUS
☐ PRIMARY
☐ SECONDARY
☐ EARLY LATENT

EPIDEMIOLOGIC NOTE: TO MINIMIZE SPREAD, PROMPT CONTROL MEASURES ARE ESSENTIAL. PLEASE PHONE REPORTS FOR INFECTIOUS CASES.

NON-INFECTIOUS
☐ LATE LATENT
☐ NEUROSYPHILIS, ASYMPTOMATIC
☐ NEUROSYPHILIS, CLINICAL
☐ CARDIOVASCULAR
☐ OTHER LATE
☐ CONGENITAL SPECIFY

REMARKS

REQUEST MORBIDITY BOOKS | NUMBER | NAME AND ADDRESS

DEPARTMENT OF PUBLIC HEALTH

Figure 15–1. Morbidity Report Form. *Top,* Front side of form. *Bottom,* Reverse side.

not only to civil judgments (negligence per se) and professional and social sanctions but also to criminal charges; the same is applicable to the reportable conditions listed in the next section.

15–2. OTHER REPORTABLE CONDITIONS

The following conditions are reportable in a sufficient number of states that requirements should be checked locally. This list is not necessarily comprehensive.

Reportable Condition	**Reportable to:**
A. Abortions (about half of states)	Local Health Department
B. Births (live or stillborn)	Local Health Department
C. Bites, animal	Local Health Department or local animal control agency
D. Child abuse (all states)	Local Health Department or specified agency
E. Controlled substances (drugs)	
1. Narcotics lost, destroyed, stolen	District Director of Internal Revenue
2. Change of address by physician with Bureau of Narcotics and Dangerous Drugs (BNDD) number	District Director of Internal Revenue

Reportable Condition	Reportable to:
3. Treatment of a narcotic addict	State Narcotics Agency
4. Prolonged treatment with narcotics	State Narcotics Agency
F. Deaths	
1. Noncoroner's cases	Local Health Department
2. Coroner's or Medical Examiner's cases	Coroner's office
G. Epilepsy or episodic unconsciousness	Local Health Department
H. Homicide threats	Local Police Department
I. Pesticide exposure	Local Health Department
J. Suspected criminally caused wounds (any reasonable suspicion) or battery, including rape (*14*)	Local Police Department

16. Serum Sensitivity and Desensitization

Animal antiserum should never be used unless a human antiserum is not available. Although hypersensitivity of the skin to animal serum does not necessarily parallel systemic hypersensitivity, intradermal (intracutaneous) skin tests should always be done before injections of animal antisera of any type are given. The injection must be made into, and not through, the skin and must not draw blood. A syringe containing 1 ml of 1:1000 epinephrine hydrochloride (Adrenalin) should be available for immedate use; deaths have occurred from anaphylactic reactions *(24–1)* to diluted antitoxin used for skin tests. Ophthalmic tests for sensitivity to antisera should never be used—severe reactions may result in permanent eye damage. Scratch tests are of no value.

If an indurated wheal (with or without pseudopods) is present 20 minutes after intradermal (intracutaneous) injection of 0.1 ml of 1:10 dilution, the test should be considered positive, and the need for passive protection by antitoxin should be reevaluated very carefully. If indicated, the following desensitization procedure may be carried out as a considered risk:

Inject	0.01 ml of antitoxin subcutaneously
20 minutes later	0.02 ml of antitoxin subcutaneously
20 minutes later	0.04 ml of antitoxin subcutaneously
20 minutes later	0.10 ml of antitoxin subcutaneously
20 minutes later	0.25 ml of antitoxin subcutaneously
20 minutes later	0.58 ml of antitoxin subcutaneously
Total	1.00 ml

Twenty minutes later, 1 ml of antitoxin may be injected subcutaneously or intramuscularly, accompanied by 0.5 ml of a 1:1000 solution of epinephrine HCl (Adrenalin) subcutaneously.

Following this desensitization procedure, large amounts of antisera can be given with relative safety, provided no local erythema, urticaria, asthmatic breathing, nausea, vomiting or chills have occurred. If such reactions do develop at any time during the procedure just outlined, the last dose should be repeated after a 20-minute wait; two reactions make further attempts at administration of the particular antiserum (usually equine or bovine) inadvisable. Similar skin testing with available antisera derived from other animals (e.g., bovine instead of equine and so forth) may be practical. As an alternative, benzathine penicillin G (Bicillin) and tetracycline therapy have been reported to be effective. Human tetanus immune globulin (TIG) should always be used in place of equine tetanus antitoxin (see *20, Tetanus Immunization*).

Oral administration of an antihistaminic (preferably in sustained action form) at the time the antitoxin is given and daily for 10 days thereafter may prevent, or decrease the severity of, serum sickness (*24–4*).

17. Suicide and Suicide Attempts

Reporting of Suicide

Cases of successful suicide—like all homicides—are reportable to the closest law enforcement agency, and suicide attempts are reportable in jurisdictions that still follow common law on the subject or are so codified (though today it is not generally considered a crime).

Patients at High Risk of Attempting Suicide

Patients who especially need close surveillance and consideration concerning suicide are those who detail suicide methods or confirm suicidal intent; are generally severely depressed; have previously attempted suicide; are extremely lonely or have suffered loss of loved ones; are experiencing the anniversary date of the loss of a loved one (i.e., departure, divorce, death); have sustained substantial loss in finances, position or esteem; or are seriously ill, elderly or dependent on drugs or alcohol. ANY PERSON KNOWN TO HAVE ATTEMPTED SUICIDE, OR SUSPECTED OF THE ATTEMPT, SHOULD BE KEPT UNDER IMMEDIATE CLOSE OBSERVATION WITH A PHYSICALLY ABLE ATTENDANT IN THE ROOM AT ALL TIMES WHILE THE PATIENT IS UNDER EMERGENCY MEDICAL CARE.

Measures to be Taken Following Attempted Suicide

If toxic substances in any form are known or suspected as the means of attempted suicide, ALL BODY CAVITIES ACCESSIBLE TO THE PATIENT (especially the rectum and vagina) SHOULD BE EXAMINED AS SOON AS POSSIBLE AND EMPTIED IF INDICATED. (See also *53, Poisoning*.) A specimen of any suspect material obtained from each site (including the stomach and bladder)—as well as a blood specimen—should be collected and placed in a labeled container for immediate qualitative and quantitative toxicologic examination. The blood alcohol level should be determined routinely.

The majority of suicide attempts are induced by alcohol, drugs, or both; great caution must be exercised not to compound the situation iatrogenically, which may occur in an attempt to quiet a hostile or semidelirious patient through prescription of medication that may have a detrimental additive or synergistic effect.

Note: Though often patients will indicate—when they are able to communicate—that their overdose was accidental or unintentional, sitting down with the patient and reviewing major life sectors will generally bring to light unresolved problems that make it clear that this was not the case; appropriate resolution then can commence.

Treatment

- Provide supportive care in the hospital and specific treatment as described in 32 *(Coma)* and 53 *(Poisoning)*.
- Give specific treatment of any wounds.
- Obtain psychiatric consultation and follow-up care.
- Provide whatever type of psychiatric service and environment are needed to control the situation until the patient makes the transition from self-destructive to self-preservative attitudes (see also *54–8* and *54–14*).

18. Surgical and Emergency Procedures and Techniques

This chapter describes procedures that are helpful to master for use in various stages of emergency care and some comments that can be of aid concerning the more common procedures.

18–1. RESUSCITATION TECHNIQUES *(See 5–1)*

18–2. ANESTHETIC TECHNIQUES *(See 12)*

18–3. ARTHROCENTESIS

The skin must be thoroughly cleaned with Betadine or a comparable antiseptic. Sterile technique is used with drapes and gloves; after cleaning, the skin is anesthetized with topical Fluori-Methane or ethyl chloride or with injected lidocaine. An 18-gauge needle is preferable for aspiration of larger joints such as the knee. Specimens should be taken for Gram stain and cell count (immediate, if bacterial infection known or suspected) and other laboratory examination and culturing. If one purpose of aspiration is to reduce fluid, a broad compression bandage may be applied (but not too tightly) to slow reaccumulation; circulation should be monitored if this is done.

18–4. BANDAGING

Purposes

- To approximate wound (e.g., with "butterfly" bandage and/or Steri-Strip; see Figs. 59–1 and 59–2).
- To secure placement of dressings (to protect wound from environment).
- To compress wound for control of bleeding and reduction of edema (use broad soft material to reduce tissue injury and ischemia).
- To support parts and restrict movements with or without splints (see Figs. 47–1 and 47–2).
- To secure placement of splints.

General Principles in Bandaging

- Use bandage material and size appropriate to purpose.
- Use sterile or cleanest bandage available when securing wound dressings; can wash and boil for 10 to 15 minutes or iron when sterility is necessary.
- Leave fingers and toes exposed or open to inspection after any circular wrapping, so that one is able to periodically check for excess compression or ischemia, edema, whitish (pale) or bluish (cyanotic) color, decreased pulse or cold tissue, or numbness or tingling.

- Secure bandage adequately from start to finish, to reduce loosening and slippage. When wrapping cylindrical surfaces, start wrapping at an angle, cover about 60% of the prior wrap with each successive wrap, and finally apply a piece of tape perpendicular to the bandage layers if much motion will be occurring.
- Pad bony prominences.
- Place part to be bandaged in as comfortable and functional a position as possible. When bandaging across joints, put parts in anatomical position or slightly flexed position if possible.
- Avoid elastic bandage compression dressings when more swelling will occur, unless prepared to observe and loosen prn and patient is competent to aid in process.
- When replacing bandages encrusted with dried blood, remove with care after softening with small amounts of sterile saline or half-strength hydrogen peroxide, so as not to disturb wound healing.

Materials

In addition to the various types of cotton gauzes, tubular gauzes (varying sizes used with applicator tube), multitailed and roll elastic bandages, tubular elasticized net bandage of appropriate varying sizes has great value in affixing dressings to large, difficult-to-secure areas, such as the shoulder, hip, trunk and head. Cuts are made in the tubular elasticized net bandage at angles and lengths proportionate to the body part to be covered.

18–5. CARDIAC (OR CHEST) COMPRESSION (External Heart Compression [EHC] *(See 5–23)*

18–6. CATHETERIZATION (Bladder)

Insertion of any type of tube into the bladder invites infection; therefore, a clean catch or second glass specimen should usually be used for routine diagnostic purposes. If acute retention *(41–24)* or need for minute-by-minute determination of kidney function (as in cases of shock [57] requires catheterization, careful sterile technique should be used.

Suprapubic

If bladder distention is acute with inability to voluntarily void and there is (a) accompanying urethral trauma, (b) inability to pass a urethral catheter, (c) no urethral catheterization equipment available or (d) sepsis, the bladder can be adequately emptied with a suprapubic catheter. In order of decreasing preference, the following can be used: commercial suprapubic catheter (Ingram trocar catheter or Cystocath—insertable tubing can be left in for continuing drainage), No. 14 central venous pressure catheter, No. 18 3-inch spinal needle (insert and withdraw with each use).

Procedure

1. Palpate and outline the urinary bladder.
2. Cleanse the suprapubic area from the umbilicus to the pubic bone and drape around the lower midline.
3. Inject a local anesthetic (e.g., lidocaine) in the area to be punctured.
4. Insert the needle well within the confines of the palpable bladder, perpendicularly into the bladder—this is in the midline, 2 to 3 fingerbreadths above the pubis. Withdraw the stylet periodically to check time of entry into the bladder.
5. After urine is obtained, the small, sterile polyethylene catheter is inserted through the needle bore and taped to the abdomen after the needle is removed. The free end of the catheter is connected to a closed reservoir system for continued bladder drainage.

Contraindications to suprapubic bladder needle insertion are inability to palpate the bladder and prior suprapubic or lower abdominal surgery.

Urethral

Male

1. Cleanse the penis thoroughly with soap and water and surround the penis with a sterile towel.
2. Put on sterile gloves.
3. Insert a well-lubricated (soluble sterile lubricant as K–Y jelly) sterile catheter by using gentle, steady pressure and holding the dorsum of the penis upward toward the abdominal wall when the catheter reaches the prostatic urethral area to straighten the urethral curve.

If obstruction is encountered so that the bladder cannot be entered on two or three gentle attempts, or if there is bleeding, a sedative should be given and the patient referred for urologic care. If bladder distention is acute and urologic care is not immediately available, the bladder can be decompressed by using the suprapubic sterile technique just described.

4. Fill the retention balloon to specified degree once catheter is well within the bladder.
5. Send a collected urine specimen for routine analysis and any special analysis necessary, plus for culture and sensitivity studies of any significant organism growth.
6. Attach the free end of the catheter to a reservoir bag if continued use if planned. Preferably, use a closed system with periodic cleaning irrigation.

Female

In female patients, urethral catheterization can be done easily, preferably by a female nurse, using a sterile nonbreakable catheter and sterile technique, as described for male patients.

18–7. CENTRAL VENOUS PRESSURE (CVP)

Measurement of CVP is of great aid as a guide to adequacy of volume replacement and as an index of blood vessel tone, circulating blood volume and status of the heart as a pump; it should be used any time there is significant impairment in these areas—particularly when the patient's reserves are low and there is little margin for error. See Table 57–4 for interpretations. Hypervolemia, CHF, pneumothorax, mechanical ventilators and improper catheter position may cause a high CVP.

The accuracy of CVP measurement is dependent upon the patency of the catheter, the patient being recumbent in the supine position and the accurate location of the catheter tip in determining an external zero-point baseline. Whether the CVP line is placed by the antecubital, jugular, subclavian or jugular vein route, the tip is usually placed in the superior vena cava, close to the right atrium. See also *18–36, Venous Cannulation.*

18–8. CRANIAL TREPHINATION *(See Fig. 44–2)*

18–9. CULDOCENTESIS

This rapid diagnostic procedure is of value in women in evaluating for pelvic inflammatory disease, ruptured ectopic pregnancy or presence of intraperitoneal bleeding of any cause, after initial bimanual pelvic examination has aroused the suspicion.

After the patient is in the lithotomy position, a vaginal speculum is inserted for visualization of the posterior fornix, which is cleaned with povidone-iodine (Betadine) solution. To best expose the posterior fornix, the posterior cuff of the cervix is grasped with a tenaculum and gently pulled distally and upward.

A 4-inch 18-gauge needle (affixed to a 10-ml syringe with finger control) is inserted with a quick motion in the midline, 1 cm posterior to the junction of the cervix and vaginal wall and parallel to the posterior vaginal wall (rather than caudally toward the rectum) and to a depth of approximately 2 cm while aspiration is applied with the syringe. Instead of a 4-inch needle, a 2-inch butterfly needle held with a tenaculum and affixed to a small catheter and syringe may be used. Aspiration of blood or purulent material (send to the laboratory for culture, smear and Gram stain) indicates the presence of a disease state. Note whether the bloody aspirate clots or not.

18–10. ENDOTRACHEAL INTUBATION *(See 5–18)*

18–11. GASTRIC LAVAGE

When emetics are ineffective or contraindicated, washing the stomach may be necessary unless also contraindicated. Since the object of lavage is rapid, complete emptying of the stomach, as large a tube as possible should be used. Even small children will tolerate passage through the mouth of relatively large tubes. Attempted lavage through an intranasal tube is unsatisfactory. Uncooperative or uncontrollable children can be mummified in a tightly wrapped sheet and quartered on the left side with the head turned to one side and the hips (or foot of entire table) slightly elevated to aid control and prevention of aspiration. The lavage tube should be smooth and well lubricated with a water-soluble preparation. If the patient has taken large amounts of petroleum distillate or is sedated or comatose, a cuffed endotracheal tube should be in place to prevent aspiration if gastric lavage is being done. A large syringe or funnel or an irrigating can suspended above the patient's head and equipped with a two-way stopcock is satisfactory for introduction of the solution (in adults, tap water or half-normal saline and in children, normal saline). Repeated washings with small amounts of solution (20 to 50 ml in children and approximately 200 ml in adults) should be done until the return solution is clear. Overfilling of the stomach should be avoided because of the danger of regurgitation and aspiration. The tube should be pinched off, or gentle suction retained, during removal to prevent aspiration. In cases of suspected or known poisoning, a specimen of vomitus or stomach washings should be collected, marked for identification and saved for possible later analysis. Following emptying of the stomach, a specific antidote *(53–10)* or activated charcoal *(53–8)* and cathartic (such as Mg citrate) may be instilled. Do not give combinations, of course, where there is adverse interaction; e.g., do not give charcoal, which interferes with n-acetylcysteine action, as an antidote for acetaminophen poisoning.

18–12. GRAM STAIN

The Gram stain is an essential emergency procedure for the assessment of bacterial infectious diseases. It rapidly helps in establishment of the gross presence or absence of organisms and the differentiation of gram-positive from gram-negative bacteria as an aid to antimicrobial medication *(33–83)* and provides an index of the type and magnitude of leukocyte response.

Gram-Staining Technique

1. Use a clean, dry, labeled slide.
2. Make a smear of the specimen on the slide thin enough so that individual cells are separated.
3. Dry the smear with very gentle warming—the slide should feel no more than comfortably warmed against the volar forearm skin.

4. Cover the slide with methanol and allow to dry before proceeding.
5. Cover the slide with a copious amount of buffered crystal violet solution for 60 seconds. Add 2 to 3 drops of $NaHCO_3$.
6. Wash the crystal violet solution off with iodophor mordant; then allow the slide—covered with a copious amount of iodophor mordant—to set for another 60 seconds.
7. Drain the slide and rapidly drop the acetone across the upper end of the tilted slide until the solution reaching the other end is colorless—takes about 10 seconds (the leukocytes should be colorless at this stage).
8. Rinse the acetone off with water and shake the water off the slide.
9. Cover the slide with safranin for 60 seconds, then wash off with water.
10. Examine the slide under the microscope with oil immersion.

18–13. INTERCOSTAL NERVE BLOCK *(See 31–16)*

18–14. INTRAGLOSSAL INJECTIONS (Rare use)

In an unconscious patient in a state of shock whose veins are collapsed or impossible to locate without a cutdown, a small amount (up to 2 ml) of a vasopressor drug injected into the tongue muscle is rapidly absorbed without residual ill effects; intravenous injection through the lingual vein on the interior surface of the tongue can be used if it can be easily cannulated (apply pressure afterward to prevent prolonged bleeding). Enough effect can usually be obtained to allow location of a peripheral vein for conventional venous infusion. It is more common now to give epinephrine, for instance, via the endotracheal route *(18–16)* if an IV line is not available.

Technique

1. Grasp the tongue by the tip and pull it upward toward the nose.
2. Using a short bevel, 20- or 22-gauge needle, inject the solution IV or into the muscles on the underside of the base of the tongue, avoiding injury to the large veins on each side of the midline.
3. Only rapidly absorbable, nonirritating medications should be used, as rather severe temporary tongue swelling and pain can occur with irritating substances.

18–15. INTRAOCULAR PRESSURE TONOMETRY

Gentle ballottement of the eyeball with the two index fingers (tactile tension) gives a rough index of intraocular pressure; normally, the globe is semifirm and may be slightly indented, whereas in patients with glaucoma, the globe is firm to hard. The standard instrument for accuracy, however, is the Schiøtz tonometer, which is rested on the anesthetized cornea to determine the eye's resistance (normal = 14 to 21 mm Hg). In addition to being sure the tonometer is clean, ascertain that no drops of cleaning fluid are on the plunger ready to drop onto the cornea—preferably use an ultraviolet light sterilizer.

18–16. INTRATRACHEAL (ENDOTRACHEAL) INJECTIONS

Some medications may be injected endotracheally in emergency conditions when there is no IV route available (or as with lidocaine when an additional local effect for severe bronchospasm reduction may be desired). Injection is given through the cricothyroid membrane (see Fig. 5–6) with the patient in a horizontal position. Epinephrine, lidocaine and atropine are medications that may be given this way; naloxone and diazepam have also been effectively given in animal experimentation. Aerosol pressure increases dispersal and absorption area. Dose effect is less predictable and slightly less rapid than with the preferred IV route, and slightly higher medication doses may be required for comparable effect.

18–17. "LIFE LINES"

This term applies principally to tubes inserted into the body for administration of fluid, blood, electrolytes and medication plus monitoring of vital functions. Especially in complex cases, it is helpful to *label* all tubes into and from the body as to the functional use.

18–18. NASAL PACKING

Anterior

Several methods are satisfactory. Topical anesthesia with 4% cocaine often is required.

1. Pack tightly with petrolatum gauze coated with neosporin ointment. Do not use iodoform gauze.
2. Pack firmly with a gauze strip moistened with 1:1000 epinephrine HCl (Adrenalin); watch dose, because drug is absorbed.
3. Use an inflatable device such as the Foley catheter or the Nasostat. This may be combined with partial gauze packing put in before inflation of the device.

Posterior (Nasopharyngeal)

Many times posterior nasopharyngeal packing can be avoided with use of inflatable anterior tubing (Nasostat) and anterior packing, or by insertion of a Foley catheter (see below).

Gauze Packing

1. Give a preliminary injection of morphine sulfate or diazepam (Valium) to older children and adults to allay apprehension. A pentobarbital sodium (Nembutal) suppository may be substituted in children less than 10 years of age. Topical anesthesia may be indicated in hypersensitive persons.
2. Pass a small (No. 10 or 12), soft catheter through each nostril and into the pharynx.
3. Grasp the slotted end of each catheter with forceps and bring it out through the mouth.
4. Attach to the slotted end of the catheter the ends of a 12-inch length of No. 0 or 2-0 silk suture of ⅛-inch umbilical tape, to the middle of which is fastened a piece of soft, nonmedicated selvage-edge gauze attached to another 12-inch length of suture that can be either taped to the side of the mouth or cut short to be visible and reachable in the posterior pharynx.
5. Pull the gauze gently but firmly into the posterior nares by withdrawing the catheter entirely from the nose.
6. Unfasten the catheters and tie the ligatures extruding from the nostril loosely together over a thick, soft piece of folded gauze placed on the upper lip below the nostrils to reduce pressure on the columella to prevent irritation and necrosis. Tape the mouth string to the side of the cheek. (An alternative technique is to bring both strings through the same nostril and avoid columellar pressure, but posterior pressure is not as uniform.)

Foley Catheter

Insertion of a Foley catheter with filling of the tip reservoir with air and application of gentle traction may suffice as an alternative to gauze packing.

The patient should be hospitalized for observation and continued analgesia and sedation, as well as treatment of any coagulation disorders *(45–7, 45–8)* and hypertension *(29–14)*.

18–19. NASOGASTRIC (NG) TUBE

Passage of a nasogastric tube is a common, simple procedure.

1. Select a tube of appropriate length and diameter for the patient. To determine appropriate length, if feasible, elevate the patient's head.
2. Lubricate the distal third of the tube with a water-soluble jelly and insert it through the floor of the most patent nasal passage (located by the patient's breathing through each nostril separately).
3. After the tube is in the pharynx, advance it slowly until a swallowing reflex is elicited and back off slightly unless the tube has advanced with swallowing. Give the patient some ice chips to aid swallowing if feasible. Advance the tube as swallowing occurs. If the reflex is not initiated, try externally rubbing the trachea up and down gently between the thumb and index finger to initiate the swallowing reflex, then advance the tube into the stomach.
4. Absence of breath sounds and choking generally indicate the tube is in the stomach, and this is confirmed by auscultation of loud sounds over the abdomen following air instillation or by aspiration of gastric contents.
5. Send appropriate samples to the laboratory for examination and, after irrigating the stomach as needed, attach suction to the external end of the NG tube.

18–20. NASOTRACHEAL INTUBATION *(See 5–20)*

18–21. PACEMAKER *(See also 29–13, Heart Block, Complete; 29–17, Pacemaker Failure)*

Emergency cardiac pacemakers are indicated for symptomatic bradyarrhythmias, prophylactically in acute inferior MI with Type II 2° AV heart block (Mobitz II), and in cases of new bifascicular block or new bilateral bundle branch block. A standby pacemaker should also be available for new onset of 2° AV block (Type I or II) in acute anterior MI. Finally, pacemakers may be used for overdrive pacing and atrial or ventricular tachyarrhythmia. Efficiency of pacing is considerably greater in complete heart block unresponsive to medications than in cardiac arrest with asystole and slow idioventricular rhythms.

Temporary pacemakers are placed 90% of the time via the subclavian, internal jugular, brachial or even the femoral vein; placement is most easily accomplished when there is bloodflow to propel the balloon tip of the pacemaker along to the right atrium and ventricle. Passage may be blind, but fluoroscopic control is preferred. When there is cardiac arrest, the placing of a transmyocardial pacing stylet from the epigastric area (see Fig. 18–1) into the left or right ventricle is generally preferable and much easier. Rhythm should be continuously monitored on ECG and all ACLS equipment at hand during placement.

18–22. PERICARDIAL SAC ASPIRATION *(See also 29–18, Pericardial Effusion)*

The only equipment needed for this procedure, which may be lifesaving if cardiac tamponade *(31–4)* is present, is a 3- or 4-inch 18-gauge short-beveled hypodermic needle with a metal hub, a medium Luer syringe and ECG

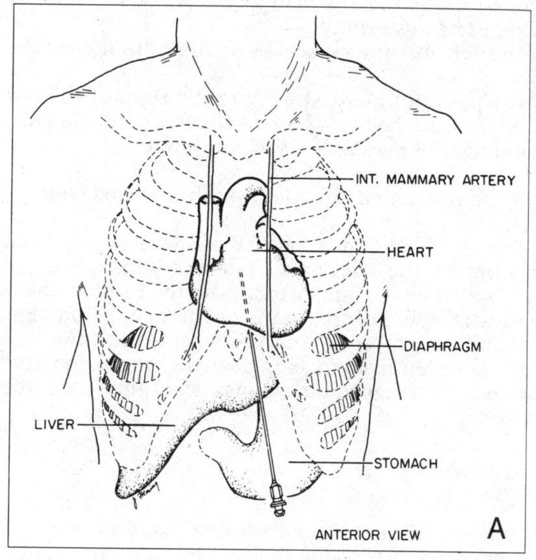

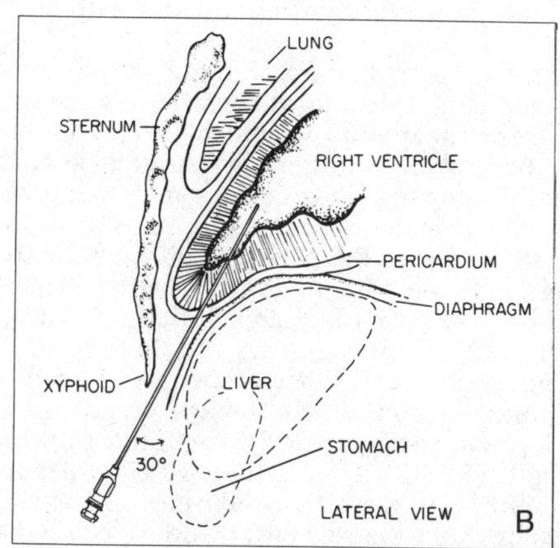

Figure 18–1. Transthoracic pacemaker into right ventricle via the subxiphoid approach. (See *18–21, Pacemaker.*) (From Roberts, J. R., and Greenberg, M. I.: Ann. Emerg. Med., 10:600, 1981.)

monitor. (For electrocardiographic monitoring for position of the needle tip, see *29–18*.)

Sites of Aspiration (In order of desirability)

1. Slightly to the left of the xiphoid process of the sternum with the needle directed superiorly and posteriorly.

2. Through the left 4th interspace ½ inch to the left of the sternocostal junction.

3. Through the posterior chest slightly to the right of the inferior angle of the left scapula. This method transverses the lung and should not be used if there is any possibility of pericardial sac empyema.

Technique

1. Cleanse the selected area thoroughly with soap and water and paint with Ioprep or Betadine.

2. Insert a short-beveled 3-inch long 18-gauge needle attached to a 10- or 20-ml syringe through the chest wall into the pericardial sac, using ECG precautions outlined in *29–18*, and aspirate gently. Either fresh or defibrinated blood may be obtained. Relief from tamponade may be obtained by removal of as little as 5 ml. The procedure may be repeated as often as necessary for relief, but immediate thoracotomy is indicated if aspiration gives no relief, if no blood is obtained or if signs and symptoms of tamponade recur in spite of repeated aspirations.

18–23. PERITONEAL ASPIRATION *(Diagnostic for intra-abdominal injury. In women, see also 18–9, Culdocentesis)*

Peritoneal aspiration is an adjunctive technique to provide indication of effects of intraperitoneal injury due to blunt trauma (and equivocal penetrating wounds) and to aid in assessment of patients with equivocal abdominal findings.

After a nasogastric tube and a Foley catheter are inserted, shave the abdomen and the umbilicus. Inject local anesthesia with epinephrine into the inferior umbilicus (may make stab wound with No. 11 blade along lateral rectus 2 to 3 cm below umbilicus if there is a surgical scar in midline). Insert trocar at 45° angle, aiming caudad, being careful that the momentum of fascia penetration does not cause perforation of viscus. Remove stylet and advance catheter gently toward the pelvis. Aspirate with 20-ml syringe. If 20 ml of blood is aspirated, the present tap is positive. If less than 20 ml is aspirated, rapidly infuse Ringer's lactate solution (20 ml/kg up to 1 liter) by gravity drainage through IV tubing. After the fluid is in, roll the patient (if possible) gently from side to side. Place empty bottle on floor and allow fluid to drain from abdomen. Results of the lavage procedure are positive if (a) newsprint cannot be read through the IV tubing (25 ml blood/liter), (b) the level of red blood cells (RBC's) is more than 100,000 per ml, (c) the level of white blood cells (WBC's) is more than 500 per ml in the absence of gross blood (if at least 3 hours have elapsed post trauma), or (d) the level of amylase in lavage fluid is greater than 200 Somogyi units/ml.

18–24. PERITONEAL DIALYSIS

This relatively simple procedure is of great value in the treatment of certain types of poisoning (see *53–4*) and in systemic diseases such as hepatic coma *(32–10)*.

Technique

1. Prepare a site on the abdomen by shaving and by presurgical skin preparation. The patient should be supine and in bed. The usual site of choice is in the midline 4 cm below the umbilicus; however, the umbilical area is relatively avascular, and a trocar can also be angled distally through the inferior border of this area into the peritoneum. Any scarred areas should be avoided because of the probability of adjacent intra-abdominal adhesions. The urinary bladder should be empty.

2. After anesthetizing the area, insert a No. 22 paracentesis trocar through a stab wound. In the absence of ascites, 500 ml of air should be injected preliminarily; if there is ascites, this is not necessary.

3. Push the trocar with obturator in place through the peritoneum; remove the obturator and substitute a previously prepared dialysis tube—a 12-inch section of plastic intravenous tubing with elliptical holes cut at frequent intervals in the distal 4 inches is satisfactory. Gently work the dialysis tube into the pelvis.

4. Remove the trocar and suture the skin around the dialysis tube.

5. Connect the dialysis tube to a piece of tubing at least 36 inches long. The tubing, in turn, should be connected through a three-way stopcock or double Y connectors to three flasks, containing the following solutions (if commercial dialysate solutions are not available):

Normal saline, 1000 ml.
Dextrose, 5% in water, 1000 ml.
Sodium bicarbonate (100 ml of 10% solution) in 1000 ml of 5% dextrose in saline.
(Potassium, 5 mEq/liter, is added or deleted according to the clinical problem.)

Note: Special problems require special dialysates (e.g., hypernatremia), and osmolarity must be a consideration.

6. With the solution bottles elevated on an intravenous stand, adjust the flow so that 1¼ to 1½ hours are required for all to empty into the abdomen. (Two liters of commercial dialysate solution may be substituted for the solutions specified earlier and used according to the manufacturer's directions.)

7. When about 20 ml remain in each bottle, remove them from the intravenous stand and place them on the floor and allow the fluid from the abdomen to run out by gravity.

8. Collect specimens of fluid for analysis as required.

9. Substitute new solution bottles and elevate to the intravenous stand.

10. Repeat the procedure just described as needed, governed by the patient's clinical condition and analysis of the returned dialysis fluid.

11. Keep an accurate input-output record.

18–25. PNEUMATIC (MILITARY ANTI-SHOCK) TROUSERS (MAST)

This valuable emergency device is particularly indicated in prompt treatment of hypovolemic shock states (750 to 1000 ml of blood can be directed to the circulating volume), treatment of neurogenic shock, stabilization of femoral and pelvic fractures, and control of intra-abdominal bleeding. Patients are candidates for MAST when the BP gets down to 90 mm Hg or lower as a result of hypovolemic shock; however, if the injury is above the diaphragm, use of these trousers is controversial.

The most important contraindications to use of MAST are pulmonary edema and cardiogenic shock. Furthermore, abdominal chamber inflation is generally best avoided when there is abdominal evisceration, a partially impaled abdominal object that should not be removed, or pregnancy beyond the 2nd trimester. Color-coding of tubes helps assure their proper connection. Disadvantages include inability to check the abdomen and skin color under the suit, and sudden severe and possibly fatal shock should the pneumatic trousers suddenly deflate. However, the latter is a rare occurrence, and in general the disadvantages are largely outweighed by the advantages. Fluid replacement should at least keep up with shifts that will occur as suit pressure is reduced. Pressure readjustment is needed during air transport.

18–26. REDUCTION OF DISLOCATIONS *(See 47–6)*

18–27. RING REMOVAL FROM FINGER *(See also 43–1)*

See Figure 63–1. The swollen finger is wrapped with string as shown (or one can start at the proximal interphalangeal joint if desired) until the ring is reached. Then the proximal end of the string is looped under the ring, after which the proximal end is pulled distally in the direction of the fingernail. The ring is gradually removed as the string unwinds; soap aids sliding.

If this is unsuccessful, ring cutters must be used.

18–28. SKULL TRACTION

Reliable stabilization-traction of the cervical spine following cervical fracture-dislocation is readily achieved by applying traction on the skull using Gardner-Wells traction tongs. A CT scan may be used to check the integrity of the spinal canal.

1. The scalp and tong points are cleaned with povidone-iodine (Betadine); shaving of the scalp is not necessary.
2. Inject lidocaine with epinephrine into the scalp and periosteum of the ridge of the temporal bone above the posterior border of the pinna.
3. Insert the needle-sharp tongs into the scalp at the anesthetized area, with the points directed toward the line of pull.
4. The traction tongs are screwed in until 30 lb of pressure are indicated on the spring-loaded clamp or the indicator extends 1 mm beyond the hole at the distal end of the screw knob.
5. After the tongs are well set, attach a rope to the tongs and attach about 20 to 30 lb (or 10 lb plus 5 lb for each cervical level of the fracture above C5) of weight initially to the other end of the rope, which has first been slid through a pulley to afford pull in the direction of the general axis of the spine.

18–29. SPINAL (SUBARACHNOID; LUMBAR) PUNCTURE

Although spinal puncture usually has no use as a therapeutic measure in emergency situations, it is a valuable diagnostic adjunct in conditions in which intracranial or spinal cord disease is suspected. The principal contraindication is evidence of increased intracranial pressure thought to be due to an intracranial mass (unless preparations have been made for immediate remedial surgery). Spinal puncture is necessary in the presence of acute fulminating infections with signs of meningeal irritation so that the offending organism can be identified and prompt treatment begun (see *33–40*). For normal values of cerebrospinal fluid, see Table 18–1.

Technique

1. Place the patient on his or her side with the knees drawn up to reverse the normal lumbar lordosis and spread the spinous processes.

Table 18–1. CEREBROSPINAL FLUID—NORMAL VALUES

Amount (adults)	100–140 ml
Appearance	Clear, colorless
Pressure (on side, relaxed)*	
Newborn	30–80 mm of CSF
Children	50–100 mm of CSF
Adults	70–200 mm of CSF
Specific gravity	1.003–1.009
pH	7.35–7.40
Total cell count	
Infants	0–20 per cu mm (no PMNs)
Adults	0–10 per cu mm (no PMNs)
Proteins, total	20–45 mg %
Glucose	50–75 mg %
Chlorides (as NaCl)	120–130 mEq/L

*Apprehension, excitement, straining, crying or excessive flexion of the neck or trunk may give above normal readings that should not be interpreted as indicating organic disease.

2. Scrub the skin over the full width of the back from the lower thoracic to midsacral area with povidone-iodine, paint with Ioprep and drape.

3. Inject a local anesthetic into the space between the spinous processes of the 4th and 5th lumbar vertebrae. The space between the 3rd and 4th vertebrae may be used in adults but not in infants and children.

4. Insert a short-beveled No. 22 spinal puncture needle between the spinous processes in the midline with the obturator in place, keeping the bevel of the needle in the plane of the long axis of the body to minimize dural tears (see *30–26, Spinal Puncture Headaches*). A definite resistance will be felt as the tip of the needle passes through the dura.

5. Remove the obturator stylet, connect the manometer and record the initial cerebrospinal fluid pressure in millimeters.

6. Collect a total of 5 to 6 ml of cerebrospinal fluid (CSF) in three sterile vials and observe for color, viscosity and translucency. Send the collected specimens at once to the laboratory for necessary tests—for example, cell count (RBC's, WBC's and differential), smears for microorganisms, cultures and sensitivity tests, chemistry [chlorides (such as NaCl), glucose and total proteins] and Kolmer complement-fixation test.

7. Note variation in the manometer column with respiration.

8. Test for evidence of block by the Queckenstedt maneuver (digital external compression of jugular veins) if spinal subarachnoid block is suspected (absence of column rise is indicative of block).

9. Record the final manometric pressure in millimeters of CSF.

10. Disconnect manometer and remove needle gently. Apply a sterile pad over the puncture site.

11. If signs and symptoms of acute meningeal irritation are present and the spinal fluid is grossly purulent, start massive systemic antibacterial therapy and symptomatic and supportive care at once without waiting for complete laboratory results (see *33–40, Meningitis*). Do a Gram stain at once as a guide to therapy.

12. Keep the patient prone for 1 hour to minimize gravity seepage of cerebrospinal fluid. If postpuncture cephalgia develops (incidence, 10–20%), treat as outlined under *30–26, Spinal Puncture Headaches*.

Note: Cisternal puncture may be required when lumbar puncture cannot be done. The aseptic techniques are as above, but the suboccipital area of the back of the head must also be prepared. With the neck flexed and the patient on his side, the needle is inserted obliquely cephalad in the exact midline of the upper neck. It is first advanced into the occipital bone near the foramen magnum and then "walked" anteriorly (mm by mm until no resistance is obtained) until it is in the foramen magnum; continue to advance a mm at a time until fluid is obtained.

18–30. SPLINTS *(See 47–2, Immobilization)*

18–31. SUBCLAVIAN VEIN CATHETERIZATION *(See 18–36)*

18–32. SWAN-GANZ CATHETER

The flow-directed catheterization technique combined with a balloon-tipped catheter (Swan-Ganz) has greatly aided the bedside monitoring of hemodynamics (arterial pressure, pulmonary artery and/or pulmonary capillary wedge pressure, cardiac output). Among the conditions these aid in diagnosing, monitoring and treating are hypovolemia, heart failure (left and right ventricles), pulmonary hypertension, pulmonary congestion and cardiac tamponade. Skill in insertion and improved design help reduce the incidence of complications such as knotting, rupture of the pulmonary artery, pulmonary infarction and arrhythmias.

18–33. THORACENTESIS AND THORACOSTOMY

The skin is first cleaned with an antiseptic agent such as povidone-iodine (Betadine) and anesthetized with 2% lidocaine for both procedures.

Thoracentesis is performed with the patient in the sitting position and at the site most likely to facilitate removal of the fluid found by clinical and x-ray means.

The posterior axillary line in the 8th interspace on the left or the 5th to 6th on the right is often favorable. Insert the needle over the superior margin of the nerve (see Fig. 18–2 for technique). Advance the needle slowly and aspirate frequently, to avoid puncturing the lung.

Thoracostomy technique is shown in Figure 18–3. The free end of the tube may be attached to an underwater seal bottle or a chest drain valve (Heimlich valve), depending on the volume of aspirate involved.

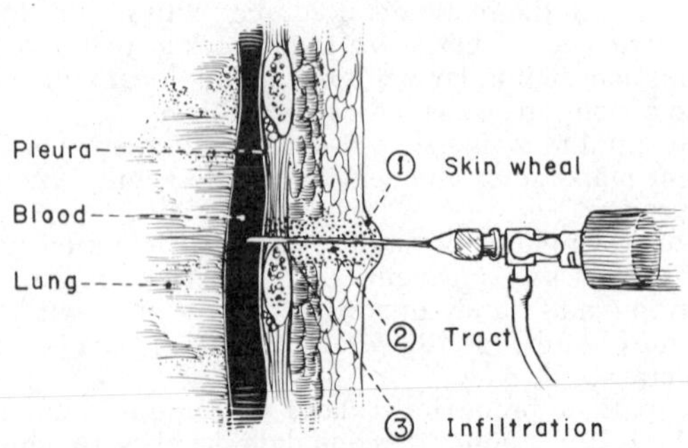

Figure 18–2. The technique of thoracentesis. (From Zuidema, G. D., Rutherford, R. B., and Ballinger, W. F.: *The Management of Trauma,* 3rd ed. Philadelphia, W. B. Saunders Co., 1979.)

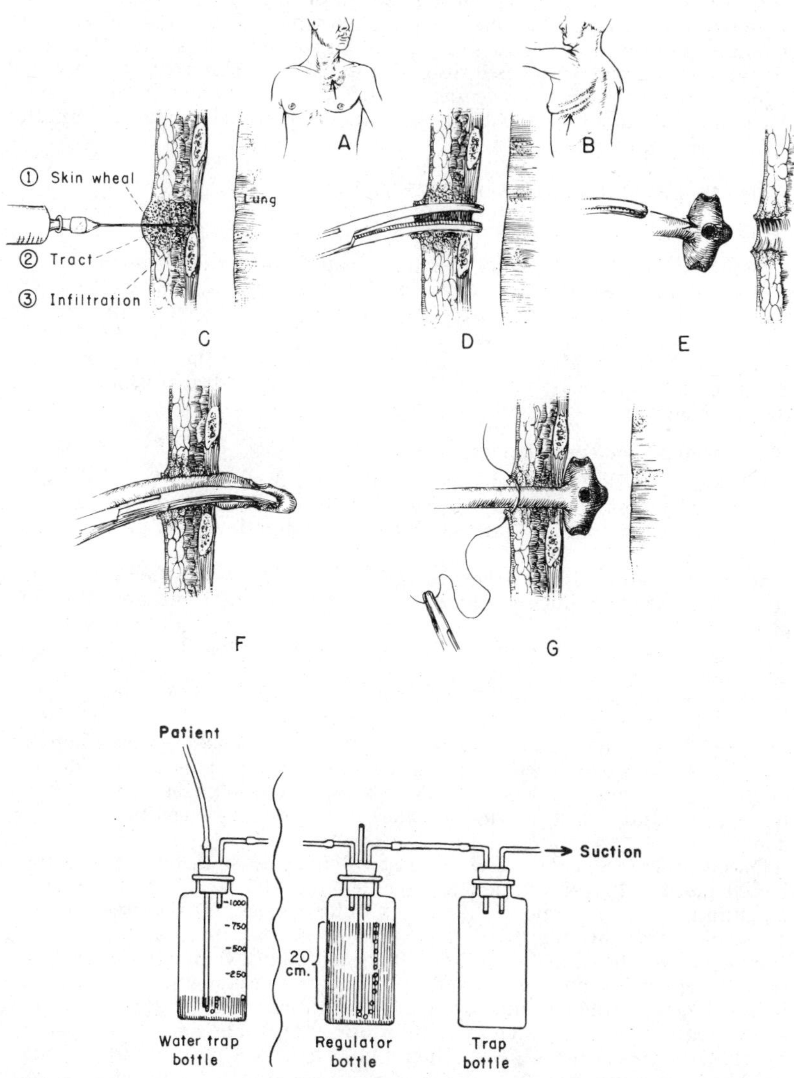

Figure 18–3. The technique of closed tube thoracostomy. The second interspace in the midclavicular line *(A)* is selected for the removal of air and the 6th or 7th intercostal space in the posterior axillary line *(B)* for the removal of fluid. Water-trap bottle is shown on the near right—respiratory excursions in intrapleural pressure promote egress of pleural contents. The simple suction apparatus shown here or a pump may be used to further aid withdrawal of fluid. (From Zuidema, G. D., Rutherford, R. B., and Ballinger, W. F.: *The Management of Trauma,* 3rd ed. Philadelphia, W. B. Saunders Co., 1979.)

Open thoracotomy (usual location, Fig. 18–3*B*) indications include persistent thoracic hemorrhage (greater than 200 ml/hour from chest tubes); rupture or penetration of major vessels, heart, esophagus, bronchi, diaphragm; persistent leakage of large volumes of air; and for control of gross distal bleeding. It is also sometimes performed through the left anterolateral 6th intercostal space as an emergency procedure in the ED to accomplish aortic cross-clamping in cardiac arrest patients who are not responsive within 5 minutes of full resuscitative measures.

18–34. TRACHEOSTOMY *(See 5–10, 5–19 and 5–20)*

18–35. TRANSFUSIONS *(See also 57, Shock)*

Transfusions of whole blood, when indicated, are an efficient physiologic means of maintaining and increasing blood volume and oxygen-carrying ability, replacing toxic circulating blood (exchange transfusion) and enhancing blood coagulation. In emergency situations, the urgency of the need for blood modifies the details of administration but *never* the need for careful labeling and identification. See 57–5 for discussion of transfusions in blood volume restoration.

Hazards of Blood Transfusions

Acidosis. The pH of bank (storage) blood varies from 6.4 to 7.2. This can be controlled by monitoring pH and by IV injection of sodium bicarbonate solution as needed; avoid alkaline state, however. Potassium level also rises in stored blood.

Acute Respiratory Distress Syndrome (ARDS) *(see also 55–4).* Microfiltration of stored blood helps reduce the incidence of this condition, but also filters out platelets.

Air Embolism. Sixty to 80 ml of air is required to stop the heart—smaller amounts are usually well tolerated. (See *63–11, Venous Air Embolism.*)

Allergic Reactions *(see also 24).* IV diphenhydramine and/or steroids may be of benefit.

Bacterial and Viral Contamination. See comments in *33–28* regarding hepatitis and in *33–2* regarding AIDS. At present the plan by some to use "directed donors" is officially considered by blood banks not to increase safety and may have a crippling effect on vital supplies of community blood for emergency use.

Coagulopathy *(see Table 45–1).* Platelet deficiency or thrombocytopathy in stored blood, DIC (45–5), deficiency of Factor VIII (45–7) and low serum calcium (*46–14*) are among the factors to be considered. Use fresh blood in subsequent transfusions.

Citrate Intoxication *(see also 53–214).* This occurs most frequently in exchange transfusions in erythroblastotic infants or in multiple transfusions for massive hemorrhage. It can be treated by IV administration of 10% calcium gluconate as needed according to calcium monitoring (*46–14*). The need for supplemental calcium and clotting factors should be considered after administration of approximately every 5 to 10 units in adults. Less problem is encountered with packed RBC's.

Hemolytic Reactions. Hemolytic reactions are usually dangerous only if more than 250 ml of incompatible blood have been given. In all instances, the first 100 ml of blood should be given under close observation. If there is evidence of hemolysis (fever, chills, sacral/low back pain, hypotension, apprehension, bleeding, hemoglobinuria), the transfusion should be stopped at once. Give 80 mg furosemide IV and initiate large IV fluid volume to increase urine flow. Obtain urinalysis and serum creatinine or BUN.

Hypothermia. These reactions (62–3) can be avoided by carefully warming the blood to room temperature before and during administration, while also warming the patient.

Overtransfusions. Serial central venous pressure determinations may be of assistance in avoiding this problem. Sumida's blood deficit nomogram (based on CVP and KgBW) may be a helpful adjunct in estimating blood replacement requirements following whole blood loss events.

Pyrogenic Reactions. Pyrogenic reactions most often are due to nonbacterial pyrogens and are characterized by malaise, chills and a rapid temperature rise of up to 40°C (104°F). Full recovery in a short time is to be expected, but the transfusion being given should be discontinued. Consider leukocyte-poor blood transfusion if there is recurrence.

Runaway Catheters. See *39–11, Foreign Bodies in the Venous System.*

Autotransfusions

Rapid bleeding of massive volumes of blood into closed compartments of the patient's body (usually the thorax or occasionally the peritoneum) can rapidly exceed the supply of bank blood, and demise may be imminent; in these situations, reprocessing of this collected blood warrants the hazards involved. A specialized system (such as a Bentley-100 Autotransfusion System) can be used to collect, filter, defoam and reinfuse the blood into the patient. Alternatively, blood is drained (also using 12 to 15 cm water suction) from the chest tubes into a 1-liter bottle containing 400 ml of normal saline and reinfused into the vein after passage through a blood administration filter that removes particles over 40 microns in size.

Autologous blood is used in the following situations: when there is acute loss of 1000 ml of blood into a satisfactory compartment (usually the chest); when massive bleeding exceeds homologous supply; and when massive bleeding and religious tenents preclude use of homologous blood. Relative contraindications are a wound that is more than 4 to 6 hours old; gross contamination of blood; known hepatic/renal insufficiency; and the presence of malignant lesions in the wound area. Complications are hematologic (mostly involving platelets, clotting factors and hemolysis), bacteremia, air embolism, microparticle embolism and potential sepsis.

*Blood Substitutes**

Basic and clinical research and early clinical trials of perfluoro (Fluosol DA), a chemical blood substitute developed in Japan, continue. In the United States, the FDA has approved limited clinical use of this substitute in patients with anemia of marked degree who refuse homologous blood transfusion on the basis of religious conviction. The current need for close proximity to a freezer and oxygen tank has limited its consideration for field use. Clinical research for use in acute MI is also being conducted.

Research and development of synthetic hemoglobin solutions are currently under way, but these substances are not anticipated to be ready for clinical use until the late 1980's.

18–36. VENOUS CANNULATION

Venous cannulation for infusions may be done at sites such as those indicated in Table 18–2, which outlines some of the advantages and disadvantages of each. The following information concerning the various venous

---

*Also referred to as "artificial blood"—although not scientific, this term is common in lay use.

Table 18–2. ADVANTAGES AND DISADVANTAGES OF VARIOUS VENOUS CANNULATION SITES

Venous Cannulation Site	Advantages	Disadvantages
A. Peripheral Vein Arm (Fig. 18–4) Saphenous (Fig. 18–5)	• Ease of technique • Administration of IV drugs during cardiac arrest without interference with CPR measures	• Difficult to find during circulatory collapse • Phlebitis and pain develop with hypertonic/irritating solutions
External Jugular Vein (Fig. 18–7)	• Ease of technique. With training and skill can also insert central catheters and guidewires into subclavian vein	• See C *(Internal Jugular Vein)* and D *(Subclavian Vein)*, below. *Note:* Injury much less likely with external jugular vein
B. Femoral Vein (Fig. 18–6)	• Does not interfere with CPR • Often can be cannulated when peripheral veins are collapsed	• If femoral artery pulse absent, may cannulate artery in error, with subsequent injury to extremity from vasopressors • Hematoma, thrombosis
C. Internal Jugular Vein (Figs. 18–7, 18–8) *D. Subclavian Vein* (Figs. 18–8, 18–9)	• Rapid access to vein and central circulation even if peripheral veins are collapsed • With internal jugular vein can see/control hematomas better than with subclavian vein; also easier to insert balloon-tipped flow-directed pulmonary artery catheter on right • Subclavian route permits more neck motion	• Damage to apical pleura with pneumothorax, plus chance of lymphatic duct and nerve damage • Hematomas can be difficult to control and hazardous if bilateral in neck (obtain chest x-ray immediately after procedure)

cannulation sites, including most diagrams, is patterned after the American Heart Association's *Textbook of Advanced Cardiac Life Support*; this publication should be consulted for further resource and references.

A. PERIPHERAL VEIN CANNULATION

Since the largest visible superficial veins of the arm are in the antecubital fossa (Fig. 18–4), these may be selected initially if the patient is in circulatory collapse. However, if accessible, preferably the more distal veins of the forearm or next, those of the dorsum of the hand, should be used. Similarly, the long saphenous vein at the medial malleolus may be used (Fig. 18–5); this has the advantage of constancy of location, and it can be entered at any point along its course. Often a point between the junction of two veins is chosen for entry, since here the vein is more stabilized and venipuncture is more easily accomplished. In infants, a scalp vein can be used.

The steps for initiating IV therapy of the arm or leg vein are as follows:

1. Apply tourniquet (TK) proximally.

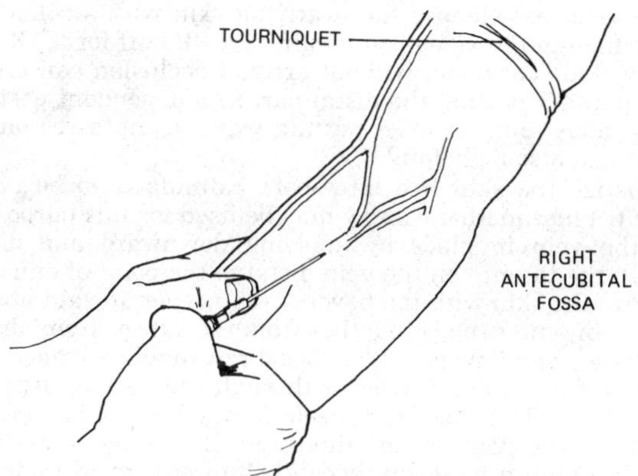

Figure 18–4. Forearm—antecubital venipuncture. (From *Textbook of Advanced Cardiac Life Support.* American Heart Association, Dallas, 1981, p. XII-4).

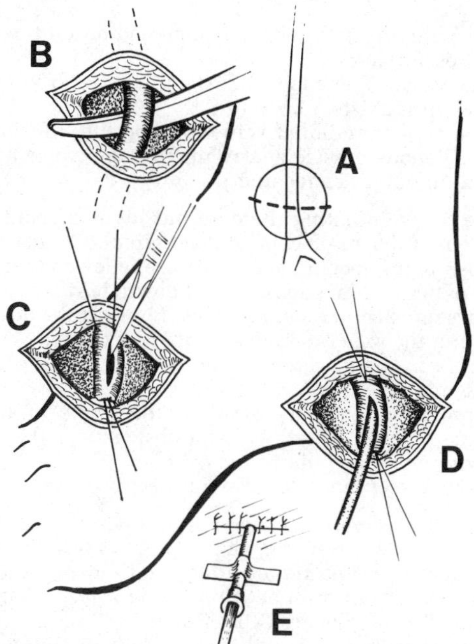

Figure 18–5. Saphenous vein "cutdown" cannulation. *A,* Make a short transverse incision through the skin proximal and lateral to the medial malleolus. *B,* Locate and isolate vein (distended by proximal tourniquet) with blunt dissection. *C,* Place distal ligation of vein and proximal loop of suture material for lifting vein and bleeding control; make longitudinal vein wall incision. Release tourniquet. *D,* Insert sterile catheter into vein lumen. Insert IV tubing into catheter. Tie proximal ligature firmly without occluding catheter. *E,* Secure catheter to skin; suture skin; apply antibacterial ointment over incision/catheter site; cover with dressing.

2. Locate vein and cleanse the overlying skin with alcohol or povidone-iodine. When finding the veins is difficult: If a BP cuff for a TK is inflated at 40 mm Hg, venous occlusion without arterial occlusion can often be better assured; temporarily putting the distal part in a dependent position, sharply patting the venous area, or even putting warm compresses on the area (if time permits) can also be helpful.

3. Anesthetize the skin if a large-bore cannula is to be inserted in an awake patient; Fluorimethane spray may be used for this purpose.

4. Hold the vein in place by applying downward and distal traction pressure (with the thumb) on the vein distal to the point of entry.

5. Puncture the skin with the bevel of the needle upward about 0.5 to 1.0 cm from the vein; enter the vein either from the side or from above.

6. Note slow, even flow of venous blood return and advance the needle or catheter intraluminally either over or through the needle, depending on the type of catheter-needle device being used. (Large-bore catheters, near the size of IV line tubing, or even IV line tubing itself—which is sterile inside and outside—put through a cutdown, accept a full stream of IV fluid.) Remove tourniquet. See *B, Femoral Vein Cannulation, Step 6,* for description of guidewire use; see also Figure 18–5.

7. Withdraw and remove the needle and attach the infusion tubing.

8. Secure the catheter with a loop of tape just distal to the hub, and tape to the skin.

9. Cover the puncture site with povidone-iodine ointment and a sterile dressing. Tape dressing in place.

10. Usually a second IV line is established, particularly if shock is present or if the potential for it exists.

11. At times, a well-cannulated vein will stop the infusion of fluid for no apparent reason. Venous muscle spasm may be the cause and is relieved by infusion of 1 to 2 ml of 0.5% lidocaine.

The procedure for cannulating the external jugular vein is similar to that for peripheral veins (above), except that no circular tourniquet is used and the following positioning recommendations are followed (see also Fig. 18–7):

1. Place the patient in a supine, head-down position to fill the visible external jugular vein; turn the patient's head toward the opposite side.

2. After cleaning the skin (and anesthetizing if patient is conscious), align the needle-cannula in the direction of the vein with the point aimed toward the ipsilateral shoulder.

3. Make venipuncture midway between the angle of the jaw and the midclavicular line, "tourniqueting" (distal obstruction) the vein by applying light pressure with one finger above the clavicle.

4. Proceed as with technique for arm and leg, above.

The steps for cannulation of a scalp vein in infants are as follows:

1. Shave the scalp over a major vein, apply a circumferential headband (forehead to occiput) for tourniquet effect and cleanse the skin as above. *Caution:* Differentiate vein from accompanying artery; scalp location for IV is generally unsatisfactory during CPR efforts.

2. Stretch skin overlying vein and identify flow direction for needle insertion.

3. After checking to ensure patency, insert butterfly needle, bevel up, into vein until blood flows freely into tubing. Release headband tourniquet. Secure needle with tape applied to skin coated with tincture of benzoin. Evacuate any air in tubing and connect infusion.

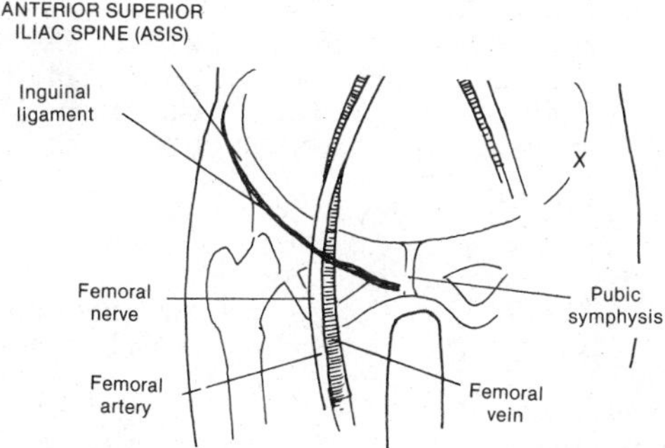

Figure 18–6. Anatomy of femoral vein, which lies medial to femoral artery, below inguinal ligament. (Modified from *Textbook of Advanced Cardiac Life Support*. American Heart Association, Dallas, 1981, p. XII-6.)

B. FEMORAL VEIN CANNULATION (See Fig. 18–6)

Cannulation techniques are similar to those outlined for peripheral veins, with these additional comments:

1. The region may have to be shaved for aseptic technique.
2. Anesthetize the injection site with lidocaine if the patient is awake.
3. Make the puncture with the needle (attached to a 10-ml syringe) medial to the palpated femoral artery pulsations (felt midway between the anterior superior iliac spine (ASIS) and pubic symphysis) about two fingerbreadths below the inguinal ligament in an adult (one fingerbreadth in infants), directing the needle cephalad at a 45° angle with the skin until the needle will go no further. (*Note:* Some prefer to enter at a 90° angle.)
4. Maintain suction on the syringe and pull the needle back slowly until blood appearing in the syringe indicates the vein lumen has been entered.
5. Lower the needle more parallel to the frontal plane, remove the syringe and insert the catheter.
6. An alternative to Step 5, particularly used in pediatric patients, is as follows: A guidewire is placed into the needle and the needle is properly advanced into the vein, as described above. A small incision is then made in the skin around the needle, using a #11 blade. While placing gentle pressure on the groin, remove the needle, leaving the wire in place. A catheter or introducer is then advanced over the guidewire, using a twisting motion as it enters the vein. Next, the guidewire is removed, all air is carefully evacuated, an infusion set is attached and the catheter is taped securely.

C. INTERNAL JUGULAR VEIN CANNULATION (After AHA)

Specific Indications for Internal Jugular and Subclavian Venipuncture

Since the internal jugular and subclavian veins remain patent when peripheral veins are collapsed, their cannulation allows emergency access to the venous circulation when IV therapy is urgently required. Cannulation of these veins is also used to gain access to the central circulation for measurement of central venous pressure (CVP; see *18–7*), for administration of hypertonic or irritating solutions, and for passing catheters into the heart and pulmonary circulation.

Anatomy: Internal Jugular Vein (Figs. 18–7, 18–8)

The internal jugular vein emerges from the base of the skull, enters the carotid sheath posterior to the internal carotid artery, and runs posteriorly and laterally to the internal and common carotid artery. Finally, near its termination, the internal jugular vein is lateral and slightly anterior to the common carotid artery.

The internal jugular vein runs medial to the sternomastoid muscle in its upper part, posterior to it in the triangle between the two inferior heads of the sternomastoid in its middle part, and behind the anterior portion of the clavicular head of the muscle in its lower part, where it ends just above the medial end of the clavicle by being joined by the subclavian vein.

Technique: General Principles (Internal Jugular and Subclavian Veins)

The steps for initiating IV therapy of the internal jugular and subclavian veins follow:

1. A needle at least 6 cm long with a 16-gauge catheter at least 15 to 20 cm long is usually selected for the adult. (For pediatric equipment, see data in Table 18–3.) If the catheter is to be inserted through the needle, the needle must be 14-gauge. If the Seldinger technique is employed, a thin wall 18-gauge needle will accept a standard guidewire. (See guidewire technique under *B, Femoral Vein Cannulation, Step* 6.)
2. Determine the depth of catheter placement by measuring from the point of insertion to the following surface markers on the chest wall (Fig. 18–8).
3. Place the tip of the catheter above the right atrium for administration of fluids.
4. Cleanse the area around the site of puncture with povidone-iodine and drape it as for any surgical procedure. Wear sterile gloves. Ideally, a face mask and a hair cover should be worn as well.
5. If the patient is awake, infiltrate the skin with lidocaine.

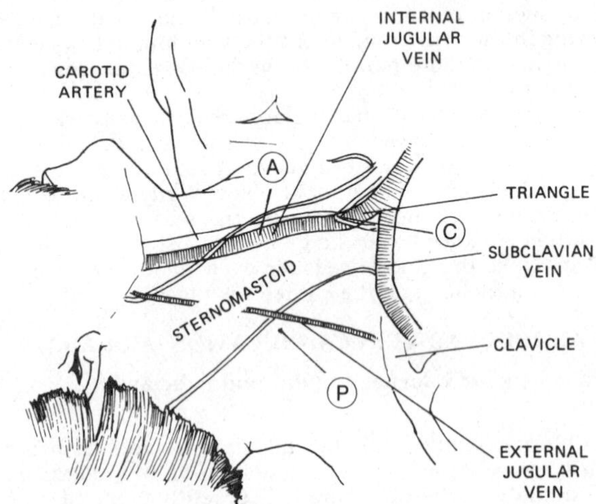

Figure 18–7. Anatomy of internal jugular vein and three sites for cannulation: *P,* posterior; *C,* central; and *A,* anterior (push the anterior border of sternomastoid muscle posteriorly to expose the vein). (See also Fig. 18–9.) (Modified from *Textbook of Advanced Cardiac Life Support.* American Heart Association, Dallas, 1981, p. XII-7.)

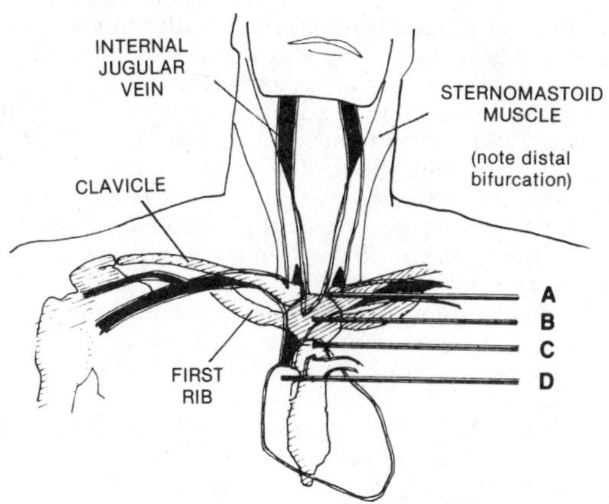

Figure 18–8. Anatomy of chest wall, with surface markers shown to determine depth of catheter placement: *A*, sternoclavicular joint–subclavian vein; *B*, midmanubrial area–brachiocephalic vein; *C*, manubrial-sternal junction–superior vena cava; *D*, 5 cm below manubrial-sternal junction–right atrium. (Modified from *Textbook of Advanced Cardiac Life Support*. American Heart Association, Dallas, 1981, p. XII-8.)

6. Mount the needle on a 5- or 10-ml syringe containing 0.5 to 1.0 ml saline solution or lidocaine. After the skin as been punctured with the bevel of the needle upward, flush the needle to remove an occasional skin plug.

7. Place the patient in a supine, head-down position (Trendelenberg) of at least 15° to distend the veins and reduce the chance of air embolism. Extend the patient's head and turn it away from the side of venipuncture. (*Note:* The neck may be further hyperextended by placement of a towel roll under the shoulders. An assistant is necessary for restraining when the procedure is performed in infants and children.)

8. As the needle is slowly advanced, maintain negative pressure on the syringe. As soon as the lumen of the vein is entered, blood will appear in the syringe; advance the needle a few millimeters further to obtain a free flow of blood. *Rapid spontaneous backward movement of the plunger and the appearance of bright red blood indicates that an artery has been entered. Completely remove the cannula and apply pressure, to the puncture site for at least 10 minutes.*

9. Occasionally, the vein will not be entered despite the fact that the needle has been inserted to the appropriate depth. Maintain negative pressure on the syringe and slowly withdraw the needle; blood may suddenly appear in the syringe, indicating that the needle is now in the lumen of the vein. If no blood appears, completely remove the needle and reinsert it, directing it at a slightly different angle depending on the site of venipuncture.

10. Remove the syringe from the needle, with the finger occluding the needle to prevent air embolism. (A 5-cm water pressure difference across a 14-gauge needle will allow the introduction of approximately 100 ml of air per second.) If the patient is breathing spontaneously, remove the syringe during exhalation. If the patient is being artificially ventilated either with a bag-valve unit or with a mechanical ventilator, remove the syringe during the inspiratory (positive pressure) cycle. Quickly insert the catheter or guide-wire through the needle to a predetermined point and remove the needle.

11. If the catheter is inserted through the needle, *never pull the catheter backward through the needle*, as the sharp end may shear off the tip of the catheter, producing a catheter-fragment embolus.

12. It is occasionally impossible to advance the plastic catheter despite the fact that the needle tip is within the vein. Since the catheter must not be withdrawn through the needle, the needle and the catheter must be removed together and the venipuncture attempted again. The use of the flexible straight or J-tipped guidewire should eliminate this problem. Insert the guidewire through the needle into the vein. If the guidewire does not pass freely into the vein, remove the guidewire, attach the syringe and, while maintaining negative pressure on the syringe, reposition the needle until it is in the vein; remove the syringe and insert the guidewire once again. If the guidewire passes freely into the vein, remove the needle and then pass the catheter over the guidewire into the vein.

13. Where feasible, affix the catheter to the skin with a suture, making certain that the catheter is not compressed by the suture.

14. Attach infusion set to the catheter, but do not start the infusion. Lower the IV reservoir below head level. When blood backs up freely into the IV tubing, start the infusion. If blood is not visible in the tubing, assume the catheter is not in the vessel and adjust.

15. Apply povidone-iodine ointment and sterile gauze to the puncture site and tape the catheter in place.

Technique: Internal Jugular Vein

The right side of the neck is preferred for venipuncture for three reasons:

1. The dome of the right lung and pleura is lower than the left.
2. There is more or less a straight line to the atrium.
3. The large thoracic duct is not endangered. Three alternate approaches will be described: posterior, central, and anterior. In trained hands, each is an effective means to cannulate the internal jugular vein. The route chosen depends upon the experience and the preference of the operator. In general, the central approach is the easiest to learn and to teach. The following three approaches assume that the patient is in the supine, head-down (Trendelenburg) position as described above.

Posterior Approach. The steps for initiating the posterior approach to internal jugular cannulation follow (Fig. 18–7):

1. Introduce the needle under the sternomastoid muscle near the junction of the middle and lower thirds of the lateral (posterior) border (5 cm above the clavicle or just above the point where the external jugular vein crosses the sternomastoid muscle).
2. Aim the needle caudally and ventrally (anteriorly) toward the suprasternal notch at an angle of 45° to the sagittal and horizontal planes and with 15° forward angulation in the frontal plane.
3. The vein should be entered within 5 to 7 cm.

Central Approach. The steps for initiating the central approach to internal jugular cannulation follow (Fig. 18–7):

1. Locate by observation and palpation the triangle formed by the two heads (sternal and clavicular) of the sternomastoid muscle and the clavicle. It may be helpful to have the awake patient lift his head slightly off the bed to make the triangle more visible. In some patients with large or obese necks, it may be difficult to identify the triangle. Palpate the suprasternal notch and slowly move laterally, locating first the sternal head of the sternomastoid muscle, the clavicle, the triangle itself, and finally, the clavicular head of the sternomastoid muscle.

2. Occasionally the carotid arterial pulse will be palpable within the triangle. Place two fingers along the artery and retract it medially. This maneuver identifies both the location of the artery (so that inadvertent puncture is avoided) and the position of the internal jugular vein, which is lateral to the artery.

3. Insert the needle at the apex of the triangle formed by the two heads of the sternomastoid muscle and the clavicle.

4. Direct the needle caudally and laterally, parallel to the medial border of the clavicular head of the sternomastoid muscle toward the ipsilateral nipple at a 45° to 60° angle with the frontal plane.

5. If the vein is not entered after the needle has been inserted a few centimeters, slowly withdraw the needle, maintaining a negative pressure on the syringe. If the vein is still not entered, withdraw the needle completely; reinsert it, directing it 5° to 10° more in the lateral direction. If still unable to enter the vein, direct the needle more in line with the sagittal plane. However, do not direct the needle medially (across the sagittal plane), since the carotid artery will be punctured.

Central Approach for Newborns and Infants. In newborns and infants the "high" central approach appears safer. Catheters can be introduced as above either by the Seldinger technique or with a through-the-needle catheter. With the Seldinger technique the appropriate sizes for cannulation devices are as noted in Table 18–3.

Table 18–3. PEDIATRIC VENOUS CANNULATION EQUIPMENT

Age, yr	Equipment
<2	Steel needle—thin walled 21-gauge Guidewire—0.018 in Catheter—3.0 F Teflon
>2	Steel needle—thin-walled 20-gauge Guidewire—0.021 in Catheter—4.0 F Teflon
With the catheter through-the-needle technique the appropriate sizes are:	
<2	Catheter (19-gauge) with 17-gauge needle
>2	Catheter (16-gauge) with 14-gauge needle

After the vein has been entered, remove the syringe and advance the catheter as previously described.

Great care must be taken with the catheter through-the-needle technique not to withdraw the catheter through the needle, causing it to shear off and act as an embolus. If difficulty is encountered in advancing the catheter, the entire assembly—needle and catheter—should be withdrawn as a unit and another insertion attempt made.

Anterior Approach. The steps for initiating the anterior approach to internal jugular cannulation follow (Fig. 18–7):

1. Place the left index and middle fingers (if from the right side) on the carotid artery and retract it medially away from the anterior border of the sternomastoid muscle.

2. Introduce the needle between the index and middle fingers at the

midpoint of this anterior border (5 cm above the clavicle and 5 cm below the angle of the mandible).

3. Forming a posterior angle of 30° to 45° with the frontal plane, direct the needle caudally toward the ipsilateral nipple and toward the junction of the middle and medial thirds of the clavicle.

Anatomy: Subclavian Vein (See Fig. 18–9)

The subclavian vein, which in the adult is approximately 3 to 4 cm long and 1 to 2 cm in diameter, begins as a continuation of the axillary vein at the lateral border of the first rib, crosses over the first rib, and passes in front of the anterior scalene muscle. The anterior scalene muscle is approximately 10 to 15 mm thick and separates the subclavian vein from the subclavian artery, which runs behind the anterior scalene muscle. The vein continues behind the medial third of the clavicle, where it is immobilized by small attachments to the rib and clavicle. At the medial border of the anterior scalene muscle and behind the sternocostoclavicular joint, the subclavian unites with the internal jugular to form the innominate, or brachiocephalic, vein. The large thoracic duct on the left and the smaller lymphatic duct on the right enter the superior margin of the subclavian vein near the internal jugular junction. On the right, the brachiocephalic vein descends behind the right lateral edge of the manubrium, where it is joined by the left brachiocephalic vein which crosses over behind the manubrium. On the right side, near the sternal-manubrial joint, the two veins join together to form the superior vena cava. Medial to the anterior scalene muscle, the phrenic nerve, the internal mammary artery, and the apical pleura are in contact with the posteroinferior side of the subclavian vein and the jugulosubclavian junction. In a sagittal section through the medial third of the clavicle, both the apical pleura and the subclavian artery can be seen immediately posterior to the subclavian vein (Fig. 18–9).

Subclavian Vein Cannulation in Newborns and Infants

Catheterization of the subclavian vein in newborns and infants, although described in the pediatric literature, carries such a high risk of complication that it cannot be recommended except under unusual circumstances.

Techniques: Subclavian Vein

For general principles of technique, see above, under *Internal Jugular Vein*.

Two approaches for cannulation of the subclavian vein will be described: the direct intraclavicular subclavian puncture, and indirect cannulation of the subclavian vein via the external jugular vein with a guidewire.

Direct Technique: Infraclavicular Subclavian Approach. The steps for initiating the direct intraclavicular subclavian puncture follow (Fig. 18–9):

1. The patient must be in a supine, head-down position of at least 15°.
2. Introduce the needle 1 cm below the junction of the middle and medial thirds of the clavicle.
3. Hold the syringe and needle parallel to the frontal plane (the plane of the back of the patient).
4. Direct the needle medially and slightly cephalad, behind the clavicle toward the posterior-superior aspect of the sternal end of the clavicle.
5. Establish a good point of reference by firmly pressing the fingertip into the suprasternal notch to locate the deep side of the superior aspect of the clavicle, and direct the course of the needle slightly behind the fingertip.
6. Once the lumen of the vein has been entered, rotate the bevel of the

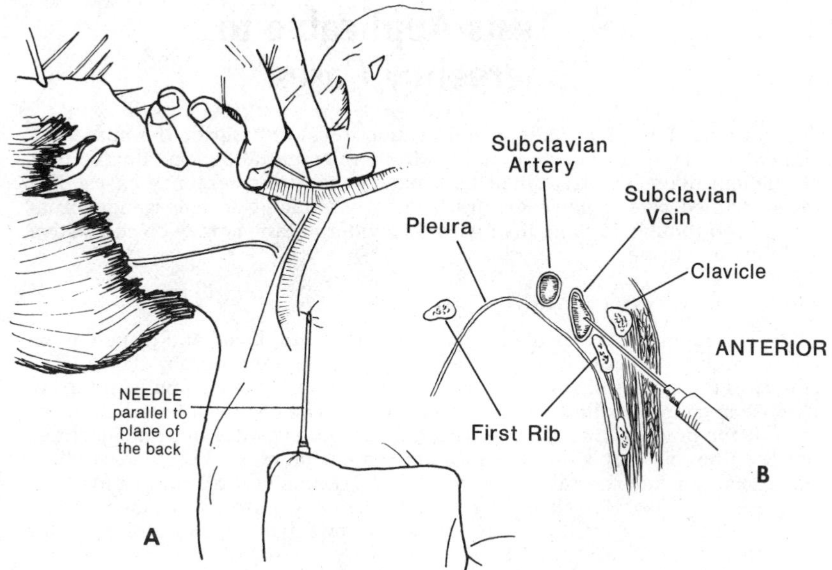

Figure 18–9. *A,* Infraclavicular subclavian venipuncture. *B,* In sagittal section through the medial third of clavicle (right), both apical pleura and subclavian artery can be seen immediately posterior to subclavian vein. (*A* modified from *Textbook of Advanced Cardiac Life Support.* American Heart Association, Dallas, 1981, p. XII-10; *B* Redrawn from Davidson et al.: Lancet, 2:1140, 1963. Used by permission.)

needle caudally and clockwise 90°, thus facilitating the downward turn that the catheter must negotiate into the brachiocephalic vein.

Indirect Technique: Cannulation of Subclavian Vein via the External Jugular Vein With a J-Wire. The steps for initiating indirect cannulation of the subclavian vein by way of the external jugular vein with a guidewire follow:

1. Prepare the patient and make the venipuncture into the external jugular vein as described previously. Use a needle through which the J-wire will pass.
2. Insert a flexible J-tipped wire that fits through both the needle and the catheter (this should be tested before the venipuncture is done) and advance the J-wire into the external jugular and subclavian veins. Gentle manipulation may be necessary to pass the device through venous valves and tortuous vessels. At no time should the wire be forced.
3. With several centimeters of wire still protruding from the distal end of the needle, remove the needle from the vein. Hold the wire near the skin insertion site as soon as it appears, to prevent the wire from being inadvertently pulled out of the vein.
4. Make a small skin incision with a scalpel to facilitate insertion of the catheter through the skin.
5. Slide the catheter over the wire up to the point of insertion. Make certain that several centimeters of wire are protruding from the other end of the catheter. Slowly advance the catheter and the wire into the vein. As soon as the catheter is in place, remove the wire.
6. Affix the catheter, and dress the insertion site as previously described.

19. Tests Applicable to Emergency Cases

No attempt has been made in this section to list or describe the numerous clinical and laboratory tests that constitute an essential and invaluable part of efficient diagnosis, treatment and management of emergency cases. The tests outlined below, however, are peculiarly valuable in emergency situations, even though in some instances their interpretations may be suggestive and not conclusive.

19–1. ALCOHOL INTOXICATION TESTS

Measurements of the alcohol content of the breath, blood and urine can be made without difficulty and are of approximately equal accuracy. The admissibility of the results of chemical tests for alcohol as evidence and its interpretive use in courts is still a source of controversy. The results of breath analysis tests at the present time are not accepted as legal evidence in some localities but may be of great value to law enforcement officers. Where admissible, their accuracy and the validity of their interpretation are still subject to cross-examination. Tests for alcohol content of the breath are often made by law enforcement officers without any signed authorization. Drawing of blood for determination of the alcohol level requires a signed and witnessed authorization (*69–2*). In many localities, refusal to submit to a breath, blood or urine alcohol test results in automatic revocation of the license to operate a motor vehicle. Audiovisual documentation of speech, behavior and coordination is also being performed.

BREATH ANALYSIS

Various modifications of breath analyzers are used: the Breathanalyzer (Borkenstein), the Drunkometer (Harger), the Intoximeter (Forrester) and the Alcometer (Greenberg). All four types depend upon the analysis of expired alveolar air collected in a plastic or rubber balloon. Breath forced into the balloon is generally considered to contain 5/8 alveolar air and 3/8 corridor air (from the nares, mouth and nasopharynx). Since the alveolar air–blood ratio for alcohol is known (about 1:21000) and the alveolar air contains about 5.5% carbon dioxide, by weighing the amount of carbon dioxide and determining the amount of alcohol in a given specimen, the blood alcohol concentration can be determined very accurately.

BLOOD ANALYSIS

- A semiquantitative and qualitative test for presence of alcohol has been developed using a "dip stick" that has adequate specificity and sensitivity for *clinical* purposes and should soon be commercially available.
- All other tests for alcohol in the blood depend upon a complex chemical analysis of blood obtained from a vein by a technique that avoids possible contamination with alcohol from outside sources.
- Interpretation of the results of blood alcohol tests is given in Table 19–1.

Method of Obtaining Blood Specimen

- On request of a patient, his or her legal guardian or a law enforcement officer, blood may be drawn by a physician for blood alcohol determination,

Table 19–1. INTERPRETATION OF RESULTS OF BLOOD ALCOHOL TESTS

Per Cent Alcohol in Blood (by weight)	Mg of Alcohol per 100 ml of Blood	Clinical Effect (Average)	Slowing of Reaction Time (Average)	Legal Interpretation: Under Influence of Alcohol?*
0.01 to 0.05	10 mg/100 ml 50 mg/100 ml	None	Possibly slight	No
0.06 to 0.10	60 mg/100 ml 100 mg/100 ml	Decreased coordination and visual fields, blurred vision, impaired control and restraint, euphoria, slurred speech, impairment of special senses	2 ×	Possibly
0.11 to 0.30	110 mg/100 ml 300 mg/100 ml	Staggering, mental confusion, stupor	4 ×	Definitely
0.31 to 0.45	310 mg/100 ml 450 mg/100 ml	Respiratory and circulatory impairment, subnormal temperature, coma, sometimes death	Total loss	Completely
0.46 up	460 mg/100 ml	Complete respiratory and circulatory paralysis, death†	Total loss	Completely, often terminally

*The constitutional applicability of blood alcohol levels in determining intoxication was recently reevaluated in some courts and found valid in final analysis.

†Lethal dose is 5–8 g/kg in adults; approx. 3 g/kg in children.

provided the permission of the patient or the legal guardian is obtained in writing without misrepresentation or coercion. For a satisfactory permit form, see 69–2. Before the permission is signed, the patient or guardian should be informed in simple nontechnical language of the purpose of the test. It is the physician's responsibility to determine that the patient is sufficiently in possession of his or her faculties at the time of signature to understand the reason for, purpose of and possible consequence of the test. Tacit permission for withdrawal of blood for the test is assumed if the patient, after having been given this information, makes no active attempt to prevent completion of the procedure.

- No alcohol, or substance containing alcohol, should be used in cleansing the skin.
- Syringes, needles and vials used in collecting the blood specimen must have been sterilized by a nonalcohol technique.
- Special containers, marked for identification, must be used. These should be labeled carefully for identification and initiated by at least two witnesses before being sent to the laboratory for analysis.
- The exact time that the specimen is taken should be indicated on the container.

CLINICAL EXAMINATION FOR ALCOHOL INTOXICATION

History and Habits

- Occupation. (Deep-sea or sports divers, caisson workers, those exposed to narcotic or inebriating gases at work, and others working under certain conditions may show symptoms characteristic of alcoholism, thereby confusing the issue.)
- Injuries or diseases that might modify interpretation of results of tests.
- Medications, especially narcotics, hypnotics, sedatives, mood modifiers, muscle relaxants and antihistaminics.
- Consumption of alcoholic beverages: Does patient have the habit of daily or periodic drinking? What is the average daily amount consumed?
- Time, kind and amount of last drink.
- Treatment in past for acute or chronic alcoholism, delirium tremens, addictions to any substances or neuropsychiatric complaints.

Physical Examination

A fair and accurate conclusion regarding alcohol intoxication requires comparison of the original examination findings with the results of previous examination or of reexamination several hours later, preferably by the same physician. Presence of any of the following signs should be noted:

- Odor of alcoholic beverages on the breath. In spite of the claims of the manufacturers of various proprietary compounds, this odor cannot be masked completely by any known method.
- Red ("bloodshot") or watery eyes.
- Impairment of speech (indistinctness, slurring)—test for by having person recite alphabet rapidly.
- Unbuttoned, stained, unclean or disarrayed clothing.
- Evidence of vomiting, bowel or bladder incontinence or seminal emission.
- Mental alertness and attitude (euphoria, sullenness, belligerence, depression, etc.).
- Evidence of recent trauma—especially head injuries (*44*).
- Impairment of muscular coordination:

  Gait—broad base, straddling, unsteady.

  Balance—ability to walk a straight line and to execute rapid turns.

  Joint sense—finger to nose or ear, foot to opposite knee, and so forth. Have person touch thumb tip to each finger tip rapidly in succession.

  Specialized motions—picking up pins or coins; comparison of person's handwriting with previous or subsequent samples.
- Evidence of unrelated injuries or of local or systemic conditions that could be mistaken for alcoholic intoxication.

Raising and Lowering of Blood Alcohol Levels

- 1 ml/kg of 50% (100 proof) ethyl alcohol will raise the blood alcohol level by 50 mg% in 2 hours.
- In a 75-kg adult, blood alcohol level rises by 25 mg% after consumption of any one of the following: 1-oz (30 ml) of whiskey; a 6-oz glass of wine; a 12-oz container of beer.
- In a normal 75-kg adult, blood alcohol level *decreases* by 10 to 35 mg% per hour (avg = 15 mg%/h).

Modifying Factors

The amount of alcohol necessary to produce the different stages of intoxication just outlined may be modified by:

- Individual sensitivity (constitutional tolerance, age, sex).
- Acquired tolerance from habitual intake.
- Mental condition.
- Environment and circumstances (climate, temperature, exercise, type of work).
- Diet—recent intake of food.
- Medications (extremely important!).
- Unrelated organic disease, including metabolic disturbances, such as diabetic hypoglycemia, acidosis, uremia, effects of increased barometric pressure, etc.; pulmonary diseases, such as emphysema with carbon dioxide retention; myocardial infarction; angina pectoris; hypertension; senility; postsurgical and postanesthetic reactions; intracranial disease.

19–2. BLOOD, TESTS FOR PRESENCE OF

Blood from the gastrointestinal (GI) tract is suspected by gross appearance if there is reddish or black coffeeground emesis and if the feces have a tarry appearance. Confirmation of gross or occult blood is made by the benzidine test.

Blood in the urine has a reddish appearance if from gross bleeding; in the case of hemolysis, the urine is brownish. The benzidine test will confirm the presence of hemoglobin. Among commercial reagent strips for blood detection are Hemastix, Labstix and Multistix.

19–3. DOPPLER TEST

The Doppler ultrasound device is available in a portable unit practical for use in ambulances or emergency departments to evaluate arterial pulsation, flow rates, pressures and location when clinical assessment is difficult. Blood pressure can be determined in noisy locations, and the efficacy of CPR (5) and the extent of arterial injury can be more easily assessed. Detection of persistence of arterial flow in the scrotum helps in distinguishing epididymitis from testicular torsion and helps in evaluating whether to continue nonsurgical or surgical methods for treatment of early compartment syndromes. It is also of valuable assistance in determining the presence of fetal heart tones.

19–4. FIBRINOGEN COAGULATION TEST

A bedside test can aid in estimation of the blood fibrinogen level and the extent of fibrinolysis. Failure of a clot to form in a test tube within 15 minutes is indicative of critical fibrinogen shortage or fibrinolysis. Normally, a formed clot continues to contract and become firmer; disintegration of the initial clot in 30 to 60 minutes is abnormal, and quantitative tests for fibrinogen and fibrin split products should be obtained.

19–5. NARCOTIC ADDICTION TEST

For clinical signs of addiction, see 7–4.

For signs and symptoms of acute intoxication from overdosage, see *53–340, Heroin*, and *53–455, Morphine*.

Naloxone Hydrochloride (Narcan) Test

1. Have the patient (or patient's legal guardian if he or she is a minor or mentally incompetent) give written permission for the test in the presence of two witnesses. The permission form must include a statement that the purpose of the test has been explained to, and is understood by, the signer and that no coercion has been used in obtaining the signed permission.

2. Measure the size of the patient's pupils, using a piece of cardboard pierced or marked in 0.5-mm gradations from 0.5 mm to 3 mm.
3. Inject 0.4 mg naloxone hydrochloride (Narcan) IV or IM, having means at hand for combating sudden severe withdrawal symptoms (step 6 below).
4. Wait 10 minutes.
5. Remeasure the size of the pupils with exactly the same amount of light present as in step 2.
6. Treat withdrawal symptoms if necessary by subcutaneous or intravenous injection of an effective amount of morphine sulfate.
7. Interpret the results of the test as follows:

Pupillary Size	Using Addictive Narcotics?
Decreased	No
No change	Occasionally (or normally has small pupils)
Increased	Yes (addict)

19–6. OPIUM DERIVATIVES TEST

For therapeutic or medicolegal reasons, rapid identification of drugs found on an emergency patient may be important. Opium and its narcotic derivatives (heroin, hydromorphone and morphine) may be identified as follows:
1. Place a drop of concentrated nitric acid on a glass slide or in an evaporating dish.
2. Scrape a few particles from the suspect tablet into the acid.
The formation of a cherry-red color indicates the probable presence of a derivative of opium. Synthetic nonopiate narcotics show no characteristic color change. The results of this test should always be confirmed by a qualified laboratory.

19–7. SALICYLATE INGESTION TEST

Because of the delay in the development of signs and symptoms, such as hyperpnea, after ingestion of salicylates and because of the too frequent uncertainty on the part of parents as to what their child may have swallowed, the following simple, rapid test is of value for emergency use:
1. Heat a specimen of urine gently to rule out presence of acetone bodies.
2. To 5 ml of urine add 1 ml of 10% ferric chloride solution.
3. Shake gently and observe the color. Development of a purple color indicates presence of acetylsalicylic acid (aspirin), methyl, phenyl or sodium salicylate or phenol derivatives.
Presence of a purple color will indicate the ingestion of as little as one 0.3-g aspirin tablet between 30 minutes and 12 hours before examination. The test is not quantitative.

19–8. SEMINAL FLUID TEST

This test is essential for complete examination for rape *(14)* and is based on the presence of acid phosphatase in seminal fluid. The test should be done on intravaginal specimens and on dried secretions on the vulva and upper thighs.

Technique

1. To a solution of the suspect material add 2 drops of a solution of sodium alpha naphthol phosphate.

2. Add 1 or 2 drops of naphthanil diazoblue B.

A characteristic purple color indicates the presence of acid phosphatase and is considered as legal evidence of the presence of seminal fluid; usually these tests are done by the laboratory.

19–9. VENTILATION TEST (Snider)

As an index of expiratory volume and flow rate, the following match test is of value in estimating changes in respiratory physiology in potentially progressive conditions if a spirometer is not available.

1. Have the patient remove dentures if present.
2. Hold a lighted half-burned book-type match 6 inches from patient's mouth.
3. Instruct the patient to blow out the match. (Several positions should be used to compensate for facial weaknesses, etc.)
4. Inability to blow out the flame indicates a forced expiratory volume of less than 1000 ml and a flow rate of less than 120 liters per minute.

Another index of ventilation is the ability to breathe through the nose with the mouth closed. This is generally indicative of a satisfactory tidal air level.

Most emergency rooms have small portable spirometers to measure tidal air, vital capacity, PEFR (peak expiratory flow rate) or FEV_1 (forced expiratory volume in 1 second), and these should be used when available.

20. Tetanus Immunization*

Because of the omnipresence of durable tetanus bacterial spores, and because the overall mortality from established generalized tetanus *(33–68)* remains near 50%, protective measures should be undertaken immediately following soft tissue injuries, beginning with as efficient a wound toilet as possible (see *59–1, Soft Tissue Trauma)* and proceeding with active or passive tetanus immunization, or both. Failure of the physician to institute proper protective and therapeutic measures at once may be actionable *(71–1)*. Many cases of active tetanus follow minute or unrecognized breaks in the skin and occur in children and elderly persons. Even older wounds may appear insignificant, as tetanus organisms are not pyogenic.

20–1. CONDITIONS REQUIRING IMMUNOLOGIC PROTECTION AGAINST TETANUS (Tetanus-prone Wounds)

All wounds in which the protective skin is penetrated require immunologic protection against tetanus. The following are examples of such injuries:

- All penetrating wounds *(59–27)* and all puncture wounds, even if minute.
- All animal, bat, snake or spider bites *(27)*.
- All open (compound) fractures *(47–6)*.
- All wounds that are deep, crushing or grossly contaminated with dirt, dust or soil, especially if possible contamination with animal excreta is present.
- All friction and pavement burns *(28–16)*.
- All cold injuries with local necrosis *(62–2)*.
- All gunshot wounds *(59–9)*.
- All penetrating injuries involving the central nervous system.

---

*See also *16, Serum Sensitivity and Desensitization*, and *33–68, Tetanus*.

- All wounds (including minute abrasions and lacerations) in which firearms or explosives of any type (dynamite, fireworks, gunpowder, cap pistol ammunition) may have been factors.
- All wounds with necrosis due to vascular insufficiency, including decubitus and stasis ulcers.
- All wounds in which adequate debridement (*59–1*) has not been possible because it would involve sacrifice of essential structures (nerves, major blood vessels, tendons, joint cartilages, etc.) or in which complete obliteration of dead spaces has not been accomplished.
- All home or other nonhospital deliveries in which the umbilical cord has been severed under unsterile conditions.
- All wounds for which treatment has been neglected, inadequate or delayed beyond 24 hours.

20–2. INDICATIONS FOR USE OF HUMAN TETANUS-IMMUNE GLOBULIN (TIG) (Passive Protection)

Table 20–1 gives indications for passive immunization with human tetanus-immune globulin (TIG), which has supplanted equine antitoxin, unless TIG is unavailable, in patients in whom active immunization is not current and complete. A complete initial active tetanus immunization series is considered to be two or three toxoid injections at 2-month intervals followed by a booster in 8 to 12 months.

A history given by the patient of "tetanus shots" may mean only a prior skin test or an injection of antitoxin given for temporary passive protection following an injury, or both of these measures.

Immediate TIG protection is required following injury and possible or actual

Table 20–1. TETANUS IMMUNIZATION SCHEDULE

	Clean Minor Wounds		All Other Wounds	
Previous Immunization*	*Tetanus-Diphtheria Toxoid*	*Tetanus Immune Globulin*	*Tetanus-Diphtheria Toxoid*	*Tetanus Immune Globulin*
No previous immunization or uncertain	Yes†	No‡	Yes†	Yes
One previous injection of T or D, T or D, T, P	Yes†	No‡	Yes†	Yes, if > 24 hr
Two previous injections of T or D, T or D, T, P	Yes†	No	Yes†	Yes
Three or more previous injections of T or D, T or D. T. P.	No§	No	No‖	No

*T = tetanus toxoid; D = diphtheria toxoid; P = pertussis vaccine.

†The series should be completed. See diphtheria toxoid comment, *20–3*.

‡Even though a wound appears clean and minor when seen by a physician, it does not assure that it will stay that way—consider also the patient's activities, occupation and general hygiene. In patients with no, or uncertain, active tetanus immunization, it may be wise to consider defining a "clean minor wound" in the context of a clean sterile needle penetrating cleansed skin (a healthy immune reaction system also being present); the usual concepts of a clean minor wound prevail in other situations.

§Unless more than 10 years have elapsed since the last booster.

‖Unless more than 5 years have elapsed since the last booster.

(Modified from *Morbidity and Mortality*, *30*(33):420, 1981.

contamination in unprotected individuals. Since passive protection from TIG lasts for a limited time only (probably not adequately effective after 21 days), further injections may be necessary if a grossly infected, tetanus-prone wound remains present despite debridement. In addition, benzathine penicillin G (Bicillin), 1,200,000 units intramuscularly for 5 days, or oxytetracycline (Terramycin), 1 to 2 g orally for 7 to 10 days, may be indicated in prophylaxis; if shock is present, intravenous antibiotic administration is preferable.

Human tetanus-immune globulin should always be given intramuscularly. The dose, *which is not age or weight related,* is 250 units under usual circumstances and up to 500 units for treatment of more contaminated wounds or wounds plus shock. With massive contaminated wounds, a several-fold increase in TIG dosage is advisable. No intradermal, ophthalmic or other tests for sensitivity are required before an injection of TIG. Anaphylactic and allergic reactions are rare, but if they do occur, they should be treated as outlined in *24, Allergic Reactions.*

Active immunization should be begun or continued, the tetanus toxoid being given in a different extremity from the TIG, with specific instructions to the patient regarding completion of the series.

Use of TIG in active or suspected tetanus is discussed in *33–68.*

20–3. INDICATIONS FOR USE OF TETANUS TOXOID (Active Protection)

An injection of 0.5 ml of tetanus toxoid, preferably alum-precipitated and usually combined with diphtheria toxoid (unless patient is allergic to diphtheria toxoid, or if immunization is current), should be given IM as indicated in Table 20–1.

20–4. INDICATIONS FOR USE OF EQUINE OR BOVINE TETANUS ANTITOXIN

Equine and bovine antitoxins are rarely used now and only when human TIG is not available. Preliminary serum sensitivity testing *(16)* is required, and desensitization is necessary if a reaction is present. Allergic reactions *(24)* are common. The total dose of equine tetanus antitoxin is 3000 to 5000 units IM.

If injections of TIG and toxoid are given at the same visit, different extremities should be used, i.e., arm and opposite thigh.

21. X-Rays and Other Imagery

21–1. INDICATIONS

A surprisingly large percentage of injury cases requiring emergency care present potential medicolegal problems, especially if occupational or industrial coverage *(75)* or liability or subrogation factors *(67)* are involved. Malpractice actions *(68)* are all too frequently based on the first treatment received by the patient. Therefore, to protect the patient, the attending physician and the hospital, x-rays should be taken whenever bony injuries or other conditions demonstrable roentgenologically are reasonably suspected, provided that moving and positioning the patient will not be harmful.

In all head injuries and in other injuries in which the presence of a neck injury is suspected, a cross-table lateral using portable x-ray equipment should be taken and examined before any movement of the neck is allowed. Normal ("negative") x-rays may have as much medicolegal value as those showing trauma or other pathology.

The frivolous taking of x-rays, on the other hand, increases patient expense and radiation exposure and is time consuming. In the absence of any specific positive physical findings in a thorough examination, the physician does not—just because there is a history of trauma to the area—have to order x-rays to be exercising prudent judgment and due care.

The taking of x-rays strictly for the purpose of providing answers to realistic clinical questions that are likely to be resolved by roentgenographic study with the assistance of radiology algorithms and agreed-upon guidelines, constitutes the most appropriate use of radiology services. Thoughtful clinical judgment must prevail in the final analysis, as guidelines cannot cover every situation. Even the well-considered Food and Drug Administration Guidelines concerning skull x-rays have been found wanting in some cases. However, in general, good guidelines can be a useful aid in making clinical decisions.

21–2. ORDERING VIEWS

When a radiologist is available, a review of difficult clinical problems in person or in a detailed written request helps in ordering the most beneficial x-ray views and also assists the radiologist in interpretation.

Some helpful considerations are as follows:

X-Ray View	Comment
Skull:	Cross-table lateral film first with a cervical spine film. Check lateral cervical film before doing skull exposures if neck injury is also possible.
Facial bones:	Waters' view should be included.
Long bones:	If fracture is strongly suspected or found at one end of a long bone, get an x-ray of the other end also.
Epiphysis injury:	Radiograph the comparable opposite side whenever there is a question or confusion concerning the diagnosis.
Patella:	Include a sunrise view.
Elbow:	Look for "fat pad sign." If fat pad is not in the olecranon fossa but is displaced, producing a posterior lucency, there is a fracture generally causing bleeding into the joint.
Wrist:	The carpal bone that commonly fractures is the navicular bone. Such fractures may be very difficult to see, requiring "navicular views" or follow-up films.
Scapula:	Lateral view included.
Abdominal aorta:	Anteroposterior and lateral view of abdomen.
Bronchial foreign body:	Inspiration and expiration chest films.

21–3. INTERPRETATION

To avoid oversight, it is helpful to examine x-ray films with a *high expectation of finding something wrong* (or pathologic).

The attending physician's interpretation of the recently developed films must often be used as a basis for emergency therapy and disposition. The presence or absence of pathology can be determined by the emergency physician with reasonable accuracy and a working diagnosis established. For better communication, it is preferable for the emergency physician to attach a notation of the initial interpretation to the requisition. If resolution of interpretation on an important issue is not possible in the emergency situation (e.g., no roentgenologist is available), proceed in a conservative manner (for example, cast an equivocal fracture and have the patient return the next day for reevaluation). The original interpretation of the x-rays should be confirmed or modified by a qualified roentgenologist as soon as possible (with immediate notification of the treating physician if there is any significant discrepancy in interpretation), and a report of the final interpretation of the films should be incorporated in the patient's record.

21–4. TRANSFERRAL OF X-RAYS

X-rays that are essential to definitive care should be sent with the patient whenever transfer to any hospital is arranged. If referral to another clinic physician's office is made, the films should be held awaiting this practitioner's request, except in those instances in which adequate treatment requires their immediate presence (fractures, dislocations, head injuries, etc.). If x-ray films for any reason leave the direct control of the physician by whom they are ordered, a receipt should be signed by the person to whom they are consigned for transportation. Return of the x-rays as soon as possible should be required, with careful follow-up in a reasonable time.

21–5. OWNERSHIP OF X-RAYS

No matter who pays for them, x-ray films are the property of the hospital or clinic in which they were obtained and not of the patient, other medical attendants, attorneys, insurance companies or other interested persons, except in special situations of contractual agreement. Since the films (not the reports based on them) must be produced when designated by due process of law *(73, Subpoenas)*, they must be safeguarded in the same manner as the clinical record *(66, Emergency Case Records)*.

21–6. FLUOROSCOPIC EXAMINATION

Fluoroscopy is of assistance in some emergency cases in which the presence of cardiopulmonary or gastrointestinal tract disease must be determined. It is also used on occasion in the reduction of complex fractures. Fluoroscopy should almost always be done by a radiologist or, when indicated, by a qualified specialist, such as an orthopedist, adequately trained to properly use special fluoroscopic equipment.

21–7. PROTECTION OF GONADS

Although the danger from gonadal radiation has been greatly overemphasized in the lay press, shielding of the lower abdomen and external genitalia is a simple procedure and should be done whenever practical, especially in children, in men and women of reproductive age and particularly in women during the first trimester of pregnancy.

21–8. X-RAY BURNS *(See also 28–34)*

Unless there has been a gross miscalculation of dosage or a defect in the operation of calibration of the equipment, radiation burns usually result from x-ray therapy rather than from x-rays taken in diagnostic evaluation. In this instance, the temporary uncomfortable erythema and subsequent atrophic changes represent a calculated risk of which the patient had been, or should have been, informed. For treatment, see *28–34*. (See also *3–5, Evaluation and Treatment of Radiation Injuries.*)

21–9. SPECIALIZED STUDIES

Radiocontrast studies of arterial and venous blood vessels, hollow structures (from urethra to esophagus), and organs (e.g., intravenous pyelogram for renal function) can greatly aid clinical diagnosis and treatment of an emergency problem. Digital subtraction angiography, still quite specialized, is a newer technique that is faster and safer and gives more complete information about vascular structures.

Computerized tomography has revolutionized emergency and routine evaluation of numerous problems, particularly intracranial disorders. In some communities, these units are mobile so they can go to individual hospitals as needed.

21–10. ALTERNATIVES TO X-RAY

Ultrasonography B scan has greatly aided clinical evaluation, particularly in the area of obstetrics. The fiberopticoscope is a major advancement for direct visualization of problems. Another noninvasive diagnostic technique is radionuclide imaging, which gives valuable information about organ anatomy and function, as well as blood flow pattern (including detection of such problems as infarct, embolus, thrombus, aneurysm and tumor). Total body scanning with this method in cases of fever of unknown cause may help detect abscesses. Single Photon Envasion Computerized Tomography (SPECT or ECT) causes about one-third less radiation than regular CT and offers more depth perception and tissue pathology definition. Nuclear magnetic resonance (NMR) imaging is likely to be an important diagnostic tool in the future.

Emergency Treatment of Specific Conditions

22. Abdominal Pain

22–1. GENERAL CONSIDERATIONS

Distinguishing an acute surgical abdomen from less serious or less fulminating conditions may require laboratory procedures for confirmation and precise identification. However, in a high percentage of cases, a tentative diagnosis can be made from the history and physical examination; certainly, from the history and clinical picture the attending physician should be able to determine whether or not immediate hospitalization is indicated. Unless a definite diagnosis of a nondangerous condition has been established, persons with persistent or recurrent severe abdominal pain may benefit from hospitalization for thorough examination, diagnosis and treatment.

Besides the manner, rate and location of onset of pain, it is of value to consider whether the pain is somatic or visceral in type. *Somatic pain* is generally rather readily distinguished by fairly rapid localization of the pain, caused by stimulation of nerve endings in the abdominal wall or in the parietal, peritoneal or retroperitoneal spaces. The pain is usually strongly felt as tearing, burning, sharp, stabbing or squeezing. *Visceral pain* is much less easily localized and lower grade in character, usually described as a feeling of pressure or aching. *Referred pain* is more easily identified by its sharp, "shooting" nature and its location in the same dermatome from which the viscera developed at the embryonic state.

Initial instructions to the patient pending evaluation and diagnosis should be as follows:

- Avoid eating anything.
- Avoid fluids (except possibly for a few ice chips).
- Limit medications to those immediately specified; avoid taking a laxative or enema unless specified.

22–2. DIAGNOSTIC AIDS IN DISTINGUISHING THE SURGICAL FROM THE NONSURGICAL ABDOMEN

History

- Evaluate features of the diagnoses listed in Table 22–1 by using the techniques for evaluation of different pathogenic mechanisms shown in Tables 22–2 and 22–3. Various poisons may also cause abdominal pain (Table 22–4).
- Onset (rapidity—sudden, rapid, gradual, interrupted).
- Progression (initial location, subsequent locations, rate of change).
- Accompanying specific events and signs and symptoms occurring with onset and their progression.

Text continued on page 146

Table 22–1. SOME CONDITIONS IN WHICH ABDOMINAL PAIN MAY BE A MAIN SYMPTOM*

Condition	Usual Site of Pain	Condition	Usual Site of Pain
Abdominal epilepsy	G	*Obstruction of the gastrointestinal tract (*40–3*)	G
Abdominal wall injury	F	Orchitis, traumatic (*41–3*)	8
Accumulation of gas (splenic flexure)	LUQ	*Ovarian cyst with torsion of the peuicle (*42–16*)	LQ
Addisonian crisis (*36–1*)	G	Pancreatitis, acute (*40–17*) or traumatic (*59–26*)	5
*Aneurysm (*63–5*); any quadrant plus back pain	—	Parathyroid crises (*36–8*)	G
**Appendicitis (*40–8*)	RLQ (starts in 5)	*Peptic ulcer with perforation (*40–4*)	1, 2, 3
Arthritis	D	*Pericardial trauma (*31–4, Cardiac Trauma*)	1, 3
Bladder retention/distention (*41–24*)	8	*Peritonitis, acute (primary, from trauma or infections)	G
**Bladder/ureter perforation (*41–1*)	8	Pleurodynia (*33–50*)	UQ
*Bowel obstruction (*40–3*)	G	Pneumonia (*56–16;* also *33–51*, *Interstitial Pneumonia*)	UQ
Caisson disease (*26–3*)	G	Poisoning, acute (see Table 22–4)	G
*Cholecystitis (*40–9*); radiation to shoulder	RQ	Porphyria (*46–24*)	G
Cirrhosis of the liver	RUQ	*Premature separation of the placenta (*50–11*)	5, 8
Constipation with fecal impaction (*40–3*)	G	Pyelonephritis (*41–23*, *Nephritis*) plus back pain	4, 5, 6
Coronary disease and infarction (*29–15*)	1, 3	Pyloric stenosis (*40–13*, *Gastrointestinal Obstruction*)	1, 5
Cystitis (*41–11*)	8	Rectus abdominis muscle hemorrhage	F, 1, 5, 8
Decompression sickness (*26–4*)	G	Renal colic (*41–20*) unilateral, radiation to 8 and back	4, 5, 6
Diabetes (hyperglycemia and ketoacidosis) (*32–3*)	G	Round ligament spasm during pregnancy	8
**Dissecting extending aneurysm (*63–5*)	—	**Rupture of a viscus	G
Diverticulitis (*40–11*)	LLQ	Salpingitis (*42–12*, *Pelvic Inflammatory Disease*)	8
Dysentery (*40–10*)	G	Sickle cell crisis	G
**Ectopic pregnancy, ruptured (*50–7*)	7, 8, 9	*Subdiaphragmatic abscess (*23–30*)	1, 2, 3
Enteritis, acute bacterial or regional (*40–10; 40–21*)	G	Tabes dorsalis (*33–66*)	G
Epilepsy, abdominal	G	Tetany (*46–25*)	G
*Esophageal perforation (*40–4*)	1, 3	Thrombosis or thrombophlebitis, portal or hepatic vein	RUQ
Fecal impaction (*40–3*)	G	**Torsion of testicle (*41–8*)	8
Fractures of spine (*47–28*), dermatomal level	—	Trauma, direct—focal plus generalized if penetrating	F, G
Foreign bodies (*39–7*)	—	Tubal pregnancy (*50–7*)	8
*Gallbladder disease (*40–9*) radiation to shoulder	RUQ	*Tubo-ovarian abscess (*42–12*)	LQ
Gastroenteritis (*40–14*); progresses to all quadrants	UQ	Tumors, space consuming or malignant	—
		Uremia (*32–16*)	G
		Ureteral stone (*41–26*); pain greater on side of lesion	LQ
		Uterine pathology (back pain also)	8

Hepatitis, acute *(33–28)*	RUQ
Hepatic trauma *(59–23)*	RUQ
Hernia—diaphragmatic *(52–5)*; femoral, inguinal *(40–6)*; umbilical	F
**Hernia—incarcerated and irreducible	F
Herniation of an intervertebral disk *(47–13)*	D
Herpes zoster *(30–14, 49–13)*	D
Hypoglycemia *(46–15)*	G
Ileus obstruction, nonmechanical *(40–3)*	G
**Infarcts of abdominal viscera	G
Infections, acute systemic	G
Intestinal obstruction *(40–3)*	G
Intestinal parasites *(40–18)*	—
**Intestinal perforation *(40–4)*	—
**Intraperitoneal perforation *(40–4)*	G
*Intussusception *(40–6)*	LQ
Irritable bowel syndrome	G
Kidney stones *(41–26)*	LQ
Leptospirosis	G
Leukemia	G
Liver disease *(59–23, Liver Injuries)*	RUQ
Lupus erythematosus (systemic)	—
Mediastinitis *(40–4, Perforation)*	1
Mesenteric adenitis and lymphangitis (in children)	LQ
**Mesenteric thrombosis and embolism	5
Migraine *(30–22)*	—
Mittelschmerz *(42–11)*	LQ
Myocardial infarction *(29–15)*	1, 3
Nephritis *(41–16)*	4, 5, 6
Neuritis, intercostal; dermatomal level	—
Urinary bladder retention and distention *(41–24)*	8
Vascular purpura (Henoch's purpura)	—
*Volvulus *(40–23)*; greater in lower quadrants	—
Withdrawal symptoms, narcotics	G

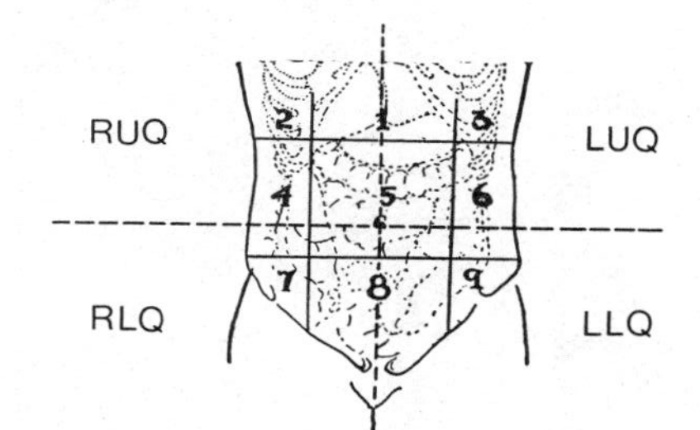

Figure 22–1. Regions of the abdomen bounded according to the standard system: 1, epigastric;2, right hypochondriac; 3, left hypochondriac; 4, right lateral (or lumbar); 5, umbilical; 6, left lateral (or lumbar); 7, right inguinal (or iliac); 8, pubic (hypogastric); 9, left inguinal (or iliac). Dashed lines divide major quadrants: *RUQ,* Right upper quadrant; *RLQ,* right lower quadrant; *LUQ,* left upper quadrant; *LLQ,* left lower quadrant. (Modified from *Dorland's Illustrated Medical Dictionary,* 26th ed. Philadelphia, W. B. Saunders Co., 1981, p. 2.)

**Key to abbreviations and symbols:*
**—Acute surgical evaluation is necessary.*
***—Immediate surgical procedure is usual; pain usually sudden in onset.*
G—Generalized pain.
F—Focal pain in area of lesion.
D—Dermatomal distribution.
Numbers (1 to 9) and quadrants (LUQ, RLQ, etc.) under "Usual Site" refer to designations in Figure 22–1.
Dash (—) indicates pain is too variable to specify location.

Table 22–2. DIAGNOSTIC CLUES IN GASTROINTESTINAL ABDOMINAL PAIN (BY PATHOGENIC TYPE)*

Findings: Signs/Symptoms	*Inflammation* (Peptic Ulcer)	*Hemorrhage* (Peptic Ulcer)	*Perforation* (Peptic Ulcer)
Pain Onset	Gradual, often early A.M., interprandial	Variable, often absent	Sudden, severe
Pain Location (See Table 22–1) Initial	Epigastrium (1) and adjacent area	Same as ulcer inflammation	Diffuse
Later	Into back with penetration	May ↓ with bleeding	Increased in RLQ; one or both shoulders
Pain Type	Gnawing, burning, aching; "hunger pain"	Same as ulcer inflammation	Steady, severe
Abdominal Tenderness	Some epigastric	Variable, not prominent	Severe, may ↓ later
Abdominal Distention	Usually not present unless obstruction	Variable	Gross; ↑ later
Abdominal Wall Rigidity	Usually not present unless there is penetration/perforation	Absent	Intense
Bowel Sounds	Active	Active, may ↑	Marked ↓ or absent
Intestinal Function Status (ileus/diarrhea, constipation, etc.)	Usually normal	Increased activity	No defecation; cessation, ileus
Nausea	Common	Common	Usual
Vomiting	Occasional	Hematemesis (see Fig. 40–1)	Often present
Fever	Infrequent	Low-grade	Present, increasing
Shock	No	Rapid onset if bleeding severe	Present, increasing
Other Comments	Pain relieved by food, antacids, histamine H_2 receptor blockers (cimetadine), sucralfate Diagnosis confirmed by x-ray/gastroscopy Avoid caffeine, tobacco, salicylates	Pass NG tube: remove blood, lavage Replace blood volume losses Surgery required if recurrent massive bleeding (e.g., 6 transfusions in 24 hours)	Liver dullness is decreased or absent X-ray: free peritoneal air often in upright or lateral decubitus position

*For diagnostic clues in gastroenteritis, see Table 40–1; for diagnosis of poisoning/toxicity, see Table 53–1.

Table 22–2. DIAGNOSTIC CLUES IN GASTROINTESTINAL ABDOMINAL PAIN (BY PATHOGENIC TYPE)* *(Continued)*

Obstruction (Incarcerated Hernia, Volvulus, Intussusception)	*Infection* (Appendicitis)	*Inflammation* (Acute pancreatitis)	*Inflammation with Obstruction* (Acute Cholecystitis with or without Common Duct Stone)
Rapid to sudden	Usually gradual	Rapid	Usually gradual
Focal	Periumbilical	Upper abdomen	RUQ; epigastrium
Generalized	RLQ (RUQ in late pregnancy)	Back pain	Below right scapular blade
Intense cramping to steady	Cramping, aching; later steady	Colicky to severe intractable; relieved by sitting	Aching, cramping; later, steady ache of moderate to severe degree
Focal	Present unless retrocecal (do rectal exam)	Intense tenderness	RUQ
Moderate to severe	Moderate	Occasionally present	Variable
Focal splinting	Present; common at McBurney's point	Occasionally present	RUQ
Early: ↑ Later: ↓	Early: Normal Late: ↓	Usual ↓	Usually present, but decreased
Function ↓ Gas proximal ↑ Gas distal ↓	Usually only 1 BM near time of onset; diarrhea infrequent	Function; bleeding may occur	Present, but often diminished
Usual	Common	Common	Usual
Gastric contents; presence of bile (green-yellow) followed by fecal matter if vomiting is prolonged	Few episodes common; may not occur	Common	Usual
Later	Low-grade usual	Low-grade usual	Low-grade usual
Later sign	After rupture (peritonitis)	Present in severe attacks	Uncommon except with rupture; sepsis generalized
X-ray reveals signs of obstruction	↑ WBC, PMN's Positive psoas sign Hyperesthesia of abdominal skin Surgery required	Pain relieved by sitting; increases with movement and breathing Increased WBC, serum amylase Rectal exam normal Jaundice may occur with or without stones	Pain occurs in early A.M. X-ray: stones may or may not be present Radionuclide scan with HIDA confirms presence or absence of acute cholecystitis Gallbladder echoscan often helpful

Table 22–3. DIAGNOSTIC CLUES IN ABDOMINAL PAIN

Findings Signs/Symptoms	*Vascular* (Sup. Mesenteric Art. Thrombosis)	*Vascular* (Aortic Aneurysm Dissection)	*Ureteral Stone*
Pain Onset	Sudden	Sudden	Sudden
Pain Location Initial	Mid-abdomen	If thoracic: neck, epigastrium	Flank
Later	Generalized	If below L subclavian: back & abdomen	Radiation to testicle/groin Abdomen (ureteral course)
Pain Type	Severe, steady	Severe	Severe episodic (renal colic)
Abdominal Tenderness	May be intense	Over aneurysm	Usually absent
Abdominal Distention	Variable	Later	Common (ileus)
Abdominal Wall Rigidity	May be intense, with spasms	Occurs with abdominal aneurysm	Absent, may be reflex spasms
Bowel Sounds	Decreased	Hypoactive	Present; may be decreased
Intestinal Function Status	Decreased; often blood in feces	Decreased (later)	Decreased secondary to ileus
Nausea	Common	Common	Common
Vomiting	Common	May occur	Common
Fever	Later, low-grade	Not a feature	Later, fever and chills common
Shock	Common	Cardiac and/or hypovolemic	No
Other Comments	X-ray shows ileus, widening of intestinal wall, pneumatosis intestinalis Much milder course with inferior mesenteric artery thrombosis	BP in legs often much lower than in rt arm, pulses ↓ or ≠ Diagnosis made by x-ray, ultrasound, angiogram	Emergency infusion IVP establishes diagnosis Hematuria Urinary frequency

Physical Examination of Abdomen

In addition to checking vital signs and making a general evaluation, do the following:

- Inspect for wounds, distention, herniations, skin and vascular changes.
- Palpate for masses and organ enlargement, including pelvic and rectal examination. Evaluate for focal, referred and rebound tenderness and rigidity. Record femoral pulses, and palpate femoral and inguinal rings.

Table 22–4. POISONS THAT MAY CAUSE ABDOMINAL PAIN*

Antimony *(53–81)*	Lead *(53–386, Lead Salts)*
Arsenic trioxide *(53–92)*	Methyl alcohol *(53–426)*
Aspidium *(53–100)*	Morphine *(53–455)*
Barium *(53–111)*	Mushrooms *(53–462)*
Bichloride of mercury *(53–124)*	Organic phosphate pesticides *(53–497)*
Botulism *(53–142)*	Phenolphthalein *(53–535)*
Cadmium *(53–158)*	Physostigmine *(53–547)*
Carbon tetrachloride *(53–176)*	Solanine *(53–644)*
Chromates *(53–206)*	Spider venom *(53–649;* see also *27–28, Spider Bites)*
Colchicine *(53–220)*	Squill *(53–650)*
Copper salts *(53–224)*	Staphylococcal food poisoning *(53–314)*
Croton oil *(53–230)*	Sulfapyridine *(53–660, Sulfonamides)*
Cyanides *(53–232)*	Thallium *(53–692)*
Diethylstilbestrol *(53–264)*	Tung nuts *(53–729)*
Ergot *(53–291)*	Turpentine *(53–730)*
Fluorides *(53–311)*	Veratrum viride *(53–740)*
Formaldehyde *(53–315)*	Viosterol *(53–743)*
Gasoline *(53–323)*	
Kerosene *(53–379)*	

*Incomplete list; see also 53.

- Check psoas sign (place thigh in extension and resist flexion—increase in pain indicates psoas tenderness as occurs with appendicitis. Check obturator sign (flex thigh and knee both approximately 90° and then rotate hip externally; increased tenderness of obturator internus (and occasionally piriformis) is a sign of inflammation, as may occur with appendicitis, diverticulitis, and pelvic inflammatory disease.
- Percuss for fluid or gas distention.
- Auscultate for bruit and bowel sounds (frequency, duration, pitch and intensity); in difficult cases, frequently recheck and record bowel sounds as well as tenderness findings. Lungs should also be checked.

Laboratory Tests

- Draw blood as needed for complete and differential blood counts; determination of blood sugar, blood urea nitrogen (BUN), creatinine, electrolyte, amylase and calcium levels; and additional tests, according to the specific diagnosis suspected. If surgery appears imminent, draw blood for blood type and crossmatch and coagulation defect.
- Urinalysis.
- Analysis of feces and nasogastric aspirate for appearance and blood content. Culture feces and blood if high fever and/or diarrhea is present.
- If poisoning as a cause of abdominal pain is suspected (Table 22–4), consider collection of specimens for qualitative and quantitative evaluations and treatment according to condition.

Radiologic and Other Visual Tests

- Routinely obtain flat plate and lateral decubitus views of the abdomen, plus an upright posteroanterior view of the chest for evaluation when a surgical abdomen is suspected. If possible, have the patient in an upright or sitting position for 4 to 5 minutes (to permit rising of free air) before the upright film is taken. Obtain a lateral abdominal view if, for instance, an aneurysm or penetrating foreign body is suspected.

- Emergency examinations, such as radiocontrast studies of the upper urinary tract, upper and lower gastrointestinal series fiberoptic laparoscopy and enteroscopy, radioisotope scans, CAT scans (particularly for locating blood, air and pus), and ultrasound scans, are done on special indication. A urethrogram should be performed in severe pelvic injuries in which urethral avulsion is suspected prior to an attempt to pass a catheter into the bladder.

Other Common Procedures

- Culdocentesis (*18–9*).
- Nasogastric aspiration for volume, appearance and type of contents.
- Peritoneal aspiration (*18–23*).

22–3. MANAGEMENT

If after a careful history and physical examination and utilization of available laboratory tests the emergency physician is unable to determine the cause of persistent or recurrent abdominal distress, or if the patient needs surgery or inpatient medical care, the patient should be hospitalized. Because of the possibility that they will mask signs and symptoms, no opiates or synthetic narcotics of any kind should be given for control of pain or relief of apprehension until a definite diagnosis has been established; even then, narcotics in only small doses are preferable. Narcotic effect can also be relieved with naloxone (Narcan).

A detailed summary of all laboratory tests, observations and findings, especially changes in condition, and of all treatment should be sent with any patient having abdominal pain who is being transferred to a hospital or referred to a private physician's office. To protect the patient and themselves, emergency physicians should be sure that the patient understands the need for further medical or surgical care.

23. Abscesses

23–1. GENERAL CONSIDERATIONS

- Evaluate for the underlying cause of the abscess, e.g., infection secondary to puncture wound or foreign body; exposure to unusually pathogenic organisms; faulty or overwhelmed immune reaction system; presence of hyperglycemia; bacteremic spread from another focus; development of a deep abscess in badly contused muscle tissue in which there was no preceding penetration of skin.
- All patients with abscesses should have an assay of blood sugar level and complete and differential blood counts.
- Purulent material should have a Gram stain examination and the specimen should be sent for culturing (both aerobic and anaerobic) and sensitivity testing before any antibiotic treatment is started.
- Blood cultures should also be drawn if the patient is febrile and the abscess is septic, or if bacteremic spread is suspected.
- Ultrasonography or x-ray films may provide information on the size, location and presence of any gas in the abscess.
- In unusual cases, an "abscessogram"—injection of radiopaque dye (Renografin-60) into larger abscess cavities—may be necessary to outline perimeters and aid in localization of any embedded foreign body.

- Cellulitis without localization or fluctuation should be treated by frequent local application of warm moist heat plus antibiotics as indicated. Many will be absorbed under this regimen; others will localize in a short time.
- Warn the patient not to try decompressing the abscess by squeezing, as dangerous spread can occur.
- Adequate surgical incision and drainage of all pockets of infection constitute the primary therapy for localized abscesses (identified by central "pointing," fluctuance or softness, and change from diffuse redness of cellulitis).
  —*Small superficial abscesses* may be incised and drained under lidocaine or carbocaine block anesthesia. If a central whitish core is present, it should be removed.
  —*Large deep abscesses* require that the patient be hospitalized for treatment by wide drainage, usually under general anesthesia. Maintenance of drainage is aided by a rubber dam drain or iodoform gauze packing.
  —*Postsurgical measures*: See *59–3*.
- It is important to protect other people and other portions of the patient's body from the purulent drainage. Placing of contaminated dressings in impervious plastic bags (which are then preferably burned) in addition to handwashing after contact is important.
- Treat pain (*12*). Usually a codeine type drug is needed for a few days.

ABSCESSES OF SPECIAL TYPE*

23–2. ALVEOLAR (DENTAL) ABSCESSES

Alveolar abscesses arise from infection at a tooth root or root fragment(s) and may be exquisitely painful (although occasionally they are asymptomatic). With periapical, periodontal or pericoronitis abscesses (especially if there is fever or lymphadenopathy), oral analgesics (acetaminophen with codeine) and antibiotics (penicillin V, 250 mg q 6 h) should usually be administered and the patient immediately referred to a dentist. If swelling, fluctuation or pointing is present, an intraoral incision (after local anesthetization) is often done.

- A *periapical abscess* is the most likely type to be seen in an emergency room, because of the intense pain. There may be no apparent swelling. The tooth is normally very sensitive to slight percussion and is often thermally sensitive as well. The pulp has been compromised, and pain and/or infection radiate from the foramen at the root apex. Endodontic (root canal) therapy or extraction by a dentist is indicated.
- A *periodontal abscess* usually presents with swelling but with no significant percussion sensitivity. Tooth mobility is not uncommon. Drainage via incision is often provided with subsequent referral to a dentist or periodontist.
- *Pericoronitis* results from erupting molar teeth, particularly mandibular third molars, and is most often seen in the 18 to 26 year age group. This inflammation can develop into a serious infection. Trismus is often present. The patient should be referred to a dentist or oral surgeon.

23–3. ANORECTAL ABSCESSES

Anorectal abscesses may be superficial or deep, but all require incision and drainage. Local lidocaine block is sufficient for superficial abscesses, but deep lesions require that the patient be hospitalized for general or low spinal anesthesia.

---

*Management *in addition to* measures described under "General Considerations."

23–4. BARTHOLIN'S GLAND ABSCESSES

Bartholin's gland abscesses may be severely painful. If the abscess is fluctuant and large (3 cm or greater), an incision should be made, with drainage *on the mucosal side* into the vagina, and a Word catheter should be inserted, or the patient should be referred to a gynecologist for this procedure. Occasionally marsupialization is needed.

23–5. BOILS *(See 23–1)*

23–6. BRAIN ABSCESSES

Brain abscesses may follow head injuries (especially fractures), otitis media or mastoiditis. Suspicion of the presence of a brain abscess is an indication for immediate hospitalization and neurosurgical evaluation.

23–7. BREAST ABSCESSES

Breast abscesses may give severe pain, with general malaise and elevated temperature.

- Have the patient wear an oversize brassiere for support.
- Onset frequently occurs within several weeks of the patient's having been in a hospital, so antibiotics should be effective against penicillin-resistant organisms (usually staphylococcal) that may be causing the infection.
- If the patient is nursing, discontinuation of lactation depends on the physician's judgment.

23–8. CARBUNCLES

Carbuncles are multilocular abscesses with multiple individual compartments. If surgical drainage becomes necessary, the incision(s) must enter each of the compartments.

23–9. COLD ABSCESSES

Cold abscesses are usually due to attentuated organisms following antibiotic therapy or to tuberculosis and are rarely encountered as an emergency unless sudden spontaneous drainage occurs. Fluctuation may be present, but the usual signs of inflammation (redness, local heat, tenderness) are absent. No emergency treatment is needed, but the importance of adequate medical care should be stressed to the patient, and referral should be made.

23–10. COLLAR-BUTTON ABSCESSES

Collar-button abscesses are infections in the webs between the fingers that cause acute palmar tenderness and swelling but that point on the dorsal surface of the hand. They may also develop in the palm or dorsum of the head or in the plantar area or dorsum of the foot.

Treatment

EARLY

- Immobilization with a position-of-function hand-forearm splint and sling.
- Frequent hot soaks.
- Control of pain by elevation.
- Systemic antibiotics.

ADVANCED

- Incision and drainage through two incisions, a curved incision along the edge of the volar swelling and a small incision over the dorsal web. This procedure should be done in a hospital under nerve block or general anesthetic. Cultures and sensitivity tests should be obtained.

- Insertion of a rubber dam drain.
- Application of a position-of-function hand-forearm splint and sling.
- Administration of appropriate antibiotics.
- Careful and frequent follow-up care.

23–11. DENTAL ABSCESSES *(See 23–2)*

23–12. EPIDURAL ABSCESSES

Epidural abscesses in the spine are characterized by low back pain, progressive spinal cord compression with flaccid weakness of the legs, urinary retention, fever and chills. They represent an acute emergency, and immediate hospitalization for drainage is mandatory.

23–13. FELONS (Whitlows)

Felons or whitlows require immediate drainage through a "hockey-stick" incision on the nonpinch (ulnar) side, if possible, or a vertical incision through the pod of the fingertip; if it is necessary to go across the flexion crease, use a zigzag incision with a horizontal cut in the flexion crease or, if possible, use two incisions—one distal to and one proximal to the flexion crease. Care must be taken to open every infected compartment. Digital nerve block at some distance above the infected area is usually adequate for anesthesia.

23–14. GAS ABSCESSES *(See also 59–42, Soft Tissue Infections)*

If crepitus, foul odor and tenderness, together with severe systemic signs and symptoms, develop in a previously comfortable wound 2 to 4 days after injury, immediate hospitalization for exploration and removal of necrotic tissue is required. X-rays or an ultrasonogram may confirm gas location. Penicillin in massive doses (up to 12 million or more units a day) is indicated, with large doses of tetracyclines. Treatment with gas gangrene antitoxin is of no value in these cases.

23–15. ISCHIOANAL ABSCESSES

These abscesses can develop suddenly, with extreme pain, fever and chills; a feeling of fullness in the rectum; and urinary retention. For superficial ischioanal abscesses, see treatment measures listed in *23–1*. Deep extensive abscesses with severe toxic signs and symptoms require hospitalization for surgical drainage under general anesthesia. Late fistulectomy is often necessary.

23–16. MIDDLE EAR ABSCESSES *(See 35–18)*

23–17. NASAL SEPTUM ABSCESSES

Nasal septum abscesses may follow trauma or operative procedures. Spread of the infection and permanent perforation are possible risks. Antibiotic therapy should be started at once and the patient referred immediately to an otolaryngologist for incision and drainage, to help avoid permanent perforation.

23–18. PALMAR SPACE ABSCESSES *(See 23–10, Collar-button Abscesses; 43–5, Cellulitis of the Hand)*

23–19. PARONYCHIA

Throbbing pain accompanied by redness and swelling adjacent to the border of a finger or toenail can be relieved only by incision and drainage. This can often be done without anesthesia, or after a digital block is performed. The incision into the abscess can be made by pushing against the nail bed into the affected areas with a No. 11 Bard-Parker blade.

23–20. PERIANAL ABSCESSES *(See 23–15)*

23–21. PERINEAL ABSCESSES

Perineal abscesses require emergency incision and drainage if pressure causes partial or complete urinary retention. All cases should be referred to a urologist or gynecologist for care.

23–22. PERITONSILLAR ABSCESSES (Quinsy) *(See also 61–16, Tonsillitis-Pharyngitis)*

Signs and symptoms consist of agonizing pain on one side of the throat, acute dysphagia, high temperature, extreme general malaise and bulging in the supratonsillar fossa.

Treatment

If the abscess is fluctuant and can be accurately localized:

- Aspiration with a large-bore needle (after spraying area with an anesthetic) *or* infiltration of the medial mucous membrane only, with 1% lidocaine followed by incision with a #11 blade with several layers of adhesive tape wrapped around the blade 3/8 inch from the point as a guard against too deep penetration. Gentle opening of the abscess inside with a forceps.
- Irrigation with warm saline dripped by bulb syringe or nozzle on forming abscesses. Place affected side down so fluid can drain out the mouth.
- Administration of antibiotics after Gram staining and sending of a specimen for cultures and sensitivity tests.
- Referral to an otolaryngologist for follow-up or, in severe cases, for primary care, particularly if the abscess is deep and no area of fluctuation can be determined (see below).

If the abscess is deep and no area of fluctuation can be determined:

- Refer the patient to an otolaryngologist.
- *Do not* attempt to *explore* the throat. Deaths have occurred from uncontrollable hemorrhage from the ascending pharyngeal, external carotid and internal carotid arteries and from the internal jugular vein.

23–23. PERIURETHRAL ABSCESSES

Periurethral abscesses arise from acute urethritis or from infection of the glands in the area and usually point near the base of the shaft of the penis. The patient should be referred to a urologist for further care.

23–24. PILONIDAL ABSCESSES

Treatment consists of incision and drainage under local, spinal or general anesthesia, depending on extent of involvement. The central pore should be excised with as small a circular cut as possible (not larger than 3 mm), and then a linear incision should be made into the abscess parallel and lateral to the natal cleft. Avoid incisions in the midline or removal of large areas of skin.

23–25. PULMONARY (LUNG) ABSCESSES

Lung abscesses may present with sudden rupture of copious, purulent, unpleasant- to foul-smelling material into the bronchus that is followed by coughing up of the drainage for days to weeks. Frequently the patient will have had prior chills and slow resolution from bacterial pneumonia for 1 to 2 weeks. Obtain Gram stain and culture for both aerobes and anaerobes (putrid odor), and institute antibiotics accordingly. A physical or respiratory therapist should be engaged to instruct the patient and help provide adequate postural drainage (aiding by "cupping") on a multiple daily basis. Immediate bronchoscopy is not needed; arrange for close follow-up.

23–26. RETROPERITONEAL ABSCESSES

Retroperitoneal (anterior, posterior [perinephric] and retrofascial) abscesses require immediate hospitalization for surgical drainage.

23–27. RETROPHARYNGEAL ABSCESSES

These abscesses may be seen directly as a bulging of the posterior pharyngeal wall or indirectly on lateral x-ray film of the neck. Do not palpate, as rupture and aspiration may occur. Refer immediately to an otolaryngologist (transport the patient in the semiprone position) for evaluation and incision and drainage; if an otolaryngologist is unavailable and rupture is imminent, local cocaine anesthesia and syringe aspiration through a long large-bore needle may provide partial relief.

23–28. STITCH ABSCESSES

Stitch abscesses may be superficial or deep and can be drained easily by removal of the offending stitch (cutting it close to the uninfected side). Spreading of the incision may be necessary.

23–29. SUBURETHRAL ABSCESSES

These abscesses should not be opened externally if this can be avoided. Reference to a urologist is indicated as soon as the diagnosis has been made.

23–30. SUBDIAPHRAGMATIC ABSCESSES

Hospitalization for treatment is required if a subdiaphragmatic abscess is suspected by clinical course, fever, thoracoabdominal pain, decreased diaphragmatic excursion, x-ray studies or sonogram.

23–31. TENDON SHEATH ABSCESSES (Tenosynovitis) *(See 43–5)*

23–32. TUBO-OVARIAN ABSCESSES *(See 42–12)*

23–33. WHITLOWS *(See 23–13)*

24. Allergic Reactions

A bracelet or necklace providing information regarding special medical problems, such as heart trouble or allergic reactions to drugs or other substances, may be lifesaving. Additional emergency information can be obtained by telephone on a 24-hour basis from the central agency.*

Patients with known severe allergy who are at risk of unavoidable allergen reexposure, such as individuals with insect sting sensitivity or those susceptible to severe reactions to certain foods such as seafoods, nuts, olives or products containing sulfites, are well advised to have at all times a small kit containing a predrawn calibrated syringe of stabilized epinephrine and antihistamine tablets† on their person or immediately nearby (e.g., home, car, boat, knapsack). Oral antihistamines may be taken before sensitive patients go into high-risk areas to offer partial prophylaxis by helping deter histamine binding.

Four types of acute allergic reactions require immediate, sometimes lifesaving, emergency measures. These are anaphylactic shock, acute angioedema, asthma with acute bronchospasm, and serum shock. In immediate hypersensitivity reactions, the body's IgE antibody combines with calcium and the specific introduced allergen, which in turn activates a specific esterase. This enzyme then acts on the mast cell within which histamine and slower-acting anaphylaxis-producing substances are released that in turn cause shock *(57)* and bronchospasm *(56–4)*. The combination of IgG and specific allergens can affect the complement system in such a way as to cause slow histamine release and a slower hypersensitivity reaction.

24–1. ANAPHYLACTIC (ANAPHYLACTOID) SHOCK

Anaphylactic shock usually develops within a few seconds or minutes of exposure to the allergen but may be delayed for a few hours. Its onset may be overwhelming, and death may occur from rapid respiratory and circulatory collapse before any treatment can be given.

Treatment

- Immediate injection of epinephrine hydrochloride (Adrenalin) at the first evidence of anaphylaxis. In cases of sudden severe collapse, if a vein for intravenous administration is not immediately available, no further time should be spent looking for an available vein. Instead, 10 ml of 1:10,000 epinephrine hydrochloride should be injected endotracheally (see *18–16, Intratracheal Injections*). Repeat every 5 to 20 minutes until the evidence of vascular collapse or cardiorespiratory failure lessens. Establish an IV fluid route with normal saline; give IV epinephrine slowly (dilute 0.5 to 1.0 ml of 1:1000 aqueous epinephrine to 10 ml with physiologic normal saline or distilled water) and monitor for arrhythmia and response. For less severe cases, give 0.3 ml of 1:1000 epinephrine SC.
- If the anaphylactic reaction results from an injection or an insect sting *(60)* 0.1 to 0.25 ml of 1:1000 epinephrine should be injected into and around the site of entry of the antigen. Application of ice may slow absorption. A

---

*Medic Alert, P.O. Box 1009, Turlock, California 95380; telephone number (209) 632–2371.

†ANA-KIT, Hollister-Steir Laboratories, Division of Cutter Laboratories, Inc., Spokane, Washington 99220.

temporary tourniquet may be applied proximally on an affected limb for 15 to 20 minutes pending administration of medication.

- Establish a clear airway by use of suction and positioning and support of the angles of the jaw.
- Assist ventilation *(5–1)* via mouth-to-mouth or bag-valve-mask resuscitation or endotracheal airway as necessary; do not attempt endotracheal tube passage without being prepared to perform a tracheostomy. In the presence of severe laryngeal spasm, edema or both, an emergency cricothyrotomy *(5–19)* may be necessary.
- Remove or neutralize the drug-allergen if known or suspected.
- Treat shock *(57)* by IV injection of dopamine HCl (Intropin) followed by levarterenol bitartrate (Levophed) if hypotension is extreme (see 57–5C). Hydrate with IV fluids and electrolytes to restore volume.
- IV injection of 200 mg hydrocortisone sodium succinate (Solu-Cortef) or 80 mg methylprednisolone sodium succinate (Solu-Medrol). Repeat as necessary.
- IV injection of an antihistaminic drug, such as diphenhydramine hydrochloride (Benadryl), 50 mg or 25 mg, as soon as available.
- For treatment of bronchospasm, see *56–4, Asthma.*
- After the measures just described have been taken, the patient should be hospitalized and kept under close observation for at least 24 hours.

24–2. ANGIOEDEMA

In addition to the measures outlined in *24–1,* it may be necessary to perform a conventional tracheostomy *(18–34)* to replace the previously performed cricothyrotomy.

Hereditary angioedema (HAE) and acquired angioedema with carcinoma are often recurrent and relatively resistant to the treatment just described; oral administration of danazol (Danocrine), 200 mg tid, may aid therapy. Draw blood for complement profile (C1 esterase inhibitor and C4) and refer to allergist.

Give danazol or fresh plasma prophylactically before surgery (even minor) if patient has known hereditary angioedema.

24–3. ASTHMA WITH ACUTE BRONCHOSPASM *(See 56–4)*

24–4. SERUM REACTIONS

Serum Disease

Onset

Seven to 12 days after injection of antiserum in patients not previously sensitized. Drugs, particularly penicillin, and horse serum are the most common offenders.

The clinical picture of serum disease consists of severe headache accompanied by a high temperature; diffuse erythema; urticarial wheals; severe itching; marked edema, including the airways; nausea; vomiting; abdominal cramping; generalized adenopathy; and severe joint and muscle pain. On rare occasions, peripheral and central neuritis and varying degrees of cardiac ischemia may occur.

Treatment

Mild Cases

- Control of itching by sodium bicarbonate paste or calamine lotion or Caladryl. Colloidal oatmeal (Aveeno) tub baths help in relieving pruritus.

- Hydroxyzine hydrochloride (Atarax), 25 to 50 mg orally every 6 hours and buffered salicylates.

Severe Cases

- Follow measures described under Anaphylactic Shock *(24–1)*.
- Administer steroids IV or PO.

Prognosis

There is usually complete recovery, although uncomfortable and sometimes disabling symptoms may persist for 10 to 14 days.

Serum Shock

Onset

Immediately following injection. As in anaphylactic shock, death may occur in a few minutes from respiratory and circulatory collapse. For immediate treatment, see *24–1*.

Prophylactic Treatment

- Prevention is the only sure effective treatment. Intracutaneous (intradermal) tests for sensitivity *(16)* should always be done before antiserum of any type is given, although the absence of dermal hypersensitivity does not always indicate that there will be no general hypersensitivity reaction. If the intracutaneous test is positive, the method for desensitization as outlined in *16* should be used if administration of antitoxin is essential and no other animal or human antiserum is available. Preliminary oral intake of a sustained release capsule of an antihistaminic may prevent or decrease the severity of the hypersensitivity reaction.
- Any person who has had a severe systemic reaction to an insect sting should carry, and be familiar with the use of, an emergency kit as mentioned in the introduction in this section. Hyposensitization to insect venom allergens is effective.
- Hospitalize the patient for observation and following treatment of the initial shock. This applies even if complete recovery apparently has taken place.

Prognosis. Full-fledged serum shock may be overwhelming and rapidly fatal, but if the patient survives for 5 minutes or more, there is a good chance of complete recovery.

24–5. LESS SERIOUS ALLERGIC REACTIONS

Less serious allergic reactions are common and may cause varying degrees of edema, urticaria and pruritus.

Treatment

- Remove from contact with or stop intake of the offending agent if known or suspected.
- Inject epinephrine hydrochloride (Adrenalin), 0.3 to 0.5 ml of 1:1000 solution SC or IM. For home administration, a 1:100 solution used with a nebulizer may be prescribed, with specific instructions regarding its use.
- Prescribe hydroxyzine, 25 to 50 mg PO 3 to 4 times a day for swelling, wheals and severe itching, unless the offending drug is an antihistamine *(53–80)*.
- Apply calamine lotion or Caladryl to the itching areas.
- Refer severe or stubborn cases to an internist or allergist for follow-up care.

25. Asphyxiation*

25–1. ASPHYXIA

Asphyxia, or suffocation, is caused by lack of oxygen, hypoxemia, increased carbon dioxide in the blood and rapidly increasing acidosis. It is characterized by rapidly worsening signs and symptoms of air hunger: acute anxiety, dyspnea, tachypnea, tachycardia and later dysrhythmia, increasing lividity, cyanosis, coma and death, if the chain is not broken by prompt and adequate therapy.

Treatment

- Remove victim from toxic exposure (e.g., carbon monoxide, carbon dioxide, hydrogen sulfide or other gases that have replaced oxygen) or from the suffocating substance (water, grain bins etc.). In many situations, extreme caution and adequate preparation (e.g., special protective suits and self-containerized breathing units) need to be employed by the rescuers also, so that they do not become similarly incapacitated.
- After the above has been accomplished, resuscitation proceeds as outlined in 5, *ABC's of Resuscitation.*

25–2. ASPHYXIA NEONATORUM *(See 52–1)*

25–3. DROWNING (NEAR DROWNING)

- Rapid relocation of the submerged body is essential. Some communities have specially trained under-water rescue units (professional and/or voluntary) equipped with SONAR units. Cold water (<20°C [68°F]) hypothermia combined with bradycardia associated with the "diving reflex" may help preserve organ function: drowning victims recovered as long as 20 and even 40 minutes after submersion have been successfully resuscitated without cerebral deficit. Clarity of water, absence of current, and systematic swim-look-feel efforts in a grid-type pattern aid rescuers.
- Mouth-to-mouth resuscitation (5) administered *while* an unconscious apneic person is being brought to shore (if distant) may be lifesaving. If the airway is blocked with water, the abdominal thrust (5–*13*) may relieve the problem.
- As soon as the apneic victim has been removed from the water, assure emptying of airway water (over 85% of drowning victims aspirate fluid in amounts ranging as high as 20 ml/kg of body weight). This is effectively achieved by the abdominal thrust, Heimlich maneuver (victim's head can be to the side if only water or fluid is being evacuated). The prone Schafer method is also effective, but may be more injurious. The victim's apnea minimizes aspiration of gastric contents if gastric emptying also occurs with maneuvers.
- Proceed with resuscitation in the field and during transport as outlined in 5.
- Administer oxygen for hypoxemia by nasal cannula, bag-valve-mask ventilation or volume ventilator with endotracheal tube and with enough positive end-expiratory pressure (PEEP) to obtain an oxygen partial pressure

---

*See also 5, *ABC's of Resuscitation* (esp. Tables 5–2 and 5–3); 32, *Coma;* and 55, *Pulmonary Edema.*

(pO_2) of 80 mm Hg. (See also pulmonary edema management in 55–4, *ARDS*.)

- Arrange for transportation to a hospital, even if apparent improvement has taken place. Prolonged immersion in either fresh or salt (hypertonic) water for lengthy periods can result in delayed ventricular fibrillation (29–25) and pathologic alteration of the surfactant properties of the tracheobronchial tree.
- In fresh water drowning, massive hemolysis from osmosis may necessitate transfusions of packed red blood cells. VF is slightly greater with fresh water drowning, whereas pulmonary edema is generally worse with salt water. Lower nephron nephrosis is also a serious complication.
- The possibility of a preliminary heart attack, an acute neck injury or an overwhelming toxic or allergic reaction (24) to some type of marine life (60, *Stings*) should be considered in all drowning persons.
- Sodium bicarbonate should be given intravenously to combat metabolic acidosis. The initial dose is 0.5 to 1.0 mEq/kg of body weight, followed by a dose of 0.5 mEq/kg after 5 to 10 minutes and repeated as necessary.
- Frequent pulmonary wedge, central venous pressure (CVP) and blood gas monitoring should be done, and the patient should be kept under close observation for 24 to 72 hours to avoid such potential problems as pulmonary tissue reaction (delayed drowning).
- Pulmonary and cerebral edema (55) may require treatment consisting of fluid restriction, hypothermia (slowed rewarming) and diuretics, such as furosemide (Lasix), 20 to 40 mg PO, IM or IV, and 30% nebulized ethyl alcohol aerosol. In initial treatment of cerebral edema, give dexamethasone (Decadron), 10 mg IV, and 4 mg q 6 h thereafter, according to response. Consider also mannitol and hyperbaric oxygen.
- The degree of purity or contamination (by toxins, bacteria, etc.) of water in which the person was submerged affects survival; antibiotics and other measures (53) may be required.
- Drowning in cold water helps protect the metabolism and viability of vital organs for longer periods and improves hope of recovery. The usual criteria for determining time of death (8–2 to 8–5) may not apply in these cases because of core hypothermia (62–3) and the "diving reflex."
- Recurrence of coma after initial apparent improvement indicates a poor prognosis.

25–4. SMOKE INHALATION

Inhalation of smoke by persons trapped in burning buildings and by firemen causes acute symptoms (air hunger, cough, bronchospasm); fatalities are usually the result of acute carbon monoxide or toxic fume poisoning or thermal damage to the respiratory tract below the vocal cords (usually from steam inhalation). The first measure, of course, is removal for exposure (28–*1*). Often the inhalation is accompanied by significant burns of the upper body and face (28). For treatment, see also 53–*175*, *Carbon Monoxide*, and 28–*19*, *Mucous Membrane Burns* (Burns of the Respiratory Tract).

Injury from smoke inhalation is principally due to chemical irritation from materials in the smoke. Plastics cause a particularly damaging type of smoke inhalation; cyanide poisoning may occur. Fumes in closed spaces are most likely to cause contact that is overwhelming. Treatment is aided by knowing the type of smoke exposure and the circumstances of exposure.

Signs and Symptoms

The presence of burns, ashes and soot about the face and nares, oral mucosa burns, coughing with blackish sputum, hoarseness, rhonchus or decreased breath sounds, and cyanosis are indicative of inhalation injury. Stridor with hoarseness indicates significant (about 70%) airway obstruction. Onset of serious complications and deterioration may be delayed for several days. Vital capacity and FEV_1 (or PEFR) should be promptly assessed.

Treatment

- Maintain a clear airway and start high concentrations of oxygen by mask or nasal cannula.
- Extensive external signs—particularly mucosal burns—as described above are an indication for early intubation, which should be left in for 3 to 4 days and extended according to clinical judgment. Although prolonged intubation carries the risk of vocal cord injury, it is generally preferable to tracheotomy, which creates a fertile field for bacterial entry.)
- Early bronchoscopy may help to define the extent of the problem and help to guide management, as do routine ABG's (55–4), COHb and evaluation of ratios of PaO_2 to FIO_2 (fractional inspired oxygen concentration). If the ratio of PaO_2 to FIO_2 is > 400, this is normal; if < 300 increase oxygen concentration and flow rate; if < 250, intubation/IPPB/PEEP are probably needed; and observe closely.
- If there are signs of respiratory distress or above signs, initiate high flow of 100% moisturized O_2 followed accordingly with IPPB and PEEP via endotracheal tube. (See *55–4, ARDS*.)
- Repeat ABG's q 4 to 6 h (or more often) as indicated.
- Chest x-ray should be taken on admission, but may appear normal for several days. Lung scans can be considered if other indices are inadequate.
- Assays of central venous and pulmonary wedge pressures in more serious cases aid monitoring of pulmonary edema and rate of fluid administration.
- Infusion of human serum albumin (Albumisol) to reduce lung congestion remains controversial.
- Steroids are not recommended for burn patients because of their association with a greater incidence of infections in the lungs and urinary tract as well as generalized edema. Antibiotics are advised in response to specific culture results and infections, but not for use prophylactically.
- Hospitalization is indicated with abnormality of above tests or physical signs. Because some problems resulting from smoke inhalation may be delayed, caution and observation are the preferable direction.

26. Barotrauma

Changes in atmospheric pressure—both decreases and increases—can cause or aggravate numerous conditions that may require emergency care. The three most important gas laws that account for the physiologic effects in humans experiencing significant changes in atmospheric pressure are:

Boyle's Law: Volumes and (absolute) pressures of a given gas are inversely proportional. As the gas is compressed, its volume decreases as the pressure increases, and vice versa. Interference with or slowness of normal equalization of pressure between air spaces of the body and ambient pressure creates problems.

Henry's Law: The quantity of a gas dissolved in a liquid increases in direct relationship with the pressure exerted on the liquid. This is of importance in understanding the benefits of hyperbaric oxygen (HBO) in oxygenating tissues in a severely anemic person and the ill effects from gas bubbles and gas embolization following too rapid decompression.

Dalton's Law: The pressure exerted in a space by each gas of a gas mixture is independent of the other gases in the mixture; adequate pO_2 is critical to living tissue.

26–1. ACUTE MOUNTAIN SICKNESS (AMS)

Although individual tolerances vary, at altitudes greater than 8000 to 10,000 feet many persons develop signs and symptoms from hypobaric pressure plus hypoxemia, ranging from increased pulse and respiration and euphoria to gradually decreasing mental and physical efficiency with eventual loss of consciousness. Symptoms such as headache, sleeplessness, lethargy, anorexia, nausea, vomiting, mild dyspnea, slight ataxia, tinnitus and deafness are common but usually clear spontaneously in several hours if the patient descends to a lower level of altitude; at the same altitude, symptoms may remain for 2 to 3 days before clearing. Some individuals, however, develop progressively severe problems, such as HAPE and HACE (see under severe AMS, below), with oliguria being an ominous preliminary sign; immediate descent is necessary.

MILD AMS

Acute mountain sickness is more common among people who (a) are under 21 years of age, (b) begin trips at an altitude greater than 10,000 feet without acclimatization before climbing and (c) ascend at a rate greater than 1000 feet per day when over 10,000 feet. Signs and symptoms increase with increasing altitude but are also related to the patient's prior acclimatization and individual tolerance.

Prevention

Acute mountain sickness may be prevented by slow ascent (at altitudes greater than 10,000 feet one should ascend no more than 1000 feet per day, and for every 3000 feet an extra day should be taken to acclimatize). If an unanticipated necessity for more rapid change should present itself, prophylactic treatment with acetazolamide (Diamox), 250-mg tablets taken orally q8h for 1 to 2 days prior to and after ascent, may forestall illness.

Treatment

Mild acute mountain sickness is treated by minimizing activity to the extent of bed rest if necessary and waiting for symptoms to resolve before continuing. If symptoms still do not resolve, the patient must be evacuated to a lower altitude. Adequate intake of oral fluids, but minimal salt intake, is usually helpful. Intestinal edema, characterized by malabsorption, cramps and flatus, can be treated with light diet and administration of digestive enzymes and phenothiazines (Phenergan, Compazine).

SEVERE AMS

The two principal life-threatening disorders of altitude sickness are high altitude pulmonary edema (HAPE) and high altitude cerebral edema (HACE). The pathophysiology is not clearly understood. HAPE and HACE may occur concomitantly. Descent is the only proven treatment.

High Altitude Pulmonary Edema (HAPE) *(See also 55, Pulmonary Edema)*

Signs and symptoms include coughing as an early sign, followed by orthopnea, severe dyspnea, rales and hemoptysis.

Treatment

1. Immediate return to a lower level at which the patient was asymptomatic; the vast majority recover with a descent of 1000 feet.
2. Furosemide (Lasix), 40 mg IV; may be repeated 1 to 2 times according to the patient's condition. Digitalis is not useful.
3. Oxygen administration, if available. Intermittent positive pressure breathing with positive end-expiratory pressure (or pursed-lip expiratory breathing) may be needed.

High Altitude Cerebral Edema (HACE)
(See also 44–7, Cerebral Edema)

Unremitting headache, confusion and loss of judgment are earlier signs and may be followed by ataxia, weakness, stupor, unconsciousness and seizures. In some patients hemiparesis, hemiplegia, or cranial nerve palsy—particularly of the sixth—may occur. There may be hypothermia *(62–3)*, and papilledema may or may not be present. Retinal hemorrhages are not diagnostic of HACE, as they may occur in asymptomatic mountaineers.

Treatment

1. Immediate return to a lower level, at least to where the patient had been asymptomatic. (Recovery may occur with descent of 1000 feet or even less.)
2. Oxygen and diuretic administration.
3. Dexamethasone, 10 mg IV, followed by 6 mg IV every 6 hours.

26–2. BENDS *(See 26–4)*

26–3. CAISSON DISEASE *(See 26–4)*

26–4. DECOMPRESSION SICKNESS (Bends, Caisson Disease, Compressed Air Sickness)

Decompression sickness may occur on too rapid ascent in divers who breathe compressed air or oxygen through any type of mechanical equipment and in persons who work in air locks under increased atmospheric pressure. It can occur in those in an aircraft with inadequate pressurization or sudden cabin decompression at high altitude or in patients under therapy in a hyperbaric chamber who are brought out too rapidly. SCUBA divers should preferably not fly within 12 hours of diving (see 26–7).

Under increased compression circumstances (1 additional atmosphere of body pressure for each 33 feet of depth in water or its equivalent), nitrogen and other gases are forced into the blood and tissues in increased amounts. With gradual ascent, the dissolved nitrogen comes out of solution at a rate the body can eliminate through respiration. However, if decompression is not gradual, bubbles of nitrogen are released into the blood and tissues and produce a variety of signs and symptoms; onset can be in minutes, though usually within 1 to 3 hours and infrequently up to 12 hours.

The most common of these signs and symptoms is severe throbbing pain that shifts its location frequently and especially involves muscles, joints and bones. This is caused by the expanding gas molecules. Abdominal pain may be acute enough to be confused with an acute surgical abdomen. Intense pruritus and mottling and erythema of the skin may be present ("skin hits"). If only pain is present, the problem may be categorized as Type 1 decompression sickness.

Involvement of the central nervous system (CNS) is considered Type 2 decompression sickness. Vertigo *(49–21)* is often severe enough to cause staggering that may be mistaken for drunkenness. Also among frequent nervous system symptoms are numbness and tingling of the extremities and bizarre paresthesias. In serious situations in which the CNS has been "hit," which are, fortunately, uncommon, the following may occur: hemiplegia, paraplegia, quadriplegia, strabismus, nystagmus, diplopia and paresis.

Though occurring in only about 1 to 2% of decompression sickness cases, a most serious problem is "chokes" (probably gross nitrogen bubble embolization in the pulmonary vasculature, with increased permeability and large third compartment losses). Coughing, burning substernal discomfort, a reddened pharynx and a pleuritic type of pain are earlier manifestations, and severe dyspnea, hypoxia, unconsciousness and death may ensue. Serious cardiac arrhythmias, bradycardia and hypotension/shock leading to death can occur with decompression sickness. Acute dyspnea may occur several hours after apparently successful recompression and decompression and may be followed by collapse and unconsciousness.

Caution: Divers breathing compressed air must not hold their breath during ascent, or the expanding gas pressure may rupture alveoli (overinflation syndrome), causing sudden pneumothorax, mediastinal emphysema and hemoptysis, which in turn lead to gas embolization and possible unconsciousness and death. Air embolism *(63–6)* is to be especially suspected with immediate or rapid onset of unconsciousness and the presence of pneumothorax *(56–17)*.

Treatment

Recompression and gradual decompression constitute the only definitive treatment of any value. See *26–6* for information on locating hyperbaric chambers. While transfer is being arranged, the following supportive measures may be of assistance:

- Continuous artificial ventilation by any feasible method *(5–21)* as necessary—mouth-to-mouth and mechanical resuscitation are the most satisfactory.
- Inhalation of 100% oxygen initially at 5 to 6 liters per minute.
- General supportive care and intravenous fluids (given cautiously).
- Dexamethasone, 10 mg IV, in the presence of CNS involvement *(44–7)* that is rapidly evolving, particularly if it is not responsive to recompression. Variable benefits found with use.

26–5. DIVING HAZARDS *(See also 26–4, Decompression Sickness)*

The problems, limitations and hazards of deep water diving with air hose, suit and metal helmet have long been recognized. Commercial divers are required to be in good physical condition and are trained and instructed in accordance with stringent safety regulations. In contrast, the development and wide use of various types of self-contained underwater breathing apparatus (commonly abbreviated to SCUBA) by inexperienced, untrained, unsupervised and unlicensed persons diving for sport has resulted in the need for recognition and treatment of various physical, metabolic and mental disturbances resulting from exposure to an unfamiliar and potentially dangerous environment.

Skin divers (who can remain under water only as long as they can hold their breath) are subject only to the usual well-known hazards of diving and swimming. Prior hyperventilation should be avoided by all swimmers and divers, as the reduction of the CO_2 level of the blood may be sufficient to cause loss of stimulus to breathe, resulting in unconsciousness ("shallow water blackout"). Snorkel swimming near the surface with a 12-inch tube presents no unique barotrauma problems.

Diving in cold water causes a vagal response bradycardia ("diving reflex") that is especially hazardous to persons with preexistent heart disease.

The principal immediate diving hazards are listed in Table 26–1.

General Principles of Management and Care

- Artificial respiration—expired air respiratory assistance *(5–21)*—to dyspneic, cyanotic, unconscious or "near-drowned" divers, continued not only during rescue and en route to the pressure chamber but also in the chamber during recompression, may be lifesaving.
- Knowledge of the location of, the shortest route to and the indications for use of the closest pressure chamber equipped for recompression and gradual decompression.
- Recompression and slow supervised decompression of any seriously ill, stuporous or comatose diver who has been using any type of air- or gas-filled diving apparatus, no matter how long an interval has elapsed since the dive, even if very shallow. Recompression and gradual controlled decompression in a pressure chamber is harmless not only to the diver but also to an attendant, and under certain circumstances may prevent serious, permanent, even terminal after effects. *When in doubt, recompress!*
- The conditions listed in Table 26–1 are related directly or indirectly to underwater pressure or subsurface environment and may require emergency management.

26–6. HYPERBARIC OXYGEN THERAPY (HBO)

Hyperbaric oxygen chamber therapy, in either a large recompression chamber or a single monoplace chamber, also has value for emergency conditions other than those caused by the aforementioned barotrauma and air embolism *(63–6)*. Chief among these are carbon monoxide poisoning *(53–175)*, cyanide poisoning *(53–232)*, gas gangrene *(59–42)*, compromised grafts or skin *(59–43)* and extreme blood loss anemia *(45–6)*.

If the location of the nearest hyperbaric recompression chamber is not known, assistance and advice on a 24-hour basis can be obtained from the U.S. Air Force at (512) 536-3278 or the Navy Duty Officer at (904) 234-4355 or 4351. "DAN" (Diving Accident Network) at Duke University Medical Center (919) 684-8111 also offers 24-hour advice regarding SCUBA diving accidents.

For signs of oxygen toxicity see *53–503*.

26–7. RESTRICTIONS ON AIR TRAVEL

Although modern commercial aircraft are equipped with pressurized cabins that limit the effects of barotrauma to those caused by ascent to and descent from a maximum of 8000 feet, persons with certain physical ailments may develop uncomfortable, possibly serious, symptoms if they travel by air. Among the conditions that may require special consideration and preparation for flight or with which flight should be avoided are the following:

- Valvular heart disease or other severe or decompensated cardiac conditions, extreme hypertension, angina pectoris, coronary disease and, particularly, recent myocardial infarction that could be seriously aggravated by altitude

Text continued on page 168

Table 26–1. DIVING HAZARDS

Condition	Type of Diver: *IA: Snorkel IB: Skin*	Type of Diver: *IIA: SCUBA IIB: Helmet*	Cause	Signs and Symptoms	HBO Chamber?	CPR Often?	Other Treatment and Comments
Air embolism	No	Yes	Holding breath during ascent	See 26–4, *Decompression sickness*	Yes	Yes	Sedatives; analgesics for pain. Permanent sequelae may occur
Anoxia (hypoxia)	No[1]	Yes[2, 3]	Failure of breathing apparatus	Unconsciousness without apparatus	Yes	Yes	SCUBA "buddy sharing" of O_2 if possible; if rapid ascent, see 26–4
Bends	No	Yes	Decompression sickness	Pain in joints and/or abdomen	Yes	No	Sedatives; narcotics for pain. See 26–4
CO_2 poisoning	No[1]	Yes: IIA[2] No: IIB	CO_2 absorbent inadequate	Rapid breathing, unconsciousness	Yes	Yes	Prevention: Routine maintenance of equipment Treatment: See *53–173*
CO poisoning	No	Yes: IIA No: IIB	Impure air in cylinder	Sudden loss of consciousness	Yes	Yes	Prevention: Routine maintenance of equipment Treatment: See *53–175*
Chokes	No	Yes	Decompression sickness	Dyspnea, cough, chest pain, hemoptysis	Yes	Yes	Recompress immediately. See 26–4
Conjunctival hemorrhage	Yes	Yes	Tight goggles; excessive depth	Bleeding may be retrobulbar	No	No	Symptomatic treatment only. Recovery complete
Decompression sickness	No	Yes	Rapid ascent from long or deep dives	Onset may be delayed for many hours; see 26–4	Yes	Yes	Sedatives and anodynes for pain. Immediate recompression

Drowning	Yes	Yes	Hypoxia, neck injury, entanglement	Unconsciousness, absent vital signs	±[4]	Yes	Any "drowned" diver using any type of gas-containing breathing apparatus requires recompression at once. For treatment, see 5; 25–3
Eardrum rupture	Yes	Yes	Barotrauma, previous disease	Pain, hearing loss	No	No	Stop diving. Nothing into ear. Small holes usually close spontaneously
Emphysema	No	Yes	Air embolism	Crepitus of soft tissues, dyspnea	Yes	Often	Subcutaneous emphysema clears; mediastinal often recurs after decompression
Epistaxis	Yes	Yes	Barotrauma, previous disease	May vary from slight oozing to severe hemorrhage	No	No	Symptomatic treatment only
External ear squeeze	No	Yes	Nonequalizing air-containing apparatus	Redness, bleb formation, bleeding	No	No	See 35–4; recovery complete in short time
Hemoptysis	Yes	Yes	Usully air embolism; possible decompression illness	Bloody froth indicative of respiratory tract damage	Yes	Yes	Type I A/B divers: Supportive therapy Type II A/B divers: Recompress immediately
Hypocarbia	Yes	Yes	Voluntary hyperventilation or faulty gas regulation	Paresthesias, decreased ventilation, unconsciousness	No	No (usually)	Avoid hyperventilation before diving; check equipment

[1]Unless syncope occurs, as following hyperventilation.
[2]IIA, closed circuit.
[3]IIB, air supply cut off.
[4]±, varies with circumstances.

Table 26–1 continued on following pages

Table 26–1. DIVING HAZARDS *(Continued)*

Condition	Type of Diver: *IA: Snorkel IB: Skin*	Type of Diver: *IIA: SCUBA IIB: Helmet*	Cause	Signs and Symptoms	HBO Chamber?	CPR Often?	Other Treatment and Comments
Hypothermia	Yes	Yes	Low water temperature	Shivering; slowed functions	No	±[4]	Shivering makes holding mouthpiece difficult. Mental errors. For treatment, see *62–3*
Neurologic disturbances (*Note*: May occur with any type of diving if caused by envenomation from marine life (*65*) or CNS injury from trauma)	No	Yes	Usually dives below 30 feet	Onset may be hours after apparent recovery from other conditions; see *26–4*	Yes	±[4]	Neurologic abnormalities in a diver who has descended >10 ft using any type of breathing apparatus require that recompression be done at once
Otitis externa	Yes	Yes	Infection, wetting	Pain, redness, tenderness of pinna or external canal	No	No	Drying after each dive is indicated; see also *35–17*
Otitis media	Yes	Yes	Frequent wetting, irritation	Pain, tinnitus	No	No	See *35–18*
O_2 poisoning (hyperoxia)	No	Yes	Excessive depth, excess O_2 proportion	Vertigo, nausea, muscle twitching, followed by convulsions	No	No (usually)	Usually complete recovery if rescued before complications (e.g., drowning, air embolism) occur

Pneumothorax	No	Yes	Usually air embolism but may occur independently	Dyspnea, cyanosis, chest pain	Yes	±[4]	After reexpansion in pressure chamber symptoms may recur when pressure is lowered
Respiratory arrest	Yes	Yes	Air embolism, decompression sickness, CO or CO_2 intoxication	Not breathing	Yes	Yes	Immediate CPR, continued during transportation. Cardiac arrest (5–2) is more uncommon
Sinusitis, "sinus squeeze"	Yes	Yes	Mucosal edema, gas contraction and expansion	Pain, tenderness, fever, sinus opacity	No	No	See 56–23. Begin ENT equilibration procedures

[4] ± = varies with circumstances.

sickness *(26–1)*, air sickness *(26–4)* or motion sickness *(49–11)*. Patients with cardiac pacemakers should avoid microwave oven areas and passenger surveillance electronic body scanners unless these devices are specifically designated as safe.

- Conditions under which the normal expansion of body gases (1.75 at 8000 feet, compared with 1.0 at sea level) might be detrimental. Among these are glaucoma, acute or chronic sinusitis, nasopharyngitis and otitis, large unsupported hernias, intestinal obstruction, acute appendicitis, peptic ulcers or postoperative conditions (e.g., eye surgery, pneumonectomy, intestinal anastomosis) in which increased gas volume might cause acute complications. All patients who have or are prone to have gastrointestinal dilatation during air evacuation are safer and more comfortable if a nasogastric tube and rectal tube are either inserted or ready for insertion. Patients with subcutaneous crepitation and gas may require special management during gas expansion occurring at higher altitude (see *59–42, Soft Tissue Infections*).
- Fractured jaw. Unless some method of quick release in case of vomiting has been substituted for the usual wiring or a person knowledgeable in the use of wire cutters is accompanying the person during air ambulance transportation, persons with broken jaws should not travel by air.
- Conditions in which slight hypoxia (90% arterial oxygen saturation at 8000 feet, compared with 96% at sea level) might be detrimental; among these are shock, status asthmaticus and severe respiratory conditions with limited respiratory reserve, due to either diminished ventilatory power (all conditions with muscular paresis, including myasthenia gravis) or impaired gas exchange. It should be remembered that the oxygen masks available above each seat on commercial aircraft have a flow rate of only 1.5 liters per minute—far less than the flow rate (5 to 10 liters per minute) necessary for treatment of acute hypoxemic states. Prearrangements can be made with airlines for use of special portable baby incubators (e.g., Ohio Air-Vac) or ventilatory assistive devices with self-contained power reserve and adaptive plugs that use the aircraft's electrical power system.
- Conditions associated with profound anemia. These include the presence of S and C hemoglobins in some blacks; sickling and hemolysis may occur with reduced oxygen tension.
- Psychoses and severe neuroses—especially those related to closed spaces and altitudes.
- Communicable diseases during communicable period.
- Pregnancy beyond the 32nd week—unless written clearance for flight is obtained from a physician within several days.
- Individuals who have been diving under compressed air conditions (e.g., SCUBA divers) should avoid air flights within 12 hours because of the increased likelihood of decompression sickness *(26–4)*; if the cabin is unpressurized and the patient had long underwater exposure, a 24-hour delay is safer, although a shorter time period is allowable if the plane can fly at a low altitude. (*Note*: If a person is already ill, the benefits of rapid air evacuation to a recompression chamber may take precedence over these considerations; helicopter is ideal for relatively short distances.)
- The pressure in pneumatic trousers (MAST) increases during ascent and drops with descent; monitoring and adjustment is required.
- Though commercial airlines are gradually stocking a better variety of medical emergency drugs in flight, people with known potential problems should obtain recommendations for carrying supplies until on-board supplies are standardized.

27. Bites

This section should be read in conjunction with *Soft Tissue Injuries, 59–1* to *59–3*. It should be recognized that envenomation does not occur with each bite from poisonous members of the animal kingdom. Also see *60, Stings*.

27–1. GENERAL TREATMENT CONSIDERATIONS

The principal issues in the treatment of animal bites are as follows:

- Prompt cleaning of the wound. Management of any possible envenomation.
- Management of the mechanical aspects of the soft tissue injury (*59–1* to *59–3*). Tetanus immunization (*20*) should be made current within about 24 hours. Human bites and other dirty bites generally should not have primary repair, but disfiguring facial bites can be an exception. Most dog bites can be closed primarily, except for severe hand and deep puncture wounds, which are preferably left open. Prophylactic antibiotic treatment is generally not necessary, except for hand and puncture wounds, for which one should administer penicillin V, 500 mg PO qid (or cephalexin or dicloxacillin).
- Obtaining of culture for aerobes and anaerobes when signs of infection are already present or if the wound is badly contaminated.
- Consideration of whether rabies treatment should be started (see *33–54*). The prototype of the bite not requiring immediate initiation of rabies treatment is the bite from a healthy domestic animal that has had rabies immunization, was threatened or teased into a provoked bite and is under observation. Bites from small animals such as hamsters, rabbits, squirrels, chipmunks, gerbils, guinea pigs, mice and rodents in general are not considered to present a risk of rabies. Human rabies has not been reported from human bites. Unprovoked bites by ill domestic animals that cannot be located or those by wild animals (particularly the bat, skunk, monkey, fox and raccoon) that usually fear and avoid human contact and cannot be located are indications for rabies treatment. Other manifestations of rabies in animals are vicious and/or agitated activity, "dumb," paralytic behavior and behavior peculiar to that animal.
- Notification of the local Health Department or animal control agency (*15*) of the bite so that proper investigation can be made and any needed assistance given in locating and observing the animal, where indicated. The Health Department should also be notified of the presence of insects (mosquitoes, fleas, mites) when their bites are spreading communicable diseases, so that abatement procedures may be instituted.

TREATMENT OF SPECIFIC BITES*

27–2. ANT BITES AND STINGS *(See also 27–13)*

The bites or stings of many ants can cause transient discomfort. The venom of the fire ant is injected not by its jaws but by an abdominal stinger, sometimes causing severe localized reactions and systemic effects that can even be lethal.

27–3. BARRACUDA BITES

These voracious fish (in the Caribbean) have tremendously long jaws armed with large, sharp, serrated teeth that can inflict serious lacerations requiring extensive

---

*Management in conjunction with 27–1, *General Treatment Considerations.*

debridement and repair. However, humans can usually swim among them unmolested (but should avoid wearing shiny metals). (Don't eat large Caribbean barracuda.)

27–4. BAT BITES

Certain varieties of carnivorous and insectivorous bats may be rabid *(33–54)*. In addition, they may carry other infectious viruses in their salivary glands. Orchitis, oophoritis and aseptic meningitis have been reported following bat bites.

27–5. BEDBUG BITES

The bedbug *(Cimex lectularius)* gives multiple bites, causing a series of locally irritating hemorrhagic lesions, usually discovered by the patient on arising in the morning. Only symptomatic treatment is needed except in the case of sensitivity reactions.

27–6. BLACK WIDOW SPIDER BITES

The female of this genus *(Latrodectus)*—often identifiable by an hourglass-shaped (sometimes a single or double spot), bright (orangish, red, white) coloration on the abdomen—is responsible for many toxic effects. The bite of the small male cannot penetrate the skin.

In spite of wide publicity to the contrary, black widow spider bites are rarely fatal. The bite has little local reaction. The toxic picture (developing within 2 hours after the bite) is characterized by headache, pain, muscle cramps, increase in blood pressure, fasciculations and cramping of the abdomen and large muscle groups of the extremities, nausea, vomiting and a hypertensive response. The intense local abdominal pain may be severe enough to be mistaken for an acute surgical abdomen. Treatment consists of the following:

- Intensive supportive care (see 57, *Shock*) as needed.
- Administration of antivenin in severe cases of envenomation, in patients with cardiac disorders and in younger (under 16) and older (over 65) patients; these patients should also be hospitalized. If antivenin is to be given, inject 0.02 ml intracutaneously to test for sensitivity. If no wheal or indurated area is present after 20 minutes, give 1 ampule (2.5 ml diluted to 15 ml in saline) slowly IV.
- Control of the characteristic acute myalgia by intravenous methocarbamol drip or diazepam. Injection of 10 ml of 10% calcium gluconate solution may also be effective, and a repeat in 4 to 8 hours may be necessary.

27–7. BROWN SPIDER BITES

The venom of a brown spider (genus *Loxosceles*, brown recluse) contains complex chemicals and is quite toxic. The brown recluse spider is identified by a violin-shaped mark on its cephalothorax.

Milder reactions to brown spider bites are characterized by slight discomfort (less than a bee sting) at the time of the bite and for up to several hours after the bite, following which pain may gradually increase. Bleb formation surrounded by an area of intense ischemia develops, followed in 24 to 48 hours by formation of a tough black eschar surrounded by purplish induration. On removal there is a deep, irregular, necrotic-based ulcer that heals very slowly with extreme scarring and usually with surrounding permanent pigmentation. There is no effective antivenin.

Treatment

- Early local excision of the bite area, if done within 8 hours after the bite.
- Analgesics *(12)* for pain, as necessary.
- Early administration of corticosteroids such as prednisone or initially dexamethasone, 4 mg q 6 h, may reduce tissue reaction. Consider use of dapsone or colchicine.

Severe reactions are indicated by a generalized morbilliform eruption, fever up to 40°C (104°F), recurrent fainting spells, severe arthralgia, shock and hemoglobinuria.

Treatment. Treat as for milder reactions (above); in addition, patient should be hospitalized for symptomatic and supportive therapy.

Prognosis. Prognosis for recovery is good unless a massive dose of venom has been received. Ulcers are slow to heal and require daily attention and soaks; disfigurement by scars and pigmentation is common, and plastic surgery may be needed.

27–8. CAMEL BITES

Because of the tremendous leverage resulting from the unusual shape of the jaws and the peculiar dentition (long incisors in the upper jaw that imbricate with the canines) of these vicious animals, camel bites usually result in fractures and dislocations in addition to extensive crushing, tearing and avulsion of soft tissues. Extensive reconstructive surgery is often required.

27–9. CAT BITES

Cat bites and scratches, even if minute, may cause a benign low-grade infection (cat-scratch fever). Because of their long, slender, sharp incisors, cats can penetrate deeply into soft tissues, including into joint spaces on the hand, and seed a potentially serious deep infection with only a minimal surface wound; these should be observed closely and may require surgical intervention. Local treatment is the same as for dog bites *(27–11)*.

27–10. CHIGGER BITES *(See also 58–12, Pruritus)*

The small larvae of thrombiculid mites (chiggers), which often are parasitic to birds and reptiles, may cause uncomfortable but rarely serious local irritation, especially in children. Infestation usually occurs from playing in damp, swampy areas of scrub vegetation and is characterized by papules and vesicles at the site of the bite (usually located where clothing presses against skin). Itching, redness and swelling, lasting 3 to 5 days, may occur, with secondary cellulitis and lymphadenitis or, occasionally, bacteremia from scratching. Cautious temporary focal application of a lotion containing 1% gamma benzene hexachloride will kill the mite.

27–11. DOG BITES

Dog bites vary in extent from slight contusions, superficial abrasions and fang puncture wounds to deep tearing lacerations if the animal or the victim attempts to pull away.

Treatment

- See 27–1, *General Treatment Considerations,* and 33–54, *Rabies.*
- Contusions usually require no treatment, provided the skin is not broken.
- Whenever possible, the dog should be kept under observation by the appropriate animal control agency. If the animal has been killed, the body should be turned over to the local health authorities for disposition. Under no circumstances should the body be destroyed.

27–12. EEL BITES

Large eels, such as the Moray eel, have sharp teeth and strong jaws that can cause substantial soft tissue injury *(59)*.

27–13. FLEA BITES

Flea *(Siphonaptera)* bites may cause severe local reactions with surrounding edema, wheals, cellulitis and intense itching. In addition, these parasites are important vectors of diseases such as typhus.

Treatment

- Cold compresses.
- Application of sodium bicarbonate paste, calamine lotion or medium-potency corticosteroids.
- Oral administration of chlorpheniramine or hydroxyzine (Atarax) for further relief of symptoms.

- Referral to an allergist for possible desensitization in extreme cases.
- Abatement measures to eradicate the source.

27–14. FLY BITES

The subclass Diptera includes biting flies such as the deerfly, sandfly, horsefly and tsetse fly that can cause a painful, irritating small lesion. More important, flies are the vectors for many types of serious illness, such as human sleeping sickness from trypanosomes of infected tsetse flies.

27–15. GILA MONSTER BITES

Gila monster bites cause severe local reactions but rarely cause systemic reactions.

27–16. HORSE BITES

Severe horse bites are rare because of the shape of the front teeth. If the skin is broken, treatment is the same as that outlined for dog bites *(27–11)*, except that the need for rabies prophylaxis is rare. Small bones of the hands or feet or of a child's extremities can be broken.

27–17. HUMAN BITES

Human bites often result in severe infections. Treatment consists of thorough debridement and irrigation, with the wound left open to heal by primary intention, assisted by daily cleansing to reduce infection. If infection occurs, after obtaining a culture (including an assay for the presence of anaerobes and starting sensitivity studies), start appropriate antibiotics *(59–42)*. Wounds into bone or joint spaces require surgical debridement and immediate antibiotic treatment. Tetanus immunization *(16)* should be made current because of possible later contamination.

27–18. INSECT BITES

Although severe systemic diseases—e.g., malaria *(33–38)*, yellow fever *(33–81)* and typhus *(33–74)*—may be transmitted by insect bites, local reactions are usually mild. Systemic allergic reactions, however, may be extremely severe and require immediate and extensive care (see *24*). Treatment of milder problems usually consists of relief of pruritus *(58–12)*, treatment of secondary infections and elimination of the insect to prevent recurrences. If the insect is found, it should be brought in for expert identification, as necessary.

27–19. KISSING BUG BITES

These cone-nosed bugs, *Triatoma protracta*, can cause painful local bites and allergic reactions *(24)*. In some areas, they are vectors of diseases such as trypanosomiasis.

27–20. LLAMA BITES

Llama bites have the same peculiarities and characteristics as camel bites *(27–8)*.

27–21. LOUSE BITES *(See 33–47, Contagious and Communicable Diseases, Pediculosis)*

27–22. MITE BITES *(See 33–61, Contagious and Communicable Diseases, Scabies; 27–10, Chigger Bites)*

27–23. MOSQUITO BITES

Therapy is the same as that given for flea bites *(27–13)*. See also 33–38, *Malaria;* 33–81, *Yellow Fever.*

27–24. OCTOPUS BITES

The cephalopods have a pair of horny jaws, a form of tooth and venom apparatus. Although the octopus is generally timid, the strong jaw mechanism can cause deep penetration associated with envenomation, which, on rare occasion, has been fatal.

27–25. RAT BITES

Persons (particularly infants) living in squalid surroundings may be injured severely by rat bites. For treatment, follow the guidelines outlined in *27–1*.

Severe systemic conditions, such as bubonic plague *(33–49)*, may be transmitted by rat fleas. Rat-bite fever, caused by introduction of *Streptobacillus moniliformis* into the wound, is treated with penicillin.

27–26. SHARK BITES

The savage, capricious attacks of these territorial predators make the shark one of the most feared members of the animal kingdom. Attacks have been noted to occur more often in daylight and in shallow water, with initial bites located somewhat oftener on the lower extremities and buttocks than on the forearms and hands. The shark's powerful jaw mechanism (a biting pressure of 18 tons per square inch has been recorded) is aided by "teeth" that are capable of sawing and shearing (in addition, there are four to five rows of reserve dentition) and further abetted by rapid, violent torque movements of the head and body; this can result in enormous avulsion and amputation injuries. Approximately 70% of bites are fatal in humans. Extrication of the victim, control of bleeding *(45)* and soft tissue injury management *(59)* may require heroic efforts.

27–27. SNAKE BITES

"Bites" of poisonous snakes are not caused by closing of the jaws but by strikes or thrusts with the mouth open, with introduction of the venom through needle-like fangs. Not all bites of venomous snakes result in envenomation. There may be no reaction or only local reaction without systemic toxicity. Systemic toxicity may occur either progressively after local reaction or very rapidly with minimal local reaction.

Three of the four kinds of poisonous snakes inhabiting North America (rattlesnake, copperhead and water moccasin or cottonmouth) are pit vipers and can be identified by the presence of a triangular head, elliptical pupils, pits posterior to the nostrils and enlarged anterior maxillary teeth or fangs. The fourth kind—the coral snakes—are most frequently recognized by series of alternate black and red bands, each separated by a yellow stripe (although this is not true for all coral snakes). By far the most common is the rattlesnake (tail rattles), which may vary in length (from 6 inches to over 6 feet) and in color and markings with its environment. Snakes in the fer-de-lance group—the tropical rattler, the cantril and the bushmaster—are common in tropical Central and South America. Many varieties of cobras and kraits occur in southeastern Asia and India. Several varieties of sea snakes are extremely toxic.

Snake venoms contain biologically active substances in varying proportions and amounts depending on the species. Antivenins are available for some, but not all, snakes in the areas in which the snakes are found.

Signs and symptoms of rattlesnake bite consist of fang marks—usually 2 distinct punctures. A row of small superficial wounds from the upper teeth may be present or, on rare occasions, from the lower teeth. Envenomation is characterized by rapid (within minutes) onset of local pain and progressive swelling, with ecchymosis and hemorrhage occurring 1 to 12 hours later; the rapidity and degree of these local signs vary considerably, dependent on several factors (including type and amount of venom). After the bite of some species, a systemic toxic reaction may be heralded in minutes by paresthesias such as numbness and tingling including the mouth and the tongue, which may also sense a peculiar taste. Progressive respiratory and circulatory depression and neurologic signs and symptoms, depending upon the toxic properties of the venom, may develop. The presence or absence of envenomation is generally evident by 30 minutes and at least within an hour.

The venom of the coral snake may cause rapid onset of drowsiness, paresis with drooping lids and difficulty in speaking and breathing, and gross sweating and salivation; however, there is less pain and swelling than with the rattler venom.

Treatment

- Transport the patient to a hospital for care as soon as possible; initial treatment can continue en route. The single most important aspect of treatment is immediacy of antivenin administration if envenomation has occurred.
- For pit viper bites, apply a constriction band about 2 inches proximal to the bite or swelling if on an extremity, tight enough to occlude the lymphatics but not tight enough to shut off the arterial or venous blood supply (it should be possible to slip a finger into the band). The constriction band should not be removed until the patient can receive definitive care, but it can be loosened slightly every 20 to 30 minutes for a minute and advanced as necessary to keep it 2 inches proximal to the swelling extending from the bite (later recordings of extremity circumference at several proximal levels are advisable to document swelling change). Continue until antivenin has been given.
- If more than 40 minutes from a hospital, incise the bite (including the fang marks) linearly about 0.5 cm and about 0.3 cm deep, going just into the fat and extending slightly beyond each fang mark (do not go through nerves and tendons; the fang penetration is superficial). Do not make any cruciate incisions. Suction should be applied immediately by suction cup or other means. Incision and suction are of value only if initiated within the first 5 minutes. Mouth suction can be used, but may result in secondary infection of the incised area. (The venom is of low toxicity and not poisonous to the person sucking, but it should be spit out.) Suction of some type should be continued for about 30 minutes; this can be done during transport to the hospital.
- Keep the patient as calm and quiet as possible. Splint the bitten area and keep the extremity in a slightly dependent position. Excessive activity may result in more rapid spread of the venom. If possible, kill the snake and bring it in for identification, or give a comprehensive accurate description.
- Keep the patient warm and support the circulation as necessary (see also 57–5, *Treatment of Shock*).
- Give codeine orally or other analgesics cautiously for severe pain and apprehension. Pain is not usually severe during the first few hours but may develop later with the onset of edema.
- Antivenin is indicated only in treatment of bites with more than trivial envenomation. Assistance concerning antivenin can be obtained from the Arizona Poison Control System, (602) 626–6016, on a 24-hour basis. After testing for sensitivity to horse serum *(16)*, inject antivenin in adequate amounts as soon as possible, even if the victim is moribund. Pit viper polyvalent antivenin is available for the rattlesnake, copperhead, moccasin, fer-de-lance, cantril and bushmaster. It is not effective against coral snakes, cobras, kraits and poisonous sea snakes. An antivenin against coral snake venom is available in the United States. In other parts of the world, special types of antivenin effective against indigenous poisonous snakes are prepared and available, usually through local public health authorities. With rare exceptions, land snake antivenins are ineffective against sea snake venoms. In adults, minimal toxicity cases are treated with 5 vials of antivenin given IV; moderate to severe cases require 10 to 30 vials. Children may require twice the adult dose. No antivenin need be given locally around the bite. Decrease in edema (include serial circumferential measurements) and reversal of progressive clinical signs and symptoms guide the amount given.
- Inject human tetanus-immune globulin (TIG). Tetanus toxoid may be indicated if the patient has never been actively immunized *(20)*.
- Give broad spectrum antibiotics if infection is present.
- Transfer all patients to a hospital as soon as possible for antivenin, necessary supportive therapy and close observation. In severe cases, laboratory studies, including those advised for treatment of shock *(57)* and evaluation of hematologic problems *(45)*, should be done and typing and cross-match performed. An electrocardiogram (ECG) may be advisable, and a urinalysis should be obtained. Dangerous relapses may occur after apparent marked improvement as long as 3 days after the bite.

Table 27–1. DIFFERENTIATION OF TICK PARALYSIS FROM BOTULISM

	TICK PARALYSIS	BOTULISM	
		Adults	*Infants*
Exposure	Outdoors	Improperly canned foods	Enteric organism
Age	Young children	Adults more commonly	Infants under 6 months
Incidence	Usually individual cases	May be a group of people	Usually individual cases
Onset	Gradual progressive muscle weakness	Rapid onset of muscle weakness and later gradual regression	Gradual onset of muscle weakness and response to treatment
Paresthesias, areflexia	Common	Not common	Not common
Motor nerve conduction	Velocity usually decreased	Velocity usually unchanged	Velocity usually unchanged

- DO NOT cauterize the punctured area with acids, potassium permanganate crystals, iodine or hot metallic objects. Alcohol-containing drinks are of no therapeutic value, although they may result in a beneficial temporary decrease in anxiety and activity. Corticosteroids and antihistaminics are of disputed value in the emergency treatment of snake bite. Ice immersion or cold application is not recommended because of frequently unskilled use, resulting in severe frostbite *(62–2)*—even requiring amputation on occasion.
- Treatment for known nonpoisonous snake bites consists of primary wound management *(59)* and assurance of tetanus immunity *(20)*.

27–28. SPIDER BITES

Except for the 3 kinds listed below, spider bites usually result in mild local reactions only and require no specific therapy.

Black Widow Spider. The female is characterized by an hourglass-shaped bright marking on the belly *(27–6)*. The male is smaller and harmless.

Brown Spider. Characterized by a violin-shaped darker brown or black coloration on the cephalothorax *(27–7)*.

Tarantulas. Characterized by large size and hairiness of legs and body *(27–29)*.

27–29. TARANTULA BITES

Tarantula bites cause few systemic reactions, but locally there may be swelling and edema. The bite area should be cleansed thoroughly. Human tetanus-immune globulin (TIG) or toxoid *(20)* should be given routinely if immunity is not current.

27–30. TICK BITES

Tick bites are characterized by burying of the head of the tick; since awareness of the bite is unusual, this is best detected by routine daily skin and scalp inspection when in infestation areas. The following procedures may be necessary to release the head from the tissues: application of kerosene, turpentine, petroleum jelly (Vaseline), gasoline or a drop of clear nail polish; careful approximation of the glowing end of a cigarette close to the buried head of the tick—so the tick backs out; or excision of the buried head under local anesthesia.

Rocky Mountain Spotted Fever *(See also 33–57)*. This disease is transmitted by both the wood tick and the dog tick, is endemic in the United States and represents an often overlooked cause of severe local and general symptoms (fever, chills, rash, prostration, myalgia, headache, edema). Treatment is as follows:

- Frequent inspection for and removal of ticks, especially from the scalp.
- Hospitalization for rapid-identification immunofluorescent tests, agglutination tests and definitive therapy, if the clinical picture is suggestive of Rocky Mountain spotted fever.

Tick Paralysis *(See also 49–14, Paralysis/Paresis)*. Bites of certain varieties of wood ticks *(Dermacentor andersoni)* and dog ticks *(Dermacentor variabilis)* may cause severe, even fatal, paralysis. Some type of powerful neurotoxin absorbed from the head of the gravid female tick apparently is the toxic agent. Tick paralysis is often ascending and progressive and can be distinguished from the paralysis of anterior poliomyelitis and Guillain-Barré syndrome only by the absence of fever and spinal fluid changes. Differentiation between tick paralysis and botulism may be aided by the information in Table 27–1. Treatment consists of the following:

- Surgical removal of the buried head of the tick. Except in moribund patients, this will result in progressive improvement starting 2 to 3 days after excision, with ultimate complete recovery.
- Energetic supportive therapy until improvement begins.

28. Burns

Of the approximately 9 million thermal injuries that occur yearly in the United States, about 2 million require medical treatment, and approximately 5% of patients with these injuries are hospitalized. Of those requiring hospitalization, about 12% die. Prevention and proper early treatment help reduce morbidity and mortality.

GENERAL PRINCIPLES

28–1. PRINCIPLES OF MANAGEMENT AT THE SCENE OF INJURY AND DURING TRANSPORTATION

The following should be done to the extent possible with available equipment:

- Separate the patient from the offending burning agent. Extinguish any flames or embers; decrease oxygen source with blanket wrap or body rolling, etc., if no water is available. Use caution.
- Neutralize any continuing progressive effects of the burn agent. Immediate copious dousing with water usually has the following effects: puts out any fire and cools embers, reduces ill effect of thermal reaction on the skin, dilutes and washes away any chemicals and is comforting to the skin. Remove burned clothing that is not adherent.
- Cool all affected areas of skin with water for several minutes for cleaning and comfort. Cooling is important for tar burns until the tar has hardened. Do not continue to cool much more than 10% to 20% of BSA at any time thereafter with anything as cold as iced water. Do not use dry ice or ice.
- Establish and maintain an airway; ventilate as necessary. Give oxygen if there is smoke inhalation or carbon monoxide poisoning or if the injury is a moderate burn or worse; give 8 to 14 L/min of 40–100% O_2; humidify as soon as possible.
- Evaluate for and treat any other concurrent injuries, such as fractures and major soft tissue injuries (which may occur in falls following unconsciousness due to electrical shock or during vehicular accident); also, correct cardiac arrhythmias, which may occur following electrical discharge through the body. Consider underlying causes of fire (e.g., possibility of patient's having been on alcohol or drugs), and manage accordingly where indicated.
- Wrap in a clean or sterile sheet; if chilling is occurring use a blanket to cover unaffected areas. Keep burned arms or legs slightly elevated.
- Start one or more intravenous lines and infuse Ringer's lactate solution if injury is more than a slight or minor burn.
- Assess the extent (Table 28–1) and depth (Fig. 28–2) of the burn and other complicating factors.
- All patients who have more than a slight burn should be immediately transported to a burn center if within approximately ½ hour transportation time. Otherwise, an interim emergency department should be sought if closer. Give notification of pending arrival and status of patient.
- Evaluate for and treat any shock (57).

DO NOT:

- Apply salves, ointments or creams anywhere if injury is more than a slight burn. Do not remove adherent clothing or tissue.

- Use narcotics, especially if there is also a head or abdominal injury; preferably use a benzodiazepine preparation for sedation as necessary.
- Give any food or liquids in the presence of nausea, vomiting or ileus. Clear water or electrolyte supplement solution (such as ERG) may be given in sips if no vomiting or ileus is present and circumstances dictate.

Measures for Self-Preservation in Evacuating from Burning Buildings

Evacuation of others from a confined burning area, particularly a multiple-story building, is highly hazardous and should always be left to trained fire fighters if imminently available. However, there are general principles of self-preservation applicable to everyone, as follows:

- Assess alternate escape routes on entry into any building.
- Count doors or passageways from known exits before entering any room.
- Feel doors before opening—if hot, leave closed.
- Remember to take keys to self-locking room doors, since retreat to the room may be necessary if hallways and stairwells—where most deaths occur—are blocked by fire and/or dense smoke. It is best to always leave keys in same location, so that they may be found quickly.
- Before closing door into stairwell, be sure it can be reopened from inside.
- Remove synthetic flammable material/clothing.
- Diminish smoke exposure by taking the following measures: move or crawl close to the floor; cover the nostrils with a wet rag or towel; if trapped in a room, close vents and block door and vent cracks with wet material as available; cover bodies with wet, nonsynthetic materials; breathe with nose close to window cracks.

DO NOT:

- Open doors that feel hot.
- Walk upright into smoke or breathe it voluntarily.
- Use any elevator.
- Return to retrieve personal possessions.

28–2. PRINCIPLES OF EVALUATION

Emergency therapy, disposition and prognosis in all types of burns are based on the following factors, which must be considered at the first evaluation of the patient.

Percentage of Body Surface Affected

The total body surface area (BSA) of an average-sized (70 kg or 154 lb) adult is about 1.73 square meters or 18½ square feet. Disposition of treatment (particularly fluid administration) and prognosis depend upon the estimation of the amount of body surface involved (see Fig. 28–1 and accompanying Tables 28–1 and 28–2). In addition to skin surface damage, there may be major respiratory problems resulting from smoke inhalation (25–4), as evidenced by soot and burns in and around the mouth and nostrils, coughing, huskiness of voice and stridor (indicating airway occlusion of 70% or greater).

Depth

Accurate estimation of the exact depth of burn is impossible on first examination, but the guidelines in Figure 28–2 serve to help differentiate.

Location ("PHEEFF")

Shock (57) is much more common and severe pain may be present if highly specialized or sensitive areas such as the *p*erineum, *h*ands, *e*ars, *e*yes, *f*ace, and *feet* (PHEEFF) or freely movable areas (such as flexion creases or joints) are involved. All but slight burns of these areas are relative indications for hospital treatment, independent of total BSA burned.

Time Elapsed Since the Burn

The danger of shock and infection is directly related to the interval between injury and start of treatment, with shock usually occurring in the first few hours and infection occurring as a later complication. Infection may change lesser burns to full-thickness burns.

Age and General Physical Condition

Children less than 5, and especially less than 2 years of age, elderly persons and all individuals whose resistance is less than normal for any reason are especially susceptible to the systemic complications of burns that affect all organs. In these individuals, a 10% BSA burn may be considered critical, and hospital management is indicated.

Type of Burn Agent

Prominent causes of burns are thermal (flash, flame, steam, contact), electrical, chemical and radiation (solar, ionizing and non-ionizing) agents. Electrical devices may give an electrical or thermal burn, or both. Electrical burns (28–*12*) are deceiving, since they may cause greater damage than is superficially apparent. See discussions of specific types of chemical burns and 28–*24*, *Radiation Burns*. In addition to the type of burn agent, the proximity and duration of exposure are highly significant. Thermal burns occurring in closed areas increase the likelihood of inhalation injury (see 25–*4*, *Smoke Inhalation*, and 28–*19*, *Mucous Membrane Burns*). Chemicals in smoke may cause methemoglobinemia (53–*12*) in addition to carbon monoxide poisoning (53–*175*).

Overall Categorization

No single listing is adequate for therapeutic grouping of burns, but additional usable guidelines are as follows:

Slight or Minor Burns (Usually treat victim as an outpatient)

- First-degree burns.
- Partial-thickness burn areas of less than 15% of BSA* in adults (and less than 10% in children).
- Full-thickness burn area of less than 2% of BSA.*

Moderate Burns (Hospitalize patient for observation and therapy)

- Partial-thickness burn area of more than 15% and up to 25% of BSA (10 to 20% in children).
- Full-thickness burn area of between 2% and 10% of BSA.
- If complex factors are present, treatment in a burn center is preferable; also, the community standard may be to care for all hospitalized burn patients at a burn center.

Major Burns (Admit or transfer patient to burn center)

- Partial-thickness burn area of greater than 25% of BSA in adults (and 20% in children).
- Full-thickness burn area of more than 10% of BSA.
- Presence of any of the following complex factors:
  —Electrical burns.

---

*Applicable if complex factors are absent; if not, hospitalize.

Table 28–1. GROSS ESTIMATION OF BODY SURFACE AREA (BSA) BURNED (RULE OF NINES)*

% BSA	Part of Body
9	Head, face and neck
9	Right arm, forearm and hand
9	Left arm, forearm and hand
9	Thorax—front
9	Thorax—back
9	Abdomen—lower ribs to inguinal
9	Back—lower ribs to subgluteal
9	Right thigh, leg and foot—front
9	Right thigh, leg and foot—back
9	Left thigh, leg and foot—front
9	Left thigh, leg and foot—back
1	Genitalia
100%	

*Palm surface of patient's hand equals approximately 1% of BSA. Small spot burn areas are estimated by using fractions or multiples of this percentage.

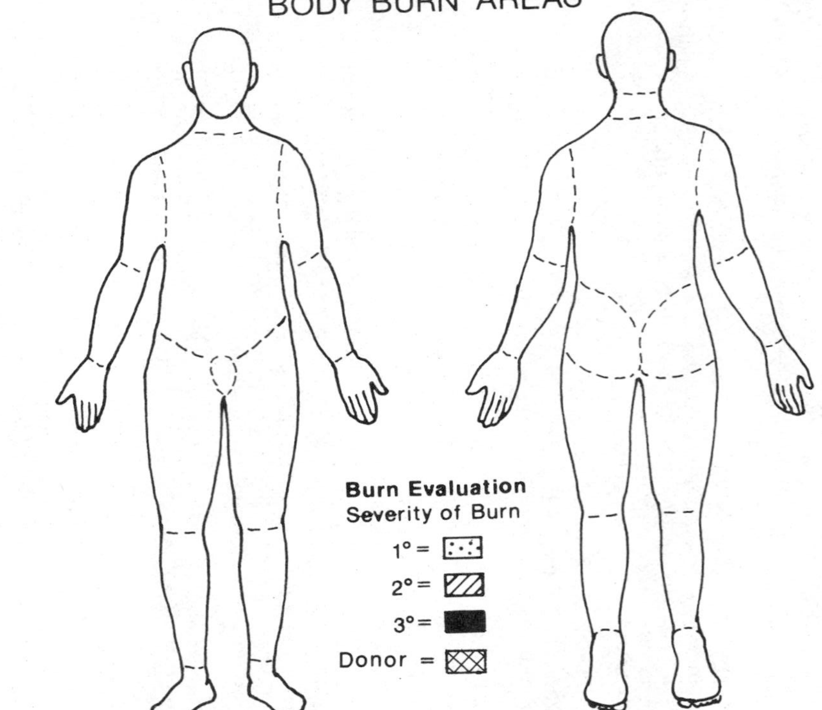

Figure 28–1. Figure for diagramming burned BSA. (Redrawn from Artz, C. P., and Montcrief, J. A.: *The Treatment of Burns*, 2nd ed. Philadelphia, W. B. Saunders Co., 1969.)

Table 28–2. CHART FOR TABULATION OF PERCENTAGES OF TOTAL AMOUNT OF BODY SURFACE AREA BURNED (LUND AND BROWDER)

Area	Infant	Ages 1–4	Ages 5–9	Ages 10–14	Age 15	Adult	Partial	Full	Total	Comment
Head	19	17	13	11	9	7				
Neck	2	2	2	2	2	2				
Ant. Trunk	13	13	13	13	13	13				
Post. Trunk	13	13	13	13	13	13				
R. Buttock	2½	2½	2½	2½	2½	2½				
L. Buttock	2½	2½	2½	2½	2½	2½				
Genitalia	1	1	1	1	1	1				
R.U. Arm	4	4	4	4	4	4				
L.U. Arm	4	4	4	4	4	4				
R.L. Arm	3	3	3	3	3	3				
L.L. Arm	3	3	3	3	3	3				
R. Hand	2½	2½	2½	2½	2½	2½				
L. Hand	2½	2½	2½	2½	2½	2½				
R. Thigh	5½	6½	8	8½	9	9½				
L. Thigh	5½	6½	8	8½	9	9½				
R. Leg	5	5	5½	6	6½	7				
L. Leg	5	5	5½	6	6½	7				
R. Foot	3½	3½	3½	3½	3½	3½				
L. Foot	3½	3½	3½	3½	3½	3½				

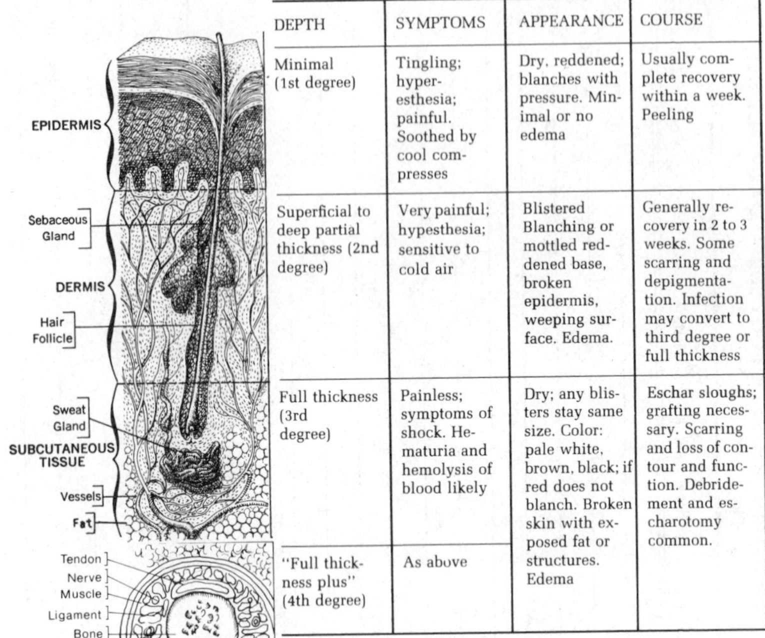

DEPTH	SYMPTOMS	APPEARANCE	COURSE
Minimal (1st degree)	Tingling; hyperesthesia; painful. Soothed by cool compresses	Dry, reddened; blanches with pressure. Minimal or no edema	Usually complete recovery within a week. Peeling
Superficial to deep partial thickness (2nd degree)	Very painful; hypesthesia; sensitive to cold air	Blistered Blanching or mottled reddened base, broken epidermis, weeping surface. Edema.	Generally recovery in 2 to 3 weeks. Some scarring and depigmentation. Infection may convert to third degree or full thickness
Full thickness (3rd degree)	Painless; symptoms of shock. Hematuria and hemolysis of blood likely	Dry; any blisters stay same size. Color: pale white, brown, black; if red does not blanch. Broken skin with exposed fat or structures. Edema	Eschar sloughs; grafting necessary. Scarring and loss of contour and function. Debridement and escharotomy common.
"Full thickness plus" (4th degree)	As above		

Figure 28–2. Diagnosis of burn depth. (Modified from Sako, Y.: Hosp. Med., 1(2), 1964.)

—Third-degree burns of *p*erineum, *h*ands, *e*ars, *e*yes, *f*ace, and *f*eet (PHEEFF).

—Pulmonary inhalation injury (fumes from burned synthetics are quite noxious).

Respiratory infection or smoke inhalation, fractures, major soft tissue injury, extremes of age and preexistent significant illness complicate the treatment and increase mortality and morbidity of burn victims.

28–3. PRINCIPLES OF INITIAL TREATMENT AT SITE OF DEFINITIVE CARE OR IN THE EMERGENCY DEPARTMENT

The following measures should be carried out:

- Check the status of all previously mentioned measures and progress with further treatment for them if there is any change or greater need.
- Reclean the skin with copious cool water or saline using gentle spray pressure (syringe or Water Pik) for clearing of debris as needed. A one-half strength povidone-iodine solution (Betadine) may be used for further antiseptic cleaning, such as a 20-minute tub soak, for more extensive burns; rinse with saline or water afterwards. For treatment of tar burns, see 28–6.
- If the burn is *minimal or slight*, and the victim can be treated as an outpatient, do the following:
  —Apply silver sulfadiazine (Silvadene) to affected areas.
  —Cover affected areas with a fine mesh gauze or fluffy protective dressing, or both, to help avoid further trauma.

—Prescribe simple analgesics and a few days' supply of a sleeping medication such as flurazepam hydrochloride (Dalmane) in case needed.
—Arrange follow-up in 24 to 48 hours for reevaluation and dressing change (patients may continue silver sulfadiazine application 1 to 2 times daily at home). Start exercise program and arrange physiotherapy if needed.

- If the burn is *moderate to critical*, continue with the following after more detailed assessment of involved BSA (Table 28–1 and Fig. 28–1) and burn depths (Fig. 28–2).
- Assess for smoke inhalation and injury (25–4) and proceed accordingly. Obtain carboxyhemoglobin (CoHb) and methemoglobin (MHb) blood levels, respiratory blood gas and arterial pH levels; perform blood studies such as complete and differential cell counts; and obtain blood urea nitrogen (BUN), creatinine and electrolyte values.
- Establish 2 to 3 intravenous fluid lines in severe cases; also consider use of lines for testing central venous pressure, and a Swan-Ganz catheter for pulmonary artery wedge pressure to evaluate fluid and colloid therapy, partial pressure of oxygen (pO_2) and cardiac output/failure, as needed. Remember that each line is a potential portal of entry for bacteria and only the minimum essential number of therapeutic and diagnostic lines should be used.
- Administer fluid (Table 28–3). Use method of preference and experience. If administering Ringer's lactate solution intravenously according to the generally preferred Parkland schedule in thermal burns, the total 24-hour volume *from time of burn* = body weight in kilograms × % BSA burned × factor (which varies from 2 to 4 ml/kg of BSA—generally the latter.) For example, if an 80-kg person has a 30% BSA second degree burn: 80 kg × 30% BSA × 4 ml/kg BSA = 9600 ml in 24 hours. Give one half of the total 24-hour volume (4800 ml) in the first 8 hours and one quarter of the total volume (2400 ml) in each of the second and third 8-hour periods. Clinical considerations such as probable fluid tolerance and monitored response (including urine volume and vital signs) (see Table 57–4, Guidelines for Degree of Severity of Shock) help to establish which factor (2 to 4 ml) to

Table 28–3. ADMINISTRATION OF FLUIDS*

Formula†		First 24 Hours	Second 24 Hours	Total
Brooke	‡Colloid §Electrolyte D/W	1.5 ml/kg/% burn 0.5 ml/kg/% burn 2000 ml	0.75 ml/kg/% burn 0.25 ml/kg/% burn 2000 ml	(70 kg—40% burn) 12,400 ml fluid 1694 mEq Na
Evans	Colloid Electrolyte D/W	1.0 ml/kg/% burn 1.0 ml/kg/% burn 2000 ml	0.5 ml/kg/% burn 0.5 ml/kg/% burn 2000 ml	12,400 ml fluid 1736 mEq Na
Parkland**	Colloid	None	‖None to 500 ml as needed	
	Electrolyte D/W	4 ml/kg/% burn None	None Ad lib (sufficient to maintain urine output)	13,200 ml fluid 1716 mEq Na

*Modified from Schwartz, G. R., Safar, P., Stone, J. H., et al. (eds.): *Principles and Practice of Emergency Medicine*. Philadelphia, W. B. Saunders Co., 1978.
†Use form of preference and experience.
‡Colloid = Plasmanate, plasma, dextran.
§Electrolyte = Ringer's lactate.
‖If urine output cannot be maintained with D/W alone, give 500 ml colloid as necessary.
**Preferred.

continue. Colloid solutions (plasma, blood) are generally not started until the second 24-hour period in the Parkland schedule (because of capillary leak of colloids the first 24 hours) but may be given as volume of body weight in kilograms × % BSA burned × factor (0.25 to 0.5 ml/kg BSA) (for example, 80 kg × 30% BSA × 0.25 ml/kg BSA = 600 ml) if hypovolemia-shock is not being corrected by other fluids.

- Insert a nasogastric tube and apply gentle suction. Restrict oral intake until any nausea, vomiting and ileus have subsided. Give antacids and consider cimetadine for ulcer prevention.
- Monitor as for shock (57). Insert a Foley catheter for monitoring urine output; a catheter is also essential in all perineal and genital burns. An output of 30 to 50 ml/hr (½ to ⅔ ml/kg/hr) should be assured. Obtain periodic urine specimens for a urinalysis and determination of specific gravity and urine hemoglobin and myoglobin content.
- Assure that tetanus immunity (20) is current.
- Systemic antibacterial therapy is indicated if the wound is contaminated; otherwise use depends on the physician's judgment. Use of penicillin should be particularly considered in major burns.
- Use no pillows, especially when there are ear burns. Use pads to protect special areas. Position to decrease edema. Prepare splints for functional positioning.
- Apply silver sulfadiazine (Silvadene) to affected areas (mafenide acetate cream [Sulfamylon] may be preferable for ear burns), unless the patient is being further transferred to a burn center nearby, in which case obtain the center's preferences or protocol in addition to outlining and discussing management to date. Digits should be individually wrapped or, in less severe cases, an oversize sterile surgical glove may be worn, after the silver sulfadiazine has been applied.
- Exposed muscles, tendons, ligaments and nerves must be kept covered and moist with saline until grafting can be arranged. Obtain urine myoglobin levels when there are third- and fourth-degree burns or electrical burns.
- Analgesics may be given as necessary, including narcotics in small doses if there are no contraindications.
- Check rectal temperature; paradoxically some patients may have been cooled and chilled into an unfavorable hypothermic state (62–3).
- Performance of escharotomy requires consideration in full-thickness burns in which progressive edema of third compartment areas causes impedance to thoracic excursion for breathing or decreased peripheral pulses by palpation of Doppler instrument testing. Escharotomy is performed on the trunk or in the midcoronal section of the extremities (including the digits if necessary) with use of a cautery instrument or scalpel, going just deep enough to obtain release of tissue tension and extending from normal tissue to normal tissue where possible.
- For comfort, protection and promotion of healing, early coverage should be considered in the following situations: to cover exposed nerves, arteries, tendons or joints; to treat deep burns of any area greater than 2.5 to 3.0 cm in breadth; to treat deep burns of the hands, feet and flexion areas.
- Amniotic membranes, often more readily available than other biologic coverings such as skin, may be used as an emergency temporary biologic dressing for deep or contaminated wounds to aid healing and provide pain relief.

Preparation of amniotic tissue is accomplished by removing the amniotic membranes from the placenta immediately after delivery (use only if there has been no infection or contamination). Wash 4 to 5 times with normal saline before and after a single washing with 0.25% sodium hypochlorite, removing any clots or surface substances with gentle agitation in the process. Membranes may be stored for 4 to 6 weeks in individual sterile containers at 4° C (39.2° F) for later use. Apply the membrane as smoothly and directly adherent to the wound as possible and change in 24 to 48 hours, depending on the degree of wound contamination. For partial-thickness wounds, apply the amnion surface (shiny) toward the wound; in full-thickness wounds, apply the chorion surface (dull) toward the wound.

BURNS REQUIRING SPECIAL MANAGEMENT CONSIDERATIONS*

28–4. ACID BURNS

Treatment

- Wash immediately and thoroughly with running water for a lengthy time (e.g., 10 to 15 minutes) at the scene as soon as possible after contact with acid. In areas where acid is being used, foot-operated shower and bubblers should be immediately adjacent.
- Manage as indicated under *28–3*. See also *28–14, Eye Burns; 38–31, Conjunctival Injuries; 38–32, Corneal Injuries; 53–33, Acids*. For treatment of hydrofluoric acid burns, see *53–351*.

28–5. ALKALI BURNS

Treatment

- Wash immediately and thoroughly for a lengthy time with running water until all alkali is removed.
- Manage as outlined under *28–3*. See also *28–14, Eye Burns; 38–31, Conjunctival Injuries; 38–32, Corneal Injuries; 53–45, Alkalies; 53–401, Lye*.

28–6. ASPHALT, BITUMEN, PITCH OR TAR BURNS

Treatment

- Apply cool running water immediately; continue to run water over affected areas until substance has hardened and cooled—then stop to avoid causing hypothermia. (Do not attempt to remove substance from the skin in the field.)
- Adherent tar must be removed, since infection occurs underneath. This is done as follows:
  —Mechanically remove tar pieces adherent to blistered tissue in the course of debridement. Cooling of pieces of the substance (as with ice or ethyl chloride or fluoromethane spray) has been found helpful in some cases.
  —Nontoxic dissolving-emulsifying agents such as petrolatum, mineral oil and antibacterial ointments (e.g., Bacitracin, polysporin; *note:* may be painful) may be applied and are preferable when the tar is firmly adherent. Mayonnaise has also been found to to be successful, and has the advantages of being comfortable and bacteria retardant. Apply a generous layer of ointment—1⁄16″ to 1⁄8″ thick—over the affected areas and cover with gauze. At intervals of 6 to 8 hours, remove gauze, use tub soak or whirlpool as needed, and reapply ointment and gauze. Six to eight repetitions may be necessary for complete removal. When all the substance is removed, proceed with usual treatment.
- Hospitalize if the congealed asphalt or tar covers a large portion of the body or if complex care is needed. Hot asphalt and tar burns are usually much deeper than first examination would seem to indicate.

---

*These special measures are to be done in addition to following the general principles outlined in *28–1, 28–2*, and *28–3*.

28–7. ATOMIC RADIATION BURNS *(See 3–5)*

28–8. CAUSTIC BURNS *(See 28–5)*

28–9. CEMENT OR CONCRETE BURNS *(See 28–5)*

28–10. CHEMICAL BURNS *(See 28–4, Acid Burns; 28–5, Alkali Burns; or specific entries in 53, Poisons, for the particular chemical involved)*

28–11. EAR BURNS

Of the Soft Tissues. Treat as outlined in 28–3, except that open treatment without bandaging is often practical. Avoid pressure of pillows. Mafenide acetate (Sulfamylon) ointment helps decrease bacterial colonization.

Of the Canals. These injuries are usually from hot slag or metal. After removal of the foreign body *(39–1)*, a topical antibiotic, such as polymyxin B solution (Lidosporin Otic Solution) may be instilled 4 times daily. The patient should be warned against putting foreign bodies or plugs of any type into the ear canal.

Of the Eardrums. If slight, removal of the foreign body *(39–1)* and treatment of the canal is all that is required. If the foreign body is burned in or has perforated the drum, cover the ear with a pad and refer the patient to a specialist for further care.

28–12. ELECTRICAL BURNS *(See also 32–5, Electrical Shock)*

Passage of an electrical current through living tissues often does far more damage than is apparent on superficial examination. Immediate death from ventricular fibrillation *(29–25)* may occur. Respiratory failure requiring artificial respiration *(5–21)* is common. Low-voltage currents are usually more dangerous than high-tension, and alternating current is more lethal than direct current; document these factors, if possible. High-voltage direct current lightning injury, because of "flashover," can result in a lesser degree of internal injury than high-tension alternating current. Remember that electricity may cause thermal burns, electrical burns, or both. Contusions and fractures can occur secondary to falls and blows.

Treatment

- The electrical source, if continuing, and victim must be separated with great caution, so that the rescuer does not get in the conduction pathway. If possible, switch off the source at a circuit breaker, or unplug. Professional rescue is necessary for downed high-tension lines; use of long boards to move wires when the ground is wet can be unsafe.
- If the patient is in coma or in circulatory or respiratory collapse, defer all local treatment until the measures outlined under 5, *Resuscitation*, and 32–5, *Electrical Shock*, have been carried out and the patient's condition has stabilized.
- Identify the points of entrance and exit of the current (the latter often is overlooked). By estimation of the path of the current, some idea of the organs that may have been damaged can be obtained. Destruction along arteries and nerves is more likely to occur than destruction of other soft tissue and bone. Delayed bleeding from blood vessels may occur.
- Debride both the entrance and exit wounds thoroughly with the patient under local anesthesia, removing all charred or devitalized structures. Close with loose, interrupted, nonabsorbable sutures and apply sterile dressings. Relaxing incisions and skin grafting may be necessary. Further necrosis may have occurred than is apparent.
- Hospitalize for observation for at least 48 hours if the patient has been unconscious, if cardiac irregularities have been noted or if the burned areas are deep, extensive or likely to involve important structures.
- Use of a slowly infused bolus of IV fluoroscein (15 mg/kg) followed in 20 minutes by wood lamp exposure reveals fluorescence of viable areas and none in nonviable areas.

28–13. ESOPHAGEAL BURNS *(See also 28–19, Mucous Membrane Burns; 53–401, Lye)*

Immediately have the patient drink generous amounts of a diluting and cleansing neutralizing substance such as orange juice, milk or water. Do not attempt to make the person vomit. Early esophagoscopy can delineate the extent of injury and guide therapy. A piece of string, long enough to reach to the stomach, may be swallowed and the end taped to the side of the mouth; this serves as a guide to the tissue plane of the esophageal canal, if needed later. Strictures requiring dilatation may occur.

28–14. EYE BURNS *(See also 38–31, Conjunctival Injuries; 38–32, Corneal Injuries. Consider use of irrigating contact lens.)*

Acid, Alkali or Caustic Burns

- Irrigate for at least 30 minutes with tap water, sterile water or normal salt solution. Never attempt to use neutralizing solutions in the eyes unless experienced in their use or under an ophthalmologist's direction. Be sure to irrigate the fornix area well, using lid retractors (see Fig. 38–2) for later irrigation and inspection.
- Instill 2 drops of 0.5% tetracaine (Pontocaine) solution to control pain and facilitate examination.
- Apply an eye patch. Refer at once to an ophthalmologist.

Hot Asphalt, Tar, Slag or Metal Burns

- Cool and rinse with copious running water.
- Instill 2 drops of 0.5% tetracaine (Pontocaine) solution.
- Remove any loose or superficially embedded foreign bodies *(38–31; 38–32)*. If deep or firmly adherent, do not attempt mechanical removal.
- Apply an eye patch. Refer at once to an ophthalmologist.

28–15. FLASH BURNS

Nuclear Fission Bomb Flash Burns. These are characterized by involvement of the side of the body toward the point of explosion and by bizarre patterns of several depths resulting from the varying absorbabilities of different clothing fabrics. Immediate removal of irradiated clothing is essential. The treatment is the same as outlined under 28–3.

Welder's Flash Burns (Photophthalmia). See *38–31, Conjunctival Injuries.*

28–16. FRICTION BURNS

Friction burns usually involve the palmar surface of the hands ("rope burns") or those portions of the body not protected by heavy clothing (see *28–22, Pavement Burns*). Friction burns may range in severity from slight superficial abrasions to shredding and avulsion of charred and blackened tissues. Embedded material must be thoroughly removed.

28–17. GASOLINE (DISTILLATE, FUEL OIL, KEROSENE) BURNS

Treatment

- Remove all contaminated clothing at once.
- Wash the affected areas thoroughly as described under *28–3.*
- Apply a bland ointment to areas of erythema. Second degree burns are not common, but if present they should be dressed with petrolatum gauze or Xeroform gauze.
- Watch carefully for evidence of upper respiratory tract irritation caused by aspiration or inhalation of fumes or flames; if present, antibiotic treatment followed by hospitalization is indicated. See *53–323* for further information.

28–18. MAGNESIUM BURNS *(See also 53–402)*

Treatment

- Irrigate with copious amounts of tap water.
- Paint the burned area with 5% copper sulfate solution; irrigate thoroughly afterwards, to prevent complication of copper toxicity *(53–224)*.
- Remove superficially embedded particles of metal by sharp dissection, using local anesthesia or regional nerve blocks if necessary.
- Watch carefully for development of crepitation, ulceration or sloughing.

28–19. MUCOUS MEMBRANE BURNS

Mucous membrane burns are usually mild, but in some instances they may result in extreme edema and severe pain. Three sites are common: mouth, throat and respiratory tract.

In the mouth and throat (except for acid burns *[28–4]* and alkali burns *[28–5]*), burns are usually caused by swallowing extremely hot foods or drinks. As a rule, these burns are more uncomfortable than serious. Symptomatic treatment is all that is required. Oral lidocaine (Xylocaine Viscous) swished around in the mouth, then swallowed or applied focally with applicators for 1 to 2 minutes, aids eating (soft bland foods or clear liquids are preferable; use caution, as swallowing reflex may be altered).

In the respiratory tract, burns are caused by the inhalation of flame or hot gases (see 25–4). Symptoms of acute carbon monoxide poisoning *(53–175)* may be present.

Treatment

- Administration of sedatives. In severe cases, small doses of narcotics for control of reflex spasm may be necessary.
- Insurance of an adequate airway by removal of secretion by postural drainage and suction. If marked edema, dyspnea or cyanosis is present, emergency endotracheal intubation, cricothyreotomy or tracheostomy *(18–34)* may be necessary.
- Prescription of a soothing cough mixture.
- Immediate hospitalization if evidence of lung damage is present. Terminal pulmonary edema *(55)* may occur, usually as delayed development.

In the vagina, the use of strong caustic medications as douches or in attempts to induce abortions (see 53–569, *Potassium Permanganate*) may cause mucous membrane injury ranging from slight edema to necrosis and perforation. Direct irrigation and inspection using a speculum are necessary to assure that all areas are adequately cleansed and particulate matter removed.

Treatment

- Mild cases require only sedation and copious, frequent, nonirritating douches.
- Moderate cases require adequate frequent careful cleansing to prevent secondary infection.
- In severe cases with extreme edema and ulceration or perforation, the patient must be hospitalized at once. Surgical debridement and repair under general anesthetic may be necessary.

28–20. MUSTARD GAS BURNS *(See 53–746, Mustard Gas; 3–10, Poisonous Gases)*

28–21. NAPALM BURNS

Spraying of burning gasoline or distillate mixed with a contact adhesive is now a common offensive weapon in war and results in severe burns with the characteristics of hot asphalt burns *(28–6)* and upper respiratory tract burns *(28–19)*.

28–22. PAVEMENT BURNS

Persons thrown from moving vehicles often slide along abrasive surfaces with considerable momentum. Friction and abrasion, with grinding into the skin, subcutaneous tissues and underlying structures of multiple small foreign bodies, can result in injuries peculiarly susceptible to infection, tattooing and permanent scarring. Thorough removal of embedded material to prevent infection and permanent tattooing may have to be done under general anesthesia.

28–23. PHOSPHORUS BURNS *(See also 53–545, Phosphorus)*

The use of rockets and flares in modern warfare has resulted in a large number of serious second and third degree burns from phosphorus, which has the physical property of igniting spontaneously, even in the tissues, on exposure to air. Systemically, absorption of phosphorus may result in liver and kidney damage and depression of the blood-forming organs.

Treatment

- As soon as possible after injury, flood with large quantities of water or 2% sodium bicarbonate solution.
- Coat with 5% copper sulfate applied directly to the phosphorus particles to reduce continued burning; then irrigate.
- Debride all necrotic or loose tissue at once, removing all particles of phosphorus by forceps or sharp dissection. The severity of systemic reactions is directly proportionate to the amount of phosphorus left in the tissues.
- Irrigate the wound thoroughly with normal saline solution to remove excess copper, which in itself may give serious toxic effects *(53–224)*.
- Apply sodium perborate solution or mafenide acetate (Sulfamylon) cream directly to the burned areas. Keep wound moist/wet.
- Transfer for prompt and adequate follow-up medical care for systemic effects—ecchymoses, gastrointestinal bleeding, jaundice, hypoglycemia, hematuria and blood changes.

28–24. RADIATION BURNS *(See 28–34, X-ray Burns; 3–5, Wartime Emergencies, Nuclear Bombs)*

28–25. RESPIRATORY TRACT BURNS *(See 25–4, Smoke Inhalation; 28–19, Mucous Membrane Burns)*

28–26. ROPE BURNS *(See 28–16, Friction Burns)*

28–27. SCALP BURNS

Mild cases require only application of a soothing lotion. In severe cases, after clipping the hair and shaving the area around the burn, treat as outlined under *28–3*.

28–28. SLAG BURNS

In the Ear. See *28–11*.
In the Eye. See *28–14; 38–31, Conjunctival Injuries; 38–32, Corneal Injuries.*

28–29. SUNBURN

Mild cases require only sedatives or analgesics and local application of a soothing lotion. These may be commercially obtained, or a paste may be made of crushed aspirin tablets mixed with an antacid and applied once on the involved skin.

Severe cases with bleb formation should be treated as outlined under *28–3*. Hospitalization may be required if more than 40% of the skin surface (less in children—see *52–14*) is affected. Death can occur from extensive severe sunburn with involvement of a large percentage of the body surface.

For systemic effects, see *62–9, Sunstroke.*

28–30. TEAR GAS BURNS *(See 53–746, War Gases)*

28–31. TITANIUM TETRACHLORIDE BURNS *(See also 53–708)*

Do not use water for original treatment, unless copious amounts are applied.

28–32. VAGINAL BURNS *(See 28–19, Mucous Membrane Burns; 53–569, Potassium Permanganate)*

28–33. WAR GAS BURNS *(See also 53–746)*

Tear gas burns respond well to early use of topical steroids.

28–34. X-RAY BURNS

Roentgen therapy in large doses *(21–8)* may result in an uncomfortable erythema. Industrial use of x-ray equipment (determination of defects in metals, etc.) is resulting in an increasing number of x-ray burns. Monitoring and shielding machines to control radiation, together with employee use of exposure badges, is essential.

29. Cardiac Emergencies*

Definitive therapy for acute cardiac disease varies with the etiologic background of the illness or injury and usually requires more than brief treatment under emergency conditions. There is, however, a distinct group of cardiac emergencies in which prompt and rational action on the part of the attending physician may be the deciding factor in the patient's chance for survival. When life-threatening heart conditions, resulting from either mechanical or electrical failure, are present or circumstances conducive to their development occur, the patient must be given immediate emergency supportive therapy, continued during careful and safe transportation to a well-staffed and adequately equipped intensive or coronary care unit.

29–1. ACUTE VENTRICULAR RUPTURE

Occurring to some degree in 10 to 20% of fatal myocardial infarctions, ventricular rupture may cause sudden death, although in some instances ventricular septal ruptures may be amenable to corrective surgery if detected early. Cardiac tamponade *(29–18)* may occur.

In the early postmyocardial infarction period, exacerbation of chest pain, increase or appearance of congestive heart failure *(29–10)* or shock (57), development of a coarse systolic murmur or progressive change in electrocardiographic vector should alert to the possibility of ventricular septal rupture or rupture of the chordae tendineae. Echocardiography and right heart catheterization aid in diagnosis. Referral for surgical evaluation and possible emergency intervention (closure of septal rupture, placement of a prosthetic valve or prosthetic chordae replacement) is indicated in such situations.

29–2. ANGINA PECTORIS

Classic angina pectoris is characterized by rapid onset of substernal or precordial pain, usually squeezing or burning in character, which is generally

*See also 5, *Resuscitation;* 55, *Pulmonary Edema;* 57, *Shock;* and 63, *Vascular Disorders.*

associated with increased cardiac work from exercise or emotional stress as a precipitating cause. Angina at rest is ominous.

This acute discomfort usually clears in not more than 15 minutes with no treatment except rest in the supine position. More rapid relief can be obtained by sublingual absorption of glyceryl trinitrate (nitroglycerin), 0.3 to 0.6 mg, repeated every 5 minutes. If 3 doses do not cause marked relief of symptoms, the patient should be evaluated for possible myocardial infarction *(29–15)*. Smaller doses of nitroglycerin may be indicated if hypotension or severe throbbing headaches develop. Nitropaste is one form of nitroglycerin that offers ongoing relief by gradual absorption of the drug, which is applied topically.

Note: Glyceryl trinitrate (nitroglycerin) tablets gradually deteriorate and lose their effect on exposure to air and should be replaced approximately twice a year.

Variant angina pectoris (Prinzmetal angina) is identified by similarly located chest pain and T_1 to T_6 dermatome distribution, which comes on at rest, often lasts more than 30 minutes and is accompanied by ST segment elevation on the electrocardiogram (ECG) during pain. Patients with this condition are at risk of fatal arrhythmias and generally should be hospitalized and monitored and should receive angiographic assessment. Calcium-blocking drugs (e.g., Verapamil) have revolutionized the therapy of vasospastic angina and are effective adjuncts in Prinzmetal angina.

29–3. ATRIAL FIBRILLATION

If it occurs with a rapid ventricular rate, atrial fibrillation (Fig. 29–1*G*) may cause acute pulmonary edema *(55)*, shock *(57)* or both from ventricular failure. Treatment under these circumstances is most readily managed with direct current cardioversion (using lower dosages such as 25 to 50 watt seconds).

However, if the rapid ventricular rate is tolerated and the patient has not been previously digitalized, rapid intravenous digitalization with digoxin, in divided doses, is indicated; usually a total of 0.6 to 1.0 mg digoxin is required in a 70-kg adult. Digitalis preparation can be hazardous in converting rapid atrial fibrillation in the presence of accelerated conduction or preexcitation syndromes.

29–4. ATRIAL FLUTTER

This condition usually demonstrates a rapid regular atrial rate of about 300 per minute and may have a variable atrioventricular (A-V) block, usually 2:1 (see Fig. 29–1*F*). It may occur during the course of treatment of atrial fibrillation with quinidine. The acuteness of the problem varies with the cause, degree of block and ventricular rate. As with atrial fibrillation (to which atrial flutter may revert during treatment), basic treatment consists of electrical cardioversion or rapid intravenous digitalization with digoxin (Lanoxin). Quinidine, sometimes recommended, should not be used unless the patient is fully digitalized.

29–5. ATRIAL PARAOXYSMAL TACHYCARDIA *(See Fig. 29–1I and 29–24, Supraventricular Tachycardia)*

29–6. BACTERIAL ENDOCARDITIS, ACUTE

Usually secondary to a primary streptococcal, staphylococcal or pneumococcal focus elsewhere in the body, this endocardial and valvular infection is

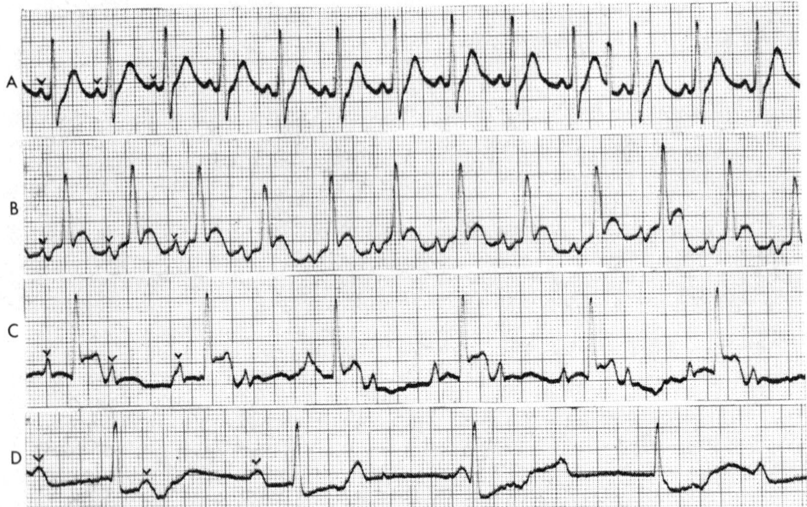

Figure 29–1. Electrocardiographic tracings. *A,* Sinus tachycardia. *B,* First degree A-V block. *C,* Second degree A-V block. *D,* Third degree A-V block.

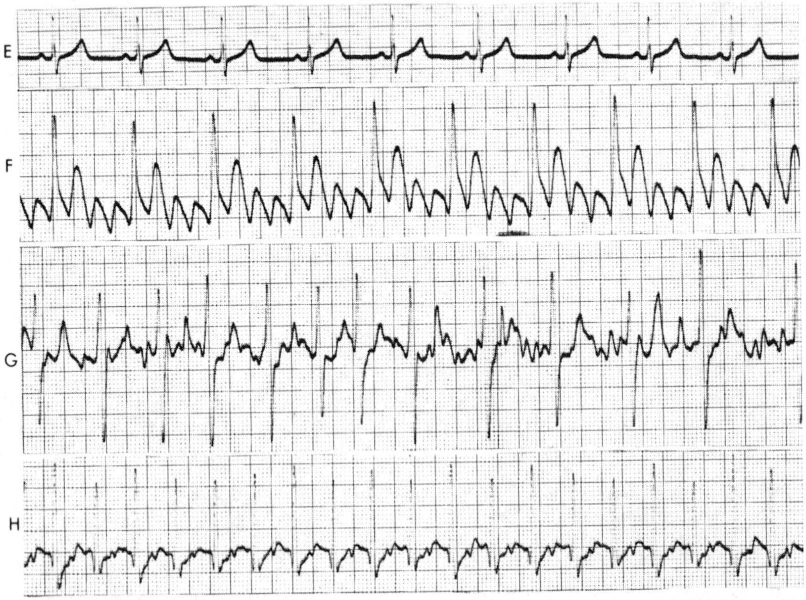

Figure 29–1. *(Continued). E,* Normal sinus rhythm. *F,* Atrial flutter. *G,* Atrial fibrillation. H, Supraventricular tachycardia, nodal.

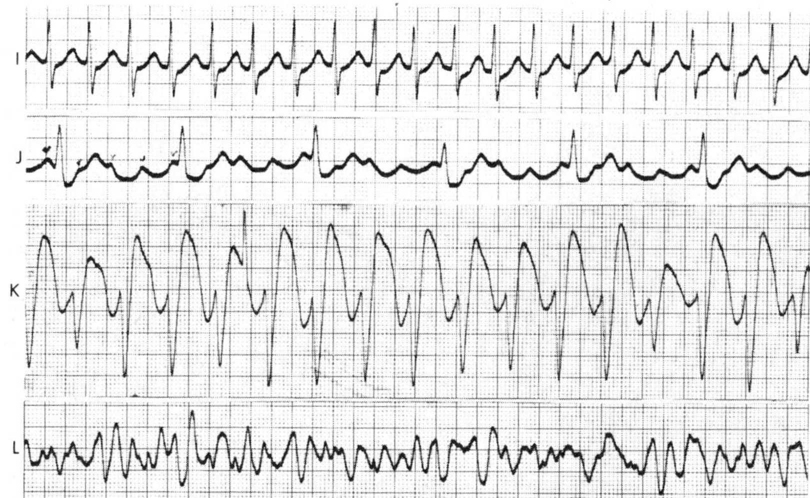

Figure 29–1. *(Continued). I,* Supraventricular tachycardia, atrial. *J,* Atrial tachycardia with 4:1 A-V response. *K,* Ventricular tachycardia. *L,* Ventricular fibrillation. (Tracings *B, C, F, H, I and J* made from instructional rhythm strip tapes available from the Physiologic Training Company, San Marino, California.)

suggested by septicemia, murmur, diffuse electrocardiographic ST-T changes, bacterial growth in blood cultures and signs of emboli.

Treatment

- Obtain three to six blood cultures rapidly, within several hours.
- Start massive antibiotic therapy parenterally based on the probable cause of the primary infection without waiting for results of cultures and sensitivity tests. For appropriate antibiotics, see *33–83.*
- Check for primary focus.

29–7. BRADYCARDIA

Bradycardia, defined as a pulse of less than 60 beats/min, may be of several types, presented here in order of increasing seriousness.

Sinus Bradycardia. A 1:1 conducted sinus mechanism with a pulse of less than 60 beats/min (even in the 40 to 50 beats/min range) can be entirely normal in well-conditioned people. Variable slowing of rate with inspiration (sinus arrhythmia) is usual. This type of person is asymptomatic and shows an appropriate increase in heart rate with exercise and rapid recovery after exercise; no treatment is indicated. Athletes can benefit from having a baseline ECG taken while they are healthy, as there are frequent deviations from the average that may be misinterpreted during illness. Yogis may also demonstrate remarkably slow rates with relaxation techniques.

If the patient is symptomatic with activity and has inadequate levels of CO,* check for presence of responsible drugs (e.g., digitalis; beta-blockers such as propranolol), which should then be reduced in dosage, or presence of myxedema or hypothyroidism. If the patient has acute symptoms from the decrease in CO, give atropine, 0.01 to 0.02 mg/kg to a maximum initial dose

*Cardiac output

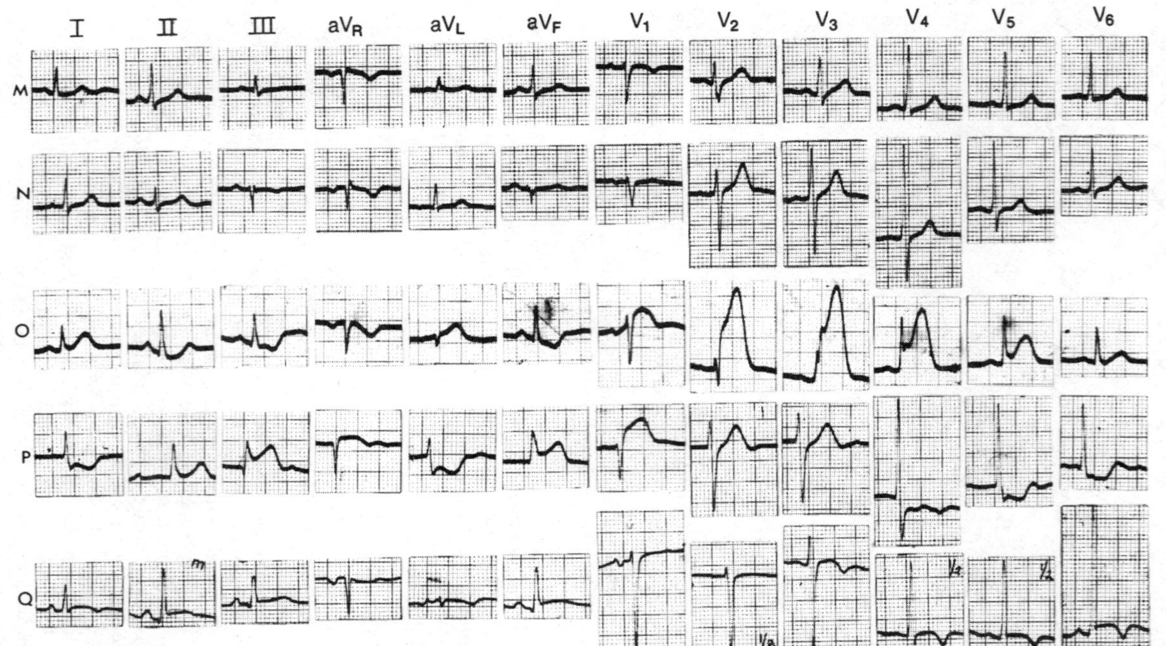

Figure 29–1. *(Continued). M,* Normal electrocardiogram, intermediate position. *N,* Normal electrocardiogram, horizontal position. *O,* Acute anterior myocardial infarction. *P,* Acute inferior myocardial infarction (plus third degree atrioventricular block). *Q,* Pericarditis (typical limb leads; T wave of precordial leads usually upright early and invert later).

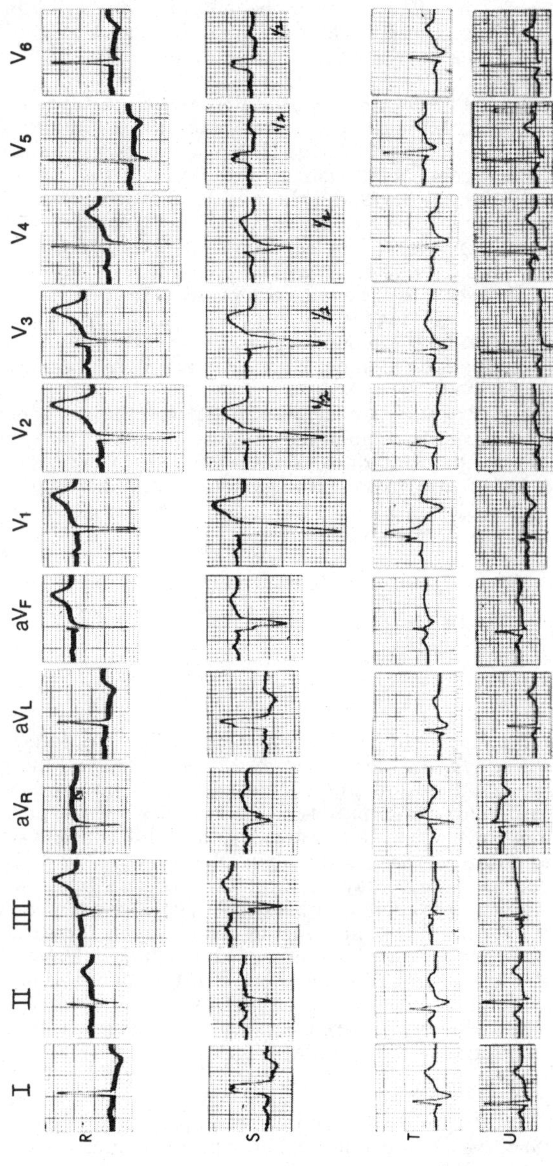

Figure 29–1. *(Continued). R*, Left ventricular hypertrophy (plus first degree atrioventricular block and q wave in aV_F due to probable old inferior myocardial infarction). *S*, Complete left bundle branch block (r wave in V_1 and V_2 may be absent). *T*, Complete right bundle branch block. *U*, Incomplete right bundle branch block.

of 0.5 to 1.0 mg. Failure to respond with an increase in heart rate is indicative of "sick sinus"; proceed to treat with isoproterenol infusion, and if no response proceed to use of a temporary pacemaker *(18–21)*.

Sinus Arrest. Intermittently P waves will be absent and there will be a junctional or nodal escape. These patients are more refractory to medication than are those with sinus bradycardia, and are more likely to require a temporary pacemaker to prevent Stokes-Adams attacks *(29–23)*.

Partial Atrioventricular (A-V) Block. In this condition, not all P waves result in a ventricular contraction. Patients are described as having either Type I (Wenckebach or Mobitz I) or Type II (Mobitz II) A-V block, as discussed below.

TYPE I. The P-R interval gets steadily longer until finally a P wave does not result in excitation of the A-V node and there is no ventricular contraction. Pulse rates are usually slowed to 40–50 beats/min. If the patient is on digitalis, reduction of dosage may give relief. The condition may improve with atropine or isoproterenol, but temporary pacing may still be needed.

TYPE II. With this condition there are even slower rates: 30–40 beats/min with 2:1 or 3:1 A-V block due to damage to the bundle of HIS. Patients with Type II block are more likely to be symptomatic than those with Type I, are more refractory to the medications cited under Type I and are more likely to require a temporary pacemaker.

Complete Heart Block. P waves are conducted beyond the A-V node, but disease of the intraventricular conduction system results in a very slow variable infranodal rhythm, with rates of 20–40 beats/min being common. Drugs are generally ineffective, and a transvenous pacemaker is preferable to a transthoracic pacemaker in emergency therapy (see *29–13*). Use atropine and isoproterenol while readying pacing.

29–8. CARDIAC ARREST *(See 5, Resuscitation, especially 5–2)*

29–9. CARDIAC TRAUMA *(See 31–4)*

29–10. CONGESTIVE HEART FAILURE *(See also 55–4 for differentiation from Noncardiogenic Pulmonary Edema [ARDS])*

This serious condition is due to pump failure of the ventricles (left, *forward failure;* right, *backward failure*) and is characterized by gradual increase in intra- and extravascular fluid volume, increased venous pressure, delayed circulation time (arm to tongue; arm to lung), pulmonary rales, edema of the liver and extremities, orthopnea, paroxysmal nocturnal dyspnea, exertional dyspnea, decreased effort tolerance and tachycardia.

Causes of the cardiac failure may be complex (coronary atherosclerosis, hypertension and fibrosis, myxedema, thyrotoxicosis, constrictive pericarditis, vitamin deficiency, valvular or septal defect or combinations thereof). Hospitalization may be required for definitive studies and appropriate treatment of the primary cause. Clinical and ECG monitoring in the more seriously ill is aided by the use of flow-directed catheterization with a flexible balloon-tipped catheter (Swan-Ganz catheter) to serially measure cardiac output and left ventricular filling pressures at the bedside.

General Measures in Treatment

- Rest; decrease in cardiac work demand until compensated. Use position of maximum comfort, which is usually a semi-upright sitting (semi-Fowler) position.
- Low sodium.

- Oxygen (moisturized) by mask, nasal cannula, partial rebreather or nonrebreather mask according to PaO_2 as determined by blood gases; can start with 30–40% O_2 at 6 L/min, unless patient has COPD, in which case start at 1–2 L/min. IPPB via endotracheal tube helps reduce pulmonary edema in severe cases. Also see *56–4* for use of aminophylline to relieve bronchospasm.
- Furosemide (Lasix), 40 to 80 mg orally in a single dose, or 20 to 40 mg IM or IV and repeated as necessary. Alternatively, sodium ethacrynate (Edecrin), 0.5–1.0 mg/kg diluted in 50 ml D5W, may be given slowly IV over 5 minutes for rapid diuresis.
- Morphine sulfate, 10 to 15 mg in 10 ml of sterile water, given slowly intravenously until pain and anxiety decrease, numbness around the mouth begins or respirations slow. Minimal doses only should be used in patients with kidney disease, chronic pulmonary pathology or hypothyroidism *(36–12)*. Use of opiates and synthetic narcotics is contraindicated in the presence of severe COPD, unless naloxone is readily available and the patient is closely monitored.
- Digitalization (unless interrogation indicates recent use) for adults: *Slow:* By digoxin, 0.5 mg orally, then 0.25 mg every 8 to 12 hours until signs of adequate digitalization are present. Slow digitalization is preferable in elderly or debilitated patients.
  Intermediate: By digoxin, 0.75 to 1.0 mg orally, followed by 0.25 to 0.5 mg every 8 hours until patient digitalized.
  Rapid: By digoxin, 0.5 to 1.0 mg intravenously, in a first injection with subsequent supplements, or (preferably) in smaller divided doses, with one quarter to one half given initially, then one eighth of the original dose given at 4-hour intervals until the patient is digitalized. *Digitalizing doses for children:* See Table 29–1.
- Correction of electrolyte imbalance, particularly hypokalemia.
- "Bloodless phlebotomy" by application of blood pressure cuffs (at 60–80 mm Hg) serially to the most proximal portions of 3 to 4 extremities with periods of release of 1 tourniquet at a time for 15 minutes. This method is not preferred, because it may initiate deep venous thrombosis. On infrequent occasions, actual phlebotomy with removal of 250 to 500 ml of venous blood may be an advisable adjunct—particularly in the presence of polycythemia.
- Consider use of sodium nitroprusside (Nipride) to reduce cardiac afterload and preload if the measures just described are not successful; monitor patient with Swan-Ganz catheter to evaluate response.
- Consider use of a mechanical pump—left ventricular assist device (LVAD)—in refractory cases (e.g., due to acute MI or ventricular septal or papillary muscle rupture).

29–11. DIGITALIS TOXICITY *(See also 53–265)*

The latitude between therapeutic and toxic doses of digitalis is small. Toxicity may result from overdosage, low tolerance (as in elderly patients) or disturbances in renal digitalis excretion or electrolyte balance (low serum potassium level especially).

Patients taking digitalis preparations who have previously had atrial fibrillation and who convert to a regular rhythm (i.e., complete atrioventricular block with regular nodal rhythm take-over) have digitalis toxicity until proved otherwise and require serial evaluation with electrocardiograms. Right carotid sinus pressure for 5 seconds may assist in determining the presence of early

Table 29–1. DIGOXIN SCHEDULES IN CHILDREN* †

	Premature Infants; Weight Under 2.5 kg (mcg/kg)†	Under 1 month; Weight Over 2.5 kg (mcg/kg)	Under 2 Years, Over 1 Month; Weight Under 30 kg (mcg/kg)	Under 2 Years; Weight Over 30 kg (mcg/kg)	2 to 5 Years (mcg/kg)	Over 5 Years (mcg/kg)
Route of Administration for Initial Digitalization IV, IM, SC	20 to 30	40	50	40	40	30
Oral	–	–	70	60	60	45
Range* Approximately total daily maintenance dose	6 to 10	8 to 12	12 to 20	10 to 18	8 to 12	6 to 10
Approximately every 12 hours maintenance dose	3 to 5	4 to 6	6 to 10	5 to 9	4 to 6	3 to 5

*Maintenance doses in the range of 15 to 20 mcg per kilogram per day, as may be needed, for example, with left to right shunts with congestive heart failure such as with ventricular septal defect, are best administered with the assistance of a pediatric cardiologist.

†Notations to use:

1. In converting mcg to mg, divide by 1000 or move the decimal 3 places to the left. Also, 1 mcg% = 10 nanogram (ng) per milliliter.
2. Give one half the total dose immediately, one fourth the total dose 4 to 8 hours later and one fourth the total dose 8 to 16 hours after first dose. Use the longer periods if less urgency.
3. Give a maintenance dose of digoxin every 12 hours, commencing 12 hours after last digitalizing dose.
4. Onset of digoxin effect is 5 to 10 minutes for IV route, 15 to 60 minutes for IM and SC routes and 2 hours for the oral route. Maximum digoxin effect occurs 2 to 4 hours after IV route and 4 to 6 hours after other routes.
5. Arrhythmias having onset after digitalization must be considered as related to digoxin toxicity until proved otherwise.
6. The therapeutic blood level in adults (0.07 to 0.18 mcg %) is not generally as helpful in children. Clinical response is a more reliable therapeutic guide. The therapeutic range in infants is often considered to be 0.14 to 0.28 mcg% and in children 0.05 to 0.18 mcg%.
7. The blood level of digoxin causing toxicity is lower when the potassium level drops below 3 mEq/L.

toxic states. The electrocardiographic signs of toxicity in the following description may increase during the period of carotid stimulation.

Signs (In order of increasing severity)

- Mild malaise, anorexia, occasional unifocal premature ventricular contractions on ECG.
- Nausea, vomiting, diarrhea, blurred vision, cephalgia and an increase in electrocardiographic findings—first-degree conduction block (see Fig. 29–1*B*), wandering pacemaker, frequent unifocal premature ventricular contractions.
- Disorientation, partial heart block (especially paroxysmal atrial tachycardia with 2:1 block and atrioventricular dissociation), complete heart block, multifocal premature ventricular contractions and ventricular fibrillation *(29–25)* or ventricular tachycardia *(29–26)*.

Treatment

Mild Overdosage

- Withholding of digitalis preparation for several days or up to 3 weeks, depending on the excretion rate of the particular drug in use and the observed clinical improvement.
- Correction of any potassium deficit.
- Reinstitution of a lower maintenance dose.

Severe Toxicity

- Hospitalize at once.
- For details of treatment, see *53–265*.

29–12. ELECTROMECHANICAL DISASSOCIATION

Common causes and treatment of this condition are presented in Figure 5–2.

29–13. HEART BLOCK, COMPLETE

Third-degree atrioventricular block is diagnosed electrocardiographically, (see Fig. 29–1*D*) and suspected clinically by the presence of slow ventricular rate (approximately 30 to 40 per minute) with unappreciable increase with activity, and is often heralded by syncope (Stokes-Adams attack). Administration of isoproterenol (Isuprel) IV, by drip infusion of 2 mg in 500 mg of 5% dextrose in water, or SL, 10 to 15 mg every 4 to 6 hours; institution of any necessary resuscitative measures *(5)*; and hospitalization for insertion of a temporary or permanent cardiac pacemaker are indicated. (*Note:* Use of isoproterenol diminished greatly once pacemakers became widely available.) In some urgent situations, in which there has been adequate oxygenation, pending arrival of alternatives, a series of precordial thumps may act as a pacemaker. Check the pulse before each thump.

29–14. HYPERTENSIVE CRISES AND ENCEPHALOPATHY

Significant further increments in diastolic blood pressure, particularly in an individual with a background of chronic diastolic hypertension and associated degenerative effects, may precipitate cardiac failure *(29–10)*, coronary ischemia *(29–15)*, severe headaches, nausea, vomiting, confusion, coma and focal cerebral neurologic signs. These clinical signs and symptoms may be due to edema, major vessel vasospasm or hemorrhage (see *63, Vascular Disorders*). Appropriate diagnostic tests must be performed.

Treatment

- Reduction of diastolic blood pressure toward normal at a rate and degree consistent with maintenance of effective arterial perfusion pressure of vital organs.
- Antihypertensive medications. When immediate reduction in blood pressure is essential, administer IV, by microdrip regulator, sodium nitroprusside (Nipride) (a 50-mg vial diluted in 500 ml or dextrose in water gives a concentration of 100 μg/ml) initially at 0.5 μg/kg/min and increase the dose progressively until the clinically desired blood pressure is attained. Though high doses are tolerated, a dose of more than 10 μg/kg/min is not advised by the manufacturer. Reversal of blood pressure reduction can occur in several minutes following cessation of sodium nitroprusside. Monitor thiocyanate blood levels if continued use is necessary.

  Alternatively, give 20 to 40 mg of furosemide (Lasix) IV followed by 1 to 3 mg/kg, up to 150 mg, of diazoxide (Hyperstat) IV (in less than 30 seconds); a drop in blood pressure will occur in a few minutes; may repeat treatment in 5 to 15 minutes. Keep norepinephrine at hand if blood pressure drop is too great. Another medication that can be considered if the IV diazoxide is unavailable is hydralazine hydrochloride (Apresoline). Maintenance therapy is usually necessary after establishment of a satisfactory blood pressure level.

  Neither guanethidine nor methyldopa should be used in the presence of pheochromocytoma *(36–2)* or in association with monoamine oxidase inhibitors such as isocarboxazid (Marplan), phenelzine sulfate (Nardil) and tranylcypromine sulfate (Parnate).
- Lumbar puncture (see *18–29, Spinal Puncture*). This procedure not only may be of diagnostic value but also in some instances may be of assistance in control of convulsions and severe cephalgia. See also *44–7, Cerebral Edema.*
- Limitation of sodium intake and thiazide administration.

29–15. MYOCARDIAL INFARCTION, ACUTE

Acute myocardial infarction should be particularly suspected in people who have intense substernal chest pain with or without radiation to the jaws or upper extremities; abdominal pain; spontaneous nausea; and vomiting and signs and symptoms of shock *(57)*. The onset may be "silent," though usually there is accompanying substantial fatigue and malaise.

Confirmation of the diagnosis can be made by single or serial electrocardiogram results (see Fig. 29–1,*O*), serum enzyme levels (creatine phosphokinase, serum glutamic-oxaloacetic transaminase, lactic dehydrogenase), vectorcardiogram and radionuclide scanning or scintiscanning. Common treatable sequelae of myocardial infarction that can occur are: arrhythmia, shock *(57)*, congestive heart failure *(29–10)*, aneurysm and rupture *(29–1)* pericarditis *(29–19)* and cardiac arrest *(5)*.

Whenever possible, persons with suspected or proved myocardial infarction should be started on treatment while arrangements for hospitalization are being made.

Treatment

- Have the patient remain quiet in a position of comfort.
- If the patient is not in shock *(57)*, mix morphine sulfate, 10 to 15 mg in 10 ml of distilled water, and inject 1-ml portions slowly IV until acute pain and apprehension lessen or respirations slow or numbness is perceived around the mouth.

- Keep the intravenous portals open by slow infusion of 5% dextrose in water.
- Start oxygen 3–5 L/min (1–2 L/min in patients with COPD) by intranasal catheter or face mask.
- If acute pulmonary edema develops, treat as outlined under *29–10*.
- If evidence of shock *(57)* is present, start an IV infusion of dopamine. It is generally best to avoid IM injections during shock states, as they may not be absorbed; they may also complicate enzyme studies.
- Transfer the patient to the hospital by a well-equipped ambulance, not by private auto, continuing supportive and any resuscitative therapy (supervised by trained personnel) en route; attach monitoring equipment if available. Smooth and safe transportation, not excessive speed, should be emphasized.
- On arrival at the hospital, confirm diagnosis with standard ECG and move the patient ASAP to the coronary care or intensive care unit. Start electrocardiographic monitoring immediately.
- If symptoms of shock *(57)* progress, or congestive heart failure occurs, start a second infusion line containing dopamine (Intropin) (see *57–5C*). This infusion should be given slowly for its inotropic effect rather than for its peripheral vasoconstrictive effect and titrated to give an adequate carotid pulse and a urinary output of about 1 ml per minute. Frequent blood pressure determinations are indicated, and central venous pressure monitoring is of assistance, especially in elderly persons. In more severe cases, use of a Swan-Ganz catheter is of great value. Also consider use of an IV crystalloid "fluid challenge." If intravenous infusion of smaller amounts of a plasma volume expander (e.g., 250 ml of low molecular weight dextran) appears to be indicated, as in postsurgical shock with hypovolemia, watch carefully for early signs of pulmonary edema *(55)*.
- For treatment of serious premature ventricular beats (5 or more per minute, 2 or more in a row or any premature ventricular beats occurring in the T waves), give 50 to 100 mg (5 to 10 ml of 1% solution) of IV lidocaine, repeated in 5 minutes if necessary, followed by IV infusion of 1000 to 2000 mg of lidocaine in 1000 ml of 5% dextrose in water at an initial rate of 1 to 3 mg per minute (1 to 3 mg/kg/hr).
- Treat cardiac arrest as indicated in 5–2; see also 5–*21, Breathing-Ventilation,* and 5–*23, EHC Techniques.*

29–16. NODAL PAROXYSMAL TACHYCARDIA

Differentiating this condition from atrial tachycardia *(29–5)* by clinical and electrocardiographic examination (see Fig. 29–1*H*) may be difficult. Both may be grouped together for treatment under supraventricular tachycardia *(29–24)*. Particularly dangerous are those attacks with heart rates of 250 to 300 per minute in which the low ejection volume may cause cerebral hypoxemia, syncope and cardiac failure. Rates in nodal tachycardia are generally slower. Treatment is directed at two objectives: (1) reducing the excessively rapid ventricular rate by decreasing the excitability and propagation of the atrioventricular node; and (2) preventing recurrences of the attacks. Digitalis toxicity must be evaluated. Dilantin may be useful in reducing episodes.

29–17. PACEMAKER FAILURE

As the prevalence of implanted cardiac pacemakers increases, so does the frequency with which physicians encounter problems associated with occasional ineffective operation. Episodic or complete malfunction may be caused by mechanical factors (wire breakage, loss of adequate contact, penetration of leads through the myocardium) or failure of the battery. An altered heart rate (more than 5 beats per minute for fixed-rate pacemakers [use practically extinct now]; more than 10 beats per minute for demand pacemakers) over the usual established heart rate (approximately 70 per minute) may be a sign of pending battery failure, as may be a relative decrease in voltage of ventricular complexes on the electrocardiogram. Use of an Avionics-Holter electrocardiocorder may help to determine whether any malfunction of the pacemaker is occurring during episodic syncopal attacks or during periods of pulse alteration or absence. Sometimes a pacer may overdrive ("runaway pacer"), and rate-related ischemia can occur. If a defective pacemaker is suspected or proved, referral for definitive care, including replacement, is indicated, with any necessary intervening supportive treatment (see *5, Resuscitation; 29–13, Heart Block*). Patients should have with them at all times data concerning the pacemaker implant (model, manufacturer, serial number, rate/programming, pulse generator site, name of physician who inserted). Generator life has been enhanced fortunately by introduction of the Lithium model.

29–18. PERICARDIAL EFFUSION/CARDIAC TAMPONADE

- Diagnosis and treatment of the primary cause (septic, aseptic, viral, traumatic) and treatment of pain are usually of greatest importance. Occasionally, signs of cardiac tamponade may appear; these include increasing venous engorgement with inspiratory filling rather than collapse; increased heart rate; decreased pulse pressure and heart tones; pulsus paradoxus; abnormal Valsalva response (no slowing of heart rate within 9 to 10 beats after 15 seconds of Valsalva's maneuver); decreasing voltage of ventricular complexes of electrocardiogram or electrical alternans; characteristic abnormal echocardiogram pattern.
- If signs of cardiac tamponade are appearing, an emergency pericardiocentesis *(18–22)* is indicated for drainage. This is most safely performed by attaching the V lead of the ECG to the hub of a Luer-Lok syringe with a 3-way stopcock in between and using a 4-inch 20-gauge needle; the tip of the needle becomes an exploring electrode and an enormous *current of injury pattern* will appear immediately on the electrocardiogram if the needle touches the epicardium. If this occurs, the needle is then withdrawn a few millimeters until the ST segment elevation disappears. The pericardial effusion is removed as adequately as possible and a specimen saved for any necessary diagnostic tests (cytology, cultures, smears). If septic pericardial effusion is present, infusion of antibacterial solution through the same needle at the time of the procedure may be advisable. Rapid recurrence of effusion with tamponade is an indication for surgical referral regarding pericardiotomy and a draining procedure. A Teflon catheter may be left in place to redrain fluid in the event of recurrence pending definitive surgical treatment.

29–19. PERICARDITIS (*See Fig. 29–1Q*)

Inflammation of the pericardial sac is usually characterized by precordial pain and friction rub plus low-grade fever at times; it may develop slowly or rapidly and may be due to:

- Septic causes (pneumococcus, meningococcus, tuberculosis).
- Viruses (particularly Coxsackie).
- Fungi.

- Aseptic causes (uremia, myocardial infarction, collagen diseases, postpericardiotomy).
- Trauma (chest crush injuries, particularly compression from steering wheels).

Days to weeks after a pericardiotomy or myocardial infarction, a syndrome of pericardial and pleural friction rub effusion plus fever and arthralgia (Dressler's syndrome) may present, which often must be distinguished from acute MI by absence of cardiac enzyme rise; treatment is symptomatic, with use of indomethacin or ASA. Corticosteroids are not frequently indicated.

Treatment

- Appropriate antibiotics after Gram staining and obtaining of specimens for cultures if from a septic cause.
- Discontinuation of anticoagulants if being used, e.g., as in treatment of myocardial infarction.
- Use of a nonsteroidal antiinflammatory drug (NSAID such as indomethacin [Indocin] 25 mg PO qid). If additional pain relief is needed, see *12*.
- Intercostal nerve blocks with lidocaine or alcohol may be required for persistent and severe pain.
- Prednisone, 40 to 80 mg in divided daily doses and tapering off over a 7- to 10-day period, is an adjunct in aseptic or viral cases with severe pain.
- Prompt removal of pericardial fluid *(29–18; 18–22)* if cardiac tamponade is occurring (although this is rare).

29–20. PULMONARY EDEMA, ACUTE

For signs and symptoms of pulmonary edema due to congestive heart failure compared with noncardiogenic pulmonary edema (ARDS), see *55–4* and Table 55–1. For treatment of congestive heart failure, see *29–10*; for treatment of noncardiogenic pulmonary edema, see *55–4*.

29–21. SINUS TACHYCARDIA *(See Fig. 29–1A)*

Sinus tachycardia occurring at rest infrequently is an emergency situation in and of itself, but attention must be given to diagnosis and treatment of the underlying cause (infection, anemia, hyperthyroidism [*36–11*], shock [*57*], congestive heart failure [*29–10*], myocardial infarction [*29–15*], anxiety states [*37*].

29–22. SHOCK, CARDIOGENIC *(See 57)*

29–23. STOKES-ADAMS SYNDROME *(See also 5, Resuscitation; 29–13, Heart Block; 29–25, Ventricular Fibrillation; 29–26, Ventricular Tachycardia)*

Sudden intermittent unconsciousness—due usually to periods of ventricular standstill, complete atrioventricular block or, occasionally, ventricular fibrillation or tachycardia—may revert spontaneously to a cardiac rhythm consistent with life, or, alternatively, complete collapse and sudden death may occur. The number of fatalities can be reduced by immediate supportive measures given in accordance with a preconceived plan (see *5, Resuscitation; 29–13, Heart Block)* pending definitive defibrillation or external or internal cardiac pacing.

29–24. SUPRAVENTRICULAR TACHYCARDIA (SVT) *(See also 29–11, Digitalis Toxicity; 29–16, Nodal Paroxysmal Tachycardia)*

This condition is characterized by sudden onset of rapid heart rate of 180 or greater, accompanied by sensations of shakiness, weakness and nausea and associated with pallor and occasionally fainting and even shock. It may last for minutes, hours or even days and can subside as rapidly as it appeared. Various forms of stress may underlie the onset of attacks.

Treatment of Acute Attacks

Nonmedicinal

The following nonmedicinal measures may be effective:

- Have the patient rest in a recumbent position with the feet higher than the head. Put an ice compress on the forehead or face. Combine with relaxation techniques (*12*).
- Have the patient sit up in bed with the head bent forward as far as possible between flexed knees; have the patient breathe slowly and deeply.
- Have the patient perform the Valsalva maneuver by expelling a deep breath against a closed glottis or blow into a sphygmomanometer tubing to maintain a pressure of 40 mm of mercury for 15 to 30 seconds. With short intervening rest periods, this procedure may be repeated several times.
- Another simple method of invoking the vasovagal reflex in patients who are generally healthy is to have the patient intermittently put his face into a pan of cold water (19° C or less) while holding his breath; monitor pulse response and discontinue when pulse is slowed, when the patient becomes comfortable or if repeated trials have not been fruitful.
- Perform carotid sinus massage. *Note:* This is potentially hazardous in some patients, and the precautions listed below should be instituted first:
  —Have the patient lie supine, preferably with equipment for cardiopulmonary resuscitation immediately available. Have IV line running.
  —Keep a syringe containing atropine sulfate, 0.4 to 0.6 mg, at hand for immediate intravenous injection if excessive vagal stimulation occurs.
  —*Do not massage both sides of the neck at the same time.*
  Begin carotid sinus massage by using gentle pressure. Massage the right carotid sinus area (over the middle portion of the carotid artery at the level of the hyoid) for several seconds, monitoring the heart rate. If a satisfactory decrease in rate is not obtained, the duration of massage may be increased to 10 seconds and the pressure may be increased but not enough to occlude blood flow in the carotid artery. Massage of the left carotid sinus may be tried but not simultaneously with massage of the right carotid.

Medicinal

- Verapamil (Isoptin), 5–10 mg IV bolus, is the preferred initial medication in uncomplicated SVT. It is contraindicated with heart block or severe CHF and must be used with caution in digitalized patients. Dose may be repeated in 10–20 minutes if needed.
- Increase peripheral arterial pressure through reflex vagal stimulation by intravenous injection of 5 to 10 mg of methoxamine hydrochloride (Vasoxyl) diluted in 10 ml of solvent, monitoring response. This approach is preferably limited to young people with low blood pressure.
- If the patient has been on digitalis therapy prior to the acute episode of tachycardia (or if the history regarding prior use of digitalis is indefinite), propranolol hydrochloride (Inderal) can be given orally but should not be given intravenously for this condition. Consideration may be given to use

of edrophonium chloride (Tensilon), but this must be used with particular caution in elderly patients and those with suspected sick sinus syndrome.

- Digitalize by administration of digoxin orally, initial dose, 1 mg, followed by 0.25 mg every 4 hours until patient is digitalized (see Table 26–1 for dosages in children). The route of administration used will depend upon the rapidity of effect required.
- Direct current cardioversion (0.25 to 1.0 joules/kg initially) should be considered in infrequent cases refractory to the more common methods just outlined, particularly if cardiac decompensation is occurring because of the rapid heart rate and if digitalis toxicity *(29–11)* is not present.

Prevention of Recurrences

- Provision for adequate graduated physical conditioning accompanied by physical and emotional rest.
- Limitation of use of tobacco and alcohol.
- Quinine, procainamide hydrochloride (Pronestyl) or oral propranolol hydrochloride may be used instead of digitalis if repeated attacks still occur.

Differentiation of Supraventricular Beats with Aberrant Ventricular Conduction from Ventricular Tachycardia

The following features are characteristic of supraventricular beats with aberrant conduction (Marriott, H.J.L.: *Practical Electrocardiography*, 6th ed. Baltimore, Williams & Wilkins, 1977). The differential is important, as it governs between therapies of SVT *(29–24)* and VT *(29–26)*.

ECG

- Preceding P′ wave.
- RBBB pattern (80%).
- Triphasic contour in lead V_1 (rsR′) and reciprocal in V_6 (qRs).
- Initial vector identical with that of flanking conducted beats.
- Only the second in a group of rapid beats shows an anomalous pattern.

Clinical

- First heart sound constant in intensity.
- No cannon waves or no regular cannon waves.
- Slowing with vagal stimulation maneuvers.
- Procainamide IV produces temporary A-V block and atrial rhythm more visible.
- Consider hypoventilation with secondary ischemia as a correctable cause of the conditions.

29–25. VENTRICULAR FIBRILLATION *(See Fig. 29–1L and Section 5–4)*

29–26. VENTRICULAR TACHYCARDIA

Since ventricular tachycardia (Fig. 29–1*K*) can result in ineffective cardiac output, signs of cardiac arrest *(29–8)* may appear, although not as readily as with ventricular fibrillation *(29–25)*. Although life may be maintained for long periods of time in the presence of this condition, treatment should commence as soon as it is recognized. Ventricular tachycardia may occur from various causes—myocardial infarction *(29–15)*, valvular heart disease and toxic effects of certain drugs, including digitalis *(29–11, 53–265)* procainamide *(53–578)* and quinidine *(53–591)*. Correct hypoxemia, acidosis, hypoglycemia and electrolyte imbalance.

Treatment

Treatment is aimed at restoration of normal sinus rhythm and rate; it varies with the severity and exciting cause. If there is no pulse, see Figure 5–2 (Cardiac Arrest Algorithm); if initial precordial thump has been used and there is no improvement, then the following measures may be applied:

- Treatment of non–digitalis-related ventricular tachycardia is intravenous bolus administration of 1 mg/kg of lidocaine (see Table 5–2) followed by direct current electrical cardioversion using 2.0 joules/kg, up to 200 joules (adults) initially; in children may use 0.5 to 2.0 joules/kg. If improved, follow with lidocaine infusion; if not, repeat above cycle except using 0.5 mg/kg lidocaine bolus. If still not improved and drug toxicity not a factor, use either IV procainamide or bretylium tosylate in next attempts (bretylium not indicated in children). Overdrive pacing (usually with a transvenous pacemaker initially) may follow if problems still exist.
- If digitalis toxicity *(29–11)* is a likely cause and adequate perfusion levels and urinary output are being maintained:
  —Stop digitalis intake.
  —Give an IV lidocaine bolus of 50 to 100 mg followed by drip infusion (see 5–2).
  —If the patient is hypokalemic, give an IV infusion of 40 to 80 mEq of potassium in 500 ml of 5% dextrose in water at a rate of 100 to 200 ml per hour, controlled by cardiac monitoring. Urine output should be adequate (45 ml per hour), and there should be no hyperkalemia when therapy is started.
  —Give 0.5 to 1 mg of propranolol hydrochloride (Inderal) slowly IV at 10-minute or longer intervals (total not to exceed 3 mg) until electrocardiographic monitoring shows reversion to a sinus mechanism or the rhythm present before onset of ventricular tachycardia.
  —Attempt electrical conversion with synchronized countershock in critically ill patients.

29–27. VENTRICULAR TACHYCARDIA AND VENTRICULAR FIBRILLATION PROPHYLAXIS

- Cautious use of drugs conducive to ventricular tachycardia and ventricular fibrillation.
- IV infusion of lidocaine, with loading dose of 1 mg/kg and then 500 to 1000 mg in 500 ml of 5% dextrose in water at 1 to 2 ml per minute if premature ventricular contractions are observed in pairs, runs, or superimposition on previous T wave, or are multifocal or occur at rate of more than 5 per minute, while a patient with acute myocardial infarction *(29–15)* is being monitored. Procainamide may also be used.

30. Cephalgia (Headaches)

30–1. GENERAL CONSIDERATIONS

Many types of headache may be severe enough to cause the sufferer to seek emergency medical care. Although the etiology in many instances is obscure and requires more thorough study for determination than is practical in an emergency setting, there are certain types that need to be promptly recognized to start definitive treatment, and others that require at least temporary relief on an emergency basis. The algorithm in Figure 30–1 aids therapeutic designation of the headache, and Table 30–1 outlines the major causes of headache. See also *12* for pain management, preferably non-narcotic.

30–2. ALCOHOLIC EXCESS ("HANGOVER") HEADACHES *(See also 53–295, Ethyl Alcohol)*

Administration of fluids, rest, quiet and acetylsalicylic acid (aspirin) may help. Barbiturates and all types of opiates and synthetic narcotics should be avoided.

30–3. ALTITUDE SICKNESS *(See 26–1, Mountain Sickness)*

30–4. ARTHRITIS OF THE CERVICAL SPINE

Arthritis of the cervical spine (with or without aggravation by trauma) may cause severe headaches, usually localized to the distribution of the greater or lesser occipital or the posterior auricular nerves on one or both sides. Occasionally, the pain may be frontal or postorbital. Use of the polyaxial cervical traction unit (Goodley), which avoids TMJ compression, may be valuable. Signs and symptoms of occipital nerve irritation can be relieved by nerve block.

30–5. BRAIN TUMORS

Brain tumors may cause frontal or generalized headaches, aggravated by changes in position, and are more common in the morning. A space-occupying lesion should be considered if the headache presents a disturbing new symptom and/or neurologic sign or deficit. Check the fundi for signs of increased intracranial pressure (papilledema and venous distention).

Treatment

Acetylsalicylic acid (aspirin), with or without codeine sulfate, may give temporary relief. If a brain tumor is suspected, referral to a neurologist for thorough investigation and definitive treatment is mandatory. Avoid lumbar puncture if there is papilledema.

30–6. CAFFEINE-WITHDRAWAL HEADACHES

In habitual coffee drinkers, abstinence may cause severe, sometimes completely disabling, headaches.

Treatment

Coffee by mouth, caffeine sodiobenzoate, 0.5 g IM, or oxygen inhalations can give rapid relief. Gradual reduction of caffeine intake is advisable.

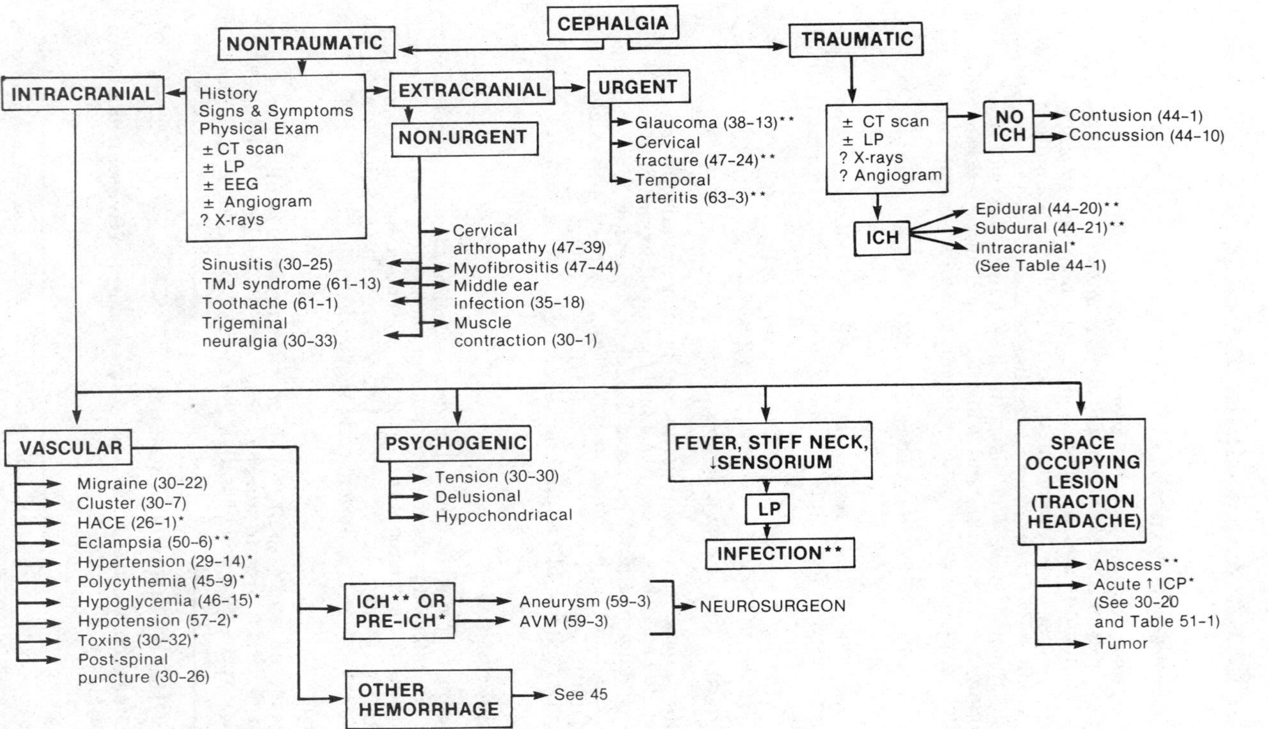

Figure 30–1. Cephalgia algorithm.

Table 30–1. DESCRIPTION OF MAJOR CAUSES OF HEADACHES (Crossover of Causes Is Present in the Algorithm Above)

Type of Headache	Presentation	Treatment
Muscle Contraction	Persistent contraction of striated skeletal muscles of the scalp, neck and face results in a steady "vise" or "bandlike," "squeezing," "pressure" headache	Reduction of muscle contraction, preferably by nonmedical means (*12*). Therapeutic exercise, counseling, biofeedback, hypnoanalysis, acupuncture are often effective. Muscle relaxant and sleeping medications may be helpful initially. Narcotics are best avoided
Traction	Traction or stretching on intracranial structures with sensory nerve endings—mainly the blood vessels and meninges. Insidious tension, as with tumor, causes low-grade, steady, dull ache noticed mostly in the morning, when sleep and other activities do not mask it. Severe, rapid stretching as with an intracranial bleed causes sharp agonizing pain	Identification of the type and location of lesion with CT scan. Follow with appropriate treatment of the primary problem
Vascular	Vascular headaches often begin with a vasospastic phase in which even focal ischemic effects are sometimes evident. Vaso vasorum involvement probably helps account for the pathologic vasodilatation and perivascular swelling (associated with pain) that subsequently occurs, probably as a result of accumulation of metabolic end-products. Catecholamines and histamines play a role	See migraine (*30–22*) and cluster (*30–15*) headaches. The same approaches effective for relaxing striated muscle contraction (above) are beneficial in breaking up the cycle of recurrent smooth (vascular) muscle constriction that initially occurs. Acupuncture may be effective in relieving even full-blown migraine attacks
Inflammatory	Inflammation—either septic or aseptic—of the blood vessels or meninges	Lumbar puncture and Gram stain needed to perform emergency evaluation of intracranial types. Treat according to diagnosis (see *33–40*, *Meningitis*; *63–3*, *Temporal Arteritis*). Urgent treatment required
Extracranial	Manifestations are of the presenting primary problem (which may be masked by the secondary headache); see list of extracranial causes in Figure 30–1	See urgent and nonurgent extracranial causes in Figure 30–1. Usually mixed type headache
Mixed	Combination of any 2 or more of the above	Treatment of each component in a balanced therapeutic approach

30–7. CLUSTER HEADACHES *(See 30–15)*

30–8. CONCUSSION HEADACHES

Concussion headaches follow direct trauma to the head, but the severity of the headache has little, if any, relationship to the intensity of the trauma. In mild cases, rest, reassurance and acetylsalicylic acid (aspirin) are all that is necessary. Give a head injury instruction sheet (*44*, [Fig. 44–1]). Severe cases require treatment as outlined under *44–1, Head Injuries*.

30–9. ECLAMPSIA *(See 50–14)*

30–10. EPILEPSY *(See 32–7, Coma; 34, Convulsive Seizures)*

30–11. EYE STRAIN

Simple eye strain is a very unlikely cause of recurrent severe headaches; all such patients—regardless of age—should be checked for glaucoma. If signs and symptoms of acute glaucoma *(38–13; 38–40)* are present, tonometry or evaluation by an ophthalmologist should be done immediately.

Treatment

Treatment consists basically of avoiding excessive use of the eyes, especially at close or fine work. Dark or tinted glasses may be of assistance if photophobia is present. Acetylsalicylic acid (aspirin) will often give temporary relief. The patient should be referred to an ophthalmologist for evaluation.

30–12. FEBRILE HEADACHES

Febrile headaches may be caused by any condition that results in a high fever. Administration of acetylsalicylic acid (aspirin), cold packs or iced saline enemas may be used to bring the fever down while serious conditions such as meningitis *(33–40)*, poliomyelitis *(33–52)* and pneumonia *(56–16)* are being ruled out by careful examination.

30–13. FOOD ALLERGY HEADACHES

Food allergy headaches may occur following the ingestion of almost any kind of food by susceptible individuals. The most common offenders, especially in children, seem to be cabbage, chocolate, garlic, green peppers and peanuts. Antihistamines may give rapid relief. Precipitating foods should be avoided. Many of these headaches are vascular or migraine in nature and should be treated accordingly *(30–22)*.

30–14. HERPES

Herpes of the posterior auricular or greater or lesser occipital nerves may cause severe localized headache with or without severe burning. The diagnosis can usually be made from the distribution of the lesions and by the type of pain.

Treatment

- Protection of the herpetic lesions from infection by petrolatum gauze or butacaine (Butyn) ointment dressings. If the lesions are on the scalp above the hair line, chlortetracycline (Aureomycin) ointment, rubbed in gently, is effective.

- Control of acute pain: *See 12, Pain Control.* Nerve block with lidocaine or bupivacaine can give rapid relief.
- Hospitalization in severe or stubborn cases or if the eyes are progressively involved *(38–14)*.

CAUTION: chronic pain is best not treated in the emergency department with narcotics that are rather rapidly habit-forming and addicting. Antidepressants and tranquilizers are preferable in these instances, and an injection of the latter should suffice for patients presenting in the Emergency Department with acute exacerbations.

30–15. HISTAMINE HEADACHES

Histamine headaches (cluster headache, Horton's cephalgia) are severe, invariably unilateral and throbbing, with a duration of 30 to 60 minutes on the average. They tend to occur in groups over a period of weeks. The pain is located about the eye, which may redden and tear. Sometimes there are constriction of the ipsilateral pupil and drooping of the ipsilateral eyelid. The ipsilateral nostril is often blocked or discharging. The attacks are often nocturnal. Alcohol is a consistent precipitating and aggravating factor. Measures such as jugular compression that raise the spinal fluid pressure and decrease the blood supply will temporarily relieve the cephalgia, as may analgesics. Ergot and other measures recommended for treating migraine headaches (see *30–22*) may be effective. Severe cases require hospitalization.

30–16. HYPERTENSIVE HEADACHES

Hypertensive headaches are usually present in the morning and wear off by noon. Acetylsalicylic acid (aspirin) will give temporary relief. Sleeping with the head elevated may prevent attacks. Appropriate treatment of the hypertension is indicated.

A new onset of severe lateralized headaches accompanied by focal neurologic signs in a patient with a history of hypertension should suggest the possibility of a hypertensive intracerebral hemorrhage *(63–3)*. Computerized tomography should reveal the correct diagnosis.

30–17. HYPERVISCOSITY CONDITIONS

Headaches associated with lethargy, seizures, coma and bleeding problems may be seen in conditions associated with observable increased blood viscosity *(45–9, Polycythemia)* or serum viscosity due to abnormal protein states (such as multiple myeloma, Sjögren's syndrome, Waldenström's macroglobulinemia). The patient should be referred to an oncologist for treatment of the primary condition and possible plasmapheresis.

30–18. HYPOGLYCEMIC ("HUNGER") HEADACHES

Hypoglycemia is suspected by occurrence between meals and is determined by a blood glucose sample taken at the time of the headache. Excessive intake of carbohydrates can cause a large output of insulin that results in hypoglycemia, and a vicious cycle can get established. Sometimes these headaches will present with a migraine-type prodrome. They are relieved by food, especially proteins, avoidance of refined carbohydrates and increased frequency of eating but ingestion of smaller meals. There may be enough time lag to require acetylsalicylic acid (aspirin).

30–19. HYPOTENSIVE HEADACHES (ORTHOSTATIC HEADACHES)

Hypotensive headaches are caused by any of the many conditions that produce a drop in blood pressure and often are accompanied by vasodepressor syncope *(63–7)*.

30–20. INCREASED INTRACRANIAL PRESSURE (IIP)

Increased intracranial pressure is suspected when headache is accompanied by retinal and focal neurologic pathologic findings. The retina early reveals bilateral blurred margins and a flattened cup; these signs are followed by the appearance of widened tortuous veins, retinal hemorrhages around a reddened disc and then gross swelling of the disc. Since many different pathogenetic mechanisms (such as tumor, abscess, hemorrhage, large areas of infection, leptomeningeal diseases, pulmonary emphysema, certain toxins and idiopathic pseudotumor cerebri) lead to increased intracranial pressure, a careful history and thorough evaluation are required.

The role of the emergency physician is to recognize the possibility of increased intracranial pressure and initiate appropriate evaluation. See *18–29, Spinal Puncture,* for Cautions. See Table 51–1 (under CNS involvement) for causes of IIP in the absence of a mass lesion.

30–21. MENINGEAL IRRITATION

Severe and persistent headaches associated with fever and stiff neck require immediate spinal puncture to determine the etiology *(33–40, Meningitis; 33–6, Arboviral Infections)*.

30–22. MIGRAINE HEADACHES

Migraine headaches can be either unilateral or bilateral. They are associated with nausea, are often preceded by visual disturbance (zig-zag lines, blurred vision, hemianopia, flashes of light) and are sometimes preceded by, or associated with, focal neurologic signs such as weakness or numbness of an arm, or a combination of the two, or difficulty with speech for a period of minutes to hours. There is usually a history of previous similar attacks and a family history of migraine.

In Adults. Relief from the acute discomfort of migraine-type head pain can sometimes be obtained through a combination of the following measures:

- Absolute rest in a darkened room.
- Ergotamine tartrate (Gynergen), 2 to 3 mg PO initially, followed by 1 mg every 2 hours by mouth. *The total oral dose should not exceed 6 mg per attack or 10 mg per week.* A slower effect can be obtained by 2 tablets of Cafergot (ergotamine tartrate, 1 mg, with caffeine, 100 mg) orally, repeated in 2 hours only once, or by rectal suppository.

Ergot in therapeutic doses has many undesirable side effects *(53–291)*, including myalgia, fatigue, nausea, vomiting, tingling and numbness of the hands and feet and even myocardial infarction. Atropine sulfate, 0.4 mg subcutaneously, will neutralize some of these side effects. Numbness or tingling of the extremities, a cold feeling or cyanosis calls for immediate discontinuance of ergot in any form.

- Pentazocine lactate (Talwin), 15 to 30 mg IM; minimize narcotic use because of danger of addiction.
- An antiemetic, such as prochlorperazine (Compazine), 5 to 10 mg IM or 25-mg rectal suppository, may be necessary in treatment of protracted vomit-

ing. Trimethobenzamide hydrochloride (Tigan), 100 mg to 200 mg IM or as a 200-mg rectal suppository, is also effective; follow manufacturer's cautions for use in children.

PROPHYLAXIS. Although it is of no value in treatment of acute attacks, methysergide maleate (Sansert), 2 mg by mouth 3 times a day, may prevent the development of migraine. The possibility of serious side effects makes careful follow-up care important. Propranolol (Inderal), 10 to 20 mg PO tid to qid is also helpful in some patients.

In earlier stages of acute onset and for prophylaxis, various forms of reflex therapy (see *12, Pain Control*), including acupuncture and biofeedback, can be effective in control.

30–23. MYOFIBROSITIS (FIBROMYOSITIS, MYOFASCITIS)

Myofibrositis of the upper portion of the neck from trauma *(47–11)*, postural strain (television headache) or infection (especially viral) may cause unilateral or bilateral headache, usually occipital with localization to the distribution of the posterior auricular or greater or lesser occipital nerves on one or both sides. Treatment of the underlying cause is necessary for permanent relief. Symptomatic relief can be given by the measures outlined for whiplash injuries *(47–11)*.

30–24. PSYCHOGENIC HEADACHES

Psychogenic headaches are characterized by complaints of a tight band around the head or a pulling sensation over the vertex and usually are caused by anxiety, depression or tension singly or in varying combinations (see also *30–30*). Patients usually fail to offer these factors initially and often deny them.

30–25. SINUS HEADACHES

Sinus headaches often can be relieved temporarily by shrinking the nasal mucous membranes, postural drainage or ultrasonic therapy. If these measures do not give relief, the patient should be referred to an otolaryngologist.

30–26. SPINAL PUNCTURE HEADACHES

Headaches occur in 10 to 20% after spinal puncture whether or not local anesthetics or the preventive measures outlined later in this section are used.

Cycle of Development

1. The cerebrospinal fluid pressure is decreased by puncture.
2. The difference between the spinal fluid pressure and intracranial venous pressure is increased.
3. Dilation of the intracranial venous structures results in increased volume of the brain with resultant stimulation of the intracranial pain centers.

Preventive Measures

1. Use of a small needle with the bevel parallel to the long axis of the body to minimize dural tears.
2. Avoidance of any motion of the spine while the needle is in place.
3. Limitation of amount of fluid removed to not more than 6 ml.
4. Maintenance of the prone position for 1 hour after completion of the procedure.
5. Intravenous administration of 5% dextrose in water (unless contraindi-

cated by some systemic condition). Caffeine sodiobenzoate, Pituitrin, ergotamine and nicotinic acid have been used empirically but probably are of no value.

Symptomatic Treatment

1. Bed rest with the head at or below the level of the feet. (This is also a preventative measure.)
2. Acetylsalicylic acid (aspirin) in mild cases; codeine sulfate in small doses if the discomfort is acute. The drugs listed under tension headaches *(30–30)* may also be of benefit.
3. Application of a tight abdominal binder, especially following puncture for obstetric spinal anesthesia.
4. Hospitalization if the headache persists or is unaffected by postural changes.
5. Homologous "blood patching" of the dural tear has been described as giving relief in the extreme or protracted case (5 ml of freshly drawn patient's blood is injected into the epidural space at the leaking area).

Prognosis

Complete recovery is the rule, although in some cases 7 to 10 days may be required for complete relief. The patient may or may not develop symptoms of spinal puncture if repeated at a later date.

30–27. SUBARACHNOID HEMORRHAGE (SAH) *(See 63–2)*

30–28. SUNLIGHT HEADACHES

Sunlight headaches are caused by peripheral vasodilation from unaccustomed exposure to bright sunlight. They often precede heat cramps *(62–5)*, heat stroke *(62–7)*, and sunstroke *(62–9)*.

30–29. SYPHILIS (Cerebral) *(See 33–66)*

30–30. TENSION HEADACHES (Psychogenic Headaches)

Tension headache is an overworked catchall for many cases of headache of mixed etiology. Such headaches are characterized by complaints of a tight feeling or band around the head, aching of the neck, a pulling sensation over the vertex, soreness behind the eyes, and tautness and tenderness of the muscles of the neck and scalp. Although extreme mental stress and strain may cause severe headaches in certain individuals, a thorough history and examination will usually disclose a specific causative factor. Many of these headaches result from spasm or tonic contraction of skeletal muscles at the back of the neck and skull. They can be relieved by cryotherapy (ice, fluoromethane, heat), massage, stretching and resolution of mental and physical stress. Persistent daily tension headaches frequently reflect an underlying depressive state. Some of the following may give relief while the basic cause is being determined:

- Acetylsalicylic acid (aspirin), 0.6 g PO every 4 hours.
- Meprobamate (Miltown, Equanil), 400 mg PO 3 times a day; diazepam (Valium), 2 to 5 mg PO 3 to 4 times daily; or chlorpromazine (Thorazine), 10 to 25 mg PO 3 times a day. (See also *30–32, Migraine.*)
- Physical therapy measures, such as warm water submersion, warm packs, deep muscle massage and isometric and relaxation exercises.
- Training in nonmedicinal approaches to relief of pain *(12)*.

30–31. TOOTHACHES OR EARACHES

Toothaches *(41)* or earaches secondary to middle ear infection *(35–18)* may cause severe headaches of focal location.

30–32. TOXIC HEADACHES

Ingestion, inhalation or absorption through the mucous membranes or the intact skin of many substances may cause severe headaches, usually frontal in location, but sometimes orbital, occipital or diffuse. Among the more common substances whose toxic pictures are characterized by headache are:

Alcohol—amyl *(53–70)*, ethyl *(53–295)* and isopropyl *(53–372)*.
Ammonia fumes *(53–61)*.
Benzene—inhalation or ingestion *(53–117)*.
Caffeine withdrawal *(30–6)*.
Carbon monoxide poisoning *(53–175)*.
Chlorine *(53–192)*.
Epinephrine hydrochloride (Adrenalin)—from overzealous use of a nebulizer or from hypodermic administration. See *53–288*.
Hydrochloric acid vapors. See *Acids, 53–350.*
Iodine–inhalation of the fumes *(53–365)*.
Kerosene fumes *(53–379)*.
Lead and its salts—from inhalation of the fumes or dust or ingestion. Chronic lead poisoning (plumbism) is often characterized by severe headaches *(53–386)*.
Metal fumes *(53–423)*.
Methyl acetate fumes *(53–434)*.
Naphthalene fumes *(53–469)*.
Nicotine *(53–478)*.
Nitrates *(53–481)*.
Ozone—in certain hypersensitive persons, inhalation of even minute concentrations of this gas will cause very severe frontal headaches *(53–505)*.
Phosphorus pentachloride fumes *(53–546)*.
Pyrethrum dust or powder *(53–584)*.
Tobacco–inhalation of dust or ingestion. See *Nicotine 53–478*.
Zinc oxide—inhalation of dust. See *Metal Fumes, 53–423*.

30–33. TRIGEMINAL NEURALGIA (Tic Douloureux) *(See 49–13)*.

30–34. UREMIA

Uremia *(32–16)* may be accompanied by a very distressing type of headache that will persist until the causative condition is remedied. Sedatives and analgesics are of limited value in treatment.

30–35. VASOPRESSOR HEADACHES

Vasopressor headaches may be caused by administration of phenylephrine hydrochloride (Neo-Synephrine), epinephrine hydrochloride (Adrenalin) *(53–288)* and other rapidly acting vasopressor drugs. Unless excessively large doses have been given or individual hypersensitivity is present, the effect is transient only and requires no emergency treatment.

31. Chest

31–1. INITIAL CONSIDERATIONS IN CHEST TRAUMA

- The usual priorities in chest injuries are as follows: establish and maintain the airway (5), cover and close all sucking chest wounds (with any available broad external dressing), relieve tension pneumothorax, stop any gross hemorrhage, relieve pericardial tamponade, externally protect and stabilize, as feasible, any flail movements of the chest *(31–8)* and treat any cardiac injury.
- Evaluate for insertion of bilateral chest tubes ("closed thoracotomy"), using local anesthesia, and connect to underwater seal drainage.
- It is best to assume that thoracic vertebral (and cervical) trauma has also occurred in severe trauma and to splint the cervical spine accordingly before any movement—even in the absence of neurologic long tract deficits. (Leave splint on until x-rays confirm that vertebrae are intact.)
- Generally do not withdraw penetrating foreign objects until in the surgical arena—preferably close off any sucking and stabilize with external tape or dressing. Avoid tight circumferential binding, which restricts thoracic cage expansion. Insofar as possible, transport with the least involved side of the thorax in a superior position.
- Administer oxygen, start intravenous fluids—particularly saline or Ringer's lactate—as necessary and relieve pain *(12)*.
- Diagnostic chest x-rays are indicated, and an echogram or CAT scan may be needed as well. Emergency bronchoscopy is valuable with suspected bronchus rupture and hemorrhage. The same applies to esophagoscopy if esophageal injury is suspected. Baseline ABG values and ECG should be obtained. An arteriogram to evaluate for aortic tear (see *31–2*) and a radioisotope scan may be needed.
- If rib fractures involve the lower thorax, also consider concomitant renal injury, in which case IVP is also advised (on occasion renal injury may be present even without accompanying hematuria); on the left also consider spleen trauma and diaphragm rupture, and on the right, liver injury.
- Acute restlessness and apprehension in a patient who gives a history of severe rib cage compression are often the only indications of intra-alveolar or mediastinal bleeding; evaluate for hypoxemia with ABG's. Even in the absence of external evidence of trauma, supportive therapy should be begun at once. Emergency bronchoscopy should be performed if the possibility of a ruptured bronchus is considered.
- Respiratory depressants, especially opiates and synthetic narcotics, should not be administered to a patient with any type of chest injury until the nature and extent of the injury have been definitely determined.
- Always consider the magnitude of the force involved (speed, mass, focal or diffuse impact, and the degree of movement of the patient after impact), as well as the possibility of injury from secondary impact. Consider the possibility of aortic rupture, fracture, myocardial contusion or infarction from substantial impact even when there is little superficial evidence of trauma.

31–2. AORTIC RUPTURE (or Rupture of Its Major Thoracic Branches or Both)

- About 10% of patients—most have been in decelerative vehicular accidents—sustaining severe blunt chest trauma with thoracic aortic rupture survive long enough to reach the emergency room. External evidence of trauma need not be dramatic; therefore, the condition needs to be routinely considered in these situations in order to initiate definitive treatment. Chest x-rays reveal the following clues: tracheal shift to the right, widened mediastinum (more than 8 cm at level of the aortic knob is indicative of mediastinal hematoma), blurring of the usual sharp aortic contour, a left mainstem bronchus angle of less than 40 degrees, obliteration of the medial aspect of the left upper lobe at the apex, obliteration of the space between the aorta and left pulmonary artery, widening of the paravertebral outline, fracture of the sternum or first rib, fracture-dislocation of the thoracic spine or posterior dislocation of the clavicle, esophageal displacement to the right, as demonstrated by positioning of a nasogastric tube or barium swallow, and hemothorax on the left side.

- Even if x-rays are normal with respect to the features just listed, on the basis of unexplained shock, massive hemothorax, contained brisk intrathoracic bleeding or strong suspicion of arterial injury following severe blunt chest trauma, including diminution or absence of peripheral pulses, the patient should have retrograde aortography or digital subtraction angiography for diagnosis and localization preparatory to prompt surgical repair of any demonstrated rupture.
- Hemorrhage into the chest can be of exsanguinating proportion, but intrathoracic hemorrhage is one of the situations in which autotransfusion *(18–35)* can be considered (if appropriate personnel and equipment are available) in addition to usual transfusions.

31–3. BULLET WOUNDS *(See 31–11)*

31–4. CARDIAC TRAUMA

Penetrating or severe concussive chest injuries may cause injury to the myocardium or endocardium and bleeding within the pericardium with cardiac tamponade (for signs and symptoms, see *29–18;* for treatment, see *18–22*). Contusions of the heart are treated similarly to myocardial infarction *(29–15)*, except that anticoagulants should not be used. If a person with chest or sternal injuries *(31–1)* or a penetrating injury to the neck or abdomen is in unexplained or therapy-resistant shock, an electrocardiogram revealing myocardial damage may clarify the picture; also order SGOT, CPK and LDH with isoenzymes. Radionuclide scanning or scintiscanning using technetium-99m pyrophosphate may also be used to obtain a very early demonstration of injury. Treat shock *(57)* according to the predominant cause—hemorrhage, cardiac (myocardial) contusion or mechanical constriction (cardiac tamponade); patients with smaller penetrating chest injuries (not more than 1 cm) are candidates for treatment of pericardial sac hemorrhage by aspiration alone. Any patient with a penetrating injury that may have been directed toward the heart and pericardium should have an immediate surgical consultation. If the external injury is larger, if shock is refractive to treatment or if tamponade recurs following aspiration, immediate intervention may be warranted. Transfer to a hospital with coronary bypass facilities may be necessary.

31–5. CONTUSIONS/CRUSHING/COMPRESSION INJURIES *(See 31–10)*

31–6. COSTOCHONDRAL SEPARATION

Treatment is similar to that outlined in *31–8*. Sometimes injection of lidocaine with a few mg triamcinolone into each joint brings relief.

31–7. DIAPHRAGM INJURY OR RUPTURE

Rupture of the diaphragm may be caused by direct nonpenetrating trauma over the lower ribs on either side or, less commonly, by penetrating wounds. Dyspnea and cyanosis may be acute. Dullness, decrease in breath sounds in the lower lobes, decrease in diaphragm excursion and, if rupture is through the left diaphragm, a mediastinal shift to the right may increase suspicion of this type of injury. Shock, usually the result of mediastinal shift, may require treatment before and during transportation to a hospital equipped for open heart surgery. Transport in the semi-sitting position. Insert a nasogastric tube with suction to decompress the stomach and bowel as much as possible before surgery. If there is "free air" in the chest and compromise of lung expansion, a chest tube may be needed initially. Small defects in the diaphragm are very difficult to detect and are potentially more dangerous than large rents because of the increased chances of obstruction and strangulation. Chest x-ray may be initially misread as showing acute gastric dilatation and elevated diaphragm.

31–8. FRACTURES

- Immediate diagnostic x-rays to evaluate for presence of pneumothorax and hemothorax as well as fracture locations are indicated.
- A patient with simple fractures of ribs or sternum usually requires no treatment except limitation of activity, control of pain and periodic deep breathing and coughing as necessary to clear secretions and prevent atelectasis. Use of a transcutaneous nerve stimulator (TNS) unit can be of value; also see *12* for other pain relief measures. Local application of cold will often decrease immediate discomfort; after 24 hours heat may give relief. Blocking of the intercostal nerves proximal to the fractures with a local anesthetic (see *31–17*) may be necessary for relief if overriding, depression or displacement is present. Tight circumferential binding or strapping of the chest may be dangerous, because it limits to some extent the aeration of the lungs and increases the possibility of the development of a traumatic pneumonitis; however, a properly applied rib belt or hemithoracic taping will give considerable relief. Encourage periodic deep breathing and clearing cough. This is especially important in elderly persons. Marked sternal depression requires immediate hospitalization.
- Multiple rib fractures in a patient with the loss of ability of the thorax to expand on inspiration may result in a flail chest with "paradoxical respiration." Establish airway. Sandbags alongside the chest wall and judicious positioning with the uninvolved side superior can aid stabilization. Immediate hospitalization is always required if paradoxical respiration is present. An NG tube should be placed for early insertion in patients with extensive rib fractures, as aerophagia, gastric distention and vomiting often occur. Surgical stabilization procedures are less frequently used now. Meticulous frequent respiratory care—tracheobronchial toilet—is essential and can greatly aid pulmonary function; the assistance of a respiratory therapist and a physical therapist can be invaluable. Intubation and volume-controlled ventilation with positive expiratory end pressure (PEEP) is indicated when the other procedures described are not providing adequate ventilation-perfusion. The measures described in the preceding paragraph should be instituted for management as indicated.
- Treatment of compound rib fractures is similar to that outlined for pleural lacerations *(31–11)*—use towel clip countertraction if paradoxical respira-

tion is present and ventilation-perfusion is being interfered with. Emergency laparotomy may be necessary as well as thoracotomy.

- Thoracic vertebral fractures require immobilization on mere suspicion and continuation of immobilization upon confirmation (see *47–14*). Decompression laminectomy is indicated with spinal cord compression, unless the magnitude of dislocation precludes spinal cord viability. With dislocation fractures, later fusion or stabilization may be needed.

31–9. HEMOPERICARDIUM

See *29–18* for signs and symptoms of cardiac tamponade; see *18–22* for pericardiocentesis; see *31–4* for other suggestions in the management of cardiac trauma.

31–10. NONPENETRATING INJURIES *(See also 59, Soft Tissue Injuries)*

Sudden forcible compression of the chest may cause serious intrathoracic damage without external evidence of injury, especially in children. Slowly progressive bleeding due to alveolar rupture may result from the "accordion action" of the resilient rib cage. Crystalloids, such as saline, in preference to colloids or plasma volume expanders, should be started intravenously if a patient with a history of possible thoracic compression is acutely and persistently apprehensive and restless. This should be done even if signs and symptoms of hemorrhagic shock *(57)* are absent and there are no other indications of intrathoracic injury. Hospitalization for careful and frequent observation for changes in vital signs and hematocrit levels is indicated for at least 24 hours after injury. Evaluate for aortic rupture *(31–2)*, particularly in victims of severe decelerative vehicular accidents. Do not overtreat with colloids or under-resuscitate; "shock lung," or ARDS *(55–4)* may develop, requiring vigorous treatment.

31–11. PENETRATING/PERFORATING CHEST INJURIES

Stab and knife wounds are most likely to be penetrating, whereas high-velocity missile injuries are more frequently perforating. Refer to considerations in *31–1* and consider possibility of esophageal, nerve, spinal cord and heart injuries, as well as injury to the mediastinum, bronchi and lungs.

Treatment

- Cover the surface entrance site (and exit site, if any) with gauze (plus an impervious material if a sucking wound) and a pressure bandage. If foreign objects are still protruding, generally do not remove at the scene but preferably seal off wound and wait until in surgical arena. Do not probe for bullets or other foreign bodies in the field.
- Treat shock *(57)*.
- If dyspnea or cyanosis is marked, give air or oxygen by face mask or intranasal catheter (or by mask-bag or nasotracheal or endotracheal tube if necessary) after cleansing the airway by suction.
- Use gentle restraint as needed. Provide pain relief *(12)*.
- As soon as possible, transfer by ambulance for hospitalization, continuing respiratory assistance in the ambulance if necessary. Put in chest tube with underwater-seal drainage when available to help reexpand the lung.
- Exploratory thoracotomy and abdominal laparotomy may be needed; obtain thoracic or general surgical consultation.

31–12. PNEUMOTHORAX, TENSION

- Pneumothorax can be of apparent "spontaneous" onset following rupture of subpleural blebs; check for preceding Valsalva-type maneuver. Pulling, pleuritic chest pain, shortness of breath, cough, tachypnea, asymmetrical hemithoracic expansion, guarded shallow respirations, decreased breath sounds and hyperresonance over the involved side plus subcutaneous emphysema and crepitations are common. Tracheal shift can be palpated in the suprasternal notch. Shock and cyanosis can follow. Obtain inspiratory and expiratory chest films. Look for mediastinal shift, pleural fluid and collapsed lung with absent lung markings from visceral to parietal pleura.
- Tension pneumothorax, caused by leakage of air from the lung or ruptured bronchus into the pleural cavity with an intact chest wall, is a very serious condition that requires immediate correction. Before transportation of the patient, if definitive care equipment is not available, a large-bore (No. 16, No. 18 or larger) needle or intracath needle with a rubber glove finger or finger cot with a small hole in the tip fastened to the needle base should be inserted into the pleural cavity on the involved side between the 2nd and 3rd ribs in the midclavicular line or as shown in Figure 31–1 to act as a flutter valve; alternatively, the finger can be placed over the needle nub during inspiration and released during exhalation. Hospitalize for placement of water seal drainage or use of Heimlich flutter valve.
- If the lateral visceral pleura is only 1 cm away or the apical visceral pleura not more than 4 cm away from the parietal pleura and the patient is not in respiratory distress, initial treatment is observation of the patient only; if the distance is greater, put in a chest tube *(18–33)*.

31–13. PNEUMOTHORAX, TRAUMATIC

Traumatic pneumothorax should be ruled out by careful clinical and x-ray examination. Its presence requires hospitalization after careful observation for, and treatment of, latent or delayed shock (57). If the injury is severe or if after aspiration *(18–33, Thoracentesis)*, air still reaccumulates, if indicated,

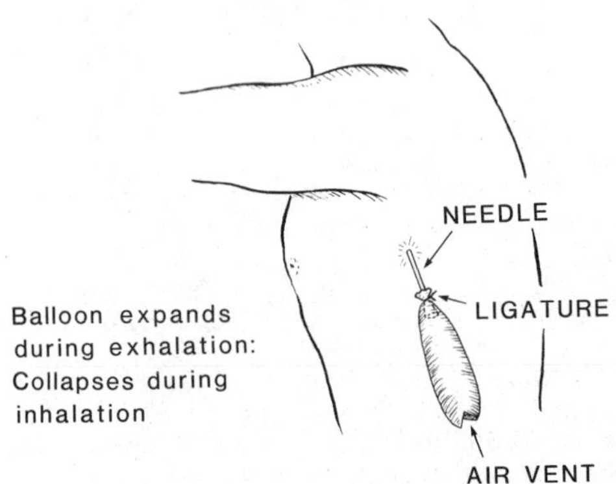

Figure 31–1. Treatment of tension pneumothorax can be aided by this approach. The collapsible device can be from a finger cot, finger portion of a surgical glove, or a balloon.

a chest tube with underwater-seal drainage or Heimlich flutter valve should be placed.

31–14. SUBCUTANEOUS EMPHYSEMA

Air in the subcutaneous spaces causes expansion of the tissues, which, when pressed, give a crepitant response. Most often, the source is air coming through a wound in the thoracic wall and pleura or coming from a pneumothorax, a rupture of a bronchus or esophagus or a leaking tracheotomy. The problem is not the subcutaneous air but rather diagnosing and correcting the source of the air—the air will then dissipate spontaneously. Use chest tube ("closed thoracotomy") as necessary.

31–15. TRACHEOBRONCHIAL RUPTURE

This serious condition is most likely to occur in severe blunt chest trauma. Location and magnitude of rupture determine whether there will be rapid death or, as in most cases, time for repair. Emergency manifestations are as follows: mediastinal and subcutaneous emphysema, tension pneumothorax, complete unilateral atelectasis, airway obstruction, pneumothorax and continuous air leak despite chest tube, and, if also associated with vascular injury, gross hemorrhage, hemoptysis and hemothorax. Emergency bronchoscopy can establish the diagnosis.

Treatment

- Treat as for airway obstruction *(5)*, tension pneumothorax *(31–12)*, traumatic pneumothorax *(31–13)*.
- Measure all fluid and blood collected from chest tubes.
- Indications for thoracotomy include the following:
  —Gross tracheobronchial bleeding.
  —Greater than 200 ml per hour blood loss via drainage tubes.
  —Continuing massive air leak despite water-seal drainage.
- Treat hypovolemic shock *(57)* and relieve pain *(12)*.
- Obtain thoracic or general surgical consultation.

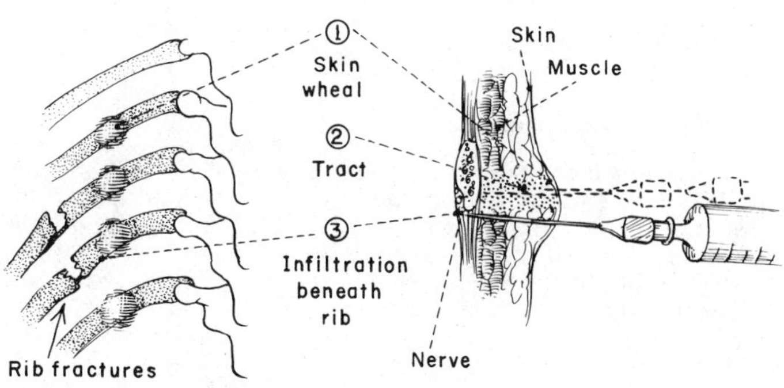

Figure 31–2. The technique of intercostal nerve block. Note that the infiltrating needle is "walked" under the lower rib margin, unlike the technique of thoracentesis. (From Zuidema, G., Rutherford, R., and Ballinger, W. (eds.): *The Management of Trauma,* 3rd ed. Philadelphia, W. B. Saunders Co., 1978.)

SPECIAL EMERGENCY THORACIC PROCEDURES

31–16. FLUTTER VALVE FOR TENSION PNEUMOTHORAX *(See Fig. 31–1)*

31–17. INTERCOSTAL NERVE BLOCK

Focal thoracic chest wall pain, whether from trauma or neuritis, can be greatly relieved by intercostal nerve blocks, which permit better thoracic excursion and ventilation. Injection of the intercostal nerve not only along the dermatome of the site of major injury (as rib fracture) but also 1 or 2 interspaces above and below will give the best results. Use 4 ml of 1% lidocaine with epinephrine injected using the technique shown in Figure 31–2. *(Note:* Iatrogenic pneumothorax can occur as a complication of this type of block.)

31–18. THORACENTESIS/THORACOSTOMY/THORACOTOMY *(See 18–33 and Figs. 18–2 and 18–3)*

32. Coma/Altered Consciousness

Common causes of coma (reduced awareness from which a patient cannot be aroused by usual stimuli, in contrast to sleep) and altered consciousness are as follows:

I. *Intracranial pathology* (see 44–3, *Localization of Injury Level*)
- Head injury
- Cerebrovascular accidents
- Convulsive disorders
- Infection
- Intracranial tumors—usually space-consuming
- Psychopathology

II. *Systemic conditions*
- Asphyxia (suffocation)
- Toxic substances (poisons, drugs, etc.)
- Cardiac pathology
- Temperature variation injuries—cold or heat
- Metabolic abnormalities

For clinical approach to management and treatment of coma of undetermined origin, see Table 32–1. Head trauma, strokes and intoxications—particularly from drug overdose—account for the majority of cases in any hospital.

See Table 32–2 for clinical gradations of coma, which can be periodically scored to evaluate improvement or regression.

32–1. ACUTE INFECTIOUS DISEASES

Especially in children, acute infectious diseases of the CNS/meninges may cause deep coma. Treatment depends upon the causative condition (see 33, *Communicable Diseases*).

32–2. CARDIAC DECOMPENSATION *(See 29)*

32–3. DIABETES MELLITUS

Two conditions directly related to diabetes may require emergency care: hyperglycemia (diabetic coma) and hyperinsulinism (insulin shock). For the differential diagnosis of these two conditions, see Table 32–3. Each may be fatal if not recognized promptly and treated adequately; however, each usually responds to proper therapy.

Determinations of blood sugar levels and carbon dioxide combining power are sometimes essential for differential diagnosis, but unfortunately, it is not always possible to perform these tests in emergency situations (even Dextrostix may not be available). Therefore, the attending physician may be forced to base the diagnosis on information obtained from family members, friends or persons who observed the onset of the condition, and on careful clinical examination and observation; see Table 32–3. If there is any doubt concerning the differential diagnosis, 2 ml/kg (up to 50 ml) of 50% dextrose should be given IV immediately; this is both a valuable diagnostic test and probably the safest initial therapeutic measure. If the coma is hyperglycemic, no harm will result; on the other hand, additional insulin and lack of glucose may be fatal to a person already in insulin shock.

Treatment of Diabetic Coma and Severe Ketoacidosis (*See also 46–1*)

When the patient is first seen outside of the hospital:

- Draw 20 ml of venous blood for determining levels of serum sugar, serum acetone, sodium, potassium, blood urea nitrogen (BUN) and HCO_3, plus arterial blood for determining pH and blood gas pressures (pO_2 and pCO_2) when facilities are available. Blood specimens must be sent with the patient to the hospital.
- Start intravenous infusion of 1 to 2 liters of normal saline over the first 2 to 3 hours (or faster if the patient is in shock). Glucose should be started if insulin is given and the blood sugar is less than 250 mg%. Patients are usually deficient in total body potassium. Potassium should be administered (a) if initial serum K is low or normal, (b) if K is initially high, but returns to normal with therapy, or (c) if glucose or $NaHCO_3$ is given. Potassium preferably is replaced as phosphate rather than chloride.
- Insulin may be given in one of several ways. IV or IM administration is preferred, because SC injections may be erratically absorbed. Ten to 15 U may be given IV followed by 5 to 10 U/hr of insulin IV or IM. The dose is then adjusted according to blood sugar response. Serum acetone determination is not of much value in monitoring the response to therapy.
- Treat for shock (*53–7*). Keep the patient warm but not hot; room temperature is satisfactory.
- Transport the patient immediately to an adequately equipped hospital.

When the patient reaches the hospital:

- Complete the blood tests specified earlier.
- Obtain a hematocrit and white blood cell and differential cell count. The WBC is considerably elevated in patients with diabetic ketoacidosis (DKA). Follow response to therapy with blood sugar, serum K and pH determinations.
- Obtain a urine specimen without catheterization if possible; otherwise, insertion of an indwelling catheter (*18–6*) is mandatory.

Table 32–1. MANAGEMENT AND TREATMENT OF COMA/ALTERED CONSCIOUSNESS OF UNDETERMINED ORIGIN

Initial Measures (as any prior resuscitation (5) continues)

- Check responsiveness to auditory and physical stimuli.
- Clear and maintain an adequate airway.
- Maintain adequate ventilation and circulation (5, *Resuscitation*).
- Draw a specimen of blood for Hb, Hmct, CBC, Diff. and basic blood chemistry determinations (levels of sugar, BUN, electrolytes [Na, K, Cl, HCO_3], serum acetone and toxins). Now give IV glucose as described in first step under Initial Specific Therapy, below.
- Use of Dextrostix and Ketostix gives rapid initial sugar/acetone level; a single Keto-diastix may be used.
- Draw blood samples accordingly if the following organ systems may be involved:
  —Liver/Heart/Brain: SGOT, CPK with possible isoenzymes
  —Pancreas (if history of abdominal pain): amylase
  —Adrenal glands: cortisol
  —Thyroid (particularly in myxedema coma): T_3, T_4, FTI
- Obtain ABG's for pH, PaO_2, PCO_2 and oxyen saturation.
- Methemoglobin and carboxyhemoglobin levels must be specifically ordered; cannot be calculated from other tests.
- Obtain blood culture (30 ml) if patient is febrile.

Initial Specific Therapy

- Administer 50 ml of 50% glucose and 100 mg of thiamine HCl intravenously, to which is added an opiate antagonist (0.4 to 1.6 mg of naloxone [Narcan]) if narcotic overdose is known, suspected or not excluded. Glucagon, 0.5 to 1.0 mg IV, can be given also in hypoglycemic events.
- Start an intravenous infusion of 5% dextrose in water or saline, preferably with a radiopaque plastic intravenous catheter or Swan-Ganz catheter for CVP monitoring if patient is in shock. Proceed with treatment of shock (57).

History and Physical Evaluation

- If no one is available to give any accurate information, delegate some person (preferably with professional experience) to trace, if possible and as soon as possible, the patient's background. This should include:
  1. Location where patient was found and the circumstances, including possible exposure to noxious gases and toxins.
  2. State of consciousness when found.
  3. Presence of medications or instructions for their use.
  4. History of prior episodes of coma.
  5. Condition and complaints before development of coma. Observe the patient closely—first fully clothed, then completely undressed—covering the following points:
     a. Clothing—mud, blood, semen, grease, grass, corrosive agents or other stains; alcohol or other odors; holes or tears; burns.
     b. Identification data—"dog tags" around neck or wrist.

c. Skin (including scalp)—puncture wounds, ticks, thermal or electric burns, contusions, ecchymoses, pallor, sweating, cyanosis of lips or fingernails, swelling, effusions, needle marks or thrombosed veins, lacerations of the genitalia, evidence of pregnancy. Also note color of skin and whether it is moist or dry, hot or cold.
d. Musculoskeletal misalignment and muscle tone.
e. Breath—alcohol, acetone, uremia, carbon tetrachloride, gasoline, the "musty" odor of hepatic failure.
f. Respiratory pattern—rate, rhythm, paradoxical respiration, use of accessory muscles.
g. The patient as a whole—make-up, tattooing, type of clothing, body hygiene, expression.

- Perform a complete physical examination and a neurologic examination covering the sensorium, cranial nerves, cerebellar and meningeal signs, motor and sensory responses and reflexes (superficial [corneal, abdominal, cremasteric and rectal sphincter], deep tendon [biceps, triceps, patellar, Achilles] and pathologic [Babinski]). *Remove any contact lenses (38–39).* Check for neck stiffness and Kernig's sign if patient is febrile, to check for meningitis, and if not febrile, to check for subarachnoid bleeding. Check for presence or absence of bowel sounds. Check the mouth, rectum and vagina as depositories for toxic substances.

Further Diagnostic and Therapeutic Steps

- Catheterize *(18–16)*; leave a Foley catheter in place and note volume output in 15 minutes. Start a 24-hour specimen collection for analysis including drugs and toxins. Obtain a specimen of urine for routine urinalysis (specific gravity; pH; levels of proteins, sugar and acetone; and microscopic examination) and porphyrin analysis.
- Lavage the stomach; save a specimen of vomitus or aspirate for later possible laboratory analysis (usually not of great value, however). Describe the aspirate. Note portions of tablets or pills if found; instill activated charcoal *(53–8)*.
- If the patient is febrile and has no focal neurologic signs suggesting transtentorial or cerebellar tonsillar herniation, perform a lumbar subarachnoid puncture (see *18–29*). Examine cerebrospinal fluid at once for pressure, color, turbidity, protein and sugar content and cells (including Gram stain). Save a specimen of cerebrospinal fluid for culture.
- Culture any wounds or aspirates for aerobes and anaerobes and start antimicrobial therapy according to Gram stain results if clinical picture dictates.
- Take an electrocardiogram for evaluation of cardiac status and for information regarding electrolytic balance. Set up ECG monitoring.
- Take x-ray films as indicated in the following outline, but only if necessary positioning will not be harmful to the patient.
  a. Skull series when indicated. One lateral should be taken on a large enough film to show any gross misalignment of the cervical spine.
  b. Chest films if signs of thoracic or pulmonary pathology have been noted.
  c. Areas of suspected injury as based on physical examination.
- Obtain a CAT or radioisotope scan on the head if focal neurological signs are present or are evolving. In the setting of head injury, CAT scanning with its excellent detection of focal hemorrhage and edema is almost always the test of choice. Also, if the cause of the coma remains uncertain despite the initial evaluation as outlined, a cranial CAT scan should be done.
- Continue observation and investigation until a definite reason for coma has been determined. More than one factor may be contributory!
- Institute specific therapy as indicated while continuing diligent supportive therapy.

Table 32–2. PROFILE OF SCORES AT THE TIME OF ADMISSION ON THE VERBAL, EYE-OPENING AND MOTOR SECTIONS OF THE GLASGOW COMA SCALE*

Best Verbal Response (e.g., ask "What year is this?")	**Eye Opening**	**Best Motor Response** (to command or pain)
—	—	—6 Obeying of commands
—5 Oriented	—	—5 Localized response
—4 Confused	—4 Spontaneous	—4 Flexion withdrawal
—3 Inappropriate	—3 To speech	—3 Abnormal flexion
—2 Incomprehensible	—2 To pain	—2 Extension
—1 None	—1 None	—1 None

*Lancet 2:81, 1974. Patients with total scores of 9 or more are considered by this scale not to be in coma. *Note*: A 0–34 scale developed at Dinderfield Hospital, Wakefield, England, is under evaluation and may offer more versatility and specificity.

- Start hourly urine volume and sugar determinations.
- Obtain an EKG, particularly in older patients, to rule out myocardial infarction as cause for the DKA. Patients should be monitored to follow changes in K level and possible arrhythmias.
- Every attempt should be made to determine the cause of the DKA. Appropriate cultures, including blood, should be obtained as indicated. Antibiotics should be started pending cultures if infection is evident or suspected. Start antibiotic therapy based on Gram stain results initially and adjust according to sensitivity determinations when available.
- Continue IV saline until the blood sugar is less than 150 mg%. Patients may have an initial total body deficit of 4 to 7 liters. Half of this should be replaced the first few hours and the rest over a 24-hour period.
- IV administration of sodium bicarbonate is necessary if (a) pH is less than 7.1, (b) the patient is hypotensive and in shock or (c) there is noncardiogenic pulmonary edema.

32–4. ECLAMPSIA *(See 50–6, Eclampsia; 50–14, Hypertensive Disease in Pregnancy)*

32–5. ELECTRICAL SHOCK *(See also 28–12, Electrical Burns)*

Severe cases are usually caused by contact with lower voltage (110 to 220V) circuits, although occasional contact with high voltage (high power lines, electronic equipment condensers, lightning strikes) occurs. Sequelae include ventricular fibrillation *(29–25)*, coma and respiratory paralysis. Once ventricular fibrillation is established, resuscitative measures must be immediately instituted; striking the chest forcibly with the fist, external heart compression *(5–23)* and expired air respiration *(5–21)* should be tried, with external defibrillation *(5–26)* as soon as equipment is available. When in doubt, defibrillate!

If there is perceptible heart action:

- Start expired air respiration *(5–21)* and continue until mechanical methods, such as close-fitting face mask, oropharyngeal airway or endotracheal tube with resuscitation bag, can be substituted. External heart compression *(5–23)* may be required as an adjunct to weak or irregular heart action. Resuscitation should be continued for at least 4 hours before the patient is

Table 32–3. DIFFERENTIAL DIAGNOSIS OF HYPERGLYCEMIA AND HYPERINSULINISM

	Hyperglycemia with Ketoacidosis (Diabetic Coma)	Hyperinsulinism (Insulin Shock or Reaction)
History	Known diabetes; increasing thirst, air hunger, sleepiness; nausea and vomiting	Rapid onset following insulin; may not have eaten usual meal before or after dose; may have taken too much insulin
Diet	Usually recent anorexia (days)	Not enough food (hours)
Nausea and vomiting	Often present	Seldom present
Fever	May be present	Seldom present
Thirst	Intense	Absent
Facies	Looks toxic	Looks pale and weak
Vision	Dim	Diplopia
Eyeballs	Soft	Normal
Mouth	Dry; ketotic fruity odor	Drooling
Skin	Dry and flushed	Moist and pale
Blood pressure	Low	Normal or low
Respiration	Rapid and deep	Normal
Abdominal pain	Common; may simulate an acute surgical abdomen	Absent
Tremor	Absent	Frequent
Mental state	Gradual development of coma	Sudden onset of delirium, deep coma and bizarre neurologic picture
Convulsions	None	Late
Infection	May bring on symptoms	No effect
Insulin	May have omitted usual dose	Always has taken dose; sometimes too much
Urine	Sugar and diacetic acid present	Sugar may be present and diacetic acid absent in 1st specimen; in 2nd specimen, both absent
Blood surgar (normal, 80–120 mg %)	Above normal (also serum acetone present)	Below normal
CO_2 combining power	10 mEq/L or less	Normal (21–30 mEq/L)
Response to treatment	Slow (see 32–3)	Rapid to IV glucose (may be delayed if protamine zinc or NPH insulin overdosage)

declared dead. The attending physician should remember that the presumptive signs of death *(8–2)* often do not apply following an electrical shock and that normal breathing and heart action have been reestablished as long as 8 hours after contact with the current.

- Do not give stimulant (analeptic) drugs; they are of no value until the breathing center has recovered and spontaneous respiration has been established. Narcotics (natural and synthetic) are contraindicated because of their respiratory depressant effects.

32–6. EMPHYSEMA AND CHRONIC OBSTRUCTIVE PULMONARY DISEASE (COPD)

Comatose patients with pulmonary emphysema and COPD are frequently and mistakenly considered to be beyond aid. (Sometimes these patients will go into coma in the ED because of imprudent use of high O_2 concentration/flow rate.) However, recognition of the condition and immediate institution of the following measures may result in restoring these persons to useful activity:

1. Cleansing of the airway by suction to remove mucous plugs from the large bronchi.
2. Ventilation by use of a volume or other mechanical respirator. Depression of the respiratory center by IV morphine sulfate may be necessary to allow the apparatus to function efficiently. Moisture should be supplied by a saline spray.
3. Maintenance of an open airway *(5–1)* and ventilation.
4. Restoration of normal fluid-electrolyte balance (see *11*).
5. Administration of broad-spectrum antibiotics.
6. Obtaining of arterial pH, pO_2, pCO_2 and HCO_3 determinations.

32–7. EPILEPSY *(See 34)*

32–8. EPISODIC OR RECURRENT UNCONSCIOUSNESS *(See Table 49–3, Differential Diagnosis Chart)*

32–9. EXCESSIVE HEAT *(See 62–6, Heat Exhaustion; 62–7, Heat Hyperpyrexia; 62–8, Iatrogenic Heat Stress; 62–9, Sunstroke)*

32–10. HEPATIC COMA

Hepatic coma results from liver disease (usually with portal system shunting of venous blood). Personality changes, including confusion, inappropriate behavior, and difficulty with judgment, are common before coma. The breath has a fetid sweet odor, and dorsiflexion of the wrists with the arms extended may produce a flapping tremor. Serum ammonia level is often elevated, but this is not a good treatment guide—i.e., lowering the ammonia level will not necessarily result in improvement.

Treatment

1. Hospitalization for treatment of shock *(57)* and hemorrhage *(45)*.
2. Reduction of body protein breakdown by IV infusion of dextrose, 800 calories in hypertonic solution per day.
3. Reduction of intestinal ammonia caused by bacterial decomposition. Give lactulose (Cephulac), 20 to 30 g PO every hour until there is a laxative effect, and then tid to qid; or may give 30- to 60-minute retention enema of 200 g (300 ml) of lactulose in 700 ml of water or normal saline every 4 to 6 hours. Also may give neomycin, 1 g PO every 6 hours.
4. Sedation with oxazepam (Serax) or paraldehyde as needed.
5. Balancing of fluid input and output, with avoidance of saline if hepatorenal symptoms are present. Protein intake should be sharply limited.
6. Administration of vitamin K (phytonadione) intramuscularly.
7. Cautious treatment of anemia.

32–11. HYPEROSMOLAR NONKETOTIC COMA

Hyperosmolar nonketotic coma usually occurs in the elderly, sometimes even when there is no past history of diabetes. It is characterized by coma or lethargy, severe dehydration, hypernatremia and hyperglycemia. The mainstay of therapy is hydration with normal or half-normal saline. The initial dose of insulin should be small (e.g., 10–15 U IV) and further administration adjusted to the initial response. Because of the advanced age of these patients, cardiac status should be monitored closely with the rapid administration of fluids. As in diabetic ketoacidosis, a source of infection should be sought. Patients should be monitored, with electrolytes—particularly Na and K—followed closely.

When diabetic ketoacidosis accompanies the hyperosmolarity (check magnitude) high serum glucose levels contribute significantly to the osmolarity, as does water loss from various causes. Water, insulin, sodium and potassium are administered, while glucose and other nondepleted salts are withheld until the condition is corrected. Total water deficit may be in the range of 10 to 12 liters and usually exceeds relative loss of sodium and potassium. As soon as adequate urine flow is established and serum potassium is less than 5 mEq/L, 20 to 40 mEq of potassium is added to each liter of half-normal saline, and ECG monitoring is performed.

32–12. INTRACRANIAL PATHOLOGY *(See 44, Head Injuries; 63–4, Intracranial Hemorrhage; and Fig. 32–1 regarding the importance of the pupil in diagnosis)*

32–13. MYXEDEMA *(See 36–12, Thyroid Emergencies)*

32–14. POISONS *(See 53)*

32–15. SHOCK FOLLOWING TRAUMA, SEVERE BURNS, HEMORRHAGE, DRUG OVERDOSAGE OR POISONING

(See 57 for treatment of shock; see also 28, Burns; 45, Hemorrhage; 53, Poisoning)

32–16. UREMIA

If uremic convulsions or coma have developed, symptomatic and supportive treatment is all that can be done. Sedatives, hypnotics and narcotics may be given in the smallest possible effective doses while hospitalization for definitive care is being arranged.

32–17. RARE CAUSES OF COMA

Rare causes of coma are brain tumors, encephalitis *(33–6, 33–20)*, malaria *(33–38)*, syphilis of the central nervous system *(33–66)* and tuberculosis (acute miliary, meningeal form) *(33–72)*.

These conditions require only supportive and symptomatic care before and during transfer for hospitalization.

32–18. PROLONGED POSTOPERATIVE COMA

Modern anesthetic techniques usually result in rapid postoperative recovery of consciousness; however, because emergency procedures sometimes do not allow complete preoperative investigation of intercurrent diseases, drug idiosyncrasies or other complicating factors, postoperative coma can be abnormally prolonged. In this case the following conditions must be considered:

Anesthesia and Medical Diseases and Drugs

Certain diseases interfere with detoxification and elimination of anesthetic agents, so that usual amounts may cause prolonged postanesthetic coma.

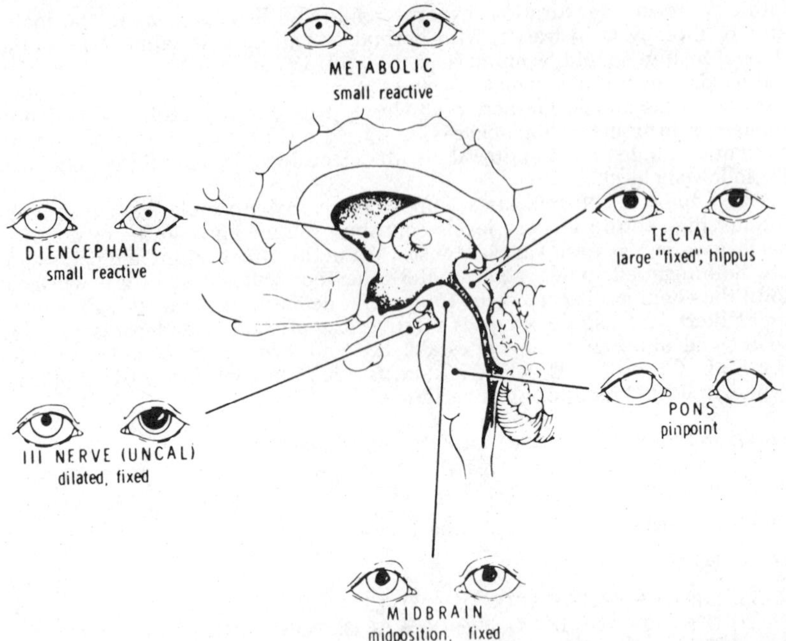

Figure 32–1. Pupils in the unresponsive patient. The state of the pupil helps the physician to discriminate between mass lesions and diffuse central nervous system disease. In general, during toxic and metabolic coma, the pupillary light reflex, though typically sluggish, is preserved until the patient's condition is terminal. In contrast, in the patient with transtentorial herniation caused by mass lesions, the pupillary light reflex is lost early. Important exceptions may give rise to diagnostic uncertainty. Overwhelming anoxia or ischemia may be associated with pupillary dilatation. Atropine and scopolamine produce dilated unreactive pupils. Glutethimide causes midposition to large irregular pupils that are unreactive to light. Opiates produce pinpoint pupils. Near-fatal barbiturate intoxication can fix the pupils. *The pupillary light reflex can be regarded as absent only after examination with a bright light and observation with magnification.* (From Plum, F., and Posner, J. B.: *Stupor and Coma,* 2nd ed. Philadelphia, F. A. Davis, 1972, with permission as reproduced in Sigsbee, B., and Plum, F.: The unresponsive patient. Med. Clin. North Am., *63*:813, 1979, with permission.)

Among these are:

- Addison's disease *(36–1, Adrenal Insufficiency)*
- Diabetes *(32–3, Diabetes Mellitus)*
- Liver disease *(32–10, Hepatic Coma)*
- Malignant hyperthermia *(62–8)*
- Muscular dystrophies
- Myxedema *(36–12)*
- Porphyria *(46–24)*
- Renal disease *(41)*

Certain drugs potentiate and prolong the action of anesthetic agents. These include:

- *Corticosteroids (53–225, Corticotropin; 53–226, Cortisone)*

- *Monoamine oxidase inhibitors* (Iproniazid [Marsilid], isocarboxazid [Marplan], nialamide [Niamid], phenoxypropazine [Drazine], tranylcypromine [Parnate])
- *Phenothiazines (53–536)*
- *Sedatives (53–110, Barbiturates; 53–146, Bromides)*

Particularly in elderly persons, a history of daily administration of some of these drugs may not be obtainable prior to emergency surgery.

Anesthetic Overdosage *(See 53–71, Anesthetics, Inhalation; 53–72, Anesthetics, Intravenous)*

Carbon Dioxide Retention

A high oxygen content in the anesthetic mixture may mask serious underventilation, which becomes apparent when postoperative breathing of air is resumed. Carbon dioxide retention is characterized by flushing, excessive perspiration, elevated pulse and hypertension. The respiration is "jerky," with a tracheal tug. Check blood gas levels and oxygen saturation. Treatment is as follows:

- Cautious hyperventilation, avoiding too rapid elimination of carbon dioxide, which may in itself cause hypotension, cardiac arrhythmias and ventricular fibrillation *(29–25)*.
- Control of bronchospasm *(56–4)*.
- Control of respiratory acidosis by IV injection of 50 ml of 8.4% sodium bicarbonate solution (1 mEq/ml), repeated if improvement does not take place.
- Monitoring with serial arterial pH, pO_2, pCO_2 and HCO_3 content determinations.

Cerebral Hypoxia

Delayed recovery of consciousness after anesthesia or delayed relapse into coma after a period of semiconsciousness may be due to hypoxic brain damage with edema (see *44–7* for evaluation and treatment). Continue adequate ventilation and life support. Draw a blood sample for determination of sugar level and give 50 ml of 50% glucose IV if hypoglycemia may be a factor contributing to the clinical picture.

Cerebrovascular Disorders

Cerebral thrombi or emboli *(63–6)*, identifiable by focal signs, occur occasionally and result in prolonged postanesthetic coma. Cerebral hemorrhage *(63–4)* is very rare, except as a concomitant condition with other traumatic or degenerative conditions.

Fat Embolism

This condition can practically never be diagnosed in an emergency situation but may occur following severe crush injuries to the soft tissues, long bone fractures, burns and decompression sickness. Orthopedic procedures and inadvertent intravenous contrast media injections are iatrogenic causes. Most of the fat globules are deposited in the lungs, but involvement of the brain, kidneys and liver does occur. The urine frequently shows free fat. Treatment is symptomatic and supportive. Prophylactically, 50 ml of 50% glucose every 8 hours IV has been reported as decreasing the incidence of fat emboli in multisystem injured patients; IV alcohol may also be considered. Corticosteroids also help to attenuate the effect of fat emboli.

Hypothermia *(See also 62–3)*

Especially in infants, elderly persons and myxedematous patients, a decrease in body temperature may result in prolonged postanesthetic coma. Treatment consists of rewarming as soon as possible.

Metabolic Acidosis *(See 46–1)*

Shock *(See 57)*

32–19. PSYCHOGENIC COMA

The patient frequently resists attempts at pulling up the eyelids. There is reaction to visual threat. The patient is often a young woman. There is often a history of some upsetting experience (e.g., family quarrel) just before onset of the "coma." The onset usually occurs in the presence of witnesses. The neurologic examination is negative except for lack of response to voice. Pain responses are present, though usually diminished.

32–20. WERNICKE'S ENCEPHALOPATHY

Severe thiamine (vitamin B_1) deficiency will result in increases in cerebral vascular resistance and reduction in bloodflow with encephalopathy (cerebral beriberi). Ataxia, nystagmus, ocular palsy, decreased mental function, coma and death can result. Thiamine, 100 mg parenterally daily, plus large oral doses, can correct this if started early.

33. Communicable Diseases (CD)

See also 58–6, *Contagious and Communicable Diseases;* 59–42, *Soft Tissue Infections (Life Threatening).*

The incidence of communicable and contagious (highly communicable) diseases in the world remains staggering. For instance the occurrence of malaria is 150 million cases per year; gonorrhea, 250 million per year; and syphilis, 50 million cases per year. An estimated 300 million people have filariasis and 200 million have schistosomiasis. With increased world travel and greater resistance of microorganisms to antimicrobials and vector carriers to pesticides, plus too often a blasé attitude on the part of the public and professionals toward communicable diseases and their control, many cases will continue to present for urgent treatment to stop the pathologic process in the individual and break the chain of dissemination.

33–1. CD OR INFECTIOUS DISEASE CONTROL TECHNIQUES

Clean Techniques

It is extremely important for medical personnel, family and other close contacts to protect themselves from the patient's CD and conversely to protect the patient and others from exposures to cross-contamination. Actions to be taken to break the CD chain include the following:

- Wash hands before and after contact with any CD sources. Be particularly thorough after exposure to excrement, discharges, drainage, etc.

- Wear disposable gloves with high-exposure direct handling of any materials connected with the infected patient.
- Protect clothes with a gown if close exposure to direct contact type CD (if gown is reused, always hang it up with the outside of gown folded inward).
- If airborne CD, particularly avoid exposure to coughing; wear a disposable mask when close to patient; provide adequate ventilation. It may be preferable, at times, to have the patient wear a mask.
- Use disposable materials—plastic eating utensils, paper towels, etc.—as much as possible.
- Place material contaminated with discharges, secretions, excretions, dressings, etc., in a plastic bag and then dispose of, preferably by burning.
- In certain disease states, strict isolation of the patient, boiling, autoclaving, burning, or chemical antisepsis treatment of all contact materials, and other stringent measures are required.
- Evaluation and treatment of close contacts who may be asymptomatic carriers (including sometimes pets) should be considered.
- Further measures to be instituted in the home depend upon the type of disease and its manifestations, and may include the following: hot laundering or dry cleaning of the patient's clothing and bedding as well as other materials contacted; airing and sunning of materials that cannot be laundered (mattress, pillows, upholstery) for 6 to 8 hours; washing of furniture with soap and water.

Control of Symptoms

Guidelines for management and control of symptoms in simple febrile illness and warning signals of possible complications are given in Tables 33–1 and 33–2.

Identification for Control (Treatment and Prophylaxis)

Cultures or specimens should be taken from all likely foci or routes of infection, including wounds, drainage, abscesses, infected sites, blood, urine, sputum and CSF. Gram stain and wet mount examinations in advance of cultures can be valuable. Aerobic and anaerobic bacterial cultures and special techniques for fungi, parasites, rickettsiae, spirochetes, viruses and worms, plus other techniques including serum, skin testing and study by electron microscope aid identification.

33–2. ACQUIRED IMMUNE DEFICIENCY SYNDROME (AIDS)

AIDS is a serious new, potentially life-threatening disease (70 to 80% mortality) that was first recognized in 1979 and was reported in 1981 for its specific defect: impairment of cell-mediated immunity and other host defenses, which results in the loss of the body's resistance against disease. These manifestations of AIDS (approximately several months to 2 years after exposure) and death occur mostly from opportunistic infections. However, there is often both justifiable and unreasonable fear concerning getting the disease, which, along with secondary diseases acquired because of the AIDS patient's decreased immunity, may present acute problems.

The disease is to be suspected when the following occur *in the absence of other common explanations:* Unexplained weight loss of more than 10 pounds within a 2-month period • enlarging firm tender lymph nodes, particularly in the neck and axillae • persistent fever/night sweats/diarrhea/cough/unexplained fatigue/dyspnea with minor exertion • recent-appearing skin rashes—slowly enlarging discolored small nodules, papules or growths on the skin or

Table 33–1. THERAPEUTIC MEASURES IN VIRAL RESPIRATORY INFECTIONS (AND EARLY NONSPECIFIC FEBRILE STATES)

- Abundant rest during time of fever. (Patient is probably benefited by reduction of usual activity for 24 to 48 hours after cessation of fever.) Avoid becoming overly fatigued for 1–2 weeks after recovery from a severe bout.
- Drink 1½ to 2 times normal daily fluid input (e.g., adults should have 12–15 glasses of fluid: water, tea, broth, carbonated beverages, etc.). Avoid milk products. Eat lightly during the illness: soup, broth, jello, sherbet, soft boiled eggs, toast, crackers or any foods appropriate for age in infants. Adequate fluid intake is especially important in loosening phlegm and decreasing cough. Benefit of vitamin C in large doses (e.g., 100–1000 mg qid) remains controversial.
- Relieve generalized aching and fever in adults as needed with aspirin (two 5-grain tab PO q 4 h) or acetaminophen (one or two 325-mg tab q 4 h to max 12/day).
- Take periodic rectal temp in children < 8 yr. If fever is low-grade and the child is comfortable, acetaminophen and baths need not be given.
- In children under 16 years, acetaminophen is preferable to aspirin (see *Reye's Syndrome*, 33–55). See Table 12–1 for recommended doses.
- If fever doesn't respond to aspirin or acetaminophen, soaking for 20 minutes or more in a luke-warm tub bath or sponge bath (tepid water without alcohol) may be effective. Use particularly in children/infants with rising temp over 103°F rectally. In children, the general condition is usually more important than the degree of fever.
- Sore throat may be relieved by gargling with hypertonic salt water (½ tsp NaCl in ¾ glass H_2O) every 2 or 3 hours, or by use of nonprescription lozenges (e.g., Chloraseptic).
- Steam is very helpful in loosening secretions and decreasing congestion—preferably use a vaporizer. Normal saline drops aid loosening of nasal secretions, which can then be removed with a soft nasal bulb syringe in infants; there is no "rebound" congestion with saline.
- Decongestants (without antihistamine) may be given to relieve obstruction, but are not intended to decrease normal drainage and secretions. Topical adult spray or drops or pediatric drops (e.g., nonprescription oxymetazoline [Afrin]) used bid offer quicker relief, but rebound congestion can occur; limit periodic use as directed to 1–3 days. Oral OTC and prescription decongestants can cause ↑ BP, ↑ HR in certain individuals, but have longer duration and less rebound. Pseudoephedrine (Sudafed) is available OTC in 30-mg tablets or in 60-mg tablets for use 3 or 4 times/day.
- Irritative, nonproductive cough may be relieved by OTC Robitussin or, in more severe cases, by dihydrocodeinone (Hycodan), 1 tsp q 4–6 h prn. (Avoid any voluntary/involuntary tobacco smoking to reduce compounding respiratory irritation [and while at it, might as well quit altogether].)
- Antibiotics are not indicated for viral infections unless there is a secondary bacterial infection, in which case a penicillin or tetracycline might be ordered after preliminary culture.
- Return to work or school and other outside activities is guided by recovery rate and overall condition.
- See Table 33–2 for evidence of complications or surfacing of other conditions that require medical attention.

mucous membranes inside the mouth, anus, nasal passages or eyelids • slower than usual healing of wounds/infections • neurologic manifestations, including focal weakness, sensory loss, painful paresthesias, SIADH, personality changes, hallucinations, seizures, progressive dementia and coma. It is now recognized that there may be earlier and milder manifestations of AIDS.

The cause of AIDS is not known, but there are strong indications that it involves a transmissible agent—possibly a blood-borne virus. Also, in part it may be an exhaustion phenomenon of the immune system.

The United States Public Health Service (USPHS) reports that approximately 2000 cases have occurred nationwide since 1981, with 95% of these occurring in males (primarily ages 25 to 45) in 4 major groups:

Table 33–2. SIGNS AND SYMPTOMS IN FEBRILE ILLNESSES THAT SHOULD REDIRECT PATIENT TO MEDICAL ATTENTION

- Worsening of symptoms with no response to treatment.
- High fever, accompanied by deteriorating condition, that persists despite aspirin or acetaminophen and sponge bath, or seizure *(34)* occurs.
- Labored or obstructed breathing (see Table 5–2) or difficult swallowing with drooling (URGENT SITUATION).
- Coughing produces thick, yellow/green sputum.
- Persistent vomiting or diarrhea (especially if bloody); inability to keep food/medications down.
- Evidence of dehydration (dry mouth, decreased urination, decreased tearing and/or sunken eyeballs, weakness).
- Inability to fully flex neck, especially when associated with lethargy or decreased responsiveness; pain on moving neck and legs.
- New rash (particularly if on pressure blanching there is pinpoint or larger bluish-black area); increase in tissue/skin redness, swelling and tenderness or other signs of speading infection.
- Weakness or paralysis of muscles, loss of coordination, inability to stand or walk.
- Severe or steady intensification of pain in any location (e.g., abdomen, flank).
- Yellowing skin, darkening of urine, stool color changes (whitish, black, bloody).

- Sexually active homosexual and bisexual men with multiple sex partners (75%).
- Present or recent past IV drug users (17%).
- Hemophiliacs who received Factor VIII blood administration (8%).
- Haitian aliens in the USA (5%).

The incidence appears to be accelerating, with a doubling of the number of AIDS patients seen about every 6 months. The exact status of many infants and children with immune deficiency states (including offspring of AIDS victims) is under reevaluation.

Diagnosis is further clarified by demonstration of lymphopenia, leukopenia, ↑ IgG (more often than ↓ IgG), ↑ IgA, and particularly an inverted T_4 (helper-inducer) cell to T_8 (suppressor) cell ratio. Serious rare opportunistic diseases, such as Kaposi's sarcoma and a difficult-to-treat protozoan pneumonia due to *Pneumocystis carinii*, may appear. Other opportunistic diseases that may develop are cryptococcosis *(33–15)*, non-Hodgkin's lymphoma, candidiasis *(42–17)*, herpes simplex *(33–29)*, CMV *(33–16)* and toxoplasmosis.

Treatment

Prevention is the best treatment; recommended precautions are as follows:

- Direct contact with the blood of AIDS patients should be avoided, and gloves should be worn when dealing with trauma cases involving them.
- General contact of a nonsexual type, accompanied by good hygiene, appears not to present a risk. As yet, no health care personnel* caring for AIDS patients have become ill with AIDS; gown and gloves should be worn when in contact with feces, blood, discharges; use bedside needle disposal.
- People in the high-risk groups mentioned should, of their own initiative, forego being blood donors while formal screening/restrictive measures are developed.
- A high risk to homosexual men is presented with oral/anal and anal intercourse contact with multiple or promiscuous sexual partners; they

*That is, who did not have other risk factors.

should be guided accordingly. Effectiveness of condom use in preventing AIDS is not yet established.

- IV drug users, if they must temporarily continue, should avoid any exchange of paraphernalia that has had blood contact (e.g., needles, syringes), even if boiled.

Treatment of AIDS to date consists of treating the secondary problems listed above and referring the patient to a specialist for ongoing care. Interferon has not yet demonstrated its value. Trials with interleukin-2 are underway. Treatment with radiation, medications and surgery may offer assistance while research is ongoing for a definitive cure. An important part of treatment is maintenance of excellent hygiene by AIDS patients.

The USPHS has established a toll-free AIDS Hotline: 1-800-342-AIDS. From Washington DC, call 1-800-646-8182, and from Hawaii/Alaska call collect: 202-245-6867.

33–3. AMEBIASIS *(See 33–46)*

33–4. ANAEROBIC INFECTIONS *(See 59–42 and Table 59–2)*

33–5. ANTHRAX (Malignant Pustule, Wool Sorters' Disease)

Usually anthrax occurs in industry in persons who handle, cure or process animal hides. The incubation period is 1 to 7 days. No quarantine is required, but the patient should be isolated until drainage from superficial lesions clears. Anthrax is managed by symptomatic treatment plus large doses of penicillin G; penicillin-sensitive patients should be given erythromycin or a tetracycline.

33–6. ARBOVIRUS AND ARENAVIRUS INFECTIONS

The arboviruses are arthropod-borne (principal vectors are the mosquito, the sandfly and the tick through bites), and humans and a variety of other vertebrates are hosts. Arenaviruses are rodent-borne, and there is person-to-person transmission.

Syndromes

- ***Encephalitis and aseptic meningoencephalitis (33–20)*** caused by numerous viral strains, among which are the following:

Eastern equine	Louping ill (British Isles)
Western equine	Murray Valley (Australia)
St. Louis	Congo-Crimean
California	Kyasanur Forest disease (India)
Powassan	Hong Kong
Japanese B	Lymphocytic choriomeningitis

- ***Dengue-like fevers*** *(33–17)* are of 3 to 7 days' duration and may include rash and lymphadenopathy.

Colorado tick fever
Sandfly fever
Chikungunya and o'nyong-nyong fevers (Africa)

- ***Hemorrhagic fevers***

Hemorrhagic fevers of South Asia, Congo-Crimea, Argentina and Bolivia
Kyasanur Forest disease (India)
Yellow fever *(33–81)*

Treatment

No specific therapy is available. Antibiotics are of no value and should be used only in the presence of bacteriologic complications. Efficient symptomatic and supportive care is often effective.

33–7. BALANITIS (IVD) *(See 41–20)*

33–8. BOTULISM *(See 53–142; see also 27–30, Tick Paralysis; 53–314, Food Poisoning)*

Infant botulism, occurring mostly in infants between about 1 and 6 months of age (but occasionally seen in those up to 18 months of age), should be considered in the presence of constipation, decreased sucking and eating, lid ptosis, generalized weakness leading ultimately to respiratory insufficiency and a limp, "floppy" state. The toxin comes principally from *Clostridium botulinum* spores growing in the infant's intestine. Honey may be a source. Treatment requires excellent supportive care, particularly including respiratory monitoring and ventilation.

33–9. CHANCRE (Hard Chancre)

This primary lesion of syphilis appears from 10 to 60 days (usually about 3 weeks) after exposure. No medication or treatment that might block the diagnosis should be prescribed, or be allowed to be applied, until a diagnosis by darkfield examination has been done. A baseline serum sample should be drawn for Venereal Disease Research Laboratory (VDRL) or Rapid Plasma Reagin (RPR) testing, together with a fluorescent treponemal antibody (FTA) test or a microhemagglutination assay for *Treponema pallidum* (MHA-TP). When the diagnosis of syphilis has been established, treatment should be commenced as outlined in *33–66*.

33–10. CHANCROID (Soft Chancre)

The incubation period of this common, painful, localized disease due to *Hemophilus ducreyi* organisms is several days. Skin papules enlarge and often form coalescing ulcers. Enlarging tender inguinal nodes may form a fluctuant mass (bubo) that will drain to the skin surface; if present, needle aspiration drainage from the side through adjacent normal skin (rather than lancing) may help to prevent a sinus tract from forming. The patient should be placed on oral tetracycline, 0.5 g qid for 2 weeks.

33–11. CHICKENPOX (Varicella) *(See Table 33–5)*

Treatment of chickenpox is as follows:

- Isolation of patient for 10 days or until all lesions have "scabbed over."
- Sedation as required, with close observation regarding development of interstitial pneumonia *(33–33)*. Avoid aspirin (see *33–55*).
- Measures to relieve itching (see *58–12, Pruritus*). Treat any cellulitis *(59)*.
- Consider use of acyclovir, VZIG for high-risk patients.

33–12. COCCIDIOIDOMYCOSIS *(See 33–44, Mycotic Infections)*

33–13. COMMON COLD (Rhinovirus, Coryza) *(See also 56–7, Croup)*

General malaise, fever, sore throat, chest tightness, nasal catarrh and cough are the usual presenting features. This common viral malady involves the entire respiratory tract down to the trachea and bronchi. In a previously healthy person it should not last more than 5 to 7 days. It is less severe than influenza. Patients with LTB and bacterial complications usually have higher fever, purulent exudate and greater appearance of toxicity.

There is as yet no definitive prevention or cure for the common cold, but supportive and symptomatic care as described in Table 33–1 can appreciably reduce its miserable effects.

33–14. CONDYLOMA ACUMINATUM (Genital Wart, Venereal Wart, Verruca Acuminata, Verruca Vulgaris)

Perianal and genital warts due to a virus grow over a period of many weeks and months. From small, grayish to pink, rough nodules they become multiple pedunculated, broad, vegetating lesions (not flat like secondary syphilis lesions) with a foul odor. Moisture enhances the growth. If treatment with 25% podophyllin in tincture of benzoin does not provide relief after multiple applications on alternate days for 6 hours before being washed off, surgical or dermatologic referral may be necessary for removal. Daily applications of a 5% solution of 5-fluorouracil may be used for vaginal lesions. Laser ablation and fulguration may also be utilized.

33–15. CRYPTOCOCCOSIS *(See 33–44, Mycotic Infections)*

33–16. CYTOMEGALOVIRUS INFECTION (CMV, Cytomegalic Inclusion Disease)

The incubation period of this herpes group virus that can pervade all tissues is about 1 month. Infection may be dormant or cause signs and symptoms of pharyngitis, pneumonitis, hepatitis, neuritis and lymphadenopathy with a syndrome similar to that of infectious mononucleosis. Fetal mortality and neurological impairment in infants may occur.

Identification requires tissue culture or specific antibody tests. As yet, there is no specific treatment, but good supportive care and personal hygiene aid recovery and help decrease dissemination.

33–17. DENGUE (Dandy Fever, Breakbone Fever)

This acute but rarely fatal viral infection is transmitted by mosquitos of the genus *Aedes*. Although it is more common in tropical climates, it has been reported in temperate zones. The incubation period is 5 to 10 days.

Signs and symptoms include a sudden rise in temperature—39.4 to 40.6°C (103 to 105°F)—associated with a slow pulse. There is usually an intense headache with general malaise and prostration, often associated with severe myalgia and arthralgia, especially of the muscles of the back. A cyanotic, blotchy appearance of the face and soreness behind the eyeballs with severe pain on eye movements are characteristic. There is usually generalized adenopathy with splenic enlargement and deferred appearance of a generalized morbilliform rash, usually starting on the back of the hands and feet. Leukopenia is usually present.

Treatment is supportive, and hospitalization may be necessary. Complete recovery usually occurs in from 10 to 14 days.

33–18. DIPHTHERIA

This febrile upper respiratory tract disease causes predominantly a severe sore throat, dirty gray tonsillar pseudomembrane (with bleeding underneath when removed), laryngeal obstruction and cervical lymphadenopathy. Neuritis and myocarditis are later findings.

The disease affects chiefly children between 1 and 10 years, mostly those 2 to 5 years. Incubation period is 2 to 5 days. Spread by direct and indirect contact. With widespread DPT vaccination in infancy, diphtheria is rarely seen in the United States.

Clinical differentiation from infectious mononucleosis *(33–31)*, streptococcal pharyngitis *(33–27)* and Vincent's angina *(61–15)* may be difficult, and diagnosis may be dependent upon laboratory and culture findings.

Treatment

- Immediate administration of adequate doses of diphtheria antitoxin is imperative if the clinical findings are suggestive of diphtheria. This applies even if smears are negative or inconclusive. Dosage is 20,000 to 40,000 units. Before administration check for sensitivity *(16)*.
- Erythromycin, 500 mg PO every 6 hours for 7 days. Penicillin G and rifampin are also effective. Contacts: Give erythromycin; update immunization.
- Supportive care and bed rest are essential. Monitor ventilation to assess need for intubation or tracheostomy. Check electrocardiogram (ECG) for evidence of myocarditis and arrhythmia.
- Serious cases require hospitalization. Mild cases may be treated at home with quarantine until two consecutive nose and throat cultures taken at 24-hour intervals show no diphtheria bacilli.

33–19. DYSENTERY (Bacillary) *(See Table 40–1, Common Causes of Acute Bacterial Diarrhea)*

This disease complex covers a range of diarrhea states from occasional liquid feces to severe, repetitious watery, bloody, mucoid stools accompanied by tenesmus, profound prostration, dehydration and toxicity, which, if untreated, may result in death. Incubation period is 1 to 9 days (usually less than 4 days). Isolation is indicated until stool cultures no longer show the bacilli responsible. Fluid and electrolyte replacement *(11)* are essential (usually by IV route in more severe cases) and are the cornerstone of treatment. Many times the patient will be in hypovolemic shock *(57)*. Ampicillin, sulfamethoxazole/trimethoprim and chloramphenicol are important therapeutic agents. Stool cultures may reveal disappearance of the pathogen from the stool without antibacterial therapy. This disease entity in food handlers must be reported *(15)*.

33–20. ENCEPHALITIS AND ASEPTIC MENINGOENCEPHALITIS

Many conditions that have been reported to be due to infectious viral organisms are grouped together under this general heading (see *33–6, Arbovirus and Arenavirus Infections*, and *33–21, Enterovirus Infections*, which frequently cause meningeal involvement but with less encephalitic components, and may also cause paralysis). A toxic form of postinfectious encephalitis unrelated to these viruses can also occur. In addition, the following clinical entities are among those that may manifest themselves as encephalitis: chickenpox *(33–11)*, measles *(33–39)*, mumps *(33–43)*, herpes simplex *(33–14; 33–29)*, lymphogranuloma venereum *(33–37)*.

Laboratory investigation is necessary to determine the etiology, since, in general, all are characterized by high fever (often to 41°C [106°F]), general malaise, acute restlessness, severe headache, severe generalized myalgia and sometimes palsies. Delirium convulsions (especially in children) and coma may be present. EEG is generally abnormal.

The cerebrospinal fluid (CSF) findings are at first more suggestive of a mycotic or bacterial meningitis than they are later but should not cause confusion in the total analysis. Early, there may be a faint ground-glass, colorless, but not purulent, appearance. Though at first white cell counts occasionally may be over several thousand (usually less than 500 per cubic millimeter) and neutrophils are frequent or predominate (compared with nearly all lymphocytes later), the Gram stain is negative on spun specimen, the protein level is generally normal or only slightly elevated and, unless the patient is also hypoglycemic (check level), the CSF glucose value will be normal. On rare occasions, recheck of the CSF in 8 to 12 hours (or depending on condition) may be needed to help clarify the situation.

Blood and CSF specimens for identification of viral stains must be refrigerated, packed in special containers and sent at once to a properly qualified laboratory.

Treatment is attentive supportive care, and hospitalization is usually required unless the condition is mild and there is a good supportive home environment. Ventilatory assistance is needed in some cases. Adenine arabinoside or acyclovir is of value in Herpes simplex encephalitis.

33–21. ENTEROVIRUS INFECTIONS

Echovirus, coxsackievirus and poliovirus constitute the enteroviruses.

All of the enteroviruses may cause a febrile illness with paralysis, aseptic meningitis, myocarditis, pericarditis, gastroenteritis and respiratory involvement, though certain strains may show a greater predilection for a particular clinical manifestation. An erythematous maculopapular rash, appearing on the upper thorax, neck or face, is occasionally seen with strains of echovirus or coxsackievirus. Coxsackievirus is most likely to cause herpangina; epidemic pleurodynia *(33–50)*; and hand, foot and mouth disease in which vesicles form on the buccal membrane of the mouth and between the fingers and toes.

Treatment is rest and symptomatic and supportive care, which may need to be sufficiently intensive to be lifesaving in some instances. Recovery in 1 to 2 weeks is usual. Immunity through vaccination for all available strains (poliovirus) should be kept current.

33–22. ERYSIPELAS *(See 58–6A)*

33–23. FILARIASIS

This disease-producing thread-like nematode worm is found in the tropics and is carried by mosquitos that disseminate it to humans by biting them. The incubation period is 2 to 3 months, and the febrile prodrome is not characteristic, but inflammation of the lymphatics, including elephantiasis, is. The worm may be identified in lymph or blood and is treated with diethylcarbamazine citrate (Hetrazan), 2 mg/kg PO 3 times daily for 3 weeks.

33–24. GERMAN MEASLES *(See 33–58 and Table 33–5)*

33–25. GONORRHEA (GC) *(For prophylaxis, see 33–67)*

No matter what history is given by the patient, if a urethral discharge is present in a male, a smear should be taken by the attending physician and stained and examined for the presence of gram-negative intracellular and/or extracellular diplococci. Transmission may occur from heterosexual or homosexual contact. Additional smears or cultures should be sent to a laboratory for examination. The same applies to females who have profuse whitish vaginal discharge or are suspected of being asymptomatic carriers of infection. Cultures from the anus and pharynx may be necessary when combinations of oral-anal-genital sexual activity have occurred. If the clinical picture and Gram stain indicate the presence of gonorrhea, treatment should be started without waiting for further confirmatory laboratory findings.

Treatment

- Aqueous procaine penicillin G, 4.8 million units IM (2 sites), plus probenecid (Benemid), 1 g PO; or ampicillin, (3.5 g) or amoxicillin (3.0 g) plus probenecid, 1 g PO, is adequate for most uncomplicated gonococcal infections.* Patients who are allergic to penicillins may be given tetracycline hydrochloride by mouth, 0.5 g 4 times daily for 7 days; spectinomycin hydrochloride (Trobicin), 2.0 g IM, may be given in a single dose to those who cannot take tetracycline or penicillin. Avoid giving tetracycline to pregnant women.
- If penicillinase-producing *Neisseria gonorrhoeae* organisms are present, patients and their sexual contacts should be treated with a single IM injection of 2 g of spectinomycin hydrochloride (Trobicin) instead.
- Complicated gonococcal infections, such as those with dissemination (arthritis, bacteremia), require 10 million units of penicillin daily, and with pelvic inflammation, the dose is increased to 20 million units daily.
- Follow-up cultures and evaluation should be carried out 3 to 7 days after completion of treatment.

33–26. GRANULOMA INGUINALE (Donovanosis)

Development of the proliferative, painless (until secondarily infected), round, smooth, bright reddish granuloma generally in the groin, prepuce, perineum, vulva or perianal region is slow, beginning from 1 week to 3 months after exposure. The granuloma may ulcerate and is slow to heal. Biopsy or tissue smear reveals encapsulated gram-negative bipolar rods within mononuclear cells. Treatment is with tetracycline, 2.0 g PO daily in divided doses for 2 to 3 weeks.

33–27. HEMOLYTIC STREPTOCOCCAL INFECTIONS *(See Table 33–5)*

These organisms may cause septic sore throat, a diffuse erythematous rash, scarlet fever (characterized by circumoral pallor, strawberry tongue and Pastia's lines—dark, reddened skin creases) and various other serious conditions. Incubation period is 1 to 5 days; it is spread by both direct and indirect contact. Communicability starts from first symptoms. Recovery from a condition caused by one type of hemolytic streptococcus does not result in immunity to other types. The affected area should be cultured prior to starting an antibiotic, but treatment may then be started on clinical basis. See also *66–16, Tonsillitis–Pharyngitis.*

Treatment

- Bed rest and symptomatic care. Use precautions against oral secretions and isolate patients with purulent discharge.
- Penicillin or erythromycin in large doses (e.g., penicillin V, 125 to 250 mg PO qid) for at least 10 days, followed by reculturing.

---

*Follow with tetracycline, 500 mg qid × 7 days for commonly concurrent *Chlamydia* infection.

33–28. HEPATITIS, VIRAL

Clinically the early phases of acute hepatitis caused by hepatitis A, hepatitis B and non-A, non-B hepatitis virus are not distinguishable. The disease process starts with a low-grade febrile prodrome with symptoms of anorexia, malaise and aching for 3 to 14 days. Alanine transferase (ALT) and aspartate transferase (AST) levels are increased for about 1 week before the onset of jaundice; darkened urine and lighter stools may also precede jaundice by several days. With jaundice, both direct and indirect bilirubin levels are elevated, as is alkaline phosphatase. The WBC is normal to slightly decreased. The jaundice increases for 1 to 2 weeks and then tapers over the next 2 to 4 weeks. (See Table 33–3 and Fig. 33–1 for further details on the later course of the disease, serologic differences, and management of contacts to these hepatitis viruses.)

Treatment can usually be carried out at home with precautionary measures *(33–1)* and guidelines to management of uncomplicated viral illness (Tables 33–1 and 33–2). The overall fatality rate for acute hepatitis is low (1% or less). Fulminating hepatitis, however, requires hospitalization and intense care.

33–29. HERPES SIMPLEX *(See also 38–14, Ophthalmic Herpes)*

All adults probably have latent infection. Uncomfortable, clear, fluid-filled vesicles may form when the body's resistance is low for any reason or after a direct stimulus such as bright sunlight. Subsequent drying, crusting and healing occur over approximately 3 weeks. Genital herpes can occur by sexual contact. Presence of herpes in the birth canal in term pregnant women may be cause for cesarean section. Encephalitis *(33–20)* can be a serious complication, especially in children.

Treatment

- Local application of zinc oxide or other ointment to prevent cracking and secondary infection.
- Use of alcohol or camphor for exudative lesions, or glycerin (Gly-Oxide) for intranasal or intraoral mucosal lesions.
- Use of acyclovir, topically, 6 times a day for 7 days for first attacks. (Effectiveness of oral acyclovir is currently under evaluation.) An IV preparation of acyclovir is available.
- Referral to an internist or dermatologist for further care as needed.
- If the eyes are involved *(38–14)*, referral to an ophthalmologist is necessary.
- Acute encephalitis *(33–20)*, if it develops, requires immediate hospitalization.
- Use of corticosteroids is contraindicated.

33–30. IMPETIGO *(See 58–6B)*

33–31. INFECTIOUS MONONUCLEOSIS

This febrile viral disease (caused by Epstein-Barr virus) is probably spread by close oral contact and simulates many other illnesses. Usual signs and symptoms include malaise, sore throat, headache, chilliness, diffuse lymphadenopathy, and, by 1 to 2 weeks, an elevated WBC count, lymphocytosis, increased incidence of atypical lymphocytes, and decrease in neutrophils (2000–3000/mm^3). About 50% of patients have splenomegaly that requires caution during examination, to avoid rupturing. About 10% of patients have hepatomegaly, and 5% have jaundice. There may be a rash (see Table 33–5),

Table 33–3. VIRAL HEPATITIS AND PROPHYLAXIS FOR CONTACTS

Hepatitis Virus (HV): Type	Incubation Period (Days)	Serology Tests and Interpretations	Dissemination Methods (Contact Exposures)	Prophylaxis for Contacts/Other Comments
A	15–49	Anti-HVA (IgM) / Anti-HVA (IgG): + / + } Active disease + / − } Active disease − / +: Immune state − / −: Incubating or no HAV HB_sAg: Negative	Fecal-oral route; includes contaminated food and water (household, sexual or intimate contact).	ISG: 0.04 to 0.06 ml/kg up to 5 ml IM. Give 0.02 ml/kg to people going to or just returning from epidemic areas (Asia, Africa, Middle East, Central or South America).
Characteristics: RNA virus. IgM appears/leaves early; IgG ↑ later, lasts lifetime. Subclinical to moderate disease usual. Mortality rate 0–0.2%. No chronic liver disease or carrier state.				
B	25–160	HB_sAg (HBV surface Ag): Positive = infectious state HB_cAg (HBV core Ag): Positive in liver HB_eAg (origin unknown): Positive = chronic infectious hepatitis; find with HB_sAg Anti-HB_sV: Ab indicates HBV reinfection resistance Anti-HB_cV: Ab indicates early or past HBV infection Anti-HB_eV: Ab suggests decreasing infectivity	Blood products; also present in saliva, semen and urine of patients in early (infectious) phase of HBV (percutaneous, sexual or intimate contact).	HBIG: 0.06 ml/kg to max 5 ml IM. Repeat dose in 1 month. High-risk exposures include homosexuals, bisexuals, IV drug users, hemodialysis patients, leukemic patients. Treat close contacts with HBIG. Vaccinate.
Characteristics: DNA virus. Generally more common than A type. Mortality 0.3% up to 15% in older people in prior poor health. Chronic carrier states vary from about 1 to 10% depending on geographic area (higher in Europe and Asia than in U.S.) 10% develop chronic liver disease (hepatitis, cirrhosis, cancer).				
NON-A NON-B	15–160	All above HAV/HBV serologic tests negative but similar to acute viral hepatitis	Blood products (percutaneous; possibly sexual contacts).	ISG: 0.04 to 0.06 ml/kg IM to max 5 ml. Repeat dose in 1 month.
Characteristics: ↑ chronic liver disease (> HBV); mortality rate and incidence of carrier state ≅ HBV.				

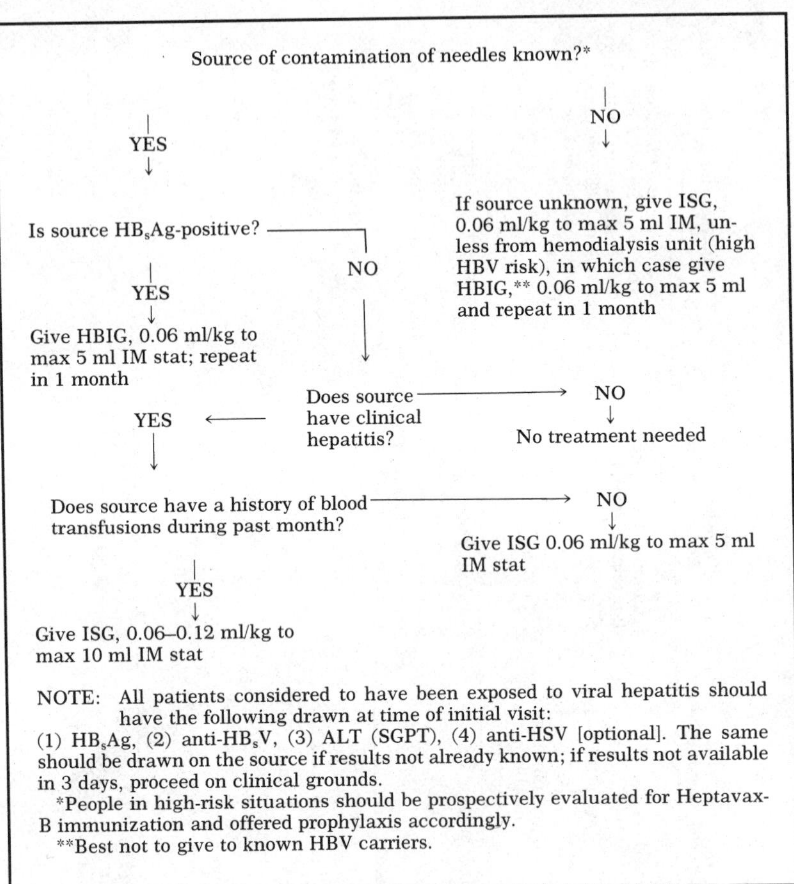

Figure 33–1. Algorithm for people punctured by contaminated needles. (Modified from Gordon, E. K., Geiderman, J. M., and Brill, J. C.: Immunoprophylaxis of viral hepatitis. Ann. Emerg. Med., *10*:216, 1981, and Seeff, L. B., and Hoofnagle, J. H.: Immunoprophylaxis of viral hepatitis. Gastroenterology, *77*:161, 1979.

the incidence of which increases to 80% among patients on ampicillin, although this is not an allergic reaction to the drug itself.

Monospot testing is negative initially, increasing to 40% within the 1st week and 80% by the 3rd week.

Treatment is supportive and preventative. Airway obstruction, hemolytic anemia and myocarditis may develop, requiring administration of 60 to 80 mg of prednisone tapered over a 10-day period.

33–32. INFLUENZA

Incubation Period: 1 to 5 days.

Signs and Symptoms: Sudden onset, usually with acute catarrhal symptoms and fever of 38.9 to 40.6°C (102 to 105°F) followed by severe, generalized myalgia; chest pain; marked pharyngitis; and purulent bronchitis, often associated with sinusitis. In children, otitis media *(35–18)* may develop. Pneumonia, usually involving both lower lobes, may occur. Acute gastrointestinal symptoms may be present in some forms. The blood may show a leukopenia. With the more virulent forms and/or occurrence in debilitated persons, death can occur and is generally preceded by delirium and coma and occasionally by convulsions.

Treatment

- Home care is usually possible except if a severe pneumonic process or other serious complication is indicated by clinical or x-ray examination.
- Supportive treatment is largely as under *33–13, Common Cold.*
- Antibiotics have no effect on influenzal conditions and should be used only for associated secondary bacterial infections.
- Amantadine hydrochloride (Symmetrel), 100 mg bid PO (in children aged 1 to 9, 4.4 to 8.8 mg/kg/day up to a maximum of 150 mg), is considered useful for treatment and prophylaxis against the influenza A viruses.

33–33. INTERSTITIAL PNEUMONIA (Viral Pneumonia) *(See also 33–35, Legionnaire's Disease)*

The causative organism for acute interstitial pneumonia may be a filterable virus or an obligate intracellular parasite *(33–35)*, or it may be unknown.

Incubation Period: 10 to 14 days.

Signs and Symptoms: Insidious onset, with systemic symptoms more marked than respiratory symptoms. Severe headaches and general malaise are usually present, with a slight intermittent temperature rise, usually not more than 38.8°C (102°F). The pulse is relatively slow. Physical signs in the lungs are usually minimal, but striking x-ray changes (increase in size of hilar shadow; soft, patchy infiltration, most marked near the hilum) are usually present. The white blood count is normal or decreased. The respiratory symptoms vary from minimal to profound, and death may occur.

Treatment

- Bed rest at home is generally adequate. Hospitalization is necessary for severe forms of the disease.
- Copious amounts of fluids by mouth or intravenously if the patient shows evidence of dehydration. Supportive care substantially as described in Table 33–1.
- Tetracyclines or erythromycin if due to mycoplasma or chlamydia.
- Oxygen therapy if dyspnea or cyanosis is present.

Prognosis. Though lassitude and weakness may persist for weeks, complete recovery usually occurs except in legionnaire's disease, which may run a devastating course with even death.

33–34. KAWASAKI'S DISEASE (Mucocutaneous Lymph Node Syndrome—MLNS)

This high febrile illness with a maculoerythematous rash, cervical lymph node swelling and pain resembles scarlatina *(33–62)* and Rocky Mountain spotted fever (33–57) in many ways. This occurs mainly in children. No causative organism has yet been identified. Death may occur from vasculitis and cardiomyopathy. Treatment is supportive and includes aspirin administration to reduce cardiac complications. Use of corticosteroids is controversial.

33–35. LEGIONNAIRE'S DISEASE

This increasingly found serious illness causes severe myalgia and pneumonia in all lobes and is fatal in about 20% of cases. Malaise, chills, fever and cough are early signs; headache, confusion, diarrhea and chest pain may occur also, with liver and renal damage present later. Smokers and older people are more susceptible.

Chest x-rays reveal a diffuse interstitial to nodular pattern. An immunofluorescent stain test of sputum or body tissues helps to identify the disease. Electrolyte imbalance occurs with hyponatremia and hypophosphatemia, leukocytosis and elevation of liver enzymes and bilirubin.

The responsible gram-negative pleomorphic bacterium is most susceptible to erythromycin but is also responsive to tetracycline. Diligent supportive care is also needed.

33–36. LEPROSY

The incubation period is very long; the method of transmission is not fully known but may be by a very close prolonged respiratory route. Quarantine in specially designated hospitals is no longer required, but this disease is reportable (*15*), and the person must be under treatment, generally with a sulfone such as dapsone.

33–37. LYMPHOGRANULOMA VENEREUM (Lymphopathia Venereum)

Formerly believed to be caused by a virus, this condition is now known to be caused by obligate intracellular parasites, *Chlamydia trachomatis*, which are spread by sexual contact and become clinically manifest about 1 to 4 weeks after exposure.

Signs and Symptoms. Minute (often undemonstrable) lesions at site of entry, development of reddened skin and enlarged painful lymphatic nodes ("buboes") that may suppurate and become fistulous. Scarring and stricture of the rectum may develop. Systemic illness with fever, chills, diffuse aching, anorexia and vomiting may occur. Diagnosis is confirmed by complement fixation test. Lymphogranuloma venereum is a reportable disease (*15*).

Treatment

- Instruction regarding sterilization of bedding, clothing, towels and dressings.
- Tetracycline, 1 g PO initially, then 0.5 g 4 times daily for 3 weeks; or sulfisoxazole (Gantrisin), 4 g PO initially, followed by 1 g every 4 hours for 3 weeks. Use topical antibacterial ointment on lesions.
- Arrangement for further medical care or referral to a public health clinic.

33–38. MALARIA

This is one of the most common serious communicable diseases in the world. It is produced in humans by any 1 of 4 protozoan parasites transmitted by the bite of the infected anopheline mosquito. Episodic severe chills coincident with release of new merozoites into the circulation followed by high fever are common. Headache, nausea, vomiting, splenomegaly, anemia and leukopenia are common. The parasite may be identified in red blood cells of peripheral blood or bone marrow, using Wright's stain. Quarantine or isolation is not required. Incubation period: 14 days.

Treatment

- *Plasmodium falciparum:* Chloroquine phosphate, PO, 600 mg base initial dose, followed by 300 mg base of the drug at 6, 24 and 48 hours. *Note:* Chloroquine is not an effective treatment for falciparum malaria acquired in Panama, South America, and Asia east of Pakistan. If chloroquine resistance is suspected, use quinine sulfate, 650 mg, every 8 hours for 10 to 14 days, with pyrimethamine, 25 mg, twice daily for 3 days and sulfadiazine, 500 mg, every 6 hours for 5 days; a single dose of 2 to 3 tablets of Fansidar can also be used. In severe or complicated falciparum malaria, especially with cerebral complications, immediate treatment with quinine hydrochloride dissolved in 500 ml of isotonic saline solution should be begun IV, infused slowly over a period of 8 hours and repeated every 8 hours until the patient is able to tolerate oral medication.
- *P. vivax, P. ovale* or *P. malariae:* Chloroquine for 3 days, as noted previously. Follow with primaquine phosphate, 15 mg base, daily orally for 14 days.
- Prophylactic treatment of persons going into endemic areas should be considered. Prophylaxis is achieved with chloroquine, 300 mg base every week, unless the individual is going to an area where *P. falciparum* is prevalent, in which case 1 tablet of Fansidar (500 mg sulfadoxine plus 25 mg pyrimethamine) once weekly is *added* to the chloroquine regimen. These once-a-week doses should be continued for 6 weeks after leaving the endemic area.

33–39. **MEASLES** (Rubeola) *(See Table 33–5)*

Treatment is symptomatic, including relief of conjunctival irritation with dark glasses or darkened room. Early recognition and treatment of complications such as otitis media, bronchopneumonia and encephalitis is essential. Prophylactic injection of gamma globulin should be done for contacts under 1 year of age, or if immunity is compromised. Vaccinate on exposure.

33–40. **MENINGITIS, BACTERIAL** *(See also 33–6, Arboviral Infections; 33–21, Enterovirus Infections; 33–20, Aseptic Meningitis; 33–44, Mycotic Infections)*

Bacterial meningitis is characterized by a rapidly progressive febrile illness leading to a toxic state with delirium, coma and convulsions. In addition, there are signs of meningeal irritation causing resistance to meningeal stretchings by straight leg raising and subsequent further aggravation by dorsiflexion of the foot, by extension of the knee when the hip is flexed 90° (Kernig's sign) and by flexion of the neck by bringing the chin to the chest—this latter maneuver may also cause the hips and knees to flex (Brudzinski's sign).

The cerebrospinal fluid (CSF), which is generally under increased pressure (and in the absence of papilledema), is grossly cloudy or has a ground glass appearance and may even be whitish with particulate matter. The protein level is elevated and the glucose level is diminished. The Gram stain *(18–12)*, done immediately, reveals the pathogenic bacteria (intracellular, extracellular, or both), which guides treatment (see *33–83*).

Meningitis from *Neisseria meningitides* and *Streptococcus pneumoniae* infections can occur at any age. Enteric organisms such as *Escherichia coli*, *S. faecalis*, Group B *Streptococcus* and *Listeria monocytogenes* are most prevalent in neonatal meningitis (52–17). *Haemophilus influenzae* is frequently responsible for causing the disease in children from age 2 months to 10 years. *Staphylococcus aureus* and *Proteus* and *Pseudomonas* organisms are occasional offenders.

Treatment

- Antibiotic treatment in conjunction with the information just discussed, plus see 33–83, *Antibacterial Drugs of Choice*. For treatment of neonates, see 52–17.
- Control of convulsions (34).
- Reduction of high fever by sponging, fanning and other available means.
- Maintenance of clear airway and ventilation.
- Intensive supportive care including intravenous (IV) administration of fluids and electrolytes.

33–41. MENINGOCOCCEMIA

The septic state from *N. meningitides* may be so fulminant that the person dies before meningitis develops. Moment to moment outcropping of petechiae (the periphery may blanch somewhat, but the telltale pinpoint or larger center does not) can occur anywhere on the body, but most often this starts in the distal extremities. Acute adrenal insufficiency (Waterhouse-Friderichsen syndrome) can occur with bacteremia, most often with meningococcemia, and requires treatment for shock (57).

Large doses of penicillin or chloramphenicol IV should be used (see 33–83, *Antimicrobial Drugs of Choice*). Rifampin, 600 mg, orally twice a day for 4 doses is given to family contacts. Exposure of hospital attendants is not an indication for prophylaxis with rifampin unless mouth-to-mouth resuscitation is done or there is a significant break in clean technique.

33–42. MOLLUSCUM CONTAGIOSUM

Large intracytoplasmic inclusions within epidermal cells are caused by a pox virus. They result in multiple asymptomatic, pink- to flesh-colored, dome-shaped papules with central umbilication that vary in size from 2 to 30 mm in diameter but usually are 2 to 5 mm. Spread occurs through close or sexual contact. The core of caseous material can be removed with a needle or treated with cryotherapy, topical cantharidin application or electrosurgery.

33–43. MUMPS (Epidemic Parotitis)

Fever, malaise and pain with swallowing and eating usually precede parotid gland swelling by a day or two. Oral secretions are communicable from 2 days before parotid swelling appears until the swelling subsides. The incubation period is 12 to 26 days, with 16 to 18 days being the norm.

Treatment

- Bed rest in isolation until the liver and glandular swelling subside.
- Ice packs to swollen areas.
- Careful mouth hygiene.
- Early recognition and treatment of complications (orchitis, pancreatitis, meningoencephalitis). Early administration of corticosteroids (prednisone)

orally, 60 mg at once, then 20 mg 3 times a day, may relieve symptoms and possibly prevent sterility from pressure necrosis of the testicles. Gradual tapering off of the steroid should accompany decrease of edema.

- Vaccinate susceptible or unprotected close contacts.

33–44. MYCOTIC INFECTIONS

Patients infected with systemic mycoses do not generally present for emergency treatment unless there is either an exacerbation in conjunction with worsening of the underlying disease that weakened the host's resistance to the fungus in the first place or the presence of a rarer form of the fungus that has caused rapid progression.

Usually there is gradual onset of low-grade fever, anorexia and weight loss, malaise plus chills, sweats and sometimes blurred vision.

Accelerated onset may occur with the following: phycomycosis, causing blindness and CNS destruction in patients with diabetic ketoacidosis; cryptococcosis (*Torula* infection), leading to pulmonary infection and meningitis; histoplasmosis, with pulmonary and hepatic involvement (hepatosplenomegaly); and progressive coccidioidomycosis, with disseminated spread including severe and often fatal meningitis.

Diagnosis is confirmed by morphologic identification in involved tissues and fluids and culture.

Treatment consists of therapy for any underlying disease, supportive care and, for the progressive disseminated forms, amphotericin B intravenously and sometimes intrathecally; combination therapy such as oral flucytosine with amphotericin B is valuable.

33–45. NONGONOCOCCAL URETHRITIS

This disease may occur in conjunction with or without gonococcal urethritis (which it closely resembles clinically) and may account for as much as 60% of infectious urethritis. Dysuria and mucopurulent discharge from a reddened meatus are common. Women may be asymptomatic or also have pelvic and vaginal pain and involvement. Cultures reveal the presence of *Chlamydia trachomatis* organisms in about 50% of cases. Tetracycline, 250 to 500 mg PO qid for 7 days, is generally adequate, with a 2- to 3-week course indicated for relapses.

33–46. PARASITIC INFECTIONS *(See 40–18)*

33–47. PEDICULOSIS *(See 58–6E)*

33–48. PERTUSSIS *(See 33–80)*

33–49. PLAGUE

The incubation period for both the bubonic and pneumonic forms, which are highly contagious, is 3 to 7 days. Quarantine until complete recovery is mandatory. Streptomycin intramuscularly is the drug of choice for treatment *(33–83)*; tetracycline and chloramphenicol are alternative drugs. Prophylaxis with tetracycline is indicated for face-to-face contacts.

33–50. PLEURODYNIA, EPIDEMIC *(See also 56–15, Pleuritis)*

Caused mostly by a coxsackievirus *(33–21)*, pleurodynia may be encountered as an emergency because of the sudden onset of high fever associated with rapid breathing and acute chest pain. In children, acute abdominal pain may simulate a surgical emergency. Myalgia, headache, sore throat and pericarditis also occur. Treatment is supportive and symptomatic.

33–51. PNEUMONIA *(See 56–16)*

33–52. POLIOMYELITIS *(See also 33–21, Enterovirus Infections)*

Three causative viral strains have been identified. Spread is by both direct and indirect contact. Incubation period is from 3 to 35 days (usually 7 to 14 days). Vaccination has fortunately made this dread disease rare; however, a recent outbreak in South Africa emphasized the need for continuing immunization.

Treatment

- Immediate hospitalization for supportive therapy and spinal puncture *(18–29)* to help establish the diagnosis if the history and clinical examination suggest the possibility of poliomyelitis. (See also *33–8, Botulism; 27–30, Tick Paralysis.)*
- Isolation for 1 week from the onset of first symptoms or while patient is febrile.
- Artificial respiration by mechanical or other methods *(5–21)* and emergency tracheostomy *(18–34)* may be needed for respiratory distress.

33–53. PSITTACOSIS (Ornithosis, Parrot Fever)

A history of contact with birds (e.g., parrots, parakeets, lovebirds, pheasants, barnyard fowl, laboratory birds) or animals infected with the disease is essential for a provisional diagnosis of psittacosis. The causative organism is an obligate intracellular parasite, *Chlamydia psittaci.*

Incubation period is 5 to 21 days.

Signs and Symptoms: Acute onset with chills, general malaise and fever to 40.6°C (105°F). The pulse remains relatively slow. The patient usually complains of a splitting headache and of photophobia. There is usually nausea and vomiting, herpetic skin lesions and acute sore throat. Pulmonary involvement with persistent cough and signs of patchy consolidation may develop in a few hours. Severe cases may show pinkish oval papular lesions of the trunk and may develop diplopia, hallucinations and stupor.

Treatment

- Supportive treatment and prescription of analgesics *(12)* for pain relief.
- Tetracycline hydrochloride, 250 mg PO every 4 hours.
- Hospitalization if patient is acutely ill.

33–54. RABIES (Hydrophobia)

This acute infectious disease has been reported in badgers, bats (insectivorous and vampire types), cats, coyotes, dogs, domestic farm animals, foxes, jackals, mongooses, raccoons, skunks, squirrels, weasels, wildcats and wolves. All bites of wild animals should be regarded as from a rabid animal. It may be transmitted to human beings in the following ways:

- The bite of a rabid animal (see also 27, *Bites*).
- Licking of any superficial abrasion of the skin by a rabid animal.
- Contact of oral secretion from a patient suffering from rabies with any break in the attendant's skin.
- Exposure to (possibly inhalation of) dust in caves infested with rabid or rabies-carrying bats.

Local health department authorities should be consulted for presence of rabies in specific sites and species in the area. In the United States, bites from rodents (such as the rat, mouse, guinea pig, gerbil, chipmunk, hamster or rabbit) cause rabies extremely rarely, if at all, and prophylactic treatment would rarely, if ever, be needed. Likewise, bites from livestock are considered on an individual basis, and treatment is rarely required.

Incubation period: 2 weeks to 12 months (usually 15 days to 5 months).

Prophylactic Treatment After Exposure

If there is no suspicion or proof that the animal is rabid, the treatment should consist of the following:

- Immediate local cleansing. Lacerations should be thoroughly washed with soap and water or saline, followed by 1 or 2% solution of benzalkonium chloride (all soap should be removed before application of quaternary compounds).
- Provision for current tetanus immunity *(20)*.
- Institution of measures to control bacterial infection as necessary.
- Immediate reporting of the incident to the proper local authorities for impounding, observation and possible postmortem examination of the animal. As a general rule, impounded animals are kept under observation for 10 days; if they show no evidence of illness during this period, the danger of rabies is negligible; if any signs of rabies develop during the 10 days, treatment with human rabies immune globulin (RIG) and human diploid cell vaccine (HDCV; 5-shot series) is started promptly. The animal should not be destroyed by the victim or the victim's family or friends unless it is wild and will escape; if it has been killed, the body must be saved and turned over to the proper public health authorities as soon as possible.

If the animal is known or suspected to have rabies (exposure to bites of any of the previously indicated wild animals or those of an unknown dog or cat or on advice from local health department officials), treatment should consist of the following:

- Initial measures as in steps listed above. Use RIG plus HDCV (or DEV [duck embryo vaccine] if HDCV not available) according to USPHS guidelines as in the following step (discontinue use if immunofluorescent studies of animal are later found to be negative). Lacerations should be spread and the depths of the wound washed thoroughly. Puncture wounds should not be probed or extended surgically because of the danger of spreading the virus.
- Human RIG, 20 IU per kilogram of body weight. A portion of the RIG should be used to infiltrate the wound and the remainder administered IM gluteally. (If locally unavailable within 24 hours, delivery from the producer can be obtained by calling anytime to 214-631-6240, or 415-276-8200.) If RIG is not available, give equine antirabies serum, 40 IU per kilogram, after checking for sensitivity *(16;24)*. Hyperimmune serum should be given as soon as possible; it is ineffective if given 72 hours after bite.
- HDCV is given in a series of five 1-ml injections IM into the deltoid or gluteal area starting on the day of exposure and repeated on days 3, 7, 14 and 28. If inadequate antibody response is found on checking the serum 3 weeks after the last dose, give a sixth 1-ml booster.

If the only exposure is not from a bite (licking of open wound, scratch or abrasion) from an unknown or escaped, healthy-appearing domestic dog or cat, serum need not be given, and only HDCV is advised because of the very low risk. If the skin is intact, the exposure is considered nil by WHO standards.

33–55. REYE'S SYNDROME (RS)

This increasingly recognized, etiologically enigmatic, pediatric (occasionally seen in adults) syndrome of liver dysfunction and fatty degeneration of the liver and other viscera plus acute encephalopathy often occurs several days after a seemingly minor viral illness. Aspirin and other salicylates have been shown to have a reasonably likely significant contributing effect on RS, and the current recommendation is to avoid use of these agents in children under 16 with viral illnesses, particularly varicella and influenza. Acetaminophen may be used safely instead and may even have a protective effect.

Severe nausea and vomiting shortly precede onset of combativeness, disorientation, hyperventilation and hyper-reflexia. Coma, decortication, areflexia, seizures and respiratory arrest characterize Reye's syndrome, which has a mortality rate of more than 75%. The initial evaluation may involve workup as for coma *(32)*. Serum NH_3, alanine transferase and aspartate transferase levels are elevated. Intensive supportive care is required, including ventilatory assistance, correction of fluid loss *(11)* and electrolyte and pH imbalance *(46)* from the vomiting, and generous intravenous glucose administration. Consultation or possible referral to a specialty center is advisable in serious cases.

33–56. RICKETTSIAL INFECTIONS *(See Table 33–4)*

This complex of communicable febrile diseases is caused by organisms (rickettsiae) that are classified somewhere between viruses and bacteria. Continued fever of 1 to 3 weeks, maculopapular rash, vasculitis and eschar with some forms and severe headache are common findings. The presence of specific complement-fixation antibodies (IgM), a positive Weil-Felix reaction and isolation of rickettsiae from the blood help confirm the clinical diagnosis. Rickettsiae are sensitive to tetracycline or chloramphenicol, which are preferably administered early and according to disease severity.

33–57. ROCKY MOUNTAIN SPOTTED FEVER *(See 33–56)*

33–58. RUBELLA (German Measles) *(See Table 33–5)*

Treatment consists of symptomatic care and keeping the patient indoors until acute symptoms subside. Complications are rare; however, an uncomfortable polyarthritis with fibrositis, paresthesias, myalgia and muscle weakness lasting as long as 2 weeks may occur. Thrombocytopenia purpura is a rare complication. Susceptible contacts should be vaccinated.

33–59. RUBEOLA *(See 33–39; Table 33–5)*

33–60. SALMONELLA INFECTIONS *(See 33–73, Typhoid Fever; Table 40–1, Acute Bacterial Diarrhea; 53–314, Food Poisoning)*

33–61. SCABIES *(See 58–6D)*

33–62. SCARLET FEVER *(See Table 33–5)*

Simple cases may be cared for at home. Toxic or septic cases require immediate hospitalization. Delirium and convulsions are complications that may require emergency treatment.

33–63. SHIGELLA INFECTIONS *(See 33–19, Dysentery, and Table 40–1, Acute Bacterial Diarrhea)*

33–64. SMALLPOX *(See Table 33–5)*

Smallpox has now been eradicated worldwide as a communicable disease; its inclusion is principally of historic interest.

Treatment

- Immediate isolation as soon as the diagnosis has been established, with sterilization of the examination room and its contents after the patient has been transferred. Whenever possible, isolation should be in a suitable single dwelling or isolation unit with controlled ventilation to reduce airborne exposure, and not in a general hospital.
- Immediate vaccination of all persons who have come in contact with the patient.

33–65. STEVENS-JOHNSON SYNDROME *(See 58–8)*

33–66. SYPHILIS

The reverse side of the standard confidential morbidity form *(15)* must be completed in all cases.

Primary Lesions (Chancres) *(See also 33–9, Chancre)*

The primary lesion, an erythroid papule, of syphilis develops about 1 month after exposure and soon forms a painless, hard-based ulcer from which the offending organism, *Treponema pallidum,* can be identified (darkfield microscopy).

The patient should be told not to apply any medication of any type prior to establishment of diagnosis and treatment program—usually this is not possible in the emergency department. Lesions should be covered with a dressing that is carefully disposed of. Patients should be referred to their physician or to a venereal disease (VD) clinic as soon as possible for confirmation of diagnosis and treatment. The VDRL or the fluorescent treponemal antibody absorption (FTA-ABS) test is often negative at this phase, as are hemagglutination tests. Primary cases are reportable *(15)*. For treatment of established cases, see the following section (secondary lesions).

Secondary Lesions

Secondary syphilitic lesions—which are often nonpruritic, erythematous maculopapules or condylomata accompanied by lymphadenopathy—are reportable *(15)* and require energetic and prolonged treatment. As soon as the diagnosis has been established, one of the following intramuscular therapy regimens should be begun:

- Benzathine penicillin G, 1.2 million units intramuscularly into each buttock (total 2.4 million units) immediately.

OR

- Procaine penicillin G, 2.4 million units at once, followed by 1.2 million units every 3 days for 2 doses (total 4.8 million units).

OR

- Aqueous procaine penicillin G, 600,000 units daily for 8 days (total 4.3 million units).

Oral administration of penicillin is not effective.

If the patient is allergic to the penicillins, a broad-spectrum antibiotic such as erythromycin or tetracycline orally should be substituted, with a total

Table 33–4. SOME IMPORTANT EPIDEMIOLOGIC AND CLINICAL CHARACTERISTICS OF RICKETTSIAL DISEASES*

Disease; Causative Organism	Epidemiologic Features: *Geographic Occurrence*	Epidemiologic Features: *Usual Mode of Transmission to Humans*	Reservoir	Usual Incubation Period (Days)	Rash or Eschar: *Distribution*	Rash or Eschar: *Type*
TYPHUS GROUP						
Primary louse-borne typhus *R. prowazeckii*	Worldwide	Infected louse feces rubbed into broken skin or as aerosol to mucous membranes	Humans	12 (8–15)	Trunk to extremities	Maculopapular; no eschar
Murine typhus *R. prowazeckii* var. *typhi*	Scattered pockets, worldwide	Infected flea feces spread as above	Rodents	12 (6–14)	Trunk to extremities	Macular; maculopapular; no eschar
Brill-Zinsser disease *R. prowazeckii*	Worldwide	Recrudescence months or years after a primary attack of louse-borne typhus	—	—	Trunk to extremities	Macular, maculopapular; no eschar

SPOTTED FEVER GROUP						
Rocky Mountain spotted fever *R. rickettsii*	Western Hemisphere	Tick bite	Ticks, rodents	6 (2–12)	Extremities to trunk; palms and soles	Macular; maculopapular, petechial; no eschar
Tick typhus *R. conorii* *R. sibirica*	Mediterranean littoral, Africa, Asia	Tick bite	Ticks, rodents	12 (7–18)	Trunk, extremities, face, palms, soles	Macular, maculopapular, petechial; frequent eschar
Rickettsialpox *R. akari*	USA, USSR, Korea	House mouse, mite bite	Mites, mice	12 (9–24)	Trunk, face, extremities	Papular, vesicular; frequent eschar
Scrub typhus *R. tsutsugamushi*	Japan, SW Asia, W/SW Pacific	Mite bite	Mites, rodents	11 (6–21)	Trunk to extremities	Maculopapular; frequent eschar
Q FEVER *C. burneti*	Worldwide	Inhalation of infectious dried dusts	Ticks, mammals	14 (9–20)	None	None; no eschar

*Modified from Beeson, P. B., and McDermott, W.: *Textbook of Medicine*. Philadelphia, W. B. Saunders Co., 1979.

dosage of 40 g given in divided doses every 6 hours over a period of 15 to 20 days (0.5 g every 6 hours for 15 to 20 days).

Syphilis of More Than One Year's Duration

If late syphilis or cardiovascular or neurosyphilis is present, give benzathine penicillin, 2.4 million units IM in 3 weekly doses, with follow-up, including spinal fluid examinations before and after treatment. Another regimen for neurosyphilis is to give penicillin G, 10 to 12 million units IV for 10 to 14 days.

Lightning pains and gastric crisis (after ruling out a surgical abdomen) require symptomatic care in tabes dorsalis—avoid narcotics if possible. Flare-ups of paretic mental disturbance usually respond to chlorpromazine (Thorazine).

Coexistence of syphilis and gonorrhea, which should always be searched for, requires that adequate additional antibiotic also be given to treat the gonorrhea if the syphilis was treated with long-acting penicillin.

33–67. SYPHILIS/GONORRHEA PROPHYLAXIS AFTER EXPOSURE TO KNOWN CASES*

Gonorrhea

The patient should urinate to help clear the urethra and should wash the external genitalia with soap and water as soon after exposure as possible. The patient should go to his or her physician or to a VD clinic as early as feasible for the same treatment as given for known gonorrhea (33–25).

Syphilis

A history of exposure to infectious syphilis in the 90 days previous to examination requires treatment as for early syphilis.

33–68. TETANUS (Lockjaw) *(See also 20, Tetanus Immunization)*

The incubation period of tetanus is from a few days to 3 weeks or longer and the average period is 5 to 10 days. Although about 50% of cases follow puncture wounds and lacerations, cases have been reported following injections, abortions, animal kicks, gum and tooth infections and animal bites. The diagnosis of tetanus is based on clinical findings. Early signs are abdominal and paravertebral muscle spasm, trismus, risus sardonicus and difficulty in swallowing. Stimulation of the posterior pharynx with a tongue blade produces characteristic masseter spasm.

Treatment

- Protection from unnecessary stimuli in a private, quiet, but not excessively darkened, room.
- Efficient and painstaking nursing care, with minimal handling.
- Lessening of spasm and reflex irritability in severe cases by administration of muscle relaxants (diazepam [Valium], up to 10 to 20 mg IV q 2 to 4 h, with ventilatory assistance); milder cases may be controlled with about half this dosage, taken orally. A combination of a muscle relaxant and a sedative (such as chloral hydrate) can be more effective and less toxic than either one separately. Narcotics should be avoided generally because of their respiratory depressant effect.

---

*Or probable cases when the contact cannot be located for further evaluation.

- Human tetanus-immune globulin (TIG), 5000 units IM in divided doses given at several sites, including adjacent to the wound, may be of value. Tetanus toxoid *(20)* is ineffective in treatment of established tetanus.
- Wide surgical excision of the site of infection with removal of all potentially traumatized or infected tissues. The operative site should be left open and irrigated or compressed daily with half-strength hydrogen peroxide.
- Penicillin, 30 million units the first day, followed by 10 million units/day for 10 days. If penicillin allergy is present, tetracycline IV should be substituted in an initial dose of 500 mg followed by 250 mg q 4 h.
- Tracheostomy *(18–34)* if airway obstruction from acute laryngospasm is present (as is almost always the case) or if the patient is developing difficulty in clearing secretions from the pharynx. Emergency endotracheal intubation is difficult and aggravating unless a high degree of muscle relaxation is obtained; use of succinylcholine chloride, 1 mg/kg IV, may be needed. A sterile tracheostomy set should be available at bedside at all times; early elective provision for a patent airway is best. Artificial ventilation may be necessary. For treatment of acute bronchospasm, see *56–4*.
- Daily monitoring of serum and urine electrolytes, with replacement *(11)* as indicated. Adequate potassium replacement is important. Continuous ECG monitoring is a valuable adjunct to therapy. If tachycardia and arrhythmias are present, check that oxygenation (arterial pO_2) is adequate; propranolol may aid control.
- Careful supportive therapy to prevent complications that in themselves may act as irritating stimuli to the underlying condition. Among these are urinary retention, fecal impaction, gastrointestinal tract bleeding, thrombophlebitis and secondary infections.

33–69. TOXIC EPIDERMAL NECROLYSIS *(See 58–6C)*

33–70. TOXIC SHOCK SYNDROME (TSS)

TSS is a febrile multisystem illness accompanied by shock *(57)* and all its ramifications and a progressive scarlatiniform rash that is probably secondary to staphylococcus toxins.

Major criteria for diagnosis are*

1. Fever (temperature 38.9°C or higher).
2. Rash (diffuse macular erythroderma).
3. Desquamation, one to two weeks after onset of illness, particularly of palms and soles.
4. Hypotension (systolic blood pressure 90 mm of mercury or less for adults or lower than the fifth percentile by age for children 16 years of age or under, or orthostatic syncope).
5. Involvement of three or more of the following organ systems:
   - A. GI (vomiting or diarrhea at onset of illness).
   - B. Muscular (severe myalgia or creatine phosphokinase level two times the upper limit of normal or greater).
   - C. Mucous membrane (vaginal, oropharyngeal, or conjunctival hyperemia).
   - D. Renal (BUN or creatinine level at least twice the upper limit of normal, or five or more leucocytes per high power field—in the absence of urinary tract infection).
   - E. Hepatic (total bilirubin, SGOT, or SGPT twice the upper limit of normal or more).
   - F. Hematologic (100,000 or fewer platelets per cu mm).

---

*From National Center for Disease Control: Follow-up on toxic shock syndrome. Morbid. Mortal. Weekly Rep., *29*:441, 1980.

   G. CNS (disorientation or alteration in consciousness without focal neurological signs when fever and hypotension are absent).
6. Negative results on the following tests:
   A. Blood, throat, or CSF cultures.
   B. Serologic tests for Rocky Mountain spotted fever, leptospirosis, or measles.

Despite some similarities to toxic epidermal necrolysis scalded skin syndrome (TENS; *58–8*), TSS is not clinically or pathogenically the same. It is particularly important to identify drug-induced TENS so that the offending chemical is stopped. In Kawasaki's disease *(33–34)*, which is also confused with TSS, patients are most often much younger (<6 yr) and are unresponsive to antibiotics; no causative organism for this condition has yet been identified.

Although both sexes and persons ranging in age from 6 to the 6th decade may be afflicted, the overwhelming peak incidence of TSS is found among white menstruating women, mostly under age 20. Use of high-absorbency vaginal tampons has been implicated as a cause; therefore it is advisable for women to use sanitary napkins or only a medium-absorbency tampon with several daily changes and, at least at night, alternation with sanitary napkins. TSS is also seen with skin and soft tissue infections and postoperative wound infections.

Laboratory studies may reveal the following abnormal findings: ↑ WBC, ↓ Hb, ↓ platelets; ↑ BUN, CPK, AST, LDH, bilirubin (total and direct); ↓ Ca, K, P, PT, PTT and indications of nephritis (urinary casts, protein, WBC; ↑ creatinine). DIC *(45–5)* may develop.

Treatment

- Remove any tampon at first sign of any febrile infection.
- Culture tampon, cervix and vagina; blood, urine, pharynx and any other focus of infection should be cultured if source is in doubt.
- Treat as a hypovolemic–third compartment leak type shock *(57)*. Penicillinase-producing *Staphylococcus* bacteria are more likely to be present, and therefore an antibiotic such as nafcillin (IM or IV) or a cephalosporin is more likely to be beneficial. Antibiotics also can decrease the chance of recurrence.
- Dobutamine hydrochloride or dopamine may be needed to treat shock *(57)*. Reduce fluids when urine flow is adequate. Treat any ARDS *(55–4)* or DIC *(45–5)*. Vigorous attentive supportive care is needed to combat the approximately 10% overall mortality rate.

33–71. TRACHOMA

This very infectious conjunctivitis is due to an obligate intracellular parasite, *Chlamydia trachomatis*, spread by personal contact. It may cause severe scarring and blindness. Treatment consists of instructions to the patient regarding disposal of infected handkerchiefs, towels, etc.; oral and topical tetracycline *(33–83)*; tetracycline ophthalmic drops; and referral to an ophthalmologist.

33–72. TUBERCULOSIS (TB)

Though commonly indolent in onset, miliary TB is fulminating and can involve the kidneys, pericardium, bone and commonly the meninges in addition to the lungs. The organism may be identified on acid-fast stained smears or cultured from sputum, gastric washings, bone marrow or urine. Treatment is given in single daily doses of isoniazid, 3.0 to 5.0 mg/kg (up to a total of

300 mg) plus either ethambutol, 15 mg/kg/day, or rifampin, 9.0 to 20 mg/kg (up to 600 mg).

33–73. TYPHOID FEVER

Fever, toxicity and relative bradycardia are usual; diarrhea is an unimportant feature, and constipation is as prevalent. Severe epistaxis may occur. Except in large outbreaks—usually through contamination by a chronic carrier of the disease—the condition presents as a fever of unknown origin.

Incubation period of *Salmonella typhosa* is 10 to 15 days. Acute cholecystitis requiring surgical attention may occur.

Treatment

As soon as the diagnosis is established or suspected, the patient should be hospitalized for confirmatory diagnosis, chloramphenicol, ampicillin or sulfamethoxazole-trimethoprim therapy and careful supportive treatment. Reporting *(15)* and restriction, particularly of food handlers, is required until two consecutive negative stool cultures have been obtained.

33–74. TYPHUS FEVER *(See also 33–56, Rickettsial Infections)*

This rickettsial disease is transmitted from one individual to another by the human body louse, with the human as the reservoir of infection or, in certain instances, by chiggers or other mites carried by rodents and other wild animals. The usual incubation period is 12 days, but the disease may occur years after the patient has left a known typhus area. Treatment consists of control of hyperpyrexia and pain, prevention of complications and administration of large doses of tetracyclines or chloramphenicol (Chloromycetin), preferably intravenously. Penicillin is ineffective in treatment, and sulfonamides are contraindicated. Although convalescence may be slow, permanent ill effects rarely occur.

33–75. UNDULANT FEVER (Brucellosis)

This acute febrile illness with myalgia and arthralgia has an incubation period of 5 to 21 days, occasionally longer. Quarantine is not required.

33–76. VARICELLA *(See 33–11; Table 33–5)*

33–77. VARIOLA *(See 33–64; Table 33–5)*

33–78. VENEREAL DISEASES (VD)

The variety and frequency of sexually transmitted diseases continues to gradually increase in the United States and world-wide. Oral-genital-anal contact has contributed significantly to the greater variety of diseases, and difficulty in detecting and controlling carriers has aided frequency, as has the increased resistance of organisms to antibacterials and the involvement of a wider age range of the population at risk. Efforts continue to de-stigmatize VD and make necessary treatment easier to obtain.*

---

*Laws regarding reporting cases in minors to their parents vary from state to state; e.g., in California certain venereal diseases when suspected in minors age 12 and over no longer require parental knowledge or approval for diagnostic and therapeutic measures when the minor patient seeks professional help. These include candidiasis, chancroid, condyloma acuminatum, *Gardnerella vaginalis* vaginitis, cytomegalovirus, gonorrhea, granuloma inguinale, *Hemophilus* vaginitis, herpes, molluscum contagiosum, nongonococcal urethritis, pediculosis, scabies, syphilis and trichomoniasis.

It is important that the sexual partner(s) be treated concomitantly in all instances. The penetrating male should wear a condom during any periods of contagious exposure if abstinence is not adhered to, and oral-genital and oral-anal contact should be avoided by all partners. Personal hygiene must be excellent to prevent autoinoculation as well as interpersonal contagion. *All patients should be tested for syphilis* in addition to any other sexually transmitted disease detected.

Of interest in addition to the diseases listed below which are spread by sexual contact, it is widely considered that squamous cell cervical intraepithelial neoplasia (CIN), a precursor of cervical carcinoma, is a venereal disease and is controllable in these early stages by condom use.

The following is a list of the more common sexually (heterosexual and homosexual) transmitted diseases. In some, the most urgent aspect is stopping the tissue inflammatory and destructive process; in others, it is making the correct diagnosis in order to break the chain of transmission. Any contagious disease is more easily spread during intimate contact. (See also MMWR supplement, "Sexually Transmitted Diseases," August 20, 1982, Vol. 31, No. 25; and The Medical Letter: *Handbook of Antimicrobial Therapy,* revised ed., 1984.)

Acquired immune deficiency syndrome (AIDS) *(33–2)*
Amebiasis (Table 40–2)
Balanitis *(33–7)*
Candidiasis *(42–17)*
Chancroid *(33–10)*
Chlamydia trachomatis infection *(33–45)*
Condyloma acuminatum *(33–14)*
Gardnerella vaginalis vaginitis *(42–17)*
Cytomegalovirus *(33–16)*
Donovanosis *(33–26)*
Genital warts *(33–14)*
Giardiasis *(40–18)*
Gonorrhea *(33–25)*
Granuloma inguinale *(33–26)*
Hemophilus vaginitis *(42–17)*
Hepatitis *(33–28)*
Herpes *(42–17, 33–29)*
Lambliasis *(40–18)*
Lymphogranuloma venereum *(33–37)*
Molluscum contagiosum *(33–42)*
Nongonococcal urethritis *(33–45)*
Pediculosis *(58–6E)*
Proctitis (multiple causes)
Reiter's syndrome
Salmonellosis (Table 40–1)
Scabies *(58–6D)*
Shigellosis *(33–63)*
Syphilis *(33–66)*
Trichomoniasis *(42–17)*

Text continued on page 265

Table 33–5. COMMON EXANTHEMS—DIFFERENTIAL DIAGNOSIS

CONDITION	INCUBATION (Days)	PERIOD OF COMMUNICABILITY	SYMPTOMS AND SIGNS	SITE	ERUPTION—ONSET, DURATION AND CHARACTER
Chickenpox (Varicella). For treatment, see **33–11**	12–21	From 1 day before onset of symptoms until about 6 days after appearance of rash	Chills, moderate fever, headache, malaise	Usually 1st on trunk, later face, neck and extremities; infrequently on palms and soles	Develop day after onset of symptoms; persist for 1 to 2 weeks. Lesions discrete; progress from macules to papules to vesicles which rupture and form crusts. Appear in crops—various forms may be present simultaneously
Drug rash	History of use of drug	None	Variable, including fever, malaise, arthralgia, nausea, photophobia, pruritus	Generalized; sometimes restricted to exposed surfaces	Varies in time of onset and duration—may be morbilliform, scarlatiniform, erythematous, acneform, vesicular, bullous, purpuric, or exfoliative
Exanthema subitum (Roseola infantum)	Probably 7–10	Unknown, although blood and washings from the throat may be infective during the first day of rash	Infants affected. High fever, usually postoccipital lymphadenopathy	Chest and abdomen, with moderate involvement of face and extremities	This diffuse macular or maculopapular rash appears on the 4th day, usually at the same time the temperature drops to normal; lasts 1 to 2 days
German measles (Rubella). For treatment, see **33–58**	14–21	From 1 day before onset of symptoms until 1 day after disappearance of rash	Malaise, fever, headache, rhinitis, postauricular and postoccipital lymphadenopathy	Face, neck, spreading to trunk and limbs	Develop 1 to 2 days after symptoms; lasts 1 to 3 days. Fine pinkish macules that become confluent
Infectious mononucleosis. See **33–31**	5–15	Undetermined	Malaise, headache, fever, sore throat, splenomegaly and generalized lymphadenopathy	Most prominent over trunk	In about 15% of cases, a morbilliform, scarlatiniform, or vesicular rash appears 5 to 14 days after symptoms; lasts 3 to 7 days
Measles (Rubeola). For treatment, see **33–59**	7–15	From 2 to 4 days before appearance of rash until 2 to 5 days thereafter	Fever, coryza, cough, conjunctivitis, photophobia, Koplik's spots, pruritus	Forehead, face, neck, and then spreading over trunk and limbs	Develop 3 to 5 days after symptoms; lasts 4 to 7 days. Maculopapular; brownish pink; irregularly confluent
Scarlet fever (Scarlatina). For treatment, see **33–62**	3–5	Usually from 24 hours before onset of symptoms until 2 to 3 weeks thereafter; longer if complications occur; shorter if treated with antibiotics	Chills, fever, sore throat, vomiting, strawberry tongue, cervical lymphadenopathy, circumoral pallor	Face, neck, chest, abdomen, spreading to extremities. Entire body surface may be involved	Develops on 2nd day; lasts 4 to 10 days. Diffuse pinkish red flush of skin, with punctate "gooseflesh" feel. Positive blanching reaction
Smallpox (Variola).* For treatment, see **33–64**	10–14	From 1 to 2 days before onset of symptoms until all crusts have disappeared	Abrupt onset with chills, fever, rapid pulse and respiration, nausea, vomiting, severe headache, backache and pains	First face, neck, upper chest, hands. Most on exposed surfaces; may involve palms, soles, pharynx	Develops on 3rd or 4th day; persists for 2 to 5 weeks. Shot-like papules changing to vesicles and umbilicated pustules which enlarge and become confluent. Usually only 1 crop of lesions

*Now eliminated worldwide as a communicable disease.

Table 33–6. ANTIMICROBIAL DRUGS OF CHOICE*

Infecting Organism	Drugs of First Choice	Alternative Drugs
BACILLI		
Acid-fast		
Mycobacterium tuberculosis (*33–72*)	Isoniazid plus rifampin	Ethambutol, streptomycin, kanamycin, pyrazinamide, paraminosalicylic acid (PAS), capreomycin, cycloserine
Gram-negative		
Enterobacter	Gentamicin, tobramycin, netilmicin	Amikacin cefotaxime, carbenicillin
Bordetella pertussis (*33–80*)	Erythromycin	Ampicillin, trimethoprim-sulfamethoxazole
Donovania granulomatis (granuloma inguinale) (*33–26*)	A tetracycline	Chloramphenicol; streptomycin
Escherichia coli	Gentamicin, tobramycin, or neomycin If severely ill may add ampicillin, carbenicillin, ticarcillin, mezlocillin, piperacillin, azlocillin or a cephalosporin	Amikacin, ampicillin, carbenicillin, ticarcillin, mezlocillin, piperacillin, or azlocillin; a cephalosporin, trimethoprim-sulfamethoxazole,‡ a tetracycline† or chloramphenicol
Fusobacterium (Vincent's infection, *61–5*)	Penicillin G	Metronidazole; clindamycin; chloramphenicol
Hemophilus ducreyi (chancroid, *33–10*)	Trimethoprim-sulfamethoxazole or erythromycin	A tetracycline; streptomycin
Hemophilus influenzae		
epiglottitis (*56–8*)		
respiratory infections (*33–32*)	Ampicillin or amoxicillin	Sulfamethoxazole/trimethoprim
meningitis (*33–40*)‡	Chloramphenicol	A tetracycline; ampicillin
Proteus mirabilis	Ampicillin	A cephalosporin, gentamicin
Proteus (indole-positive)	Gentamicin, tobramycin	Amikacin, cefotaxime, carbenicillin
Pseudomonas aeruginosa	Carbenicillin with gentamicin	Amikacin with carbenicillin
urinary infections	Carbenicillin or ticarcillin	Piperacillin, tobramycin, gentamicin
Salmonella typhi (*33–73*)	Chloramphenicol	Ampicillin; trimethoprim-sulfamethoxazole
Salmonella (other)	Ampicillin or amoxicillin	Chloramphenicol, trimethoprim-sulfamethoxazole
Shigella (*33–63*)	Trimethoprim-sulfamethoxazole	A tetracycline, ampicillin, chloramphenicol
Vibrio cholerae (cholera)	A tetracycline	Trimethoprim-sulfamethoxazole
Yersinia pestis (bubonic plague, *33–49*)	Streptomycin	A tetracycline; chloramphenicol; gentamicin

Gram-positive		
Bacillus anthracis (*3–5, Anthrax*)	Penicillin G	Erythromycin; a tetracycline
Clostridium tetani (*33–68*)	Penicillin G	A tetracycline
Clostridium welchii (perfringens) (gas gangrene, *23–14; 59–42*)	Penicillin G	A tetracycline; chloramphenicol; clindamycin; metronidazole
Corynebacterium diphtheriae (*33–18*)	An erythromycin	Penicillin G
COCCI		
Gram-negative		
Gonococcus (*33–35*)	Penicillin G or amoxicillin followed by a tetracycline	A tetracycline; ampicillin; spectinomycin; cefoxitin
Meningococcus (*33–44*)	Penicillin G	Chloramphenicol; cefuroxime, cefotaxime; a sulfonamide
Gram-positive		
Enterococcus (severe)	Ampicillin with gentamicin	Vancomycin with gentamicin or streptomicin
Pneumococcus (*56–16*)	Penicillin G or V	Erythromycin; clindamycin; vancomycin
Staphylococcus aureus		
non-penicillinase producing	Penicillin G or V	Cephalosporins; clindamycin; vancomycin
penicillinase producing§	A penicillinase-resistant penicillin	Cephalosporins; vancomycin; clindamycin
Streptococcus anaerobius	Penicillin G	Erythromycin; clindamycin; a cephalosporin
Streptococcus faecalis	A penicillin with streptomycin	Vancomycin with streptomycin or ampicillin with streptomycin (if endocarditis is present)
Steptococcus pyogenes groups A, C and G	Penicillin G or V	Erythromycin; cephalosporins; vancomycin
Streptococcus viridans	Penicillin G with or without streptomycin	Cephalosporins; vancomycin
FUNGI		
Coccidioides immitis (*33–44*)	Amphotericin B	Ketoconazole, miconazole
Cryptococcus neoformans (*33–44*)	Amphotericin B	Ketoconazole, miconazole

Table continued on following page

Table 33–6. ANTIMICROBIAL DRUGS OF CHOICE* (continued)

Infecting Organism	Drugs of First Choice	Alternative Drugs
OBLIGATE INTRACELLULAR PARASITES		
Chlamydia venerii (lymphogranuloma venereum, *33–37*)	A tetracycline or erythromycin	A sulfonamide
Chlamydia psittaci (psittacosis, *33–53*)	A tetracycline	Chloramphenicol
Chlamydia trachomatis		
Trachoma (*33–71*)	Oral and topical tetracyclines	Oral and topical sulfonamide
Inclusion conjunctivitis (*38–26*)		
Mycoplasma (atypical viral pneumonia, *33–33*)	A tetracycline	Erythromycin
RICKETTSIA (Rocky Mountain spotted fever, *33–57;* typhus, *33–74;* Q fever)	A tetracycline	Chloramphenicol
SPIROCHETES		
Leptospira	Penicillin G	A tetracycline
Spirillum minor (rat bite fever)	Penicillin G	Erythromycin; tetracycline
Treponema pallidum (syphilis, *33–66*)	A penicillin	Erythromycin; a tetracycline
Treponema pertenue (yaws)	A penicillin	A tetracycline

*Modified from The Medical Letter: *Handbook of Antimicrobial Therapy*, revised edition, 1984.

†Tetracyclines are best avoided in pregnant women and children under 8 years of age.

‡Cephalosporins are generally an effective alternative for penicillin-allergic patients, but only newer drugs cross the blood-brain barrier to treat meningitis or can be used against anaerobes; cross-sensitivity to penicillin is possible.

§Cloxacillin and dicloxacillin, orally, and oxacillin, methicillin or nafcillin, parenterally, are effective against most penicillinase-producing staphylococci. If strains are resistant to these antibacterials, they are usually also resistant to cephalosporin.

Comment: Aminoglycosides are excellent for gram-negative bacilli, but must be monitored for ototoxicity and nephrotoxicity. Chloramphenicol, because of serious side effects, should be used only when less hazardous drugs are not effective. Penicillins may produce serious allergic reactions; check history and use safe alternatives.

33–79. VINCENT'S ANGINA *(See 61–15)*

33–80. WHOOPING COUGH (Pertussis)

Caused by a gram-negative bacillus, *Bordetella pertussis*, whooping cough usually lasts for about 6 weeks. Its incubation period is usually 7 to 10 days, but it may be as long as 21 days. It is communicable from about 7 days after exposure (when symptoms appear to be those of a common cold) until 3 weeks after onset of the typical spasmodic cough. Vaccinate susceptible contacts.

Treatment

- Cautious sedation for rest and control of the paroxysmal cough by oral codeine sulfate in small doses (0.2 mg/kg) or phenobarbital (0.5 to 2.0 mg/kg) every 8 hours.
- Insurance of a patent airway, air humidification and supplemental oxygen therapy if evidence of hypoxia is present.
- Supportive care; frequent oral intake of small amounts of fluids.
- Erythromycin or ampicillin for approximately 1 week. Vaccinate.
- Early recognition and treatment of complications such as otitis media, bronchopneumonia, gastric tetany or rectal prolapse following paroxysms of coughing or vomiting, and encephalitis *(33–20)*.

33–81. YELLOW FEVER

In this age of rapid transportation when intercontinental travel within the 3- to 6-day incubation period is not only possible but common, the physician must be aware of this very serious virus infection transmitted by the *Aedes aegypti* mosquito. Yellow fever is still endemic in parts of South America and Africa.

Incubation Period: 3 to 6 days.

Quarantine Period: *Patient*—3 to 5 days after development of acute symptoms; *all contacts*—6 days.

Signs and Symptoms: Chills, fever, myalgia, jaundice, nausea, vomiting and oliguria. As fever goes up to 40°C (104°F), pulse goes down. A crisis usually occurs on the 6th or 7th day; either the patient dies or the beginning of recovery is indicated by a rapid fall in body temperature and increased urination.

Treatment: No specific therapy is known. Immediate hospitalization is indicated, since the outcome will depend to a considerable extent upon adequate supportive therapy and nursing care.

33–82. COMMON EXANTHEMS—DIFFERENTIAL DIAGNOSIS *(See Table 33–5)*

33–83. ANTIMICROBIAL DRUGS OF CHOICE *(See also 59–42, Antibiotics for Bacterial Anaerobes)*

Before any of the antimicrobial agents specified in Table 33–6 are administered, the manufacturer's brochure or a pharmacology text should be consulted for method of administration, dosages, toxicity and side effects.

Smears and cultures for identification and sensitivity tests should be taken before an antimicrobial agent is given for definitive treatment, but emergency therapy based on clinical findings, as a rule, should not await laboratory results. See *18–12, Gram Stain,* for bacterial staining technique. See Appendix for table on usual starting doses of common antimicrobial drugs.

34. Convulsions/Seizures*

Types

Convulsions, seizures, epilepsy and "fits" are all terms used (some imprecisely) to describe short episodes of sudden onset in which the patient has uncontrolled motor activity, altered states of consciousness, paresthesias, visual or olfactory hallucinations or peculiar behavior due to temporarily altered cerebral function.

Convulsions are categorized as partial, generalized, unilateral or unclassified. An electroencephalogram (EEG) taken electively or within 6 hours of the seizure (if sedatives have not been given) can be a most useful electrodiagnostic aid for classification. Documentation of the exact observations before, during and after the seizure assists diagnosis and classification. The following should be considered: precipitating causes (such as fever, alcohol, excitement, stimulation, hypoxemia, trauma), aura, focal or generalized seizure, tetany or myoclonic movements, biting of tongue, loss of bowel or bladder control, postictal confusion and lethargy.

Age Group Factors

Persons of any age may develop convulsive seizures either for the first time or on a recurrent basis. Subsequent episodes are usually, though not invariably, related to prior causes.

The underlying factors responsible for convulsions vary with age.

Neonatal and Infant Age Group

Hypocalcemia (see *52–11*)
Hypoglycemia (see *52–10*)
Birth injury
Developmental abnormalities
Bacterial and viral central nervous system infections

Children and Adolescents. Same as for infants, with the addition of trauma *(44, Head Injuries)* as a frequent cause, and a rarer incidence from hypoglycemia and hypocalcemia. Idiopathic causes are also frequent in this age group.

Adults

Trauma *(44, Head Injuries)*
Neoplasms
Heat stroke *(62–4)*
Metabolic abnormalities *(46)*, e.g., hypoglycemia *(46–15)*
Effects of drugs and poisons *(53)* and alcohol withdrawal *(54–7)*
Toxemias of pregnancy, eclampsia *(50–6)*
Vascular conditions, particularly intracranial arteriovenous malformation; see also *63–4, Intracranial Bleeding*
Infectious diseases of the central nervous system (see *33*)
Hyperventilation *(37–10)*
Idiopathic causes
Conversion reactions (i.e., hysterical seizures), which can present a diagnostic challenge; close observation is essential.

---

*See also *37, Excitement States.*

Treatment of Acute Generalized Convulsions (Grand Mal Seizures)

The vigor with which emergency treatment is applied will depend largely on the state of the patient at the time he or she is first seen by the physician, since frequently the acute episode will have subsided. Treatment measures include the following:

- Protection from injury by gentle restraint and maintenance in a lying position at a safe level. (Keep calm. The person is usually not suffering or in danger.)
- Maintenance of an unobstructed airway during the postictal state. The patient should be placed in a prone or semi-prone position with the head turned to one side (Fig. 4–5*A*). A folded handkerchief or padded tongue blade slipped between the teeth can help protect the tongue. Do not put fingers between the patient's teeth.
- Institution of direct cooling measures by sponging, tepid tub baths and cool water enemas if the convulsions are caused by hyperpyrexia.
- Administration of salicylates when the convulsive seizures are associated with hyperpyrexia.
- Avoidance of unnecessary light, sound or contactual stimulation.
- Active seizures in an adult can be treated with diazepam (Valium), 5 to 10 mg diluted to 10 ml with normal saline for slow, cautious IV administration (this may be repeated up to every 10 to 15 minutes to a maximum of 30 mg/hr in adults, but it is preferable to give diazepam *once* and follow with phenytoin). In children, the IV dosage should not exceed 0.25 mg/kg given over 3 minutes and can be repeated in 15 to 30 minutes if phenytoin is not available. Alternatively, slow IV administration of a dilute solution of lorazepam (Ativan), 0.044 mg/kg to a maximum dose of 4 mg, may be given, or an IV barbiturate administered. Support ventilation (*5*). Avoid combinations of diazepam and phenobarbital—particularly in children—because of their extreme synergistic depressive effect on respiration.
- Patients having serial seizures (status epilepticus), if no prior phenytoin has been taken, should receive phenytoin (Dilantin) IV, 150 mg to 250 mg, at a rate not to exceed 50 mg/min, and supplemented with 100 to 150 mg 30 minutes later if necessary; more severe cases may require a higher dosage, but this should not exceed a total of 500 mg in adults. (Dosage for children is 250 mg/m^2 [see Fig. 9–1]; IV administration rate is proportionately slower than that for adults.)
- Inhalation anesthesia and intubation and oxygen administration may be necessary in more severe cases. Hypothermia may also be helpful.
- Correction of any acidosis or electrolyte or sugar imbalance.
- Paraldehyde, 5 to 10 ml rectally or PO, or 5 ml IM, or chloral hydrate, 0.5 to 1.0 g PO or by retention enema. These drugs can be valuable if respiratory depression must be avoided.
- Phenytoin sodium (Dilantin), 150 to 250 mg IV, but not to exceed a rate of 50 mg per minute and supplemented with 100 to 150 mg 30 minutes later if necessary, for prophylaxis against further episodes in adults. Oral administration initially can be given at 5 mg/kg in 3 or 4 divided doses to an average total dose of 300 to 400 mg/day or a maximum total dose of 600 mg/day. Blood levels guide therapy; therapeutic blood levels are 10 to 20 μg/ml, and toxic levels are over 25 μg/ml.
- Treatment of causative condition (see Age Group Factors, above).

(date)

_______ County Health Department Officer

Dear Sir:

The following individual has been diagnosed as having a disorder characterized by lapses of consciousness as designated in the Health and Safety Code, Paragraph 410, and in the California Administrative Code, Title 17, Section 2572.

Name of patient ________

Address ________

____

Date of birth ________

Medical Record No. ________

This report is being filed in accordance with the above statutes.

Very truly yours,

Distribution: Addressee
Chart
Patient

________ M.D.

Figure 34–1. Form for reporting convulsive seizures.

Further Evaluation

Any person with convulsions of undetermined origin should have a thorough investigation, including the following:

- History of medications, alcoholic intake and stressful events.
- Family history.
- Complete physical and neurologic examination as outlined under Table 32–1, *Coma of Undetermined Etiology.*
- Lumbar puncture *(18–29, Spinal Puncture),* unless contraindicated by the possibility of increased intracranial pressure.
- Sugar and calcium level determinations of blood specimens taken at the time of the convulsion. If the patient is already on an anticonvulsant medication, blood must be drawn for drug level determinations before subsequent modified doses of the medication can be administered.
- Electroencephalogram and CT scan.

Further Management

- Definitive care. This will depend upon the type and the cause of the convulsions and may require trial of several regimens for control.

- Caution the patient regarding using hazardous equipment (particularly motor vehicles) and being in precarious places until adequate control (medically and in accordance with jurisdictional standards) has been established.
- Report convulsive seizures in accordance with jurisdictional requirements (*15*; see also Fig. 34–1). Inform the patient of the report and consider advising the patient to go to the Department of Motor Vehicles and turn in his or her driver's license (showing responsibility for doing this voluntarily may ease return of the license later). Failure of the physician to report on a patient who has had a seizure may result in professional, civil and criminal penalties.

35. Ear Conditions

35–1. GENERAL CONSIDERATIONS

In the course of examining the ear, it is often helpful to obtain and record a rough index of hearing acuity, such as ability to hear the ticking of a watch, a tuning fork or a whispered voice.

- Perform the Rinne test: Using the tuning fork, check to see whether air conduction is better than bone conduction (normal). If the reverse is noted on the affected side, there is a conductive hearing loss (perforated tympanic membrane, fluid in middle ear). With sensorineural hearing loss, air conduction is still greater than bone conduction, but both are diminished in intensity.
- With the tuning fork held in the middle of the forehead (Weber test), normally the tone is heard equally in both ears. In conductive hearing loss, the tone sounds louder on the affected side; in sensorineural hearing loss, the tone is heard best on the unaffected side.
- Tympanometry evaluates mobility and patency of the tympanic membrane, functional condition of the middle ear and ventilation capacity of the eustachian tube.
- Direct observation with the otoscope and a clean speculum reveals patency of the canal (see *35–6, Cerumen*), inflammation, bleeding, perforation, or bulging or inflammation of the tympanic membrane. With a pneumatoscope, one can also check tympanic membrane mobility (decreased with middle ear fluid/pathology).

35–2. AEROTITIS *(See also 35–18, Otitis Media)*

This acute form of otitis media occurs most commonly in patients with precedent respiratory tract congestion who undergo rapid barometric change such as occurs in airplane travel or diving. An acute decrease in hearing, pain, inflammation or even a hemorrhage of the drum may occur. Treat with nasal and systemic decongestants (see *56–6, Coryza*) and advise periodic Valsalva maneuvers and swallowing. If continued flight is mandatory, be sure the patient is awake and doing short Valsalva maneuvers and swallowing (infants may be given a bottle to suck on in addition to a nasal decongestant) from the start of descent. Prophylactic use of an oral decongestant about 45 minutes before flight time can be helpful, as can use of an over-the-counter nasal spray containing pseudoephedrine or oxymetazoline.

35–3. BLEEDING FROM EARS

Following blunt trauma to the head, bleeding from an ear is suggestive of basilar skull fracture *(44–12)*. Hospitalize at once for care of the head injury. No attempt should be made to cleanse the ear canal. A sterile pad may be applied over the ear, but *nothing* should be inserted into the external auditory canal. In the hospital, blood may be cleared from the canal with a sterile "brain suction" tip, but no irrigation should be performed.

In the absence of head trauma, the most common cause of bleeding is otitis media *(35–18)* with perforation or, if a ventilating tube is in place, from inflammation and possible polyp erosion; treat with topical corticosporin suspension and systemic antibiotics.

35–4. BULLOUS MYRINGITIS

Bullous myringitis causes acute ear pain and fever and is distinguished by clear, fluid-filled blebs on the tympanic membrane. In adults, evaluate for underlying malignancy. The cause is often a viral infection and as such would need no antibiotic treatment, but *Hemophilus* organisms, *Diplococcus pneumoniae* and *Mycoplasma* infections are usually clinically indistinguishable and require ampicillin or erythromycin therapy; *Mycoplasma* is the most common source of infection, and erythromycin is preferable. Cautious puncture of the blebs may relieve pain. Auralgan otic drops may be helpful. Oral analgesics may be needed (7).

35–5. BURNS *(See 28–11)*

35–6. CERUMEN

For adequate examination, the ear must be cleared of cerumen, which can also cause a decreased hearing acuity and an uncomfortable stuffiness of the ear. The condition of the drum should be known—any evidence of perforation is an absolute contraindication to irrigation or instillation of any liquid into the ear canal. If the drum is intact, removal of impacted wax can be accomplished by the following method:

- Fill the external auditory canal with triethanolamine polypeptide oleate-condensate (Cerumenex) drops.
- Plug with cotton for 15 to 30 minutes.
- Irrigate with warm water, using a large syringe.
- If perforation of the drum is a possibility but not established, remove cerumen under direct vision using a speculum (ear or nasal) and wire loop. If acute perforation is found, refer at once to an otolaryngologist.

35–7. COLD INJURIES (Frostbite and Hypothermia) *(See 62–2)*

35–8. CONTUSIONS

The marked cosmetic blemishes caused by bleeding into the helix, concha and lobule ("cauliflower ears") can often be prevented by immediate aspiration and flushing out of residual blood particles with normal saline or by surgical drainage of the hematoma. This should be followed by gentle counterpressure over and behind the ear with bulk padding or a small dressing held in place by a collodion-soaked felt pad molded over the helix before drying to form a splint.

35–9. DEAFNESS (Rapid Onset)

Diminished acuity often occurs after barometric changes (see *35–2, Aerotitis; 39–2, Foreign Bodies in the Ear)* or as a result of water trapping behind excessive cerumen *(35–6)* or eustachian salpingitis *(35–18)*. Rapid onset of presbycusis can also occur from sensory (or cochlear) pathology as can follow acute trauma, inflammation (usually associated with vertigo as in viral labyrinthitis or Meniere's syndrome [49–7]) or ingestion of ototoxic drugs. Rapid neural or acoustic 8th nerve loss is more likely to occur from hematoma from head injury *(44)* than from cerebellar pontine angle tumor complications. Treatment consists of managing the underlying cause. Inflammation from viral labyrinthitis can be relieved by tapering doses of prednisone, starting with 45 to 60 mg/day.

If caused or aggravated by concussion (e.g., from explosions) or by sudden or prolonged exposure to intense noise (from jackhammers, amplified modern music, riveting, etc.), only symptomatic treatment of the acute acoustic neuritis is indicated. The patient should be referred to an otolaryngologist for examination and care.

35–10. EARACHE, NONSPECIFIC

Acute bacterial earache can often be relieved by analgesics and treatment of underlying infection of the middle ear and upper respiratory tract with broad-spectrum antibiotics. Pain in the ear may be referred from tooth, pharyngeal, mandibular and temporomandibular joint disease. Persistent earache requires care by an otolaryngologist.

35–11. EUSTACHIAN SALPINGITIS *(See 35–18)*

35–12. FOREIGN BODIES *(See 39–2)*

35–13. HEMATOMAS *(See 35–8)*

35–14. LACERATIONS *(See 59–16)*

35–15. MASTOIDITIS

This complication of otitis media *(35–18)* has become rather rare since the advent of antibiotics, but still occurs in cases in which treatment has been inadequate. If mastoiditis is proved or suspected, immediate hospitalization is indicated for intensive antibiotic treatment with the assistance of an otolaryngologist. Coalescent mastoiditis occurs in most cases no sooner than 1 to 2 weeks after the onset of otitis media. Most commonly now posterior auricular swelling in a febrile patient represents a posterior auricular lymph node abscess or cellulitis.

35–16. MENIERE'S DISEASE *(See 49–7)*

35–17. OTITIS EXTERNA *(See also 26–5, Diving Hazards)*

Inflammation of the external auditory canal is often very painful because of edema in the confined area and should be distinguished from middle ear involvement (see *35–18, Otitis Media*). Posterior traction on the pinna usually exacerbates the pain of otitis externa. Culture drainage as indicated. A combination antibiotic and anti-inflammatory otic solution (Cortisporin) instilled into the ear, initially hourly, then 3 to 4 times daily, may control infection. *(Note:* If the tympanic membrane is perforated, Cortisporin Otic

Suspension is preferable, as the solution burns with perforation.) A cotton ear canal wick will help get the medication in contact with the inflamed tissues. Analgesics with codeine are prescribed for relief of more severe pain. Application of heat from warm compresses, a hot water bottle or even from blowing warm cigar smoke in the ear (finally one good use for tobacco!) may aid pain relief. Prevent recurrence of "swimmer's ear" by prescribing a thimbleful of a solution of half rubbing alcohol and half white vinegar to be poured into each ear immediately after each shower or time in the pool. The patient should be advised to consult an otolaryngologist if irritation of the canal persists.

35–18. OTITIS MEDIA

Acute inflammation of the middle ear is often encountered as an emergency in children. Formerly uncommon in adults, it is now seen fairly often in sports divers *(26–5)*.

Treatment

Treatment is palliative, with control of infection by antibiotics, aimed at preventing secondary complications such as meningitis, mastoiditis, decreased hearing and cholesteatoma. Specific treatment measures are as follows:

- Ampicillin, 50 to 100 mg/kg/day up to usually 2 g daily for 10 days by mouth or initially parenterally if necessary. Alternatively, erythromycin plus sulfisoxazole, 150 mg/kg/day, or Septra or Ceclor.
- No medication should be introduced into the canal unless there has been rupture of the drum with drainage of frank pus; in this case, Cortisporin Otic Suspension may be of benefit.
- Aspirin, 0.06 to 0.3 g, depending on age or weight *(9)* every 4 hours. Codeine sulfate PO or SC, or pentazocine lactate (Talwin) PO or IM may be necessary for control of severe pain (dosage determined by age, weight or skin surface *[9]*).
- Tympanocentesis or paracentesis of the drum is now infrequently necessary with adequate early antibiotic treatment. If an emergency procedure is needed for pain relief in the first 24 to 48 hours or for diagnosis, the external canal should be cultured and then cleaned. Topical anesthesia should be applied. Decompression under topical anesthesia can be achieved with syringe aspiration through a No. 18 spinal needle inserted through the anterior-inferior to inferior membrane if the fluid is sufficiently liquid. An incision may be required to permit evacuation of inspissated purulent material. Cultures should be obtained and sensitivity testing done, and appropriate antibiotic therapy instituted *(33–83, Antimicrobial Drugs of Choice)* initially according to the results of Gram stain.
- Warmth from a heating pad on a low setting placed over the external ear may give comfort.
- Complete control of the infection is essential in all cases of otitis media. Inadequate therapy, especially with antibiotics, may result in apparent alleviation of acute symptoms with later development of a suppurative mastoiditis.

35–19. OTORRHEA

Drainage of cerebrospinal fluid from the ears is definitive evidence of basal skull fracture *(44–16)*. Unless massive, it usually clears spontaneously. Guard against retrograde infection via canals.

35–20. TINNITUS

Tinnitus may be severe enough to require analgesics or phenothiazines; avoid narcotics. Discontinue aspirin if it is causative. All patients with severe or persistent tinnitus should be referred to an otolaryngologist.

35–21. VERTIGO *(See 49–21)*

36. Endocrine Emergencies

ADRENAL

36–1. ACUTE ADRENAL CORTICAL INSUFFICIENCY

This severe, life-threatening situation, manifested by profound fatigue and general weakness, nausea, vomiting, trunk and extremity pain, hypotension and shock, stupor and frequently high fever, occurs in previously undiagnosed persons—usually first recognized by their hyperpigmentation*—or in diagnosed chronic adrenal insufficiency patients who omit their maintenance dose or who fail to increase their dose of hydrocortisone to meet the requirements of added stress of some type. In addition, marked extracellular fluid depletion (20% loss or more) is a prominent feature. Primary acute cases may be associated with or precipitated by rampant infections such as meningococcemia *(33–41)* and adrenal hemorrhage. ECG may show signs of hyperkalemia (see Fig. 46–1), low QRS voltage and prolonged PR and QT intervals. Prominent laboratory features are: ↑K > 5 mEq/L (see *46–8*); ↓Na < 130 mEq/L (see *46–18*); ↓FBS < 60 mg/dl; ↓WBC; ↑eosinophils; ↑Hmct/Hb's. Test for serum ACTH level (usually increased unless there is also lowered pituitary function) and cortisol (decreased) prior to initiating treatment.

Treatment

- Inject up to 100 mg of hydrocortisone sodium succinate IV initially.
- Give 50 to 100 mg hydrocortisone IV q 6 h for the first 24 hours; can dilute in D5NS infusion.
- D5NS should be administered vigorously IV (to replace both volume and salt loss). Up to 3 liters may be required in the first few hours.
- No mineralocorticoid is necessary during the acute stage of adrenal failure.
- Treat precipitating cause for the adrenal crisis.
- Dose of hydrocortisone could be reduced by 50% the second day if patient is stable, with further reduction depending on the clinical response. Maintenance dose of hydrocortisone is 20 to 30 mg daily given in 2 doses: A.M. and between 2 and 3 P.M. Maintenance mineralocorticoid may or may not be required.
- Glucose should be administered if hypoglycemia is present.
- Instruct patient to: (1) double or triple the usual dose of steroid under stress; (b) have an injectable preparation of steroid available for emergency (dexamethasone, 4 mg/cc); (c) wear MEDI-Alert bracelet indicating that patient is on steroids.
- Arrange for follow-up care with an internist or endocrinologist.

36–2. PHEOCHROMOCYTOMA

The urgent hypertensive complications that occur with this catecholamine-producing tumor may be spontaneous, stress-induced (e.g., by infection or

---

*A sign of primary adrenal insufficiency.

unrelated surgery) or related to investigation of or surgical procedures for the tumor. Provocative testing for pheochromocytoma is rarely needed and should be considered an exception. A histamine-provocative test may elicit a profound hypertensive episode, requiring administration of either sodium nitroprusside (Nipride), 100 to 200 mg/L, by closely monitored IV infusion, or phentolamine (Regitine), 2 to 5 mg IV, repeated at 10- to 20-minute intervals as needed. Propranolol, 2 to 4 mg IV, may also be needed for cardiac arrhythmias.

During surgical excision of the tumor, epinephrine or norepinephrine may be released, and the resultant hypertension may necessitate similar therapy. The hypovolemia occurring with surgical removal of the pheochromocytoma will usually not respond well to pressor agents. Massive fluid replacement should be administered while monitoring central venous and pulmonary wedge pressures; plasma or blood transfusions may be required. All patients undergoing surgery for pheochromocytoma should be continuously monitored with intra-arterial blood pressure lines, Swan-Ganz catheters, and so on. Pretreatment of these patients with an alpha-adrenergic blocking agent such as phenoxybenzamine can reduce the intraoperative complications; however, some controversy exists with regard to the advisability of such preoperative preparation.

36–3. HYPERALDOSTERONISM

Aldosterone's mineralocorticoid effect is to cause sodium and water retention and potassium loss, which can result in hypertension *(29–14)* and manifestations of hypokalemia *(46–16)* that require prompt treatment in addition to referral for definitive correction. Secondary aldosteronism (such as that associated with cirrhosis, nephrotic syndrome or CHF) may be more clinically evident than with adenoma (Conn's syndrome).

36–4. ADRENAL CORTICAL HYPERFUNCTION

Usually this problem arises from cortisol hypersecretion (Cushing's syndrome) due to increased ACTH secondary to increased function of the anterior lobe of the pituitary, adrenal adenoma or carcinoma, iatrogenic administration or ectopic ACTH. The syndrome is recognized most readily clinically by the buccal fat pad ("moon face"), truncal obesity and purple striae, upper thoracic-cervical fat pad ("buffalo hump"), hypertension *(29–14)*, hyperglycemia, depression *(54–8)* and even psychotic states *(54–17)*. Serum ACTH and cortisol levels should be drawn. Treat presenting problem and refer for definitive care.

PANCREAS

36–5. DIABETIC COMA *(See 32–3, Diabetes Mellitus; Table 32–1)*

36–6. INSULIN SHOCK *(See also 32–3, Diabetes Mellitus; Table 32–1)*

Hypoglycemia may be secondary to excess insulin administration or islet cell tumor (manifested by coma with or without convulsions, and by prior increase in appetite and body weight). Significant hypoglycemia also may result from insulin rebound in postgastrectomy patients.

Treatment

- Treat acute symptoms (see Insulin Shock under 32–3, *Diabetes Mellitus*).
- Put patient on well-balanced, simple carbohydrate, adequate calorie diet, with 3 to 6 feedings per day.
- Refer for definitive workup and treatment.

PARATHYROID

36–7. HYPOPARATHYROIDISM

The emergency presentation of hypoparathyroidism comes usually because of the neuromuscular excitability indicated clinically by carpopedal spasm, facial muscle twitching following tapping, convulsions and laryngeal stridor (due to low ionized calcium concentration *[46–14]* and/or hypomagnesemia *[46–17]*). Hypoparathyroid crises are caused by atrophy, degeneration, fibrosis or surgical removal of the parathyroid glands; rarely they may occur in patients with end-organ insensitivity to parathyroid hormone (PTH) in pseudohypoparathyroidism. It is not uncommon for patients undergoing surgery for hyperparathyroidism to develop transient postoperative hypocalcemia; this may occur within hours following the surgery. Others may develop permanent hypoparathyroidism, which can occur within days to as long as several months after surgery. Decrease in ionized calcium levels may be caused by hyperventilation, or rarely large doses of citrate may precipitate crises in which serum Ca is as low as 7 to 8 mg/dl.

Treatment

- Perform ECG and collect a blood specimen to determine serum Ca, Mg, PO_4 level and serum PTH level prior to slow administration of calcium gluconate, 1 g IV, with 1 or 2 repetitions as needed (*note:* if the patient is digitalized, give cautiously along with electrocardiogram monitoring).
- Sedate with diazepam (Valium).
- Refer to a hospital for stabilization as necessary and institution of long-range treatment with dihydrotachysterol and calciferol together with a low-phosphorus, high-calcium diet.

36–8. ACUTE PARATHYROID INTOXICATION

Acute hyperparathyroidism with hypercalcemia can produce an emergency situation in which the patient presents with profound weakness, nausea, vomiting, and lethargy progressing to coma. See *46–6* for treatment of hypercalcemia. Definitive treatment is surgery.

PITUITARY

36–9. PITUITARY INSUFFICIENCY

Emergencies related to pituitary gland insufficiency (either anterior or posterior lobe) are rare and secondary to causative mechanisms such as pituitary hemorrhage and destruction from surgery or radiation. Decreases in circulating glucocorticoids *(36–1)* and thyroid hormone *(36–12)* occur subsequent to decreased adrenal and thyroid stimulation from hormonal deficiency of the anterior lobe (↓ACTH/↓TSH).

Destruction of or damage to the posterior lobe of the pituitary may cause diabetes insipidus (DI), which is characterized by a high urine volume with low specific gravity, polydipsia and profound hypovolemic dehydration. Destruction of the posterior pituitary lobe without damage to the hypothalamus or the pituitary stalk rarely causes permanent diabetes insipidus. The higher the site or section of the stalk affected, the greater the chance for permanent DI. Traumatic lesions may give rise to the classic triple response: initial DI followed by decreased urine output and then by permanent DI. Draw blood to determine levels of serum electrolytes, triiodothyronine (T_3), thyroxine (T_4), cortisol and adrenocorticotropic hormone (ACTH) prior to starting treatment.

Treatment of Diabetes Insipidus (DI)

- Have unlimited access to free water at all times. Patients with DI if permitted will drink as much water as is required.
- Specific therapy is with vasopressin, available in injectable and spray forms. Aqueous vasopressin has a short half-life and must be given several times during the day (5 to 10 units SC q 4 h). Vasopressin tannate in oil given IM will last 24 to 36 hours. If nasal access is possible, one of the nasal sprays can be used. Have patient inhale lysine vasopressin, 1 to 2 puffs q 4 to 6 h, or, better, give 0.05 to 0.1 ml of DDAVP intranasally bid. When administering vasopressin, particularly in a comatose patient, a close watch on intake and output is necessary to prevent SIADH. DDAVP is now also available for IV administration.
- If anterior pituitary function is involved, administer hydrocortisone, 100 mg IV q 8 h initially.
- In acute cases, hospitalize for evaluation and determination of requirements.

36–10. PITUITARY HYPERSECRETION

Elevated ACTH production by the anterior pituitary lobe results in increased cortisol production in functioning adrenal glands (see *36–3*). Excess excretion of growth hormones does not result in an emergency situation, but it is important to recognize the developing process of acromegaly and gigantism in order to direct the person to appropriate care to arrest the process. Galactorrhea may be a sign of a prolactin-producing pituitary adenoma or may be secondary to drugs such as the phenothiazines or (rarely) to primary hypothyroidism. No significant syndromes from posterior pituitary hypersecretion are evident.

THYROID

36–11. THYROID STORM

This is a very serious condition precipitated by various stresses (e.g., infection, surgery) in a previously untreated patient with hyperthyroidism. It usually occurs in a patient with Graves' disease but may also be seen in a nodular toxic goiter. Thyroid storm is a clinical diagnosis characterized by the following: (a) acute exacerbation of the symptoms of hyperthyroidism (tachycardia, fine finger trauma, restlessness, nausea, vomiting, dehydration, weight loss); (b) increase in temperature to greater than 39.4°C (100°F), or even as high as 41°C (105.8°F); (c) symptoms related to the cardiovascular, gastrointestinal and central nervous systems.

Prompt treatment should be instituted. If the patient is not known to have hyperthyroidism, thyroid function studies (including at least T_3 and T_4) should be obtained prior to treatment. Treatment must be more vigorous than for lesser hyperthyroid states.

Treatment of Thyroid Storm

Supportive Care

- Fluid and electrolyte replacement to correct losses from sweat and the GI tract.
- Treatment of hyperglycemia (due to insulin resistance from excess thyroid hormone, inhibition of insulin release, increased glycolysis and increased absorption of glucose from the gut). If the hyperglycemia is not significant

it should be merely monitored; if, however, it is markedly elevated, insulin should be administered to lower the blood sugar.

- Lowering of fever in patients with hyperpyrexia, by use of cooling blankets and administration of cooled saline (see 62, *Temperature Variation Emergencies*).
- Treatment of hypercalcemia *(46–6)* if significantly elevated (rare).
- Administration of glucocorticoids to correct adrenal insufficiency caused by the stress of thyroid storm. Initially give hydrocortisone, 100 mg IV, followed by 50 to 100 mg IV q 6 h in the first 24 hours; review periodically over the ensuing days. Steroids may also be beneficial by inhibiting the conversion of T_4 to T_3.
- Treatment of cardiac failure with digitalis, O_2 and diuretics (see *55–3*). Propranolol may be used after initial digitalization.
- Treatment of arrhythmias with propranolol administered IV at a rate of less than 1 mg/min up to 10 mg total initially, with close monitoring; repeat in 3 to 4 hours. If no response, another antiarrhythmic drug may be used as appropriate.
- Vitamin replacement has been advocated.

Decrease Production and Release of Thyroid Hormone

- *Propylthiouracil (PTU) to decrease production.* If the patient is already on this medication, it should be continued. If not, an initial dose of 900 to 1200 mg should be administered (via NG tube in unconscious patients), followed by 400 mg daily. Continue this dose until patient is euthyroid (usually 4 to 6 weeks). This dosage for thyroid storm treatment is 3 times greater than the usual treatment of less severe hyperthyroidism. If methimazole (Tapazole) is used, one tenth of the above dose should be given. Monitoring of CBC is necessary.
- *Iodine to decrease release.* Iodine should be administered about an hour after the PTU is given. Administer orally via Lugol's solution, 30 drops daily, or give 1 g sodium iodide slowly IV, repeated in 8 to 12 hours.

Block Peripheral Effects of Thyroid Hormone

Administer the following:

- Propranolol: Orally, 40 to 80 mg q 6 h; or IV, less than 1 mg (1 ml)/min up to 10 mg.
- Guanethidine sulfate: 1 to 2 mg/kg/day PO in divided doses.
- Reserpine: 1 to 5 mg IM followed by 1 to 1.5 mg IM q 4 to 6 h.

In patients with heart failure, propranolol may be given after initial digitalization with 0.5 mg of digoxin IV.

HYPOTHYROID EMERGENCIES

36–12. MYXEDEMA COMA

These patients have the classic symptoms of myxedema (e.g., dry, coarse, edematous-puffy skin; mental dullness; weakness; thinned, coarse hair), plus hypothermia (if temperature is normal usually infection is present) and stupor or unconsciousness. Bradycardia, small QRS complexes and prolonged QT interval are found on ECG. This rare, life-threatening form of myxedema is usually precipitated by stress (including infections and injuries) in a hypothyroid individual whose condition was previously unrecognized and untreated. About half the patients who go into myxedema coma do so while already in the hospital with other problems. Patients with myxedema are extremely sensitive to narcotics, and ordinary doses may cause acute respiratory depression and shock; if this occurs, give naloxone HCl (Narcan) IV as needed (see *53–10*). Draw blood studies (T_3, T_4) to confirm diagnosis before starting treatment; also perform usual studies for coma (*29*).

Treatment (General Supportive Care)

- *Hypotension:* Usually unresponsive to pressor agents until thyroid hormone is administered; must be watched closely.
- *Hypothermia:* Bring temperature up passively very gradually (*62–3*); heating blankets may be detrimental and could cause circulatory collapse.
- *Hypoglycemia:* Treat with glucose (see *46–15*).
- *Hypoventilation with respiratory acidosis:* This is not an uncommon cause of death in patients with myxedema coma. Such patients have decreased maximum voluntary respiration, decreased carbon monoxide diffusion, and decreased respiratory response to inhalation of CO_2. Frequent ABG's should be obtained, and ventilatory support given if required.
- *Hyponatremia:* Even though the total body sodium is increased, the patient with myxedema coma could have significant hyponatremia. If serum Na is less than 115 mEq/L, partial correction with hypertonic saline should be made with close monitoring.
- *Adrenal insufficiency:* Patients with myxedema coma may have associated adrenal insufficiency either as part of hypopituitarism (*36–9*) or as part of Schmidt's syndrome. All patients with myxedema coma have an impaired pituitary response to lysine vasopressin. Hydrocortisone should be given in an initial dose of 100 mg, followed by 100 mg IV q 8 h. This dose should be continued for about 1 week.
- *Thyroid hormone replacement:* L-Thyroxine is probably the preferred choice of therapy. The initial dose of 200 to 400 μg IV is followed by 50 to 100 μg IV daily.
- *Intercurrent infection:* Should be looked for vigorously and promptly treated. Give naloxone if there has been prior narcotic administration.

37. Excitement States (Anxiety)*

37–1. EXCITEMENT STATES—COMMON CAUSES

Excitement states generally occur because of one or more of the following:

- Toxic brain damage (drugs, alcohol, chemicals, infection).
- Mechanical brain damage (swelling, hemorrhage, tumor, epileptiform activity).
- Hypoxemia.
- Respiratory alkalosis (hyperventilation; see *37–10*).
- Terror and fear of situational nature (*54–3*).
- Behavioral disorders and phobias (*37–14*).

37–2. EXCITEMENT STATES—CONTROL MEASURES

Control of excitement states is achieved by one or more of the following measures (all performed with calm, firm, compassionate resolve):

- Treatment and elimination of the specific cause. (Hypoxemia in particular requires immediate treatment and should be managed before treating other problems.)
- Situational control.

*See also *54–17, Psychoses.*

- Physical control (see also 54–21, *Violent Behavior*).
- Voice control with assurance/reassurance/firmness. Hypnosis can aid.
- Medicinal control (oral, IM, IV), using any one of the following: diazepam (Valium), 2.5 mg parenterally in increments up to 10 mg; chlorpromazine HCl (Thorazine), 25 to 50 mg PO; thioridazine (Mellaril), 50 to 100 mg PO; haloperidol (Haldol), 2 to 5 mg IM, repeated every 30 to 60 minutes prn.
- Aid of family, friends, close associates.

The more common causes of acute excitement states coming for urgent evaluation are detailed in the following sections.

37–3. ACUTE SITUATIONAL REACTIONS *(See 54–3)*

37–4. ALCOHOLISM *(See also 7–2, Addiction; 19–1, Alcohol Intoxication Tests; 54–7, Delirium Tremens; 53–295, Ethyl Alcohol)*

An acute excitement state may precede the onset of somnolence or coma *(32)*; therefore, care should be used in administering any medication for control. Diazepam (Valium), 2.5 mg parenterally and in slow increments up to 10 mg, is rapid, effective and relatively safe, provided barbiturates or opiates have not been given previously. Paraldehyde intramuscularly is also of value. Preferably control the patient with firm, reasonable (and inoffensive) voice control. Physical restraint should be used only in extreme cases and while sedation is taking effect. Syrup of ipecac, 15 to 30 ml PO, usually will induce vomiting if gastric emptying is desired and in addition may have a delayed sedative effect. Gastric lavage should not be attempted unless the cooperation of the patient cannot be obtained or unless emetics do not result in satisfactory emptying of the stomach. Other causes for acute excitement must be considered in all cases of apparent acute alcoholism, as during this state the patient may have incurred a head injury or ingested a wide variety of other toxic substances. Treat withdrawal with chlordiazepoxide HCl (Librium), 25 mg PO tid, but varied response may direct larger or smaller doses.

37–5. CHEST AND PULMONARY CONDITIONS

Air hunger following nonperforating chest injuries *(31–10)*, rib fractures *(31–8)*, penetrating chest wounds *(31–11)*, cardiac tamponade *(31–4)* and severe crushing injuries of the thorax *(31–5)* may cause an acute excitement state and should be treated accordingly. Other respiratory tract conditions *(56)*, such as asthma and pulmonary edema *(55)*, can lead to severe anxiety.

37–6. DELIRIUM *(See 54–7; see also 7–2, Addiction; 19–1, Alcohol Intoxication Tests; 37–4, Alcoholism)*

37–7. DRUG EFFECT

Drugs may cause excitement states through an unusual pharmacologic effect, side effects, idiosyncratic reactions or a combination effect with other drugs; the effect of barbiturates in small children is a particularly common example. Stop the drug and see 53 under the specific agent for appropriate treatment. Among the leading offenders are drugs listed in 53–332, *Hallucinogens.*

37–8. HEAD INJURIES *(See also 44)*

Injury to the head can cause hyperactivity symptoms ranging from slight restlessness to homicidal mania. Physical restraint should be kept to a minimum; however, physical control may be necessary to prevent further injury to the patient or injuries to attendants. Immediately correct any hypoxemic states. Opiates or synthetic narcotics should generally not be used, but in certain situations (e.g., a writhing head/neck-injured patient with potential of cord transection), narcotics may be necessary, with reliance on naloxone (Narcan) to reverse any excess effect of the narcotic. See *44, Head Injuries*, for further treatment measures.

37–9. HEART FAILURE *(See 29–10, Congestive Heart Failure)*

37–10. HYPERVENTILATION (EMOTIONAL REACTION)

It is important to distinguish hyperventilation due to an emotional cause from organic hyperventilation due to underlying metabolic acidosis and hypoxemia. Severe emotional hyperventilation can cause a cyclic chain of physiologic events that causes a sincere belief of imminent demise. Initial reassurance is important, but protracted discussion of precipitating factors is best delayed till the hyperventilation is controlled. Muscle spasms and tingling occur.

Rebreathing into a paper bag held over the face or inhalations of carbogen by face mask and rebreathing bag usually will result in complete recovery in a short time. Calcium gluconate, 10 ml of 10% solution IV, may be added if prior measures are not effective after approximately 10 minutes.

In most cases, the signs and symptoms subside rapidly and the precipitating event (such as an acute situational reaction or phobia) can be assessed and follow-up measures advised as necessary. Prescription of a few days' amount of diazepam (Valium) may be appropriate. Preferably, the patient can be sent home with a member of the family. If the history suggests an acute exacerbation of chronic mental distress as a causative factor, psychiatric evaluation should be recommended.

37–11. INFECTIONS

Although infrequently an important contributory cause in adults, acute infections are a frequent cause of excitement states in infants and children. Treatment is principally directed at eradicating the offending organism and providing supportive care. In all age groups the rapid development of irritability, confusion and then delirium associated with fever should prompt testing for bacterial meningitis *(33–40)*; also consider toxic drug reactions.

37–12. MANIC STATES *(See also 54–17, Psychoses; 54–21, Violent Behavior)*

During the excitement stage physical restraint may be necessary until control possibly by adequate doses of parenteral chlorpromazine (Thorazine), 25 to 100 mg, or haloperidol (Haldol), 2.5 to 5 mg, or diazepam (Valium), IM or IV, has been accomplished. An attendant must be with the patient at all times until transfer for psychiatric evaluation and care has been completed. No patient who shows evidence of an actual or impending excitement state should ever be left alone. Users of phencyclidine (PCP or Angel Dust, 53–532) are particularly prone to unpredictable violent activity.

37–13. PHENOTHIAZINE EXTRAPYRAMIDAL REACTIONS *(See also 53–536)*

Idiosyncratic reaction to phenothiazine drugs is relatively common, especially in children and elderly persons. Rapid subsiding of the acute excitement state usually occurs as the offending medication is metabolized or counteracted (as with antihistamines and antiparkinson drugs).

37–14. PHOBIAS

This type of generally covert neurosis comes to clinical attention most commonly when the patient's inability to avoid the terrifying stimulus results in an acute excitement state. Significant alterations of judgment, thought content and insight are present, but not delusions or hallucinations. The immediate terror may be closely followed by feelings of depression and thoughts of suicide. Hyperventilation *(37–10)* and panic are common in this unique type of situational reaction *(54–3)*. Removal of the patient from the specific stimulus, stabilization, calm discussion of the dreaded object or social situation, reassurance and *later* psychiatric treatment for the deeply rooted unconscious anxiety and any other associated problems are usually adequate approaches. When phobias are combined with depression, administration of a tricyclic antidepressant such as imipramine, 25 to 50 mg tid, may help. Especially with patients with agoraphobia (literally fear of the marketplace but generally fear of any outside social contact), it is necessary to check that they are getting follow-up care.

37–15. THYROTOXICOSIS (Thyroid Storm) *(See 36–11, Hyperthyroid Emergencies, and 53–706, Thyroid)*

38. Eye Conditions

An estimate of the vision of each eye should be recorded in the patient's record before further examination is performed for any eye condition. Vision should be tested if possible by the Snellen or Jaeger test charts; if these charts are not available, finger counting, perception or reading tests are satisfactory. Visual fields may be checked grossly by confrontation test or with a wall chart. Test for increased intraocular pressure with a sterile tonometer *(18–15)*. The "swinging flashlight" test detects pupillary escape.

To prevent further damage during examination, the eye should be stabilized by holding the elevated upper lid against the supraorbital rim with the thumb or index finger. Fluorescein solution (Fluress) should be used to stain the corneal surface in order to outline, locate and evaluate corneal defects. Indirect lighting (or the use of a slit lamp) is essential. Samples of any discharge or excessive secretion should be cultured and stained.

Local medication (antibiotics and so forth) should be in the form of ophthalmic drops, not ointments. If an eye patch is indicated (Fig. 35–1), it should fit snugly.

General precautions in treatment include avoiding the following:

- Topical anesthetics (use during emergency room diagnosis procedure only).
- Topical corticosteroids singly or in combination.
- Prolonged-acting dilating drops, such as atropine. Preferably, use cautiously a shorter duration dilator, such as 2% or 5% homatropine, and do not use if patient has or may have glaucoma or narrow angles.
- Do not use ointments in the eye until you have made a diagnosis (or an ophthalmologist has done so). Weigh use of medications affecting pupillary response while neurologic evaluation is in progress.

See *38–40* for differential diagnosis of the inflamed eye ("red eye") and *38–41* for differential diagnosis of sudden vision loss.

NONTRAUMATIC EYE CONDITIONS

38–1. ANGIOEDEMA *(See also 24, Allergic Reactions)*

Treatment

- Apply cold compresses.
- Inject epinephrine hydrochloride (Adrenalin) (1:1000 solution), 0.5 to 1 ml SC; repeat in ½ hour if necessary.
- Prescribe tripelennamine hydrochloride (PBZ), 25 mg PO mouth, every 4 hours, or hydroxyzine hydrochloride (Atarax).
- Refer to an ophthalmologist if the condition persists.

38–2. BLEPHARITIS

Treatment

- Examine for and remove ingrowing or turned under eyelashes.
- Cleanse the lids and remove scales from the eyelashes.
- Prescribe antibiotic eye drops and, at night, ointment.
- Refer to an ophthalmologist if marked irritation is not lessening or is still present after 7 to 10 days.

38–3. CHALAZION

Begin intermittent warm moist compresses plus antibiotic drops (day) and ointment (at bedtime). Refer to an ophthalmologist if condition is not markedly improved after 3 weeks.

38–4. CHOROIDITIS

This condition causes no pain, but patient may present with acute visual loss and should be referred immediately to an ophthalmologist.

38–5. CONJUNCTIVITIS *(See also 38–40, Differential Diagnosis Chart)*

Treatment

- Clean eyelid edges thoroughly and frequently.
- Instill sodium sulfacetamide drops (10%) every 2 to 6 hours during the day; apply an antibiotic ointment at night.
- Prescribe warm compresses 2 to 3 times a day.
- Instruct the patient to consult an ophthalmologist if condition is not improving or is still present after 4 to 7 days.

38–6. CORNEAL ABRASIONS *(See also 38–32, Injuries to the Cornea; 38–40, Differential Diagnosis Chart, Keratitis)*

Treatment

- Determine the extent of the abrasion by staining with fluorescein, using a strip or individual sterile ampules.
- Give emergency treatment as outlined for keratitis (*38–20*).
- Instruct every patient with a corneal abrasion to report to an ophthalmologist if not healed with normal vision and comfort in 48 hours; deep abrasions should be checked sooner.

38–7. DACRYOCYSTITIS

Treatment

- *Acute:* Apply frequent hot compresses and give local and systemic broad-spectrum antibiotics; refer to an ophthalmologist if pain and tenderness are severe.
- *Chronic:* No emergency treatment is necessary. Evaluation by an ophthalmologist should be recommended.

38–8. ECTROPION (Eversion of Lid)

Tearing may occur. No emergency treatment is needed unless exposure keratitis is occurring (see *38–20* for treatment). The patient should be advised to consult an ophthalmologist.

38–9. EDEMA OF THE EYELIDS

Inflammatory (from styes, dacryocystitis, sinusitis, etc.). Apply warm compresses frequently. Control pain *(12)* as necessary. Refer for determination and treatment of the underlying cause.

Systemic (renal or cardiac). No emergency treatment is needed. The importance of complete investigation of the cause should be stressed to the patient.

Allergic. Usually due to some type of local application or medication (mascara, eye shadow, lash curlers and dyes, eye drops, ophthalmic ointments, etc.). Recovery is usually rapid after use of the offending substance is stopped.

38–10. EMPHYSEMA OF THE LIDS

Crepitus from air in the soft tissues generally means a fracture of the sinus wall if there is only focal involvement.

Treatment

- Apply a firm pressure bandage.
- Warn the patient against blowing his or her nose.
- Hospitalize immediately for head injury care.

38–11. ENTROPION (Inversion of Lid)

Treatment

- If corneal abrasion is present, see *38–20* for treatment.
- Hold the lid in proper position if possible by Scotch tape.
- Refer to an ophthalmologist for definitive treatment.

38–12. EVERSION OF THE EYELIDS *(See 38–8, Ectropion)*

38–13. GLAUCOMA *(See also 38–40, Differential Diagnosis Chart)*

Treatment

- Check intraocular tension of both eyes with sterile tonometer.
- Whenever examination indicates the possibility of increased, increasing (from prior examinations) or asymmetrically increased (greater than 5 mm Hg) intraocular tension, refer at once to an ophthalmologist.
- Rapid failure of sight, violent headache and severe ophthalmic pain, sometimes associated with nausea, vomiting and general depression, should suggest the possibility of acute angle closure glaucoma and call for immediate referral to and intervention by an ophthalmologist. Reduction of

intraocular pressure in acute angle closure may be directed by the ophthalmologist with pilocarpine and with oral and intravenous acetazolamide (Diamox), 500 mg (if no sulfa drug allergy is present), and glycerol, 1 to 1.5 g/kg PO, or mannitol, 1.5 to 2.0 g/kg IV, unless systemic osmotics are contraindicated. Restrict food ingestion in view of possible imminent surgical intervention.

38–14. HERPES

Herpes Simplex Keratitis (dendrite) (see also *33–29*). Immediate referral to an ophthalmologist if the condition is suspected or proved. Treatment with 5-iodo-2-deoxyuridine (IDU) or adenine arabinoside (Ara-A) under an ophthalmologist's direction may result in complete healing without vision loss.

Herpes Zoster Ophthalmicus. Vesicles to the tip of the nose are concomitant with nasociliary nerve involvement. Treatment is as follows:

- Control severe pain *(12)*.
- An eye patch (Fig. 38–1) is optional.
- Do NOT give steroids.
- Refer to an ophthalmologist for treatment at once.

38–15. HORDEOLUM *(See 38–24, Stye)*

38–16. INVERSION OF THE EYELASHES *(See 38–27, Trichiasis)*

38–17. INVERSION OF THE EYELIDS *(See 38–11, Entropion)*

38–18. IRIDOCYCLITIS *(See 38–19, Iritis; 38–40, Differential Diagnosis Chart)*

38–19. IRITIS (Iridocyclitis, Uveitis) *(See also 38–40, Differential Diagnosis Chart)*

Treatment

- Treat pain *(12)* with oral analgesics.
- Advise sunglasses to reduce light irritation.
- Arrange for immediate confirmation of diagnosis and treatment by an ophthalmologist, who will manage any cycloplegic or corticosteroid use.

38–20. KERATITIS *(See 38–40, Differential Diagnosis Chart)*

Treatment

- Examine thoroughly for and remove any foreign bodies.
- Use oral analgesics for relief of pain *(12)* as necessary.
- Use topical anesthetic drops for diagnosis only, not for treatment.
- An eye patch (Fig. 38–1) diminishes eyelid abrasion and aids comfort.
- Impress on the patient the need for immediate care by an ophthalmologist. Use of medium strength cycloplegics (e.g., 5% homatropine) may give the greatest relief.

38–21. PANOPHTHALMITIS AND ORBITAL CELLULITIS

Panophthalmitis is an acute inflammation (with an incubation period of a few hours) of all three coats of the eye and intraocular contents that, if not treated immediately and vigorously, may extend to cause widespread orbital cellulitis and be life threatening. Endophthalmitis is less fulminating and extensive than panophthalmitis, but treatment is similar. Onset of panophthalmitis may follow penetrating foreign bodies, global lacerations and bacteremia; orbital cellulitis may also occur as a result of extension from adjacent sinusitis.

Advanced stages are characterized by severe global tenderness and pain, redness, swelling, decreased ocular movement, fever and toxicity.

Cultures of blood, nasopharynx and any discharge (plus Gram stain) should be made, and unless an ophthalmologist is rapidly available—who will want to obtain a culture specimen from inside the eye prior to starting antibiotics—intravenous broad-spectrum antibiotics should be started immediately (see *33–83, Antimicrobial Drugs of Choice*). See also *Traumatic Eye Conditions, 38–29* to *38–38*. Hospitalize *at once* for care by an ophthalmologist.

38–22. PTERYGIUM

No emergency treatment is needed. Refer to an ophthalmologist.

38–23. SCLERITIS

Apply hot compresses and arrange for immediate care by an ophthalmologist.

38–24. STYE (Hordeolum)

Apply hot compresses for at least 20 minutes, 4 times daily. Prescribe 1% chlortetracycline (Aureomycin) ointment (at bedtime).

38–25. SYMBLEPHARON (Conjunctival Adhesions)

Refer to an ophthalmologist.

38–26. TRACHOMA

This very infectious conjunctivitis is caused by *Chlamydia trachomatis*, an obligate intracellular organism *(33–71)* that is spread by personal contact. It may cause severe scarring and (occasionally) blindness.

Treatment

- Tetracycline, 0.25 to 0.5 g q 6 h for 3 weeks.
- Tetracycline ophthalmic drops.
- Instruction regarding careful disposal of infected handkerchiefs, towels and so forth.
- Referral to an ophthalmologist.

38–27. TRICHIASIS (Inversion of Lashes)

If only a few lashes are inverted, they may be removed with cilia forceps. If multiple lashes are involved or if severe pain, lacrimation, photophobia or ulceration is present, the patient should be referred to an ophthalmologist.

38–28. UVEITIS *(See 38–19, Iritis; 38–40, Differential Diagnosis Chart)*

TRAUMATIC EYE CONDITIONS

In all cases of suspected eye injury, vision of each eye should be tested before detailed examination, by the Jaeger or Snellen chart method or by reading tests or finger visualization, and results recorded on the patient's chart. Check with glasses, if worn.

38–29. INJURIES TO THE CHOROID

Rupture of the choroid can be caused by a severe contusion of the eyeball. The diagnosis as a rule cannot be made on emergency examination, but suspicion of its presence requires immediate reference to an ophthalmologist.

Penetrating wounds may cause suppurative iridochoroiditis with exquisite pain, requiring codeine or morphine sulfate for relief. Hospitalization and care by an ophthalmologist should be arranged as soon as possible. Use an eye shield to protect against further injury.

38–30. INJURIES TO THE CILIARY BODY

Injuries of this area are in the so-called "danger zone" of the eye and not infrequently result in sympathetic ophthalmia (*38–38*). Immediate reference to an ophthalmologist is indicated if an injury to the ciliary body is suspected.

38–31. INJURIES TO THE CONJUNCTIVA

Burns (see *53–746* for "tear gas"; see also *28–14*). Thorough yet gentle irrigation with copious amounts of tap water for 5 to 10 minutes with the eyelids held open is the only treatment needed in mild cases. Moderately severe cases require cold or iced compresses and application of antibiotic ophthalmic drops after thorough irrigation. No attempt should be made to irrigate with a neutralizing solution. To adequately remove substances causing chemical burn, especially when there is particle or powder substance, it is necessary to inspect and irrigate far back under the upper lid (fornix) using a lid speculum or Desmarres retractor. Use a Luer-Lok syringe if applying irrigating stream through a needle (though streams through needles are not preferred). Copious irrigation is advised using an irrigating contact lens, if available, attached to a liter of normal saline or other ocular irrigating solution. An eye patch may be applied and arrangements made for the patient to consult an ophthalmologist within 24 hours. Severe cases, especially electrical, acid or alkali burns, require immediate referral to an ophthalmologist. A medium strength cycloplegic, such as 5% homatropine, can help relieve pain. Have the patient avoid rubbing the eye.

Foreign Bodies. Many foreign bodies are found lying on the inner surface of the upper lid and can be removed with or without 0.50% tetracaine hydrochloride (Pontocaine) anesthesia by turning back the lid (Fig. 38–2) and brushing with a cotton applicator dampened with saline. If acute conjunctivitis or corneal irritation is present, antibiotic ophthalmic drops should be prescribed. If an abrasion is present, recheck examination by an ophthalmologist should be arranged in 2 days.

With even suspicion of a penetrating injury by examination, history or both, x-rays of the orbit with soft tissue views of the anterior chamber and a Waters' view should be ordered.

Injuries Caused by Intense Light (Welder's Flash, Ultraviolet Lamp Burn, Photophthalmia). (See also *28–15, Flash Burns*). Patients' stories are often inaccurate; therefore, a thorough search should be made for foreign bodies in the conjunctival sac, under the lids and on the cornea before a diagnosis of photophthalmia is made. If none is found and the history is indicative of a "flash," the following routine should be used:

1. Apply intermittent cold (preferably iced) compresses for 5 minutes.
2. Dilate pupil with 2% or 5% homatropine for relief of intense pain and photophobia (also, sunglasses are an aid).
3. Instill artificial tear solution (e.g., Tears Naturale) periodically, as needed.

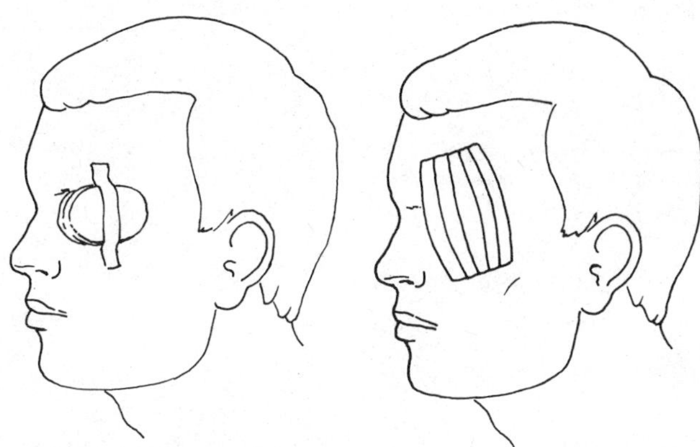

Figure 38–1. Application of an eye patch.

4. Instruct the patient to apply cold or iced compresses periodically and to arrange for further medical care in 24 hours if acute discomfort persists.

Lacerations. No attempt should be made to suture cuts in the surface of the conjunctiva. A sterile eye patch should be applied (Fig. 38–1) and the patient referred at once to an ophthalmologist.

38–32. INJURIES TO THE CORNEA

Burns. If corneal burns are small and superficial, treatment is the same as for conjunctival burns *(38–31)*; if extensive or deep, immediate care by an ophthalmologist is essential (a dilator, such as 2% homatropine, may relieve pain of secondary iritis/uveitis).

Contusions. Usually caused by some blunt object, contusions as a rule clear spontaneously (and slowly) without treatment. Internal bleeding and dislocation of the lens require immediate care by an ophthalmologist.

Foreign Bodies

1. A history of any object striking the eye makes a thorough search for foreign bodies mandatory. Fluorescein (1 or 2%) is harmless and should be used to demonstrate breaks in the external layers of the cornea. The eye should be irrigated thoroughly after examination. A fresh solution of fluorescein should always be used, preferably from individual-dose sterile ampules. Fluorescein-impregnated strips are satisfactory. Exact localization of embedded or intraocular radiopaque foreign bodies can often be obtained by special radiologic techniques (soft tissue anterior chamber and Waters' view).

2. Foreign bodies on or embedded superficially in the cornea may be removed with the patient under 0.50% tetracaine hydrochloride (Pontocaine) anesthesia, using a damp cotton applicator or an eye spud (Fig. 38–2) under magnification. An excellent eye spud can be improvised from a short-bevel 25-gauge needle. Removal of any residual rust ring requires referral to an ophthalmologist and should not be attempted as emergency treatment.

3. No attempt should be made to remove deeply embedded foreign bodies as an emergency measure. An eye patch is generally not used, as the pressure of the pad might cause further penetration. The patient should be referred at once to an ophthalmologist.

4. An electromagnet should never be used except under the direction of an ophthalmologist.

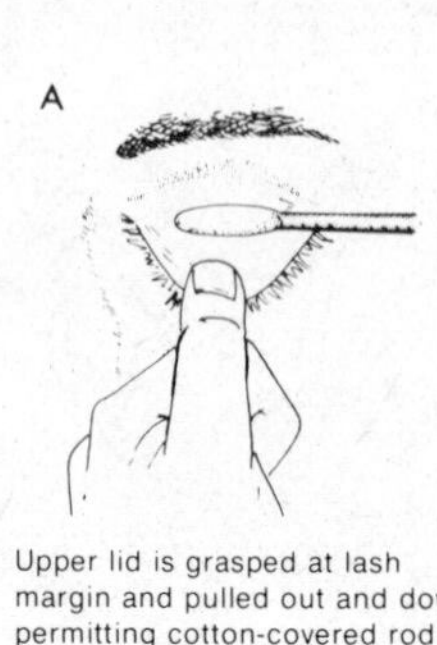

Upper lid is grasped at lash margin and pulled out and down, permitting cotton-covered rod to be placed above the tarsal fold

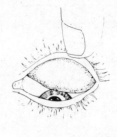

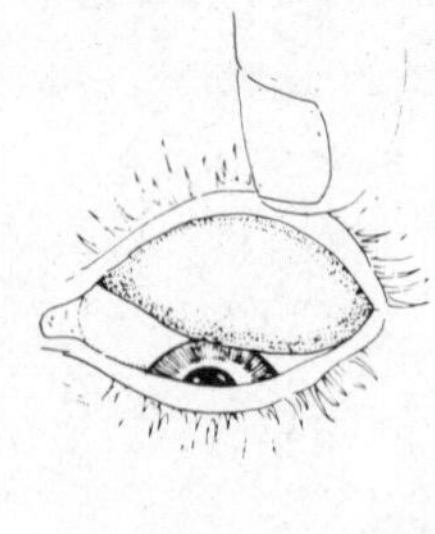

With the lid everted, a foreign body on the inside is exposed and may be wiped away

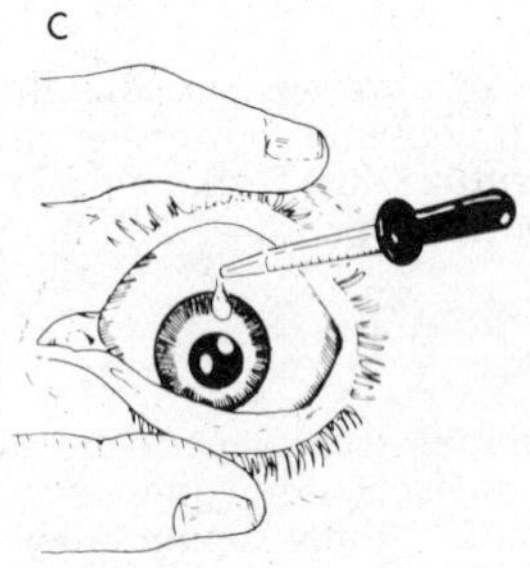

If the foreign body is on the cornea, topical anesthetic is instilled prior to removal by needle point or spud

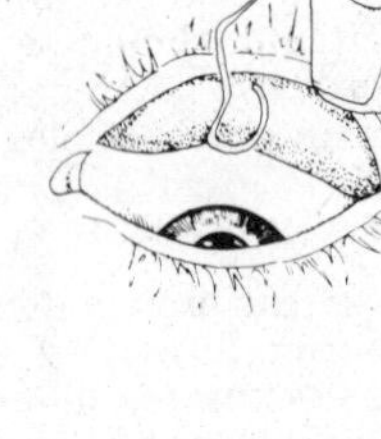

Double eversion for fornix exam is aided by Descemet's retractor or folded paper clip

Figure 38–2. Eversion of the eyelid for inspection and removal of foreign body. (Modified from Gordon, D. M.: Hosp. Med., 5:21, 1969.)

5. Defects (ulcers) of the cornea following removal of foreign bodies require application of 10% sulfacetamide (unless allergy exists) or 1% chlortetracycline (Aureomycin) eye ungt every 1 to 2 hours and referral to an ophthalmologist in 48 hours. Cycloplegic eye drops need not be used unless a definite indication (as for comfort) is present.

Wounds

SUPERFICIAL. These generally heal without complications, provided they are kept clean. The eye should be irrigated, after which antibiotic eye drops are instilled and an eye patch is applied.

PENETRATING. Immediate care by an ophthalmologist is mandatory. X-ray films should be taken to rule out or localize buried radiopaque foreign bodies.

38–33. INJURIES TO THE EYELIDS

Burns. Assume underlying conjunctival burn also (see *38–31*). Handle carefully.

Ecchymosis (Black Eye). Direct trauma in the region of the eyes severe enough to cause ecchymosis may also cause severe underlying injuries. The following conditions, which require immediate care by an ophthalmologist, should be ruled out:

- Lacerations of the cornea *(38–32)*.
- Fracture of the orbital wall (see *38–10, Emphysema of the Lids; 38–35, Injuries to the Orbit*). Special x-rays, including Waters' views, usually are necessary.
- Detachment of the retina, partial or complete (see *38–36, Injuries to the Retina*).

Treatment of ecchymosis consists of cold compresses for 24 hours, followed by hot compresses. If a fracture is suspected from clinical or x-ray examination, the patient should be hospitalized for observation and treatment.

Insect Bites (see also *24, Allergic Reactions; 27, Bites; 60, Stings*). Cold compresses are indicated for control of swelling, which may be extreme. Antihistaminics may be of value.

Lacerations. Because loss of tissues of the eyelids may result in ectropion *(38–8)* or entropion *(38–11)*, lacerations in this area should be thoroughly irrigated but not debrided before suturing. Antibiotics and tetanus-immune globulin (TIG) or toxoid *(20)* should be given if gross contamination is present.

Especially in vertical lacerations, suturing should be done with great care in order to prevent contractures. If the laceration extends through the eyelid, careful examination for damage to the eyeball should be made before suturing; this type of suturing is best done in layers with microscopic technique by an ophthalmologist (Fig. 38–3). If a through-and-through laceration is jagged or extensive, or if there is avulsion or loss of tissue, a sterile bandage should be applied and the patient hospitalized at once for operative repair and possible skin grafting.

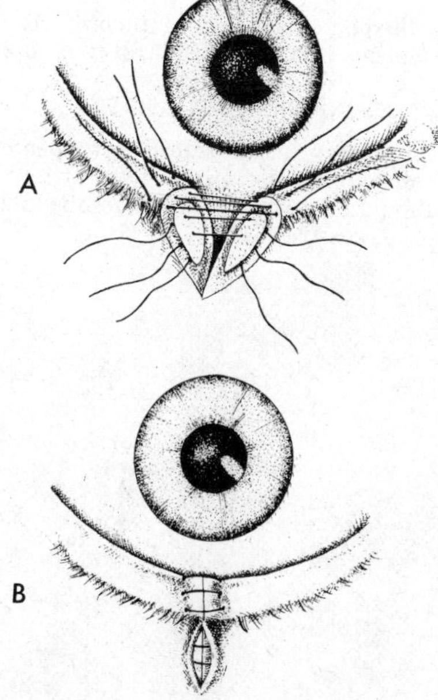

Figure 38–3. A technique of eyelid laceration repair that is best done by an ophthalmologist utilizing the operating microscope.

38–34. INJURIES TO THE IRIS

Nonpenetrating. Concussion with subsequent traumatic mydriasis is the most frequent cause. Apply an eye patch and refer to an ophthalmologist.

Penetrating. This condition calls for application of a metal eye shield and immediate referral to an ophthalmologist for care.

38–35. INJURIES TO THE ORBIT *(See also 44, Head Injuries)*

If injury to the orbit is suspected from clinical or x-ray examination, immediate ophthalmologist referral is indicated. Fractures of the margins or floor of the orbit require surgical repair to avoid impaired vision.

Protect the traumatized eye with an eye shield (cone-shaped) during transportation. If there are unstable orbital fractures through the sinuses (check for crepitus) and transportation must be by air ambulance, use a plane with a well-pressurized cabin or fly at low elevations, as retrobulbal gas expansion may cause global extrusion.

If, after severe orbital injury, global penetration or a combination of the two, the patient experiences pain and straining on trying to lift the lids (owing to increased extrusion of the eyeball due to increased intraglobal pressure), this can be relieved by causing temporary paralysis of the lid muscles with a lidocaine block of the facial nerve.

If, following a blow-out fracture, in addition to the lid droop and enophthalmos, there is decreased ocular movement, to determine if this is due to nerve or muscle injury, some combination of the two or mechanical entrapment, a forced duction test may be necessary; this is preferably done by the consulting ophthalmologist.

38–36. INJURIES TO THE RETINA *(See also 38–41, Differential Diagnosis of Sudden or Rapid Vision Loss)*

Suspected or proved incomplete or complete detachment of the retina requires immediate referral to an ophthalmologist.

38–37. INJURIES TO THE SCLERA

If injury to the sclera is suspected, the patient should be referred to an ophthalmologist *without delay* for examination and treatment. X-ray films should be taken to rule out embedded radiopaque foreign bodies if the history is suggestive (38–32).

38–38. SYMPATHETIC OPHTHALMIA

This extremely serious condition practically never occurs unless there has been a penetrating injury of the opposite eye at some time in the past. Recognition in the stage of sympathetic irritation may result in preventing total blindness. The usual signs and symptoms of this stage are marked photophobia and lacrimation, with dimness of close vision, bizarre bright and colored sensations and neuralgic pain in and around the eye.

Any person with a history of a perforating injury to an eye at any time in the past who complains of any of the signs and symptoms just listed in the uninjured eye should be referred immediately to an ophthalmologist.

CONTACT LENS REMOVAL AND DIFFERENTIAL DIAGNOSIS

38–39. REMOVAL OF CONTACT LENSES

Modern contact lenses are made of plastic and are of two types:

- *"Hard."* These cover the cornea only and measure 8 to 9 mm in diameter. These lenses usually can be identified by reflection from an edge on lateral illumination.
- *"Soft."* These extend onto the conjunctiva; usually they are 12 to 14 mm in diameter.

Removal may be necessary in an emergency situation, since either type may cause serious irritation if retained for more than 12 hours.

Methods of Removal

- *Irrigation.* With the patient supine and the head turned toward the side to be irrigated, float the lens out by gentle lavage with normal saline solution, using a soft-tipped rubber bulb syringe.
- *Suction.* With the eyelids separated, press a small suction cup designed for the purpose against the middle of a hard lens and lift it out.
- *Pinching* (soft lens only). With the eyelids separated, pinch the lens out by gentle pressure between the thumb and forefinger. Place the removed lenses in normal saline solution at once to prevent dehydration and shriveling.

38–40. DIFFERENTIAL DIAGNOSIS OF THE INFLAMED EYE ("RED EYE") *(See table on page 294)*

38–41. DIFFERENTIAL DIAGNOSIS OF SUDDEN OR RAPID VISION LOSS

Condition	Ocular Pain	Visual Perception Defect	Other Findings	Treatment *In all cases:* *a. Check intraocular pressure.* *b. Referral to an ophthalmogist.*
Acute angle closure glaucoma	Usually severe.	Unilateral to bilateral involvement. "Blurred," "cloudy," "filmy," or "smoky" loss of acuity.	Elevated intraocular pressure and generally, but not always, inflammation. Abdominal pain may occur. See also *38–40, Differential Diagnosis of the Inflamed Eye ("Red Eye")* and *38–13, Glaucoma.*	See *38–13, Glaucoma.*
Central retinal artery occlusion	No	Almost always unilateral. Only light perception if central; segmental vision if a branch. Onset very sudden.	The pupil responds sluggishly to light, if at all. The fundus is pale, the retinal arteries narrow and the macula a cherry red.	Inhalation of 5% CO_2 with 95% O_2 or rebreathing into bag. Acetylsalicylic acid, 0.3 g orally Glycerol administration, 1 ml/kg PO, or acetazolamide, 500 mg IV or IM. Judicious firm ocular pressure for 5 seconds if embolus suspected to "distalize" embolus. Ophthalmologist may perform anterior chamber paracentesis, retrobulbar tolazoline injection.
Central retinal vein occlusion	No	Almost always unilateral, general gross decrease in acuity. Onset very sudden.	The optic disc is swollen, the retinal veins are dilated and tortuous and there are many hemorrhages in the fundus.	Treat any associated glaucoma. Acetylsalicylic acid, 0.3 g orally to decrease platelet stickiness. Treat any underlying diseases.
Intracranial disease	No	Unilateral distal to optic chiasm; homonymous hemianopsia proximal.	Headache, signs of cerebral edema including occasional papilledema, other focalizing neurologic deficits. See also 63, *Vascular Disorders.*	*See 63, Vascular Disorders,* with regard to indications for neurosurgical referral.

Migraine	Usually no	Generally bilateral blurring of vision with zigzag lines.	The visual changes usually occur before any headache. Ophthalmic examination is normal. See *30–22, Migraine*.	See *30–22, Migraine*.
Nonorganic vision loss (hysteria or malingering)	Varies, usually no	More often unilateral blindness, may have "tunnel vision."	See *54–12, Hysteria*. Physical examination of anatomical parts of eye is normal. Responses inconsistent and physiologically incompatible with the stated problem are cardinal signs of the diagnosis.	See *54–12, Hysteria*. Remember the hysteric perceives the interpretation as real, while the malingerer knows the interpretation is a sham.
Retinal detachment	Generally no	Almost always unilateral. Segmental to complete loss.	Early, it may be difficult to see change; later, elevation and floating appearance of the retina are found. May see "film," "cloud," or "flashes of light."	Referral to ophthalmologist immediately. Preferred position of rest will place the detached retina in the most dependent location.
Retrobulbar or optic neuritis	Yes, plus light sensitivity	Usually bilateral central scotomata. Decrease in red color perception varies.	Optic disc swelling and hemorrhage may be present. Positive response to "swinging flashlight" test (Marcus-Gunn pupil).	See ophthalmologist or neurologist.
Trauma	Yes	Unilateral or bilateral. Degree of loss varies.	Loss varies from slight and temporary to complete and permanent and depends on severity of trauma and areas affected.	See *38–30* to *38–38, Traumatic Eye Conditions*. Immediate attention of an ophthalmologist is needed.
Vitreous hemorrhage	Generally no	Almost always unilateral, clouded vision.	Maroon appearance of vitreous and obliteration of fundus with severe hemorrhage; reddish cellular ground-glass appearance with less severe hemorrhage.	Treat increased intraocular pressure, if present. Treat any coagulation defects and other underlying causes. Avoid acetylsalicylic acid.

38–40. DIFFERENTIAL DIAGNOSIS OF THE INFLAMED EYE ("RED EYE")*

Fluorescein stain *ALL* "red eyes" for examination. Look for foreign bodies.

	Pan-ophthalmitis	Acute Glaucoma	Acute Uveitis	Keratitis and Corneal Ulcer	Conjunctivitis†
SIGNS					
Limbal flush	+++	+	++	+++	0
Conjunctival injection	+++	++ to +++	++	++	+ to +++(B)
Corneal haze	0 to +++	+++	0	+ to +++	0
Pupil abnormality	0 to +++	semidilated; ↓ reaction	small irreg. ↓ reaction	0 to small	0
Anterior chamber depth	N to ↓	↓	N	N	N
Intraocular pressure	N to ↑	↑	N to ↓	N	N
Discharge	0 to +++ bacteria	0	0	0 to +	+ to +++ (B)
SYMPTOMS Vision	N to ↓	↓ blurred	↓ blurred	↓ blurred	N
Eye pain	+ to +++	0 to +++	++ to +++	++	0
Photophobia	0 to +	0 to +	+++	+++	0 to +++ (V)
Halo	0	0 to +++	0	0	0
Itching	0	0	0	0	0 to ++ (A)
Headache	+ to +++	often, severe	often	0 to +	0
Nausea	±/toxic	often, severe	may occur	0	0

*Ruled-in areas: Serious signs and symptoms requiring immediate ophthalmologist attention.

†Types of conjunctivitis: allergic (A), bacterial (B), viral (V), including measles. N = normal range; O = absent.

39. Foreign Bodies (FB)

39–1. GENERAL CONSIDERATIONS

- Pain, obstruction, perforation, secondary infection and history (often of sudden loss of small objects or actual witnessing of a child swallowing or inserting something) are the common indications of the presence of a foreign body (FB).
- Unless actual obstruction or perforation is present (or there is imminent danger thereof), or the FB is inherently toxic, an ultra-urgent situation usually does not exist.
- Prudent rate of removal is indicated to minimize later inflammation, infection, perforation, hemorrhage, toxicity, interference with function and circulation compromise (e.g., by direct pressure, or "tourniquet syndrome").
- The removal approach should be the one that is most likely to succeed while causing the least additional physical damage and emotional distress. In some cases in which the removal of the foreign body would cause considerable trauma, whereas its presence would be relatively inconsequential (as with stray buckshot, for example), the foreign body may be left in place.
- The overall categories of removal approaches most commonly effective are as follows: • irrigation • suction • cotton applicator with or without adhesive substance • pull of gravity • mechanical jarring loose (as with a concussive slap on the back—to be done with caution, as this maneuver may turn a partial into a complete airway obstruction • compressed air expulsion (cough, sneeze, Heimlich maneuver) • magnetic extraction • surgical extraction using a spud or scalpel • digital, forceps or snare grasp or lifting • attraction of live insects with light • reduction in size as by irrigation, snipping (as with rongeurs), proteolytic enzymes for meats (caution: these digest mucosa also!) • lubricants and edema reduction to aid slipping off, or cutting to remove constrictive bands over appendages (especially digits and genitalia).
- The method used depends on the site, substance (including toxicity) and degree of penetration of the foreign body, as well as the degree of immediate difficulty and danger to the patient.
- X-rays, including use of soft tissue technique, skin markers and radiocontrast material, may aid localization. Metals, lead-base paint, and most types of glass show up well on x-ray. Detection of wood, grease and non-lead paint is aided by xeroradiography. Location of nonradiopaque substances is also assisted by ultrasonography, CT scan, and direct visualization by fiberoptic scopes. Swelling, presence of free air and fluid levels help localization also. Fluoroscopic control can be used to locate and remove radiopaque objects; it is important not to open the hemostat for grasping until it is touching and moving the foreign body, to avoid soft tissue injury.
- Caution should be exercised in evaluation, since nonradiopaque substances may be introduced along with obvious radiopaque foreign bodies.
- Operating room exploration and removal is generally preferred over removal in the office, field or ED if the foreign body (a) is not visible or cannot be located and removed readily under direct visualization; (b) is associated with other injuries that will require treatment in the OR; (c) requires exposure incisions for detection and repair (e.g., for occult or extensive lesions as from paint spray guns or when an object is impaled through vital tissue). See also *39–8*.

- The age and emotional state of the patient, as well as the circumstances surrounding the occurrence of the foreign body, are factors that are to be considered in determining the need for sedation (even anesthesia) and bodily control preparatory to removal of the object and counseling afterwards.

39–2. IN THE EARS

Examine with an otoscope. Avoid pushing the foreign body in deeper. Children frightened from previous attempts at removal often require sedation by a pentobarbital sodium (Nembutal) suppository or diazepam (Valium) before examination. If superficial, and if swelling of the wall of the external auditory meatus has not resulted from previous attempts at removal (usually at home), most foreign bodies can be removed with forceps or a plastic suction tip or by carefully inserting a curved probe behind the object and gently working it outward. Gravity may help. Dry, firm foreign bodies can sometimes be removed by pressing a cotton applicator tip moistened with collodion against the surface, holding it till the foreign body is sticky, then withdrawing it.

Substances that will not absorb moisture can sometimes be removed by syringing with a saline or soda solution and suctioning. A ceruminolytic agent (Cerumenex Drops) will soften cerumen and some other firm substances prior to irrigation. Do not attempt irrigation for beans, peas, candy, etc.; absorption of moisture and subsequent swelling can cause serious and permanent damage. Do not irrigate if there is suspicion or evidence of drum perforation.

Foxtails can usually be removed with forceps without difficulty. A few drops of any glycerin or petrolatum base ear drops instilled into the ear usually will result in immediate relief of discomfort, and spontaneous evacuation may occur if the patient sleeps with the affected ear against the pillow.

Hot slag particles usually are loose in the canal and can be removed with a cotton applicator. If particles are firmly adherent to the drum or if there is evidence of severe drum damage, treatment by an otolaryngologist should be arranged.

Insects alive and buzzing in the external auditory canal will often fly or crawl out toward a flashlight held close to the external auditory meatus. If this maneuver is unsuccessful, removal by syringing may be necessary.

Referral to an otolaryngologist generally is required if there is damage to or perforation of the drum, if the foreign body cannot be removed on 1 or 2 gentle attempts or if the cooperation of the patient cannot be obtained.

39–3. IN THE EYES *(See 38–31, Injuries to the Conjunctiva; 38–32, Injuries to the Cornea; 38–38, Sympathetic Ophthalmia; and 38–40, Differential Diagnosis Chart)*

39–4. IN THE NOSE

Foreign bodies in the nose are frequently encountered in small children; often, the person giving emergency care cannot obtain sufficient cooperation to permit removal of the object with forceps, a small wire probe or an ear curette with the tip bent into a scoop. A rapid irrigation of body-temperature sterile water or saline through the uninvolved nostril will flush water anteriorly through the involved nostril (which should be in the down and dependent position) to dislodge the foreign body. Sedation by means of a pentobarbital sodium (Nembutal) suppository or diazepam (Valium) may be tried; however, if the child struggles or resists examination, assistance of an anesthesiologist should be considered. If necessary, postponement until care by an otolaryngologist can be arranged will result in no danger to the patient.

In some instances, foreign bodies will be expelled from the nares in infants and small children by sneezing. Small children will sometimes sneeze if a puff of cigarette smoke is blown suddenly against the nose while the mouth is kept covered. An alternative method consists of blowing into the child's mouth with the uninvolved nostril closed by pinching. Preliminary shrinking of membranes with a sympathomimetic nasal decongestant (Neo-Synephrine) may be helpful. If considerable instrumentation is expected, a topical anesthetic, such as 4% cocaine, is advisable.

39–5. IN THE THROAT

If the child is cooperative, removal of small sharp objects (fish bones, splinters, sucker sticks, toy arrows, etc.) imbedded in the gums, hard palate, posterior nasopharynx or tonsillar fossae may be possible. In some cases, particularly after unsuccessful attempts at removal at home, a general anesthetic is necessary.

Retroflexion (rather than "swallowing") of the tongue may occur following severe direct trauma to the head or face, during convulsions or while the patient is in coma, causing blockage of the posterior pharyngeal airway. Treatment consists of supporting the jaw and pulling the tongue back into normal position by whatever means (e.g., tongue blade, hemostat, towel clip) are available (it is difficult to do this manually, without instruments, even in a small child). Sliding gauze around the tongue helps in grasping and pulling. If these measures are unsuccessful and the airway is severely blocked, cricothyroid puncture (*5–19*) must be done immediately.

39–6. IN THE LARYNX, TRACHEA OR BRONCHI *(See also Table 5–3, Guide to Localization of Airway Obstruction)*

If a patient has cyanosis, air hunger and absence of coughing and airway exchange, immediate action is required as a lifesaving measure. If the patient is markedly cyanotic or moribund, the following procedures should be done without hesitation:

1. Have the parents, relatives or friends clear the area unless their assistance is needed.
2. Attempt dislodgment of the foreign body by abdominal thrust (*Heimlich maneuver, 5–13*), interscapular back blow or both if there is complete airway obstruction or nearly complete obstruction with severe distress. Caution in use of external concussion must be exercised, as a partial obstruction may be changed into a total obstruction with further motion of the foreign body by this maneuver—if the condition is stable and enough air is getting in and out, maintain that status until technically prepared to handle all eventualities. If this procedure does not result in increased airway flow, an emergency cricothyroid puncture (*5–19*) or tracheostomy (*18–34*) must be considered.
3. Administer oxygen by bag-valve-mask or through the tracheostomy tube.

If signs and symptoms of irritation or obstruction are less severe and the patient has airway patency and is able to cough, do not attempt maneuvers outside the hospital to clear the airway. Have the patient sit or stand during transport to the hospital; these patients should not lie down or bend over unless they have already achieved comfort thereby. X-ray of the chest (AP and lateral views, both inspiratory and expiratory) should be taken after examination of the posterior pharynx. If a radiopaque foreign body is lodged in the trachea, its greater surface will appear in the lateral film; if it is in the esophagus, the anteroposterior film will show the greater width. Small pointed or irregularly shaped nonradiopaque foreign bodies can sometimes be demonstrated by x-ray films taken after the patient has swallowed a small cotton pledget saturated with contrast medium.

Foreign bodies lodged in the larynx that cannot be located with a laryngoscope and removed with long forceps require that the patient be transferred to a hospital as soon as possible in the sitting or semi-prone position or the position that affords the best air exchange. If the airway obstruction is severe an endotracheal tube should be inserted, unless supraglottic obstruction is present, in which case an emergency cricothyroid puncture or tracheostomy should be done before transporting the patient. Under any circumstances, the patient should be closely attended during transporation.

Patients with bronchial foreign bodies require immediate hospitalization for bronchoscopic examination, localization and removal. Emphysema, caused by the ball-valve action of the foreign body, and aspiration pneumonia may develop if the obstruction is not removed. Peanuts are especially dangerous because they contain the absorbable alkaloid arachidic acid.

39–7. IN THE ESOPHAGUS, STOMACH AND GASTROINTESTINAL TRACT

Ingestion or insertion of multiple foreign bodies may be seen in children and sometimes in adults. X-rays of the GI tract from the nasopharynx to the anus provide the most comprehensive information. Although radiopaque flat foreign bodies are most often oriented in the frontal plane of the chest film when in the esophagus and in the sagittal plane when in the trachea, both AP and lateral chest views should be obtained. Toxic effects may follow GI intake of certain foreign bodies (e.g., disc battery, ruptured narcotic-filled balloons).

In the Esophagus

Presenting signs and symptoms are usually pain and discomfort in the throat or chest, inability to swallow well and choking on saliva and ingested fluids. In small children, in addition to reduced appetite, respiratory tract problems of cough, wheezing and pulmonary infection may develop with associated fever. Large esophageal foreign bodies can cause indentation of the posterior tracheal wall and cause partial airway obstruction.

Treatment

- Foreign bodies in the oropharynx and hypopharynx can generally be visualized and removed under direct vision. A lateral x-ray of the neck taken with a sandbag under the shoulders and the neck in hyperextension usually locates radiopaque esophageal foreign bodies. If not, fluoroscopy aided by a small swallow of meglumine diatrizoate preparation (Gastrografin) will aid detection of the size, shape and site of the foreign body. History from the patient or parents of small children also can aid in knowledge of the type of foreign body present.
- Hospitalize at once and give nothing by mouth if esophagoscopy is necessary and there is complete obstruction accompanied by regurgitation, coughing and choking.
- Partial obstruction by smaller smooth foreign bodies, and unaccompanied by regurgitation and choking, can often be relieved by passage into the stomach after ingesting a bolus of clear gelatin. While a meat tenderizer (such as Adolph's) aids breakdown of protein or meat foreign bodies, it also

breaks down the esophageal mucosa, and is therefore contraindicated, particularly when esophagoscopy is likely to be required.

- Meperidine hydrochloride (Demerol) or glucagon (0.05 mg/kg) may aid relaxation of muscle spasm, particularly for the cricopharyngeal area, permitting foreign body entry into the stomach.
- Smooth-edged foreign bodies can sometimes be removed from the esophagus by gently passing a No. 12 to 16 Foley urethral catheter with a 5-ml balloon beyond the obstruction (under sedation and fluoroscopic control, if necessary), inflating the reservoir within comfort and withdrawing the catheter gently with the foreign body in front of it. This technique can be hazardous, and endoscopy is usually a far superior approach.
- Clinical evidence of failure to progress in 12 to 14 hours, severe pain, respiratory distress, substantial obstruction or perforation (or likelihood of perforation) are indications for prompt hospitalization, nothing by mouth and consultation for removal.
- Disc battery ingestion presents special problems (see also following discussion on stomach). These batteries, when larger than 17 mm (dime-sized), are most likely to lodge in the esophagus. At present, these batteries are not adequately sealed, and their caustic alkaline contents can cause severe mucosal erosion. Immediate removal is necessary by esophagoscopy or by Foley catheter technique. *Do not* induce emesis in an attempt to dislodge these batteries. For special assistance and case reporting, call collect to the National Capital Poison Center (202-625-3333).

In the Stomach

If the object is small enough to pass through the esophagus into the stomach and does not have any extremely sharp points, it will generally pass through the small and large bowel without difficulty.

- Anteroposterior and lateral x-ray films of the abdomen should be made. Nonradiopaque foreign bodies in the stomach can sometimes be visualized by x-ray films taken immediately after the patient has swallowed a few ounces of a cold carbonated beverage. Any space-occupying object will cause a defect in the gas shadow caused by the released carbon dioxide.
- Bobby pins and needles in the stomach (or duodenum of children less than 2 years old) should be removed at once by adherence to a magnet passed orally by a person skilled in the technique.
- Patients with large open safety pins should be hospitalized immediately for consultation with an endoscopist and possible gastrotomy.
- Small open pins, large glass fragments, needles, straight pins and other sharp objects require close observation. They may pass through the intestinal tract safely or require endoscopic surgical removal.
- No changes in diet should be made and no laxatives or cathartics given.
- If careful screening of all stool specimens for 3 days indicates that the foreign body has not passed through the gastrointestinal tract, further x-ray studies should be made. Lack of progression and clinical evidence suggestive of perforation are indications for evaluation for gastroscopic or surgical removal of sharp objects or large rounded objects (usually more than 1 to 1½ inches in size) in children.
- Disc batteries in the stomach and distally do not present a mechanical problem, but their passage must be intermittently monitored to detect toxic effects of alkaline and mercury if rupture or leakage occurs (see also preceding discussion on esophagus).
  —Unhindered passage will probably occur.

—If the patient is well and the battery intact, give a cathartic and monitor stools; if the battery is not found, repeat x-ray in 5 to 7 days.
—If the battery is disintegrating, obtain blood and urine heavy metal levels (see *53–418, Mercury Poisoning*); repeat cathartic or give an enema if the battery is is in the lower GI tract.
—Failure to pass infrequently occurs, but necessitates surgery.

In the Intestine

Treatment

- Close observation is usually all that is required. Any object that will enter and leave the stomach will almost always go the rest of the way.
- Rectal foreign bodies, of course, may be introduced through the anus with much greater ease than removal once pain and sphincter spasm have resulted. Digital exam and anoscopic observation generally are adequate for assessment. A narcotic analgesic or even spinal anesthesia may be required to permit removal. If perforation has not occurred, removal can often be achieved through the anoscope using a grasping or hooking device. To reduce suction caused by pulling the object against an encompassing muscle spasm, it may help to lay a catheter alongside the foreign body to break the air seal.
- Severe pain, abdominal rigidity and clinical and x-ray signs of obstruction or perforation are indications for immediate hospitalization and evaluation for surgical intervention.

39–8. IN THE MUSCULOSKELETAL STRUCTURES

Whether the foreign bodies are wood (splinters), plastic (spicules of plastic toys), steel or other metals (industrial accidents, household and auto accidents, bullets, needles), dirt, gravel or rock (explosions, falls, auto accidents), glass (household injuries, auto accidents) or semisolid matter (graphite, grease), the general principles of treatment are the same:

- Careful cleansing and irrigation.
- Exploration to determine the extent of penetration. This should be done with great care under direct vision if possible and with extension of the entrance tract under local anesthetic if necessary. In the feet, a new incision in a non–weight-bearing area (distant from the weight-bearing entry site) may be preferred because of a less painful scar area.
- X-ray films (anteroposterior and lateral). Skin markers should be placed for reference before the films are taken if the presence of an easily overlooked radiopaque foreign body that cannot be located by direct vision or palpation is suspected.
- If the foreign body is superficial and easily accessible, it should be removed by splinter forceps or a pointed scalpel. The extent and depth can sometimes be silhouetted by placing a strong penlight or fiberoptic light against the folded adjacent skin after turning the room lights down. Deeper foreign bodies require sharp dissection and debridement, followed by thorough irrigation and primary closure if within 6 hours of injury; after a longer period, the wound should be debrided but should not, as a general rule, be sutured. See *59–22, Lacerations*.

Deeply embedded foreign bodies usually can be treated conservatively by tetanus-immune globulin (TiG) or toxoid (*20*), local treatment of point of entry, and observation. Antibiotic therapy may be indicated.

Musculoskeletal foreign bodies require hospitalization under the following circumstances:

- When there is severe or persistent bleeding that cannot be controlled by pressure.
- If the location of the foreign body or its point or course of entry, together with clinical examination, indicates perforation of the pleura, pericardium, peritoneum or viscera or vascular injury that may temporarily not be bleeding.
- If the foreign body lies within the skull.
- If there is evidence of severe or extensive bone damage.
- When evidence of nerve pressure or severance is present.
- If x-ray or clinical examinations indicate that the foreign body lies within a joint.

39–9. IN THE URETHRA *(See 41–9, Urethral Injuries)*

39–10. IN THE VAGINA *(See also 33–70, Toxic Shock Syndrome)*

- Retained pessaries, tampons, dislodged intrauterine contraceptive devices and so forth may require use of a speculum for localization and removal. Larger entrapped objects often require anesthesia for removal.
- Metallic or other objects inserted into the vagina or cervix in attempts to induce an abortion, for sexual excitement, or by intoxicated or criminally or mentally deranged persons require removal and counseling. A thorough examination to rule out perforation should be made. When examining young children, the mother as well as the nurse should be present, if possible.
- Institute rape *(14)* and/or child abuse protocol when indicated.

39–11. IN THE VENOUS SYSTEM

Runaway broken intravenous catheters (and occasionally intravenous needles) present a true emergency. (The best therapy, of course, is prevention, by ensuring that the catheter is firmly secured to the skin.) As soon as the condition is recognized, the following steps should be taken:

- Prevent any motion of the extremity.
- Apply a venous tourniquet proximal to the site of entry (upper arm usual).
- Take scout x-ray films. If the catheter is not radiopaque, a venogram should be done.
- Immediate removal of the foreign body by cutdown under local anesthetic if in an available site, usually in an extremity (frequently at anterior shoulder). If more central, immediate arrangements should be made for operative removal under general anesthesia; try to trap the catheter in or before the right heart. The patient can be placed with the head and upper trunk slightly lowered and in the left lateral decubitus position.

40. Gastrointestinal Emergencies*

40–1. GENERAL CONSIDERATIONS

The evaluation procedures in 22–2 (Diagnostic Aids in Acute Abdominal Pain) are also applicable to gastrointestinal emergencies. Table 22–2 helps to distinguish among some of the more common types of gastrointestinal disorders.

---

*See also 22–2, Diagnostic Aids in Distinguishing the Surgical from the Nonsurgical Abdomen.

40–2. INFECTION/INFLAMMATION

Infectious processes in the GI tract are usually heralded by fever, nausea, anorexia, variable vomiting, pain (varying from steady to cramping), abdominal tenderness with or without peritoneal inflammation, and primary or secondary alteration in bowel function. The initial location of the pain and subsequent associated developments aid diagnosis. The inflammatory process may be secondary to a bacterial or nonbacterial (e.g., viral, chemical) condition. The processes may affect the peritoneum, lymph nodes, solid organs (pancreas, liver, spleen) and hollow organs (stomach, gallbladder, small and large bowel), individually at first or in combination.

40–3. OBSTRUCTION

Nausea, anorexia and cramping or colicky abdominal pain are symptoms of intestinal obstruction of gradual onset. Repetitious, sometimes fecal, vomiting; abdominal distention with tympanitic percussion (if obstruction is lower); diffuse tenderness; high-pitched tinkling or absent bowel sounds; decreased elimination and progressive dehydration are the most common signs. Always check the rectum. Diagnostic aids include anteroposterior (AP) and upright abdominal x-rays (look for distention and air-fluid levels), barium enema, sigmoidoscopy, laparotomy and, on occasion, laparoscopy and ultrasonography.

Treatment is directed at correcting the primary cause and alleviating the pathophysiologic effects of progressive obstruction, which include decompression of bowel distention and replacement of fluid and electrolyte loss; strangulation, infection, perforation and peritonitis are treated with surgery and antibiotics.

Mechanical

Intraluminal

- Intussusception. Precipitous onset of signs and symptoms of intestinal obstruction (especially vomiting and colicky abdominal pain), usually in children less than 2 years of age, and rectal bleeding of currant jelly consistency are prime features of intussusception. Occasionally, the intussusception mass may be felt, often in the right upper quadrant. Referral is indicated for an immediate diagnostic barium enema, which also may be therapeutic in reducing the intussusception; if unsuccessful, surgical correction is necessary.
- Fecal impaction. If the patient is in acute discomfort from partial or complete obstruction and rectal examination demonstrates a mass of hard-packed feces producing gross rectal wall distention, an attempt may be made to remove the mass with the gloved finger. Efforts with enemas (including lactulose or oil retention) have usually not been productive when this extreme situation is present. In elderly women, posterior and downward digital pressure through the vagina may cause sufficient dilation of the sphincter ani to allow the impacted mass to pass. These procedures are usually very painful and often unsuccessful. Premedication, such as with rapid-acting barbiturates or pentazocine lactate (Talwin) or meperidine (Demerol), is advisable. Morphine sulfate and other opiates contract the sphincter ani and therefore are contraindicated. Hospitalization for general anesthesia may be necessary if an attempt at digital removal is unsuccessful or is too painful to be tolerated. In less severe cases in which obstruction is

not complete, the patient can be sent home with instructions regarding adequate water intake, activity, reduction of inhibiting drugs (e.g., narcotics), fecal softeners (e.g., lactulose, Doss), enemas and diet.

- Foreign bodies. See *39–7;* includes bezoars.
- Gallstones *(40–9, Cholecystitis).*
- Malignancies and polypoid tumors.
- Acquired strictures and congenital atresia or stenosis.

Extraluminal

- Adhesions, usually postoperative. These particularly affect the small bowel. Small bowel obstruction results initially in periodic cramping mid-abdominal pain that subsequently becomes steady and intense. Vomiting progresses from gastric contents and bile to fecal material if the obstruction is not too high. Abdominal distention is present, and there is increased peristalsis. Plain abdominal films show distended loops of bowel and gas-fluid levels; barium swallow should quickly outline the level of involvement. Nasogastric suction and fluid and electrolyte replacement *(11)* should be started pending operative correction.
- Anatomic defects *(40–6).*
- Hernia, incarcerated *(40–6).*
- Malignancies. See *40–5, Hemorrhage.*
- Abscesses.
- Volvulus *(40–23).*

Nonmechanical (Paralytic Ileus)

Nonmechanical obstruction may be the result of inflammation or chemical effect (enzymes, organisms, poisons, medications—especially those with parasympatholytic effect), or ischemia (mesenteric or vascular occlusion), or reflex action following surgery or trauma. Check for electrolyte imbalance, including low potassium.

Treatment

- No food by mouth (NPO).
- Discontinue contributory drugs; correct other causes of obstruction.
- Hydration and electolyte replacement parenterally *(11, Fluid Replacement).*
- Nasogastric tube and suction.
- Treatment of shock *(57–5),* as necessary.
- Referral for hospital care.

40–4. PERFORATION

Esophageal. Breaks in the walls of the esophagus may be caused by corrosives *(53–33, Acids; 53–48, Alkalies; 53–401, Lye),* foreign bodies *(39–7),* instrumentation, forceful wretching and vomiting, or blunt or penetrating trauma, and may result in severe abdominal or chest pain, shock *(57)* and mediastinitis. Mediastinal air may be seen in chest x-ray. Water-soluble contrast material may demonstrate perforation.

Intraperitoneal (gallbladder, intestines, spleen, stomach). Intraperitoneal perforation may be caused by foreign bodies *(39–7)*; medications such as phenylbutazone (Butazolidin), enteric-coated potassium tablet combinations and steroids; trauma; and ulcerative processes. Abdominal pain and rigidity, local or generalized tenderness and shock usually are present. Upright x-ray films may demonstrate free air in the abdomen.

Treatment

- NPO.
- Nasogastric tube and suction.
- Treatment of shock.
- Analgesics after diagnosis and treatment course have been established.
- Hospitalization for definitive care, usually surgical.

40–5. HEMORRHAGE

Severe bleeding from any point along the enteric tract can present a serious life-threatening situation. Gastrointestinal tract bleeding may be frankly evident from blood in the emesis or stool or may be occult, with the patient initially presenting in a state of hypovolemic shock *(57)*.

Blood in the stool, whether bright red or changed, represents a potential emergency until its source (Fig. 40–1) can be determined. If gastrointestinal tract hypermotility is present, blood from the respiratory and upper gastrointestinal tracts may appear hardly changed in the rectum. Conversely, retention of blood from the colon may cause blackish alteration that is falsely suggestive of a lesion of the upper portion of the tract. In addition, ingestion of brightly colored substances—beets, red ink or paint, gelatin (Jello), strawberries and so forth—can mimic bright red blood in the stool or emesis. Similarly, iron, bismuth (Pepto-Bismol), licorice, spinach and other products can cause a blackish appearance of the stool. A guaiac test confirms the presence or absence of blood. See also specific areas for treatment. See Table 22–2 for diagnostic clues in hemorrhage from peptic ulcer.

Treatment

- Start therapy for shock *(57)*, including rapid administration of normal saline solution, colloid solution, or both. Do type and crossmatch for blood transfusions.
- Evaluate for bleeding and clotting defect *(45)*.
- Obtain a rapid history from patient and relatives to determine causes contributing to hemorrhage, i.e., use of anticoagulants, salicylates or other nonsteroidal anti-inflammatory agents; overuse of alcohol; inadequate diet; and familial conditions, such as hemophilia. (*Note:* There is still some controversy regarding whether or not steroids cause GI bleeding.)
- Hospitalize for thorough clinical and laboratory investigation, observation and treatment, even when bleeding and anemia appear to be mild, if this is the first bleeding episode. Urgent endoscopy (e.g., esophagoscopy, gastroscopy, duodenoscopy, sigmoidoscopy) and angiography are of value in locating bleeding sites in patients with persistent hemorrhage. Radiologic examination with barium is of little value for establishing the specific site of bleeding.
- Nasogastric tube for decompression and evaluation of rapidity of bleeding.
- The benefit of iced saline gavage for reduction of upper gastrointestinal bleeding remains controversial.
- For bleeding of esophageal varices, give intravenously injectable vasopressin (Pitressin), 0.1 to 0.4 units/min until bleeding slows, then taper dose as long as bleeding has ceased; while giving vasopressin, perform continuous blood pressure and electrocardiogram (ECG) monitoring. If bleeding continues to be severe and has not been controlled within about 30 minutes, consider use of a Sengstaken-Blakemore tube, weighing benefits and identified risks. (*Note:* Use with caution in patients with known hypertension

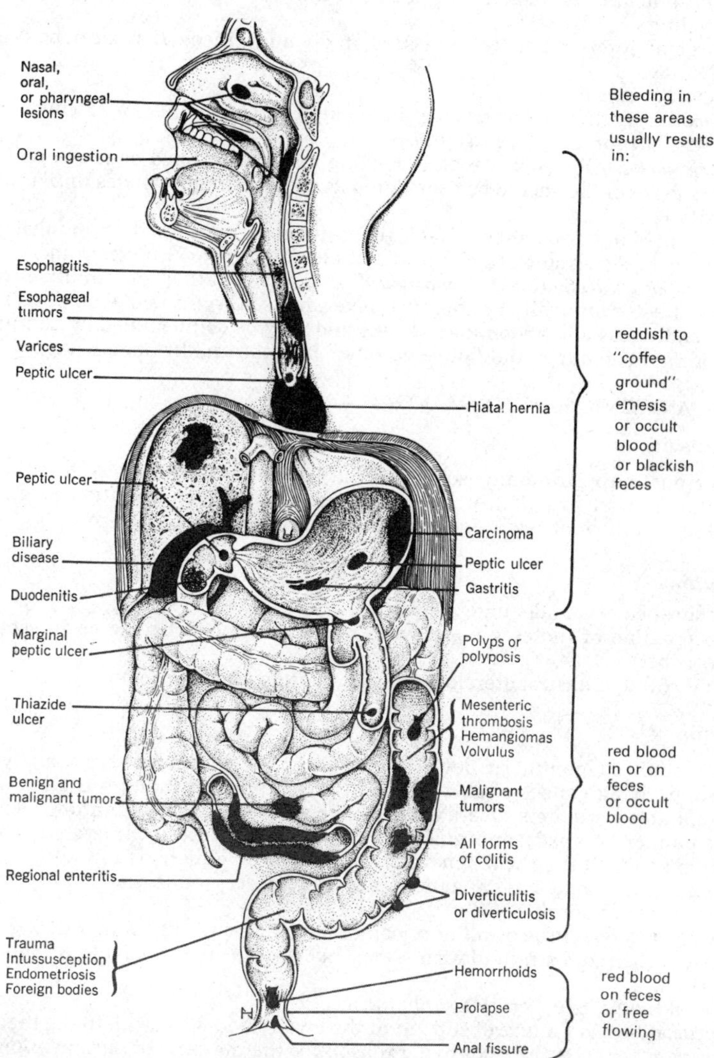

Figure 40–1. Some important causes of blood in the stool. (Modified from Turell, R.: Hosp. Med., Vol. 4, No. 6, 1968.)

or coronary artery disease.) Endoscopic injection of a sclerosing agent into varices is now being performed at many medical centers.

- Cimetidine (Tagamet), 300 mg IV q 6 h, may be given slowly initially if excess acidity is a factor, although it has not been proved to stop acute bleeding.
- Surgical intervention is necessary if vigorous medical treatment is not adequate.

Rectal Bleeding (See *40–7*).

Hemorrhoids. Loss of blood may be enough to cause anemia or shock (See also *40–7, Anorectal Conditions*)

Malignancies. All cases of rectal bleeding of undetermined cause, especially in persons over 50, should be considered as possible malignancies until proved otherwise.

Poisons. Many substances that can be ingested, absorbed or inhaled can cause severe gastrointestinal and rectal bleeding. (See 53, *Poisoning*.)

Ulcerations, Infection and Inflammation. This group of pathologic conditions may be manifested clinically by anorexia, fever, nausea, vomiting, abdominal pain and tenderness and abdominal masses and may be compounded by alteration of normal evacuation and fluid/electrolyte balance and by hemorrhage.

40–6. ANATOMIC/FUNCTIONAL DEFECTS

Achalasia

Persons with an atonic esophagus may develop sudden distress with dysphagia from obstruction or respiratory difficulty from aspiration of gastric content overflow or regurgitated food.

Treatment

- Insurance of an adequate airway.
- Evacuation of the esophagus with an Ewald tube or by use of an esophagoscope.
- Referral to a gastroenterologist for evaluation and treatment.

Hernia

Although congenital or developmental structural weaknesses usually are the underlying causes of all types of hernias, direct or indirect trauma often precipitates symptoms severe enough to require emergency attention. Hernias that cannot be easily and quickly reduced or that are incarcerated require surgical consultation and generally surgical intervention. Trauma (including strain) and congenital weakness are the most prominent factors in the appearance of hernias.

Femoral Hernia. Protrusion of a loop of bowel through the femoral ring with incarceration and strangulation is rare but does occur, usually in infants and children.

Hiatal Hernia. See *Reflux Esophagitis* (p. 308).

Inguinal Hernia. Failure of support of the lower abdominal wall in the inguinal regions represents the underlying reason for the majority of hernias. Congenital structural weaknesses of the supporting structures are commonly present. Herniation of bowel or other intra-abdominal contents may occur spontaneously—generally in infants—or be precipitated by lifting, straining, coughing or any other mechanism that increases intra-abdominal pressure in older individuals. Both direct and indirect inguinal hernias may be aggravated by occupational factors.

Treatment

- Strangulation of a hernia is an urgent condition requiring immediate hospitalization for surgical intervention.
- Incarceration. Reduction can sometimes be accomplished by sedation and gentle manipulation with the patient supine. If reduction cannot be done or if incarceration recurs after reduction, the patient should be referred for surgical consultation.
- All other patients should be advised regarding surgical repair and application of support and warned of the possible development of incarceration or strangulation.

Umbilical Hernia. This is by far the commonest type of infantile hernia. Incarceration and strangulation practically never occur. Repeated reassurance of the parents is often the most important part of therapy. Spontaneous closure without treatment usually occurs.

Ventral Hernia. Herniation of fat, omentum or abdominal content through a weakness in the abdominal wall may be congenital or the result of penetrating injuries; however, usually it is at the site of previous operative procedures. For treatment, see *Inguinal Hernia.*

Industrial or Occupational Hernias *(See also 75, Workers' Compensation [Industrial] Cases).* At the first visit, a thorough and complete history *must* be taken on every case of claimed hernia when the condition is alleged to have arisen out of or to have been caused by the patient's work. The precipitating work factors and any non-industrial factors must be given in detail. A Doctor's First Report of Work Injury should be made.

Neonatal Conditions

Neonatal conditions, often associated with severe feeding problems, respiratory distress, abnormal elimination and signs of obstruction, may require emergency care. Among these are diaphragmatic hernia, imperforate anus, intestinal atresia, megacolon, annular pancreas with duodenal compression, pyloric stenosis and tracheoesophageal fistula. All require immediate hospitalization for surgical evaluation and possible intervention. (See also 52.)

Prolapse of the Rectum

In infants and children this condition is not rare. It is probably the result of congenital defects in the firmness of the connective tissue between the muscular layers of the rectum.

Treatment

- Preliminary sedation.
- *Reduction at once* by manual replacement. The sooner this is accomplished, the easier the procedure. Delay results in shutting off the blood supply by sphincter spasm, with resultant extreme edema.
- Elevation of the foot of the bed.
- Application of cold packs to decrease edema.
- Tight strapping of the buttocks.
- Hydration, a high-fiber diet and stool softeners to avoid obstipation/constipation.
- Immediate hospitalization for reduction under general anesthesia if the measures just described are unsuccessful.

In adults prolapse generally results from lesions (hemorrhoids, proctitis, polyps) that cause excessive straining at stool. Reduction by the methods just outlined is generally much more difficult in adults than in children and recurrence is more common. The patient should be hospitalized if replacement cannot be obtained on one or two attempts, if there is discoloration of the prolapsed structures indicative of circulatory embarrassment, if marked edema is present or if the prolapse recurs spontaneously after reduction.

Reflux Esophagitis ("Heartburn")

This condition may be responsible for a variety of symptoms severe enough to require emergency treatment, including dyspnea, cyanosis (infants) and chest pain which in adults may be mistaken for acute myocardial infarction. This condition occurs even in the absence of diaphragmatic hernia.

Treatment

- Symptomatic and supportive care. Elevation of the head of the bed with 6″ blocks and administration of liquid antacids help to relieve nocturnal distress. Cimetidine reduces hyperacidity.
- ECG and even hospitalization on occasion may be necessary in ruling out myocardial infarction *(29–15)*.

40–7. ANORECTAL CONDITIONS

This area of the body is particularly prone to develop inflammatory conditions that are extremely painful and likely to be accompanied by bleeding.

Cryptitis

Inflammation of the crypts of Morgagni may cause anal spasm and pain, pruritus, and bleeding. Treatment consists of the sitz baths, dilatation of the sphincter, administration of an antibiotic after appropriate cultures, and suppositories.

Fissures *(See also Proctitis, later in this section)*

A small break in the continuity of the mucous membrane of the rectum or of skin around the anus may cause itching, pain and bleeding on defecation. See *58–14, Pruritus Ani.*

Treatment

- Warm sitz baths.
- Fecal softeners (Colace, Surfak), or bulking agents (bran or Metamucil), or both; high-residue diet.
- Sedation and analgesics as necessary.
- Thorough cleansing of all fecal material (which is both irritative and infective) from perianal skin after each defecation.
- Generous application of petroleum jelly (vaseline) or medicated rectal ointment to lubricate and protect the entire anal canal and perianal area; this is particularly important for those who will be sweating and walking or running for long periods. Suppositories with hydrocortisone may reduce irritation and symptoms.
- Referral to a proctologist if symptoms are severe or persistent.

Hemorrhoids (Piles)

Not Thrombosed. If not thrombosed but prolapsed or protruding, replacement using a lubricated gloved finger should be attempted. If this cannot be done because of acute pain or strangulation, inject a total of 2 to 3 ml of 0.5%

procaine into the swollen tissues at 3 or 4 different points. After a short wait, painless and complete replacement can usually be accomplished. Ethyl aminobenzoate (benzocaine) suppositories and other "-caine" suppositories may be sensitizing; therefore hydrocortisone-containing suppositories are preferred. Sitz baths at home should be prescribed. The patient should be instructed to arrange for further care if the symptoms persist or recur.

Thrombosed. If thrombosed, severe pain can be relieved by injection of a small amount of 1% procaine or lidocaine (Xylocaine) into the mucous membrane and evacuation of the clots through a small incision. Suturing is not necessary. The patient should be advised to take sitz baths until the acute inflammation subsides and to obtain further medical care if not completely relieved.

Proctitis

An increasing proportion of cases of proctitis are sexually transmitted. Ulcerative colitis and regional enteritis are common nonsexual causes as is schistosomiasis in the Orient.

Painful defecation, diarrhea with blood, polymorphonuclear cells, mucopurulent discharge and repetitious defecatory impulse are frequent. The anus is reddened and often edematous.

Cultures and tests for venereal diseases should be obtained in all suspected cases.

Treat identified causes with specific therapy. Preferred treatment of gonococcal proctitis is 2.4 million units of procaine penicillin G IM in each gluteal muscle, plus 1 g probenecid PO given once. Injection of spectinomycin hydrochloride (Trobicin), 1 g IM in each gluteal muscle, has been effective for gonococcal proctitis if penicillin is contraindicated. Corticosteroid suppositories, one twice daily (bid) rectally, help decrease inflammatory response. Muscle spasm is relieved by anticholinergics. See *12* for pain medication.

Prolapse *(See under 40–6)*

Pruritus Ani *(See 58–14 and Fissures, earlier in this section)*

Rectal Stricture

Stricture of the rectum may occur following rectal surgery; more often, it results from infections such as lymphogranuloma venereum *(33–37)*. No emergency treatment is indicated unless acute infection is present or complete obstruction has occurred. For acute infection, antibiotics and hot sitz baths may give relief; for complete obstruction the patient should be hospitalized.

Rectal Bleeding *(See also 40–5, Hemorrhage; 45–1, Control of Bleeding)*

Bright red bleeding is usually indicative of a bleeding site in or beyond the lower colon (Fig. 40–1). Most frequently in the emergency situation, bleeding is from ruptured hemorrhoidal vessels (see *Hemorrhoids*, earlier in this section) or trauma; particularly consider angiodysplastic lesions, ischemic colitis or diverticulitis in older individuals. For treatment, see the area or cause involved.

40–8. APPENDICITIS (Acute) *(See also Table 22–2)*

The pain from appendiceal inflammation may start rapidly, though progressive increment over a period of hours is most common. Location of pain may be anywhere in the abdomen, but migratory pain from the midabdomen to the right lower quadrant is characteristic except in later pregnancy in which right upper quadrant pain is also likely. Persons of any age may be afflicted. Nausea and vomiting are not always present, although anorexia almost always precedes pain. Slight diarrhea occasionally occurs. Fever and leukocytosis generally increase later as progression occurs.

Highly focal pain with abdominal palpation at site of appendiceal inflammation is found early; localization at a site one-third the distance from the anterior-superior iliac spine to the umbilicus (McBurney's point) is classic; further irritation and pain may be elicited with rectal digital examination, referred tenderness from palpation elsewhere in the abdomen and passive hyperextension of the thigh (psoas sign). Generalized rebound tenderness, muscle guarding, and hypoactive or absent bowel sounds are later signs indicative of peritonitis and pending or actual appendiceal rupture. WBC is usually elevated.

Hospitalization for close observation and possible surgical intervention is indicated whenever the clinical picture suggests the possibility of acute appendicitis.

If the clinical picture is ambiguous after repeat assessment and laboratory studies (see 22, *Abdominal Pain*), consider emergency barium lower gastrointestinal study (without prior enema preparation). Visualization of the appendiceal lumen is indicative of no obstruction, and appendicitis is highly unlikely; nonvisualization is most consistent with appendicitis but does not eliminate other disease as the cause of the pain and the clinical picture. In addition to helping avoid surgery in some cases, the study may aid the incisional approach for the surgical abdomen. Once the diagnosis is made or strongly suspected, treatment is surgery.

40–9. CHOLECYSTITIS (Acute) *(See also Table 22–2)*

Frequently, a history of prior gallbladder complaints will be obtained, particularly fatty food intolerance and increased discomfort after eating. Obstruction of the biliary tract from gallbladder stones, from inflammation following passage of a stone or from infection may precede involvement of the gallbladder. Generally, pain and tenderness are present in the right upper quadrant of the abdomen. Pain may radiate to the right shoulder and back along the scapular vertebral border. Decreased appetite, nausea and vomiting are usual. The gallbladder itself may or may not be palpable. Increases in WBC and amylase and bilirubin levels are common. Calculi in the biliary system are usually not radiopaque, but may be delineated by ultrasonography. Radionuclide biliary scanning with Tc^{99m}–HIDA is proving to be a superior technique for identifying gallstones and distinguishing non-gallstone pancreatitis.

Treatment

- Referral for hospitalization and decision regarding immediate surgical evaluation.
- NPO.
- Start suction generally; administer fluids IV.
- Meperidine (Demerol), 50 to 100 mg q 3 to 4 h prn for severe pain.
- Consider use of an antibiotic after blood cultures are drawn.

Table 40–1. COMMON CAUSES OF ACUTE BACTERIAL DIARRHEA AND GASTROENTERITIS*

Disease and Causative Organisms	Diarrhea	Fever	Nausea	Vomiting	Abdominal Cramps	Seizures	Therapy and Remarks (See also *33–83, Antimicrobial Drugs of Choice; 11, Fluid Replacement; 57–7, Shock; 46, Metabolic Disorders*)
Shigellosis							
Shigellae	S	S	M	M	S	M	Sulfamethoxazole/trimethoprim; ampicillin/tetracycline. Supportive care. No opiates. Stools: watery, relatively odorless, mucus, blood streaking. Meningismus, repiratory symptoms occur.
Salmonellosis							
Salmonellae (nontyphoidal)	S	S	S	S	S	±	Supportive unless bacteremic, then ampicillin or amoxicillin. Contaminated poultry/eggs common source; freezing does not eliminate.
Typhoid fever							
Salmonella typhosa	±	S	M	M	M	±	Chloramphenicol and supportive care. Slow pulse for fever; abdominal tenderness, rose spots, splenomegaly, constipation, leukopenia occur.
Escherichia coli diarrhea							
E. coli	M	±	±	±	M	±	Supportive care. If severely ill or bacteremic, then gentamicin, tobramycin or ampicillin. Toxigenic strains commoner in U.S. than invasive strains.
Food poisoning							
Staphylococcus aureus	±	±	S	S	±	±	Abrupt onset. See also *53–314, Food Poisoning*. Supportive care. Toxin in under-refrigerated dairy products, chopped meats or "frozen" foods.
Clostridium perfringens	M	±	±	±	M	±	Supportive care. Toxin generally in meats.
Vibrio parahaemolyticus	S	±	M	M	M	±	Supportive care. From raw or undercooked ocean fish. Toxigenic and invasive.
Cholera							
Vibrio cholerae	S	S	S	S	S	±	Tetracycline and supportive care. Essentially nonexistent in the Western Hemisphere.
Campylobacter enteris (jejuni and coli)	S	M	M	±	M	±	More common than any of the above causes of diarrhea. Special culture methods needed. Erythromycin effective. Illness lasts 10 to 14 days.

*Key to symbols: S = severe intensity; M = moderate intensity and frequency; ± = not common or intense. *Note:* These notations refer to average cases of the disease; great individual variance may occur.

40–10. DIARRHEA *(See also Table 40–1, Common Causes of Acute Bacterial Diarrhea)*

Diarrhea may present as an emergency situation with moderate or marked dehydration, incipient or frank shock (57), watery and bloody stools, high fever, tenesmus and toxic state. Specific bacteria (shigella and salmonella), *Campylobacter,* amebae, exogenous toxins or acute fulminant ulcerative colitis may be the cause. In instances of prior oral or parenteral antibiotic administration, evaluate for pseudomembranous colitis caused by the antibiotic. Initially, emergency treatment is massive general supportive measures; diagnostic procedures (including rectal exam and sometimes sigmoidoscopy) and specific therapy follow. Oral administration of bismuth subsalicylate (Pepto-Bismol) is an excellent adjunct in treatment.

Determination of the specific cause of the diarrhea is indicated, even in mild cases with probable specific exposure, by cultures, gross and microscopic exam, and serologic exam. Diarrhea in food handlers must be reported and the individual prohibited from working till cleared by specification.

For individuals new to an area in which certain bacteria are highly endemic, traveler's prophylactic therapy with up to 30 ml Pepto-Bismol qid in adults (avoid in children under 3 years), or doxycycline, 100 mg qd PO, may be considered. Therapy with Bactrim DS may be given: in adults dosage is 1 tablet bid PO for 5 days. Avoid prescribing Lomotil for elective use in travelers.

40–11. DIVERTICULAR DISEASE (Diverticulitis)

In adults, acute inflammation of diverticuli may cause signs and symptoms difficult to differentiate from an acute surgical abdomen. If perforation should occur with signs of diffuse peritonitis, the treatment is emergency surgery; however, subacute inflammatory conditions characterized by pain, change in bowel habit pattern, mild fever and bleeding are more common. Pain/tenderness is usually lower abdominal, more often LLQ. Diverticulosis is one of the common causes of rectal bleeding in adults over age 40.

Treatment

- In mild cases, control of the infection by antibiotics and administration of a high residue diet and fecal softeners may give relief.
- Severe acute cases require immediate hospitalization.

40–12. ESOPHAGITIS *(See Reflux Esophagitis, under 40–6)*

40–13. FOOD POISONING *(See 53–314)*

40–14. GASTROENTERITIS *(For Acute Gastritis, see Table 22–2)*

Acute gastroenteritis may result from a wide range of irritants, including bacteria (see Table 40–2), enteroviruses (usually occurring in minor epidemics; see *33–21*) and toxic substances. The factors in food poisoning *(53–314)* cause this entity of nausea, vomiting, anorexia, diffuse cramping abdominal discomfort and often later variable diarrhea. Generally the increase in WBC is not severe. The most important aspects of care are restoration of fluid and electrolyte balance, which may be profoundly disrupted, and supportive relief of symptoms.

40–15. ISCHIORECTAL OR ISCHIOANAL ABSCESS *(See 23–15)*

40–16. MESENTERIC ADENITIS

The mesenteric lymph nodes may enlarge in response most frequently to viral or *Yersinia* infection. There is moderately intense pain in the right lower quadrant (RLQ), accompanied by fever, muscle guarding to palpation in RLQ and an increased WBC. The course of mesenteric adenitis resembles that of appendicitis, from which it may be distinguished by means of serial examinations, visualization of the appendiceal lumen with barium enema, laparotomy or laparoscopy. Vomiting and diarrhea are more common than with appendicitis. Treatment is supportive.

40–17. PANCREATITIS (Acute) *(See also 59–26, Pancreatic Injuries, and Table 22–2)*

This condition may come on suddenly, although it is frequently preceded by symptoms suggestive of gallbladder disease, peptic ulcer or a history of high intake of alcohol. Pain in the midabdomen with penetration to the back or flanks may be severe. Vomiting and paralytic ileus are common. Shock may develop and is an ominous early sign. Elevated serum and urine amylase and serum bilirubin levels are clues to involvement. Serum calcium levels may drop. Radionuclide biliary scan with Tc^{99m}–HIDA or ultrasonography helps to distinguish non-gallstone from gallstone-related pancreatitis.

Treatment

- Treatment of shock *(57)*. In severe cases, large volumes of fluids and crystalloids may be needed because of "third spacing" (i.e., fluid shifts out of the intracellular and intravascular compartments into the extravascular/extracellular third compartment).
- Hospitalization for definitive care. General treatment is similar to the treatment for acute cholecystitis.
- Treatment is usually nonsurgical unless the pancreatitis is associated with mechanical obstruction or development of a pancreatic abscess or an infected pseudocyst.

40–18. PARASITIC INFECTIONS

Many parasites may cause signs and symptoms involving the gastrointestinal tract that are severe enough to require emergency medical care. See Table 40–2, Common Intestinal Parasites.

40–19. PILES *(See 40–7, Anorectal Conditions, Hemorrhoids)*

40–20. POLYPS

Polyps may be mistaken for internal hemorrhoids if located near the anus; if in the rectum, they may be associated with recurrent rectal prolapse *(40–7)*.

Treatment

- Control of infection and edema by sitz baths, lubricating and anti-inflammatory suppositories, and antibiotics.
- Referral to a surgeon or proctologist for examination and treatment. *Note:* These lesions may be premalignant.

40–21. ULCERATIVE COLITIS

Ulcerative colitis is a chronic inflammatory condition of the colon of unknown etiology; it is characterized by periodic flareups, with the worst forms

Table 40–2. COMMON INTESTINAL PARASITES

Common Name	Scientific Name *(Synonyms or Varieties)*	Distribution	Portal of Entry
FLUKES Blood	Schistosoma japonicum	Orient	Skin
	S. mansoni	Africa Latin America	Skin
Intestinal	Fasciolopsis buski Heterophyes, Echinostoma	Orient, tropics, U.S.A. (rare)	Mouth
PROTOZOA Amoebic dysentery	Entamoeba histolytica (E. dysenteriae, E. histolytica)	World-wide, especially, in moist climates	Mouth
Giardia	Giardia lamblia	World-wide, in warm climates	Mouth
ROUNDWORMS Hookworm	Ancylostoma duodenale, Necator americanus	Warm, moist climates	Skin, especially of feet
Intestinal round worm	Ascaris lumbricoides	World-wide	Mouth
	Capillaria philippinensis	Northern Philippines	Mouth
Pinworm (Seat worm)	Enterobius vermicularis (oxyuris vermicularis)	World-wide, especially in children	Mouth
Threadworm	Strongyloides stercoralis	Southern U.S.A., moist tropics	Skin, usually of the feet
Whipworm	Trichuris trichiura (Trichocephalus trichiuris)	Gulf coast, U.S.A., warm moist climates	Mouth
TAPEWORMS Beef	Taenia saginata	World-wide	Mouth
Dwarf	Hymenolepis nana	Southern U.S.A.	Mouth
Fish	Diphyllobothrium latum (Bothriocephalus latus)	Minnesota and Michigan in U.S.A., Canada	Mouth
Pork	Taenia solium	Latin America, U.S.A. (rare)	Mouth

†See "Drugs for Parasitic Infections," *The Medical Letter*, Vol. 24 (Issue 601), January 22, 1982.

Table 40–2. COMMON INTESTINAL PARASITES *(Continued)*

Source of Infection	Common Symptoms	Therapeutic Agents†
Water containing larvae of snail hosts	Dysentery, intestinal and hepatic cirrhosis	Praziquantel
Same	Same	Oxamniquine
Vegetation, fresh water snails and fish	Intestinal toxemia and obstruction	Praziquantel
Feces—contaminated water, food and fomites	Abdominal pain, dysentery, hepatitis	Diiodohydroxyquin; add metronidazole or paromomycin in symptomatic cases
Human feces	Abdominal pain, mucous diarrhea, weight loss	Quinacrine hydrochloride, metronidazole
Fecal contamination of soil	Melena, anemia, retarded growth	Mebendazole, pyrantel pamoate
Fecal contamination of soil	"Acute abdomen," colicky pain, diarrhea, obstruction of bile or pancreatic duct, intestinal blockage	Mebendazole, pyrantel pamoate
Fecal contamination of soil	Diarrhea, marasmus, emaciation	Thiabendazole, mebendazole
Eggs from contaminated fomites	Perianal itching, convulsions in children	Mebendazole, pyrantel pamoate
Fecal contamination of soil	Severe radiating gastric pain, diarrhea	Thiabendazole
Fecal contamination of soil	Nausea, vomiting, diarrhea, retarded growth	Mebendazole
Raw or incompletely cooked infected beef	"Acute apendix," severe abdominal pain, systemic toxemia	Niclosamide*, paromomycin
Eggs contaminating environment	Abdominal pain, diarrhea, dizziness, inanition	Niclosamide, praziquantel
Infected fresh water fish	Bowel obstruction, intestinal toxemia—may cause severe anemia	Niclosamide, paromomycin
Incompletely cooked infected pork	Acute abdominal pain, guarding, rigidity, systemic toxemia	Niclosamide, paromomycin

*Niclosamide (Niclocide) is the drug of choice for all tapeworms.

consisting of severe bloody diarrhea, fever, abdominal pain, tenderness and even peritonitis, and a general toxic state. Fulminant episodes require immediate hospitalization for vigorous treatment, and even then death may occur. Toxic colitis is the most lethal stage.

Treatment (Severe to Toxic Form)

- IV hydrocortisone, 4 mg/kg/day, up to 300 mg/day by continuous drip, or ACTH, 120 units/day.
- Clear liquids PO for severe cases; for toxic form: NPO and insert suction tube.
- Ampicillin, 8 to 12 g/day IV. Antibiotics are not indicated in less severe cases.
- IV fluid and electrolyte replacement, immediately and for maintenance therapy. Supplemental potassium should be given.
- Monitor weight, electrolytes, intake and output.
- May require whole blood if anemic.
- Observe for perforation. Check colon size daily with AP x-ray of abdomen until condition is in remission.
- Diversionary ileostomy and subtotal colectomy may be required if perforation or uncontrolled hemorrhage occurs.
- When condition goes into remission, consider administration of oral sulfasalazine.

40–22. VASCULAR PROBLEMS

Either arterial or venous pathologic conditions may be responsible for several types of gastrointestinal emergencies.

Mallory-Weiss Syndrome. This is caused by a mucosal tear at the esophagogastric junction—usually preceded by vigorous retching and vomiting. Iced saline gavage may slow bleeding. Most patients stop bleeding spontaneously, though surgical intervention may be needed for more severe and protracted bleeding.

Esophageal Varices. See *40–4*.

Mesenteric Vascular Occlusion. Vascular occlusion from thrombosis, embolism or severe venous stasis causes bowel ischemia or infarction with acute severe midabdominal pain, minimal or no abdominal tenderness and hyperactive bowel sounds. Ileus, shock and blood in the peritoneal space and stool are later manifestations. Peritoneal aspiration *(18–23)* and angiography may aid in diagnosis. Ischemic colitis—usually seen in elderly patients—presents with abdominal pain, fever and rectal bleeding. (See also Table 22–2.)

Treatment consists of measures to treat shock *(57–5)* and referral for surgical observation and evaluation for resection of the involved bowel.

40–23. VOLVULUS *(See also Table 22–2)*

Twisting of the small bowel usually results from improper developmental rotation of the duodenum and may cause signs and symptoms of high intestinal obstruction developing during the first few hours of life or months or years later. Volvulus is also seen in the sigmoid colon. The diagnosis cannot be made on symptoms and physical findings alone but requires thorough barium x-ray studies.

Hospitalization is indicated whenever volvulus is suspected. Operative untwisting of the distal portion of the duodenum or of other involved areas may be lifesaving.

40–24. VOMITING

Prolonged and persistent vomiting, no matter what its cause, results in acute dehydration, electrolyte imbalance (usually alkalosis) and complete exhaustion and occasionally is complicated by hemorrhage due to secondary laceration of mucosa at the gastroesophageal junction (Mallory-Weiss syndrome). Occasional regurgitation or vomiting in infants or children may be of no clinical importance other than possible overfeeding.

Treatment

Control and adequate treatment of prolonged vomiting is achieved by the following measures:

- Physiologic mechanical rest of the stomach:
  —NPO except ice chips and later clear liquids as tolerated.
  —A nasogastric tube and suction are advisable temporarily if there is obstruction.
  —Rest and quiet environment.
- Pharmacologic treatment of the stomach. This involves reducing acidity of the stomach with antacids; decreasing acid production if excessive with cimetidine (Tagamet) or ranitidine (Zantac); and administering centrally acting antiemetics such as the following:
  —Cyclizine lactate (Marezine), 50 mg PO 3 or 4 times daily or 50 mg IM 3 times a day. For children the dosage must be adjusted according to age (see *9*).
  —Dimenhydrinate (Dramamine), 50 mg PO or IM 3 times a day.
  —Prochlorperazine dimaleate (Compazine), 10 mg PO 3 to 4 times daily, or 5 to 10 mg IM (deep in buttocks) 3 times a day. In children the oral dosage should be adjusted as follows: body weight less than 9 kg—not to be used; body weight 9 to 12 kg—2.5 mg not more than twice a day; body weight 13 to 18 kg—2.5 mg, not to exceed 3 times a day; body weight 19 to 40 kg—5 mg twice a day.
  —Suppository form of prochlorperazine, 25 mg for adults or 2.5 mg for younger children (less than 40 pounds) and 5 mg for older children. In adults, trimethobenzamide hydrochloride (Tigan), in 200-mg suppositories, is also effective.
  —Meclizine hydrochloride (Antivert; OTC name is Bonine), 25 to 50 mg PO once daily (*note:* not recommended for children under 12 years).
- Intravenous fluids *(11)* and correction of electrolyte imbalance *(46)* as indicated according to clinical state and laboratory studies. Monitor as for shock *(57)* in more severe cases.
- Correction of the specific underlying cause.
- Gradual resumption of eating, starting with easily tolerated substances, such as clear fluids, gelatin or crackers, and progressing as tolerated.
- In more severe cases, hospitalization for supportive care and evaluation and treatment of underlying cause.
- For prophylactic treatment of vomiting due to motion sickness, see *49–11*.

41. Genitourinary Tract Emergencies

TRAUMATIC CONDITIONS

If injury to any part of the urogenital tract is suspected, the attending physician should perform a thorough physical examination of the abdomen, back, flanks, rectum and scrotum or perineum, followed by gross and microscopic examination of the urine for blood cells. Catheterization *(18–6)* may be necessary but should be avoided whenever possible; a "clean-catch" or second glass specimen is usually satisfactory. If there is any reasonable doubt as to the nature or extent of the injury, the patient should be hospitalized for urologic examination (including as indicated: X-rays, KUB, IVP, cystourethrogram, CT and Echo scan, renal angiography). In presence of fever considered to be due to GU infection, obtain urine culture and sensitivity, as necessary. See Figure 40–1 for guidance in evaluating post-traumatic hematuria and treatment.

41–1. BLADDER INJURIES

Trauma to the bladder may vary in degree from tears of a few fibers of the muscular wall with microscopic hematuria to large rents with extensive extravasation of urine, hemorrhage, peritonitis and shock. The most common causes are:

- Fracture of the pelvis with perforation or laceration of the bladder wall by sharp bone ends.
- Direct trauma over a distended bladder. Gross and microscopic examination of a clean-catch or second glass specimen of urine should be done if the type of injury suggests possible bladder damage. Cystourethrograms are indicated to confirm the diagnosis.
- Endurance activity participants such as marathoners with dehydration may experience gross hematuria from the "empty bladder syndrome," caused by trauma of the unfilled bladder hitting against the pubic bone; acetylation of platelets by NSAID promotes this occurrence, which is self-limiting with rehydration and relative rest.

Treatment

All patients with proved or suspected bladder damage should be transferred at once for hospitalization and care by a urologist.

41–2. KIDNEY INJURIES

A severe blow over the flank or paralumbar muscles may cause a contusion or rupture of a kidney. Suspected cases should be hospitalized for observation, diagnosis and treatment. Severe shock is common and must be treated (57) at once. IVP and renal angiography may be needed. See Figure 41–1.

41–3. ORCHITIS

Direct blows to the scrotum, as well as straddling injuries, may cause traumatic orchitis with extreme pain, rapid swelling, nausea and vomiting and complete temporary prostration. Unless fracture of the testis has occurred, hospitalization is rarely indicated, although it may be several hours before

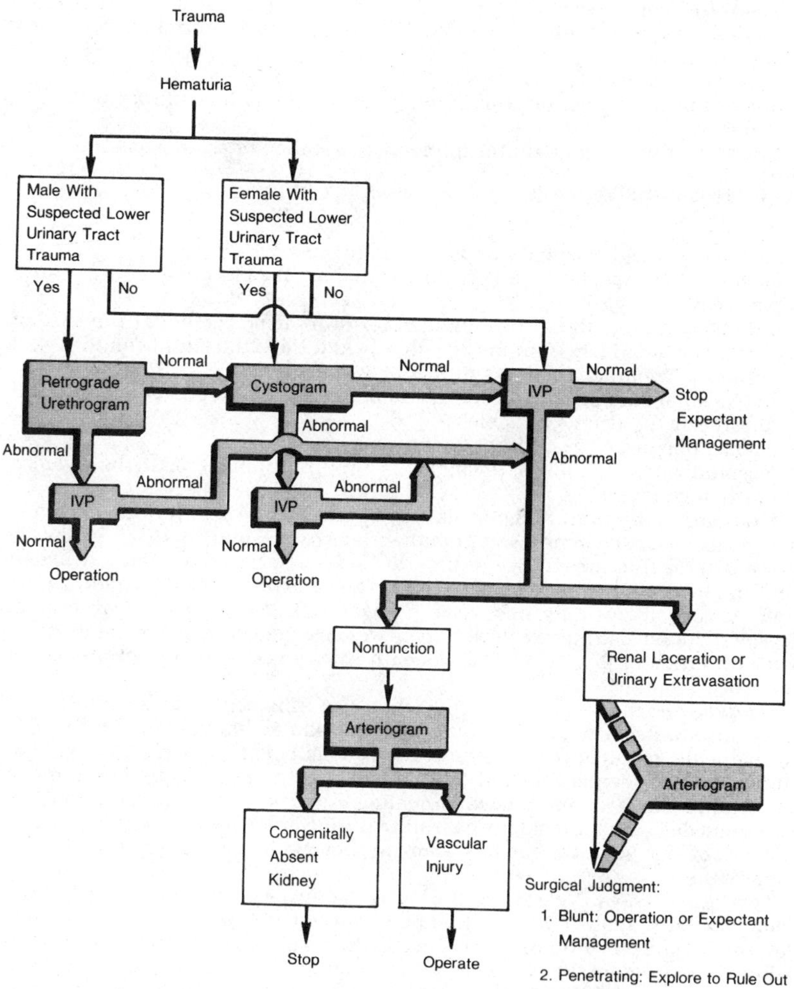

Figure 41–1. Algorithm for evaluation of the patient with post-traumatic hematuria. (From Benson, G. S., and Brewer, E. D.: JAMA, *246*: 993, 1981; copyright 1981, American Medical Association. Reprinted with permission.)

the acute discomfort and reflex nausea and vomiting decrease enough to allow any type of physical activity.

Treatment

- Control of pain and anxiety by sedatives, anodynes and narcotics. Chlorpromazine hydrochloride (Thorazine) will often help to control reflex nausea and vomiting.
- Application of cold compresses.
- Support by a T binder or athletic supporter until swelling subsides.
- Bed rest.
- Fracture of the testis requires immediate attention of a urologist.

41–4. PENIS INJURIES *(See also 59–1 and 59–2, Soft Tissue Injuries)*

Abrasions. Cleanliness will promote rapid healing.

Contusions. No special care is required; the profuse blood supply will cause rapid recovery.

Dislocation from external trauma may result in displacement of the base of the corpus beneath the symphysis pubis or into the adjacent abdominal wall or scrotum. Treatment consists of the following:

- Replacement in normal position by manipulation and traction under general anesthesia as soon as possible.
- Application of a tight-fitting athletic supporter.
- Hospitalization if there is evidence of urethral damage or if the reduced position is not stable.

"Fracture" of the shaft of the penis may be caused by direct trauma or coitus. The penis is usually bent away from the fracture site, and a bulge is generally present at the fracture site. A urethrogram is necessary to rule out a concurrent urethral injury. Treatment consists of sedation and cold packs. Hospitalization and surgery are usually necessary if the corpus cavernosum is fractured. Hospitalization also may be necessary if pressure from deep bleeding interferes with urination or if a hematoma beneath Buck's fascia is present and is not absorbed spontaneously.

Frenal Injuries may cause severe bleeding requiring control by suturing.

Lacerations. Because of the redundant loose skin and abundant blood supply of the penis, surgical repair of lacerations usually can be performed without difficulty. Debridement should be minimal. The patient should be informed in advance that scarring following healing may result in irreparable contractures and deformity, especially curvature during erections (chordee). If a large amount of skin or soft tissue has been lost, hospitalization for grafting usually is necessary.

Constrictive Lesions. Necrosis of the portion of the penis distal to a constricting band (usually applied in an attempt to control urinary incontinence or to improve sexual performance) may occur. In small babies a long hair from an adult can accidentally become wrapped around the penis and act as a constricting band. If swelling (sometimes tremendous) or the type of constricting object will not allow severance by use of a ring cutter or scissors or removal of the round-and-round constriction with the aid of a lubricant, wrapping with package cord, starting just distal to the constriction, should be tried. If this is unsuccessful, removal under general anesthesia may be necessary. Extreme distal urethral edema may require use of a retention catheter. Because of the profuse blood supply, complete and rapid recovery is the general rule unless actual gangrene is present.

Zipper Injuries. See *59–41*.

41–5. POSTCIRCUMCISION BLEEDING

Improper operative technique, especially in the use of the Gomco clamp, may result in bleeding, beginning from a few minutes to several days after circumcision. Mild bleeding or oozing generally can be controlled by pressure. Gelfoam or Oxycel held snugly over the bleeding area may be necessary. Severe bleeding requires immediate surgical control by properly placed mattress sutures.

41–6. SCROTAL ANAEROBIC INFECTION *(See also 59–42, Soft Tissue Infections [Life Threatening])*

Fournier's gangrene of the scrotum usually presents initially as a dark bluish area on both or one scrotal wall and occurs most frequently in debilitated persons, diabetics and alcoholics. This condition is a most serious urologic emergency, as involvement can double or triple within a few hours and advance up the perineum and anterior abdominal wall. Immediate referral to a urologist is indicated for surgical debridement and intensive broad-spectrum antibiotic administration.

41–7. SCROTAL INJURIES

Direct blows or straddling injuries may cause extensive bleeding into the areolar tissue of the scrotum as well as injury to the penis and the scrotal contents. Rupture of the membranous urethra or the urethra distal to this point may be heralded by blood at the meatus. Suspicion of this injury requires immediate careful physical examination; urethrograms and urologic consultation are indicated.

Treatment

- Bed rest prn until swelling subsides. Patient should wear a T binder, suspensory or athletic supporter when up.
- Application of ice bag (over a protective towel).
- Sedatives and analgesics.
- Referral to a surgeon or urologist; evacuation of a hematoma or of extravasated urine may be necessary.
- Hospitalization in severe cases; however, most patients do well on home care, provided the urethra is intact.

41–8. TESTICULAR TORSION

Testicular torsion is characterized by sudden onset of focal pain followed often by nausea and vomiting, with scrotal swelling developing soon thereafter. It usually occurs in children (although it is seen occasionally in adult men) and requires *immediate* urologist referral, hospitalization and surgical correction if the position and circulation cannot be improved by gentle manipulation. Surgical stabilization will prevent recurrence. Differentiation from inguinal hernia, epididymitis, torsion of testicular hydatid, hydrocele and hematocele may be difficult without direct inspection, even with the assistance of radioactive isotope scans or echograms. Diagnostic exploratory surgery may be necessary.

41–9. URETHRAL INJURIES

Characterized by urethral bleeding, pain and difficulty in urination, injury to the urethra may be caused by:

- Severe scrotal injuries *(41–7)*, especially those caused by straddling some hard object, with compression of the membranous urethra against the symphysis pubis.

- Displaced or comminuted fractures of the pelvis near the symphysis pubis.
- Dislocation or "fracture" of the penis *(41–4)* by direct trauma with or without associated posterior urethra injury.
- Introduction of foreign bodies into the urethra *(39–9)* by children and other adventuresome persons.
- Inexpert or injudicious attempts at catheterization *(18–6)*.

These injuries require immediate hospitalization for urologic care and evaluation, including possible urethroscopy and urethrogram, administration of analgesics and suprapubic evacuation of urine.

41–10. VAGINAL AND VULVAL INJURIES

Marked swelling and profuse bleeding may result from tears at delivery, blows, straddling injuries, forced intercourse, attempted rape *(14)*, insertion of foreign bodies *(39–10)* and caustic burns. Thorough examination after cleansing and hemostasis is always indicated.

Treatment

- Repair of small lacerations under local anesthetic.
- Hospitalization if large hematomas are present, if lacerations enter or closely approximate the bladder or rectum or if blood loss has been excessive.
- Reduction of swelling and pain by cold compresses.

NONTRAUMATIC CONDITIONS

41–11. CYSTITIS (LOWER UTI)

Characterized by dysuria, urgency, frequency of urination and bladder tenderness, cystitis rarely causes high fever or severe systemic reactions except in small children (especially girls), in whom it is one of the common causes of sudden temperature rise. If suspected, a clean-catch or second-glass urine specimen should be examined microscopically for pus and blood. Cultures and sensitivity tests should be done. Recurrences are common.

Treatment

- Maintain adequate fluid intake.
- Start on antibacterial agents that give high urinary levels, such as the sulfonamides, e.g., sulfisoxazole (Gantrisin), orally, initial dose 2 to 4 g, and maintenance dose 4 to 8 g/day divided into 4 to 6 doses; in children over 2 months: initial dose is 75 mg/kg and maintenance 150 mg/kg/day divided into 4 to 6 doses to a maximum of 6 g/day. Ampicillin is indicated if the bacteria is sulfonamide-resistant. Nitrofurantoin (Furadantin) is effective against sensitive bacteria: adults are given 50 to 100 mg PO qid. Adjust medication according to clinical response and cultures and sensitivity tests.
- Recommend bed rest until patient is afebrile.
- Prescribe bladder sedation for relief of urgency.
  Adults are given methantheline bromide (Banthine), 50.0 mg PO q 6 h; or propantheline bromide (Pro-Banthine), 15 mg PO q 6 h. For relief of dysuria (burning), add phenazopyridine hydrochloride (Pyridium), 100 to 200 mg

PO tid; warn the patient that this drug colors urine a reddish-orange, which may be mistaken for blood.

- Refer to a urologist for further care. Severe cases may require hospitalization. Dimethyl sulfoxide (50% solution) has been approved for instillation into the bladder to reduce recurrent mucosal swelling or pain in nonbacterial or interstitial cystitis.

41–12. DIALYSIS EMERGENCIES

About 10 to 15 times per month, approximately 45,000 patients with chronic renal failure have hemodialysis. As the number of home units continues to increase, modern workable artificial kidneys (WAK) become smaller and more mobile (transportable units now weigh as little as 10 pounds exclusive of ancillary equipment), and highly therapeutic group travel ventures (e.g., "Dialysis In Wonderland") become more common, EMS personnel are more likely to encounter these patients in difficulty away from their base Kidney Center. The patient with experience and excellent training is often able to assist in the diagnosis of the problem; additional help is obtained through phone contact with the patient's base Kidney Center. Finally, the special traveling groups as mentioned above generally have their own experienced medical support group. The most common problems and solutions encountered are outlined in Table 41–1.

41–13. EPIDIDYMITIS

The discomfort of acute epididymitis is often severe enough to bring the patient for emergency care. He may present with the history that the pain developed following lifting or a strain. Retrograde urine flow associated with straining during heavy lifting causes a chemical (nonbacterial) epididymitis. Investigation will generally disclose no direct trauma to be the cause, although straddling injuries with contusion of the scrotum *(41–7)* and traumatic orchitis occasionally are associated with traumatic epididymitis. Differentiation must be made to rule out idiopathic, bacterial (bacterial culture positive plus bacteria in UA and Gram stain) or mumps epididymo-orchitis. Testicular torsion *(41–8)* must always be ruled out. Obtain a urine culture in addition to routine urinalysis.

Treatment

- Bed rest prn until the acute signs and symptoms subside.
- Cold compresses and analgesics.
- Use of an athletic supporter or T binder to support the scrotum when the patient is standing; use of a scrotal bridge when patient is lying down.
- Administration of broad-spectrum antibiotics if urinalysis and culture reveal presence of a bacterial infection.
- Referral for urologic care and hospitalization as needed.
- Nonbacterial epididymitis may be treated with the measures just described plus administration of phenylbutazone (Butazolidin) for 5 days.

41–14. HERPES GENITALIS *(See 33–29)*

41–15. HYDROCELE

Even though the patient may insist that the excess fluid in the scrotal sac is very uncomfortable, drainage as a rule is not an emergency procedure. The

Table 41–1. DIALYSIS EMERGENCIES

Type of Problem	Clues to Diagnosis	Treatment
*Air embolism	↓ BP, chest pain, dyspnea, nausea and vomiting; see also *Air Embolism, 63–6*	Lay patient on left side with head down; check air bubble detectors; clamp venous line/shut off blood pump
Cardiac arrhythmias	Hypoxemia; hyper- or hypocalcemia; rapid K^+ shifts; digitalis toxicity; underlying ASHD/pericarditis	Evaluate for pO_2/calcium/ K^+/digitalis effect/ECG; treat accordingly
Depression	Psychosocial adaptation to chronic illness (see *54–8*)	Establish rapport conducive to expressing feelings; provide support during adaptive period
*Dysequilibrium	Usually occurs in first few dialyses of severely uremic patients, because amount of urea removed in plasma exceeds that removed in CSF, causing fluid shifts to balance osmolality	Gradual clearing of uremic state; closer observation and slow initiation of dialysis treatment
*Fever, chills	Bacteria, toxins in water source or artificial kidney; pyrogenic reaction; sepsis	Symptomatic treatment; blood cultures; check adequacy of treated water
*Hemorrhage	Cannula leak (reconnect if just loose); duodenal ulcer bleed *(40–5);* spontaneous retroperitoneal or subdural hemorrhage *(63–4)* secondary to excess anticoagulation *(45–8)*	Clamp cannula and apply direct pressure over it; disconnect machine if running; treat associated problem; transfuse as necessary
Hepatitis	Transmitted via blood transfusions, blood spillage or oral fecal route	Avoid blood spills; prophylactic immunization with hepatitis B vaccine; wash hands frequently
Hyperkalemia	ECG features: see Fig. 46–1; serum levels highest just prior to dialysis	STAT dialysis IV glucose plus insulin, Kayexalate resin; administer IV Ca^{++} first if patient in cardiac arrest (see Fig. 5–2)

*Hypokalemia	Serum levels lowest just after dialysis; ECG features: bradycardia, SVT, PVC's (see Fig. 46–1); ↓ BP; digitalis toxicity; seizures *(34)*	See *46–16*; treat bradycardia with 0.5 mg atropine IV; treat shock *(57)*; consider use of IV K^+
*Hypotension	Often occurs at start of treatment when blood is removed from patient to be put into dialyzer; rapid ultrafiltration; hypotensive effect of medicines taken prior to dialysis; predialysis weight near normal; nausea, vomiting; tachycardia may be absent	Put patient in Trendelenburg position; give IV boluses of saline, 100 cc, prn; IV mannitol or albumin; reduce negative pressure; if possible, avoid antihypertensive treatment on dialysis days; check Hgb/Hmct; if necessary, treat for shock *(57)*
*Hypothermia	Inadequate fluid/blood warming during dialysis	Rewarming measures *(62–3)*; emergency standby generator for power outage
Itching	Secondary hyperparathyroid state due to Ca disturbance or drug allergy (see *46–11*, *Hyperparathyroidism*); scratching may lead to skin infection	Soothing creams or lotions; antihistamines *(58–12)*
*Muscles cramps	Rapid ultrafiltration or rapid sodium and water shifts	Hypertonic saline or glucose may help
Pericarditis	Suboptimal dialysis clearances; viral infection; chest pain; pericardial friction rub; ST segment elevation	Symptomatic treatment; check blood chemistries; low-dose heparinization during dialysis; check for pulsus paradoxus and cardiac tamponade
Pulmonary edema	Weight increase of >5 lbs in 2 days; swelling of eyes/hands/ankles; dyspnea and rales	Ultrafiltration treatment with dialysis; proper dietary control of sodium and fluid intake; see 55
Seizures	Hypotension or arrhythmia; abnormal seizure threshold due to uremia; subdural hematoma *(44–21)*	Normalize cardiac output; IV Dilantin or phenobarbital *(34)*; consider cranial CT scan

*Noted most commonly during or soon after actual dialysis.

patient should be advised to consult a urologist. In children, testicular torsion *(41–8)* must always be ruled out by careful examination, even if the transillumination test is positive.

41–16. NEPHRITIS (Bright's Disease)

If glomerular, degenerative or arteriosclerotic kidney disease is present or suspected, the most common emergency measures required are:

- Treatment of convulsions (*34, Convulsive Seizures; 32, Coma*).
- Treatment of any congestive heart failure *(29–10)*.
- Arrangement for immediate hospitalization for medical workup and care.

41–17. PARAPHIMOSIS

Retraction of the foreskin can usually be reduced by application of cold compresses and steady constant manual compression of the glans penis for 10 to 15 minutes, followed by gentle traction on the prepuce. If this is unsuccessful, infiltration around the constricting ring with 1% lidocaine (Xylocaine) and incision of the dorsal ring in a dorsal slit will result in reduction—this is usually performed by a urologist. In rare instances, hospitalization for use of a general anesthetic may be necessary.

41–18. PERIRENAL (PERINEPHRIC) ABSCESS

If this condition is suspected, immediate hospitalization for care by a urologist is indicated.

41–19. PERIURETHRAL ABSCESSES *(See 23–23)*

41–20. PHIMOSIS AND BALANITIS

Basically due to chronically tight structures covering the glans penis, acute symptoms are usually brought on by trauma but occasionally may develop without known precipitating cause. If the acute swelling of the glans cannot be controlled by sedation and cold compresses, and if the constriction cannot be released by gentle manipulation, the patient should be hospitalized for surgical relief. Dorsal slits or other surgical procedures should not be done as emergency measures unless there has been prolonged constriction and delay in surgical treatment is anticipated.

Balanitis: Tissue inflammation of the prepuce or glans penis (balanoposthitis in the uncircumcised), or both, may be caused by contact with any of several of the venereal diseases, and treatment is according to specific diagnosis. Surgery may be required, including a relaxing incision because of edema.

Penile exposure to the saliva of a person with Vincent's angina *(33–79)* can initiate the same type of inflammatory process, leading to swelling, phimosis and ulcerations with a foul-smelling exudate that can even lead to gangrene. Treatment is with penicillin.

41–21. PRIAPISM

A painful, persistently erect penis—unrelated to sexual desire—that will not reduce spontaneously or with intercourse or masturbation over a period of hours becomes an emergency that usually requires urologic consultation. Ice packs and analgesics, including generally a narcotic, are indicated. Reduction may occur after amyl nitrite inhalation for 15 to 20 seconds. Needle aspiration of the corpora with a 14-gauge intracath or surgical procedures producing arteriovenous shunts may be necessary. Spinal cord lesions, leukemia and sickle cell disease are contributing factors, although most cases are idiopathic.

41–22. PROSTATITIS

Low-grade perineal pain, fever and a boggy, tender prostate are characteristic of prostatitis. Obtain urine culture. Initiate treatment with trimethoprim-sulfamethoxazole, 1 tablet bid, and arrange for follow-up care.

41–23. PYELONEPHRITIS (UPPER UTI)

Rapid onset of systemic illness with fever of 102 to 104°F, shaking chills, nausea and vomiting, flank pain and percussion tenderness in the right costovertebral angle are common. Frequency and urgency of urination may also occur. Urine microscopy shows many WBC, bacteria, casts. Urine culture is positive, and blood culture may be positive as well.

Treatment

Initial treatment with medication is started according to Gram stain findings. IV ampicillin, 150 to 200 mg/kg/24 hr, is given for 2 to 3 days, after which oral doses are given. Hospitalization is indicated for the severely ill (particularly immune-suppressed or diabetic patients), and an aminoglycoside may have to be added. Arrange for follow-up and probable IVP.

41–24. RETENTION OF URINE

This very uncomfortable condition is a common and legitimate emergency. If difficulty is encountered during catheterization *(18–6)*, the patient should be given an analgesic and referred to a urologist unless the bladder is grossly distended. In this case, suprapubic drainage *(18–6)* should be done at once. In any case, acute urinary retention is a sign of underlying pathology requiring urologic investigation. Various drugs with anticholinergic effect may initiate retention (although there may be concomitant pathology) and should be discontinued or reduced in the course of evaluation.

Passage of sounds, filiform catheters or stylet-stiffened catheters should not be attempted unless the attending physician is familiar with and skilled in their use. (For technique of catheterization, see *18–6*.). Suprapubic cystostomy may be considered as an alternative.

41–25. SOFT TISSUE INFECTIONS (DEEP) *(See 59–42)*

41–26. STONE IN THE URINARY TRACT

The severe radiating, often agonizing, pain caused by passage of a stone down a ureter is a legitimate emergency requiring immediate relief. However, because the clinical picture is chiefly subjective, it can be simulated convincingly by narcotic addicts. A careful history supplemented by review of any available previous records and by examination of a urine specimen (obtained in the presence of an attendant if circumstances are suspicious) for red blood cells is essential before narcotics are administered or prescribed. Obtain an anteroposterior (AP) x-ray film of the abdomen. A negative x-ray, however, does not rule out the presence of calculi; many are not radiopaque. An intravenous pyelogram (IVP) done on an emergency basis is the most definitive study.

Treatment

- Strain all urine. Send any specimens for chemical analysis.
- Bed rest, with application of hot stupes to the abdomen.
- Morphine sulfate, 15 mg with atropine sulfate, 0.4 mg SC, or, if the pain is very severe, IV at reduced dosages. Meperidine hydrochloride (Demerol), 50 to 100 mg, or pentazocine lactate (Talwin), 15 to 30 mg, may be substituted and given IM if the pain is of moderate intensity.
- Diazepam (Valium), 5 to 10 mg PO, for relief of secondary tension and reflex skeletal muscle spasm.

Sudden and complete subsiding of the acute pain usually, but not always, indicates that the stone has passed through the ureter into the bladder. When this occurs, reference to a urologist on a less urgent basis is still indicated. Efforts to collect the stone in the urinary filtrate should continue at home. If the pain persists, or if there is any question regarding the validity of subjective complaints and objective findings, hospitalization for observation, evaluation and treatment should be advised. Narcotic addicts will usually suddenly remember a number of apparently good reasons for refusing hospitalization, particularly if it has been suggested, directly or indirectly, that a method of hospital treatment without use of narcotics is planned (see also comments in *13, Prescription Restrictions*).

41–27. URETHRITIS (Lower Urinary Tract Infection)

Specific. See *33–25, Gonorrhea.*

Nonspecific. Acute urethritis is a very common condition, especially in girls, and is often overlooked as a cause for urinary complaints. Prescription of a mild sedative for symptomatic relief is usually all that is required initially. Thorough pediatric or medical investigation should be recommended. Some cases of nonspecific urethritis are now being found to be due to chlamydiae; these respond to tetracycline, 500 mg qid for 3 weeks.

42. Gynecologic Conditions

42–1. ABORTIONS *(See 50–3)*

42–2. AMENORRHEA (Absence of Menses)

No emergency treatment is required when amenorrhea occurs as an isolated event. However, when pregnancy is suspected, it is crucial to avoid any measures that might be harmful to the fetus: avoid pelvic and unshielded x-rays, do not prescribe potentially harmful (teratogenic) drugs, refer to a gynecologist and obtain a pregnancy test unless this is unwarranted by extremes of age or by history information.

42–3. BARTHOLIN GLAND ABSCESSES *(See 23–4)*

42–4. BATTERED FEMALE SYNDROME

This problem should be suspected in women who have multiple soft tissue injuries *(59)* [and occasionally loosened teeth *(61)* and fractures *(47)*]. The given history of an accident is often confusing or inconsistent because of fear and ambivalence on the part of the victim, and the emotional reaction is inappropriate to the proffered history, but appropriate for one who had been beaten by someone with whom there is emotional involvement. Disclaimers of being beaten are not uncommon. Reporting to local law enforcement agencies *(15)* is required in some states and is the preferable policy, particularly with serious and repeated occurrence of injuries. Discussion with the patient should be undertaken to help provide for her subsequent safety. Staying with relatives or friends may be adequate; interested groups, such as National Organization of Women through local chapters or at (202) 347-2279, have lists of special shelters. Psychiatric and social counseling is advised. As is well known to the police, persons dealing with disrupted domestic relations should use caution for their personal safety. The counterpart of this syndrome (battered male syndrome) is reported less frequently, because of less occurrence and even greater reticence to make a claim. The policy of police arrest of batterers appears to be the best deterrent to recurrence.

42–5. BREAST ABSCESS *(See 23–7)*

42–6. DYSMENORRHEA (Painful Menstruation)

Evaluate for other concurrent causes of abdominal pain *(22)*. Uncomplicated dysmenorrhea can usually be relieved with simple oral analgesics (aspirin or another NSAID such as naproxen [Anaprox] or ibuprofen [Motrin]; see *12*); tranquilizer–muscle relaxants, such as meprobamate, chlordiazepoxide or diazepam, may be added if necessary (though this is generally not encouraged). Warmth (tub bath or heating pad) can be used to reflexly aid vasodilatation and smooth muscle relaxation. Exercise is encouraged, but as usual, avoid protracted fatigue and unresolved tension conditions. If vomiting is present, relief will usually be obtained with promethazine hydrochloride (Phenergan), 25-mg rectal suppository. Refer to a gynecologist for follow-up evaluation and care.

42–7. ECTOPIC PREGNANCY *(See 50–7)*

42–8. MASTITIS/MASTOPATHY

The acute bacterial form of mastitis is treated as for breast abscess *(23–7)*. Fibrocystic disease (mastopathy) is not an urgent medical problem except for the anxiety it produces when first discovered. Evaluation between menstrual periods, aspiration of larger cysts, and gynecologic follow-up for possible biopsy are indicated. Elimination of chocolate, tea, coffee and other sources of caffeine in the diet has occasionally resulted in subsidence.

42–9. MENORRHAGIA (Abnormally Profuse Menstruation)

The need for hospitalization and immediate gynecologic evaluation is dictated by the detailed history or amount of recent bleeding, degree of current bleeding evident on pelvic examination and signs and symptoms of significant anemia and hypovolemia *(57)*. Check for coagulation disorders *(45)*. Emergency gynecologic treatment of severe cases is usually uterine curettage or hormonal therapy, or both. Patients with mild cases may be sent home for bed rest and supportive care with gynecologic follow-up; prescribe oral iron and check serum iron levels if patient is anemic.

42–10. METRORRHAGIA (Bleeding Between Periods) *(See also Table 42–1, Causes of Abnormal Uterovaginal Bleeding)*

The principles of emergency evaluation and treatment are similar to those for menorrhagia *(42–9)*. Metrorrhagia is infrequently profuse, though, and

Table 42–1. CAUSES OF ABNORMAL UTEROVAGINAL BLEEDING BY AGE GROUPS*

Age†	Cause
Newborn	Maternal estrogen; bleeding tendencies.
3 to 7 years	Foreign body in vagina; trauma; sarcoma botryoides; granulosa cell tumors.
Menarche	Precocious puberty; blood dyscrasias; emotional states; anovulation.
Reproductive age	*Organic causes:* pelvic inflammation, chronic cervicitis, polyps, fibroids, cancer of cervix or uterus, hormones, blood dyscrasias, granulosa cell tumors, intrauterine device; *Pregnancy-related causes:* abortion, ectopic pregnancy, hydatid mole, placenta previa, placenta abruptio, uterine rupture; *Endocrine causes:* thyroid disturbances, emotional states, excess estrogen, anovulation, irregular shedding; "breakthrough bleeding" (with oral contraceptives).
Menopause	Cancer of cervix or endometrium; dysfunctional uterine bleeding as with anovulation.
Postmenopause	Cancer of uterus or cervix; exogenous hormones; granulosa cell tumor; senile vaginitis; retained pessaries; benign polyps; atrophic endometrium.

*Modified from Taber, B.-Z.: *Manual of Gynecologic and Obstetric Emergencies*. Philadelphia: W. B. Saunders Co., 1979.

†Blood dyscrasias *(45)*, trauma *(58)*, infection and foreign objects may be cause at any age.

uterine malignancy may be a more ominous possible cause, depending upon age and other factors.

42–11. MITTELSCHMERZ (Pain Midway Between Periods Associated with Ovulation)

Cyclic recurrent pain, 12 to 15 days prior to menses, which may be accompanied by slight spotting or bleeding, is characteristic. Obtain complete and differential cell counts. The diagnosis may be established by culdocentesis *(18–9)* (though this is seldom necessary) revealing serosanguineous peritoneal fluid. Hospitalization is infrequently required unless there is an apparent surgical emergency, in which case laparoscopy or laparotomy is usually the next indicated diagnostic measure, along with evaluation for other causes of abdominal pain *(22)*. Differentiation from acute appendicitis *(40–8)* or ectopic pregnancy *(50–7)* is important. In cases of prolonged bleeding from a ruptured corpus luteum, shock may develop. Women on anticoagulants are more likely to have protracted ovarian hemorrhage. Sedation and analgesics (e.g., acetaminophen or another NSAID other than aspirin; see 2) will control milder cases.

42–12. PELVIC INFLAMMATORY DISEASE (Acute Salpingitis, Tubo-ovarian Abscess)

If febrile and significant signs of peritonitis are present, hospitalize at once. Cervical culture or culdocentesis revealing purulent aspirate (which should be sent for culture, including anaerobes, and Gram stain) helps establish the diagnosis along with the pelvic examination and elevated level of white blood cells. Appropriate antibiotics in large doses should be commenced and continued for at least 10 days. Gonococcus organisms *(33–25)* are commonly found, and streptococci and bacteroides are not unusual. Penicillin plus probenecid

(Benemid) or, alternatively, ampicillin or tetracycline is usually effective when given in large doses. Tetracycline is considered best for *Chlamydia* infection. Rest, avoidance of intercourse for 2 weeks or until infection is totally resolved and supportive care are necessary. Obtain gynecologic consultation. Any intrauterine device (IUD) should be removed. Milder cases may be treated at home.

42–13. POSTPARTUM BLEEDING *(See 50–12)*

42–14. RUPTURE OF OVARIAN CYST

The fluid contents released when an ovarian cyst ruptures cause peritoneal irritation with abdominal pain and shoulder pain (due to diaphragmatic irritation). Usually the pain wanes over several hours. Culdocentesis and laparoscopy may be needed to aid diagnosis, particularly when there is associated bleeding. For relief of pain, see *12*.

Table 42–2. CLASSIFICATION OF VULVOVAGINITIS*

Causes	Diseases
ORGANISMS	
Bacteria	
Donovania granulomatis (Calymmatobacterium granulomatis)	Granuloma inguinale *(33–26)*
Escherichia coli	*E. coli* vaginitis
Hemophilus ducreyi	Chancroid *(33–10)*
Gardnerella vaginalis	Nonspecific vaginitis (Table 42–3)
Neisseria gonorrhoeae	Gonorrhea *(33–25)*
Treponema pallidum	Syphilis *(33–66)*
Staphylococcus	Folliculitis *(33–37)*
Chlamydia	
Lymphogranuloma venereum agent	Lymphogranuloma venereum *(33–37)*
Genital TRIC agent	Genital TRIC agent infection
Metazoa	
Phthirus pubis	Pediculosis pubis *(58–6E)*
Mycoplasma	
Mycoplasma hominis	Genital mycoplasma hominis infection
T-strain mycoplasma	Genital T-strain mycoplasma infection
Mycoses (Fungi)	
Candida albicans	Candidiasis (Moniliasis) (Table 42–3)
Protozoa	
Trichomonas vaginalis	Trichomoniasis (Table 42–3)
Viruses	
Herpes Simplex Type II	Herpes genitalis *(33–29)*
Genital wart virus	Condyloma acuminatum *(33–14)*
Genital cytomegalovirus	Genital cytomegalovirus infection *(33–16)*
Genital moluscum contagiosum virus	Genital molluscum contagiosum *(33–42)*
ALLERGIC REACTION *(24)*	
CONTACT REACTION	
FOREIGN BODIES *(39)*	
PSYCHOSOMATIC *(54–18)*	

*Modified from Taber, B.-Z.: *Manual of Gynecologic and Obstetric Emergencies.* Philadelphia, W. B. Saunders Co., 1979.)

Table 42–3. COMMON VULVOVAGINAL INFECTIONS
(Note: Also treat sexual partners)

	Nonspeciic Vaginitis	Herpes Genitalis	Trichomonas Vaginalis	Moniliasis *(Candida albicans)*
Symptoms	Slight pain	None to burning pruritus	Variable pruritus	Gross pruritus
Vulva	Normal appearance	Normal to vesicular eruption	Normal to moderate erythema	Gross erythema common
Vagina	Normal to slight erythema	Vesicular eruptions and small ulcers	"Strawberry spots"—petechiae	Whitish patches on reddened mucosa
Discharge	Mucoid whitish-gray, foul odor	Clear, if any, without odor	Abundant, foamy, foul odor	"Cottage cheese" appearance without odor
Wet Mount	Clue cells: grainy (from adherent bacilli) epithelial cells	Nondistinguishing*	4 to 5 flagella propel trichomonads	Branching hyphae, spores
Treatment	Metronidazole (Flagyl),† 500 mg PO bid for 7 days; alternatively can give ampicillin, 500 mg PO q 6 h for 5 days	5% topical acyclovir 6 times/day for 7 days; apply with finger cot	Treat patient and sexual partner with metronidazole (Flagyl),† 2 g PO in a single dose	Vaginal miconazole nitrate (Monistat 7) cream or clotrimazole (Gyne-Lotrimin), 1 vaginal tablet or cream at bedtime for 7 days

*Diagnose by immunofluorescent staining and clinical appearance of lesions, cytology and tissue culture.
†Avoid alcohol consumption during use because of disulfiram (Antabuse)-like effect.

42–15. SALPINGITIS *(See 42–12, Pelvic Inflammatory Disease)*

42–16. TORSION OF THE PEDICLE OF AN OVARIAN CYST

This condition requires surgical correction at once. The diagnosis is usually made at diagnostic laparoscopy or exploratory laparotomy for acute lower abdominal pain of sudden onset. Pelvic examination and ultrasound scan may delineate the mass.

42–17. VULVOVAGINITIS

The multiple causes of vulvovaginitis that require prompt recognition for control of venereal spread of organisms or acute treatment are listed in Table 42–2.

The most frequently seen types of vulvovaginitis and their treatment are listed in Table 42–3. See also *58–15* for treatment of pruritus.

Since spread of the organisms is commonly venereal, communicable disease control and treatment of all sexual partners should also be done concomitantly.

43. Hand Injuries

Adequate treatment of injuries to the hand requires specialized knowledge, skill and experience—not only in the proper care of soft tissue injuries but also in traumatic orthopedics, peripheral nerve repair and plastic surgery, especially skin grafting. If the emergency physician is not sure of the proper procedures, even though the injuries appear to be minor, he or she should arrange for treatment as soon as possible by a surgeon experienced in hand injury care. Microsurgery has added important dimensions in repair, salvage and replantation. Nerve and tendon function should always be determined on initial examination and recorded in detail on the emergency chart before any anesthetic, debridement or repair is begun. See also Figure 49–1, Anatomical Locations.

43–1. HAND TRAUMA AND INFECTION: INITIAL GENERAL MEASURES*

Remove Jewelry and Other Potentially Constrictive Materials. Rings should always be removed. Tight rings are more easily slipped off after application of a clean oily or greasy material; reduce swelling with massage, ice or centripetal wrapping (see Fig. 63–1); use a ring cutter or fine saw as a final resort.

Preliminary Cleaning

- Gram stain and culture if infected.
- Cleanse the area around the wound for at least several inches. The entire hand can be washed under tap water or soaked in a pan of sterile saline or hydrogen peroxide, or both, to facilitate removal of debris, dressings or other material. See *59–1* for grease removal; see *28–6* for tar removal.
- Cover the wound with sterile gauze. Cleanse the surrounding uninvolved skin with a water-soluble iodophor (Betadine), Hibiclens Antimicrobial Skin Cleanser or soap and water.
- Remove the gauze and mechanically clean the wound with bland, nonmedicated soap and water, loosening and removing superficial foreign bodies

*For amputations, see also *59–44*.

and following with copious sterile saline irrigation using a syringe (with No. 25 needle as necessary for fine spray) or a Water Pik apparatus. Deep cleaning need not be done now. Cover wound with sterile gauze during subsequent steps (this amount of cleaning is adequate for superficial wounds).

- Tetanus immunization *(20)* can be given before or after specific procedures.

History. Obtain a detailed account of the type of injury, duration of injury preceding any infection and exposure to any substance that may require special management. Record dominant hand and occupation (functional needs may affect therapeutic approach).

Brief Examination for Other Injuries. Before attention becomes focused on the hand, rapidly check the entire upper extremity and any other body areas that may be involved.

X-ray. Unless the involvement is superficial and slight, preliminary x-ray films (AP and true lateral; special navicular views if injury suspected) of the hand are advisable; this includes views of amputated parts being evaluated for possible implantation.

Examination for Nerve and Tendon Injury. Motor and sensory function should be tested and recorded before any anesthetic use.

NERVES

1. *Sensory* (see Fig. 49–1, Anatomical Locations). The "autonomous" sensory nerve zones on the hand are as follows: tip of the little finger (ulnar), tip of the index finger (median), dorsal web space between the thumb and index finger (radial).

Two-point discrimination is a most valuable test. Unbend a paperclip so the two ends are even: Normal digit tip discrimination of the two points is 5 mm or closer—inability to distinguish farther apart is pathologic.

The "wrinkle" test can be helpful for children who cannot give reliable responses: A normal digit will wrinkle after soaking 5 minutes in sterile distilled water, whereas a denervated finger will not. Frightened children may also respond more reliably to testing with a wisp of cotton for light touch rather than a needle for sharpness.

2. *Motor function.* The simple test of holding a pencil by the eraser between the thumb and, successively, each other digit is an excellent indicator of presence of injury, from either tendon or nerve severance causing functional impairment. Gross swelling, as from massive crush injuries and fractures, impairs the validity of motor tests, and decisions on extent of damage and repair may have to be delayed until swelling subsides or evaluation is done under direct vision.

For gross differential testing purposes:

- The *median nerve* innervates singly the opponens pollicis (compare bilaterally the force needed to break through the ring formed by opposition of the thumbtip to little fingertip; if pain interferes, palpate the opponens muscle while attempting opposition.
- The *ulnar nerve* innervates thumb adduction (last ulnar nerve branch); finger adduction (compare ability to hold sheet of paper between digits); finger abduction (compare ability in both hands to separate fingers against resistance of thick rubber band looped around all the fingers); and, in the little and ring fingers, flexion of the metacarpophalangeal joints plus extension of the proximal interphalangeal joints. Finger crossing ability is also a good test.
- The *radial nerve* innervates extrinsic extensors of the wrist and digits and must function to get metacarpophalangeal extension. (Test independent extension of index and little fingers.)

TENDONS

The following are common tendon injuries likely to be missed if not carefully assessed. Check for both range of motion and motion against resistance compared with the same area of the uninjured hand if there is question of a deficit. Unless the emergency room physician is proficiently experienced in hand surgery, tendon lacerations should be referred for repair. This is particularly true for injuries in the "zone of the pulleys" (region of the volar surface of the hand from the distal palmar crease to the middle of the middle phalanx), where only the most experienced hand surgeon should venture ("no other man's land").

EXTENSORS

- *Boutonniere deformity.* Rupture or laceration of the central extensor tendon slip at the proximal interphalangeal (PIP) joint and subsequent tear of the extensor hood aponeurosis results in a flexed position of the PIP joint and loss of extensor strength and range. See *43–2* regarding repair.
- *Extensor pollicis longus (EPL).* The thumb can be extended to 0 degrees at the interphalangeal joint by the intrinsics alone, and severance of the EPL tendon will be missed if the joint is not tested for *hyperextension.* The best test is to place the hand flat on a table and have the patient lift only the thumb off the table.
- *Mallet finger.* Distal interphalangeal (DIP) joint in a flexed position at rest and there is inability to actively extend the joint. See *43–2* regarding repair.

FLEXORS

- *Flexor digitorum profundus* (FDP). While the proximal interphalangeal joint is stabilized in extension, ask the patient to fully bend the tip of the finger (flex the distal interphalangeal joint); recheck distal flexion against resistance. The same procedure applies for the *flexor pollicis longus* with stabilization of the metacarpophalangeal joint.
- *Flexor digitorum superficialis* (FDS). While the metacarpophalangeal joint and the other digits are held in extension, ask the patient to bend the middle joint of the finger (flex the PIP joint). Recheck against resistance. When PIP joint flexion is caused solely by FDS, the DIP joint should be flaccid to passive motion.

Anesthesia. See 7, *Pain Management: Analgesia and Anesthesia.* For operative and humane reasons, one or more of these methods, usually a local or regional anesthetic block *(12–3)*, should be in effect before deep cleaning and debridement are done or repair is started.

Tourniquet Control. A pneumatic arm tourniquet should be used to ensure a bloodless field when necessary. (Avoid finger tourniquets.)

1. Elevate the involved extremity for about 1 minute and empty of as much blood as possible.
2. Place a blood pressure cuff around the arm and as it is inflated, remove the thumb, compressing the brachial artery. Inflate and keep the pressure higher than 200 to 250 mm Hg to act as a tourniquet. In lengthy procedures, the tourniquet should be relaxed for a few moments after an hour, and should not be applied for longer than 1½ to 2 hours at a time without management by a specialist and at least a 15-minute period of release.

Final Cleaning for More Complex Surgery

1. Sterile operating room technique is essential for all cases. All persons in the operating room, including the patient, should be capped (with hair confined) and masked, and operating personnel should wear sterile gloves after preliminary scrubbing. A sterile operating gown should be worn and full operating room technique in effect if a lengthy or extensive repair is needed.
2. The hand is rewashed with soap and water and again copiously lavaged

with sterile saline, then wrapped in a sterile towel while the operator changes gloves. The hand is again cleaned with a water soluble povidone-iodine (Betadine) and draped for surgery.

Examination of the wound is now performed, the operator looking for severance of large blood vessels, muscles, nerves or tendons; fractures; dislocations; epiphyseal displacements; foreign bodies; hematomas; and openings into or contamination of joints, tendon sheaths or fascial spaces. Using long suture material, tag gently any lacerated tendons whose repair is beyond the skill of the operator; avoid tagging nerves. If unexpectedly severe damage is encountered, the tourniquet should be removed (or loosened and reapplied if indicated), a sterile pressure bandage applied and the patient transferred at once to an adequately equipped hospital. Administration of a sedative may be advisable.

Debridement. The object of debridement is to convert an area of traumatized and potentially infected tissue into a surgically clean wound. With a small-toothed forceps, sharp scalpel and small curved scissors, sharp dissection should be used to remove any damaged structures to a depth of 1 to 2 mm, starting with the skin and working toward the depths of the wound. If exposure is inadequate with use of nontraumatic retractors, the surface laceration should be extended, bearing in mind the areas of safe incisions in the hand (Fig. 43–1). Excise grossly nonviable, dark, noncontractile muscle. Nerves, tendons, blood vessels and articular surfaces should be preserved, as should bone fragments with periosteal and soft tissue attachments.

Distal to the flexor crease of the wrist, it is preferable to avoid subcutaneous or space-closure sutures and limit wound closure to skin only. If there is a dead space, consider applying bulky sterile gauze moistened with saline solution to the open wound with planned delayed closure. If a Penrose drain or a drain tube made from a segment of sterile catheter is used, it should preferably exit from a site other than that of the laceration itself. Bleeding not controllable by pressure should be stopped by cautery, by vessel-twisting technique or by clamping and tying with No. 000 plain catgut or polyglycolic acid (Dexon). Buried suture material, however, should be kept to an absolute minimum. Be aware that the digital nerves lie immediately *adjacent* (superficially in the digit) to the digital arteries and care must be taken not to crush or include digital nerve parts or ends with clamps or ties in the arteries.

Completely severed small sections of soft tissue (for instance, fingertips) that are not badly macerated, in some instances (especially in small children), can be carefully cleaned and debrided for suturing back in place as full-thickness grafts. Pieces of skin should be defatted. The quicker this suturing is done, the better the chance of a "take." Intact skin from amputated parts that are to be discarded can be used for grafting denuded areas.

No antibiotics, antiseptics, disinfectants, sulfonamides or other substances of any type should be painted, sprayed, insufflated or sprinkled into the wound.

43–2. SPECIFIC PROCEDURES (CLOSURE, REPAIR, INCISION AND DRAINAGE)

Repairs and Closures. These should be done within 6 hours if possible. The closure time limit may be extended to 12 hours if the wound is not deep or extensive and if there is no evidence of gross contamination or infection. Lacerations and wounds that are more than 12 hours old should be irrigated and debrided *but not sutured.*

SIMPLE CLOSURES. See *43–9* and *59–22*.

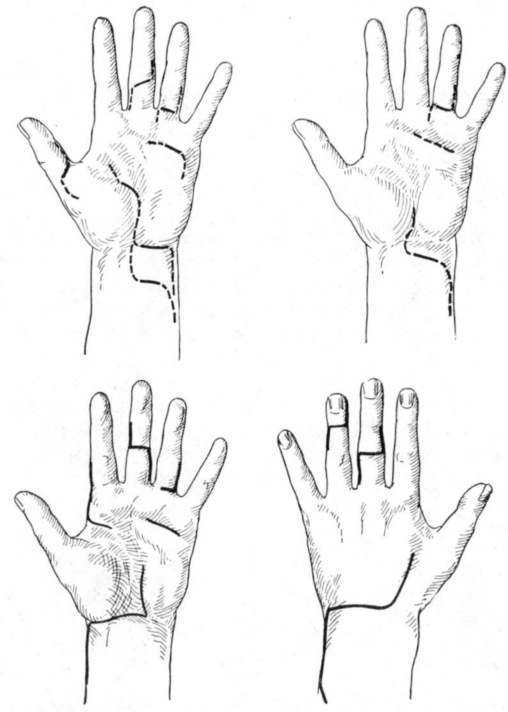

Figure 43–1. Certain general principles apply to the location of incisions on the hand. Incisions should avoid the midline; they should not cross flexion creases, but should parallel them as closely as possible and should be planned so as to produce flaps of skin and subcutaneous tissue to overlie the operative area. The same principles apply to enlargement of accidental wounds, which should be incorporated as well as possible into the general pattern of ideal incisions. Extreme caution must be used to avoid severance of the median cutaneous nerve with any incision along the radial volar aspect of the wrist. The volar zig-zag, or Bruner or "lazy S," incision (not shown), extending obliquely from one side of the finger at the flexor crease to the opposite side at the next flexor crease, affords excellent exposure for flexor tendon repair. (From Davis, L.: *Christopher's Textbook of Surgery,* 9th ed. Philadelphia, W. B. Saunders Co., 1968.)

COMPLEX CLOSURES

Grafts. See *28–3, Burns*.

Z-plasty. Usually not done as an initial procedure.

Arterial repair. See Figure 59–11.

Nerve repair. See *43–10;* Figure 59–12.

Tendon repair. See *43–12;* Figure 59–13.

Replantation. See *59–44*.

Infections (Splint and immobilize hand in all cases of infection; perform culture and sensitivity testing before selecting antibiotic)

SIMPLE

Cellulitis: Specific antibacterial administration is usually all that is required in addition to appropriate measures that are applicable as described in *59–1* and *59–3*.

Felon. See *23–13*.

Paronychia. See *23–19*.

Superficial abscess. See also *23–10, Collar-button Abscess*.

COMPLEX

1. Suppurative flexor tenosynovitis. Kanavel's four signs of tendon sheath involvement are uniform digit swelling, finger held in flexion, tenderness along the entire finger and exquisite pain with passive extension of the distal interphalangeal joint. These infections are extremely serious and require referral for urgent surgical decompression (focally and in the palm to aid circulation and to stop propagation of infection).

2. Joint infections (see *18–3* for joint aspiration). Joint infection may occur from penetrating wounds (e.g., tooth penetration of the metacarpophalangeal) and may require surgical debridement and drainage and treatment as a soft tissue infection (*59–42*), or it may be bacteremic in origin (e.g., gonococcal septic arthritis) and require appropriate treatment for the source of infection as well.

Massive infections: See *59–42, Soft Tissue Infections (Life Threatening)*, and *23–10, Collar-button Abscess*.

3. Extensor sheath infection at wrist: Focal tenderness, inflammation and pain with finger motion are present. Refer for immediate surgical and antibacterial treatment.

43–3. POSTSURGICAL MEASURES

Dressings. A small strip of sterile petrolatum gauze or a nonadherent dressing, such as Telfa, should be placed over the sutures and a pressure bandage applied to control oozing. Copious amounts of zinc oxide may be applied to a wound that would otherwise need soaks. Avoid use of tight circumferential wrapping and tubular gauze on digits. Collodion dressings should not be placed directly over a wound under ordinary circumstances because of the possibility of promoting growth of anaerobic organisms and because of the difficulty in removal. Collodion, however, can be used very satisfactorily to hold the edges of the outer dressings in place, especially on persons sensitive to various adhesive tapes.

Splints. A forearm splint also immobilizing the wrist and digits aids healing of larger and complex wounds by limitation of motion and prevention of tension on repaired structures. Immobilize in position of function [metacarpophalangeal joints in 70 degree and interphalangeal joints in 20 to 30 degree flexion and thumb in abduction-extension (grasp) position so any ensuing joint stiffness will be less disabling. Do not splint the thumb "at the side of the hand" (adducted position)]. Exposure of tips of digits permits circulation check, which should be done after the splint or cast is applied and the patient is instructed in rechecking. Circumferential wrapping with firm materials (e.g., plaster) should be avoided in acute injuries in which progressive swelling may compromise neurovascular structures. For minor injuries of the wrist, hand and fingers, volar splints may be useful initially while swelling goes down. For more severe fractures or injuries to the hand and fingers, a Bunnell-type compression pressure dressing is useful. This is accomplished by using multiple dressing fluffs on the volar and dorsal aspects of the hands and between the fingers, reinforced by Webril, plaster, and bias-cut stockinette dressing.

Elevation. Elevate the hand above the heart level with a sling (holding the hand and elbow against the chest), with pillows or with a well-padded arm board. See also Fig. 63–1 regarding later focal edema reduction.

Immunization. See *20, Tetanus Immunization; 33–28, Hepatitis Immunization.*

Antibiotics. Meticulous debridement can obviate need for routine prophylactic antibiotics. See *33–83, Antimicrobial Drugs of Choice.* Obtain a Gram stain and samples for culture and sensitivity testing in wounds that are not clean. An initial empiric antibiotic for contaminated fresh wounds, including gram-negative infected wounds, is a penicillin, a synthetic penicillin or a cephalosporin. Culture also for anaerobes.

Analgesics. See *12.* Usually aspirin or acetaminophen given alone or in combination with 16 or 32 mg of codeine is adequate.

Follow-up Care (See Table 59–1, Laceration Care). Small superficial lacerations, as well as more serious wounds, require *removal of the original bandage in 24 hours* for inspection and to allow for swelling. Compromise in circulation, gross bleeding and uncontrolled pain and spiking fever are indications for immediate recheck. Sutures are removed in 7 to 10 days except in skin areas under stress (14 days).

43–4. ABRASIONS OF THE HAND *(See 43–1)*

43–5. CELLULITIS OF THE HAND *(See 43–2; see also 59–42, Soft Tissue Infections)*

43–6. COLLAR-BUTTON ABSCESS *(See 23–10)*

43–7. CONTUSIONS OF THE HAND

Mild contusions require no emergency treatment. Cold compresses for the first 24 to 48 hours will accelerate recovery, with heat application delayed until about the 4th day with more extensive contusions. If extensive hematomas are present, the hand or digit should be immobilized on a padded splint and elevated, anodynes given and surgical or orthopedic follow-up care arranged. Severe crushing injuries may require hospitalization. Traumatic aneurysms of the palmar arteries have been reported following localized contusions.

Complications requiring special treatment measures are as follows:

- *Small hematomas* should be evacuated only if severe throbbing is present. Painless removal of the blood beneath the nail (subungual hematoma) by burning a small hole through the nail with a commercial heating unit (Thermo-Lance) or with a red-hot paper clip exposed about ⅛ of an inch below a holding forceps or with "drilling" with a 21-gauge needle gives complete relief. As a rule, no return visit is necessary unless infection develops.

- *Hematomas with associated external wounds* are potentially infected and require free drainage. A small section of the nail should be removed with sharp-pointed scissors after a preliminary drainage hole has been made (see step 1) and the blood evacuated. A dressing should be applied and protected by an aluminum or plastic fingertip guard. Recheck in 24 hours is essential.
- *Incomplete avulsion of the proximal end of the nail* may require completion of the avulsion under digital block anesthesia. Using sterile technique, the proximal portion, usually about one third of the nail, should be excised, blood removed from beneath the nail and soft tissue folds by irrigation and a stay suture of nylon inserted through the nail and soft tissue on each side. If the nail bed is lacerated in the region of the germinal matrix (Fig. 43–2), this should be repaired with fine gut (6-0, 7-0) ophthalmic suture. The nail sulcus can be maintained with Adaptic gauze, or the nail itself can be replaced (after thorough cleansing) to act as a distal splint for the repair. If the eponychium and underlying nail bed are lacerated, both must be repaired separately and kept separated by Adaptic gauze to prevent adhesions and a deformed nail. (*Note:* Check x-rays in this type of injury to be sure that open fracture of the distal tuft [47–35] is not also present.) A dressing and protective guard should be applied, tetanus-immune globulin (TIG) or toxoid given (20) and follow-up care in 24 hours arranged.
- *Contusions of the joints of the fingers* usually require prolonged splinting (*43–3, Splints*) to minimize permanent limitation of motions from fibrosis of the joint capsule. *If there is pain or instability with active or passive motion, splint!* Persistent gentle massage (inunction) of the bruised area with cocoa butter (if no open wound) will often decrease swelling and pain.

43–8. FRACTURES OF THE HAND *(See also 47–30 to 47–36; Fig. 49–1, Anatomical Locations)*

43–9. LACERATIONS OF THE HAND *(See 59–2 for simple and complex closures; see also 43–1, Initial Measures; 43–2, Repairs; 43–3, Postsurgical Measures; and Table 59–1, Laceration Care)*

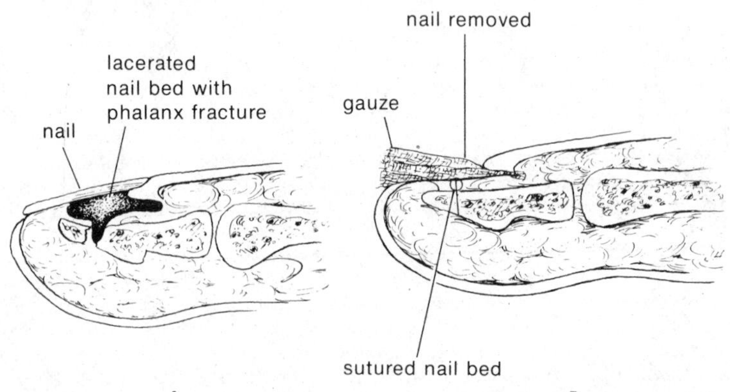

Figure 43–2. Repair of nail bed laceration. For suture of the nail bed, No. 6-0 absorbable suture is advisable.

43–10. NERVE INJURIES IN THE HAND *(See also 43–1, under Nerves, and 49–11, Peripheral Nerve Injuries)*

Primary Versus Secondary (Delayed) Nerve Suturing. Unless the emergency physician has had training in nerve repair, he or she should not attempt a primary nerve suture. If immediate referral for care by a qualified surgeon is not possible, careful debridement *(43–1)* should be performed. Since a capable surgeon will be able to identify digital nerve ends with ease, avoid tagging them, as further incurred injury may diminish the success of subsequent neurorrhaphy. Depending upon circumstances and availability of an experienced hand surgeon or neurosurgeon, the wound may be dressed open and kept moist with sterile saline or skin closure may be performed with plans for secondary nerve suture. The procedure should be explained to the patient (or parents, spouse or legal guardian). Whenever possible, and particularly when there is a question as to whether or not the deficit was caused by the injury, a baseline EMG should be made since, as a rule, denervation potentials do not develop until about 21 days after injury.

Evaluation of Motor and Sensory Deficits. Localized pressure from crushing injuries, or from a too tight tourniquet, may result in motor and/or sensory loss distal to the point of pressure. Before any anesthetic or treatment is given, motor function and sensation should be carefully evaluated and noted in detail on the emergency chart. Slow recovery of complete function usually occurs if pressure is the only causative factor in the motor or sensory deficit.

43–11. PUNCTURE WOUNDS OF THE HAND

The treatment of puncture wounds requires the exercising of good judgment and common sense by the attending physician. The method of injury, chance of infection and possibility of buried foreign bodies must be considered. Any puncture or laceration of the digital flexion creases must be highly suspect for nerve or tendon sheath laceration, because the sheaths are so superficially subcutaneous at this location; if deficits are found, they should be carefully explored (under sterile conditions) for injury using tourniquet control. All patients with puncture wounds should receive tetanus-immune globulin (TIG) or toxoid *(20)* and, if hepatitis exposure is possible, hepatitis virus immunization *(33–28)*.

Enlargement of the wound tract, thorough irrigation, careful debridement and suturing *(43–1)* are indicated for gross contamination, possible foreign bodies embedded in the soft tissue *(59–27)*, human bites *(27–17)* and indelible pencil wounds, whether or not the lead is still present. These require extensive excision of all discolored tissue as soon as possible. See *53–75, Aniline dyes.*

43–12. TENDON INJURIES IN THE HAND

In the Palm or Dorsum of the Hand. If inspection or tests of function show evidence of complete severance of a flexor or extensor tendon proximal to the metacarpophalangeal joints, immediate referral for specialized care is indicated. Partial severance without separation or loss of continuity must be recognized and repaired after irrigation and debridement, using fine Mersilene, Prolene or nylon sutures. In general, lacerations to the extensor tendons in the wrist and hand are less disabling than injuries to flexor tendons, as the extensors do not have the delicate tendon sheaths of the flexors. Occasionally, if in excellent opposition, a lacerated extensor tendon at the wrist need not be sutured; instead, the appropriate finger is immobilized in extension for 4 to 6 weeks.

In the Digits

FLEXORS. Referral for specialist care is best, if available. Repair should be done in the operating room (see Fig. 59–13).

EXTENSORS. Severed extensor tendons (except in the thumb) retract very little, and no true pulleys or tendon sheaths are present; therefore, repair can usually be accomplished at the time of emergency debridement and closure. Multiple lacerations with large wounds should be repaired in the operating room. Fine nylon or Prolene should be used, employing, for example, the Bunnell or double-right-angle stitch and splinting for 6 weeks in position of function with wrist in 30 to 40° dorsiflexion. The specialized flexible pull-out wire technique recommended by Bunnell should not be attempted as an emergency procedure unless the emergency surgeon has had adequate training and experience in this method.

Some extensor tendon injuries require special handling. One such type of injury is avulsion of the extensor tendon attachment to the proximal lip of the dorsal aspect of the distal phalanx, usually associated with tearing off of a small flake of bone—the so-called *"baseball"* or *"mallet" finger*. For treatment, see *47–35, Distal Phalanx Fractures*. Another is the *boutonniere deformity*—buttonhole splitting of the central slip of the extensor digitorum communis tendon at the proximal interphalangeal joint—which causes "paradoxical flexion." This can occur with trauma to the finger and no laceration; although it may not be obvious, pain dorsally over the proximal interphalangeal joint should make one suspicious. If no fracture of the base of the middle phalanx is demonstrated on x-ray, the treatment can be conservative with splinting. In the case of laceration, surgery should be performed by a hand surgeon. After debridement, the split in the tendon can be repaired using a simple figure-of-eight removable stitch of stainless steel wire. Splinting in continuous full extension of the metacarpophalangeal and proximal interphalangeal joints (but allowing full range of motion of the distal interphalangeal joint) for 3 to 6 weeks, followed by gradually increasing active (not passive) motion, usually results in recovery of near full function.

Traumatic and Acute Tendinitis. See *47–4*.

Stenosing Tenovaginitis (de Quervain's disease). Thickening and narrowing of the sheath of the abductor pollicis longus (and sometimes of the extensor brevis) causes severe pain and loss of function. A forearm-hand splint should be applied, analgesics given and referral made to a surgeon for further definitive care; the condition may require relief by longitudinal splitting of the sheath under local anesthesia. Injection of corticoids and acupuncture are other, nonsurgical, approaches to treatment of nonbacterial tendinitis.

Gamekeeper's Thumb. This common musculoskeletal injury is most often seen in skiing and results from a radial force being applied to the affected thumb, with specific stress placed at the metacarpophalangeal joint. The patient presents with intense pain over the ulnar portion of the metacarpophalangeal joint of the thumb. Swelling and pain of the affected area are common. X-rays are usually negative but occasionally reveal a small detached piece of the ulnar proximal phalanx. It is most important for the physician to determine the integrity of the ligamentous structures surrounding the ulnar border of this joint, using infiltration with lidocaine if necessary before stressing. If instability is demonstrated either by clinical or radiologic stress films, consideration should be given to repair of the ligamentous structures; consultation with an orthopedic specialist or hand surgeon is recommended.

44. Head Injuries*

44–1. GENERAL CONSIDERATIONS

The general condition of the patient is the primary emergency consideration in all head injuries (see *1–3*); patients who have sustained serious head injuries often have other significant accompanying injuries. Blood pressure, pulse, pulse pressure, respiration, color and especially *degree or state of consciousness* are rapid and accurate indices of the patient's condition. All should be checked as soon as possible and at frequent intervals thereafter. *Changes in condition* are the most important factors in the evaluation of head injuries; see Table 32–2, Glasgow Coma Scale. Rapid or progressive deterioration suggests a serious condition, such as an epidural hemorrhage from the middle meningeal artery (*44–20*), requiring immediate surgical intervention as a lifesaving measure (see 2, *Urgency Evaluation—Triage*).

44–2. INITIAL NEUROLOGIC EXAMINATION

The initial examination is all-important in guiding action. The first measure is to protect the neck (see sequence in *1–3*). The following points should be covered in detail and recorded in the patient's record, giving negative as well as positive findings:

- Temperature, pulse, respiration and blood pressure. Note also pattern of respirations.
- General appearance—position, condition of clothing, etc., when first seen.
- Evidence of severe or multiple injuries requiring immediate attention (2, *Urgency Evaluation—Triage*).
- Examination of the head for evidence of trauma (wounds; hematomas; depressions; bleeding from the ears, nose or throat; etc.).

State of Consciousness and Mental Status

CLEAR. Presence or absence of retrograde amnesia. Check with patient the last thing remembered before impact, and if impact itself is recalled, also check duration of unconsciousness, lucid interval, disorientation (time/place/person/events) and aphasia (fluent or nonfluent).

SEMICOMATOSE. Response to commands and painful stimuli is grossly present; patient is delirious, restless, lethargic or stuporous.

COMATOSE. Response to painful stimuli only or no response.

Speech. Clear or dysphasic. Content appropriate to circumstances.

Patient's Self-Evaluation. Any headache, nausea, vomiting?

Cranial Nerves. Evaluate all cranial nerves, with emphasis on cranial nerves II, III, IV, VII, VIII and IX; check XI and gag reflex in the unresponsive patient.

Eyes. Size and equality or nonequality of pupils, reaction to distance and light, nystagmus, diplopia, coordination of extraocular movements, funduscopic examination. Check eye movement (or lack thereof) with rotary movement of head (if no cervical fracture present); in comatose patient also check response to otic caloric stimulation if no CSF otorrhea (*35–19*).

Motor Power. Ability to move all the extremities (include hand grips and toe movements) and the facial muscles equally on both sides; note any weakness

---

*Caution: *Look for associated neck injuries.*

See also 32, *Coma* (esp. Fig. 32–1); 37–6, *Excitement States; Table 4–1, Management of Patients with Serious Head-Neck Injuries Awaiting Transportation for Hospital Care.*

or paralysis (flaccid, spastic). Note voluntary movement, movement in response to pain, decorticate movement (with arms flexed and legs extended) and decerebrate movement (arms and legs extended, neck extended, jaws tight, general rigidity).

Sensation. Variations in perception of pin prick, light touch, position and vibratory sense on the face, arms, legs and trunk.

Rectal Sphincter Tone (Anal Sphincter Reflex). Flaccidity is an indication of spinal cord injury. (*Note:* Repetitious anal intercourse may also cause some decrease in anal sphincter tone.)

Reflexes. Superficial (corneal, gag, abdominal, cremasteric, anal/otic caloric stimulation in the comatose patient) and deep tendon (biceps, triceps, radial, knee jerks, ankle jerks).

Pathologic Reflexes. Plantar response (do with the knee straight) on left and right sides—flexor (normal) or extensor (Babinski or pathologic sign); of particular note is whether there is a unilateral lack of either flexor or extensor response, which may be an early sign of pyramidal tract compromise. Unilateral Hoffman sign and clonus (either sustained or consisting of a few clonic jerks) are also pathologic signs.

44–3. LOCALIZATION OF HEAD INJURY LEVEL

Early unilateral supratentorial lesions usually cause hemiparesis and hypesia, plus agnosia (indifference) if the nondominant hemisphere is involved and aphasia if the dominant hemisphere is involved. Determination of involvement of the progressive lower levels alone is aided by utilization of Table 44–1 and Figure 32–1 (pupils in the unresponsive patient).

The oculovestibular test (30 ml iced saline flushed into the ear to the tympanic membrane) and oculocephalic test (rotating the head to each side and observing eye movement—"doll's eye" maneuver) are best delayed until after a cross-table lateral cervical x-ray has helped establish absence of a neck injury.

Computerized tomography (CT) scan, being precise, noninvasive and readily performed, is the most helpful measure in distinguishing neurosurgical patients from nonsurgical patients. Angiography is also of aid.

Voluntary efforts and responses despite unilateral supratentorial lesions (epidural and subdural hematoma, intracerebral hemorrhage—also abscess, infarct and rapidly expanding tumor) prior to the onset of unconsciousness and coma help determine the level of the lesion (and to differentiate it from metabolic encephalopathy except for possibly hypoglycemic coma and hepatic encephalopathy). After onset of coma, consider that one or both of two anatomic areas of the brain must be involved (1) the cerebral hemispheres bilaterally and (2) the reticular activating system (RAS) in the brain stem above the midpons. A unilateral supratentorial lesion must therefore either directly expand or, most commonly, cause cerebral edema (44–7) to involve these areas, causing progressive stepwise dysfunction from the hemispheres to the lower levels: thalamus, midbrain, pons and medulla. A subtentorial lesion, however, causes unconsciousness early because of rapid involvement of the RAS in the brain stem; posterior fossa subdural, epidural and intracerebellar hemorrhage, though uncommon, are amenable to neurosurgery.

Uncal Syndrome (Early Midbrain Damage)

Early midbrain involvement by herniation of the uncus (medial portion of the temporal lobe) across the cerebellar tentorium causes direct pressure on the proximal brain stem at midbrain level. This is usually due to an expanding

Table 44–1. LOCALIZATION OF INTRACRANIAL LESION LEVEL*

	Level	Consciousness Level†	Respiratory Pattern	Pupils	Oculocephalic (OC) and Oculovestibular (OV) Test‡	Movement After Painful Stimulus §
	Intact	alert	Smooth, cyclic, 12–18/minute breathing	bilaterally equal; constrict to light with slow release	OC: eyes coordinated, move toward midline OV: eyes move toward iced ear, nystagmus, pain	vigrous protective response of upper/lower extremities
Supratentorial	Early diencephalic	drowsy	early Cheyne-Stokes	as above	OC: as above OV: as above	often unilateral paresis and hypesthesia; flexor response of less affected side
Supratentorial	Late diencephalic	stuporous or unconscious	Cheyne-Stokes breathing	equal; pupillary constriction even prior to light stimulus	OC: as above OV: as above	as above, but minimal motion of less affected side
Subtentorial Brain Stem	Midbrain	unconscious	irregular tachypnea	mid sized, fixed, nondilating, early may be unilateral**	OC: no response OV: caloric stimulation of ear opposite lesion produces no medial deviation of eye ipsilateral to lesion	no response; extensor rigidity of upper/lower extremities
Subtentorial Brain Stem	Pontine-medullary	unconscious	low tidal volume, irregular, slow to apneic	nonresponsive, maximally dilated	OC: no response OV: no response	upper extremities extended/rigid; knees/thighs may flex slightly

*Modified from Plum, F., and Posner, J. B.: *The Diagnosis of Stupor and Coma*, 2nd ed. Philadelphia, F. A. Davis, 1972.
†See text.
‡OC = "doll's eyes" maneuver; OV = caloric stimulation test
§Fist rubbing of sternum; supraorbital ridge pressure—avoid slipping against eye.
**See text: uncal syndrome.

supratentorial lesion or related cerebral edema. Signs are an arousable but drowsy (may be comatose) patient; an enlarged ipsilateral pupil that responds sluggishly to light; ipsilateral medial rectus weakness; poor or no medial deviation of the eye on the involved side toward the calorically stimulated contralateral ear. Any indicated neurosurgical procedure must be done promptly.

44–4. SHOCK

Shock does not usually accompany head injuries in adults but may be encountered, for example, from a laceration of either a major cerebral venous sinus that is bleeding internally or of galeal vessels or at the end-stage of increased intracranial pressure or brain stem injury. If shock is present, it must be treated (57); at the same time, definitive therapy for other conditions is begun. Injuries elsewhere should always be looked for and treated in order of urgency (2). A gradually decreasing pulse pressure may be the only evidence of increasing intracranial pressure. Intensive treatment of gross cerebral edema (*44–7*) may be lifesaving.

44–5. ADEQUACY OF THE AIRWAY

Adequacy of the airway and ventilation is essential; head-injured patients particularly tend to develop hypercapnia and acidosis. Removal of mucus and blood by postural drainage and suction should be begun at once and continued as needed. If the patient is vomiting, the head should be lowered and turned to the side (Fig. 4–5 *A*) and frequent suction utilized to minimize the danger of secondary lung infection from aspirated vomitus. An endotracheal tube should be placed if there are signs of respiratory difficulty or stridor.

44–6. SEDATION

Sedation should be avoided unless a computerized tomography (CT) scan and evaluation indicate the absence of a clot or neurosurgical lesion and extreme restlessness or excitement (37–*8*) is present. Parenteral administration of rapid-acting drugs whose effect is of short duration is preferable, although rectal administration may be advisable in some circumstances—for instance, if a properly signed treatment permit (69–*9*) cannot be obtained. The oral route should never be used; it may cause vomiting which, in turn, may cause increased intracranial pressure with extension of intracranial damage.

44–7. CONTROL OF CEREBRAL EDEMA

Water is not compressible, and the brain is enclosed in an unyielding calvarium (except in infants and young children before closure of the fontanelles and sutures). Therefore, if the progressive cycle of edema, increased intracranial pressure and ischemia is unchecked, disastrous and many times alarmingly rapid worsening of central nervous system (CNS) function can occur.

There are as many causes of cerebral edema and increased intracranial pressure as there are of pulmonary edema; e.g., trauma, infections of many types, high altitude, tumor, hypertensive encephalopathy, numerous toxins and repetitive seizures.

Manifestations of cerebral edema and increasing intracranial pressure include headache, lethargy, vomiting, papilledema, diplopia, increased systolic blood pressure, slowed respirations and pulse and, with more advanced stages, temporal lobe herniation (ipsilateral or contralateral hemiparesis, ipsilateral pupil dilatation and cranial nerve III palsy and sometimes contralateral homonymous hemianopsia) and cerebellar herniation (midbrain signs). Of aid in establishing the diagnosis are the CT scan, the radioisotope scan, angiography and an intracranial catheter. Lumbar puncture is better avoided if diagnosis is clear but, if necessary to exclude infection, perform with small-bore needle, take only 1 manometer full of fluid and turn patient to semiprone, level position.

Treatment

In conditions that are prone to develop cerebral edema, preventive measures are the preferred treatment, as follows:

- Fluid intake, 5% dextrose with 0.25% sodium chloride, 30 ml/kg/day in children and adults. Potassium supplement as needed.
- Reduce fever.
- Control seizures.
- Treat shock and adequately ventilate.
- Lying position, lateral decubitus.
- Neurosurgical consultation.

When signs of cerebral edema are already present, consider one or more of the following measures:

- Mannitol, 2.8 to 3.0 g/kg IV initially (average adult dose = 200 g), then 0.3 to 0.5 g/kg/hr IV infusion, repeated in 4 hours if necessary.
- Furosemide (Lasix), 40 mg IM or slowly IV over several minutes.
- Passive hyperventilation to reduce pCO_2 to 25 to 30 torr.
- Dexamethasone, about 1 mg/kg up to 10 mg IV loading, and 0.4 mg/kg up to 4 mg IV q 6 h maintenance.
- Advancing case is an indication for insertion of an intracranial pressure monitor for monitoring and removal of fluid.
- Phenobarbital or thiopental sodium (1.5 to 3 mg/kg); ventilate prn.
- Possible hypothermia treatment. Consider calcium slow channel blockers.
- Consider also use of hyperbaric oxygen (HBO). DMSO given IV also has shown effectiveness but is not an approved or standard use as yet.

44–8. CONTROL OF PAIN

Opiates and synthetic narcotics are definitely contraindicated in the presence of head injuries because of the possibility of loss or modification of pupillary signs, depression of respiration or masking of signs of developing intracranial pressure. If serious injuries elsewhere in the body cause severe pain, non-narcotic and nonmedicinal approaches to pain control (*12*) can be tried; if these are not sufficiently effective, give pentazocine lactate (Talwin IM or IV in 15- to 30-mg doses; if it is found or believed that this medication is also interfering with the neurologic picture, naloxone can be administered to reverse its effect.

44–9. UNRELATED CONDITIONS

The clinical picture of acute head injury can easily be confused with certain endocrine disorders (*36*), intoxications from alcohol (*37–1; 53–295*) or drugs (*32–14*), diabetes (*32–3*) and heat stroke (*62–7*); sometimes multiple problems coexist. If the history or physical findings suggest the possibility of head injury, the patient should be kept under close observation and control until the picture has clarified.

44–10. CONCUSSION OF THE BRAIN

If details of the history or neurologic findings suggest the possibility of concussion, the patient should be kept under close observation for at least 4 to 6 hours after loss of consciousness and until the condition has stabilized before release from control. If unrelated conditions (*44–9*) that might confuse the picture are present, close observation until the possibility of brain damage can be ruled out is mandatory. Frequent examinations for changes in condition (*44–2*) should be made and recorded chronologically in the patient's record. A cross-table lateral cervical spine x-ray is indicated in every patient who has had serious head injury to rule out unsuspected cervical spine dislocation. Computerized tomography (CT) scan has proved to be of great value in evaluating acute head injuries. This technique can readily distinguish hematomas from areas of contusion. If, in the considered opinion of the attending physician, it is safe to send the patient home, specific, simply written instructions (Table 44–2) regarding observation for post-traumatic symptoms and signs should be given and explained as necessary by the physician (or a knowledgeable assistant) personally to responsible members of the family.

44–11. ACUTE EXCITEMENT STATES

Acute excitement states (*37–8*) and sometimes even mania (*54–17*), can follow brain concussion. Provided that edema, increased intracranial pressure and clot have been excluded, rapid-acting barbiturates, chloral hydrate, chlorpromazine hydrochloride (Thorazine), paraldehyde or prochlorperazine dimaleate (Compazine) may be used for mild sedation.

44–12. FRACTURES OF THE SKULL *(See 44–13 through 44–19)*

44–13. LINEAR FRACTURES WITHOUT DEPRESSION

Linear fractures without depression are surprisingly well tolerated, especially by children, provided the middle meningeal artery or its branches are not damaged (see *44–20, Extradural Hemorrhage*).

The location, not the extent, of the fracture and the condition of the patient are the most important factors to be considered in disposition. All patients with proved or suspected skull fracture should be kept under close observation for at least 12 hours; patients without neurologic signs can be allowed to go home with instructions to responsible members of the family as outlined under *44–10, Concussion*. If the general and neurologic pictures indicate that the patient's condition is deteriorating, immediate hospitalization under the care of a neurosurgeon should be arranged.

44–14. DEPRESSED FRACTURES

All scalp lacerations should be palpated with a gloved finger to examine for a depressed fracture. Depressed fractures can be confused with the edge of a scalp hematoma at times. Tangential x-ray films, CT scan, or direct observation is necessary to establish the diagnosis. Conservative treatment ordinarily is carried out. Elevation of slightly depressed fragments is not an emergency procedure unless signs of rapidly increasing intracranial pressure are present. All patients with proved or suspected depressed skull fractures should be hospitalized for close observation under the care of a neurosurgeon.

44–15. COMPOUND (OPEN) DEPRESSED FRACTURES

Treatment

- Immediate hospitalization for neurosurgical care is indicated after superficial cleansing and application of a turban-type head dressing.
- If the condition is noted during or after debridement, the galea and scalp should not be closed. Instead, after control of gross hemorrhage, a sterile dressing should be applied and the patient transferred at once to a hospital by ambulance for neurosurgical evaluation and treatment.

44–16. BASAL SKULL FRACTURES

Diagnosis usually depends upon the clinical picture since this type of fracture usually cannot be demonstrated by x-ray films. The presence of blood in the middle ear or external canal (check that it did not flow in from elsewhere) or bruising behind the pinna over the mastoid (Battle's sign) should be looked for in every case of head injury and, if present, constitutes strong evidence of basal skull fracture. The fracture itself is not associated with a high mortality rate unless there is also temporal lobe contusion or laceration. Patients with suspected basal skull fracture should be admitted for observation. See also *44–18, Middle Fossa Fractures*.

44–17. ANTERIOR FOSSA FRACTURES

Circumferential bruising around the eye ("Panda sign") is indicative of an anterior fossa skull fracture until proved otherwise.

Special Comments

- Place in a position of least drainage of cerebrospinal fluid rhinorrhea, with the draining area most superior.
- Caution the patient against blowing the nose.
- Avoid giving opiates and synthetic narcotics (*44–8*).
- Hospitalize by ambulance as soon as possible. Do not attempt to control rhinorrhea or nasal hemorrhage by packing or intranasal medication of any type. Antibiotics are not indicated. Obtain neurosurgical consultation.

44–18. MIDDLE FOSSA FRACTURES

Blood or a mixture of spinal fluid and blood from an undamaged ear canal may be diagnostic.

Observe for facial nerve injury, as this occurs in about 50% of the transverse fractures of the petrous portion of the temporal bone. Immediate paralysis is an indication for facial nerve exploration. Delayed onset of paralysis (e.g., the next morning) usually means that the nerve is in continuity but function is temporarily altered (neuronapraxia) and will improve without surgery.

Special Comments

- Warn the patient against blowing the nose.
- Cover the ear with sterile gauze and apply a turban-type head dressing. Do not attempt to cleanse the ear canal.
- Avoid opiates and synthetic narcotics (44–8).
- Hospitalize by ambulance as soon as possible for neurosurgical consultation.

44–19. POSTERIOR FOSSA FRACTURES

Unless the fracture is compound (open), the diagnosis of fractures in this area of the skull can be made only by x-rays. Anteroposterior, posteroanterior, basilar, Towne and lateral views usually are required. No emergency measures except supportive therapy, hospitalization for observation and neurosurgical consultation are indicated unless the transverse sinus is torn and an epidural hematoma (*44–20*) develops.

44–20. EXTRADURAL (EPIDURAL) HEMORRHAGE *(See also 63–4 Intracranial Hemorrhage)*

Tearing of the middle meningeal artery or separation of the sagittal sinus from the skull with tearing of the diploic veins may cause collection of blood between the dura mater and the skull. Direct trauma, sometimes very slight, is the usual cause; persons between 20 and 50 years of age represent the majority of cases.

Signs and Symptoms

Disturbances of consciousness of varying duration, a "lucid interval" lasting from one-half hour to several days (not always present; headache and vomiting may occur during this period) and rapid deterioration of condition with symptoms and signs of rising intracranial pressure, headache, vomiting, stupor succeeded by hemiplegia and slowing pulse and respiratory rate, coma and, finally, vasomotor collapse. Unilateral dilation of the pupil occurs in about 75% of cases but may be transient. Funduscopic examination is unrevealing.

Treatment

If the patient's condition is deteriorating rapidly, *immediate* evacuation of the hematoma may be a lifesaving measure (2, *Urgency Evaluation—Triage*). This should be done if possible in a properly equipped hospital by a neurosurgeon, but if a delay is unavoidable, it should be performed in any feasible emergency setting. Delay will result in irreversible brain damage from pressure. As soon as the acute compression of the brain is released, the most immediate emergency is over. Further care by a neurosurgeon should, of course, be arranged as soon as possible.

The procedure may be done with the use of a local anesthetic, injecting the successive layers that will be met, skin, fascia/muscle, periosteum of the bone. Beneath the bone is the epidural space. If a clot is found, enlarge the opening for adequate removal of clot and get further help. Continued meningeal artery bleeding requires control. Subdural hematoma may exist beneath the epidural hematoma.

The sites for trephination, which are generally located over the fracture site or as shown in Figure 44–1 (which depicts the average adult), are as follows:

- The coronal suture, 3.5 cm from midline.
- Temporal area 1.5 cm anterior to the ear and 1.5 cm above the zygoma (and anterior to the superficial temporal artery).
- Above the ear 3.5 cm and behind it 3.5 cm.
- Posterior fossa on either side of midline.

44–21. SUBDURAL HEMORRHAGE

Subdural hemorrhage may present in the acute, subacute or chronic form. The acute form presents as extradural hemorrhage (*44–20*) and should be evaluated and treated in the same manner.

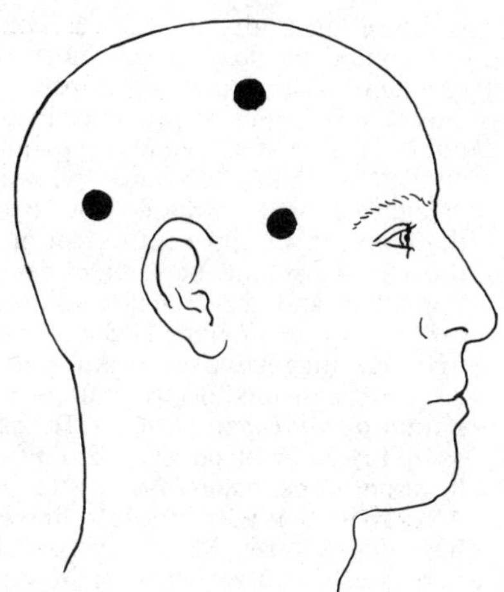

Figure 44–1. Location for craniotomy "burr holes."

The bleeding in this condition usually comes from a tear in one of the cerebral veins entering the dural sinuses, the result usually of direct trauma to the frontal or occipital regions but can be caused by trauma to any area of the head. This hemorrhage is venous and its pressure less than in extradural hemorrhage; hence, signs of brain damage may be much slower in developing—often days, sometimes weeks but rarely months after head trauma. At times, there is no history of head trauma.

In addition to the usual history of a substantial blow to the head, these patients may have severe headaches or vomiting and may have evidence of fracture behind the ears seen directly or on x-ray. CT scan readily identifies the subdural hematoma, and there may be evidence of edema and contusion of underlying brain.

Subacute or chronic subdural hematomas are characterized by persistent or recurrent headaches, personality change, periods of depressed state of consciousness, fluctuating degrees of hemiparesis, seizures, vomiting and intermittent dilatation of a pupil.

Treatment

Hospitalization for localization and definitive care by a neurosurgeon is indicated as soon as signs and symptoms suggestive of increased intracranial pressure are noted. The usual sites of entry utilized by the neurosurgeon are indicated in Figure 44–1. Trephination is a procedure that has been done since prehistoric times, and if a neurosurgeon is not and will not soon be available, a timely performed burr hole procedure done cautiously by a relatively inexperienced physician may exceed the benefits of a long-delayed operation done by the most skilled neurosurgeon. The procedure can be done with local anesthetic and under rare instances of continuing isolation and urgency should be commenced by the most able individual available.

44–22. LACERATIONS OF THE SCALP

Treatment

- After a careful history and thorough examination for evidence of intracranial damage, the area should be prepared by thorough cleansing of the surrounding scalp. Shaving is not necessary for small, clean lacerations but should be done if the laceration is jagged or extensive. Under 1% procaine or lidocaine anesthesia, the skull should be palpated with the gloved finger and, if possible, inspected. If a depression or defect can be felt or seen, a sterile nonradiopaque dressing should be applied, with x-ray studies (including tangential views) made before closure of the laceration. "Negative" x-ray films do not always rule out the presence of a fracture; therefore, if an apparent defect or variation from normal has been noted, the patient should be kept under close observation for at least 8 hours. Palpation and direct observation are often more accurate than x-rays, especially if a nondepressed linear or stellate fracture is present. Neurologic findings suggestive of brain injury, with or without evidence of skull damage, call for hospitalization, close observation and frequent determination of vital signs (*44–1*). It should be remembered that thickening of scalp layers by blood or fluid may simulate a fracture (*44–14*) and that the location of the lesion (*44–3*) is of great importance in prognosis.

- After irrigation with sterile saline and careful debridement, lacerations are best closed in two layers. Use an absorbable suture for the galeal layer for hemostasis and nylon 30 or 40 on a large cutting needle for the skin. A mattress suture is also recommended. After closure, a pressure bandage should be applied to control oozing.
- Tetanus-immune globulin (TIG) or toxoid (*20*) and antibiotics should be administered if gross contamination is present or if treatment has been delayed.
- Hospitalization is not necessary unless excessive blood loss has occurred, examination has indicated the possibility of a depressed fracture, or signs of increased intracranial pressure (*44–10*) have been noted or develop.
- All patients should be told to report to a physician for recheck examination in not more than 2 days. The patient or a responsible member of the family should be instructed in detail orally by the attending physician regarding signs and symptoms of increased intracranial pressure (*44–10*) and given a printed head injury instructions form (Table 44–2).

44–23. AXIOMS IN EMERGENCY CARE OF HEAD INJURIES
(Modified from Metcalf, S.)

Axiom 1. Initial impression of the severity of any head injury must never be regarded as final. Within 12 hours the apparently trivial head injury may become surgical, the closed head injury may turn out to be trivial.

Axiom 2. Any force of sufficient magnitude to produce either skull fracture or concussion may also have caused a cervical spine fracture. *Cross-table lateral cervical spine x-rays using a portable x-ray machine should always precede a skull series.*

Axiom 3. Except for infants and young children and except in late stages of severe brain injury, a patient with head injury who is in shock will be found to have injuries elsewhere to account for the shock. Treatment of shock takes precedence over most other diagnostic and therapeutic measures.

Axiom 4. Never send a patient to the ward with diagnosis other than "*Head Injury.*" A specific diagnosis can more safely be made when the patient leaves the hospital.

Axiom 5. Do not give narcotics or sedatives to head injury patients. Chlorpromazine hydrochloride (Thorazine) may be used for excessive restlessness after ascertaining there is no intracranial bleeding.

Axiom 6. Avoid general anesthesia whenever possible in head injury patients.

Table 44–2. HEAD INJURY INSTRUCTIONS

I. Call the Emergency Room at once if any of the following symptoms appear:
- Drowsiness or inability to be awakened
- Dizziness or clumsy walking
- Persistent vomiting
- Inequality of pupils (one larger than the other)
- Bleeding or drainage of any fluid from the nose or ears
- Convulsions or seizures (fits)
- Paralysis (inability to move) of arms, legs or face
- Severe headaches
- Fever over 100°F
- Unusual irritability or other definite changes in behavior or personality
- Change in ability to see or hear
- Slurred speech
- Progressive slowing of normal resting pulse (or pulse rate under 60/min)

II. The injured person should be checked every 2 hours for 24 hours after the injury (includes waking the patient from sleep).

Axiom 7. Lumbar punctures should not be done in cases of recent head injury. The information so gained is useless, and a lumbar puncture can be lethal if the patient has an unrecognized clot.

Axiom 8. Early airway intubation or tracheostomy may save more lives of head injury patients than any other therapeutic step.

Axiom 9. If a neurosurgeon is not available, a burr hole to let out an intracranial hematoma made within minutes by an inexperienced physician is better than one made too late by a neurosurgeon.

Axiom 10. Always beware of the combative, restless patient who may mumble and have an unrecognized aphasia. This is a sign of elevated intracranial pressure and cerebral injury, such as contusion or cerebral hemorrhage. If in doubt, a CT scan should be ordered.

Axiom 11. When discharging a patient with head injury from the hospital, always inform the family (not the patient) of the possibility of a delayed intracranial clot and its manifestations—namely, progressively severe headache, weakness of one side, visual disturbance, undue drowsiness and unequal pupils. For written form, see Table 44–2.

45. Hemorrhage and Hematologic Emergencies*

45–1. CONTROL OF BLEEDING

Mechanical Control

Control of bleeding as soon as possible is one of the chief functions of emergency personnel (2, *Urgency Evaluation—Triage*). For hemorrhage from an accessible part of the body, one or more of the following local measures may be used:

- Digital or manual pressure over the bleeding area or vessel.
- Local application of broad fluffy gauze compression bandage or packing with sterile gauze. Much the same effect is achieved by use of an air splint

*See also 57, *Shock*.

or, in the lower extremities or abdomen, by pneumatic (MAST) trousers, except that more diffuse and sustained pressure may be achieved.

- Driving the fist firmly into the suprapubic abdominal midline to compress the aorta against the sacral promontory may effectively diminish gross distal bleeding, as will knee or elbow pressure compressing the femoral artery in the inguinal region.
- Reduction of arterial hemodynamic pressure by elevation of involved area if critical flow not overly compromised (e.g., tilt-table treatment of intracranial hemorrhage).
- Clamping and tying (or twisting) or insertion of mattress sutures incorporating the bleeding vessels with good visualization (blind clamping and tying as a first aid measure can be destructive). See also 43, *Hand Injuries*, and 59, *Soft Tissue Injuries*.
- Temporary blockade of surgically inaccessible vessels with an intravascular balloon tampon or autogenous clots.
- Proper application of a tourniquet or an inflated blood pressure cuff (above systolic arterial blood pressure) proximally on an extremity. An emergency tourniquet is best applied as distally as effective on an extremity that has been or will have to be amputated. Too loose an application may cause an increase in venous bleeding. If dangerous hemorrhage has been controlled, a tourniquet should not be loosened until facilities are available for surgical control. (*Note:* Tourniquets are a last choice because of the high risk of soft tissue injury when they are applied by persons not skilled in their use.)

Chemical and Medical Control

A. Evaluation of underlying bleeding or clotting defect (see Table 45–1). History of prolonged bleeding, petechiae, purpura (personal and family). Assessment of the following: prothrombin time (PT), partial thromboplastin time (PTT), serum calcium level, platelet count, serum fibrinogen level, factor assay (as necessary), bleeding time, and quality of clot (firmness, retraction and lysis) and clotting time. A peripheral white blood cell count and a differential cell count also aid in evaluation and detection of concomitant blood dyscrasias, such as leukemia.

B. Topical Control
  1. Chemical
     - Thrombin application, 5000 US units diluted with 5 ml saline; soak absorbable gelatin sponge in solution and hold against bleeding area for 15 seconds, or spray on or use Surgicel or Gelfoam.
     - Silver nitrate stick application at the center point of bleeding
  2. Thermal
     - Ice

       Decreases swelling and venous congestion
       Decreases arterial flow to area
     - Heat

       Focal coagulation—electrocoagulation

C. Systemic Control
  1. Diminution of irritative factors, e.g., discontinuance of drugs (particularly anti-inflammatory medications such as aspirin), reduction of gastric acidity by buffering or reducing production with cimetidine (Tagamet).
  2. Correction of bleeding and clotting defects (see Table 45–1).
  3. Treatment of disseminated intravascular clotting (45–5).
  4. Treatment of hemorrhage from anticoagulant therapy (45–8).

5. Treatment of hemophilia (or deficit of Factor VIII or Factor IX, or both; see *45–7*).

45–2. GENERAL MEASURES

- Control of bleeding *(45–1)*.
- Absolute rest in a position of comfort; prevention of chilling.
- Treatment of hypovolemic shock.
- Morphine sulfate, 10 to 15 mg IM or SC to control pain, restlessness and apprehension, unless intracranial damage *(44, Head Injuries; 63–4, Intracranial Hemorrhage)* or intrathoracic injuries *(31, Chest Injuries)* are causative factors, or extreme respiratory depression is present. Pentazocine lactate (Talwin), 15 to 30 mg IM or IV, is an effective analgesic without marked respiratory depressive effect.
- Hospitalization if blood loss has been excessive, if extensive surgical repair is needed or if damage to a major blood vessel (especially an artery) is evident or suspected *(63–2)*.
- For guide to common medical hemorrhage problems, see Table 45–1.

45–3. BLEEDING, POSTOPERATIVE *(See also 45–1, Control of Bleeding; 45–2, General Measures; 57, Shock)*

In unusual cases with severe hemorrhage after discharge from the hospital, transport by ambulance for rehospitalization, preferably to the hospital where the surgery was done. Intravenous supportive therapy should be continued in the ambulance. Every possible effort should be made to get in touch by telephone with the surgeon who performed the original surgical procedure. If this is not possible, a résumé outlining all emergency treatment given should be sent with the patient. In all cases, the hospital to which the patient is being sent should be notified in advance so that there will be no delay in treatment on the patient's arrival.

45–4. BLEEDING, "SPONTANEOUS"

Although trauma is the most common cause of severe hemorrhage, spontaneous onset of bleeding of various degrees of severity may be caused by:

- Congenital structural blood vessel weakness *(63–4)*; see also *63–5, Dissecting Aortic Aneurysm)*.
- Degenerative disease processes involving the blood vessel walls *(63–3)*.
- Erosion of a blood vessel by pressure from an adjacent space-consuming or invasive tumor.
- Drugs or other agents that interfere with normal coagulation of the blood (e.g., *45–8; 53–79, Anticoagulants; 53–101, Aspirin)* or cause softening of previously formed scars *(53–226, Cortisone; 53–537, Phenylbutazone)*. See Table 45–1, Guide to Common Medical Hemorrhage Problems.
- Familial or acquired blood dyscrasias.

The known or suspected presence of any of these factors requires hospitalization after treatment of hypovolemic shock *(57–5)* for thorough investigation and treatment of the underlying condition.

45–5. DISSEMINATED INTRAVASCULAR CLOTTING (DIC) *(See also Table 45–1)*

DIC, or consumption coagulopathy, is an abnormal hematologic reaction to a wide variety of disease states and pathologic conditions. Among the more

Table 45–1. GUIDE TO COMMON MEDICAL HEMORRHAGE PROBLEMS

Class of Defect	Clues to Diagnosis	Findings or Tests	Treatment
Vascular	• Deficiency or decreased absorption of vitamin C (scurvy) • Irritative G.I. mucosa problem often due to drug ingestion • Familial history of hemorrhagic telangiectasia	• Capillary fragility, bruises, petechiae, hereditary telangiectasia lesions	• Stop causative drugs (such as aspirin and phenylbutazone) • Administer vitamin C parenterally • Improve diet, decrease alcohol intake
Clotting	• Personal and family history of spontaneous bleeding or excess bleeding secondary to trauma and surgery • Intake of chemicals (includes multiple blood transfusions) and anticoagulants that diminish production or compete with essential clotting factors • Presence of ecchymoses with induration • Severe liver disease • Poor food intake/absorption (vitamin K deficiency)	• History extremely important! • Prolonged prothrombin time, partial thromboplastin time, bleeding and clotting times • Decreased specific factors—particularly VIII [antihemophilia globulin (AHG)] and IX (plasma thromboplastin, Christmas factor) and calcium • Decreased fibrinogen • Hematomas and hemarthrosis typical a few days to 1 week after surgery or trauma	• Stop intake of interfering drug (such as heparin or warfarin) and administer antagonist parenterally (see 45–8) • Intravenous calcium gluconate 10 ml, 10% if serum calcium low • Fresh frozen plasma 10 ml/kg body weight; or see 45–7 for use of specific Factor VIII or IX concentrate to avoid volume overload; or cryoprecipitate may be used

Platelet Disorders	• History of causative drug ingestion (particularly aspirin) singly or in combination • Presence of petechiae, purpura • Presence of liver disease or hypersplenism • Presence of collagen disease, sepsis, malignancy, uremia, primary myeloproliferative disease • Healthy young women with idiopathic thrombocytopenia (ITP)	• Decreased platelets by count and presence in smear (thrombocytopenia) • Normal count of platelets but poor function (thrombopathy) • Poor clot retraction • Prolonged bleeding time	• Stop intake of caustive drug • Transfusion of platelet concentrate or platelet plasmapheresis, or both, as necessary, except treat ITP with steroids • Treat underlying problems vigorously • If acutely bleeding, treat ITP with 60–100 mg prednisone qd PO initially, in divided doses
Fibrinolytic Disorders	• As above and including also diseases causing hypoxemia, hypotension, dysthermia; pregnancy complications; prostatic surgery • Disseminated intravascular clotting (DIC)	• Low fibrogen level and usually low AHG; abnormal clot formation and dissolution, low platelet count. Increased circulating products of fibrin breakdown • Decrease PT and PTT. Fibrin monomer present with DIC	• As above for platelets • Monitor fibrinogen, platelets, and fibrin breakdown products, fibrin monomer • May include plasma, fibrinogen or Factor VIII treatment, aminocaproic acid (Amicar) • Heparin use for DIC therapy rarely indicated (see *45–5*)

common of these stressor states are the following: severe infections of all types, postsurgical state, obstetrical conditions (such as toxemia, abruptio placentae, intrauterine fetal death), shock, neoplasia (especially acute leukemia), hemolytic transfusion reactions and trauma. Near drowning in fresh or salt water may precipitate DIC. Clinically, DIC should be suspected in the advent of generalized hemorrhage, unexplained thrombocytopenia, fibrinolysis or unanticipated acute renal or respiratory failure ("shock lung"). Increased fibrinolysis is a bodily defense mechanism against the increased microvascular clotting; increased fibrin split products (FSP) and fibrin monomer, increased PT and PTT and decreased fibrinogen are detected in the blood.

Treatment

- See Table 45–1 under "Platelet Disorders" and "Fibrinolytic Disorders." Diligent treatment of the underlying problem is foremost.
- Fresh frozen plasma, 10 mg/kg, platelets and cryoprecipitate aid replacement; closely monitor clinical and laboratory response.
- Heparin is considered to inhibit the microvascular clotting, leading to diminution of the excessive fibrinolytic response, but must be used with great caution, reservation, clinical observation and repeated laboratory tests. Intravenous continuous heparin drip infusion of 200 to 500 units/kg/day. See *45–8* if bleeding increases with heparin use.

45–6. HEMOLYTIC ANEMIA

Acute manifestations are usually recognized by the presence of signs and symptoms of anemia of rapid onset, jaundice (nonobstructive), brownish urine due to hemoglobin metabolism products and reticulocytosis. Except for the hemoglobinopathy of sickle cell disease *(45–11)* and blood transfusion hemolytic reactions *(18–35)*, the emergency physician is most likely to see acute hemolysis from extracorpuscular causes such as severe infections of all types, autoimmune hemolysis (idiopathic or secondary as with neoplasia or some collagen diseases), vegetable poisons (e.g., fava beans *[53–305]*; castor beans *[53–180]*), animal poisons (snake venoms, 27–*27;* certain spiders, e.g., brown spider, 27–7), chemical agents or medications due to dosage or sensitivity (as with glucose-6-phosphate dehydrogenase deficiency), physical causes (e.g., burns *[28]* or cold *[62]*) or microangiopathic causes (DIC, 45–5).

Treatment

- Identify, remove whenever possible and treat the underlying cause(s).
- Rest, oxygen, hospitalization.
- Transfusion may complicate the problem and probably should not be considered until the hemoglobin (Hb) level is in the range of 6 g/dl. In autoimmune hemolytic anemia, identified by direct Coombs' test, avoidance of transfusion is best whenever possible; however, corticosteroid therapy may be beneficial. If transfusion must be done, give the most compatible blood unit (weakest cross matching reaction), observe meticulously and cease if condition worsens.
- Hemolytic disease in the newborn requires hospital referral and consultation from a pediatrician or neonatologist. A "bilirubin lamp" is used in milder cases, whereas more severe cases may require exchange transfusion.

45–7. THERAPY FOR HEMOPHILIA AND FOR DEFICIENCY OF FACTOR VIII OR IX, OR BOTH

- Specific factor concentrate (instructed patients may also keep at home for parenteral use according to schedule).

Bleeding Status	Dose of Factor VIII or IX
Minimal (gums/early joint pain)	10 units/kg of body weight
Moderate (obvious bleeding)	20 units/kg and repeat every 12 hours as needed
Severe (includes head trauma and major surgery)	40 units/kg initially, then 20 to 30 units/kg q 12 h until controlled

- Cryoprecipitate (cryoprecipitated antihemophilic factor) (about 1 bag/10 kg) also may be used for hemophilia or von Willebrand's disease (platelets also may be required for the latter).
- Fresh frozen plasma, 3 to 5 ml/kg, up to 10 ml/kg IV. (Plasma is not generally used unless additional blood volume is needed.)

45–8. HEMORRHAGE FROM ANTICOAGULANT THERAPY AND HYPOPROTHROMBINEMIA *(See also 53–79, Anticoagulants)*

Signs and symptoms include generalized ecchymoses; hematuria; hemorrhage from the nose, gums or gastrointestinal tract; menorrhagia; and extreme weakness from secondary anemia. Look for retroperitoneal hemorrhage if the site of blood loss is not apparent.

Treatment

- Stop the anticoagulant. If a large amount has been ingested recently, empty the stomach.
- If caused by bishydroxycoumarin (Dicumarol, *53–258*) or warfarin sodium (Coumadin, *53–79*), give an aqueous solution of phytonadione—vitamin K_1 (AquaMEPHYTON) parenterally. Initial dosage usually is 2.5 to 10 mg (up to 25 mg with more severe bleeding), preferably SC or IM—the lowest effective dose is preferred. If bleeding is extremely severe and the intravenous route is absolutely necessary, dilute solution to 10 ml for slow, cautious infusion. Doses are repeated according to clinical observations and repeat determinations of prothrombin time. Blood or plasma transfusion may be necessary in severe cases.
- Neonatal hemorrhage due to hypoprothrombinemia is treated with 1 mg of phytonadione intramuscularly. Other causes of hypoprothrombinemia include gastrointestinal disorders (obstructive jaundice, biliary fistula, hepatic disease and malabsorption problems such as occur with inflammation and resection) and other drugs (such as antibacterial preparations, salicylates, propylthiouracil).
- If caused by heparin (*53–337*), inject not more than 50 mg of protamine sulfate IV slowly (over 2 to 3 minutes) and repeat in 10 to 15 minutes if the desired effect has not been obtained. An overall guide is 1.0 mg of protamine sulfate for each 100 units (1 mg) of heparin given IV within the past 30 minutes; use half this dose of protamine sulfate for heparin given more than 30 minutes previously. Neutralization of the effects of long-acting

depot heparin may require several injections of protamine sulfate. Transfusions of whole blood and fluid replacement may be necessary.

45–9. POLYCYTHEMIA

An urgent situation requiring phlebotomy exists when impending or progressive end-organ ischemia or infarction is occurring because of vascular thrombosis and occlusion related to severe polycythemia. Premonitory symptoms are related to vascular stasis and congestion and ultimately to obstruction and thromboembolic effects. The patient may complain of a congested feeling, malaise, headache, skin burning or itching. The liver and spleen often will be palpably enlarged. Distended retinal veins without papilledema may be seen. WBC and platelet increase are often seen in addition to the elevated RBC mass.

Treatment

- The patient should be hospitalized and a hematologist consulted.
- Platelet or thrombocyte counts 3 to 4 times greater than normal and a hematocrit of more than 60% in conjunction with the clinical picture are strong indications for emergency phlebotomy. Occasionally acute lowering of platelets is done with platelet pheresis or cytotoxic agents.
- If the phlebotomy is being done prior to emergency surgery, collect the blood for storage and reuse in surgery if need be—replacement of just the red blood cells (RBC) may be preferable.

For secondary erythrocytosis alone, in the presence of the same type of clinical picture as just described, phlebotomy may also be therapeutic, but decrements of smaller amounts of blood, close clinical observation and preservation of blood for reinfusion if worsening occurs are advisable.

45–10. SEVERE GRANULOCYTOPENIA AND AGRANULOCYTOSIS

This clinical entity, which can cause rapid demise from sepsis, usually is identifiable earlier by the presence of severe sore throat; exudative tonsillitive oral ulcerations; profound fatigue or prostration; and extreme reduction of granulocytes in the blood (to even less than 500 to 1000 cells/ml). Most cases are secondary to medications or to bone marrow failure as in acute leukemia.

Treatment

- The urgency is to identify, withdraw and prohibit the use of any causative agent (except possibly in malignancy treatment, in which later close titration with similar medication may be necessary). Hospitalize for evaluation of other causes.
- Vigorous broad-spectrum antibiotic therapy (e.g., gentamicin plus a cephalosporin) after obtaining cultures.
- General supportive treatment, including treatment of shock (53), as indicated.
- Aplastic anemia presents the same type of problems as just outlined, in addition to the severe anemia that requires blood transfusions and usually bone marrow transplant.

45–11. SICKLE CELL CRISIS

This acute, severe malady occurs in those of the black population with Hb S-S disease and also in rare situations of extreme deoxygenation in those of Mediterranean descent with S-A trait.

Stress situations in conjunction with metabolic acidosis are the events most likely to precipitate a crisis; infection is a common precipitating cause. The crisis is heralded by microvascular occlusion in any organ or muscle, with fever, severe pain and organ damage and dysfunction secondary. A blood smear reveals slim sickle cells that are pointed at both ends, and during crisis, neither a sodium metabisulfite nor a Sickledex test is ordinarily required to demonstrate them. The presence of sickle cells does not establish the problem as solely a sickle cell crisis.

Treatment

- Rest and hospitalization.
- Cultures, including blood cultures, in the presence of fever or infection. Appropriate vigorous treatment of any infection, identified or suspected, in view of generally poor resistance.
- Hydration and treatment of any shock.
- Correction of moderate to severe metabolic acidosis with sodium bicarbonate or lactate *(46–1).*
- Oxygen therapy, particularly in the presence of cardiopulmonary or brain involvement.
- Treatment of pain *(12).*
- Transfusion (or partial exchange transfusion) should be considered with continuing severe pain and crisis or progressive cerebral involvement and preoperatively before major surgery.

45–12. THROMBOCYTOPENIA *(See Table 45–1, Platelet Disorders)*

Thrombocytopenia is usually considered when ordinary bleeding is not controlled, petechiae or purpura are present, or a decreased number of platelets is noted on blood smear. Platelets may be destroyed mechanically by prosthetic heart valves or consumed in certain conditions such as DIC *(45–5),* idiopathic thrombocytopenic purpura (ITP) and hypersplenism. Also platelet function may be impaired (thrombopathy) or platelet production diminished by the taking of certain drugs.

46. Metabolic Disorders*

Diagnosis of metabolic problems is usually suspected on the basis of the presenting signs and symptoms and accompanying disease process. A basic overview of acid-base imbalance is presented in Table 46–1. The ECG can aid in identifying Ca and K imbalance particularly (see Fig. 46–1). Confirmation of deficits or excess can be established by ABG's and blood/urine electrolyte determinations.

46–1. ACIDOSIS, METABOLIC *(See Table 46–1; see also 32–3 for treatment of diabetic ketoacidosis)*

Formation or accumulation of acid products in the body more rapidly than removal or neutralization can take place results in a characteristic train of

*See also 36, *Endocrine Emergencies;* 11, *Fluid Replacement in Emergencies;* 57, *Shock.*

Table 46–1. ACID-BASE IMBALANCE AND CORRECTIVE MEASURES

Acid-Base Problem and Causes	Anion Gap	pH	$PaCO_2$ (mm Hg)	HCO_3	Compensatory Mechanism and Treatment (Rx)
ACIDOSIS *Metabolic Acidosis*	±	<7.35 ↓	<40 ↓	<24* ↓	↑ R/R; ↓ CO_2; $PaCO_2$ initially normal Pulmonary disease may compromise compensatory mechanism *Rx* • Treat renal disease • Dialysis • Counteract hypoaldosteronism with mineral corticoid (Florinef) • ↓ Acetazolamide/NH_4 administration • Treatment of primary metabolic disorder • $NaHCO_3$ in severe cases (pH < 7.2; bicarbonate < 10) • Consider dialysis for poisons, renal failure • Anion gap (see 53–2) • Correct primary GI/GU problems
• ↓ ability to excrete dietary load of H, e.g.:					
—Renal failure	+				
—Distal RTA	−				
—Hypoaldosteronism	−				
• ↑ H^+ load					
—DKA	+				
—Lactic acidosis	+				
—Drugs, poisons (53–2)	+				
—Starvation	+				
—Seizures	+				
• ↑ HCO_3 loss					
—GI loss (diarrhea, small bowel fistula)	−				
—GU loss	±				
Respiratory Acidosis ↑ $PaCO_2$ due to hypoventilation from any of the problems listed in Table 5–2 (items 1–4)		<7.35 ↓	>45* ↑	N > 32 N or ↑	Renal; HCO_3 level normal initially *Rx* • Treat renal disease, which may compromise compensation • Correct according to corresponding advice in Table 5–2, items 1 to 4.
Combined Metabolic Acidosis/Respiratory Acidosis		↓	N or ↑ *	↓ *	Renal, respiratory *Rx* • Correct individual metabolic acidosis and respiratory acidosis problems; may require $NaHCO_3$ initially

ALKALOSIS					
Metabolic Alkalosis • ↓ H^+ from GI loss • ↓ H^+ from renal loss • ↑ HCO_3 administration	–	>7.45 ↑	>40 ↑	>28* ↑	↓ R/R; $PaCO_2$ initially normal *Rx* • Correct vomiting/gastric drainage or compensate for Cl losses with NH_4Cl in severe cases or NaCl in less severe cases • Decrease or discontinue diuretics • Correct hyperaldosteronism • Correct any K deficit
Respiratory Alkalosis • ↓ $PaCO_2$ due to hyperventilation from: —Emotional factors —Mechanical factors —Hypoxemic response —CNS stimulation		>7.45 ↑	<35* ↓	N < 24 N or ↓	Renal; HCO_3 initially normal *Rx* • Correct primary cause of hyperventilation (e.g., adjust ventilator) • Sedate patient • Increase dead air space • Carbogen inhalation
Combined Metabolic and Respiratory Alkalosis		↑	↓*	↑*	Renal, respiratory *Rx:* Correct for individual metabolic alkalosis and respiratory alkalosis problems
MIXED					
Combined metabolic acidosis/respiratory alkalosis		↓ N ↑	↓*	↓*	Renal, respiratory *Rx:* Correct cautiously for individual metabolic acidosis/respiratory alkalosis
Combined metabolic alkalosis/respiratory acidosis		↓ N ↑	↑*	↑*	Renal, respiratory *Rx:* Correct cautiously for individual metabolic alkalosis/respiratory acidosis

*Primary acid-base defect.

symptoms. This disturbance may be caused by interference with respiration by asthma, bronchitis, pneumonia, emphysema or other pulmonary conditions, cardiac decompensation, high concentration of carbon dioxide in the air or deep narcosis; immediate improvement in ventilation mechanics and oxygen administration is indicated plus correction of any associated metabolic acidosis. Metabolic acidosis may be caused by alkali deficiency, excessive acid production due to altered metabolism or decreased acid urine excretion, as seen in diabetes mellitus or kidney failure. Respiratory mechanisms compensate for metabolic acidosis, and renal physiologic changes compensate for respiratory acidosis.

SIGNS AND SYMPTOMS may be modified, masked or intensified by the causative condition but, in general, consist of headache, drowsiness, generalized weakness, pain in the abdomen and extremities, tachycardia, rapid respiration (later becoming weak and shallow), fruity odor to the breath, progressive stupor and coma. Acetone and diacetic acid are present in the urine, and their presence in serial dilutions should be assessed. Determinations of arterial pH, serum bicarbonate and electrolyte levels, and blood gas pressures (pO_2 and pCO_2) are of great assistance in determining the type and severity of acidosis; obtain as soon as possible.

Look for an anion gap (the sum of serum sodium minus serum chloride and carbon dioxide content) as well as lowered pH and base deficit (carbon dioxide content and extracellular fluid bicarbonate concentration are lowered). The largest elevation in unmeasured anions is likely to occur with diabetic and alcoholic ketoacidosis, renal failure, lactic acidosis and poisoning, such as from salicylates *(53–614)*, ethylene glycol *(53–300)* and methanol *(53–426)* and is usually more than 13 mEq/L in magnitude; see 53–2.

Treatment

- Keep the patient comfortably warm.
- Correct fluid deficit by administering fluids IV; start D5W unless diabetic ketoacidosis (DKA) is present, in which case start normal saline (NS).
- Inject 50 ml of sodium bicarbonate solution (44.6 mEq of sodium) IV (about 0.7 ml/kg of body weight) in acute life-threatening acidosis (as with pH less than 7.2 or serum bicarbonate levels of <10 mEq/L) repeated cautiously as necessary. In severe cases, this may be followed by an infusion of diluted sodium bicarbonate solution; sodium bicarbonate must always be used with caution and close monitoring. The mEq of bicarbonate needed to correct a base deficit can be estimated by multiplying the plasma base deficit (normal bicarbonate or CO_2 level minus the patient's observed level) times 20% of the patient's body weight. Example: 21 mEq/L base deficit × 20% factor × 70 kg body weight = 294 mEq of sodium bicarbonate. Initial *partial* correction along with monitoring is safest rather than an attempt at immediate total replacement; monitor ABG's.

  Corrective solution should be more rapidly given and should be monitored frequently along with other electrolytes, particularly potassium, until the plasma bicarbonate level is between 10 and 15 mEq/L.
- When time and circumstances permit, peritoneal dialysis *(18–24)* is an alternative therapeutic approach.
- Start treatment of the underlying causative condition as soon as identified.
- Hospitalize for acid-base balance determinations and definitive therapy. (See also *18–24, Peritoneal Dialysis; 32–3, Diabetic Coma; 56–4, Asthma.)*

46–2. ADDISONIAN CRISIS/ADRENAL INSUFFICIENCY *(See 36–1)*

46–3. ALKALOSIS *(See Fig. 46–1 and Table 46–1)*

Elevated blood pH may be due to respiratory alkalosis or metabolic alkalosis. Causes of respiratory alkalosis may be hyperventilation *(37–10)* caused by high temperature—body or external (see 62–3 to 62–7), hysteria *(54–11, 54–12)*, encephalitis *(33–20)*, hyperpnea due to high altitudes *(26–1, Mountain and Altitude Sickness)* or anesthesia. See *37–10* for treatment of anxiety-related hyperventilation and respiratory alkalosis; adjustment down of mechanical ventilation equipment and normalization of gas content is indicated if that is the problem source.

Metabolic alkalosis due to excessive loss of acid-chloride ions (1) as a result of prolonged vomiting or gastric suction, (2) via the feces, (3) from overzealous administration of alkaline substances or (4) as a consequence of congenital metabolic variations from normal may cause a similar clinical picture. Table 46–2 distinguishes saline-responsive and saline-resistant types of metabolic acidosis.

Signs and Symptoms: Restlessness; irritability; excitability; slow, deep respirations (the rate may be as low as 5 per minute during compensatory periods); and signs of neuromuscular irritability, principally due to lowered ionization of calcium (see *46–14, Hypocalcemia*). The arterial carbon dioxide combining power is increased in metabolic alkalosis (in contrast to its lowering in respiratory alkalosis).

Treatment

- Discontinue any alkali therapy and either discontinue gastric suction if feasible or more vigorously replace electrolyte losses, particularly sodium, chloride and potassium. (See Table 46–2 and corresponding advised treatment.)
- Force fluids by mouth or give 500 to 1000 ml of normal saline IV. In severe cases (e.g., chloride levels < 30 mEq/L) ammonium chloride IV may be given. Correct any potassium deficits *(46–16)*.
- Give calcium gluconate, 10 ml of 10% solution IV slowly over 15 or more minutes if signs of neuromuscular irritability are present.
- Hospitalize as needed.

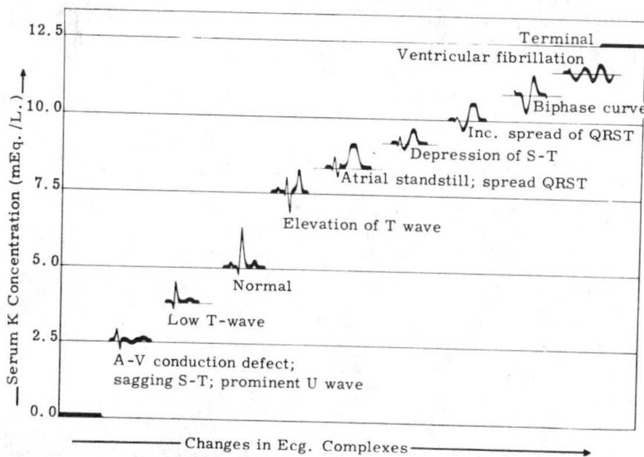

Figure 46–1. Correlation of the serum potassium concentration and the electrocardiogram (providing there is no parallel change in Na and Ca). (From Krupp, Sweet, Jawetz, and Armstrong: *Physician's Handbook,* 15th ed., Los Altos, CA, Lange Medical Publications, 1968.)

Table 46–2. METABOLIC ALKALOSIS

Saline-Responsive Types	Saline-Resistant Types	Treatment of Saline-Resistant Type
Vomiting	Mineralocorticoid excess	Give mineralocorticoid antagonist: spironolactone, 25 mg tid, up to 50 to 75 mg tid PO.
Nasogastric suction	Severe hypokalemia	Potassium replacement (see *46–16*)
Diuretics	Edema states	Acetohexamide, 250 mg tid PO; use of NH_4Cl is contraindicated with renal or hepatic disease
Post hypercapnia	Renal failure	Dialysis

46–4. DIABETIC COMA *(See 32–3)*

46–5. GOUT

Acute, totally disabling swelling and pain in the joints, especially of the feet, may occur with gouty arthritis and represent a true emergency. Presence of low-grade fever, WBC and erythema of the joint area may cause confusion with bacterial infection or thrombophlebitis. Gout is distinguished from these other conditions by the fact that the blood uric acid level is elevated and urate crystals are present in the joint aspirate. Thiazide drugs should be discontinued if being administered.

Treatment

- Codeine phosphate, 60 mg SC, or pentazocine lactate (Talwin), 15 to 30 mg IM. Morphine and other addictive narcotics should be avoided.
- Colchicine, 4 ml (2 mg), diluted with 0.9% NaCl *without preservatives* to 20 ml IV and given over 5 minutes, followed in 4 hours by 0.6 mg PO every hour for 8 doses or until nausea or diarrhea becomes troublesome. Effective alternatives are indomethacin (Indocin), 50 mg orally every 6 hours, and ibuprofen (Motrin), 800 mg every 8 hours initially, cutting dosage in half with decrease in acute symptoms.
- Dextrose, 5% in saline, 500 to 1000 ml IV.
- Referral for complete medical check-up after relief of acute symptoms and signs. Hospitalization is rarely necessary.

46–6. HYPERCALCEMIA

Symptoms of hypercalcemia are very vague and include polyuria, polydipsia, dry mouth, depression, obstipation and constipation. Severity of symptoms depends on both the degree and rate of increase in the serum Ca^{++}. With further increases, nausea, vomiting, lethargy, and finally coma may result.

The causes of hypercalcemia are very varied. Most commonly it is due to primary hyperparathyroidism *(36–8)* and metastatic bone disease. Other causes include multiple myeloma, sarcoidosis, vitamin D toxicity and hyperthyroidism.

Treatment

- IV fluids. Saline diuresis as tolerated by patient; 1000 ml of normal saline may be given rapidly over 2 to 3 hours initially. Administration of 40 to 60 mg of furosemide (Lasix) will enhance the Ca^{++} excretion. Lasix may be administered with each liter of saline. After the first 200 ml of saline, 40 mg of Lasix may be administered and then repeated 3 to 4 times a day.

- Close monitoring of serum K^+ is critical to the above regimen. The amount of K^+ in the urine can be assessed by measuring the urinary K^+ and correcting the total loss to the volume of urine passed.
- Intake and output should be monitored closely.
- Steroids are usually effective in cases of hypercalcemia due to vitamin D intoxication, sarcoidosis or multiple myeloma. In hypercalcemia crises, hydrocortisone or prednisone may be used at a dose of 100 to 300 mg.
- Calcitonin, 4 IU/kg SC or IM q 12 h up to the usual maximum of 100 IU q 8 to 12 h initially may be beneficial.
- Mithramycin, 15 to 25 μg/kg, may be given IV on a daily basis for 3 or 4 days.
- A low-calcium diet should be used.
- If patient is on thiazide diuretics, they should be discontinued.

46–7. HYPERINSULINISM *(See 32–3)*

46–8. HYPERKALEMIA

Acute adrenal crisis may be associated with hyperkalemia. In older patients the use of potassium-sparing diuretics is not an uncommon cause of hyperkalemia. Older diabetic patients may have mild hyperkalemia as a result of hyporeninemia or hypoaldosteronism (treat with 0.1 mg fludrocortisone [Florinef] PO qod).

Elevated serum potassium levels are most frequently associated with poor renal function, lower urine output, excess potassium administration and acidosis. The most telling effects of hyperkalemia are on the heart (see Fig. 46–1 for electrocardiographic changes with varying K^+ levels), though skeletal muscle paralysis also can occur. Levels of serum electrolytes and gases and blood pH should be determined immediately.

Treatment

- Treatment of underlying cause; stop potassium administration; discontinue use of any potassium-sparing diuretics.
- Urgency of treatment is dictated by electrocardiographic findings, which should be monitored. Infrequently normal sinus rhythm (NSR) may be present without T wave increase with potassium levels of 7 to 7.5 mEq/L.
- If potassium level is less than 6.5 mEq/L, hydration with 5% dextrose in normal saline, correction of any acidosis with 44 to 88 mEq of sodium bicarbonate as necessary and assurance of a high urine output if feasible (it may be preferable to test initially with 5% dextrose in water if renal shutdown is apparent) will often suffice if good urine flow commences.
- With electrocardiographic abnormalities present or pending, the following are indicated along with constant monitoring:
- Correction of acidosis *(46–1)*.
- One liter 5% dextrose in normal saline IV plus calcium administration for correction of any hypocalcemia *(46–14)* or as necessary for antagonistic effect on the heart—use extreme caution if patient is also on digitalis.
- Ion exchange resin administration: retention enema of sodium polystyrene sulfonate (Kayexalate), 50 g in 50 ml of 70% sorbital diluted to 200 ml with water; oral route may be used with one-half this concentration and amount if tolerated. If fluid overload present, can use calcium resin instead.
- Fifty ml of 50% glucose plus 10 units of regular insulin IV.
- Prepare for hemodialysis (preferable to peritoneal dialysis) if potassium level dangerous and not responding to the measures just outlined.

46–9. HYPERMAGNESEMIA

Renal failure with decreased excretion and excess administration, either parenterally in therapy or orally (laxatives/antacids), can cause the magnesium level in the plasma to rise above 2.2 mEq/L. Depression of respiration, blood pressure, deep tendon reflexes, sensorium and the heart (progressing to cardiac arrest with severe elevation) occur. ECG changes are similar to those of hyperkalemia *(46–8)*.

Treatment

- Treat the cause and discontinue intake.
- Hydrate and aid high urine volume.
- Furosemide (Lasix), 40 mg IV.
- Calcium gluconate, 10 ml of 10% solution IV slowly over 15 minutes, greater caution if digitalized; monitor with ECG.
- Hemodialysis if severe and unresponsive.

46–10. HYPERNATREMIA

Either an absolute or a relative excess of sodium in relation to water, resulting in a hyperosmolar condition (see also *32–11, Hyperosmolar Coma)* and serum level greater than 150 mEq per liter, can be caused by excess sodium intake relative to water or water losses that exceed sodium losses. Both of these conditions are more likely to occur in infants and children—the excess water losses being more common and usually in conjunction with gastrointestinal disorders and the presence of scanty urine with high specific gravity (SG). Water loss through failure of the kidney to concentrate results in high volume, low SG urine. The hyperosmolar condition is associated with central nervous system (CNS) agitation of varying degrees, including seizures as well as coma; look also for intracranial venous thrombosis and subarachnoid hemorrhage.

Osmolarity as well as blood and urine electrolyte studies and urine SG and output should be monitored. For children, obtain the assistance of a pediatrician or neonatologist.

Treatment

- Hyperosmolar, hyperglycemic coma—see *32–11* for treatment.
- For water loss from inappropriate renal diuresis due to diabetes insipidus, give treatment as under *36–9, Hypopituitary Function*. For children, give 5 IU and for infants 2.5 IU or less of IM vasopressin tannate in oil. DDAVP is available as an IV preparation.
- If in the diuretic phase following renal shutdown, use measurement of urine electrolytes and fluid losses to guide replacement after balance achieved with 5% dextrose in water (D/W).
- In adults, 5% D/W IV or oral fluids, if tolerated, will correct most conditions, unless hyperosmolar hyperglycemic coma is present. For this condition, half normal saline will gradually correct the relative serum sodium excess that is present despite total body sodium loss.
- Gradual correction over 2 to 3 days in infants and young children is best with attention to correction of water deficit.

Commence with IV infusion of 0.25% or 0.50% normal saline (plus 12.5 to 25 ml of sodium bicarbonate—11 to 22 mEq of sodium if indicated by pH of less than 7.2). Add potassium and calcium according to replacement need and ongoing requirement and reduce sodium to 40 mEq/L with establishment of renal output.

If condition is rapidly deteriorating, consider hemodialysis or peritoneal dialysis with high osmolar content solution and about 120 mEq/L sodium content.

46–11. HYPERPARATHYROIDISM *(See 36–8, Endocrine Emergencies, Parathyroid)*

46–12. HYPERPOTASSEMIA *(See 46–8)*

46–13. HYPERTHYROID CRISES *(See 36–11)*

46–14. HYPOCALCEMIA *(See also 52–11, Pediatric Emergencies, Hypocalcemia)*

Hypocalcemia can result in irritability, depression, psychosis, convulsions and tetany or neuromuscular irritability that can be demonstrated by various tests: Erb's sign (muscular weakness to a very weak galvanic current), Chvostek's sign (twitching of the facial muscles brought on by tapping the skin just anterior to the external auditory meatus), Trousseau's sign (an "obstetrical position" of the hand and fingers brought on by constriction of the arm above the elbow plus pedal spasm). These occur progressively as the serum calcium level drops further below 9 mg/dl (or 4.5 mEq/L). Prolongation of the QT interval on the ECG is characteristic.

Treatment

- IV administration of 10 ml of 10% calcium gluconate over 15 minutes or more. Use with great caution and with ECG monitoring if the patient is digitalized. Further supplemental calcium can be given by adding 2 g of calcium gluconate to a liter of IV fluid—check that any other contents do not precipitate with added calcium.
- Treat underlying problem.
- See 52–*11* for treatment in infants.
- Treat any associated hypomagnesemia and hypokalemia.
- In patients with hypoparathyroidism *(36–7)* of any cause, start administration of vitamin D, 50,000 units/day PO, or calcitriol (Rocaltrol), 25 μg/day.

46–15. HYPOGLYCEMIA

Although often used synonymously with hyperinsulinism *(32–3)*, hypoglycemia is a much broader term. Among the causes of this condition are abnormal functioning of the islets of Langerhans *(36–6)*; liver, pituitary and adrenal insufficiency *(36–1)*; "dumping syndrome" after gastric resection *(36–6)*; and administration of excessive amounts of insulin or inadequate food intake after the usual dose of insulin. Occasionally, oral hypoglycemic agents may cause an acute picture. Onset of pregnancy in a diabetic can result in significant hypoglycemia in the first trimester of pregnancy. Tumors producing either insulin or NSILA may cause fasting hypoglycemia. Reactive hypoglycemia will almost never present as an acute hypoglycemia requiring emergency treatment. Organic hyperinsulinism due to either insulin production or NSILA may be treated by frequent feedings, diazoxide, 200 to 300 mg PO bid or tid, or prednisone, 30 to 40 mg/day.

Idiopathic hypoglycemia of infancy *(52–10)* is another cause.

Signs, symptoms and treatment are the same as outlined for hyperinsulinism *(32–3, Diabetes Mellitus)*. Give sugar-containing fluid, orally if patient is conscious and not vomiting, or 2 ml/kg 50% DW IV (to 50 ml) if patient is unable to take orally.

46–16. HYPOKALEMIA

As the serum potassium level drops to 3.5 mEq/L and below, smooth, striated and cardiac muscle loses excitability and contractility, and weakness and organ dysfunction result (including kidneys losing their concentrating function and paralytic ileus developing). See Fig. 46–1 for ECG changes with low potassium.

Treatment

- Treat the underlying cause.
- Correct via the oral route if time and circumstances permit (oral potassium supplements, 1 to 2 mEq/kg/day. Bananas and oranges contain considerable potassium. However, to correct the hypochloremic alkalosis that usually accompanies hypokalemia (especially after thiazides), both oral and IV treatment should initially be in the form of potassium chloride. Potassium "piggyback" drip infusion ("K series") at 10 to 20 mEq/hr may be given. If the hypokalemia is severe, with muscle paralysis and cardiac arrhythmias, larger doses of intravenous potassium chloride should be given (up to 80 mEq/hr in extreme cases) with continuous ECG monitoring. Get serum level and check ECG. Give cautiously if urine output is not well established.

46–17. HYPOMAGNESEMIA

Magnesium deficiency (less than 1.5 mEq/L in plasma) is most commonly seen with poor intake, malabsorption syndromes, chronic alcoholism and renal dysfunction. It causes leg cramps, tremors, painful paresthesias, fasciculations, weakness, nausea, vomiting, seizures and tetany *(46–14)*. ECG changes resemble those due to low potassium and calcium levels. Obtain magnesium, calcium and potassium levels.

Treatment

- Oral magnesium salts or, if severe lowering, magnesium sulfate IV, 1 to 2 mEq/kg over a 4- to 6-hour period, or IM.
- Treat primary problem and any associated low calcium or potassium level.
- Monitor ECG and electrolytes if administration is rapid.

46–18. HYPONATREMIA *(See also 62–5, Heat Cramps)*

Total body deficit of sodium with hypo-osmolarity (serum level less than 280 mOsm/kg of water) and sodium concentration in the serum of less than 135 mEq/L causes, progressively, headache, lightheadedness, weakness, lethargy, decreased appetite, nausea and vomiting, plus manifestations of the underlying problem (e.g., diarrhea, hemorrhage, renal disease). Urine sodium concentration is less than 30 mEq/L unless the loss is renal [diuretic therapy, Addison's disease *(36–1)*, adrenal disease].

Treatment of this form of hyponatremia consists of management of the underlying disease, cessation of any diuretics and IV administration of normal saline or 500 ml of 3% saline in more severe cases. Correct other concomitant electrolyte losses.

Dilutional hyponatremia, in contrast, is associated with normal or excess total body sodium and an even greater proportion of total body water accompanied by "puffiness" (as with myxedema) or edema. Urine sodium concentration is low—less than 10 mEq/L.

Excess body salt and extracellular fluid, as with congestive heart failure *(29–10)* or various causes of hypoalbuminemia, are treated with salt and water restriction plus diuretics and other modalities for the primary disease.

In hyponatremia with normal total body sodium—as with the syndrome of inappropriate antidiuretic hormone (SIADH), seen secondary to drugs and various central nervous system (CNS) and pulmonary disorders, and cortisol deficiency—the management is principally water restriction plus treatment of the primary disorder. Severe water intoxication (serum sodium 105 to 110 mEq/L or less) with seizures, stupor or coma warrants administration of 3 to 5% saline IV, and dialysis should be considered.

Malignancy-associated SIADH that is nonresponsive to fluid restriction may be treated, in addition to the usual measures, with doxycycline, 300 mg tid.

46–19. HYPOPARATHYROID CRISES *(See 36–7)*

46–20. HYPOPOTASSEMIA *(See 46–16)*

46–21. PANCREAS *(See 32–3, Diabetes Mellitus; 36–5, Diabetic Coma)*

46–22. PARATHYROID CRISIS *(See 36–8, Intoxication)*

46–23. PITUITARY *(See 36–9 and 36–10)*

46–24. PORPHYRIA, ACUTE INTERMITTENT

Acute intermittent porphyria may cause signs and symptoms requiring emergency care in adults of both sexes. Drugs such as alcohol, barbiturates, phenylbutazone and sulfas may initiate attacks. Abdominal pain, often severe enough to be mistaken for an acute surgical abdomen, may be the presenting complaint, but a wide variety of neurologic complaints of extreme severity may be confused with poliomyelitis *(33–52, 49–13)* encephalitis *(33–20)* or acute poisoning *(53)*. The most characteristic laboratory findings during the clinical attack are the change in color of the urine to dark red or even black on exposure to sunlight and the presence of urinary porphobilinogen. Hyponatremia with volume expansion (from SIADH) and postural hypotension (from associated neuropathy) are characteristic of porphyria; adrenal insufficiency *(36–1)* is distinguished from this clinically by volume contraction.

Treatment

- Control of severe pain by meperidine hydrochloride (Demerol) or codeine.
- Assistance with respiration *(5–21)*. In severe cases, endotracheal intubation *(5–8)* may be necessary.
- Use of diazepam for any seizures *(34)*.
- Sedation by chloral hydrate, paraldehyde or chlorpromazine hydrochloride (Thorazine). Barbiturates should never be used.
- High carbohydrate intake and cautious fluid replacement. Give IV 10% hypertonic glucose if associated with SIADH.
- Hospitalization during the usually prolonged recovery from severe acute episodes. Precipitating causes (e.g., infection) must be treated.

46–25. TETANY *(See also 46–14, Hypocalcemia)*

Caused by hypocalcemia *(46–14)*, respiratory alkalosis or occasionally hypomagnesemia *(46–17)*, hyperphosphatemia and hypokalemia *(46–16)*, and characterized by neuromuscular excitability; Erb's, Chvostek's and Trousseau's signs *(46–14)* are pathognomonic.

Signs and Symptoms of acute tetany are spectacular and consist of carpopedal spasm; spasm resulting from involvement of the autonomic nerve supply of the iris, bronchi, diaphragm, heart, gastrointestinal tract and bladder; and convulsions of varying degrees of severity. These convulsions may be generalized, unilateral or confined to isolated muscle groups. Muscle contractions in strychnine *(53–659)* and organic phosphate *(53–497)* poisoning as well as those in tetanus *(33–68)* are generally more violent and sustained.

Treatment

- Treatment of the underlying condition.
- Carbogen inhalations or paper bag rebreathing if tetany is due to hyperventilation *(37–10)*.
- Calcium gluconate, 10 ml of 10% solution intravenously given slowly over 15 minutes or more.
- Blood studies, unless hyperventilation *(37–10)* is the causative condition.

The patient should be referred for medical evaluation and definitive treatment of underlying problems.

46–26. THYROID *(See 36–11* and *36–12)*

47. Musculoskeletal Disorders

47–1. GENERAL CONSIDERATIONS *(See also Tables 49–1 and 49–2)*

Disorders of the musculoskeletal system are common in any age group. Although many of these disorders are traumatic in nature, infections and arthritis can often mimic traumatic presentations. For this reason an adequate history from the patient or a reliable family member, in addition to a careful physical examination, is mandatory.

Transportation of a victim sustaining a serious musculoskeletal injury must be carried out with extreme caution. Adequate prior immobilization of obvious or suspected fractures is essential and particularly critical with injuries to the vertebral column (see *4*, Table 47–1 and Fig. 47–1). Ice, particularly when applied early, helps decrease swelling of the injured part. Ambulance transportation is indicated with more severe injuries.

Pain medication relief for injuries of the musculoskeletal system should be administered, preferably after a physician has taken a history and examined the patient. When surgical intervention is under consideration, analgesics such as aspirin that inhibit blood clotting should be avoided. Narcotics may interfere with accurate histories and physical examinations and ability of the patient to comprehend an informed consent. Also, medication should not be so potent that the patient is unable to participate in monitoring of the injury.

Thoughtful use of laboratory and x-ray facilities *(21)* many times aids in diagnostic determination of musculoskeletal disorders. CBC, including diff. and ESR, is most helpful in the diagnosis of arthritides and infections. If increased bone activity is suspected, elevated alkaline phosphatase levels add further evidence. In cases of gout, uric acid levels may be present, although the diagnosis of gout is confirmed by detection of crystals in the joint fluid. Only necessary x-rays should be taken *(21)*. Although comparison views of opposite extremities are often helpful in the diagnoses of fractures in children, the taking of routine comparison x-rays should be avoided. Special x-ray studies such as tomograms or computerized tomography are usually helpful in delineating difficult spinal fractures and outlining the extent of the injury or lesion. Computerized tomography (CT) is often used in determining the boundaries of tumors and occult fractures of the acetabulum and spine.

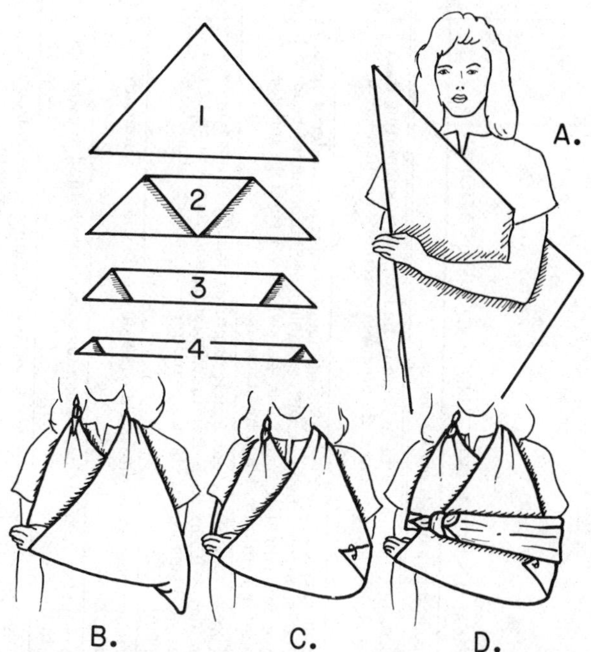

Figure 47–1. Steps 1 to 4 present folding of a triangular bandage (1) into a cravat (4). For an adult, the base of the triangular bandage is usually about 56″ long, with each of the sides about 38″. Steps A to D present formation of a sling and swathe (Velpeau bandage) from a triangular bandage and cravat. If no safety pin is available for the elbow, an overhand or "piggy tail" knot may be substituted.

Occasionally myelography is necessary to determine the integrity of the spinal canal.

Extensive effusion of the joint may require arthrocentesis *(18–3)* for relief of pain and swelling and for examination for bacteria (infection), fat (fracture) and crystals (gout). If infection is suspected, fluid from the joint should be examined by Gram stain immediately and three test tubes sent for further evaluation: (1) a sterile tube for culture; (2) a heparinized tube for qualitative and quantitative cell counts; (3) a regular clot tube for protein compliment and glucose. The color, turbidity and amount of fluid should be documented.

Splinting initially (for the first 48 to 72 hours) is usually as effective and safer than casting. Adequate splints totally immobilize joints and also allow for swelling. Circular casting of injured parts doesn't allow for swelling, which can cause neurovascular damage to the injured part. The patient and family should be instructed to do neurovascular checks *(47–2)*. Elevation is extremely important and should be carried out well above the heart. Ice is very useful in eliminating swelling and pain for the first 24 to 48 hours. Analgesia and muscle relaxation may be required. For upper extremity injuries, slings should not be used for 2 to 3 days, as they keep the extremity in a dependent position and swelling persists.

Follow-up evaluation should be carefully arranged. Reevaluation within 24 to 72 hours is usually necessary in other than minor musculoskeletal injuries. It is at this time that splints are often changed to circular casts and dressings

Table 47–1. INITIAL IMMOBILIZATION FOR OBVIOUS OR SUSPECTED FRACTURES AND DISLOCATIONS*

Location	Immobilization Methods and Precautions
Mandible	Use Barton type bandage, which goes vertically from top of head around the lower jaw, supporting it, and horizontally from behind the occiput around the chin and back. Be prepared to remove or cut away if vomiting occurs
Cervical Spine	First apply hard cervical collar and then short board (see Fig. 4–3). Add long board if remainder of spine at risk. If boards (or facsimile) are not available, support the neck with sandbags or "immobilize" head with hands using gentle neutral traction. Leave any helmet on (see Table 4–2) whenever possible and use adhesive tape binding from helmet to board to help immobilize head and neck
Ribs	See *31–8* for management regarding use of rib belt, tongs, etc. Single fractures usually do not require emergency immobilization except for comfort. With multiple fractures, stability and comfort can be improved by crossing upper extremity of affected side across chest so hand rests on opposite shoulder and then bind there with bandages and elbow support
Scapula	Immobilize shoulder girdle by using sling on upper extremity of affected side and swathe to bind arm closely to chest (Velpeau bandage; see Fig. 47–1)
Clavicle	Immobilize as for scapula, or use figure-of-eight bandage (loop of bandage goes from behind neck around both clavicles and under axilla and ties in the back)
Thoracolumbar Spine	Secure in supine position on long board/door or other firm, sturdy, level, body-length structure. Caution: "log roll" position does not adequately immobilize the spine for carrying if fracture is present
Shoulder Joint	Same as for scapula
Humerus	Bind 1 or 2 full humerus lengths of splint material to arm. Use a sling or wrist support and bind arm to thorax

Elbow	Bind splint material from shoulder down to the wrist if elbow is straight. If elbow is bent, maintain that position by binding splint material obliquely from the humerus to the forearm, thus forming a triangle with the elbow at apex
Forearm (Radius/Ulna); Wrist/Hand	Bind 2 pieces (lateral and medial) of splint material to forearm from elbow to metacarpophalangeal joints. Splint hand in position of function. Use sling
Finger	Bind finger(s) to adjacent unaffected finger, or temporarily use tongue board as splint. Can include in wrist/hand splint
Pelvis	Same as for thoracolumbar spine. Bind lower extremities together and bind to long board. Use MAST if available
Hip	Bind long board laterally to body from axilla to ankle and shorter board from groin to ankle, or use "well-limb splint" by tying lower extremities together, or use femur traction splint (e.g., Thomas or Hare). Carry patient on long board or firm stretcher
Femur	Same as for hip
Knee	Similar to elbow
Leg (Tibia-Fibula)	Similar to forearm
Ankle/Foot	Cardboard or other firm splint immobilized from foot to mid-calf, or use pillow splint. Put foot in neutral position
Toes	Same as for fingers

*"Splint 'em as you find 'em" (unless there is neurovascular compromise, which requires immediate reduction of the fracture/dislocation [if medical worker is sufficiently skilled]). Splint joints above and below the site of injury.

are changed. In addition, follow-up x-rays may be required to monitor unstable fractures.

47–2. IMMOBILIZATION

Splinting is essential for obvious or suspected skeletal fractures and is helpful in giving relief to traumatized or painful musculoskeletal parts in addition to helping to prevent shock effects. Circular casting done early doesn't adequately allow for swelling expansion, which can lead to neurovascular and skin damage from compression (see also *47–60, Compartment Syndromes*). See Table 47–1 for recommendations for musculoskeletal immobilization. Use maximum support and minimal motion while applying splints.

Splinting Materials

TEMPORARY: Any reasonably firm material of adequate length and circumference (rolled newspaper, magazines, branches, pillows, boards, cardboard, air splints, MAST); binding of affected upper extremity to thorax; binding of affected extremity to unaffected extremity ("well limb" or "buddy" splint).

SEMI-PERMANENT: Metal or plastic preformed splint, fiberglass, layered plaster strips, specific braces. Avoid circumferential plaster wrapping in acute injury when progressive swelling may compromise neurovascular structures.

Following splinting or casting, the patient and/or family should be instructed as follows:

- Do periodic neurovascular checks at least every hour for 24 hours; if abnormalities or symptoms of compartment syndrome *(47–60)* occur, seek immediate medical reevaluation, as these pathologic findings require immediate decompression. (*Note*: These checks should be done even if the patient is sleeping.)
- Use provided crutches or alternate transportation if weight-bearing should be avoided.
- Elevate the involved extremity above heart level.
- Apply ice *(12–2)* in a plastic bag to outside of splint to reduce swelling and pain during the first 24 to 48 hours.
- Analgesics, muscle relaxants and NSAID may be needed *(12–2)*.
- Call promptly for further advice if cast or splint becomes too tight, loose or broken; causes painful rubbing or pressure pain (may feel like a "rock" or burning); or causes fingers or toes to become discolored, painful, numb or difficult to move.
- Avoid the following: getting cast wet, removing padding of cast, altering cast, wrapping tape of any kind on plaster cast (as it becomes soft from retained moisture) or sticking a coat hanger (or other implement) down cast to perform scratching if itching occurs (an ice bag may be applied to the cast for relief of itching).
- Return for reevaluation in 1 to 3 day(s) (Specify).

47–3. SPRAINS/STRAINS/CONTUSIONS *(See Figs. 47–3 to 47–15)*

Soft tissue damage causes signs and symptoms as indicated in Table 47–2. Definition of the terms used is as follows:

Strain: Stress injury to muscle/tendon (stretching of fibers and bleeding may occur), but ligament and joint structure are still essentially intact.

Sprain: The varying degrees of injury to ligament(s) are outlined in Table 47–2.

Contusion: Bruising of tissue secondary to blunt trauma. May have minor or severe consequences depending on whether bleeding also occurs into or applies pressure onto vital structures or organs; considerable supportive and surgical treatment may be needed if the latter occurs.

Table 47–2. DEGREES OF SPRAINS*

Finding	First-Degree	Second-Degree	Third-Degree
Pain	None to minimal; onset may be delayed	Moderate to severe; immediate onset	Usually severe; with extensive tears may be slight; immediate onset
Active ROM	Full ROM	Moderate decrease	Minimal to no ROM
Ligament change	Minimal tear(s)	Incomplete tear(s)	Complete tear(s) Capsule tear also possible
Hemorrhage evident?	None	None to moderate	Gross
Swelling	None to slight	Moderate	Severe
Tenderness	Slight	Moderate	Severe
Function	Normal to minimal guarding	Present, but reduced	Gross impairment
Stress test†	No laxity	None to marginal laxity	Abnormal passive ROM
Traumatic arthritis?	No	Yes	Yes
Treatment (see also Table 47–3)	Early mobilization program or brace or cast; no surgery	Usually brace or cast and early mobilization; surgery may be considered but is often avoidable	Surgery indicated followed by joint support/cast

*X-rays may reveal also fracture or avulsion fracture.
†May have to be done after injection of lidocaine anesthetic locally into joint.

Treatment

- Type and intensity of treatment varies according to the magnitude of the injury. However, the measures in Table 47–3 may be of benefit in management (see also *12–2* for further details).
- Avulsion-type fractures should be ruled out by x-ray in third-degree and severe second-degree injuries. Views of the opposite nonaffected side in the same position for comparison may be valuable in determining the patient's normal anatomy, but need not be routinely done.
- If operative repair of damaged ligamentous structures is necessary, it should, if possible, be done within 24 to 72 hours.

47–4. TENDON INJURIES *(See also 43–12, Tendon Injuries in the Hand)*

Lacerations, stab wounds and other puncture wounds should be checked carefully for tendon damage by tests of function as well as for nerve and artery damage. A severe contusion may cause severance by compression of a tendon against a bony prominence. Tendons (especially the biceps, supraspinatus, plantaris-gastrocnemius-soleus, and tendo Achillis near its insertion) may rupture as a result of sudden severe muscle contraction or strain.

Treatment

Cases of suspected or proved tendon severance should be referred for

Table 47–3. MANAGEMENT OF MUSCLE/TENDON/LIGAMENT INJURY

- Restriction or modification of use of affected body part for several days (even with minor injury), plus appropriate mechanical support (see Table 47–1). Initial immobilization as needed. See text on specific body part involved for further discussion. With severe injury, these measures may need to be continued for 4 to 6 weeks.
- Postural drainage by elevation of affected part for the first 24 to 72 hours. Rigid adherence to this principle reduces recovery time.
- Cryotherapy; ice preferable the first 48 hours (see *12–2*); can follow with heat.
- Assistive devices such as crutches or a cane are indicated if weight-bearing structures are significantly involved.
- Analgesics (medicinal/nonmedicinal; see *12–2*) and muscle relaxants.
- Anti-inflammatory agents—may double as analgesics (see *12–2*)
- Physical therapy can be of great value.
- Consider DMSO, as appropriate, for reduction of swelling; may also improve healing (better hemodynamics to area) and relieve pain.
- Avoid circumferential wrapping in the first 72 hours, when progressive swelling in a fixed compartment can compromise neurovascular function.
- Avoid excessive restriction of general activity. Even with immobilization of affected part(s), general activity and productivity of the uninvolved parts should be encouraged as feasible. Muscle stimulators can be placed beneath casts to reduce atrophy.
- When tension from pain and anxiety from dysfunction and restriction are factors, consider use of a short-acting sleeping medication (e.g., Restoril, 30 mg) for a few days in addition to a narcotic analgesic.

orthopedic surgical care, with the exception of:

- Obvious minor incomplete severance—these can usually be treated by immobilization or repaired under local anesthesia, depending on the location and extent of damage.
- Extensor tendons (dorsiflexors) of the 2nd to 5th digits of the foot without retraction.
- Severance of the palmaris longus tendon. No repair is necessary, because this tendon is vestigial and serves minimal function in the wrist or hand. However, check for median nerve damage, since the nerve lies immediately below the palmaris longus tendon.
- Severance of the flexor tendons of the 2nd to 5th digits of the foot. These do not require repair.

Acute Tendinitis (Without External Trauma)

Acute tendinitis may occur at many locations. The treatment measures outlined in Table 47–3 are generally helpful.

Tendinitis of the shoulder from overuse is common. With biceps tendinitis there is pain in flexion and abduction plus focal tenderness over the long head of the biceps tendon; peritendinous injection of lidocaine and triamcinolone (10 to 15 mg) can give relief. With calcific tendinitis of the supraspinatus tendon, ROM is decreased with point tenderness posteriorly and just distal to the acromion; injection may be necessary for relief. Tendinitis of the foot (most often the anterior or posterior tibialis tendons), although not common, may benefit from addition of a posterior splint and limited weight-bearing for several days. Avoid injection of corticoids into weight-bearing tendons, particularly the Achilles.

Stenosing Tenovaginitis (de Quervain's Disease) *(See 43–12, Tendon Injuries in the Hand)*

47–5. EPIPHYSEAL INJURIES AND FRACTURES

Many of these displacements (or slips) reduce spontaneously. Examination for localized tenderness, fluoroscopic examination for excess mobility and comparative x-rays of the uninjured side are often necessary to establish the diagnosis. See Figure 47–2 for Salter and Harris classification of epiphyseal injuries and fractures. Class IV and Class V fractures carry a high incidence of permanent disability. With certain exceptions (see following list), if a loose epiphysis is in satisfactory position, a well-padded plaster splint or cast can be applied and the position confirmed by periodic x-rays—slippage may occur when a decrease in swelling results from loosening of the cast. Always inform parents in writing that future growth plate disturbance may result.

Application of a temporary splint, control of pain and immediate transfer for orthopedic care are particularly indicated when:

- Associated fractures are present.
- There is marked displacement of the epiphysis.
- Any of the epiphyses around the elbow joint are involved. Special orthopedic evaluation is indicated in all injuries of this type.
- The capital epiphysis of the femur is involved; this condition requires operative intervention.
- Reduction is unstable.
- Sufficient cooperation for proper reduction and application of a cast cannot be obtained.

47–6. FRACTURES/DISLOCATIONS

Injury to the skeletal system may cause the following: acute onset of focal intense pain after trauma or stress, obvious alignment deformity, function and ROM impairment, muscle spasm, swelling, tenderness or hemorrhage. Some of the different types of fractures are shown in Figure 47–2.

Treatment

- Immediate immobilization (see *47–2* and Table 47–1); follow the common rule of "Splint 'em where they lie," or "Splint 'em as you find 'em." Immobilization is the first measure to be taken before proceeding to treatment of pain and shock.
- X-rays for documentation prior to definitive treatment.
- Measures as described in *12, Pain Management,* and Table 47–3 for additional relief of pain. Usually with fractures and dislocations a narcotic and a muscle relaxant are needed for pain relief prior to reduction. Hematoma block may be helpful.
- Management of shock *(57)* may of necessity include consideration of IV crystalloids or blood transfusions. Blood loss within the first 4 to 6 hours can be substantial, particularly with injuries to larger bones. Estimations of blood loss may be aided with the following guidelines (for adults): pelvis, 1000–2000 ml; one femur, 500–1000 ml; combinations of tibia-fibula or radius-ulna, 250–500 ml. Approximately 100–125 ml of blood is lost with each rib fracture; if lower ribs are fractured, also consider liver/spleen laceration and bleeding. Fluid loss associated with shock increases as the time from injury (document time interval) and may involve many more liters.
- Open or compound fractures require tetanus immunization *(20)* and measures to prevent or control infection *(59–42)*.
- All severe bone injuries should receive *immediate* orthopedic consultation and management. Reductions are much more difficult 24 hours after injury, when swelling and muscle spasm are advanced. Open reduction and

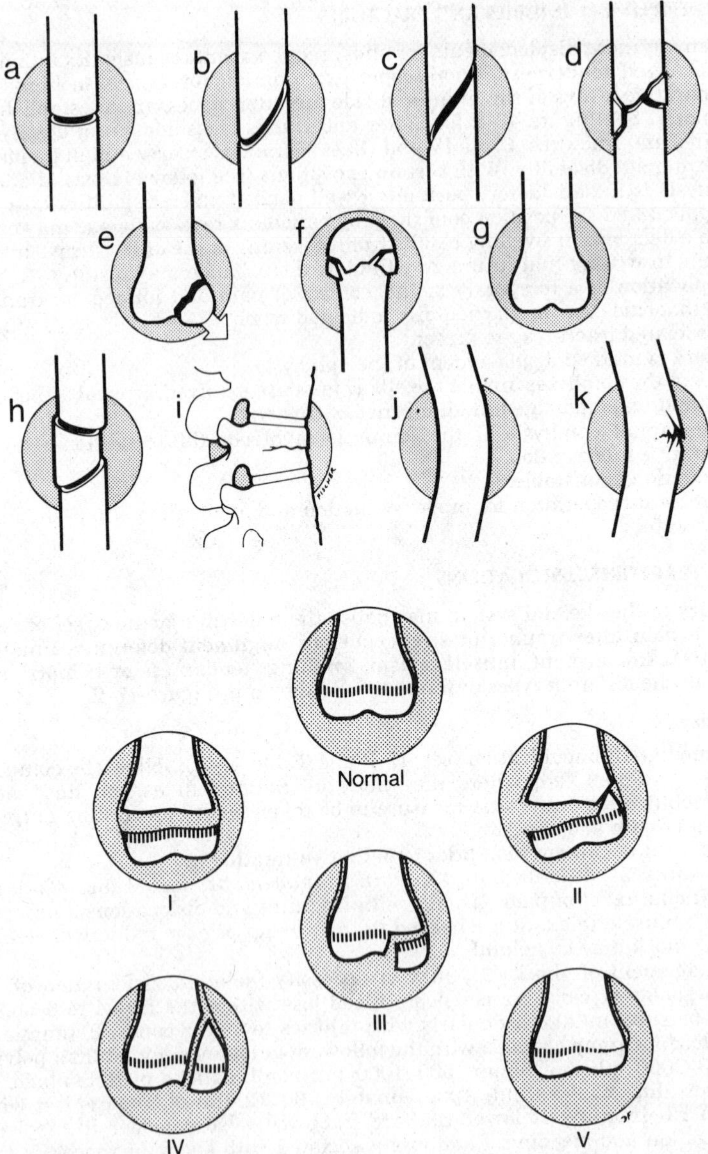

Figure 47–2. Types of fractures and epiphyseal injuries. *A,* The semantics of fractures: a, transverse; *b,* oblique; c, spiral; *d,* comminuted; *e,* avulsion; *f,* impacted; *g,* torus; *h,* segmented; *i,* compression; *j,* bending; *k,* greenstick. *B,* The Salter-Harris classification of epiphyseal injuries. (*A* from Committee on Trauma/American College of Surgeons [A. J. Walt et al. (eds.)]: *Early Care of the Injured Patient.* Philadelphia, W. B. Saunders Co., 1982, pp. 283, 284. *B,* from Salter, R. B., and Harris, W. R.: Injuries involving the epiphyseal plate. J. Bone Joint Surg., *45A*:587, 1963.)

internal fixation (ORIF) may be required. Techniques in external fixation are advancing.

- Even with stabilized disposition to home, recheck in 24 hours is advisable [or earlier if frequent checks *(47–2)* for neurovascular compromise indicate problems].
- Avoid circumferential plaster wrapping of acute injuries, since progressive swelling can compromise neurovascular structures.
- Healing time in uncomplicated cases will vary from 3 weeks for a phalanx to as long as 16 to 32 weeks for a tibial shaft.

Greenstick Fractures *(See Fig. 47–2)*

In these cases, malalignment and angulation of the buckled periosteum is minimal and can generally be corrected without difficulty by manipulation after injection of 1% procaine or lidocaine around the fracture site. Position after reduction and application of plaster should be checked by x-rays. Circulation and sensation should be monitored during the first 24 hours. Plastic deformation contributing to permanent bowing is frequently noted in the young despite anatomic reduction of fracture ends.

HEAD

47–7. FRACTURES OF THE NASAL BONES *(See 48–5)*

47–8. TEMPOROMANDIBULAR DISLOCATIONS

These dislocations are usually unilateral and, because of spasm of the powerful muscles controlling the jaw, are difficult to reduce. If heavy pressure downward and backward (with the operator's thumbs well padded) does not cause reduction, the patient should be referred to an oral surgeon. General anesthetic may be necessary for reduction.

47–9. FRACTURES OF THE UPPER OR LOWER JAW WITHOUT DISPLACEMENT OR DISTURBANCE OF DENTAL OCCLUSION

These require only control of pain and application of a Barton type bandage (Table 47–1) to support the mandible. The patient should then be referred to an oral surgeon for definitive care.

NECK

47–10. FRACTURES AND DISLOCATIONS OF THE NECK

For initial splinting, see *4*; for discussion of management of suspected or actual neck injuries, see *49–17*, spinal cord injuries with compression; see also Figure 47–3.

47–11. SEVERE STRAINS ("WHIPLASH" INJURIES) OF THE NECK

A sudden jerk or acceleration hyperextension-flexion injury to the neck may cause extensive soft tissue damage and acute symptoms, often deferred for 12 to 48 hours, that apparently are out of proportion to the trauma alleged to have been sustained. Acute soft tissue injuries often cannot be differentiated from fracture or dislocation and may require hospitalization for observation and special x-ray studies. Mild cases can be treated for a few days at home by partial immobilization by a cervical collar, with application of heat (or

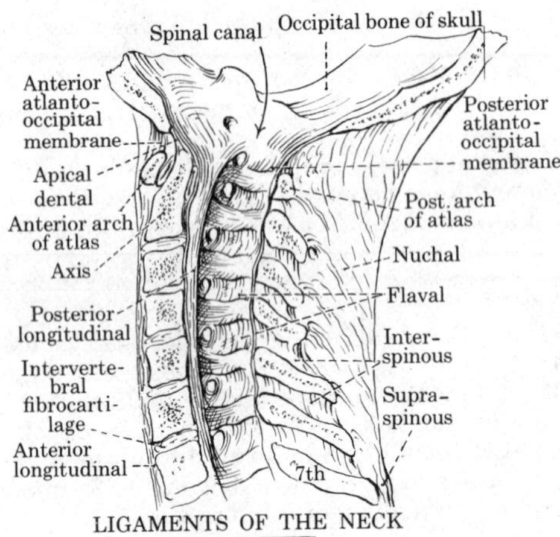

Figure 47–3. Ligaments of the neck. (From *Dorland's Illustrated Medical Dictionary*, 26th ed., Plate 24. Philadelphia, W. B. Saunders Co., 1981.)

cold) and gentle massage. (See Table 47–3 for general guidelines in management.) Traction by means of an over-the-door water bag/pulley/head halter system (or Goodley polyaxial cervical traction, which avoids pressure on the temporomandibular joint) may be beneficial.

Post-traumatic symptoms (neck pain, limitation of cervical and shoulder girdle motion, headache, dysphagia, dizziness) may persist for a lengthy time after cervical strains and require prolonged treatment for relief. After a short period of rest, recovery is aided by gradual institution of cervical range of motion, joint mobilization and isometric exercises.

BACK

47–12. BACK STRAINS AND SPRAINS *(See also 47–3 and Figure 47–4)*

Back strains and sprains are extremely common injuries that are often related many times to arduous work (which must be at least temporarily modified or curtailed) but also may be caused by improper body mechanics, inadequate general physical conditioning and chronic strain from poor posture, requiring specific stretching and strengthening exercises. Orientation and instruction in these areas abet convalescence and limit recurrence. Strains may bring attention to previously asymptomatic and undetected pars interarticularis defect.

Onset of steady aching back pain may occur suddenly after heavy or awkward lifting or bending, or may be delayed until the next day. In the absence of radicular pain or neurologic deficit, strain is more likely than herniated nucleus pulposus.

In uncomplicated back strain there is usually guarding in trunk movements, flattening of the lumbar curvature and inability to perform normal forward and lateral bending of the thoracolumbar spine. Scoliosis secondary to muscle spasm may be present with disparity of the scapular tip and pelvic brim levels. Involved muscles are tight and tender on palpation. Straight leg raising may be restricted somewhat owing to hamstring tightness, but meningeal signs and neurologic deficits are absent.

Sudden onset of low back pain can occur while doing awkward movements (such as rotary twisting of the trunk while lifting) and be accompanied by immediate scoliosis and guarded gait, focal tenderness in a unilateral facet region (commonly the T12–L1 or thoracolumbar hinge area), and referred tenderness over the midposterior brim of the pelvis—this suggests impingement of sensitive soft tissue at the facet; the joint becomes more "out of play" (due to splinting) than "out of place." Dramatic rapid relief can occur with simple mobilization and manipulation (usually a rotary motion in the direction of the pain source).

Treatment

- See Table 47–3 for general measures and principles in management.
- Because postural muscles are physiologically very slow to relax when irritated, rest in a recumbent position for at least a few days, plus muscle relaxants (Robaxin, Soma, Flexeril), is advisable in more severe cases. Sitting is stressful, but if permitted there should be opportunity to alternate with walking and lying at desired intervals. Avoid bending/lifting.
- After ice is used initially (if tolerated), lying in a tub of hot water (or hot tub) for 15 to 30 minutes, followed by gentle stretching exercises (knees to chest; shoulder and opposite knee approximated toward each other, pelvic tilts, back extension, etc.), several times a day can be helpful.
- If lateral pelvic tilt is present, use a temporary heel lift of appropriate leveling height placed inside the shoe of the "short side."
- As much as feasible, have patient stand stationary and slowly come to a full erect position before walking, rather than starting to move outright with a gross stooped position that is further aggravating.
- The most helpful and comfortable type of back support, if needed, is a firm, one piece, elasticized abdominal support "corset" in which can be placed a piece of thermolabile plastic ("Warm and Form") that can be easily custom-molded to the contour of the patient's lower back.
- Patients may return to tolerable levels of modified work as soon as reasonable, even though regular activities must await further recovery. It is extremely important for all concerned to indicate clearly from the initial visit what the probable periods of any temporary total and partial disability will be and what restrictions from regular work may be required.
- Physical therapy is beneficial; it is best for the patient to lie down during transportation if sitting is bothersome.
- When the patient has recovered sufficiently, attending a back care class may be beneficial in preventing recurrences.

47–13. HERNIATED NUCLEUS PULPOSUS (HNP, "Herniated Disk")

"Herniated disks" occur principally in the lumbosacral region following single or repetitious strain (though less frequently cervical HNP may cause radicular pain in the upper extremities and long tract signs—either unilateral or bilateral; thoracic HNP is rarely diagnosed).

Intense radiating pain (plus hypesthesia and anesthesia) in the dermatome of the involved nerve root(s) (see Fig. 49–1) is commonly increased by one or more of the following: lifting, moving, coughing, sneezing, defecation and straight leg raising (SLR) with foot dorsiflexion. SLR usually causes back and leg pain by 30 to 40 degrees of elevation. Focal muscle weakness and fasciculation and later atrophy plus decrease or loss of ankle or patellar deep tendon reflexes on the involved side are further indicators of HNP. Muscle spasm usually is intense, leading often to acute scoliotic curvature and flattening of the lumbar curvature, which does not bend or curl with forward flexion. Lower back movements, particularly extension and flexion, are greatly reduced, and all body movements are slow and guarded to avoid painful jarring. Firm interspinous pressure with a digit at the level of the HNP ("poor man's myelogram") may cause a great increase in pain.

Massive central disk herniation is a surgical emergency requiring immediate metrizamide myelogram with or without CT scan and decompressive laminectomy. The massive central HNP may result in urinary difficulties (slow stream, initiation of decreased force, incomplete emptying and bladder distention), saddle hypesthesia, decreased anal sphincter reflex and muscle tone, bilateral lower extremity weakness and intense pain.

Treatment

- In the absence of either bowel or bladder deficit (see preceding discussion of massive central HNP, management is usually nonsurgical for at least 7 to 10 days. The patient may remain at home, but if there are management or care problems, hospitalization is advised.
- Complete bed rest is essential for the first 7 days or so; preferably a bedside commode should be used. Crutches can ease short-range walking.
- Traction, as tolerated, is of possible value for lumbar HNP and of definite value for cervical HNP.
- The therapeutic principles cited in Table 47–3 are applicable. IV methocarbamol, 2 g (20 ml) in 500 ml D5W by drip infusion over several hours may reduce intense muscle spasm prior to using oral maintenance.
- Metrizamide myelogram with or without CT scan is generally done to aid localization for surgery (or chymopapain injection) or to solve a differential diagnosis problem.
- After 7 days, an electromyogram (EMG) may establish the extent of nerve root compromise.
- Failure of the above measures to improve the condition is an indication for hospitalization for further management, observation and surgical consultation.

47–14. THORACIC AND LUMBAR DISLOCATIONS *(See also 49–17, Spinal Injuries with Cord Compression, and initial immobilization measures for the spine outlined in 4, Transportation)*

These severe injuries are usually associated with high velocity accidents, complications of seat belt injuries (which may also cause internal abdominal injury if belt is not applied firmly on the pelvis) or falls from a distance. Like cervical dislocations, all may be associated with fractures and potential permanent paralysis; these require extreme care and firm immobilization from the beginning (see *4*). Hospitalization and surgery for nerve/spinal cord compression or instability are required.

47–15. FRACTURES OF TRANSVERSE PROCESSES

Fractures of transverse processes of the lumbar vertebrae are always painful but rarely serious in and of themselves; however, injury to nearby intra-abdominal organs (*59–4*) must always be thoroughly evaluated, and general surgical consultation is advisable. Partial immobilization by strapping or application of a lumbosacral belt or snug-fitting plaster body jacket may decrease the pain. The site of the fracture may be infiltrated with 1% lidocaine (Xylocaine). The patient should be instructed to sleep on a nonsagging bed. Analgesics (*12*) and muscle relaxants as needed are in order, since any motion of the back may be very painful for 7 to 10 days after injury. See Table 47–3.

47–16. SACRAL AND COCCYGEAL FRACTURES

Coccygeal fractures can be confirmed and reduced via rectal examination. Some sacral and coccygeal fractures may require hospitalization for a few days for control of acute pain and evaluation for any associated internal or nerve damage. Usually, however, strapping the buttocks together or prescription of a U-shaped cut-out foam rubber cushion (to relieve coccygeal pressure) to be carried around for use during sitting will allow home care. Ice compresses initially and then sitz baths may be of benefit.

THORAX AND SHOULDER*

47–17. FRACTURES OF THE RIBS AND STERNUM *(See also 31, Chest)*

Linear fractures of the sternum or fractures of one or two midthoracic ribs without displacement usually require only analgesics, ice initially and possibly a low-positioned (regardless of the fracture level) rib belt; x-rays are elective. Unilateral strapping of the chest is effective but if overly restrictive could limit ventilation and foster infection. Infiltration near the site of the fracture with 1% lidocaine will lessen discomfort on breathing, as will blocking of the intercostal nerves *(31–16)* proximal to the fractures.

Marked displacement, multiple unstable fractures *(31–8)* or evidence of traumatic pneumothorax *(31–13)* requires immediate surgical evaluation and hospital care. With fractures of the 1st and 2nd ribs (see Fig. 18–9), consider concomitant injury to adjacent neurovascular structures; with low rib fractures, consider concomitant spleen, liver and renal injuries. For a lateral view of the vertebral column, see Fig. 47–4.

47–18. STERNOCLAVICULAR FRACTURES AND DISLOCATIONS

These injuries are uncommon and usually heal satisfactorily if partially immobilized by tight adhesive strapping over a pressure pad and use of a sling. Severe cases require operative repair for reduction and intramedullary fixation. Posterior dislocations can cause neurovascular, brachial or esophageal damage. Anterior dislocations may leave a bump, but little disability.

47–19. FRACTURES OF THE CLAVICLE

Examination usually reveals a painful defect in the clavicle, most often in the mid-shaft, or distal bone. Reduction of closed transverse or diagonal fractures of the medial three-quarters, even with considerable displacement or overriding, can generally be obtained by proper application of a clavicular cross or figure-of-eight bandage. This can easily be made out of bias tubular stockinette if more sophisticated clavicular braces are not available. The figure-of-eight bandage is left on for 4 to 6 weeks. Fractures of the distal or lateral quarter may require only a Velpeau bandage or a snug sling, but if they are displaced, surgical reduction and fixation may be required. Check x-ray films should be taken in 24 hours and should be followed by any modifications in immobilization necessary to improve the position. Compound (open) and severely comminuted clavicular fractures may require hospitalization. Fractures of the clavicle are usually treated nonsurgically unless there is tenting of the skin from a bone spike or concern for lung puncture.

---

*See also *31, Chest,* and Figure 47–5 (anatomy of the shoulder girdle and upper extremity).

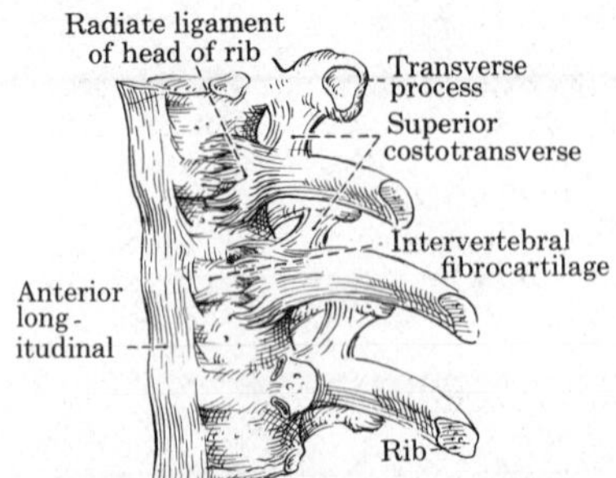

Figure 47–4. Ligaments of the ribs and back: lateral view, vertebral column. (From *Dorland's Illustrated Medical Dictionary*, 26th ed., Plate 24. Philadelphia, W. B. Saunders Co., 1981.)

47–20. ACROMIOCLAVICULAR (SHOULDER) SEPARATIONS

Complete acromioclavicular (A-C) separations are clinically apparent, but more often lesser degrees of separation can be demonstrated only by tenderness over the A-C joint, or by comparative x-rays of the shoulder girdles taken with a heavy weight in each hand. See Table 47–4 for differentiation of grades of A-C separation and treatment.

47–21. SCAPULAR FRACTURES

Scapular fractures are relatively uncommon, and usually not serious. Pain, tenderness, swelling and increased discomfort with ROM call attention to the lesion(s) that can involve various scapular areas. Fracture of the acromion process, coracoid process (seen on axillary view), neck of the scapula or glenoid fossa can usually be treated with a sling and swathe immobilization for 4 to 6 weeks, as can scapular body fractures, unless there is gross displacement and instability. With major fractures, look for associated injuries.

SHOULDER AND UPPER EXTREMITY*

47–22. SHOULDER/HUMERUS DISLOCATION

Shoulder subluxations and dislocations, along with acromioclavicular separations, are common musculoskeletal injuries in young people. Falls in football and skiing with the arm abducted and extended are a frequent cause; 90% of these dislocations are anterior. The patient presents holding the arm close to the side, and physical examination reveals a severely tender shoulder joint that is "squared off" when palpated rather than having the normal rounded contour; there is gross limitation of ROM. The head of the humerus can often be palpated in the subglenoid or subcoracoid position anteriorly. With anterior subluxations, there is a rare incidence of axillary paralysis and numbness over the deltoid muscle.

All persons with known or suspected shoulder dislocation should be checked carefully before and after reduction for evidence of nerve and/or vascular compromise (even though these complications are rare; if found, they should be recorded in the chart and the patient notified of the problem before reduction) and for fractures around the glenoid.

*See Figures 47–5, 47–10 and 47–11.

Table 47–4. GRADES OF ACROMIOCLAVICULAR SEPARATION

Grade	Findings	Treatment
I	Point tenderness over acromioclavicular (A-C) joint; strain of A-C joint and coracoclavicular ligament.	Sling or shoulder immobilizer for 2 to 4 weeks; then isometrics and progressive ROM exercises.
II	As above plus stretching of coracoclavicular ligament. No differential findings by x-ray with weight in hand between Grades I and II.	Same as above, plus use of ice and analgesics with all grades of separation.
III	"Upriding" clavicle above A-C joint on physical examination. Increased distance between coracoid process and clavicle when compared to unaffected side; x-ray shows further increase with weight in hand on affected side.	Controversial; usually excellent functional recovery after 4 to 6 weeks in shoulder immobilizer. Other experts believe early surgical intervention to restore normal anatomy hastens rehabilitation and "better" long-range strength.

Whenever possible, x-rays (AP view of shoulder, lateral view of scapula, and occasionally an axillary view) should be taken before reduction of a dislocated shoulder is attempted. If the films show a fracture—usually of the rim of the glenoid or greater tuberosity—and the reduction requires general anesthetic, hospitalization is indicated. If no fracture is demonstrated, reduction may be attempted by one of several methods. Pain and apprehension should be controlled by a preliminary injection of morphine sulfate, meperidine or diazepam (Valium). Nitrous oxide, 50% with oxygen, can be self-administered as needed during procedures as an adjunct.

Treatment

Arm-Weight Traction Method (Stimson) (Preferred)

1. After preliminary administration of a combination muscle relaxant–analgesic (e.g., IV Sublimaze and diazepam), place the patient face down on a narrow examination table with the arm on the injured side hanging down; tape 10-pound weight to hand; elevate scapula.
2. Apply prolonged firm gentle traction on the wrist with alternating gentle external and internal rotation. If after 15 to 20 minutes reduction has not been accomplished, other methods can be tried, with assistance from an orthopedic specialist as needed.

Traction-Countertraction Method (Two Operators)

1. Place the patient in a supine position. Distal traction is applied by one operator after grasping the wrist of the patient's upper extremity on the involved side, which is horizontally abducted 45 to 60 degrees.
2. At the same time, direct in-line countertraction is applied by another operator pulling on the ends of a long towel or folded sheet material that has been placed around the chest under the axilla of the dislocated shoulder.

Postreduction Measures

1. Confirm reduction with repeat x-rays.
2. Apply shoulder immobilizer for 4 to 6 weeks.
3. Institute supportive measures as appropriate (Table 47–3).
4. Warn that chance of later recurrence is high, and that if there are several recurrences, surgery may be required.
5. Check for neurovascular compromise.

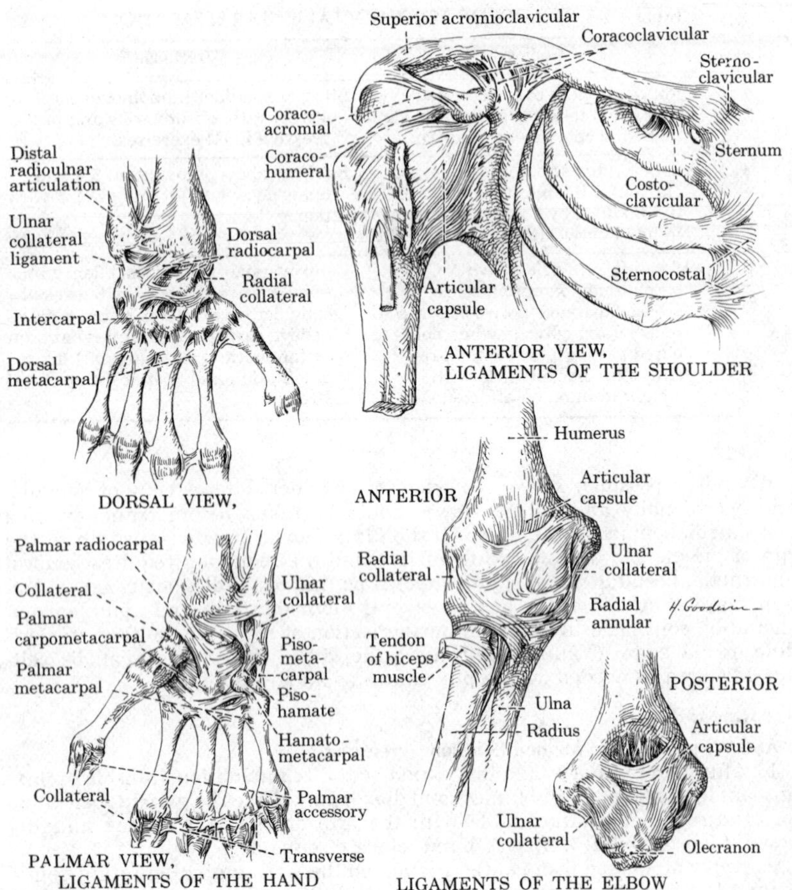

Figure 47–5. Right shoulder girdle/upper extremity skeletoligamentous anatomy. (From *Dorland's Illustrated Medical Dictionary*, 26th ed., Plate 24. Philadelphia. W. B. Saunders Co., 1981.)

47–23. HUMERUS FRACTURES

Humeral Head and Neck

Fractures involving the humeral head and neck are most often impacted and nondisplaced and can be treated in a sling for 4 to 6 weeks. Occasionally, children have fractures through the growth plate of the proximal humerus, and if enough displacement is present (usually greater than 30 degrees), closed reduction may be necessary under anesthesia. Elderly people with impacted fracture of the neck of the humerus require a sling for 3 weeks followed by early motion; assistance of a physical therapist can be valuable.

Humeral Shaft

Fractures involving the humeral shaft are quite common. Although most of these fractures are relatively undisplaced and require little, if any, reduction, care must be taken on physical examination to document the integrity of the radial nerve. This is most commonly injured in spiral fractures of the mid to distal third of the humerus. Usually radial nerve palsies resolve spontaneously, *but those injured during reduction need to be surgically explored.*

Fractures of the humeral shaft are commonly treated with slings or hanging arm casts. (*Note:* In elderly people, hanging arm casts may "overpull" the fracture and cause non-union; therefore a sling should be used in these cases.) Treatment of humeral shaft fractures is usually carried out for 3 to 6 weeks and then early motion is started.

47–24. ELBOW FRACTURES

The elbow joint is quite vulnerable to injury, especially in young children, with most injuries occurring from falls and blows. Certainly supracondylar fractures are among the worst of all fractures in children. There is an extremely high incidence of injuries to the growth plate with subsequent malunion and growth plate disturbances. Vascular injuries can be catastrophic and cause Volkmann's contracture. Orthopedic consultation is advisable for all condylar and supracondylar fractures. Fractures involving the supracondylar region can be single or a combination of the "T" variety, transverse, medial, lateral condylar or epicondylar. Fractures of the elbow without displacement are best treated initially with posterior splints or double sugar tong splints.

Physical examination in this area often reveals diffuse swelling, severe tenderness, resistance to joint motion and occasionally vascular compromise, which requires close evaluation. It is important that the x-rays obtained clearly show the extent of the fracture; comparison views of the unaffected elbow are often useful. All x-rays in children should include a lateral view with the elbow at 90 degrees so that the radial head is in a straight line with the capitulum of the humerus. Fractures involving the elbow joint in the adult more commonly involve the epicondyles of the humerus, the radial head or olecranon. X-rays may reveal an effusion of the elbow joint with an elevated fat pad in addition to the associated fracture.

Displaced fractures must be reduced; this is usually best completed in the OR. In addition, the parents of children with supracondylar fractures should be told that possible growth plate disturbances may occur later. It is worthwhile to document this warning in the emergency chart. Neurovascular monitoring should be carried out throughout the entire pre- and postreduction phases of treatment of displaced joints. Admission to the hospital for 24 to 48 hours is often advisable.

Displaced fractures of the olecranon require open reduction and internal fixation. Tension band wiring now enables ROM exercises to be started immediately. Fractures involving the lateral or medial epicondyle usually require internal fixation if displacement is greater than several millimeters.

The term "pitcher's elbow" is used to describe a condition in which there is pain in the area of insertion around the medial or lateral epicondyles or olecranon; this may be from tendinitis, but often x-rays will reveal small avulsion fractures in these areas. Usually these minor disorders resolve after 3 to 6 weeks of splinting.

47–25. ELBOW DISLOCATIONS *(See also 47–26 and 47–27 Radial Head Subluxations and Fractures)*

Provided no fractures are present, dislocations of the elbow can sometimes be reduced with the patient under heavy sedation but without anesthesia by the following method:

1. Have the patient lie supine on a narrow table.
2. Apply gentle downward traction and supination on the wrist, to reduce the olecranon and radial head.
3. Check for complete reduction by palpation, comparison with the uninjured side and x-rays.
4. Immobilize with a Velpeau bandage (see Fig. 47–1), with the wrist supinated.
5. Ascertain immediately that circulation, sensation and motor function are intact. Instruct the patient on checking, and arrange for a check-up in 24 hours. If reduction cannot be obtained in two attempts, the patient should be hospitalized for reduction under general anesthesia.

47–26. RADIAL HEAD SUBLUXATIONS

Partial subluxation of the proximal end of the radius from the sling formed by the orbicular ligament occurs almost exclusively in small children at the toddling age, although it may occur in injudiciously handled infants. The mechanism of injury is usually a sudden jerk on the outstretched arm by an adult leading or lifting the child by the hand; this mechanism has led to the eponym "nursemaid's elbow."

Signs and Symptoms. Severe pain plus tenderness over the radial head and neck, with inability of the patient to fully extend the forearm, is characteristic. The child usually holds the arm with the elbow slightly flexed and the forearm pronated and resists any attempts at examination or motion. X-rays are usually normal unless injury is severe, in which case dislocation or displacement of the epicondylar epiphyses may be seen.

Treatment

If the injury is recent, complete reduction can usually be accomplished without anesthesia by:

1. Gentle traction on the forearm with countertraction against the upper arm.
2. Pressure over the radial head with the thumb.
3. Gradual extension and supination of the forearm. A palpable (sometimes audible) click or snap occasionally accompanies reduction.

Use of a splint or sling is not required in isolated subluxations. Explain the mechanism of the injury to family members so that recurrence can be prevented.

47–27. RADIAL HEAD FRACTURES

If the fracture of the radial head involves more than a third of its surface, surgical excision of the fragment or entire head may be required; a prosthetic replacement may be considered.

47–28. RADIAL AND ULNAR SHAFT FRACTURES

These common fractures frequently result from falling on the outstretched arm or direct trauma to the forearm. Physical examination reveals swelling and deformity in the forearm and difficulty in moving the wrist or elbow because of increased pain. X-rays must be taken in the anteroposterior and lateral views; both wrist and elbow views should also be taken, even if these joints seem uninvolved. With regard to the lateral view, more significant displacement may be accepted in the child than in the adult (but slight displacement or "bayonetting" may be acceptable in the adult). However, very little displacement in the anteroposterior views (valgus or varus) is acceptable in either the child or the adult. While one of the two bones in the forearm occasionally will be intact and help to splint the adjacent fractured bone, it may also interfere with adequate reduction. Fractures involving the radial and ulnar shaft in the adult should be reduced with very little displacement in either plane and often require rigid plate fixation. Ulnar shaft fractures with radial head dislocation (Monteggia's fracture) usually require open reduction in adults, and closed manipulation by an orthopedist in children.

Reduction of fractures involving the radial and ulnar shaft requires sufficient analgesia. This may sometimes be done in the Emergency Room with intrahematoma lidocaine, IV analgesia or regional anesthesia, but often general anesthesia is required. Placing the fingers of the affected side in Chinese finger traps to hold the hand and forearm vertically and suspending a well-padded handle of a bucket of water (or sandbags and stockinette) from around the arm will give proximal traction at the flexed elbow and will aid the physician in manipulating and splinting the fracture. Adequacy of reduction must always be confirmed by x-ray. Use of an image intensifier is helpful if available; a special permit may be required for use of this instrument. Elevation and constant neurovascular checks are essential with these fractures.

47–29. FRACTURES OF THE DISTAL RADIUS AND ULNA

Fractures of the distal radius and ulna with wrist swelling are extremely common in the young and in elderly people following falls. Attempted motion is quite painful. Displaced fractures of the distal radius and ulna are most often seen dorsally (Colles' fracture), producing the so-called "dinner fork deformity." Less commonly the distal radius and ulna may be displaced in a volar position (reversed Colles' or Smith's fracture), but after reduction, the wrist is still held in flexion with ulnar deviation.

X-rays are most important in documenting the degree of displacement, comminution and joint involvement. Torus or buckle type fractures of the radial and ulnar cortex are most often seen in children, whereas comminuted interarticular fractures of the distal radius are much more common in adults. Epiphyseal injuries (47–5) are also quite common in children.

If severe comminution, angulation, displacement, misalignment or distortion of the articular surface of the radius is present, accurate reduction is essential for a satisfactory functional result. Preprocedure analgesics and muscle relaxants are helpful. Injection of 1% lidocaine into the joint and at the fracture site (hematoma block) usually gives satisfactory anesthesia. Restoration of the correct angle of the articular surface and length of the radius is necessary; suspension by the hand fixed in Chinese finger traps to an overhead fixture, such as an intravenous (IV) standard, can aid realignment. If realignment cannot be obtained under local anesthesia and confirmed by postreduction x-rays, splinting should be done and the patient transferred to an orthopedist for possible reduction under general anesthesia.

If a satisfactory reduction (as verified by x-ray) is obtained, a double sugar tong splint with a long arm extension for undue swelling (with the pressure points well padded) extending from the upper third of the humerus to the proximal metacarpal heads should be applied with the elbow at 90 degrees and the forearm in slight pronation; there is no need for circular casting. If an adequate, stable reduction has been obtained, the wrist should be immobilized in optimum grasping position—i.e., slight flexion and slight ulnar deviation—which allows the dorsal periosteum to maintain the position of the reduced fracture and the radius to be held at greatest length. After the splint has set, sensation and circulation should be checked carefully and x-rays taken. Tests of sensation and circulation must be monitored repeatedly in the first 24 to 48 hours, as postreduction swelling is common. In all cases, follow-up care should be arranged so that in adults the cast can be shortened in 7 to 10 days to allow active motion of the thumb and fingers after pain, spasm and swelling have subsided. Shortening of the cast is not necessary in children. Ice and elevation are important (see Table 47–3). Slings should be discouraged.

47–30. CARPAL (NAVICULAR) SCAPHOID FRACTURES

This type of fracture usually occurs as a result of falling onto the dorsiflexed, outstretched hand. Decreased ROM, wrist pain, swelling and particularly point tenderness in the "snuffbox" area (between the thumb extensor and abductors) should prompt x-ray evaluation with wrist and navicular views. Nondisplaced fractures may not be evident on x-ray for several days to a few weeks. Specific tenderness of the snuffbox area after trauma or evidence of a fracture are indications for splinting.

If marked comminution or displacement is present, a temporary volar splint should be applied and the patient referred at once for orthopedic care. If the position is satisfactory, a padded short arm splint or cast extending from just below the elbow to just proximal to the metacarpophalangeal joints of the fingers and to the tip of the thumb should be applied with the wrist in slight cock-up position and the axis of the thumb in line with the radial shaft. Check neurovascular status. Follow-up orthopedic care for a lengthy period is indicated because of the possibility of aseptic necrosis and nonunion. With this fracture, warn the patient of the need to immobilize the affected joint for several months and of the possibility of nonunion that could necessitate later surgery. Get repeat films in 10 to 14 days if splinted only because of snuffbox tenderness.

47–31. OTHER CARPAL BONE FRACTURES

Immobilization by a padded, short arm cast for 4 to 6 weeks is all that is necessary unless there is comminution or displacement of fragments or associated dislocations (see 47–32, *Lunate Dislocations,* and 47–33, *Perilunar Dislocations*) and/or soft tissue damage, which make hospitalization for orthopedic care in order.

47–32. LUNATE DISLOCATIONS

Severe direct trauma to the wrist may cause rupture of the ligamentous structures at the distal (scaphoid) end of the lunate bone, with subsequent partial or complete rotary displacement and possible scaphoid fracture. In evaluating this, check that the lunate is in line with the distal radius on the lateral view, and also check that there is not increased distance between the scaphoid and lunate on AP view ("Terry-Thomas sign"). Reduction and reduction maintenance may be difficult, and operative fixation of the distal end of the bone may be necessary.

47–33. PERILUNAR DISLOCATIONS

In this type of dislocation, the lunate remains in normal relationship to the radius and ulna while all of the other carpal bones are displaced. Routine x-rays may be misinterpreted, especially if associated fractures of the scaphoid or cuneiform are present. Reduction is usually difficult and requires regional block or general anesthesia, followed by immobilization for 6 to 8 weeks in a splint and then a plaster short arm cast.

47–34. METACARPAL FRACTURES *(See also 43–1 for Hand Trauma: Initial General Measures and Examination for Nerve and Tendon Injury)*

Injuries to the hand, especially in the metacarpophalangeal area of the thumb, should be radiographed prior to any handling or manipulation, to prevent converting an avulsion type of fracture to a nonreducible situation in which the extensor hood becomes interposed between the fragment and its fracture site.

The following principles are important in consideration of fractures of the metacarpals and phalanges: Valgus or vargus deformity and significant shortening in the AP view often do not give an acceptable end result. Some angulation of metacarpal fractures on lateral view may be acceptable. Often shortened or angulated metacarpal fractures can be corrected with closed reduction. Severely comminuted or shortened metacarpal fractures often require open reduction and internal fixation (ORIF). Proximal metacarpal fractures usually do not need reduction and can be placed in a "cobra cast" splint.* Angulation may be seen initially in fractures of the heads of the metacarpals, but these usually can be easily reduced by closed reduction and maintained with a short arm cast with finger splint(s) to the associated finger(s) for immobilization (put the metacarpophalangeal joint down at 30 to 45 degrees; unless specifically indicated, full finger extension is contraindicated).

Without Displacement. Apply a padded splint, take check x-rays, check for sensory and circulatory changes and refer the patient to orthopedic care in 24 hours. *Exception:* A fracture of the medial angle of the proximal end of the metacarpal of the thumb (Bennett's fracture) is unstable from muscle pull and usually requires open reduction and fixation or pinning to prevent a large permanent disability from shortening, instability and decrease in grip. If closed reduction is achieved, hold in a thumb spica and give repeated x-ray rechecks, as redisplacement can occur.

With Displacement. Multiple fractures, angulation, overriding and comminution generally require orthopedic care for reduction. Fractures of the distal ends of the 2nd to 5th metacarpals (usually the 5th) are the exception. These "boxer's" fractures (identified by a depressed or possibly absent knuckle) can usually be reduced without difficulty under local anesthesia injected near the fracture site, with correction of the volar angulation of the distal fragment by firm dorsal pressure, using the proximal phalanx flexed to 90 degrees as a lever. Direct traction in the long axis of the metacarpal is useless in fractures of this type.

47–35. PHALANGEAL FRACTURES

Proximal or Middle Phalanges. Post-traumatic pain, swelling, tenderness and decreased ROM are generally present. Check for rotary fractures by having the patient flex all the fingers; tips should all point to the same lateral (navicular) portion of the wrist. If x-rays reveal a fracture that is relatively nondisplaced, no further reduction is usually required and only immobilization is needed. However, any proximal or middle phalanx with significant angulation, comminution or intra-articular involvement requires closed reduction

---

*The "cobra cast" is a type of short arm cast (SAC) that is started just distal to the elbow and includes the wrist in a 45-degree dorsiflexed position and the metacarpophalangeal joint in 90-degree flexion. The volar aspect of the cast is brought to the metacarpophalangeal joint, and the dorsal aspect of cast continues to the proximal interphalangeal joint.

or, if this is unsuccessful, open reduction with internal fixation (ORIF). Usually reduction via manual traction reduces most phalangeal fractures without difficulty under local anesthesia. The attachments and pull of the flexor tendons should be kept in mind when splinting and applying traction. Acute flexion at the proximal interphalangeal joint may be required to achieve alignment if the fracture is distal to the attachment of the flexor digitorum sublimis tendon, after which the finger is cast in the position of function (see 43–3). Immobilization of these phalanx fractures at most require a short arm splint or cast with incorporated splint to the injured finger at a 30- to 45-degree flexion angulation. Recheck in 24 hours by an orthopedist is advisable. "Buddy taping" of fingers is to be discouraged, as in many fractures this provides inadequate immobilization. However, buddy taping after 3 to 4 weeks of treatment of a specific finger in a short arm cast with incorporated splint is often acceptable.

Another common fracture is that of the volar plate of the proximal portion of the middle phalanx sustained in a hyperextension injury. On physical examination this fracture usually shows significant swelling with decreased motion and often involvement of the proximal interphalangeal joint of the finger. Close scrutiny of the lateral x-ray view is often required to locate the volar plate fracture, which may also be volarly and proximally displaced. Despite its benign appearance on x-ray, this fracture must be treated aggressively with a short arm cast with splint to the injured finger with the finger flexed at about 30 to 40 degrees to the tip. Some experts recommend ORIF or excision of the fragment with advancement of the volar plate. Inform the patient that some stiffness and early arthritis may result from this intraarticular fracture.

Closed Distal Phalanx. Fractures of the tuft require no treatment except protection with an aluminum or plastic splint. Fibrous union, with no deformity or dysfunction, usually occurs.

Fractures of the proximal lip of the dorsal aspect of the distal phalanx at the attachment of the extensor tendon (baseball finger, mallet finger) result in inability to extend the distal phalanx and should be taped with aluminofoam tape; alternatively, an individually fitted aluminum splint should be applied, with the proximal interphalangeal joint in about 40 degrees of flexion and the distal joint in slight hyperextension (be careful not to overextend) to obtain maximum relaxation of the extensor tendon. Fitting with a "stack" type splint accomplishes this. Surgical opinion should be obtained regarding open reduction if more than a third of the articular surface is involved; surgical pinning of the fragment may be necessary.

Open (Compound) Fractures of the Digits. In open (compound) fractures of any portion of the hand, the patient should be referred to an orthopedist or hand surgeon for care, with the exception of shattering fractures of the tuft. These tuft fractures should be irrigated, debrided and closed (unless there is a "dirty" wound), saving as much length as possible and avoiding suture lines on the tactile surface of the ball. Small, loose fragments of bone not attached to periosteum or soft tissue should be removed, but larger pieces are left in place. Fibrous union often occurs with no loss of function. Antimicrobials are indicated.

Open fractures of the thumb particularly should receive the attention of a specialist. Multiple crushing fractures of the fingers associated with loss or maceration of soft tissues may require a plastic amputation, with an attempt to save as much length as possible. Amputated portions can sometimes be filleted and used as full-thickness grafts if defatted thoroughly. Every precaution should be taken to ensure satisfactory shape and thickness, with minimal scarring of the tactile surface of the stump. Digital nerve stumps are best buried in available soft tissue to prevent formation of neuromas. If the amputation is through the base of the nail, all nail matrix cells should be removed by sharp dissection and curetting.

47–36. PHALANGEAL (METACARPAL) DISLOCATIONS

Dislocations with or without associated fractures are frequently reported by the patient's accounting that "my finger popped out of joint." Even if "relocation" has been performed prior to x-ray (a procedure to be discouraged—but which is sometimes unavoidable), tenderness and swelling will persist at the involved joint.

Limited almost exclusively to the metacarpophalangeal joint of the thumb and the proximal interphalangeal joints of the other digits, these dislocations (confirmed by x-ray) can usually be reduced easily by traction and manipulation, often without anesthesia. If necessary, very small amounts of 1% lidocaine can be injected into the joint, or a digital nerve block can be done, before manipulation. By determining that the finger flexes normally into the palm, lateral or medial deviation (or slight degrees of rotation) can be avoided. After reduction, a short plaster cast should be applied (immobilize the metacarpophalangeal joint in full flexion) and the position confirmed by x-rays. Immobilization for 3 weeks, followed by institution of active motion, will usually result in regaining full function, although some permanent thickening of the capsule may result. Compressive centripetal wrappings *(63–15)* are of value in reduction of local edema.

A dislocation of the metacarpophalangeal joint of the thumb may become "locked" because of anterior protrusion of the metacarpal head through a rent in the capsule. Operative reduction is necessary.

PELVIS AND LOWER EXTREMITY DISORDERS*

47–37. ILIAC CREST TRAUMA ("Hip Pointers")

Direct blunt trauma to the iliac crest generally causes significant discomfort; athletes often refer to these injuries as "hip pointers." Often children will present with histories of jumping or running when they experience the acute onset of pain in a particular pelvic region, and they may recall hearing a "pop." Physical examination often reveals only point tenderness and mild swelling over the iliac crest region. X-rays are usually unremarkable in the adult. However, in patients 16 and under, strong, forced motions about the hip and leg may cause severe muscle contraction and subsequent avulsion of the origins of the muscles around the iliac crest region; therefore, x-rays will demonstrate avulsion of the anterior superior iliac spine associated with an avulsion of the origin of the sartorius muscle.

Treatment

Usually these bruises with avulsions around the iliac crest regions are treated with crutch-assisted partial weight-bearing, ice for 48 to 72 hours and abstinence from sports for 3 to 6 weeks. Attempts to surgically reattach these avulsed bone pieces have been disappointing.

47–38. PELVIC FRACTURES

Fractures involving the pelvis (Fig. 47–6) usually follow motor vehicle accidents and often occur with other associated injuries (e.g., back, lower

---

*See Figures 47–6, 47–7, 47–12 and 47–13.

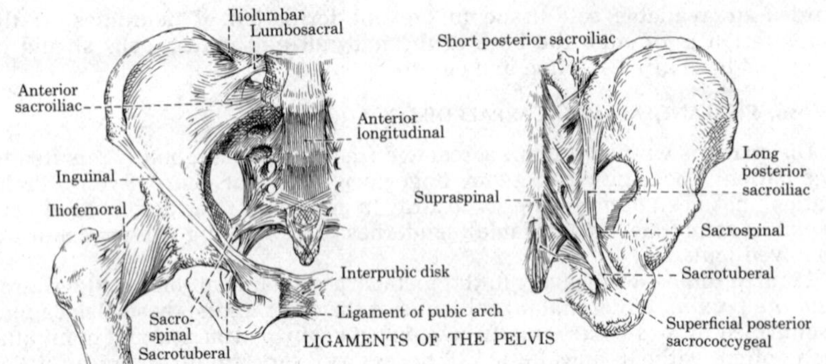

Figure 47–6. Ligaments of the pelvis. (From *Dorland's Illustrated Medical Dictionary,* 26th ed., Plate 25. Philadelphia, W. B. Saunders Co., 1981.)

extremity, internal). Physical examination requires checking the stability of the pelvis and careful examination of the lower extremities, thoracolumbar spine and abdomen. In addition, routine urinalysis should be done with suspected pelvic fractures, because of the high incidence of associated urologic injuries. If pelvic fracture is confirmed, IVP, a cystourethrogram and urologic consultation are appropriate; abnormalities may be present even in the absence of RBC's in the urine (see Fig. 41–1). Close examination of the knee areas may reveal bruises, since knees hitting the dashboard may result in acetabular fractures or hip dislocation.

An AP x-ray view of the pelvis helps to determine whether the fracture is stable or unstable, as well as showing the presence of hip dislocation or acetabular fracture. Commonly, fractures of the superior and/or inferior rami are seen, and these are considered stable by themselves. However, these fractures, when associated with disruption of the sacroiliac joint, are considered unstable, and further stabilization of the pelvic ring is usually necessary. Assess the integrity of the pubic symphysis, as this may also be affected when there is disruption of the pelvis in an unstable fashion with concurrent posterior pathology.

Treatment

- Initially immobilize on long board, with trunk, pelvis and lower extremities well secured.
- Treat shock; consider possible large blood volume loss (1 to 2 L) with pelvic fracture. Give analgesics.
- Prompt reduction of any associated hip dislocation (see *47–39*), performed by an orthopedist if pelvis is unstable or if emergency physician is unskilled in this technique.
- Urologic evaluation (see earlier comments and Fig. 41–1).
- Central acetabular fractures are among the most common of the serious pelvic fractures and require 6 weeks to 3 months of immobilization and traction in the hospital.
- Unstable pelvic ring fractures often require the use of an external fixator for adequate immobilization.
- Even stable pelvic fractures and uncomplicated hip dislocations should

usually be observed overnight, with special emphasis paid to neurovascular monitoring, urinary status, and analgesic treatment.

47–39. HIP DISLOCATIONS

Dashboard injuries to the knees and other blunt trauma to the lower extremities directed toward the pelvis may cause acetabular fractures and/or hip dislocations (with or without fracture).

Dislocation of the hip produces immediate gross positional deformity, functional loss and pain. The knee and thigh are flexed, and with posterior dislocation (90% of cases) they are inverted or adducted; with anterior dislocation (rare) they are everted or abducted. These are serious orthopedic emergencies. Check for sciatic injury with posterior dislocation. Immobilize the patient in the position in which he or she is found and transfer to a hospital for immediate reduction. The dislocated hip needs reduction quickly because of the significant risk of avascular necrosis of the femoral head. Some hip dislocations, especially those associated with fractures, require general anesthesia for proper reduction and maintenance of reduction. In cases of hip dislocation without fracture, once reduction and stability are achieved, the patient often can be ambulated within a 48-hour period, with minimal weight-bearing (e.g. 10 pounds; teach by having patient put toe pressure on a floor weight scale).

47–40. HIP FRACTURES

The femur, the longest and strongest bone in the body, usually requires a great deal of force to be fractured, unless it is osteoporotic, as in elderly people. Usually there is a history of the patient falling down and landing on the trochanteric region of the hip, but with osteoporotic bone, torsion while standing can produce fracture, and the fall is secondary.

Physical examination reveals pain with any range of motion, and often the leg is shortened and externally rotated. Fractures of the hip in the elderly are usually confirmed on x-ray and are most commonly seen in the subcapital, intertrochanteric, and subtrochanteric regions. Most often, these will require internal fixation devices or prosthetic replacements. Unfortunately, fractures involving the head and neck of the femur in young adults have a far less favorable prognosis, owing to poor blood supply to the femoral head. Any of these patients suffering fractures about the hip region are often more comfortable with appropriate analgesia and 5 pounds of traction (e.g., Buck's traction) placed on the affected leg until orthopedic consultation is obtained.

47–41. SHAFT OF THE FEMUR FRACTURES

Fractures involving the shaft of the femur are very serious orthopedic injuries and are often accompanied by other systemic injuries, since great force is required to produce them, as in motorcycle/motor vehicle accidents or falls from heights. Physical examination often reveals a deformity of the thigh with swelling and hematomatous formation. X-rays delineate the nature of the fracture, which is often comminuted, open or severely shortened.

Treatment

- Splint immediately, and apply traction; Hare or Thomas traction splints are best.
- These injuries are usually quite painful, and significant analgesia is required. The patient must be referred for orthopedic care, and open reduction with internal fixation (ORIF) may be necessary.

47–42. HAMSTRING/QUADRICEPS MUSCLE TEARS

Most commonly, tears ("pulls") of these muscles occur in the muscle bellies themselves or at the musculotendinous junction as the result of an acute burst of speed by the patient or simply muscle imbalance. However, not uncommonly, with avulsion of the origin of the hamstrings from the ischial tuberosity, the patient will complain of acute pain in the ischial tuberosity region, and a hematoma may be present. Hamstring "pull" causes significant pain with forced flexion of the knee, associated with some extension of the hip. Straightening the leg is somewhat painful.

Quadriceps muscle tears or ruptures likewise cause pain and often inability to extend the knee. Rupture of the quadriceps mechanism is relatively uncommon, but often when this injury occurs, a palpable defect can be felt in the quadriceps mechanism, usually just proximal to the patella. Hematoma may be present. Uncommonly, x-rays may reveal a gap in the soft tissues if either of these muscles is completely ruptured.

Treatment

- Patients with muscle pulls of the hamstring or quadriceps usually require crutches and partial to non–weight-bearing (see Table 47–3 guidelines on supportive assistance).
- Taping the thigh from just below the hip region to the knee region may provide comfort, but tight constriction that impairs circulation must be avoided.
- Completely ruptured muscles require crutches for non–weight-bearing, as well as strapping of the knee in a somewhat flexed position for comfort. Hamstring ruptures rarely require surgical repair.
- Complete rupture of the quadriceps tendon often requires surgical anastomosis to establish continuity and future muscle power for knee extension.

47–43. KNEE DISORDERS *(See also Table 47–5 and Fig. 47–7)*

The knee joint is vulnerable to injury not only in contact sports but also in other energetic activities, because of the tremendous torque and shearing motions to which it is often subjected.

During athletic competition especially, a most important emergency consideration is distinguishing the insignificant and tolerable injury from one that will undergo significant progressive damage from continuation of activity, as is the case with internal knee derangements (IKD). To determine whether the person has serious injury (if it is not obvious), ask the patient to point to where it hurts, then check for deformity, effusion, focal tenderness, ROM and hemorrhage, and perform the maneuvers listed below (under Tests) to further evaluate for instability. If still undecided, have person satisfactorily perform strenuous forward and lateral running or other usual lower extremity strength and agility maneuvers before permitting a return to activities (since it is sometimes possible to walk, ski, and even do easy forward running with significant IKD).

Tests

To perform the following tests, have the patient lie face up with the affected extremity over the side of a table or bench and supported by the examiner's hand beneath the knee and the other hand cupping the heel; assure patient of gentle movements and get muscles to relax.

- Gently apply varus and valgus stress with knee in full extension. Instability indicates possible capsular and collateral ligament disruption and/or posterior cruciate tear. An easy opening joint in extension indicates serious injury.

- Repeat above with knee in 30 degrees flexion—interpretation same as above (the knee may be stable in extension, but not in slight flexion). Assess collateral ligaments.
- Flex knee to 90 degrees; if possible, stabilize patient's foot on table with examiner's thigh and perform gentle passive anterior-posterior gliding "drawer" knee movement. Perform test with foot in neutral, internal and external rotation. Compare with unaffected side if increased movement; excessive motion is indicative of cruciate tear.
- A variant of the above is the Lachman's test performed with one hand supporting posterior thigh and the other the proximal tibia; the drawer maneuver is performed with knee in 10 to 20 degrees flexion. Abnormal motion is the best indicator of an anterior cruciate tear.
- With one finger and thumb in medial and lateral joint space, check for full extension of knee while rotating foot internally and externally; a "click" (and often bulge) in the joint space on the affected side represents a positive McMurray sign. Also, decreased ROM is usually indicative of a meniscus tear—usually the medial meniscus is impaired when a twisting knee motion occurs while the foot is planted.
- If large amount of effusion makes testing difficult, perform arthrocentesis *(18–3)*. Under sterile conditions, instill 15 to 20 ml of 1% lidocaine without epinephrine (adult dosage) and retest. Hematoma formation is not always synonymous with serious knee stability injury.

X-rays (AP and lateral plus "sunrise view" if patellar pathology suspected) help evaluate the presence of fracture, but with the exception of tibial spine avulsion in anterior cruciate rupture, they are not usually useful in meniscus and ligament injuries. Stress films are used by some. Arthroscopy is usually preferable to arthrograms.

Treatment

- Treat simple strains and sprains without instability as described in Table 47–3.
- A knee immobilizer or lateral knee splints (e.g., Anderson brace) may be helpful in more severe cases, in addition to crutches and restricted weight-bearing.
- Meniscus and ligament ruptures require orthopedic attention and usually operative repair if continued strenuous activity is anticipated.

47–44. PATELLAR DISLOCATIONS

Direct trauma or violent contraction of the quadriceps femoris can cause lateral dislocation of the patella, especially if the lateral parapatellar ridge is lower than normal or genu valgum is marked. Medial dislocations are very rare. With the knee straight, reduction can usually be obtained without anesthetic by a firm, medially directed thrust with the palm of the hand. Treat as in Table 47–3, after reduction with a splint or knee immobilizer (knee in extension). After 2 or 3 days, when swelling has decreased, put on a straight cylindrical cast from ankle to thigh. *Note:* Recurrent dislocations may require surgical intervention.

47–45. KNEE FRACTURES

Avulsion fractures due to partial tearing loose of the attachments of the collateral ligaments should be casted in a position that will relax the injured

Table 47–5. COMMON KNEE INJURIES*

Findings	Dislocation of Patella	Patellar or Quadriceps Rupture	Collateral Ligament Rupture	Cruciate Rupture	Meniscus Tear	Intra-Articular Fracture
Audible sound with injury	Snap	Snap/pop	Snap/pop	Bystander hears "snap"	Pop	Crack
Focal pain	Patella	Anterior knee or thigh	Medial/lateral	Internal	Internal	Diffuse
Focal tenderness	Patella	Anterior knee or thigh	Medial/lateral	Variable	Variable	Diffuse
Hemarthrosis/Effusion;† gone if capsule tear	Possible	±, with or without muscle hematoma	Variable	Yes	Yes	Yes
Pain pattern	Extension relieves pain	Active extension impaired	Initial walking pain eases	Flexion relieves effusion pain	Flexion relieves pain	Flexion relieves effusion pain
Sensation of instability	Slips in/out	On steps	Wobbles; "joint opening"	Varies	Slips in/out	—
Joint instability	No	Yes if complete	Mediolateral in extension	Positive "drawer sign" and *Lachman's* sign	Positive McMurray sign	Variable

*The injuries described may occur singly but often occur in combination. This table is a guide only to designating more serious knee injuries that will need orthopedic attention and is not a consummate presentation. Not all signs will be present in each case. Arthroscopy and x-rays may be necessary to make the diagnosis and are often preferable to arthrogram when operation is anticipated.

†The presence of hemarthrosis/effusion does not always mean that there is an internal knee derangement (IKD), nor does the absence of these assure that there is no IKD.

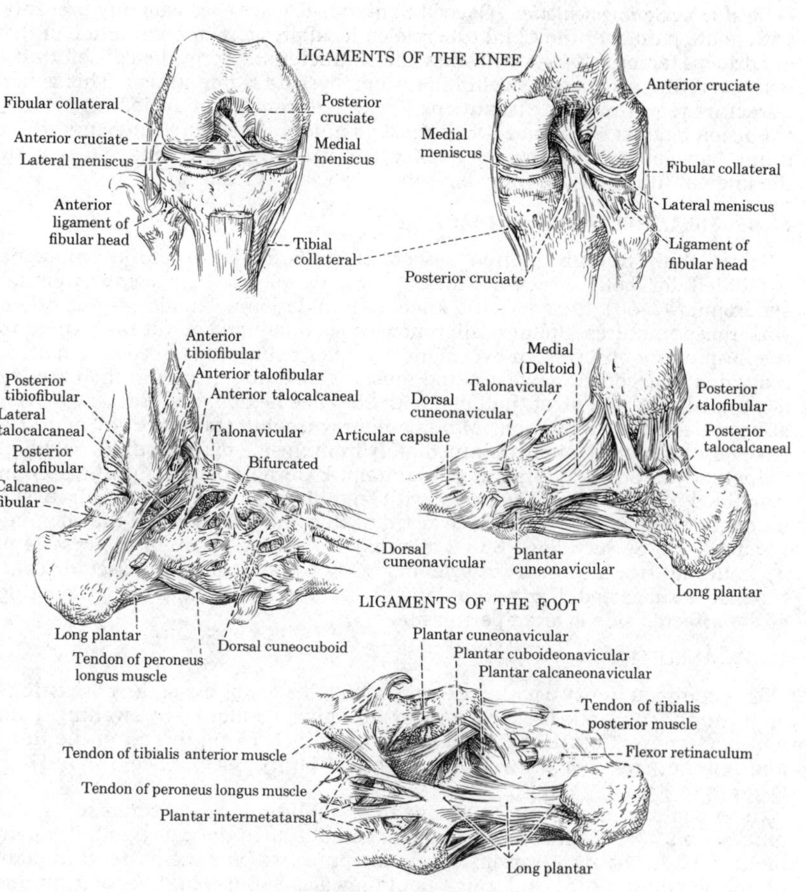

Figure 47–7. Articular ligaments of the right lower extremity. (From *Dorland's Illustrated Medical Dictionary*, 26th ed., Plate 25. Philadelphia, W. B. Saunders Co., 1981.)

ligament, using a padded cast from the groin to the toes, with the knee slightly flexed and the ankle at 90 degrees. Follow-up orthopedic care is essential.

Plateau fractures without displacement: same as avulsion fractures.

Patellar fractures without separation or displacement of fragments require a well-padded, skin-anchored walking cast (groin to 2 inches above the ankle), with the knee in full extension.

Tibial tubercle fragmentation (Osgood-Schlatter disease) occasionally presents with acute pain over the tibial tubercle on local pressure or contraction of the quadriceps femoris. X-rays will show the characteristic "crow beak" deformity with overlying soft tissue swelling plus epiphyseal fragmentation. This is not a fracture requiring acute treatment. Treatment consists of avoidance of knee extension against resistance—as is most commonly found in youngsters when riding bicycles in hilly terrain; application of a long leg cylinder cast with the knee in full extension may be utilized in some instances.

47–46. TIBIAL-FIBULAR SHAFT FRACTURES

Tibial shaft fractures, often associated with fibular fractures, must be evaluated for both direct neurovascular compromise and compartmental syndrome (47–60). X-rays of the knee and ankle joints should also be taken with these fractures. Splint if alignment is adequate and admit the patient to the hospital for observation overnight (whether reduction is needed or not). If reduction is needed, analgesics and muscle relaxants are given; then the leg is dangled off the edge of the table with 90° knee flexion, and traction/gravity assist in molding reduction. Monitor neurovascular status for 48 hours; a circular cast may be applied immediately from the toe to upper thigh, as tibial reduction can be quite difficult to maintain. External fixation may be used in combined tibial-fibular fractures with significant skin loss or soft tissue damage. The patient should be warned of this and also advised that healing in adults can be very slow (6 to 8 months). A bivalving cast for the first 24 to 48 hours may be necessary if swelling is excessive and neurovascular compromise is suspected. Early ambulation with crutches and full weight bearing of the affected side is often permissible.

47–47. ANKLE SPRAIN

This common injury usually presents with a history of the patient "twisting" or "turning" the ankle (generally inversion injury), followed by swelling, pain and tenderness. Gentle examination, including checking the tilt of the talus and anterior-posterior drawing of the talus, is necessary. (See Table 47–2, Degrees of Sprains, and Fig. 47–7.)

Inversion sprains generally involve in order of progressive seriousness, the anterotalofibular ligament; the anterotalofibular plus the calcanofibular ligament; and, in the most serious cases, the prior two plus the posterior talofibular. The anterior tibiofibular ligament may also be severed. Eversion sprains injure principally the segments of the deltoid ligament. Treatment measures are outlined in Tables 47–2 and 47–3. Except for the most serious sprains, considerable controversy exists regarding the need for surgical intervention. At a minimum, some stabilization is valuable for several weeks. The best treatment for ankle sprains is prevention, and in activities or sports associated with ankle sprains, prophylactic wearing of the T brace or taping is advisable. The T brace should also be worn to prevent recurrence.

47–48. FRACTURES AROUND THE ANKLE JOINT

Avulsion or sprain fractures should be immobilized in a splint or in a plaster short leg cast with felt pressure pads over the injured area and other pressure points and the foot in 7 to 10 degrees plantar flexion. The foot should be slightly inverted or everted to relax the particular injured collateral ligament.

Epiphyseal Injuries. Serious growth plate injuries may result from fractures with open epiphyses. X-rays reveal the type of fracture (see *47–6* and Fig. 47–2), and treatment, including any necessary reduction by an orthopedist, is given accordingly.

Malleolar Injuries. Malleolar fractures without displacement of fragments or distortion of the ankle mortise may be treated by a short leg nonwalking cast if not painful by "rotation testing"; otherwise use long nonwalking leg cast. Severe lateral bimalleolar or trimalleolar fractures require hospitalization for orthopedic reduction, as do any fractures resulting in distortion of the normal shape or width of the ankle joint. See 47–49 if dislocation is present.

47–49. ANKLE DISLOCATIONS

Ankle dislocations of any degree usually do not occur without accompanying fractures, especially of the avulsion type, and gross ligamentous damage. To prevent subsequent instability, the ankle should be splinted and immediate orthopedic consultation obtained. Surgical repair of the damaged ligamentous structures may be necessary, even if reduction of the dislocation has been accomplished as an emergency measure. Emergency reduction is required immediately at the scene (if rescue medical personnel are adequately skilled) if there is neurovascular compromise. This is accomplished by pulling distally on the foot, grasping the heel with one hand and the tarsometatarsal region with the other hand while countertraction is maintained proximally on the leg; the foot is then moved into alignment until circulation is again established. Understanding the mechanism of injury and then reversing it is the simplest guideline to satisfactory reductions.

47–50. FOOT DISORDERS

Assistance in management of acute foot problems, including trauma, can be given by both podiatrists and orthopedists. Consider use of Sorbothane sole inserts to help relieve irritation of the feet, knees and hips caused by weight-bearing pressure. Fractures of the foot, though causing a great deal of pain, are usually stable and only occasionally require closed or open reduction.

47–51. TARSAL DISLOCATIONS

Dislocations of the tarsal bones are usually of small degree but can be very painful and cause complete disability, especially in athletes. Careful comparative x-ray studies are essential for diagnosis.

Treatment consists of manipulative or open reduction with plaster cast immobilization.

47–52. OS CALCIS FRACTURES

These fractures usually follow falling from a height and landing on the heel. Swelling and hematoma follow; look also for associated vertebral compression fractures.

Incomplete or linear fractures without displacement should be placed in a padded, well-molded, short leg cast and referred for orthopedic care within 12 hours. Any comminution, subastragalar involvement or change in Boehler's angle requires orthopedic care for manipulation and reduction. Arthritis may follow.

47–53. TARSAL AND METATARSAL FRACTURES

If the bones are in good position with preservation of the normal arch, a padded plaster short leg cast with the foot plate molded to the arch should be applied. If there is overriding or malposition of the fragments, or if several fractures are present, referral for orthopedic care is in order.

47–54. GREAT TOE FRACTURES

Proximal Phalanx. These fractures often require orthopedic care, since rotation and displacement of the distal fragment, which is very difficult to reduce and control, may be present. If the fragments are stable and alignment is satisfactory, a short leg cast with a heavy platform sole may be applied and arrangements made for orthopedic care within 2 to 3 days.

Distal Phalanx. A cut-out shoe and metatarsal bar generally are all that are necessary. Fibrous union often occurs.

47–55. FRACTURES OF THE PHALANGES OF THE SECOND TO FIFTH DIGITS OF THE FOOT

Strapping of the injured digit to its neighbor, a cut-out shoe and a metatarsal bar will generally allow the patient to continue with normal activity.

47–56. TOE DISLOCATIONS

Toe dislocations are easily reducible by gentle traction followed by strapping to adjacent toes for 2 or 3 weeks.

NONTRAUMATIC DISORDERS

47–57. ARTHRITIS, ASEPTIC

Although the numerous conditions grouped under this general heading usually cause chronic symptoms, acute discomfort caused by fulminating infections (especially viral) or by traumatic aggravation of the underlying condition may require emergency care or hospitalization. Obtain requisite joint rest by use of a bed board, local splinting and use of crutch or cane support. See Table 47–3 for treatment and adjunctive supportive measures. Large doses of salicylates or NSAID by mouth may give relief in some types of arthritis. Short-term oral corticosteroids can be effective, but long-range use of these agents is often detrimental. Intra-articular corticosteroids may be indicated and effective in some cases. For treatment of gout, see *46–5.* In acute flare-ups of spinal arthritis in the elderly, consider the presence of osteoporosis and possible vertebral compression.

If the patient's response is not satisfactory or if there is a question of fracture or septic arthritis, obtain x-ray films of the area (include hip views also in children with knee pain) and orthopedic consultation.

47–58. ARTHRITIS, SEPTIC *(See also 59–42, Soft Tissue Infections, Deep and Anaerobic)*

Septic arthritis usually involves only one joint, which is throbbing and painful even at rest, and is accompanied by rapid onset of fever and chills. The joint (synovium and periarticular tissues) is swollen, tender, warm and reddened. The diagnosis is established by arthrocentesis *(18–3)* and purulent yellowish or greenish aspirate that contains many white blood cells (WBCs) (7500 to 10,000 per cu mm minimum and over 50% polymorphonuclear neutrophil leukocytes) and has identifiable organisms on Gram stain. The mucin clot easily disperses on shaking, and the "string test" reveals low viscosity. Cultures are most likely to grow one of the following: *Neisseria gonorrhoeae, Staphylococcus aureus, Streptococcus pneumoniae, Haemophilus influenzae* or a gram-negative coliform organism. History of exposures and other infections and the Gram stain help to predict which organism will grow.

Treatment

- Aspirate large effusions. Obtain C and S.
- Start antibiotics of choice *(33–83)* intravenously in large doses. See *33–25* regarding gonococcal arthritis. Consider HBO.
- Joint rest is important for pain relief and recovery. Splinting is helpful. See Table 47–3 for adjunctive relief measures.
- Arrange for immediate orthopedic consultation and possible surgery.

47–59. BURSITIS

Inflammation of any of the numerous bursae of the body may be very painful and severely disabling. The subdeltoid, gluteal and trochanteric bursae are particularly prone to give intense and progressively worse problems with minimal resolution until injected. If the olecranon bursa is filled with fluid, it should be aspirated and injected with a combination of lidocaine and Kenalog in the same procedure. Analgesics, including narcotics, may be necessary to control the acute pain until the patient can receive definitive treatment. If the bursa is hot, red and swollen, treat with oral nonsteroidal anti-inflammatory agents unless bacterial invasion is present, in which case treat as a soft tissue infection. Immobilization and spraying the skin over the affected part with Fluori-Methane may be of benefit. Infiltration of the painful bursa area with 0.5 or 1% lidocaine and 10 to 20 mg of triamcinolone (Kenalog) may give spectacular relief, although the patient should be warned of the possibility of a temporary flare-up when the effect of the local anesthetic wears off. Application of ice helps to relieve such flare-ups; see Table 47–3 for other measures. Arrangements should be made for follow-up care.

47–60. COMPARTMENT SYNDROMES, ACUTE

Increased fluid/soft tissue pressure within a closed fascial area, such as the anterior tibial compartment, can reduce arterial inflow and venous egress and increase pressure on nerves, causing pain, soreness, paresthesias, numbness and, ultimately, ischemia, necrosis and paralysis of the neuronapraxia type (see Table 47–6). Tender swelling of the muscle and soft tissues of the compartment, decreased pulses to palpation and Doppler test and direct wick catheter manometer readings of increased compartment pressure help establish the diagnosis (muscle ischemia and permanent impairment can, however, occur even in the presence of some pulses and Doppler flow).

Treatment

- Cessation of aggravating factors, such as exercise, and use of dependent position.
- Reduction of swelling by elevation and ice; and when available and approved, consider topical dimethylsulfoxide for early stages of nonbacterially caused swelling.
- Advanced and advancing cases with pulse impairment constitute a surgical emergency requiring fasciotomy decompression.

Table 47–6. SOFT TISSUE INJURIES OF THE LEG

Injury	Findings	Treatment
Tear of gastrocnemius soleus muscle	Exquisite calf muscle tenderness after running or jumping.	Crutch walking for 4 to 6 weeks; non–weight-bearing activities only.
Rupture of plantaris tendon	During activities, patient feels "pop" or "shot" in calf. Hemorrhage may show later in posterior leg.	Injury not serious, but best to use crutches for 2 to 3 weeks.
Archilles tendon rupture	Pain and swelling in musculotendinous junction of tendon. Positive Thompson test: with patient prone with foot off end of table, calf squeeze produces no plantar flexion of ankle or foot.	Casting in slight to moderate ankle plantar flexion required for 6 to 12 weeks; in young athletes, surgical repair might be best.
Shin splints	Occur in athletes; radiating pain, swelling and tenderness along shin. Probable fasciitis due to muscle imbalance (relatively weak anterior tibialis).	Partial weight-bearing with crutches for a few days, along with physical therapy, stretching of heel cords, orthotics, anterior tibialis exercises.*
Stress fracture	Focal tenderness (foot, ankle, leg, hip) increases with exercise. Often too rapid build-up of hard activity on hard surface. Positive bone scan.	Partial or no weight-bearing until comfortable. Casting and internal fixation infrequently needed. Use Sorbothane shoe inserts. Slow build-up in activity.

*Can continue training with bicycle (with toe clips—concentrate on raising each pedal to exercise anterior tibialis), swimming, or Nordic Trac.

Table 47–7. ACUTE COMPARTMENT SYNDROMES OF THE LEG*

Typical Findings	Anterior	Lateral	Superficial Posterior	Deep Posterior
Decreased sensory nerve perception (see Fig. 49–2)	Deep peroneal	Superficial and deep peroneal	Sural	Tibial
Muscle weakness	Ant. tibialis and toe extensors	Peroneus longus and brevis	Gastrocnemius and soleus	Post. tibialis and toe flexors
Pain with stretch	Foot/toe flexion	Foot inversion	Foot dorsiflexion	Toe extension
Pedal pulses†	Intact	Intact	Intact	Intact

*Modified from Mobrak, S. J., *in* D'Ambrosia, R., and Drez, D.: *Prevention and Treatment of Running Injuries:* Thorofare, NJ, Charles B. Slack, Inc., 1982.

Note: Patients complain of intense (ischemic) pain in area unless obtunded.

†Absence of pulse indicates advanced stage.

47–61. EPICONDYLITIS

Lateral epicondylar focal tenderness (at the insertion of the extensor muscles) that often radiates distally and is increased by forced wrist extension or pronation against resistance is characteristic of this problem. The acute pain from this condition (usually a localized fascitis or fibrositis from strain) can sometimes be relieved by spraying with Fluori-Methane, use of ice compresses or deep friction massage. Analysis should be made of the particular mechanical use causing strain (usually the wrist is dorsiflexed, as in screwing, or extension maneuvers are made, as in hammering or improper tennis swing). Instruction should be given in improved biomechanical methods and temporary rest advised. Temporary (sometimes permanent) relief follows infiltration of the painful area with a local anesthetic. Local heat may be of benefit in some cases; it may make others worse. Application of a forearm band or volar splint to control rotation of the forearm as well as elbow and wrist motion may be necessary. Since the discomfort is often acute and intense, analgesics and NSAID may be warranted. Physical therapy, including ultrasound (and phonophoresis with 10% hydrocortisone), deep friction massage across the tendon and graduated isotonic wrist extension exercise, is helpful. Corticoid injections and acupuncture are later considerations.

47–62. HIP PATHOLOGY WITHOUT EXTERNAL TRAUMA

It must be determined whether acute hip pain is due to pathologic involvement of bone and soft tissues around the hip or to referred pain from the low back, adjacent structures or knee.

Local hip joint structures are aggravated by hip flexion, forced internal rotation of the femur or hyperextension of the leg; pain tends to be anterior in the groin. Pain in the hip radiating from low back structures or musculus piriformis involvement with sciatic nerve irritation is usually posterior, is not made worse with the maneuvers just described but is aggravated by trunk extension, rotation and flexion and straight leg raising (SLR) followed by dorsiflexion of the foot. Sacroiliac pain is also posterior and is made worse (like hip joint pathology itself) with resisted flexion, abduction and external rotation (FABER maneuver) of the hip.

Trochanteric bursitis causes exquisite tenderness to pressure and may cause pain radiation down the lateral thigh, as may inflammation of the musculus tensor fasciae latae—except that the tenderness is greater in the latter. SLR is not aggravating, and local injection of lidocaine relieves the pain.

Ischial bursitis is made worse with sitting and local pressure over the ischial tuberosity. Stretching of the tender origin of the hamstring on SLR may mimic sciatica. Pain is relieved by local injection.

The combination of fever, limp and hip or knee pain—particularly in children—should be carefully evaluated for the serious emergency condition of septic arthritis of the hip (47–58).

On the following pages (Figs. 47–8 to 47–13) are illustrated the muscles of the trunk and of the upper and lower extremities, for easy reference.

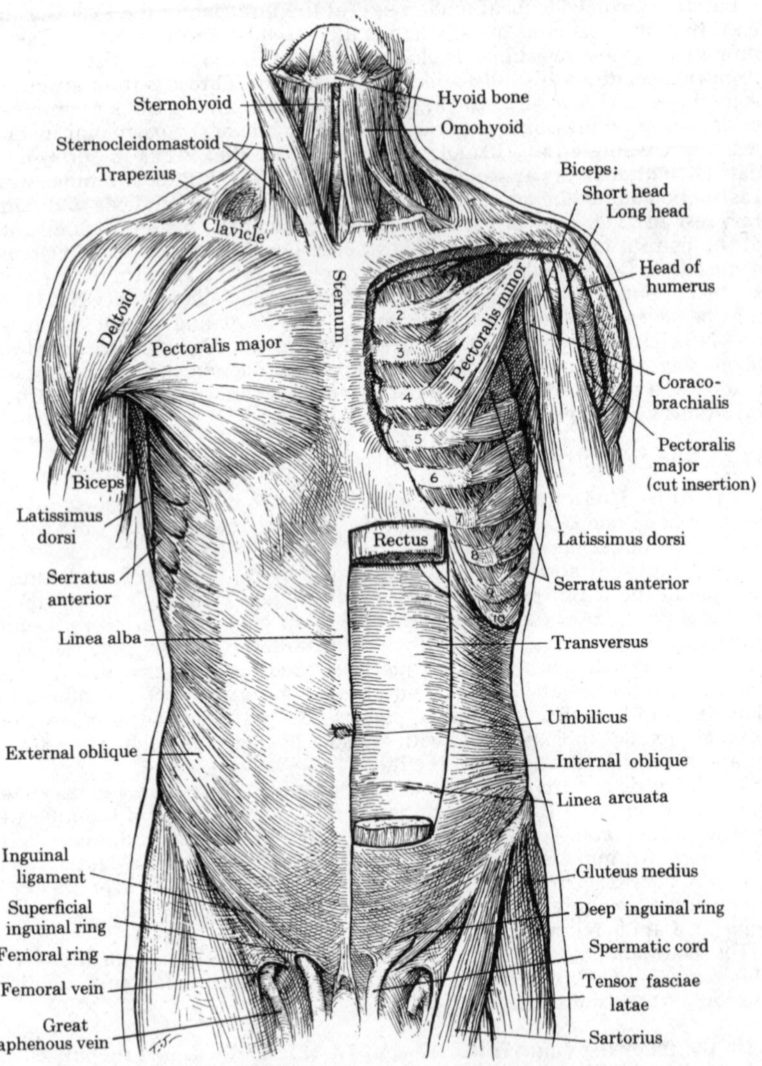

Figure 47–8. Muscles of the trunk (anterior view). The left sternocleidomastoid, pectoralis major, external oblique, and a portion of the deltoid have been removed to show underlying muscles. A portion of the rectus abdominis has been cut away to expose the posterior part of its sheath. (Jones and Shepard, in *Dorland's Illustrated Medical Dictionary,* 26th ed., Plate 30. Philadelphia, W. B. Saunders Co., 1981.)

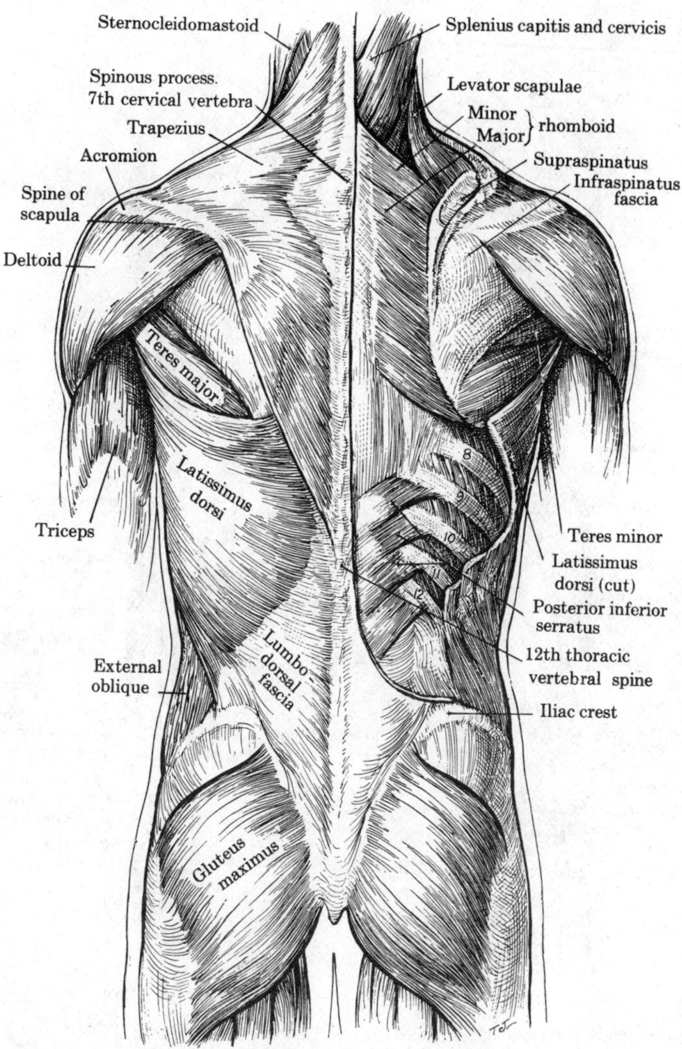

Figure 47–9. Muscles of the trunk (posterior view). The latissimus dorsi and trapezius on the right side have been cut away to expose the underlying muscles (Jones and Shepard, in *Dorland's Illustrated Medical Dictionary,* 26th ed., Plate 31. Philadelphia, W. B. Saunders Co., 1981.)

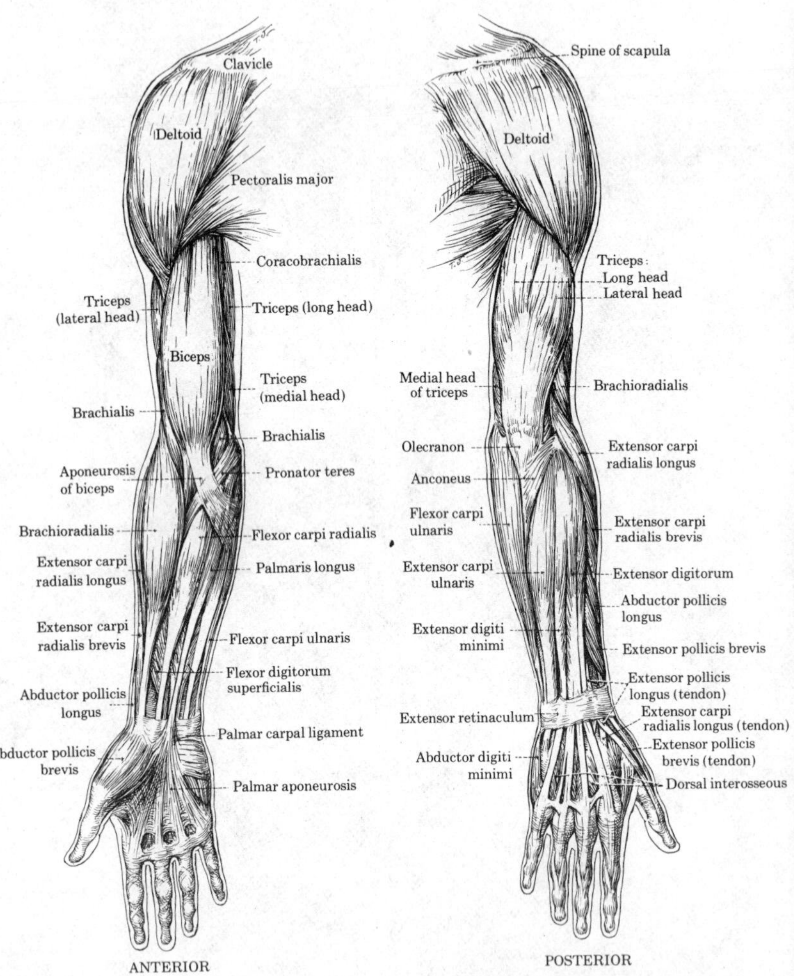

Figure 47–10. Superficial muscles of the right upper extremity. (See also Fig. 47–11 for cross sections and deep muscles.) (Jones and Shepard, in *Dorland's Illustrated Medical Dictionary*, 26th ed., Plate 32. Philadelphia, W. B. Saunders Co., 1981.)

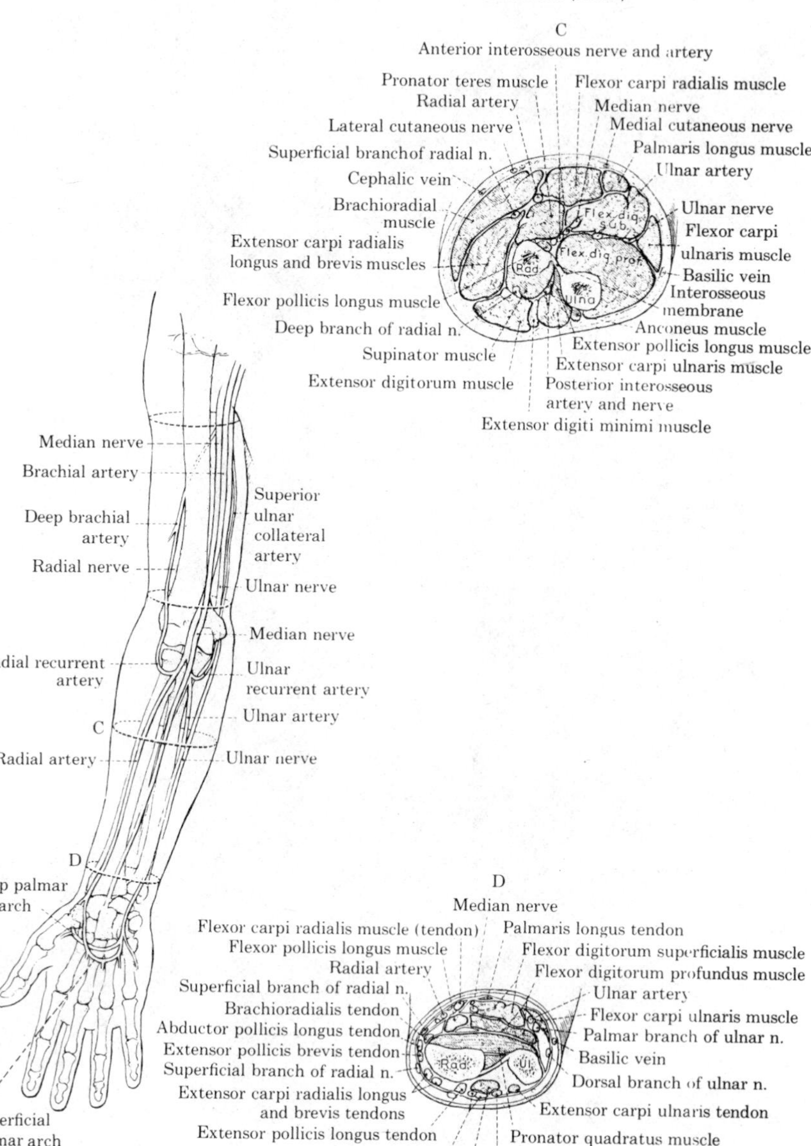

Figure 47–11. Structures of right upper extremity. Front view shows principal nerves and arteries in relation to the bones. *C* and *D* are cross sections made at levels indicated on drawing at left. (Jones and Shepard, in *Dorland's Illustrated Medical Dictionary*, 26th ed., Plate 39. Philadelphia, W. B. Saunders Co., 1981.)

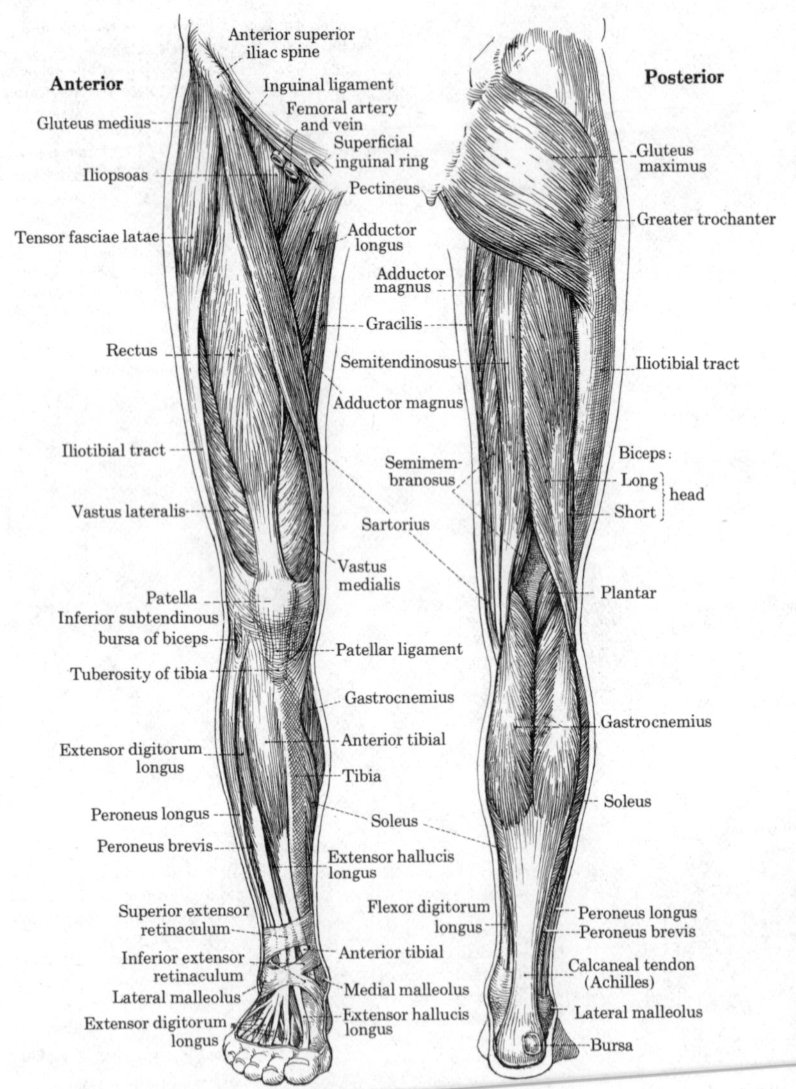

Figure 47–12. Superficial muscles of the right lower extremity. (See also Figs. 47–14 for cross sections and deep muscles.) (Jones and Shepard, in *Dorland's Illustrated Medical Dictionary*, 26th ed., Plate 33. Philadelphia, W. B. Saunders Co., 1981.)

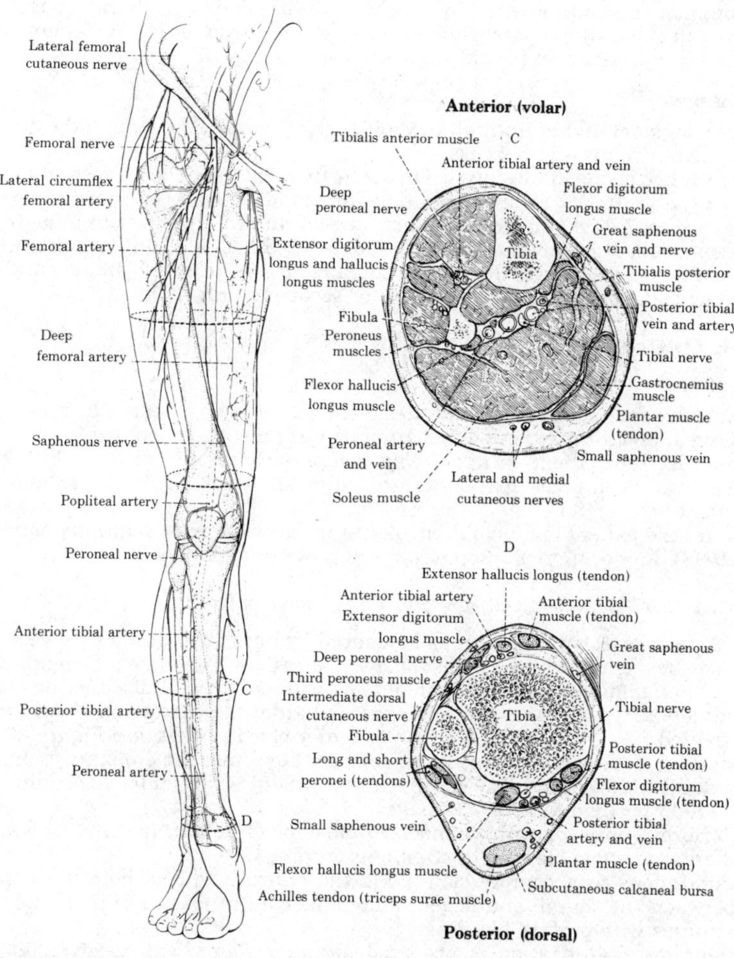

Figure 47–13. Structures of the right lower extremity. Front view shows principal nerves and arteries in relation to the bones. *C* and *D* are cross sections made at levels indicated on drawing at left. (Jones and Shepard, in *Dorland's Illustrated Medical Dictionary*, 26th ed., Plate 40. Philadelphia, W. B. Saunders Co., 1981.)

48. Nasal Conditions

48–1. AEROSINUSITIS (Sinus Squeeze)

Common in sports divers *(26–5)*, this painful condition, characterized by collection of bloody exudate within the sinuses, is due to the effect of increased barometric pressure on partially blocked ostia.

Treatment

- Avoidance of diving until all evidence of infection and edema have disappeared—usually 4 to 6 weeks.
- Insurance of adequate sinus drainage by frequent use of decongestant nasal spray, e.g., 0.05% oxymetazoline hydrochloride (Afrin) (but not for longer than 5 to 7 days) and/or short-term use of an oral decongestant, such as pseudoephedrine hydrochloride (Sudafed). Sinus washing or drainage should not be done. Ultrasonic therapy to the affected areas may be beneficial. Antibiotics may be used for secondary infection.

48–2. CONTUSIONS

Treatment

- Rule out fractures of the skull, nasal cartilages or nasal bones by thorough clinical and x-ray examination. Hematomas must be evacuated.
- Instruct the patient to apply cold compresses or an icebag at frequent intervals during the first 24 hours; after 24 hours local heat should be substituted.
- Refer the patient to an otolaryngologist if the swelling or deformity persists after 5 days or if crepitation of the soft tissues is present.

48–3. EPISTAXIS (Nosebleed) *(See also 45–1, Control of Bleeding)*

Nontraumatic Epistaxis. This may be caused by brittle arteriosclerotic vessels, varicosities, telangiectasias, nasal polyps, abrasions from nose picking, tuberculosis, malignant disease, hemophilia, acute infectious diseases or other conditions. Hypertension makes epistaxis harder to control and should also be treated *(29–14)*. For the location of major blood vessels, see Figure 48–1; posterior bleeding tends to be more copious, flows into the oropharynx and is more difficult to control. The emergency treatment is similar for all conditions:

- Upright position to allow drainage.
- Perform gentle blowing of nose to clear clots before applying pressure; thereafter avoid blowing or strenuous sniffing.
- Continuous firm compression along the entire length of both nasal alae between the thumb and flexed index finger for at least 5 to preferably 20 minutes with profuse bleeding.
- Cautious cauterization of observed bleeding points with a silver nitrate stick.
- Wedging of a pad of gauze, cotton or paper tissue between the upper teeth and the upper lip for persistent lower anterior septal bleeding if the above measures are not effective.
- Sedation as needed. Morphine sulfate may be required prior to packing procedures.
- Topical application of 5% cocaine solution for anesthetic and vasoconstrictive effects (maximum dose 3 mg/kg). Use in preference to 1:1000 epinephrine, which is rapidly absorbed and may aggravate hypertensive status.

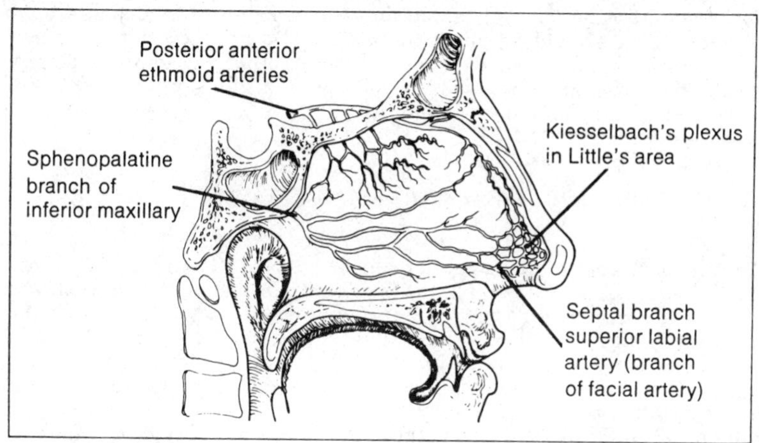

Figure 48–1. Landmarks in the nose: the location of vessels most often responsible for both anterior and posterior nosebleeds are illustrated here. Ninety per cent of nasal bleeding originates in Kiesselbach's plexus. (From Norman, F. W.: *Patient Care,* January, 1972. Copyright © Miller & Fink Corporation, Darien, Connecticut. All rights reserved.)

- Packing of the anterior nares with a neosporin (polymyxin B sulfate, neomycin sulfate, bacitracin) coated sterile gauze strip or petrolatum gauze *(18–18)* if other measures have not been effective. An inflatable device (Nasostat or Surgitek Reuter Epi-Tek) may be used in conjunction with the gauze if bleeding is severe. Leave pack in for 48 hours. Do not use iodoform gauze.
- Insertion of a posterior nasal pack for bleeding not controlled by above measures. (For technique, see *18–18.)* Since any type of nasal packing results in nasopharyngeal obstruction and edema, alteration of airway resistance in the entire pulmonary system occurs with PO_2 depression (activation of nasopulmonary reflex). Obtain blood gas values for all patients with posterior nasal packs. Administer oxygen. Hospitalize for close observation and sedation. The packing generally must be left in place for 4 or 5 days. Use of a systemic antibiotic (e.g., ampicillin, 250 to 500 mg PO qid initially, then 500 mg daily) is warranted to help prevent sinusitis.
- Questioning of patient regarding recent intake of anticoagulants or aspirin and treatment of any underlying bleeding and clotting defect *(45–2).*
- In patients with known clotting disorders, packing of the nose with Gelfoam soaked in topical thrombin. Avoid gauze packing if possible.
- Blood loss may be sufficient to require treatment of shock *(57–5)* before transportation for hospitalization. Baseline and periodic hemoglobin values should be obtained; be sure to obtain a hemoglobin value about 12 hours after cessation of severe bleeding.

Traumatic Epistaxis. If there is any possibility that the drainage from the nose following injury is a mixture of blood and spinal fluid, no packing or medication of any type should be inserted into the nostrils. The case should be treated as a skull fracture and the patient hospitalized at once. The presence of rhinorrhea can sometimes be confirmed by placing a drop of the bloody fluid on a white blotter; the presence of a light pink area around a darkened center indicates the presence of spinal fluid.

Post Epistaxis. After control of bleeding, to help prevent recurrence, the following advice should be given the patient: Do not pick the nose; avoid aspirin, smoking, strenuous exercise, alcohol or other vasodilators for about a week; keep anterior nasal septum moist with a thin layer of vaseline for about a week, and use a room humidifier.

48–4. FOREIGN BODIES IN NOSE *(See 39–4)*

48–5. FRACTURES OF THE NASAL BONES AND CARTILAGES

Treatment

- Simple displaced fractures can usually be restored to normal alignment by digital manipulation. If depression is present, the fragment can be elevated by pressure with a blunt padded instrument within the nostrils. Reductions preferably should be done immediately, before swelling occurs, but if this is not feasible, postponement for 5 to 10 days for decrease of edema usually results in a better reduction. An ice pack applied at once and kept on during transportation helps delay swelling.
- Comminuted, compound (open) or depressed fractures, especially those that result in marked septal deviation or distortion, should be immediately referred to an otolaryngologist for reduction and follow-up care.

48–6. HEMATOMAS

If untreated or if treatment is delayed, hematomas may result in permanent saddling of the bridge. The patient should be referred to an otolaryngologist for drainage as soon as presence of a hematoma (usually septal or between the lateral cartilages and the nasal bone) is recognized. If a delay in treatment is anticipated, prophylaxis against tetanus *(20)* and antibiotics are indicated.

48–7. LACERATIONS

See *59–1* for general principles of treatment. Since the nose is in the "danger zone," prophylaxis with antibiotics should be given routinely and tetanus prophylaxis *(20)* insured.

48–8. SEPTAL INJURIES

All patients with acute septal deviation or distortion require care by an otolaryngologist; early reduction may be achieved.

48–9. SINUSITIS *(See 56–23)*

49. Neurologic Disorders*

49–1. GENERAL CONSIDERATIONS

The outline of the acute neurologic evaluation is considered in detail in *44–2*, and particular reference to head injury is made in *44*. If the emergency condition involves coma or altered consciousness of unknown cause, see Table 32–1; some of the more common specific causes are listed in *49–6*. If

*See also *30, Cephalgia; 34, Convulsions/Seizures;* and *44, Head Injuries.*

neuropsychiatric manifestations of acute organic brain syndrome are presented, see *49–2* and *54–17*. Distinction of muscle paralysis or paresis due to upper or lower motor neuron disease or acute myopathy is presented in Table 49–1; a brief guide to motor function and weakness is covered in Table 49–2.

49–2. ACUTE ORGANIC BRAIN SYNDROME

Discussion of the various causes and extreme neuropsychiatric manifestations of this syndrome due to acute impairment of function of brain tissue is presented in *54–17, Psychoses*. However, it should be recognized that any psychiatric manifestation along the range of normal–neurosis–psychosis may occur (see Table 54–1). Organic disease is particularly prone to present with amnesia, depression, delirium (and coma), dementia, seizures and occasionally with excitement states *(37)* and euphoria (e.g., due to amphetamines, PCP and steroids).

49–3. ARTERITIS, TEMPORAL (CRANIAL) *(See 63–3)*

49–4. BRAIN DEATH

The presence of at least two physicians (at least one being a neurologist, and none representing an organ transplant team) is required in certification of brain death. (For criteria, see *8–4*.)

49–5. COMA OF UNDETERMINED ORIGIN *(See Table 32–1)*

49–6. COMA DUE TO SPECIFIC CAUSES

The following are among the common causes:

Acidosis, severe *(46–1)*
Acute infectious diseases *(32–1, 33, Contagious and Communicable Diseases)*
Cardiac pathology *(29)*
Cerebrovascular Emergencies *(63–4, Intracranial Bleeding; 63–6, Embolism; 63–9, Thrombosis)*
Diabetes mellitus *(32–3)*
Drug overdose *(53, Poisoning)*
Eclampsia *(50–6)*
Electrical shock *(32–5; 28–12, Electrical Burns)*
Emphysema *(32–6)*
Encephalitis *(33–6, Arboviral Infections; 33–20, Viral Encephalitis)*
Epilepsy *(32–7; 34, Convulsive Seizures)*
Episodic unconsciousness *(49–20, Differential Diagnosis Chart)*
Excessive heat *(62–6, Heat Exhaustion; 62–7, Heatstroke; 62–8, Iatrogenic Heat Stress)*
Head injuries *(44)*
Hemorrhage *(45; 57, Shock)*
Hepatic coma *(32–10)*
Hypertensive encephalopathy *(29–14)*
Insulin shock *(32–3, Diabetes Mellitus)*
Intracranial pathology *(44, Head Injuries; 63–4)*
Malaria *(33–38)*
Myxedema *(36–12, Thyroid Emergencies)*
Poisons *(53)*
Shock *(57)*
Uremia *(32–16)*

49–7. MENIERE'S DISEASE

A sensation of fullness in the ear (due to sudden hydrops of labyrinth of unknown cause) usually precedes attack, which is followed by decreased hearing acuity, tinnitus, vertigo and GI tract upset. Usually there is a history of prior attacks. Examination of the ear reveals no gross inflammation.

Mild Cases

Treatment

- Sedation.
- Administration of oral meclizine hydrochloride (Antivert), 25 mg tid, or diphenhydramine hydrochloride (Benadryl), 25 to 50 mg tid or qid or dimenhydrinate (Dramamine), 50 mg by mouth tid helps to relieve vertigo, nausea and vomiting.
- Low sodium diet and diuretics may be helpful.
- Referral to an otolaryngologist.

Severe Cases

Treatment

- Hospitalize.
- Start IV line for fluid and electrolyte replacement.
- Parenteral administration (IV or IM) of 10 to 20 mg diphenhydramine hydrochloride helps to relieve severe vomiting, whereas the rectal suppository form helps to relieve milder vomiting. Parenteral prochlorperazine (Compazine) and diazepam (Valium) are also effective antiemetics.

49–8. MENINGITIS *(See 33–40, Meningitis, Bacterial; 33–6, Arboviral Infections; 33–20, Encephalitis)*

49–9. MENINGOCOCCEMIA *(See 33–41)*

49–10. MIGRAINE *(See 30–22, Migraine Headaches)*

49–11. MOTION SICKNESS

Certain individuals who are particularly prone to air, sea or train sickness do not follow the usual course of rapid complete recovery following cessation of the motion. Nausea, vomiting and dizziness may be severe or persistent enough to bring the patient for emergency treatment. Any normal human being can be made sick by motion. The mechanism of causation appears to be principally excessive motion of small otoliths, leading to excessive labyrinthine vestibular stimulation; training diminishes susceptibility. Vertical (rise and fall—elevators, ships, planes, buses, cars), linear (forward and backward, stop and go—cars, buses, planes, playground and carnival swings, etc.) or angular acceleration (the normal rhythmic pitch, yaw, and sway of moving vehicles) or any combination of all three may be the precipitating agent that may be reinforced, facilitated and enhanced by special sense stimuli, such as sound, sight, taste, smell and perception of vibration. Undoubtedly, psychologic and emotional states contribute to and exaggerate motion sickness.

Signs and Symptoms. Restlessness, general malaise, hypersensitivity to sensory stimuli, lassitude, yawning, pallor and difficulty in breathing. Waves of nausea and vomiting may be present followed by acute depression, apathy and generalized prostration. Vague and inconstant objective signs, such as increased pulse rate and blood pressure, are transient only.

Treatment (prophylactic, symptomatic and definitive)

- Avoidance of eating or drinking just before starting a trip.
- Proper selection of a vehicle and location therein:

—As large a vehicle as possible.
—A central seat or cabin to minimize roll (sideways motion) and pitch (end-to-end, up-and-down motion).
—Smoothly driven vehicles—a bus is more stable than a passenger car, a jet more stable than a propeller-driven aircraft.
—In a bus or passenger car, avoidance of a seat over the rear axle—the site of maximum up-and-down motion.

- Focusing the eyes on a distant object; looking at close objects should be avoided.
- Antinauseants (preferably commenced before attack in susceptible individuals). The following are the most effective drugs for prevention and treatment of motion sickness of any type (air sickness, car sickness, seasickness). Dimenhydrinate (Dramamine), cyclizine hydrochloride (Marezine) and meclizine HCl (Bonine) are available without prescription; oral or parenteral prochlorperazine (Compazine), trimethobenzamide HCl (Tigan) and scopolamine (Transderm-Scōp) require prescription. See *40–24;* for doses of these antiemetics. Transderm-Scōp placed on the skin behind the ear is convenient because the anticholinergic is absorbed gradually through the skin over 3 days with 1 administration.
- Inhalation of cold air, as right in front of a car air conditioner, and rubbing the skin over the cricothyroid membrane can help forestall vomiting and nausea on occasion.
- Replacement therapy *(11, Fluid Replacement).*

Prognosis. Complete recovery without residual ill-effects always takes place after cessation of motion, although symptoms may persist for several days in severe cases.

49–12. MYASTHENIA GRAVIS

Progressive paresis of facial, oculomotor, pharyngeal and respiratory muscles may occur. Skeletal muscles are involved in advanced states. Marked fatigability is common, with aggravation of symptoms by mental as well as physical stress; sometimes a psychiatrist is the first physician to see the patient. Symptoms requiring emergency care are usually related to acute infections, aspiration of food or respiratory failure.

Overdosage from neostigmine in established cases is noted by its nicotinic side effects (muscle cramps, fasciculations and weakness) and its muscarinic effects (nausea, vomiting, diarrhea, abdominal cramps, increased salivation and bronchial secretions, diaphoresis and miosis—these are usually counteracted with atropine, 0.5 mg).

Treatment

- Place the patient in the recumbent position.
- Clear the airway and support ventilation (*5–21*).
- In known myasthenia gravis patients in whom neostigmine overdosage is not suspected, give neostigmine methylsulfate (Prostigmin), 1 ml of 1:2000 solution (0.5 mg) IM or SC if patient unable to take a 15-mg tablet orally.
- As a diagnostic measure, 2 mg of edrophonium chloride (Tensilon) is given initially IV in adults, and if no response in 15 to 30 seconds, an additional 8 mg is given IV. In children weighing less than 75 pounds, the initial test dose is 1 mg IV, and if no response in 45 seconds, 1-mg increments are given IV every 30 to 45 seconds until response or 5 mg is given. In children weighing more than 75 pounds, the initial dose is 2 mg IV, with increments as for lighter children up to a maximum of 10 mg. These test doses usually

will result in improvement in a myasthenia gravis crisis but will cause no significant lasting change in symptoms caused by neostigmine overdosage. If improvement occurs after 2 minutes, slowly give an additional 7 mg edrophonium chloride for treatment. If no improvement occurs, treat as neostigmine overdosage in known cases and/or evaluate for other causes of clinical problem—usually in the hospital under close observation.

- Improvement with large doses of steroids during crises has been noted; if used, the problem is sufficient to warrant hospitalization. Other immunosuppressive drugs have been used also.
- Plasmapheresis is now an accepted treatment for severe myasthenia gravis in which respiratory function is impaired despite use of anticholinesterase drugs and high-dose alternate-day steroids.

49–13. NEURITIS (Neuralgia)

Although many conditions (infections, trauma, toxins, viruses, poisons, pressure, etc.) may cause irritation and pain along the course and distribution of various nerves, the discomfort in most cases is not severe enough to bring the patient for emergency treatment. The chief exceptions are as follows:

Alcoholic Neuritis

Burning pain and paresthesias in the extremities related to toxic nutritional factors in chronic alcoholics may require emergency care, followed by prolonged institutional therapy. Control of pain and sedation as indicated under *37–4, Delirium Tremens*, is all that is indicated as an emergency measure. Vitamin and nutritional treatment is important in follow-up care. (See also *49–21, Wernicke's Encephalopathy.*)

Arsenical Neuritis *(See 53–90, Arsenic)*

Bell's Palsy (Peripheral Facial Nerve Paralysis)

The clinical picture (inability to close the eye, wrinkle the forehead or elevate the corner of the mouth on the affected side and drooling of saliva from the mouth) usually develops following chilling or injury of the involved side. Most cases are of nontraumatic origin, but if complete facial nerve paralysis *immediately* follows trauma, surgical exploration is indicated. (Otherwise surgical decompression is rarely needed.)

Treatment of Nontraumatic or Delayed Post-traumatic Type

- Oral administration of a loading dose of 60 mg of prednisone, followed by 20 mg of prednisone tid for 2 or 3 days, then gradual tapering off over a 7- to 10-day period. Steroids are not indicated in all cases.
- Application of an eye patch with a bland ophthalmic ointment.
- Protection of the involved side from wind and cold.
- Instruction in measures to prevent loss of facial muscle tone (upward massage, taping, etc.) Electrical stimulation may be of some aid to recovery in paretic state. If the nerve is not excitable and muscle contraction does not occur, this indicates severe nerve injury. These patients should be referred to an otolaryngologist for evaluation for nerve decompression, and steroids can be withheld.

Causalgia (Reflex Neurovascular Syndrome)

Severe causalgia following trauma has a reflex neuritic component. The single most effective measure is to restore function through active motion; this also diminishes the disuse component induced by pain. Mechanical reduction of edema is important (e.g., by elevation, compressive wrapping [*63–16*], Jobst pump, acupuncture); use of DMSO may also be of benefit. TNS units are often more aggravating than helpful in this type of problem. Relief of severe discomfort can sometimes be obtained by parenteral administration of tolazoline hydrochloride (Priscoline), 25 to 50 mg every 4 hours, but pentazocine lactate (Talwin), 15 to 30 mg intramuscularly, or opiates may be necessary. Severe cases may require sympathetic blocks or serial amputations.

Herpes Zoster *(For eye involvement, see 38–14, Herpes Zoster Ophthalmicus)*

Treatment

- Protection of lesions from infection by petrolatum gauze or dibucaine hydrochloride ointment (Nupercainal) dressings or dusting with thymol iodide (not in eyes!).
- Control of pain, if moderate, by sedation and analgesics; if severe, by pentazocine lactate (Talwin) IM or IV or codeine phosphate or morphine sulfate SC. Large doses of corticosteroids or segmental nerve blocks may be required.
- Administration of antibiotic therapy only if bacterial infection is a complicating factor.
- Hospitalization if the pain is severe or the lesions extensive.

Peripheral Neuritis During Pregnancy

This condition is usually associated with hyperemesis gravidarum *(50–13)*.

Retrobulbar Neuritis *(See also 39–41, Sudden Vision Loss)*

Signs and Symptoms. Headache and discomfort in the eye on the affected side with increase of ocular pain on eye motion or pressure are accompanied by rapid impairment of vision—blurring and central scotomata. The direct pupillary response to light is abnormal (abnormal response to swinging flashlight test). No acute disc changes are seen, but occasionally injection and blurring of the disc margins occur. Optic pallor is a late development.

Treatment

- Prednisone, 60 mg PO in a loading dose, then daily in divided doses, tapering the dosage downward as soon as improvement begins.
- Referral to an ophthalmologist or neurologist (about half of all cases are associated with multiple sclerosis).

Sciatica

Pain along the course of the sciatic nerve may be severe and totally disabling. Causative orthopedic pathology in the low back, including degenerative disk disease and disk herniation, is often present. Musculus piriformis spasm, felt in conjunction with tenderness in the posterolateral vaginal vault or pararectally near the sciatic notch, may cause sciatica, dyspareunia, urination distress and occasionally reflex abdominal pain; progressive intense pain in the back, buttocks and legs with sitting is characteristic.

Treatment

- Local application of heat or cold as tolerated. Reduce activity; bed rest may be required.
- Application of a lumbosacral belt.
- Muscle relaxants every 4 hours by mouth or parenterally for relaxation of spasm (see *12–2* and Table 47–3). Injection of 5 ml of 1% lidocaine into the musculus piriformis—being careful to avoid injecting the adjacent sciatic nerve by using, preferably, a nerve stimulator-locator—may bring rapid relief if muscular impingement on the sciatic nerve is the cause.
- Relief of pain (see *12*).
- Avoid traction for sciatica due to diffuse neuritis (in contrast to root irritation from herniated "disk"), as it can be aggravating.
- Epidural steroids with lidocaine may be helpful in some cases.
- Hospitalization if the pain is intractable and severe for determination and treatment of the causative condition, which is usually orthopedic in nature.

Trigeminal Neuralgia (Tic Douloureux)

Trigeminal neuralgia is characterized by episodic intense radiating pain in one or all of the 3 branches of the trigeminal nerve; see Figs. 49–1 and 49–2.

Treatment

- Control of pain by pentazocine lactate (Talwin), 15 to 30 mg IV or IM, or by the smallest possible effective dose of morphine sulfate IM. Sedatives, hypnotics and muscle relaxants are of little value. Because of its extreme toxicity, trichlorethylene therapy should not be attempted as an emergency procedure.
- Referral to a neurologist. Long-term medical control is often achieved with the use of oral medications, particularly carbamazepine (Tegretol), starting with 100 mg bid; close monitoring is required because of this drug's hemopoietic and cardiovascular effects. Phenytoin is also effective.

"Whiplash" Injuries of the Neck *(See also 47–10 and 47–11, Neck Injuries; 49–17, Spinal Injuries with Cord Compression)*

Severe neuritis of the cervical nerves supplying the neck, head, shoulders, arms and hands may follow sudden jerking motions of the neck. In addition, irritation of the nerve vasorum may cause apparently unrelated pain through reflex mechanisms. Development of pain may be delayed for several days after injury. See *47–11* for treatment.

49–14. PARALYSIS/PARESIS

Loss of muscle power, partial or complete, sudden or progressive, may result in a situation requiring emergency management. No matter what the etiology may be, persons showing evidence of recent, progressive or extensive paralysis (except those who respond to simple emergency measures) should be hospitalized as soon as possible and receive appropriate supportive therapy en route. Antibiotics may cause a generalized form of neuromuscular weakness. Table 49–1 helps to distinguish 3 forms of muscle weakness. Table 49–2 gives a brief guide to motor function and location of strength (or weakness).

Table 49–1. DIFFERENTIAL DIAGNOSIS OF ACUTE MUSCLE PARALYSIS OR PARESIS

Item	Upper Motor Neuron*	Lower Motor Neuron, Peripheral Lesion	Acute Myopathy
Onset	May be sudden (e.g., from trauma or CVA) or insidious (e.g., from tumor/abscess/hematoma)	Gradual to rapid (with acute infection or sudden trauma)	Usually gradual
Muscle tone	Increased (spastic)	Decreased (flaccid)	Decreased (flaccid)
Fasciculations	Absent	May present 2–4 weeks after lesion	Absent
Deep tendon reflexes (DTR)	Increased or hyperactive	Decreased, hypoactive or absent	Present despite profound weakness
DTR/strength ratio	DTR much greater than strength	Strength, if any, > DTR	DTR > strength
Weakness/atrophy ratio (later)	Weakness > atrophy	Atrophy ≅ weakness	Weakness ≅ atrophy
Pathologic reflexes†	Present usually	Absent	Absent
Sensory loss	Often present, but may be minor	Often present and may be major	Absent
CPK, IgM, IgG	Usually normal	Usually normal	Greatly elevated
EMG	Decreased or absent interference pattern anytime No fibrillation generally	*Early:* Decreased or absent interference pattern with voluntary contraction attempt *After 10–15 days:* Positive sharp waves; insertion fibrillations *Later:* Spontaneous fibrillations, low-amplitude polyphasics	Number of potentials near normal but motor unit action potential decreased in amplitude and duration. Faster firing rate may occur

*Frequently after sudden onset, the initial response for a few days is flaccid weakness simulating lower motor neuron disease.

†Such as positive Hoffman, Oppenheim, Gordon, Babinski signs, or Clonus.

Table 49–2. BRIEF GUIDE TO MOTOR FUNCTION AND STRENGTH*†

A. QUALITATIVE STRENGTH

Active Motor Function	Major Muscle Involved	Cord Level(s)	Nerve(s)
Shoulder shrug	Trapezius	C1–5	Cervical
Neck flexion	Ant. neck	C1–4	Cervical
Neck extension	Post. neck	C1–4	Cervical
Push upper abdomen out	Diaphragm	C3–5	Phrenic
Abduct arm	Deltoid Supraspinatus	C5–6 C5	Axillary Suprascapular
Flex elbow Supinate forearm	Biceps brachii	C5–6	Musculocutaneous
Extend elbow	Triceps	C6–8	Radial
Extend wrist	ECR & ECU	C6–8	Radial
Flex wrist	FCR FCU	C6–7 C7–T1	Median Ulnar
Hand functions	See *43–1*		
Flex hip	Iliopsoas	T12–L3	Femoral
Adduct hip	Adductors	L2–L4	Obturator
Extend knee	Quadriceps	L2–L4	Femoral
Extend hip Abduct hip	Gluteus max. Gluteus med.	L4–S1	Inf. gluteal Sup. gluteal
Flex knee	Hamstrings	L4–S1	Sciatic
Dorsiflex foot Supinate foot	Ant. tibialis	L4–5	Deep peroneal
Plantar flex foot	Gastrocnemius-Soleus	S1–2	Tibial
Pronate foot	Peroneii	L5–S1	Superficial peroneal
Extend 1st toe	EHL	L4–S1	Deep peroneal
Flex 1st toe	FHL	L5–S2	Tibial

B. QUANTITATIVE STRENGTH

Grade	Rating	Explanation
5	Excellent	Full ROM against hard resistance
4	Good	Full ROM against moderate resistance
3	Fair	Full ROM, no resistance except gravity
2	Poor	Partial ROM, no resistance except gravity
1	Trace	Barely moves, gravity effect neutralized
0	None	No movement, gravity effect neutralized

*Guide to abbreviations: *ECR*, extensor carpi radialis; *ECU*, extensor carpi ulnaris; *FCR*, flexor carpi radialis; *FCU*, flexor carpi ulnaris; *EHL*, extensor hallucis longus; *FHL*, flexor hallucis longus.

†Major dermatomes involved in deep tendon reflexes (DTR): Biceps, C6; brachioradialis, C7; triceps, C8; patellar, L4; Achilles, S1.

Major dermatomes involved in superficial reflexes: upper abdominal, T8–T10; lower abdominal, T10–T12; gluteal, L4–S1; anal sphincter, S2–S4; cremasteric, L1–L2; bulbocavernous, S3–S4.

Acute involvement of the muscles of deglutition may be caused by:
Botulism *(53–142)*
Brain injuries *(44, Head Injuries)*
Diphtheria *(33–18)*
Myasthenia gravis *(49–12)*
Poisons and drug overdose *(53)*
Poliomyelitis, bulbar *(33–52)*
Tetanus *(33–68)*
High cervical injuries *(47–10, 47–11, Neck Injuries)*

Involvement of the muscles of respiration may occur in:
Anterior poliomyelitis *(33–52)*
Cervical fractures and dislocations *(47–10, 47–11, Neck Injuries)*
Head injuries involving the respiratory center in the medulla *(44)*
Guillain-Barré syndrome
Acute intermittent porphyria *(46–24)*
Familial periodic paralysis (see later in this section)
Tick bites *(27–30)*
Electrical shock *(28–12, Electrical Burns; 32–5)*
Acute poisoning *(32–14, 53)*
Ascending paralysis of Landry

Treatment

Expired air respiration or mechanical ventilation *(5–21)*, often followed by endotracheal intubation *(18–10)* or tracheostomy *(18–34)*, may be necessary as a life-saving measure. Neck injuries must be immobilized.

Paralysis of central nervous system origin may result from:
Acute demyelinative disease, e.g., multiple sclerosis, transverse myelitis
Acute poisoning *(53)*
Brain infarction or increased intracranial pressure resulting from cerebrovascular accidents *(63)*
Cauda equina syndrome
Space-consuming intracranial or cord tumors
Head injuries *(44)*
Vertebral fractures
Partial or complete dislocation of any portion of the spine *(49–17)*

Paralysis due to noncentral neuropathy may be caused by herniated intervertebral disk, neuritis (metabolic, toxic or traumatic) or cauda equina syndrome.

Familial periodic paralysis is a rare disorder of electrolyte metabolism, characterized by recurrent episodes of profound paralysis and weakness and usually associated with low serum potassium levels. There is a form of this paralysis associated with high serum potassium levels, and this condition can be differentiated by electrocardiogram (ECG) and serum potassium assay.

Treatment

- Supportive therapy, particularly ventilatory assistance.
- If serum K is low, restrict Na intake and give oral KCl, 10 to 40 mEq tid. Correct severe hypokalemia by slow (not to exceed 5 ml per minute) IV infusion of 500 ml of 5% dextrose in water containing 3 g of KCl. Electrocardiographic and serum K monitoring should be done.
- If serum K is high, restrict K administration and hydrate IV.

Hysterical paralysis *(54–12)* must always be considered if the findings are bizarre and the exact causative factor cannot be determined.

49–15. PERIPHERAL NERVE INJURIES IN THE EXTREMITIES *(See also 43–10, Nerve Injuries in the Hand; Fig. 49–1, Anatomical Locations; Figs. 47–11 to 47–15, Cross Sections of Extremity Anatomy; and Tables 49–1 and 49–2, Guides to Motor Function and Strength)*

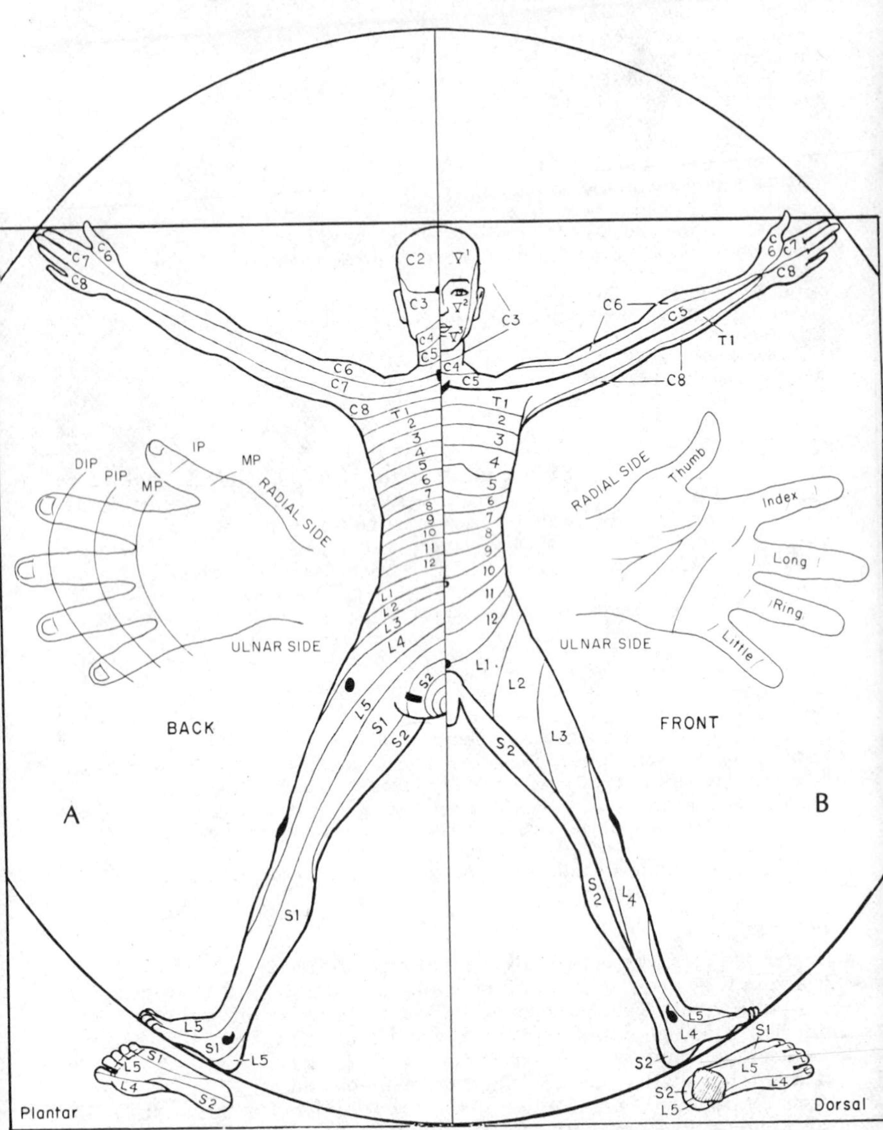

Figure 49–1. Dermatomes of human body from front (right side) and back (left side). (After Keegan and Garret from Elliott, H. C.: *Textbook of the Nervous System*, 2nd ed. Philadelphia, J. B. Lippincott, 1954.) *A,* Designation of joints of the hand. DIP, distal interphalangeal; PIP, proximal interphalangeal; IP, interphalangeal; MP, metacarpophalangeal. *B,* Nomenclature of fingers.

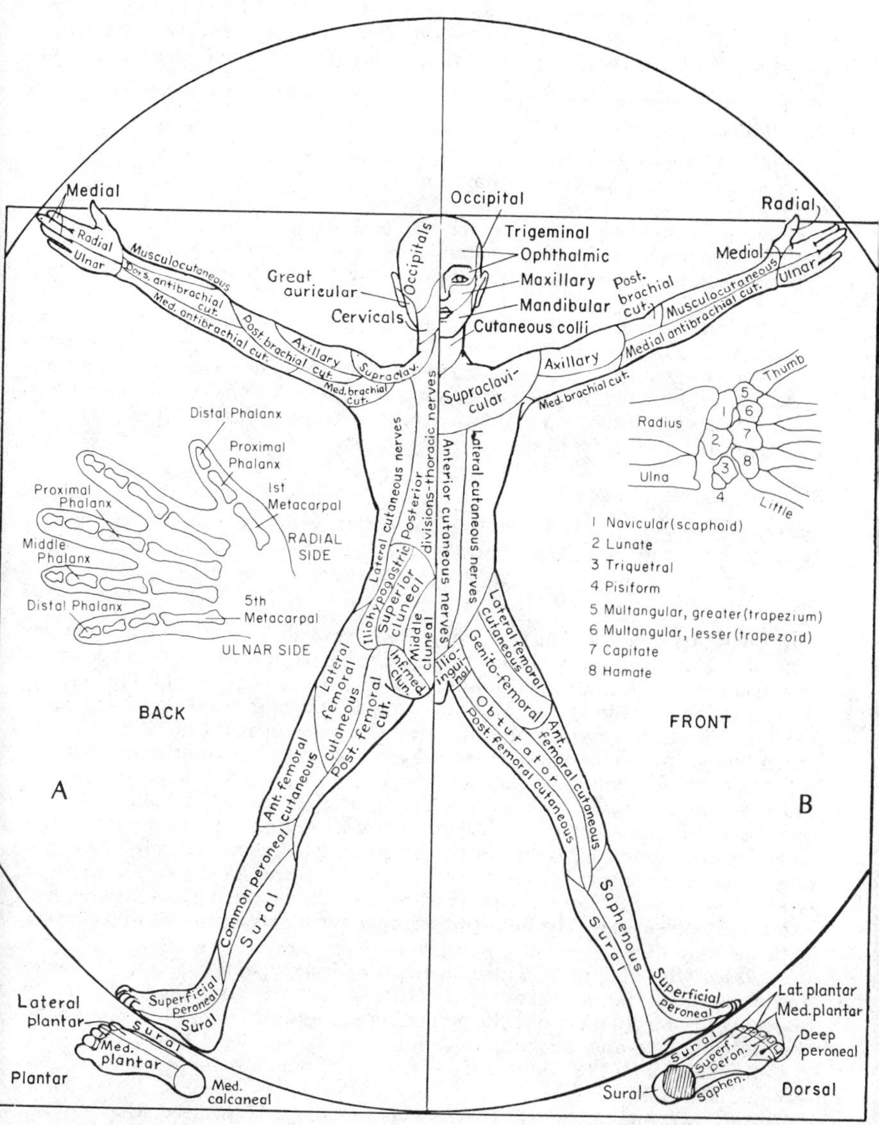

Figure 49–2. Dermal areas supplied by named nerves. Dermatomes and nerves do not coincide except where segmental structure still prevails. (After Keegan and Garret from Elliott, H. C.: *Textbook of the Nervous System,* 2nd ed. Philadelphia, J. B. Lippincott, 1954.) *A,* Phalangeal and metacarpal bones. *B,* Carpal bones.

An injured peripheral nerve can be recognized by impairment or loss of motor function or sensory perception in areas innervated by that nerve (Fig. 49–2). The location of injury can often be determined by overlying soft tissue trauma, adjacent bone fracture and displacement, and area of motor weakness (Table 49–2).

Treatment

- Splint the involved extremity.
- Control pain by analgesics or narcotics *(12)*.
- Treat soft tissue injuries *(59)*.
- Refer to a specialist surgeon for end-to-end anastomosis of completely severed nerves or decompression of severely compressed nerves. Laser beam technique holds promise for more physiologic bonding of the epineurium.
- If possible, obtain an electromyogram in all cases of peripheral nerve injury as soon as possible after injury to rule out preexistent pathology. There will be immediate loss of voluntary action potentials in complete nerve transection or reduction in voluntary units in incomplete lesions (see Table 49–1). This is particularly important in workers' compensation cases *(75)* and potential civil liability cases.

49–16. SEIZURES *(See 34)*

49–17. SPINAL INJURIES WITH CORD COMPRESSION *(See Table 4–1, Management of Patients with Serious Head-Neck Injuries Awaiting Transportation; Fig. 4–3, Head/Neck/Body Immobilization)*

All patients with obvious or suspected head/neck/back injury, with or without a history of severe direct trauma, should be treated as having possible spinal cord injuries until the condition has been ruled out by careful radiologic and neurologic examination. The following are clues that injury to the head, neck or spinal cord may be present: altered consciousness (due to trauma or other—sometimes unknown—cause); obvious awkward angulation or positioning of the spine, including palpable step-off or displaced position of spinous processes or external signs of head/spine trauma (e.g., abrasions/bruises); paralysis or paresis, especially when bilateral and nearly symmetrical (see Table 49–2); pain or burning dysesthesias in the spine or extremities, even if only transient; sensory loss level (see Figs. 49–1 and 49–2); focal swelling, tenderness and muscle spasm along the spine; unexplained hypotension/ileus/ventilatory power loss. The following approach is helpful from the first contact with the patient.

1. Assess the patient (see also *1, ABC's of Emergency Problem Analysis)* and determine whether there is an actual or potential spinal cord injury by checking for the clues cited in the preceding paragraph. Determine, if possible, the probable type and mechanics of injury.

2. Ask the patient to rest quietly while the spine is immobilized (see Table 4–1 and Fig. 4–3).

3. Airway management *(5–10)* may be an early critical need. Use the jaw lift rather than the head tilt initially, to avoid neck motion. If need be, cricothyrotomy *(5–19)* is the next step if further airway access and artificial ventilation are needed in a respiratory arrest situation. If no repiratory arrest is present, nasotracheal intubation *(5–17)* and tracheostomy *(5–20)* are preferred.

4. Start management of any shock (*57*) and other injury problems as indicated from initial survey.

5. Insert nasogastric tube and Foley catheter, if available, when paralysis is present.

6. On arrival at the hospital ED, reassess the patient's status with regard to all of the above.

7. Perform a more detailed neurologic evaluation (*44–2*), but do not remove immobilization. Obtain an immediate neurosurgical consultation if any abnormality is found.

8. Check a cross-table lateral x-ray of the cervical spine plus AP and open or closed mouth (C1, C2) cervical views to check for normalcy before any alteration of immobilized status is permitted. An adequate view of the lower cervical spine (including C7) is important, and slowly pulling the patient's shoulders down by grasping at the patient's wrists may provide adequate exposure. A swimmer's view of the area (C7, T1, T2) as well as tomograms and CT scan (with or without metrizamide myelogram) may be needed in difficult diagnostic cases, such as when extreme pain greatly exceeds the pathologic findings. If the x-rays reveal any abnormality, a neurosurgical evaluation should be immediately obtained before proceeding; if they are normal, proceed with completing cervical and any other spinal x-rays, as appropriate. Abnormalities detected subsequently on x-ray, or any finding of neurologic deficit even in the absence of x-ray abnormality, also is an indication for neurosurgical evaluation and continued immobilization.

9. If compressive myelopathy amenable to surgical decompression is found, decompression plus possible fusion or other internal fixation should be performed ASAP. Otherwise, skull traction, using Gardner-Wells tongs (*18–28*), is usually done for immobilization of the cervical spine. Lower spinal fractures or dislocations with myelopathy, if not treated operatively are immobilized externally.

10. Measures to reduce spinal cord edema are advisable. Steroid administration (e.g., dexamethasone, 0.2 mg/kg up to 20 mg IV q 6 h initially) may help, as may early cryotherapy. Experimental therapy with 10% DMSO IV (1 g/kg per day) in D5W given at a rate of 150 to 200 ml/hr in adults on 3 successive days has shown benefit, but is not approved as a standard therapy.

11. Intensive long-range supportive therapy for patients with spinal cord injuries is required; see Table 63–2 for guidelines to therapy, which should be begun as soon as feasible.

49–18. SPINAL CORD COMPRESSION WITHOUT DIRECT TRAUMA

Acute spinal cord compression may be present without any evidence of direct trauma. Spontaneous compression in these cases may be related to epidural abscess (*23–12*), insidious disc herniation (*47–13*), or collapse of a vertebra due to deterioration from advanced osteoporosis or a malignant process; occasionally compression is caused by an epidural hematoma from spontaneous hemorrhage. Treatment is as outlined under *47–17*, with transfer for hospitalization and evaluation for appropriate neurosurgical intervention. Immobilization (Table 4–1 and Fig. 4–3) should be done even in the absence of external trauma causing skeletal instability, as mechanical motion, osteophytes and other bony or ligamentous protrusions can still worsen the condition.

Table 49–3. DIFFERENTIAL DIAGNOSIS OF EPISODIC UNCONSCIOUSNESS*

	Epilepsy (Grand Mal) (See *34, Convulsive Seizures*)	Hyperventilation (See *37–10, Excitement States*))	Hysteria (See *54–12*)	Vasodepressor Syncope (Fainting) (See *63–7*)
Onset	Rapid; may be prodromal symptoms	Gradual—vertigo may be first	Slow or rapid, depending upon surrounding attention	Rapid, preceded by stretching and yawning
Duration of symptoms	Usually several minutes; may be longer	Few minutes or recur episodically	Often prolonged	2 to 3 minutes
Type, results of fall	Sudden; may result in severe injury	Gradual and slow; generally no injury	Careful; practically never any injury	Sudden; may result in injury
Unconsciousness	Total; no response to stimuli	Usually partial, brief	Partial or complete; usually respond to painful stimuli	Complete but very brief
Time or place of onset	Anywhere, even when asleep	In the presence of any situation causing anxiety	In the presence of potential sympathizers	In the presence of real or imagined severe suffering
Muscular movements	Rhythmical and symmetrical, except in focal epilepsy	Spasmodic twitching	Inconstant, irregular and bizarre	None

Recovery	Slow; confused, partially disoriented for 10 to 30 minutes	Gradual but complete	Complete at once	Usually complete in a few moments
Skin	Cyanotic from apnea	Usually normal	Normal	Pallor and sweating
Pulse	Normal	Rapid	Normal	Usually slow
Blood pressure	Slightly elevated during episode	Lower than normal	Normal	Marked transient hypotension
Neurologic changes	None except loss of response to pain; occasionally positive Babinski sign	Signs of tetany (*46–25*)	Decreased gag reflexes; resist eye lid opening by examiner; responsive to painful stimuli	None
EEG	Abnormal	Normal	Normal	Normal
Treatment	1. Prevention and treatment of injury 2. Gentle restraint 3. Sedation 4. Long-term care	1. Rebreathing (paper bag method) 2. Sedation by barbiturates 3. Investigation and treatment of cause	1. Sedation by barbiturates if necessary 2. Psychiatric care	1. Supine position 2. Aromatic spirits of ammonia inhalations 3. Treatment of injuries
Prognosis	Good for recovery from immediate attack	Complete recovery	Guarded; complete psychiatric evaluation indicated	Excellent for complete recovery

*For cases due to hypoglycemia, see Table 32–3.

49–19. UNCONSCIOUSNESS, EPISODIC *(See Table 49–3)*

Common Causes

Between 90 and 95% of the cases of transient and recurrent loss of consciousness are due to hypoglycemia *(46–15)*, epilepsy *(34)*, hysteria *(54–12)*, hyperventilation *(37–10)* or vasodepressive syncope (see *Differential Diagnosis of Episodic Unconsciousness*, below; see also 63–7, *Syncope*).

Causes of Episodic Loss of Consciousness (Complete or Partial)

- *Carotid sinus syncope*. These attacks generally follow twisting the neck in a certain way or pressure (tight collar, etc.) over the junction of the external and internal carotid arteries at the level of the upper border of the thyroid cartilage. The diagnosis can be confirmed by applying pressure *over one side only* with the patient lying down. Atropine for intravenous administration should be at hand in a syringe. This test is not without danger and should not be done unless facilities for combating cardiac arrest *(5–2)* are immediately available.
- *Cardiac arrhythmias and standstill*. See 29, *Cardiac Emergencies*.
  —Complete heart block (Adams-Stokes syncope) *(29–13)*
  —Aortic stenosis
  —Paroxysmal atrial tachycardia *(29–5)*
  —Ventricular fibrillation *(29–25)*
- *Intermittent cerebral ischemia (63–10)*
- *Accidental or surreptitious intake of causative drugs*. See 17, *Suicide*; 53, *Poisoning*.
- *Orthostatic hypotension*. Persons with this condition lose consciousness in the upright position only; they should avoid closed door phone booths or similar settings in which inability to fall horizontal could cause severe cerebral ischemia. Treat any injuries from fall.
- Vasovagal attacks. Simple faints, as from emotion, most common.

Differential Diagnosis of Episodic Unconsciousness

Distinction between the four common causes of episodic loss of consciousness requires a careful history, especially in regard to previous episodes and onset of symptoms, and detailed examination. The most important points are summarized in Table 49–3.

49–20. VERTIGO *(See also 49–11, Motion Sickness)*

Vertigo is a sensation of the external world revolving about the patient (objective vertigo) or the patient's sensation of revolving in space (subjective vertigo). It may be caused by a disturbance in any of the structures concerned with maintaining equilibrium: end-organ, vestibular nerve or nuclei (peripheral vertigo—most common) and their connections in the brainstem (central vertigo). Vertigo must be distinguished from lightheadedness, dizziness, faintness or near syncope *(63–6)*, which encompass space unsteadiness, but no whirling or rotary sensation. Severe peripheral vertigo, as seen with labyrinthitis, is usually accompanied by nausea and vomiting, but without the decreased hearing acuity or tinnitus characteristic of central vertigo.

Causes of peripheral vertigo are most often positional change, and sensitivity may be increased by physical deconditioning, toxins, drugs, allergy or idiopathic hydrops *(49–7)* in the afebrile patient (viral and bacterial etiology should be considered in the febrile patient). Bacterial infection will be detected through the primary infection site as mastoiditis or meningitis.

Central vertigo may occur as a result of trauma, vertebrobasilar artery insufficiency, brainstem vascular accidents or posterior fossa tumor, among other causes. Associated nystagmus tends to be more enduring and multidirectional.

The caloric stimulation test response is usually diminished in cases of persistent vertigo.

Treatment

Removal or treatment of the cause of the vertigo is the most important therapeutic measure. Although in some instances hospitalization is required, in many cases the following symptomatic measures will give relief:

- Rest or modified activity; avoidance of machinery and heights until the condition has passed.
- Effective anticholinergic medication for reduction of motion disturbance plus relief of nausea and vomiting (see *49–11, Motion Sickness*).
- IV administration of hypertonic dextrose solution.
- Vitamin B_6 (pyridoxine hydrochloride), 25 to 50 mg IV, and niacin (nicotinic acid), 50 to 100 mg PO, for its vasodilator effect.
- LP should be done if meningitis is suspected. Afebrile patients with persistent or intense vertigo should be referred for thorough evaluation.

49–21. WERNICKE'S ACUTE ENCEPHALOPATHY

Though this form of encephalitis is caused by chronic alcohol abuse, the problem may have precipitous onset of ataxia, nystagmus, diplopia and neuropsychiatric disorders. Vitamin B_1 specifically helps to reverse this problem if given immediately in large doses, 100 mg IV, then 100 mg IM or IV for 3 to 5 days.

50. Obstetric Emergencies

50–1. GENERAL CONSIDERATIONS

The management of emergencies related to pregnancy is dependent on multiple factors. Among these factors are:

- Maternal desires and health.
- Availability of immediate modern medical facilities and obstetrical assistance.
- Fetal status, including maturity (*50–9*) as determined by duration of amenorrhea, abdominal examination (see Fig. 50–1), weight estimation and, when necessary, sonogram (ultrasound scan) and amniocentesis studies.

Particularly during the first trimester, relative consideration must be given to the effect on the fetus of medications administered in emergencies.

Anticipation of patients with increased potential for emergency delivery problems (e.g., maternal illness, such as hypertension, diabetes mellitus or cardio-renal disease; prior cesarean section; prior premature labor and bleeding; cephalopelvic disproportion; multiple gestation; and abnormal presentations) are best managed through anticipation of their needs; the patient's consultation with a perinatologist should be considered. The trend toward home deliveries will still be fraught with dangers such as severe bleeding, endometritis and third and fourth degree lacerations, as no one can predict which "normal patient" will develop a high-risk event during labor or delivery.

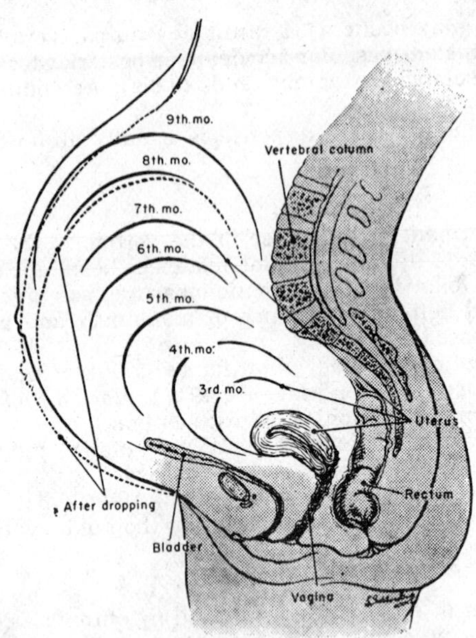

Figure 50–1. Pregnancy—uterine levels. (From *Dorland's Illustrated Medical Dictionary*, 26th ed. Philadelphia, W. B. Saunders Co., 1981, p. 1063.)

Non-complex, homelike "birthing rooms" near a well-equipped obstetric suite, to be used if needed, appear to be a satisfactory compromise.

50–2. ABDOMINAL PAIN

The pregnant woman may experience abdominal pain from any of the causes unrelated to pregnancy (see 22) as well as those related to pregnancy. Evaluation and treatment of abdominal pain in the pregnant woman requires the following special considerations:

- Avoidance of use of x-rays.
- Greater use of ultrasound and possibly laparoscopy (during early pregnancy) in diagnosis.
- Ascertainment of the stage of development and quality/viability of the fetus, using amniocentesis/amnion fluid culture and L/S ratios.

Special attention is directed to the following causes of abdominal pain specifically associated with pregnancy: ectopic pregnancy *(50–7)* • threatened abortion *(50–3)* • amnionitis *(50–4)*, with or without premature rupture of membranes *(50–19)* • pre-eclampsia and eclampsia *(50–14)* • hypertensive disease in pregnancy • pain associated with vaginal hemorrhage *(50–10)*. There is also an increased incidence of aortic dissection associated with pregnancy.

50–3. ABORTIONS *(For definition, see 65–5)*

Threatened. These patients should be hospitalized at once if uterine bleeding is excessive—by ambulance if necessary. Sedation and control of pain may be necessary; use nonmedicinal measures *(12)*. Currently no specific medications are advised for therapy of threatened abortion. IV administration of plasma volume expanders may be necessary before transfer if the patient is in shock. Treatment at home is adequate in milder cases and if the mother is not overly anxious.

Incomplete. The treatment of abortion can be expedited and much blood loss prevented by immediate speculum examination and simple removal of products of conception from the cervix by curettage. Hospitalization as soon as possible is essential if bleeding is excessive or equipment for curettage is not available in the emergency department for outpatient treatment. Excessive bleeding can sometimes be controlled by measures such as IV oxytocin (Pitocin) or ergonovine maleate (Ergotrate Maleate), 0.2 mg PO, 3 or 4 times a day for 3 days (see *50–12*). Treatment for shock *(57)* should be given before transfer if blood loss has been excessive. Observe for any complications of curettage, such as hemorrhage, lacerations, perforation and infection, and arrange for further gynecologic care.

Complete. If the attending physician is sure that no tissue has been retained and that bleeding has been controlled, home or office treatment may be feasible.

Septic. See principles of management under *59–42, Soft Tissue Infections, Life Threatening.*

50–4. AMNIONITIS

Signs and Symptoms

Amnionitis is most readily recognized when pain and tenderness of the uterus, malodorous, purulent discharge, and fever follow premature rupture of membranes (PROM) (though membranes also can be intact). Earlier signs may reveal only slight maternal fever (still always suspect amnionitis) and elevated maternal/fetal heart rate.

The risk of amnionitis is increased with lower socioeconomic groups, occurrence of intercourse late in term and poor nutrition and general health; the risk is inversely proportional to birth weight and gestational period. Frequency is probably more common than is generally suspected. Evaluate for other sources of fever and infection.

Laboratory Findings

- Rapidly rising or elevated WBC (normal elevated WBC range in pregnancy is 10,000 to 14,500), plus increased stab cells and pmn's.
- Culture results are of more retrospective value to treating the subsequent newborn than in directing clinical action during pregnancy. Endocervical cultures do not always accurately reflect intra-amniotic activity, but gram-positive cocci and gram-negative diplococci *(N. gonorrhoeae)* increase suspicion.
- If the diagnosis is debatable and delivery appears remote, properly performed amniocentesis can be of aid. *(Note:* If amniocentesis is done, also do L/S ratio.) Bacteria identified on Gram stain are the most definitive evidence.

Treatment

Fetal viability, gestational age and pulmonary maturity as well as seriousness of infection help to determine obstetrical action.

- Clearly established cases of amnionitis require immediate IV antibiotics and initiation of uterine emptying procedure. Antibiotic treatment, e.g., with a penicillin plus gentamycin or an aminoglycoside plus clindamycin, must be intensive. Generally, vaginal delivery is preferred for the mother but is favorable for the fetus only if it can be achieved readily with smooth progression of labor, and fetal weight is estimated to be greater than 2000 g. Otherwise low cervical cesarean section is preferable. In severe advanced cases, immediate hysterectomy following delivery may be necessary.

- The more borderline the diagnosis, the milder the infection, and the more immature the fetus, the more likely that IV antibiotics (e.g., ampicillin, 1.5 to 2.0 g q4h), with frequent reevaluation of the patient's condition, will satisfactorily manage the problem.

50–5. DRUGS IN PREGNANCY

Drugs administered to the mother during pregnancy also pass to the fetus, on which they may have little or no effect, a beneficial effect or a profound deleterious (teratogenic/mutagenic) effect (particularly in the first trimester) depending upon type and amount. Maternal smoking causes vasoconstriction, which adversely affects the fetus, and alcohol and caffeine also have adverse fetal effects. Therefore careful consideration of drug effects on both mother and fetus must be made. This is also true for lactating mothers, since some drugs get into the breast milk and may have harmful effects on the nursing infant.

50–6. ECLAMPSIA *(See 50–14)*

50–7. ECTOPIC PREGNANCY

Ectopic pregnancy should be suspected in any woman of child-bearing capacity who presents with abdominal pain. Concern is heightened with history of altered recent menses, vaginal bleeding, intrauterine contraceptive device (IUD) or tubal pathology. Shoulder pain can be indicative of intraperitoneal bleeding.

The ideal objective is to identify and treat before rupture and life-threatening bleeding occur. Aids in making the diagnosis are: signs of pregnancy and belief of the woman that she is pregnant, unilateral adnexal tenderness on abdominopelvic examination, a mass in either adnexa, a uterus that is palpably small for gestational size, no evidence of intrauterine pregnancy by sonogram, blood aspiration on culdocentesis and direct observation by laparoscopy. On sonogram also look for absence of "double decidual lines" yet presence of intrauterine fluid: this combination indicates ectopic pregnancy or abnormal intrauterine pregnancy. A positive pregnancy test is a valuable aid in cases of desultory onset when viewed with other prior information; it helps differentiate from pelvic inflammatory disease (PID) as will a less pronounced elevation of white blood cell (WBC) count and more normal temperature than found with PID. The pregnancy test is not always positive when symptoms begin. The preferred test is the serum radioimmunoassay pregnancy test, because of increased sensitivity and specificity plus ability to quantitate exact levels of HCG. A high suspicion of possibility of the problem is essential.

Treatment

- Obtain gynecologic consultation. If diagnosis uncertain and presenting condition of minor severity, warn patient to return immediately if pain (abdominal, shoulder or both), signs or symptoms of hypovolemia and anemia or vaginal bleeding occur. Also, return of a positive pregnancy test should prompt recall for reevaluation, which may consist of serial ultrasound and HCG examinations, culdocentesis, laparoscopy and even possibly D & C.

- Presentation with signs of severe pain and/or shock (57) and usually some vaginal bleeding is indicative of a ruptured ectopic pregnancy and necessitates vigorous intervention, including intravenous volume expanders and blood transfusions, plus preparation for prompt surgical intervention.

50–8. EMERGENCY DELIVERY CONSIDERATIONS OUTSIDE THE HOSPITAL

Adequate prenatal evaluation and preparation, early admission of likely difficult deliveries and compromise use of hospital alternative birthing centers in preference to home delivery will convert many emergencies into semielective procedures. Nevertheless, difficult deliveries will still occur at the most inopportune times and in adverse circumstances.

Decisions to be Made by Emergency Physician When Patient is at or Near Term

Is the patient approaching or in true labor? This can generally be aided by consideration of the following criteria, the last one being determinative:

- History regarding months of gestation (if a prenatal chart is available, this should be reviewed) and prior experience of the mother.
- Type, duration, strength and frequency of uterine contractures.
- "Bloody show."
- Rupture of the membranes.
- Position of the presenting part effacement and dilation of the cervix by aseptic vaginal examination. Avoid vaginal examination whenever possible in the presence of uterine bleeding, and under no circumstances should such an exam be done in cases of second and third trimester bleeding; these patients should be examined by an OB consultant.

Is there time for transportation to a hospital for delivery?

PRIMIPARAE. It is generally safe to transport primiparae in labor to a hospital for delivery—depending on time and distance unless the cervix is fully dilated and/or the presenting part lies on the perineum. On occasion, even primiparae have precipitate labor.

MULTIPARAE

In many cases, women who have had children are able to tell with great accuracy when delivery is near. Before arranging for transportation to a hospital, the physician should question the patient regarding previous precipitate labors and, if possible, review the prenatal record. Examination is helpful but can often be misleading. In making a decision regarding transfer, the physician usually should be guided more by the time since onset of pains; the frequency, strength and length of uterine contractions; the length of the patient's prior labor(s); and the patient's opinion regarding the time available before delivery than by the sole determination of cervical effacement and fetal station by examination. Delivery can frequently follow in several contractions when the cervix is dilated 6 cm or more.

Must emergency transportation to a hospital be made on an especially urgent basis because of dystocia and/or need for cesarean section (C/S)?

Modern communication systems and air ambulance transport allow greater options for rapid transfer to adequately equipped centers. Prominent causes of arrested labor and likely need for cesarean section include inadequacy of uterine contractions, cephalopelvic disproportion (CPD) and abnormal fetal presentation. Other situations frequently requiring urgent cesarean section are fetal distress and late antepartum hemorrhage *(50–11)*, and cases in which there is a viable fetus in a breech position. Current practice quite commonly is to allow a patient who has had a prior low transverse cesarean (LTC) to deliver vaginally, provided there is not a recurring indication for cesarean section, such as CPD.

All patients should be instructed to breathe through the mouth and advised against bearing down during transportation to the hospital. However, if delivery en route becomes imperative, it is much better for both the mother and the baby to avoid all delaying procedures; absolutely *do not* have the mother cross her legs or put counterpressure on the emerging head.

Narcotic drugs, natural or synthetic, should never be given under emergency conditions in an attempt to stop or slow down delivery. Their effect may be the opposite; in addition, their use may result in marked depression of the child's respiratory center.

Is emergency delivery necessary? If, in the opinion of the attending physician, sufficient time for transfer to a hospital for delivery is not available, delivery should be effected using the best possible technique that time and circumstances will allow. Spend as much time as available in speaking to reassure and calm the mother.

Difficult Vaginal Deliveries

Some deliveries of labor in progress are potentially so difficult that if labor can be safely interrupted for potential cesarean section, it should be, as mentioned in *50–18, Premature Labor*. These include apparent cephalopelvic disproportion (to prevent uterine rupture); multiple gestation; and abnormal (i.e., non-vertex) presentations.

If vaginal delivery is inevitably progressing in cases of the aforementioned fetal malpresentations in which there is no possibility of reaching a hospital, consider the following:

- Mobilize obstetric equipment *(10–4)* as available.
- Follow guidelines illustrated in Figure 50–2.
- Positions of maximum comfort for the mother are on her back with legs spread and supported in an elevated position, on her side (Sims position), or in a semiprone squat or kneeling position with the shoulders supported and elevated.
- Keep the fetal head gently flexed and the face as posterior as possible.
- If the shoulders are impacted after delivery of the head, attempt to reverse the position of the shoulders: the assistant should place his index and long fingers against the ventral surface of the fetal shoulder closest to the mother's sacrum and rotate the shoulder laterally and then up and out while giving aid to the rotary motion of the fetal body with his other hand on the abdominal aspect of the uterus ("corkscrew the shoulder out"). Be ready to intubate and do cardiopulmonary resuscitation (CPR) on the infant *(52–1)*. Shoulder dystocia often results in severe fetal depression or even fetal cardiac arrest and can occur with vertex or breech delivery; it is more frequent with large infants of diabetic mothers.
- *Breech presentations* (buttocks coming before the head) can be most difficult to manage and, if at all possible, should be handled by an obstetrician in a hospital. If this is not possible, consider the following:
  —Note that there are 3 types of breech presentations: *incomplete*, with foot presentation; *frank*, with feet by the face; and *complete*, with the fetus in a near-squat position.

—Perform a generous mediolateral episiotomy.

—Allow spontaneous delivery of breech to level of umbilicus before trying to assist delivery; watch for cord compression.

—Upper limbs can be delivered in breech delivery by reaching into the vaginal vault and sweeping one flexed arm first medially then down across the body and out and repeating for the other side.

—Permit the *flexed* head to slowly deliver spontaneously in 1 or 2 contractions if possible. If not accomplished within 3 minutes, the aider's lower hand should slide into the vagina with the palm toward baby's face, to put one finger into the baby's mouth; this hand plus the other hand slid higher on the baby's head will help to slowly guide the head down so that it doesn't pop out.

—Breech babies quite frequently have respiratory depression and may need intubation and resuscitation *(52–1)*.

- With delivery, suction fluid/secretions out of baby's nose and mouth. Preserve baby's warmth with blanket or coat, or put next to mother's body. It is not essential for the umbilical cord to be immediately clamped and severed (except in premature delivery).

Emergency Cesarean in Maternal Death

If maternal death has suddenly occurred, time is of the essence (less than 5 to 10 minutes definitely best, though longer periods are described) if a healthy viable fetus is to be delivered. Make a vertical lower abdominal midline incision from the umbilicus to the pubis with any available sharp cutting device; rapidly cutting through the identifiable layers of the skin and subcutaneous tissue, the fascia over and between the left and right musculi rectus abdominis, the abdominal peritoneum and vesicouterine peritoneal fold, down to the uterine muscle. A distended urinary bladder may be encountered and can be pushed distally or, if necessary, rapidly emptied by incision. Make a long vertical incision through the uterine corpus—avoiding cutting fetal parts. *(Note:* If not skilled, and concerned about cutting a fetal part, make a short vertical incision until in the lower uterine cavity, then place the index and long fingers through the small vertical incision and turn them palm up. While lifting up with the separated fingers, continue cutting vertically between them—using a bandage scissors if available. After wide exposure is obtained, gently deliver the baby, keeping the neck in a flexed position. As with all premature infants, immediately tie off the cord, as increased intravascular volume is not well tolerated. See also 52–1, *Resuscitation at Birth*.

50–9. FETAL MATURITY

Fetal maturity can be of importance in deciding emergency management and is usually determined by one or more of the following factors:

- *Time elapsed* since the first day of the mother's last menstrual period, measured in weeks. *Note:* Sometimes the patient's last menstrual period has occurred after the pregnancy has started (even though atypically short and of diminished flow), which throws the calculations off.
- *Observation.* See Figure 50–1.
- *Palpation.* Usually estimates are in grams, but techniques incorporate the preceding two factors as well and are subject to wide error.
- *Sonogram.* Fetal size is estimated in grams by biparietal diameter (BPD) and occasionally by abdominal circumference. Sonogram also helps to localize the placenta and indicates the presence of multiple births and fetal anomalies.

When normal delivery imminent (starting to crown):

DO

- Stay calm; help mother and others do likewise
- Spread clean sheet or newspaper if outside hospital
- Get mother comfortable in customary position
- Start D5W IV, if available
- Have mother take slow, deep breaths during contractions

DO NOT

- Let mother go to bathroom
- Attempt to hold baby back
- Push on uterus or abdomen
- Exert strong pulling pressure on fetal parts
- Have mother bear down during contractions — rather encourage slow, deep breaths

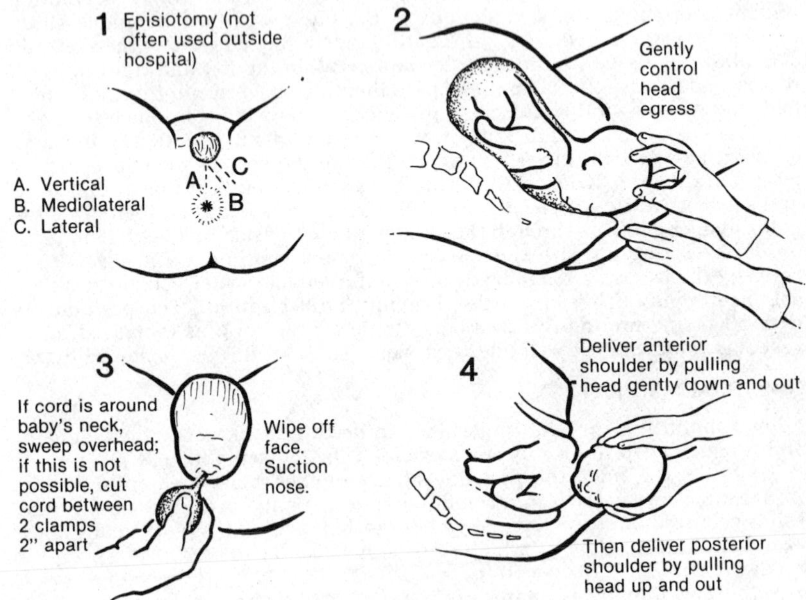
1
Episiotomy (not often used outside hospital)
A. Vertical
B. Mediolateral
C. Lateral
A
B
C
2
Gently control head egress
3
If cord is around baby's neck, sweep overhead; if this is not possible, cut cord between 2 clamps 2" apart
Wipe off face. Suction nose.
4
Deliver anterior shoulder by pulling head gently down and out
Then deliver posterior shoulder by pulling head up and out

Figure 50–2. Normal spontaneous vaginal delivery.

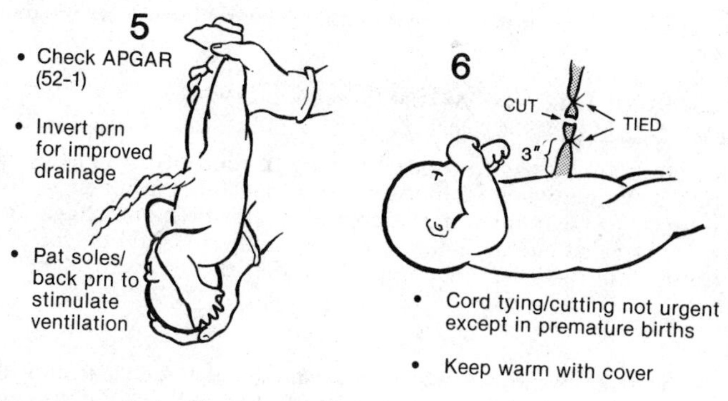

5
• Check APGAR (52-1)
• Invert prn for improved drainage
• Pat soles/ back prn to stimulate ventilation
6
CUT
TIED
3"
• Cord tying/cutting not urgent except in premature births
• Keep warm with cover

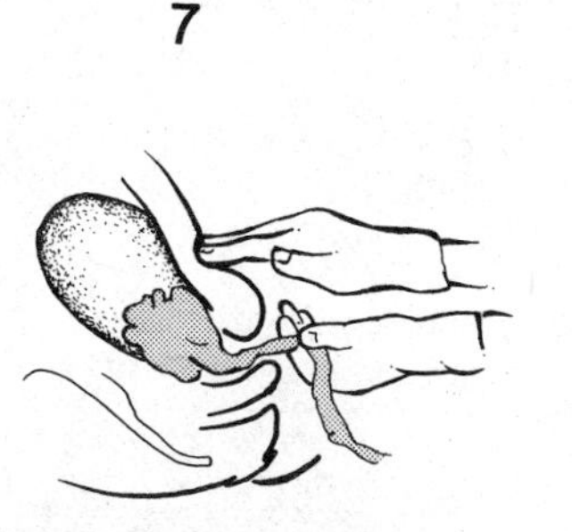

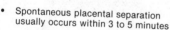

- Spontaneous placental separation usually occurs within 3 to 5 minutes
- Do not tug; if there is firm resistance to gentle pull, wait for further separation

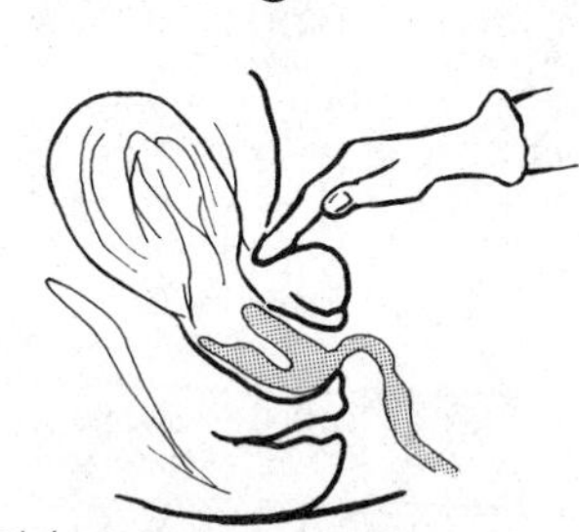

- Retain expressed placenta for exam
- Later, suprapubic massage of uterus with flat palm of hand (Credé maneuver) reduces muscle atony and bleeding

- *L/S ratio* in amniotic fluid helps to establish stage of fetal pulmonary maturity.

50–10. HEMORRHAGE, FIRST TRIMESTER

Vaginal bleeding in childbearing women sometimes first requires confirmation of pregnancy when occurring in the first trimester (use 2-minute immunologic urine pregnancy test). Furthermore, even if the patient is pregnant, bleeding may be related to other causes (see Table 42–1 and *45, Hemorrhage*).

Causes of first-trimester vaginal bleeding due to the pregnancy include the following:

- Abortion (see *50–3*). Often the fetus is defective in these circumstances.
- Ectopic pregnancy (see *50–7*).
- Coagulation defect following missed abortion. This situation requires prompt uterine evacuation with sharp curettage if the patient has been pregnant 14 weeks or less (mid- or third-trimester pregnancies require

induction of labor), accompanied by possible cryoprecipitate for fibrinogen supplement.

50–11. HEMORRHAGE LATE ANTEPARTUM *(See also Table 42–1, Abnormal Uterovaginal Bleeding)*

The more common causes of uterine bleeding in the third trimester, aside from bleeding accompanying premature labor *(50–11)*, are given in Table 50–1. Avoid rectal or vaginal examination during uterine hemorrhage unless placenta previa is ruled out by sonogram. Examination should be performed only with immediate facilities for cesarean section in the event bleeding is aggravated.

Treatment

Immediate transfer by ambulance to a hospital for obstetrical care after control of restlessness and anxiety—using a small dose of Vistaril if necessary. Measures to combat shock (57) may be necessary en route.

50–12. HEMORRHAGE, POSTPARTUM

Careful examination to locate the exact site of bleeding is essential. If from a laceration or episiotomy site, suturing to control bleeding under local

Table 50–1. LATE ANTEPARTUM HEMORRHAGE*
(See also Table 42–1, Abnormal Uterovaginal Bleeding)

	Abruptio Placentae	Placenta Previa	Uterine Rupture
Predisposition	Hypertension	Multiparity. Vaginal-rectal exam aggravates	Prior uterine surgery or abnormality
Pain	Variable to severe	Painless	Severe
Color blood	Darker red	Normal red	Variable
Degree of shock to visible blood	Disproportionately greater shock	Equivalent	Disproportionately greater shock
Clotting defect	May be severe, decreased fibrinogen (Table 42–1)	Usually normal	Usually normal
Uterus	Tender, very firm, hypertonic	Normal	Tender, decreased contractile force
Fetus	Difficult to outline	Palpable	Palpable
Fetal heart tones	Decreased or absent	Normal early†	Normal early†
Treatment*	Replace blood; prompt delivery, usually cesarean. Correct coagulation defect (45) as necessary	Replace blood. Determine amount of bleeding and assess placental position by sonogram.	Replace blood; prompt cesarean section

*Requires immediate care of obstetrician, transfer to obstetric suite area and fetal heart tone monitoring.

†Fetal heart tones (FHT) may be decreased or absent if significant bleeding from placenta previa or extensive uterine rupture is present.

anesthetic may be required. Do not reclose prior episiotomy repairs that have broken down. Check history and do any appropriate tests for coagulation disorders *(45)*; hypofibrinogenemia is not common at this stage.

Mild Cases of Uterine Bleeding

Treatment

- Limited activity, preferably bed rest; uterine massage is of value in the immediate postpartum period (see Fig. 50–1).
- Ergonovine maleate (Ergotrate Maleate), 0.2 mg by mouth 3 to 4 times a day for 3 days; initial dose may be given IM.
- Antibiotics with any evidence of infection.
- Gynecologic examination and care if bleeding persists.

Retained Tissue or Severe Uterine Bleeding

Severe cases, especially those with fever, require immediate hospitalization and a gynecologist's attention. Treatment of shock *(57)* may be necessary. If there is heavy bleeding, T and CM for possible transfusion and give IV crystalloids as NS or RL. Monitored intravenous injection of 20 units of oxytocin (Pitocin) in 500 ml of 5% dextrose solution will control hemorrhage in some instances. Uterine curettage is important for removal of any retained tissue; uterine artery ligation or hysterectomy may still be required with persistent severe bleeding. Uterine compression and massage performed between the fingers of one hand placed vaginally and the other hand cupping the uterus abdominally should be tried. Pressure on the distal aorta with the fist pushed abdominally against the lumbosacral promontory may slow brisk bleeding pending uterine artery/hypogastric artery ligature.

50–13. HYPEREMESIS GRAVIDARUM

Although of unknown cause, the weight loss and dehydration due to persistent nausea and vomiting usually occurring during the second to third month of pregnancy must be differentiated from organic systemic illness and abdominal pain *(22)*. Nondiabetic ketoacidosis may be present owing to starvation effect, and physical findings are related to that and dehydration.

Treatment

Hospitalization is advisable for persistent or severe cases. Bed rest, solitude, intravenous rehydration, correction of any electrolyte imbalance, and subsequent clear liquids and nutritious bland diet with vitamin supplement, plus psychologic evaluation, reassurance and evaluation of any domestic-social problems are fundamental. An antiemetic such as chlorpromazine (Thorazine) 25 mg by parenteral, rectal or oral route, may be necessary; ice chips, tea and soda crackers may be adequate in milder cases. Encourage small frequent feedings.

50–14. HYPERTENSIVE DISEASE IN PREGNANCY

Preeclampsia

Preeclampsia is any combination of two of the following factors: blood pressure of 140/90 mm Hg or 30/15 mm Hg rise over baseline, albuminuria or peripheral edema. The patient may also have headache, lassitude and, in severe cases, epigastric pain, impaired vision and greater degrees of albuminuria.

Treatment

- Even in mild cases of preeclampsia, patients require emergency treatment and should be referred to an obstetrician without delay. Bed rest and quiet are usually needed.
- Severe cases require the same type of treatment as does eclampsia.

Eclampsia

Limited almost exclusively to the last trimester of pregnancy, an eclamptic convulsion or coma heralds a life-threatening obstetric condition that requires immediate and expert treatment and prompt termination of pregnancy. Onset may be precipitous, but usually signs and symptoms of preeclampsia have been present.

Treatment

- Insurance of an adequate airway and administration of oxygen by face mask, nasal catheter or endotracheal tube.
- Protection against injury, especially tongue biting and musculoskeletal damage. Control of convulsions *(34)*.
- Consultation with an obstetrician should be obtained to evaluate for immediate delivery.
- Start an IV line with 5% dextrose in water (D5W) for hydration and as a route for medications to control hypertension and convulsions. Use an infusion pump (IMED or IVAC) whenever possible, for precision administration.
- Magnesium sulfate, 3 to 4 g of a 20% solution with 100 ml D5W given IV (using an infusion pump) over 5 to 30 minutes, depending on severity and response. Maintenance is required with continuous infusion of 1 g/hr, preferably monitored with the patient in or adjacent to an obstetric suite. Monitor blood pressure, urine volume, serum Mg levels and also reflexes for signs of magnesium toxicity *(46–9)*.
- If diastolic BP is 110 mm Hg or higher, initiate hypertension control with hydralazine hydrochloride (Apresoline), 5 mg IV, and monitor blood pressure (BP) every 5 to 10 minutes. Repeat in 15 minutes until the diastolic pressure is between 100 and 110 mm Hg. Seek a gradual rather than precipitous drop. Do not attempt to get BP much under 150/100. Maintenance reduction doses are necessary.

50–15. MISCARRIAGE *(See 50–3)*

50–16. NEONATAL EMERGENCY CARE *(See 52)*

50–17. PREECLAMPSIA *(See 50–14)*

50–18. PREMATURE LABOR

Bed rest, psychologic reassurance, relief from any stress and obstetric consultation are basic. Based on all factors, a decision must be made whether to encourage or discourage the premature labor.

Emergency reduction of potentially dangerous, undesired uterine contractions in immature labor (from 20 to less than 28 weeks' gestation) and premature labor (from 28 to 36 weeks' gestation) may require the following measures:

1. Use of ritodrine HC1 (Yutopar) or terbutaline SO_4 (Brethine). (*Note:* Only ritodrine is currently approved by the FDA for this use.)
2. Although not commonly used now, IV 10% ethanol may be given, infused

at a rate of 0.12 ml/kg/min, with close monitoring during the first 2 hours and proceeding at one-tenth that rate the next 4 hours; if delivery becomes inevitable, stop the infusion immediately and preferably 6 hours before delivery. $MgSO_4$ may also be given in an attempt to stop premature labor.

3. Administration of 12 mg of betamethasone IM, repeated in 12 hours, preferably initiated 48 hours before delivery, may help reduce the risk of hyaline membrane disease or respiratory distress syndrome (RDS) (see *56–10*).

50–19. PREMATURE RUPTURE OF MEMBRANES (PROM)

Spontaneous rupture of the membranes before the start of uterine contractions occurs in about 10% of deliveries.

The diagnosis may be suspected by the presence of characteristic fluid from the vagina and possibly decreased abdominal size plus easier palpation of fetal parts. A vaginal speculum exam should be performed under strict sterile conditions, in order to (1) observe for fluid passage per os and collect sample with sterile swabs for nitrazine test (amniotic fluid is alkaline), fern test (positive test confirms membrane rupture) and culture; (2) check that there is no vaginal prolapse of cord; and (3) determine amount of cervical dilatation. L/S ratio may be done from vaginal pool specimen. Additionally, the obstetrician, in difficult diagnostic cases, may perform amniocentesis under ultrasound control; besides evaluating gestational age by ultrasound and getting amniotic fluid for L/S ratio to determine fetal pulmonary maturity, injection of 0.2 to 0.4 ml of sterile indigo carmine into the amniotic sac has been performed at the same time by some investigators; PROM is proved if a perineal pad is later stained blue. Pelvic exams should be minimized if the patient is not in labor.

Treatment

Hospitalize for obstetrical management. Treatment decisions are based primarily on the presence or absence of amnionitis and fetal (pulmonary) maturity.

1. If amnionitis is present or cannot be ruled out, proceed as described in *50–4, Amnionitis*.
2. If fetal maturity is confirmed at over 36 weeks, proceed with induction of labor if not spontaneously started within 12 to 16 hours of PROM.
3. In cases of fetal immaturity (gestational age under 33 weeks), take the mother's temperature at least every 4 to 6 hours and externally check once a day for uterine tenderness and do a WBC count to check for infection until gestational age has reached 33 weeks.
4. If fetal maturity is borderline (33 to 36 weeks):

- If fetal pulmonary maturity (*50–9*) is established, proceed as #2 above.
- If low risk for amnionitis and fetal pulmonary immaturity established (or tests unavailable), proceed as described in #3 above until pulmonary maturity is established later or gestational age has reached 36 weeks.
- If risk for amnionitis is high and pulmonary maturity tests are unavailable, proceed as described in #2.

50–20. SYNCOPE *(See also 49–19)*

Pregnant women are more prone to certain types of syncopal episodes. Hyperventilation (*54–11*) is foremost as a cause. Diabetic control during pregnancy is more unstable and can further complicate an increased propensity to hypoglycemia (*46–15*) and nutritional deficiencies. Orthostatic hypotension and vasovagal syncope occur in pregnancy, as well as vena cava syndrome (*50–23*) later in the pregnancy. Accompanying hypertension and grand mal seizure point to eclampsia (*50–14*). Anemia and hemorrhage may be underlying causes of syncope. Dysrhythmias may precede syncope. Preexisting cardiac pathology, known or previously occult, may be aggravated by the increased blood volume and cardiac work of later pregnancy, and can contribute to cardiac causes of syncope.

50–21. UMBILICAL CORD PROLAPSE AND RUPTURE

Episodic fetal distress with irregular slowed heart rate should be suspected as being related to umbilical cord prolapse and compromise even when the cord is not palpably or visibly extruded. It is most common when the presentation is other than vertex. Umbilical cord rupture causes similar initial distress, and vaginal bleeding may be seen. Change of maternal position causes no significant change, however (in contrast to vena cava syndrome), and fetal distress is rapidly progressive and necessitates immediate delivery. Obtain obstetric consultation and fetal heart tone monitoring as soon as possible.

Treatment

Place the patient in the position in which quality, rate and rhythm are most normal, usually the knee-chest position (or sometimes lying on the side) if immediate vaginal delivery is not feasible. Manually elevate the baby's presenting part in the vagina with the gloved hand, to keep pressure off the cord. Do not attempt to stuff the cord back in. Delivery often can be managed from the knee-chest position. Arrange for immediate cesarean section if the fetus is viable. Give supplemental oxygen to the mother.

50–23. VENA CAVA SYNDROME

Examination of the mother in the full supine position may cause fetal weight to compress the inferior vena cava, giving rise to hypotension, syncope and subsequent fetal distress and may precipitate an abruptio placentae. Turn the patient to the left side to get the uterus off of the vena cava and routinely examine in the semi-supine/lateral position to avoid occurrence. This syndrome may be aggravated by conduction anesthesia (spinal, saddle, epidural), and it may be necessary to manually lift the uterus off of the vena cava; usually the table is tilted to the left to prevent this.

50–22. UTERINE INVERSION (After Delivery)

Fortunately this serious situation, which is usually associated with severe shock, rarely occurs. One attempt can be made to reduce by pushing cephalad on the cervical region; if this is unsuccessful, wrap the uterus with clean gauze moistened with normal saline if available. Treat hypovolemic shock vigorously (*57*). Emergency obstetric consultation and general anesthesia are usually needed to correct inversion.

51. Oncologic Emergencies

Whether they have a malignancy or not, patients who have a meaningful life or the potential for one, deserve dedication to correction of urgent remediable medical problems. Patients with malignancy may experience any type of emergency situation, but Table 51–1 deals with identification and treatment of some problems occurring more frequently in the presence of malignancy.

Table 51–1. COMMON ONCOLOGIC EMERGENCIES

Problem	Manifestations	Causes	Tests	Treatment
Airway obstruction	Respiratory distress (see also Table 5–2)	Edema and tumor causing mechanical narrowing of major airways	Chest, soft tissue x-rays, bronchogram, tomogram	Remove or bypass obstruction, see 5–21, *Artificial Ventilation; 18–34, Tracheostomy; 18–10, Intubation*. Irradiation, chemotherapy, surgery
CNS involvement				
Brain	Headache; lethargy; depression; confusion; seizures; "stroke;" focal visual and cranial nerve deficit; papilledema; hypoglycemia	IIP from metabolic/toxic infection; some vascular with normal CAT; space occupying lesion	CAT scan; EEG; RIS; x-ray; angiography; ??LP ± lethal with + CAT scan indicating IIP. Evaluate causes IIP with normal CAT scan.	Decrease intracranial pressure by corticosteroid and hyperosmolar infusion (see *44–7*). Treat primary cause. Treat seizures (*34*). Refer for irradiation, surgical evaluation
Meninges	Above plus back/extremity pain. CSF: variable increase in protein levels and decrease in level of glucose, number of malignant cells	As above. Occurs in about 5% of all cancer patients (especially lung and breast cancer, lymphoma)	As above; cautious drawing of CSF, if at all (see *18–29, Spinal Puncture*). Culture and exam for bacteria, cells	As above. Referral for intrathecal therapy and/or cranial-spinal irradiation
Spinal Cord	Pain (focal/radicular), paresthesias, focal neurologic deficits, paraparesis	Compression from extramedullary metastatic tumor or vertebral collapse	As above, plus myelogram or CAT scan; x-ray	Prompt referral for any necessary surgical decompression, irradiation and/or chemotherapy, steroids
Increased Intracranial Pressure (IIP) with CAT scan	As for *Brain*, above	↑ pCO_2, ↓ Hgb, ↑ BUN, ↑ Osm, ↑ RBC (see *45–11*), ↑ BP, CNS infection or toxicity, possibly anticancer agents	Studies as indicated under *Causes*. Check for jugular/SVC syndrome (see below, under *Vascular*) and for sinus thrombosis	See *44–7, Cerebral Edema*. Withhold steroids if already toxic factor. Treat primary cause

Electrolyte imbalance	Hypercalcemia; see *46–6*	Mainly osteolysis factors: prostaglandins, parathormone-like substance	Serum levels and electrocardiogram (See *11–2* and Fig. 46–1)	See *46–6*, *Hypercalcemia*
	Hypokalemia; see *46–16*	Diarrhea, renal tubular defect, ↑Ca, acute leukemia	As for *Hypercalcemia*, above	See *46–16*, *Hypokalemia*
	Hyperkalemia; see *46–8*	Cytolytic therapy; renal impairment	As for *Hypercalcemia*, above	See *46–8*, *Hyperkalemia*
	Hyponatremia; see *46–18*	SIADH (see *46–18*)	As for *Hypercalcemia*, above	See *46–18*, *Hyponatremia*
Hyperuricemia	Ureteral stones and colic; see *32–16*, Uremia	Increased mitosis, cell destruction from therapy, decreased excretion, dehydration	Serum uric acid, creatinine, urea nitrogen, electrolytes; urinalysis, including test for urate crystals	Allopurinol, 300 to 600 mg daily during cytolytic therapy. See *46–5* for urine volume and pH control
Vascular Embolus	Destruction of organ or extremity tissue and function	Tumor embolus or segments of thrombus	See *63–6*, *Vascular Disorders*, *Embolism*	See *63–6*, *Vascular Disorders*, *Embolism*
Hemorrhage	Acute severe vascular bleeding	Erosion of blood vessel wall. Coagulation abnormality.	Test for coagulation disorders (see Table 45–1)	See *45–1*, *Control of Bleeding* See *45–2*, *General Measures*
Pericardial tamponade	Friction rub, ↓heart sounds, ↓pulse pressure, distended neck veins, paradoxical pulse, dyspnea, chest pain	Effusion from pericardial metastasis and postirradiation pericarditis	See *29–18*, *Pericardial Effusion*	See *18–22*, *Pericardial Aspiration*. Consider intrapericardial chemotherapy, radiation, surgical window
Superior vena cava (SVC) syndrome	Neck, facial, upper extremity venous distention and edema and complications thereof; headache; IIP	Venous hypertension greatest with SVC blockage by thoracic neoplasm below the azygos vein	Clinical findings plus chest x-ray adequate. Avoid biopsy and arm venipuncture, if possible	Refer for prompt irradiation and subsequent chemotherapy

52. Pediatric Emergencies

Treatment of neonatal emergencies, and the work of neonatologists and neonatology in general, has emerged as one of the principal subspecialties of pediatrics.

The neonatal period is commonly considered to be from birth to 28 days of extrauterine life. Aspects of pediatric care beyond that period are incorporated into the general chapters. In each of the situations discussed in this chapter, assistance of a neonatologist or pediatrician should be obtained as soon as possible.

EMERGENCIES AT DELIVERY

52–1. RESUSCITATION AT BIRTH

The birth APGAR score provides a guide for determining the degree of intervention an infant will need following birth. It is determined by adding together the individual scores assigned to each of the five categories shown in the following table. An experienced physician or neonatologist should attend all high-risk deliveries, because such expertise is required for quick decisions and skillful resuscitation of the infant.

The following procedures should be used for immediate neonatal resuscitation:

	0	1	2
A Appearance (Color)	Blue, pale	Body pink, extremities blue	Completely pink
P Pulse (Heart rate)	Absent	Less than 100 per minute	Greater than 100 per minute
G Grimace (Response to nasal catheter)	No response	Grimace	Cough, sneeze
A Activity (Muscle tone)	Limp	Some flexion of extremities	Active motion
R Respiratory Effort	Absent	Slow, irregular	Good excursion, strong cry

Preliminary Measures. Place the infant on a radiant warmer (or warm blanket if unavailable), dry the skin with gentle stimulating rubbing, clear the oropharynx with suctioning and determine the APGAR score at 1 minute or less. A bulb syringe and small suction catheter may be used. If no equipment is available for suctioning, momentarily invert the infant, grasp firmly and apply mouth suction across the infant's mouth and nose after sweeping the mouth out using the finger.

Respiratory Resuscitation

- Infants with APGAR scores of 0 or 1 require immediate endotracheal intubation *(18–10)* and ventilation. Ventilate the infant using 80% inspired oxygen, a respiratory rate of 40 and a maximum pressure of 30 cm of water.

If a hand mechanical ventilator is not available, short puffs of mouth–to–mouth-nose ventilation just sufficient to cause the chest to rise 20 to 30 times per minute should be used. In infants, the neck is only minimally retroflexed to straight for mouth–to–mouth-nose ventilation and intubation, as the larynx is very anterior in the neonate. The angle of the mandible must be elevated anteriorly for more effective ventilation.

- Infants with 1-minute APGAR scores of 2 to 5 need bag-and-mask ventilation and reevaluation for improvement at 2 and 5 minutes.
- Most infants having 1-minute scores of 4 to 6 need only oxygen by mask, warmth and gentle tactile stimulation with rubbing and drying.
- Those with initial APGAR scores of 7 or greater need no therapy, just continued evaluation and supportive care—particularly warmth and drying.
- Gastric fluid and air distention should be removed via a small orogastric catheter, but routine orogastric suction should be delayed until 5 minutes after birth, to avoid vagal-induced bradycardia.

Cardiac Resuscitation

- Use external cardiac compression for asystole or bradycardia below 60 beats/min or heart rate less than 80 beats/min after 1 to 3 minutes of assisted ventilation. The operator's fingers are placed around and behind the chest (no constrictive pressure) and the thumbs used to depress the mid-lower sternum approximately two thirds of the distance to the vertebral column and to release at a rate of 100 to 120 beats per minute.
- Drugs and doses (administer intravascularly by catheterizing the umbilical artery or vein) for cardiac resuscitation include the following:

Drug	Condition	Dose
Epinephrine	Cardiac arrest (asystole)	0.1 ml/kg of 1:10,000 solution
Atropine	Persistent bradycardia	0.01 mg/kg
Calcium gluconate	Persistent bradycardia	100 mg/kg of 10% solution slowly

Metabolic Resuscitation. If APGAR score is 0 or 1 at 1 minute or less than 5 at 5 minutes, administer sodium bicarbonate for correction of acidosis. Two mEq of molar bicarbonate diluted with an equal volume of 5% dextrose is infused at 1 mEq/kg/min. *No bicarbonate is given until ventilation has been established.*

52–2. HYPOVOLEMIC SHOCK (Blood Loss Type)

Tachycardia (more than 160 beats/min), pallor, slow capillary filling, weak pulses, and hypotension based on neonatal blood pressure standards (term infant less than 50 mm Hg systolic). Placental, cord or fetal hemorrhage and birth asphyxia are common causes, as is "fetal-placental transfusion."

Treatment

Administer 10 ml/kg of type O negative whole blood typed against the mother if available. Otherwise, 10 ml/kg of 5% albumin solution or lactated Ringer's solution may be substituted. Infuse over 10 minutes and repeat if there is no improvement in diagnostic parameters.

52–3. SEVERE ERYTHROBLASTOSIS FETALIS

Dyspnea, hepatosplenomegaly, edema and extreme pallor are present.

Maternal Rh sensitization is the commonest cause. Take a sample of cord blood (for Coombs test) and maternal blood [for type, presence of anti-Rh_0 (D) antibodies] and cross match blood for infant transfusion.

Treatment

Assisted ventilation and plan partial exchange transfusion with type O-negative packed red cells; cardiorespiratory assessment [also consider giving the mother Rh_0 (D) immune globulin].

52–4. MECONIUM ASPIRATION

Thick, particulate meconium in the amniotic fluid and fetal heart rate abnormalities are clues to presence of meconium aspiration. Intrauterine growth retardation, fetal asphyxia and postmaturity are frequent underlying factors.

Treatment

Immediately after delivery of the head, the oropharynx is aspirated with a DeLee suction apparatus; if this is not available, a soft bulb syringe may be used. If thick, particulate meconium is present in the oropharynx, immediately intubate and suction via mouth-to-endotracheal tube until respirations are established. Attempt to clear all meconium within 60 seconds and initiate resuscitation if deterioration occurs. Subsequently, use postural drainage, percussion, suctioning and supplemental mist and inspirated oxygen based on arterial blood gas analysis. Aspirate the stomach if distended.

52–5. DIAPHRAGMATIC HERNIA

Dyspnea and cyanosis, shifted heart tones, decreased breath sounds on the involved side and a scaphoid abdomen occur with this developmental abnormality.

Treatment

Immediate intubation and assisted ventilation; maintenance of a head-and-chest elevated position; continuous gastric suction; radiographic confirmation; and emergency pediatric surgical consultation are indicated. Post-repair cimetidine (Tagamet) may result in improvement).

52–6. PNEUMOTHORAX *(See also 56–17, Pneumothorax; Table 5–3, Guide to Localization of Respiratory Tract Obstruction)*

Unilateral absent breath sounds and increased percussion tympany, shifted heart tones, dyspnea, cyanosis and shock-like appearance are usually found.

Aspiration syndromes, variable forms of congenital cystic lung disease and barotrauma from overzealous assisted ventilation contribute to occurrence of pneumothorax.

Treatment

1. Immediate confirmation of the diagnosis by fiberoptic transillumination of the thorax or chest radiograph.
2. If infant is severely hypoxemic or "shocky," aspirate the pleural space with an 18-gauge angiocatheter, 3-way stopcock and 20-ml syringe.

3. If the air leak is under tension, a closed-chest drainage system should be immediately established.

52–7. CONGENITAL AIRWAY OBSTRUCTION *(See also Table 5–3, Guide to Localization of Respiratory Tract Obstruction)*

- *Choanal atresia*—the infant becomes a normal pink only with crying; there is inability to pass a nasal catheter into the pharynx. Immediately intubate and consult an otolaryngologist.
- *Laryngeal atresia*—this rare condition is characterized by violent inspiratory efforts, aphonia and cyanosis. Immediate tracheostomy is required.
- *Congenital goiter* and other neck and oropharyngeal masses may cause airway obstruction resulting in dyspnea and cyanosis. Immediate intubation, tracheostomy or surgery is necessary.

CARDIOVASCULAR DISEASES

52–8. STRUCTURAL CARDIOVASCULAR DISEASE

Central cyanosis (pO_2<50 torr despite good ventilation and 100% oxygen administration) and/or congestive heart failure should lead to consideration of the presence of valvular atresias, complex cardiac anomalies and asphyxial cardiomyopathy.

Treatment

Supplemental oxygen (based on arterial blood gases—oxygen level or acidosis), treat congestive heart failure, refer immediately to tertiary (most comprehensive care status) neonatal center that, if indicated, can perform open heart surgery. Note: High oxygen inhalation may cause ductal closure in a ductal-dependent lesion.

To maintain ductal patency when ductal-dependent cyanotic heart disease is present, prostaglandin E_1 (0.1 μg/kg/min) should be started prior to and maintained during transport to a tertiary center.

52–9. PULMONARY HYPERTENSION—PERSISTENCE OF THE FETAL CIRCULATION

Dyspnea and cyanosis are noted without the presence of pulmonary or structural heart disease. Echocardiography and right radial and distal aortic blood gases may help establish the diagnosis. The most common causes of this situation are fetal or birth asphyxia, meconium or amniotic fluid aspiration, pneumonia and sepsis. Hypoglycemia *(52–10)*, hypocalcemia *(52–11)* and cold stress aggravate the condition. Serum glucose and calcium levels should be checked.

Treatment

Oxygen-assisted ventilation—including rapid ventilation (80 to 120 breaths/minute) dopamine or tolazoline may be indicated. Treat primary disease, hypoglycemia and hypocalcemia, and refer to a tertiary center.

ENDOCRINE AND METABOLIC DISORDERS

52–10. HYPOGLYCEMIA *(See also 46–15)*

Lethargy, sweating, apnea, cyanosis, jitteriness and seizures should alert to the possibility of underlying hypoglycemia, which is confirmed by the laboratory serum glucose level. Birth asphyxia, prematurity, intrauterine growth retardation, maternal diabetes with hyperinsulin effect and infection are underlying conditions that can cause hypoglycemia.

Treatment

- Treat the primary disease.
- If asymptomatic and glucose level is between 25 and 40 mg%, implement oral feeding and serial checks for blood sugar levels, as with Dextrostix.
- If symptomatic or glucose value is less than 25 mg%, infuse 10% dextrose IV at 80 to 120 ml/kg/day. Do serial Dextrostix checks.

52–11. HYPOCALCEMIA *(See also 46–15)*

Apnea, irritability and seizures occur with hypocalcemia, which is difficult to differentiate from hypoglycemia *(52–10)* except through laboratory determinations and therapeutic response to IV calcium. Leading causes of this condition are prematurity, birth asphyxia and maternal diabetes. Check serum magnesium and phosphorus also.

Treatment

- Confirm diagnosis—serum calcium less than 7 mg%.
- Therapy—if seizures, IV infusion of 100 to 400 mg of calcium gluconate slowly; maintenance using elemental calcium, 75 mg/kg daily in divided doses.

52–12. CONGENITAL ADRENAL HYPERPLASIA *(See also 36–4)*

An autosomal recessive gene is responsible for this condition, which is manifest by female virilization, salt-losing symptoms (shock) and hypertension in some patients.

Treatment

- Confirm diagnosis with serum 17α-hydroxyprogesterone, testosterone and dihydroepiandrosterone levels.
- Treat salt-losing crisis with:
  —IV salt-containing fluids.
  —Desoxycorticosterone, 2 mg IM.
  —Cortisol, 50 mg/day.

52–13. CONGENITAL THYROTOXICOSIS *(See also 36–11)*

Irritability, goiter, tachycardia, flushing and congestive failure are seen with congenital thyrotoxicosis. Transplacental stimulating immunoglobulin G (IgG) is principally responsible for this condition in infants.

Treatment

- Relieve tracheal obstruction
- Alleviate cardiovascular symptoms with propranolol, 1 to 2 mg/kg/day.
- Suppress thyroid gland activity with saturated potassium iodide (favored) or propylthiouracil.

52–14. HYPERBILIRUBINEMIA

Hyperbilirubinemia (bilirubin levels in excess of physiologic jaundice) and kernicterus [bilirubin-induced central nervous system (CNS) encephalopathy] are most frequently due to prematurity, infection, blood incompatibility and polycythemia.

Treatment

- Treat contributory factors/disease.
- Phototherapy—start at a bilirubin concentration of 5 mg/dl below expected exchange transfusion (as follows).
- Exchange transfusion (consult a pediatrician or neonatologist) is indicated in the following cases:

—Term infants—exchange when indirect bilirubin level exceeds 20 mg/dl, when bilirubin-binding assays are not available.

—Preterm infants—exchange when indirect bilirubin exceeds a level greater than 1 mg/dl for each 100 g of body weight. For example, a well-appearing, 1300-g premature infant should have an exchange transfusion when the indirect bilirubin value equals 13 mg/dl; if ill, exchange at 11 mg/dl. Use a 2 mg/dl lower indirect bilirubin value for ill premature neonates (e.g., respiratory distress syndrome, sepsis, acidosis, hypoglycemia).

—Any infants exhibiting symptoms of kernicterus (poor suck, lethargy, opisthotonus, acidosis).

52–15. RARE METABOLIC DISORDERS

Galactosemia, maple syrup urine disease, methylmalonic acidemia, hyperammonemia and other metabolic disorders can cause lethargy, poor feeding, seizures, acidosis and ketosis.

Treatment

- Nothing by mouth; use IV dextrose infusion.
- Refer to tertiary neonatal center.

INFECTIOUS DISEASES

52–16. CONGENITAL PNEUMONIA

Congenital pneumonia usually follows premature or prolonged ruptured membranes, premature labor, maternal amnionitis or perinatal distress. Signs and symptoms are respiratory distress, abnormal chest radiograph, hypotension and acidosis; absolute neutrophil count is less than 1500 or immature/total neutrophil ratio is over 0.20.

Treatment

- Specific diagnosis by endotracheal aspirate culture.
- Supportive care.
- Antibiotics: the gentamicin dose at 0 to 7 days of age is 5 mg/kg/day given in divided doses every 12 hours IV or IM. Increase to 7.5 mg/kg/day in divided doses every 8 hours after 7 days of age. The ampicillin dose is 50 mg/kg/day given in divided doses every 12 hours IV or IM at less than 7 days of age. Increase to 75 to 100 mg/kg/day in divided doses every 8 hours at 7 days of age or older.

If meningitis is also present, use ampicillin and gentamicin instead at 100 mg/kg/day and 7.5 mg/kg/day, respectively, in divided doses; obtain blood and probably cerebrospinal fluid (CSF) and antibiotic levels. Ampicillin dosage increases to 200 mg/kg/day if the patient is 1 to 4 weeks of age. Consider use of chloramphenicol only if blood levels can be monitored.

52–17. SEPSIS AND/OR MENINGITIS

The associated predisposing problems are the same as those of congenital pneumonia *(52–16)*. Likewise, the signs and symptoms are similar to those of pneumonia and include lethargy, poor feeding, thermal irritability and seizures. Blood cultures or lumbar puncture *(18–29)* confirm the diagnosis. Fontanelle taps may be used for diagnosis of ventriculitis and for checking lack of adequate therapy for neonatal meningitis.

Treatment

Treatment is the same as for pneumonia; seek immediate pediatric consultation regarding meningitis treatment.

NEUROLOGIC DISEASES

52–18. BIRTH TRAUMA

Birth trauma most often occurs with premature, breech or difficult delivery. Signs and symptoms include seizures *(52–19)* from intracranial hemorrhage, Erb's palsy due to brachial plexus injury (obtain orthopedic consultation) and dyspnea occurring with phrenic nerve injury (provide supportive care, particularly respiratory).

52–19. SEIZURES

Asphyxia, intracranial hemorrhage, intracranial anomalies, drug withdrawal *(52–21)*, infections, birth defects and endocrine and metabolic disorders, particularly hypoglycemia *(52–10)* and hypocalcemia *(52–11)*, are contributory causes.

Treatment

- Treat primary disease (e.g., meningitis, hypoglycemia).
- Seizure control: phenobarbital is the treatment of choice. Loading doses up to 10 mg/kg IV for 1 to 2 doses for seizure control. Maintenance dose of 5 mg/kg/day every 12 hours, IV, IM or PO. Diphenylhydantoin (Dilantin), drug of second choice, 5 to 10 mg slowly IV for treatment failures. Maintenance dose of 5 mg/kg/day every 12 hours, IV or PO.

Blood levels are essential in optimizing seizure control in neonates. Side effects of diazepam preclude its routine use in neonatal seizure control. Pyridoxine hydrochloride (vitamin B_6) on trial basis will aid deficiency states. Obtain neurologic or pediatric consultation.

52–20. APNEA

Prematurity, trauma, seizures, infection and metabolic factors (including maternal drugs) are causes or are associated with onset of apnea.

Treatment

Cardiac and respiratory resuscitation *(52–1)*, primary disease treatment and stimulation, such as with gentle rubbing, will aid. Biophysical monitoring of cardiac and respiratory is essential, and an at-risk assessment for SIDS should be made prior to discontinuing such monitoring. Aminophylline (2 to 4 mg/kg/day every 8 or 12 hours) or caffeine (10-20 mg/kg loading dose and 5 mg/kg maintenance given once or twice per day) can help reduce the chance of recurrence. Obtain pediatric or neonatal consultation.

52–21. DRUG WITHDRAWAL

If the mother has been providing the fetus with narcotics, barbiturates or alcohol via the placental route, the infant will often demonstrate onset of withdrawal several hours after or within the day of delivery. Methadone can cause withdrawal symptoms for from hours up to 2 to 3 weeks after birth. This is in addition to the problems of immediate toxicity noted occasionally at birth, which are partially dependent on time since the mother's last dose. Alcohol is no longer used medically to inhibit labor. (Fetal alcohol syndrome refers to the malformations caused rather than withdrawal problems). Signs and symptoms of drug withdrawal include: irritability, poor feeding, sweating, temperature instability and seizures.

Treatment

- Narcotic withdrawal can be treated with tincture of paregoric, 2 gtt/kg PO q 4 to 6 h, and/or chlorpromazine, 2 mg/kg/day IM q 6 h, or phenobarbital, 10 to 20 mg/kg/day loading dose, followed by 5 mg/kg/day divided into q 12 h doses), depending on severity.
- Barbiturate or alcohol addiction—mostly supportive care during withdrawal.

52–22. MENINGOMYELOCELE

Keep the area clean, prevent focal trauma and obtain neurosurgical consultation.

52–23. NEONATAL MYASTHENIA GRAVIS

Two forms of myasthenia gravis are seen:

- *Transient*—seen in about 12% of infants of myasthenic mothers.
- *Congenital*—rare.

Characteristic findings are feeding problems, respiratory difficulty, weak cry and hypotonia. Improvement upon therapeutic trial of neostigmine methylsulfate with atropine helps establish the diagnosis.

Treatment is maintenance on neostigmine, 1 mg, one-half hour before feedings and titrated as indicated.

RESPIRATORY DISEASES

52–24. RESPIRATORY DISTRESS SYNDROME (RDS or Hyaline Membrane Disease) *(See also 56–2, Acute Respiratory Distress Syndrome)*

Prematurity, maternal diabetes, iatrogenic early delivery, birth asphyxia, bacterial pneumonia, patent ductus arteriosus, and perinatal hemorrhage are all factors contributing to or associated with RDS. Grunting, flaring of the nares, retracting of intercostal spaces, cyanosis and reticulogranular radiographic appearance with air bronchograms are indicative of RDS.

Treatment

Supportive, including monitored supplemental oxygen; obtain pediatric or neonatal consultation. See also comments concerning prophylactic treatment in premature labor *(50–18)*.

52–25. TRACHEOESOPHAGEAL ATRESIA (AND FISTULA)

The signs and symptoms of this congenital anomaly are polyhydramnios, dyspnea, choking and inability to pass a nasogastric tube much beyond the oropharynx.

Treatment

Place the infant in a semi-upright posture, provide continuous suction of pouch, give respiratory support and obtain immediate pediatric surgical consultation.

SURGICAL EMERGENCIES

52–26. INTESTINAL OBSTRUCTION

The most common causes are atresias, volvulus, aganglionic megacolon and imperforate anus. Symptoms of obstruction include bilious emesis; delayed, scant or absent meconium passage; and abdominal distention.

Treatment

Confirm the diagnosis by radiograph. Provide nasogastric suction and intravenous fluids; obtain a pediatric surgical consultation.

52–27. ABDOMINAL WALL DEFECTS (Omphalocele or Gastroschisis)

Treatment for these conditions should commence with covering of the defect with sterile, warm, saline-soaked gauze. Provide supportive care and intravenous fluids and obtain immediate pediatric surgical consultation.

52–28. INTESTINAL PERFORATION

Obstructions and necrotizing enterocolitis are the most common causes of intestinal perforation at this age. Signs, symptoms and treatment are as for intestinal obstruction (*52–26*); also treat sepsis.

OTHER PEDIATRIC EMERGENCIES

52–29. CHILD ABUSE OR BATTERED CHILD SYNDROME

Abuse of children by parents or other custodians is common, so much so that special laws have been enacted in many localities, including all 50 states of the United States, aimed not only at protection of children but also at protection of the attending physician, who also has a legal, moral and ethical obligation to report cases of child abuse to the proper law enforcement agencies (*15*). Evidence of the battered child syndrome is usually incidental to examination for an acute condition for which the child is brought to medical attention.

The attending physician should have a high index of suspicion when examination of an infant or child discloses any of the following conditions:

- Any instance in which there is a discrepancy between the condition found and the history on onset given by the parents or other interested persons. An attempt should be made to distinguish between an accidental and an induced injury. The possibility of a contrived or prearranged accident should also be considered.

- All cases in which the history of onset given by the parents differs from that given by neighbors or other witnesses.
- All "crib deaths" (52–30, *Sudden Infant Death Syndrome [SIDS]*) Recent studies seem to indicate that a few of these deaths are in fact infanticide.
- X-ray demonstration of multiple fractures in varying stages of healing. This finding is usually considered to be conclusive evidence of child abuse.
- Severe head injuries (fractures, subdural hematomas, etc.), especially if repeated.
- Multiple bruises in different stages of healing.
- Burns, especially a series of burns with an indefinite or unconvincing history of how they occurred.
- Recurrent subluxations, especially of the elbows and shoulders.
- Malnutrition and skin infections indicative of severe neglect; unexplained failure to thrive.
- Repeat episodes of poisoning (53).
- Unusual behavior by the child, such as fawning, cowering, subservience or extreme paucity of activity when told to be still.

The responsibilities of the attending physician are primarily the same as for any other type of case—adequate diagnosis and proper treatment. Every effort should be made to keep good rapport with the persons concerned with care of the injured child, avoiding an accusatory or punitive approach. Secondarily, however, the attending physician has the direct responsibility of reporting the condition to the proper authorities and of assisting in measures for evaluating the personality of the child's attendants by a special examiner trained and skilled in this field. Lastly, the attending physician should be prepared and willing to testify in court, in case a legal action should ensue. Failure to report can result in loss of the physician's medical license, criminal charges and civil action. Authorities may direct removal of the child from the home for welfare of the child. Increasingly stringent laws and penalties pertaining to child abusers will probably be enacted. Sweden has even gone so far as to pass a law prohibiting parents or others from striking or otherwise humiliating a child, even for discipline.

52–30. SUDDEN INFANT DEATH SYNDROME (SIDS—"Crib deaths")

Every year, about 25,000 infants, usually between 1 week and 2 years of age, who appear in good health (or have only insignificant-appearing problems) when put to bed, are found dead in bed in the morning. The peak incidence is between 3 and 6 months of age with a higher incidence in males, in prematures and when there is a family history of prior cases of SIDS. Death is invariably silent, though there may be evidence to suggest a terminal convulsion, hypoxemia and struggle (defecation, urination, emesis, blood-tinged oronasal froth, blanket fibers in clenched hands), and occurs during sleep. Postmortem examination, which should be done early, usually reveals nonspecific findings; laryngospasm, pulmonary edema, hypertrophy of medial smooth muscle layers of smaller pulmonary arteries and slightly dilated right ventricle and atrium may be present. Previously undetected infection, anomalies of the central nervous or cardiovascular system or evidence to support abnormal physiologic mechanisms may be found in up to 15% of patients. Sleep apnea may be a very important underlying event. The possibility of a toxin (from *Clostridium difficile*) is under evaluation.

The emergency in these cases deals principally in management of the bereaved parents (see 54–3, *Acute Situational Reactions*). The universal reaction of the parents is to place unfounded guilt upon themselves. Assistance from local chapter members of the National Foundation for SIDS—(312)663–0650—or International Guild for Infant Survival—(202)833–2253—can be of great value and comfort.

In "near sudden death syndrome," as in "near drowning" *(25–3)*, the efforts are aimed first at resuscitation *(5–1)* and correction of metabolic acidosis *(46–1)*, then at evaluation for concomitant infection or anomalies (including testing at specially-equipped sleep apnea centers), followed by close mechanical or direct personal monitoring, or both, for incipient hypoxemic states or recurrence.

Crib deaths have been blamed in the past on numerous conditions. Among these are suffocating from bedclothes, battered child syndrome *(52–29)*, parathyroid abnormality, acute overwhelming bacterial or viral infections, hypersensitivity to cow's milk, deficient levels of immunoglobulins, toxic agents and deficits in magnesium and selenium. SIDS is a definite clinical entity whose etiology remains unknown.

53. Poisoning, Acute

53–1. DEFINITIONS

Sollmann: "A poison is any substance which, acting directly through its inherent chemical properties, and by its ordinary action, is capable of destroying life or of seriously endangering health, when it is applied to the body externally, or in moderate doses (to 50 g) internally." This definition specifically excludes injurious physical, mechanical and bacterial agents, and substances that are toxic only in very large doses.

Paracelsus (1493–1541): "All substances are poisons. There is none which is not a poison. The right dose differentiates a poison and a remedy."

53–2. INITIAL TREATMENT AXIOMS

- Remove from further toxin exposure and "decontaminate" (see *53–6* and *53–7*).
- Perform rapid "toxicological" physical examination, evaluating:
  —Mental status: evaluate response to voice and pain.
  —Vital signs: pulse, respiration, blood pressure, temperature (rectal thermometer with low scale capacity).
  —Eyes: size and reactivity of pupils, abnormal eye movements, vertical or horizontal nystagmus, eyelash/corneal reflex.
  —Skin: color, wetness, dryness, temperature, perfusion.
  —Bowel sounds: increased or decreased (frequency, intensity, duration, pitch).
  —Muscle tone and activity: flaccidity, tremor, rigidity, myoclonus.
  —Reflexes: DTR, pathologic.
- Neutralize toxins with specific antidotes *(53–10)* as available or modify ill effects. Aid excretion as much as possible without overhydrating.
- Avoid, as much as possible, compounding the initial poisoning toxicity with toxicity from therapeutic agents.
- Vigorous, immediate supportive treatment is of paramount importance (see *53–11*):
  —Airway: Maintain proper positioning (Fig. 4–5*A*); consider intubation *(53–11)*; prevent aspiration.
  —Breathing: assess and periodically reassess air exchange; ventilate as necessary; obtain arterial blood gases.
  —Circulation: Assess pulse, tissue perfusion and blood pressure; start an IV.
  —Dextrose: Every comatose or stuporous patient should be administered the following (after blood sample drawn):
  (a) 25 g of glucose, IV bolus (50 ml D50W)

(b) 100 mg of thiamine IM and 100 mg in IV bottle

(c) Naloxone hydrochloride (Narcan). (*Adults:* minimum 0.4 mg [1-mg ampule] occasional resistant cases [such as with propoxyphene or pentazocine poisoning] may require 1.6 to 2.0 mg. [4–5 ampules] or more [e.g., 4 mg] initially; *children and neonates:* start with 0.01 mg/kg IV, IM or SC in known or suspected narcotics cases.)

- Identify the toxic substance whenever possible and consider its inherent lethality. Obtain appropriate samples (blood, urine) for laboratory analysis—gastric aspirate collection is of limited value. Though blood levels of many substances can be obtained, aspirin *(53–101)*, acetaminophen *(53–19)*, theophylline *(53–694)*, lithium *(53–395)* and ethyl alcohol *(53–295)* are the principal ones in which immediate blood levels direct emergency treatment.
- Label all therapeutic lines connected to the patient. Use arterial monitoring and CVP in complex cases. Monitor I & O, BP, TPR.
- Obtain an electrocardiogram and monitor, as indicated. Also look for EKG clues, such as: long QT interval (phenothiazines, *53–536;* tricyclic antidepressants, *53–723*); wide PR, QRS complex, long QT, variable AV block (tricyclic antidepressants, *53–723;* quinidine, *53–591*); long PR interval with narrow QRS, short QT and variable IV block (digitalis, *53–265*); J wave conduction abnormality (hypothermia, *62–3*); ischemia and infarction (carbon monoxide, *53–175*).
- Obtain an abdominal x-ray (to evaluate for radiopaque substances) and chest x-ray. Common radiopaque medications and substances may be remembered by the mnemonic CHIPETS (*C*hloral hydrate, *H*eavy metals, *I*ron, *P*henothiazines, *E*nteric-coated substances, *T*ricyclic antidepressants and *S*ustained release substances).
- Order evaluations of serum Na, K, Cl, CO_2, creatinine, blood urea nitrogen (BUN) and arterial blood gases, particularly with evidence of respiratory failure or acid-base disturbance. Look for increased anion gap: $(Na)-(CHO_3+Cl)$; some causes of anion gap acidosis are: lactic acidosis (CO poisoning, cyanide, iron), alcohols (ethylene glycol, methanol), salicylates and seizures (as from tricyclic antidepressants, INH, theophylline). Record the anion gap magnitude.
- Serum osmolarity can be both measured and calculated. The formula for calculation is 2(Na) + Blood sugar/18 + BUN/2.8 = mosm/L. Osm gap = measured osm − calculated osm = 0 (normally). Ethanol is the commonest cause of elevated osm gap (20 mosm/L for 100 mg%). Other causes are isopropyl alcohol, methanol, ethylene glycol and dimethyl sulfoxide (DMSO).
- Call Regional Poison Center assistance when treating patients who have toxicity from unfamiliar substances, who are deteriorating in condition despite vigorous supportive therapy or who are in critical condition. Updated microfilm service advice is valuable where available.
- Obtain a body weight as early as practical.
- Assess for mimicking or concomitant problems, such as:
  - —Head trauma: unequal pupils, focal deficits, wounds, hematomas, seizures.
  - —Other trauma causing shock, hypoxemia.
  - —Sepsis: generalized toxemia; meningitis.
  - —Metabolic problems: abnormal glucose, sodium, potassium, BUN; liver or renal disease; etc.
  - —Hypothermia.
- Anticipate delayed effects of ingestions of certain substances, such as iron, acetaminophen and sustained-release preparations such as aspirin and theophylline.
- Remember that more than 50% of poisonings involve more than one toxin.

53–3. CLASSIFICATION

General Classifications

This chapter deals with chemical, mineral and plant poisons. See *24, Allergic Reactions; 60, Stings;* and *27, Bites,* for animal poisons.

Poisons may affect one organ system more than others. The clinical manifestations are dependent not only upon factors such as the type, dose and route(s) of administration; distribution; and excretion dynamics of the toxic agent, but also upon a multitude of variables related to the host (e.g., age, prior physical condition and organ reserve, development of resistance to the toxin or tachyphylaxis). Classification of poisons as neurotoxic and hematoxic has been discarded.

Legal Considerations

Poisonings, whether accidental or intentional, induced by others or self-induced, frequently have legal effects that must be considered. Poisonings accidentally induced by others must be reported by injured employees, and exposure to some chemicals (e.g., pesticides) must be reported to the Public Health Department; civil negligence may also be involved. If a poisoning is intentionally induced by another, criminal charges (attempted murder or murder) plus intentional civil torts are actionable; international laws even "govern" wartime use of some chemicals. Intentional self-induced poisoning is a crime under common law but no longer is a crime under state statutes. Also note that there is a distinction between attempted suicide (a serious, overt effort to kill one's self) and "self-poisoning" (a deliberate, impulsive, conscious, manipulative action that is taken to resolve an intolerable situation and that does not have loss of life as a prime objective); in either event the physician should provide the victim of self-induced poisoning with psychiatric counseling or referral to avoid liability for civil errors and omissions.

Accidental poisoning and suicide attempts each account for about one-tenth of poisoning cases; recognized criminal poisonings are responsible for only a minute fraction of cases, though probably they are much more common than suspected, and the vast remainder of cases are due to "self-poisoning."

53–4. GENERAL THERAPEUTIC CONSIDERATIONS

- If the patient reaches the hospital alive and supportive care is excellent, including removal of unabsorbed toxin, survival is likely, with the death rate usually less than 2%. Only a few specific antidotes *(53–10)* are commonly used and effective. In general: TREAT THE PATIENT AND NOT THE POISON.
- The history obtained from the patient, relatives and friends is often inaccurate as to substance, amount and time of exposure. Toxic agents are often in improperly labeled containers but save containers and any remaining contents, nevertheless.
- Overdosage, both inadvertent and intentional, is far more common than suspected. Overdosage in children is more likely to be a single toxin, whereas in adults, it tends to be multiple (with alcohol often one of the ingredients). Battered child syndrome *(52–29)* should be considered with repeat episodes of pediatric overdosage.

53–5. CLUES TO UNKNOWN TOXIC AGENT TYPE *(See Tables 53–1 and 53–2)*

53–6. REMOVAL FROM FURTHER EXTERNAL TOXIN EXPOSURE

This can be accomplished by taking the toxic source away from the patient or in instances in which the toxin covers a large geographic area, moving the patient away from the source.

53–7. REMOVAL FROM FURTHER INTERNAL TOXIN EXPOSURE

Removal from the Skin and Mucous Membranes. Wash with copious amounts of water immediately and for prolonged period. Chemical antidotes, such as baking soda for acids and vinegar or acetic acid for alkalies, are generally discouraged because of exothermic reactions.

Even though substances such as titanium tetrachloride *(53–708)* or concentrated acid (HCl or H_2SO_4) are exothermic when mixed with water, copious amounts of fluid will reduce and relieve otherwise ill effects. Contaminated clothing should be removed. Particularly when aiding victims of toxins readily absorbed through the skin, such as organic phosphates, the rescuer should wear impervious gloves for self-protection.

Removal from Wounds or Following Hypodermic Administration. Limit muscular activity. See 27–27 for treatment of snakebites.

Removal from the Alimentary and Gastrointestinal Tract. Swallowed poisons should be evacuated as soon as possible by emetics or lavage unless contraindicated (as by definite evidence of mucous membrane corrosion [e.g., from strong mineral acid or alkali], absence of a gag reflex, presence of convulsions or hydrocarbon ingestion of less than 1 ml/kg), even though there is a history of the patient having vomited and several hours or more may have passed since ingestion. Emesis should not be induced in a patient who is unconscious or losing consciousness. If it is known or suspected that the poison has been swallowed with the intent of self-destruction (*17, Suicide and Suicide Attempts*), other body cavities should be examined and evacuated if necessary. Specimens should be saved for possible chemical analysis.

Household Measures to Induce Vomiting

1. Use of syrup of ipecac, as described later, is the approach of choice if readily available. One ounce can be procured without prescription to be on hand for emergency home use.
2. Gargling with soapsuds (nondetergent) or table salt should *not* be done.
3. Such measures as swallowing of large amounts of household mustard in warm water (often ineffective) and tickling the back of the throat as with a tongue blade or fingertips should be avoided, as gastric emptying may be incomplete by these methods.
4. Drinking about 3 to 4 ounces of water may dilute any toxin but mainly provides volume for more effective emesis.

EMETICS. Measures to cause vomiting are indicated whenever a poisonous substance has been swallowed (even many hours earlier), *except* when the vomiting center is paralyzed, the gag reflex is absent, the poison is a corrosive or the patient is convulsing, extremely depressed or comatose; petroleum distillates present the added danger of aspiration pneumonia and require special care (emesis in the standing or sitting position in conscious patients or gastric lavage with use of a cuffed endotracheal tube in unconscious patients is safer). Generally, induced emesis, performed with the stomach full of fluid, is preferred over lavage. Vomiting will often result in removal of large particles that will not pass through a stomach tube and possible emptying distal to the stomach. If emetics are ineffective after 2 doses, lavage is indicated because emetic drugs in themselves have some toxicity.

ADMINISTRATION OF SYRUP OF IPECAC. This is the method of choice in initiating delayed emesis, particularly in children (a supply should be in home first-aid kits). The recommended amount of syrup of ipecac is shown in the following table:

Age	Amount of Syrup of Ipecac	Amount of Water
< 1 yr*	10 ml (2 teaspoonsful)	90–150 ml (3–5 oz)
1 to 12 yrs	15 ml (3 teaspoonsful)	180–240 ml (6–8 oz)
Teenager to adult	30 ml (2 tablespoonsful)	240–480 ml (8–16 oz)

If emesis does not occur within 20 minutes approximately, the same dose may be repeated, but only once. If emesis does not take place within 40 to 60 minutes, the ipecac should be removed from the stomach by gastric lavage. Parents of children given syrup of ipecac should be informed of its delayed depressant side action, which may last for 2 to 3 hours after an emetic dose. This depressant action is only temporary and rarely requires any treatment. Patients with cardiac abnormalities should be closely watched, as the syrup of ipecac (emetine) can produce cardiac conduction abnormalities.

Fluid extract of ipecac is 14 times stronger than syrup of ipecac and should never be used—deaths have been reported from confusion of the two preparations.

INJECTION OF APOMORPHINE HYDROCHLORIDE is not preferred, because of its secondary opiate depressant action, and *generally is to be avoided in everyone in the presence of alternatives*. It is contraindicated in deeply sedated to comatose patients. Apomorphine, in a dose of 5 mg SC for an adult (for children use 0.03 mg/kg), if used at all, is the most effective of all emetics because of its direct action on the vomiting center. Do not give if there are restrictions to emesis as previously outlined. Its secondary depressant action can be neutralized by injection of naloxone hydrochloride (Narcan), 0.01 mg/kg.

---

*It may be best to avoid use of syrup of ipecac outside the hospital setting in children under age 1; its use in infants under 9 months is controversial.

Table 53–1. CLUES TO IDENTIFICATION OF TOXIC AGENTS

System Feature	Quality	Toxins (more common)
Skin/Mucosa		
Color	Cyanosis	Cyanides, nitrates, methemoglobinemia, hypoxemia
	Flushed	Atropine and other anticholinergics (plus dry skin and tachycardia), phenothiazines, cholinergics (plus wet skin and bradycardia), amphetamines and other adrenergics, alcohol, boric acid, disulfiram
	Cherry red (?)	Carbon monoxide (red color usually absent)
	Stain	Orange: chlorine gas; green: copper salts, vanadium (affects tongue); brown: PCB's, iodine; blue: oxalic acid; yellow: nitric acid, TNT, epoxy resins; black: osmium trioxide, silver salts; dark gums: arsenic, lead, mercury
Moisture	Dry (and warm)	Atropine and other anticholinergics, phenothiazines, antihistamines, narcotics
	Moist	Cholinergics, organic phosphates, alcohol, adrenergics, amphetamines, pentachlorophenol, dinitro-*o*-cresol
Lesions	Bullae and exfoliative dermatitis	Penicillin, sulfonamides, arsenic, phenylbutazone (see also 58–8A, *Toxic Epidermal Necrolysis*), barbiturates
	Acne	Bromides, chlorinated naphthalenes, PCB, chlorobenzene, Agent Orange
Temperature	Hyperthermia	Salicylates, amphetamines, cocaine, anticholinergics, PCP, sepsis, seizures of any etiology, if repeated or prolonged, metal and polymer fumes, pentachlorophenol
	Hypothermia	Narcotics, clonidine, phenothiazines, sedative-hypnotics, ETOH, exposure
Breath Odor	Acetone	Isopropyl alcohol, methanol, salicylates, ketoacidosis
	Alcohol	Ethyl alcohol (most identifiable is the odor of digested alcohol fumes)
	Bitter almonds	Cyanides (a "silver polish" odor; undetected by some people)
	Garlicky	Arsenic, phosphorus, organic phosphates, thallium, dimethylsulfoxide
	Peanut odor	Vacor (RH-787) (rat killer)
	Pear-like	Chloral hydrate
	Pungent	Ethchlorvynol
	Wintergreen	Methyl salicylate
	Unique	Ammonia, gasoline, kerosene, petroleum distillates, paraldyhyde
Eyes		
Motion	Nystagmus	Phenytoin, barbiturates, phencyclidine (vertical), ETOH (most common), ketamine
	Ophthalmoplegia	Botulism, thiamine deficiency, hypnotics
Pupil size	Pinpoint	Narcotics, organic phosphates, phenothiazides, pilocarpine, propoxyphene, clonidine, cholinergics, sedative-hypnotics; also caused by pilocarpine (as in eye drops for glaucoma), β-blockers, heat stroke and pontine angle infarction
	Dilated	Adrenergics, amphetamines, atropine and other anticholinergics, scopolamine, glutethimide, cocaine, LSD, and any drugs leading to hypoxemia, such as tricyclic antidepressants, barbiturates and cyanide. Also seen postictally and in death

Table 53–1. CLUES TO IDENTIFICATION OF TOXIC AGENTS *(Continued)*

System Feature	Quality	Toxins (more common)
CNS (general, including respiratory centers)	Excitability	Atropine and other anticholinergics, scopolamine, cholinergics, adrenergics, amphetamines, alcohol (earlier stages), barbiturates (idiosyncratic reaction)
	Seizures	Phencyclidine, cyanide, isoniazid (INH), strychnine, phenothiazines, theophylline, antihistamines, amphetamines, hypoglycemics, chlorinated hydrocarbons, lithium, carbon monoxide, digitalis in large amounts, TCA's, cocaine
	Depression	CNS tranquilizers (phenothiazines, barbiturates and similar compounds), alcohol (large amounts), narcotics, carbon monoxide, medications leading to hypoglycemia
Cardiovascular		
Heart rate	Bradycardia	Cholinergic-type drugs, propranolol, ethchlorvynol, digitalis (variable)
	Tachycardia	Adrenergics, amphetamines, nicotine, tricyclic antidepressants, caffeine, theophylline, anticholinergics, cocaine and most toxic substances
Blood pressure	Elevated	Anticholinergics, moderate alcohol intoxication, adrenergics, amphetamines, cocaine, atropine (earlier stages), caffeine, PCP
	Decreased	CNS tranquilizers, narcotics, alcohol, antihypertensives, diuretics, neuromuscular blocking agents and most toxic substances (all at end stages)
Gastrointestinal		
Diarrhea	Severe to bloody	Arsenic, iron, cholinergic drugs, digitalis, ergot derivatives, hydrogen sulfide, iodine, heavy metals, phosphorus, thallium, paradichlorobenzene, paraquat, bacterial toxins and food poisoning
	Blue-green	Boric acid
Bowel sounds	Increased	Organophosphates, cholinergics, cathartics
	Decreased	Narcotics, sedative hypnotics
Muscle		
Increased activity	Rigidity	PCP, haldol, methaqualone, strychnine, antipsychotics (dystonic reactions), tetanus
	Myoclonic jerking	Phencyclidine, PCP
	Muscle fasciculations	Organic phosphates, strychnine, nicotine, lithium, PCP, tetanus
	Flaccidity	Narcotics, clonidine, sedative hypnotics
	Paralysis	Botulism, neuromuscular blocking agents

Table 53–2. MORE COMMON TOXIC SYNDROMES (Toxidromes)*

Medication Type	Signs and Symptoms: Agitation	Lethargy	Coma	Seizures	Heart Rate	Blood Pressure	Skin	Temperature	Pupils	Nystagmus	Bowel Sounds	Muscle Tone	Major Therapeutic Considerations (Always support ventilation [5] and circulation [57])
Cholinergics	+	–	+	+	⇊[1]	–	Wet	–	Pin-point	–	⇈	↑[2]	Give atropine (53–*10*) for muscarine receptors
Anticholinergics	+	+	+	+[3]	↑	↑	Dry	⇈	Dilated	–	↓	↓	Reduce hyperthermia (62)
Tricyclic antidepressants (TCA's)	±	+	+	+	↑	⇅	Dry	⇅	Dilated	–	↓	↓	Treat acidosis (*46*) and seizures (*34*); check ECG; see 53–723
Sedatives/Hypnotics	±	±	+	↓	↓	↓	–	↓	±[4]	+	↓	↓[5]	Support ventilation (5)
Narcotics	±[6]	+	+	±	↓	↓	–	↓	Pin-point	–	↓	↓	Give naloxone Support ventilation (5)
Stimulants	+	–	±[7]	+	↑	↑	Wet	↑	Dilated	+	↑	↑	Reduce hyperthermia (62) Control seizures (34)
Salicylates (see also 53–*614*)	+	+	+	+	↑	⇅	–	⇈	–	–	–	–	Treat metabolic acidosis, electrolyte imbalance
Insulin (see also Table 32–2)	±	+	+	+	↑	↓	Wet	–	Small	–	↓	↓	Give dextrose infusion, possibly glucagon

*The signs and symptoms presented are general guidelines, but can vary considerably depending on factors such as amount and stage of toxicity; patient age, weight and physical condition; and presence of other toxins or drugs.

[1]Initially may increase; [2]Fasciculations common; [3]Physostigmine "antidote" may induce seizures; [4]Glutethimide may dilate pupils dramatically; [5]Methaqualone may cause rigidity; [6]Increase following withdrawal or after antagonist administration in addicts; [7]Postictal state generally if present.

Common drugs in each category are as follows: *Cholinergics:* organophosphate (53–*497*), carbamate insecticides (53–*172*), physostigmine (53–*547*), mushroom poisoning (53–*462*); *Anticholinergics:* antihistamines (53–*80*), atropine sulfate (53–*103*), belladonna (53–*115*),
Amanita muscaria mushrooms (53–*462*); *TCA's:* see 53–723; *Sedatives:* barbiturates (53–*110*), ethyl alcohol (ETOH) (53–*245*), methaqualone (Quaalude) (53–*427*), benzodiazepines (53–*121*); *Narcotics:* see 7–3; clonidine (Catapres) may present a similar picture;
Stimulants: amphetamines (53–*66*), cocaine (53–*218*), hallucinogens (53–*322*), phencyclidine (53–*532*), epinephrine (53–*288*), nicotine

GASTRIC LAVAGE. Emptying of the stomach by washing with tap water or half normal saline with a large-bore tube about the diameter of the patient's little finger is indicated if the vomiting center is paralyzed (as in deep morphine or phenothiazine poisoning) and, in many cases, if ingestion of acutely toxic substances is known or suspected, provided that the danger from the toxic substance is considered to be greater than the risk of possible aspiration during lavage. The danger of aspiration can be decreased by careful positioning before and during gastric lavage (see left Sims position [Fig. 4–5*A*] for desired position), by use of a cuffed endotracheal tube, and by pinching off of the gastric tube during removal. Lavage should not be used if a corrosive poison (see *Acids, 53–33; Alkalies, 53–45; Lye, 53–401*) has been swallowed, if there is advanced strychnine poisoning *(53–659)* or if convulsions *(34)* and/or acute excitement state *(37)* are present. For technique of gastric lavage, see *18–11*. After the lavage, an antidote or activated charcoal may be instilled.

CATHARTICS. The overall value is debatable, and these substances should not be used in the presence of nephrotoxins, corrosives or electrolyte problems. The hazards from aspiration pneumonia following oily cathartics (castor oil) probably outweigh the benefits. When given, saline cathartics, such as magnesium sulfate (Epsom salts), 250.0 mg/kg, are administered by mouth or instilled through the stomach tube after lavage; adult dose is usually 20 to 30 g per dose up to 100 g total if needed. Osmotic cathartics such as sorbitol and lactulose (30–60 ml) may have fewer systemic electrolyte changes and can be used safely with repeat doses of charcoal.

ENEMA. An enema aids clearance of the toxin if the rectum was the site of instillation and might aid transit from higher in the GI tract, though it is not a routine procedure.

Removal from the Circulation

HEMODIALYSIS. Hemodialysis is a method of removal used under select circumstances. Some toxins (such as organic phosphates, haloperidol or cyanide) are so readily fixed in the tissues that dialysis is of little or no value. If the patient is severely poisoned from a still-circulating poison and (1) there is no specific antidote to the poison, (2) there is impairment of the liver or kidneys and (3) hemodialysis may substantially speed elimination of the toxin, the benefits of hemodialysis may justify and outweigh the risks, such as infection, air embolism, severe fluid and electrolyte imbalance and hemorrhage.

CHARCOAL HEMOPERFUSION. This method has been used in some centers to remove toxins such as aspirin, theophylline and *Amanita phalloides* poisoning. Because the blood of the patient comes in contact with the charcoal (or other absorbent), rapid decreases in platelet counts can occur.

PERITONEAL DIALYSIS. The indications for peritoneal dialysis are similar to those for hemodialysis, though hemodialysis, if available, is preferable, except possibly in smaller children (exchange transfusion may also be considered in this age group).

URINE PH ADJUSTMENT. In some extreme cases, acidification with ascorbic acid or ammonium chloride has been proposed to aid elimination of drugs of alkaline composition (e.g., amphetamines, phencyclidine [PCP]; this technique is still controversial, and complications may arise. Also, alkalinization with sodium lactate or bicarbonate or by continuous gastric aspiration is used in occasional difficult situations to facilitate excretion of weak acid compounds, such as phenobarbital and salicylates. Alkalinization is best suited for ion trapping in salicylate intoxication. Alkalinization of the urine may be induced by giving sodium bicarbonate, 1 to 2 mEq/kg, added to 15 ml D5½NS/kg, administered IV over a 3- to 4-hour period. The urine pH will reach 7 to 7.5 in about an hour.

Careful monitoring of blood pH and electrolyte levels is necessary. Potassium supplementation may be required. When possible, urine volume should be kept at average to higher normal levels, but caution should be exercised not to overload the system; "forced diuresis" can be hazardous and not particularly effective regarding excretion of a poison that is not eliminated in this active form or is reabsorbed by the kidneys.

GASTRIC SUCTION. Continuous gastric suction has been used to "trap" and remove toxins that are found in high concentrations in the gastric contents, such as PCP and cocaine.

PLASMAPHERESIS. This technique has been used in some difficult cases for removal of toxins such as ricin (see *53–179, Castor Bean Extract*).

53–8. ADSORPTION OF POISON

Activated charcoal suspension or slurry is the preferred substance for adsorption of most remaining toxins after gastric emptying. Fifteen to 30 g of the suspension may be given orally in a glass of water or via a gastric tube. Among the available preparations (good for at least 1 year in mixed form) are Norit A, Darco G and Nuchar C. All have the ability to absorb toxic chemicals (except cyanides [53–232]) and to retain them tenaciously while they are being passed through the bowel.

Activated charcoal should not be given before, or with, an emetic or an oral specific antidote; it may adsorb the emetic or neutralizing drug and decrease its effect. Activated charcoal has little or no adsorptive effect on the following: alkali, boric acid, cyanide, DDT, ferrous sulfate, mineral acids, *N*-methyl carbamate.

Pure activated charcoal has replaced the "universal antidote" and its household equivalents (2 parts burned toast, 1 part milk of magnesia and 1 part strong tea) because of its much greater efficacy.

Demulcents such as raw eggs, boiled starch or milk are not generally of proved effectiveness. Present evidence has shown the value of repeat doses of activated charcoal (e.g., q 6 h) in many poisonings, particularly those involving tricyclic antidepressants. Also, recent studies have demonstrated that some drugs (e.g., phenobarbital and theophylline given IV) still have significant reduction in serum half-lives (T ½) with enteric charcoal present through repeated doses.

53–9. PRECIPITATION OF THE POISON

In the past a number of substances (such as tannic acid, tincture of iodine, sodium thiosulfate, raw eggs, boiled starch, flour, and milk) were advocated for the precipitation of various poisons. However, careful evaluation has not brought forth adequate evidence to support their use and they are not now generally recommended.

Activated charcoal, as mentioned earlier for the absorption of poisons, is the only general substance advised now for that purpose. Chelation of toxins, such as Ca^{++} precipitating phosphate, can be useful in preventing enteric absorption.

53–10. NEUTRALIZATION OF THE POISON BY SPECIFIC ANTIDOTES *(See Table 53–3)*

Considering the myriad of toxic substances that exist, relatively few specific antidotes have highly significant clinical application. For practical purposes, of the six most common poisons that must be diagnosed immediately so that an appropriate specific antidote can be given promptly, three are in commercial products—(1) organic phosphates, (2) cyanides and (3) methanol—and three are medical preparations—(4) opiates, (5) insulin and (6) anticoagulants. Although other poisons have specific antidotes, occurrence of such poisoning is less common.

Caution must be exercised in the use of specific antidotes, as their overzealous or inappropriate use may complicate the initial injury, producing other confusing or detrimental forms of poisoning. Attentive general and supportive treatment aided by sensible selection and use of therapeutic drugs/antidotes is most likely to benefit the majority of patients.

53–11. SUPPORTIVE TREATMENT

In making the decision to hospitalize for observation and treatment, which is advisable in more than minimally involved poison patients, it is important to consider, among many important issues, the tendency of the poison to have delayed onset of manifestations, in addition to its half-life and the half-life of any antidotes given. For instance, the antidote atropine has a duration of therapeutic effect of approximately 30 to 60 minutes and needs to be repetitiously given in many cases of organic phosphate poisoning.

The following references concern support for most of the commonly occurring problems seen with poisoning.

Respiratory failure and circulatory failure: See 5, *ABC's of Resuscitation.*

Shock: See 57.

Convulsions: See 34. Diazepam (Valium), 0.1 mg/kg (up to 5 to 10 mg) slowly IV, or phenobarbital IV, is probably the safest initial treatment.

Table 53–3. NEUTRALIZATION OF POISONS BY SPECIFIC ANTIDOTES

Antidote/Poison(s)	Remarks
ATROPINE For: Anticholinesterases Organic phosphates *(53–497)* Physostigmine *(53–547)*	Antagonist for organic phosphate insecticides. Test dose of 2 mg (for child, 0.05 mg/kg diluted to 10 ml with normal saline is given slowly IV until symptoms of atropinism. Dose is repeated (and increased if necessary) every 10 to 15 minutes, with cessation of secretions considered adequate end point. Frequent and large doses of atropine may be required to reach this end point. Subsequent use of pralidoxime (2-PAM) is given additionally. Atropine should be used to reverse toxic effects of physostigmine.
SODIUM NITRITE SODIUM THIOSULFATE AMYL NITRITE For: Cyanide *(53–232)*	Antidotes for a rapid and lethal poison, the nitrites form methemoglobin, which has a greater affinity for cyanide than does oxyhemoglobin. Sodium nitrite 3% (10 ml) is given IV over 5 minutes; children's dosage is 10 mg/kg. Sodium thiosulfate 25% (50 ml) is given immediately afterwards IV over 10 minutes; children's dosage is 0.7 ml/kg of the 25% solution. An ampule of amyl nitrite may be inhaled at a rate of 30 seconds every minute until the sodium nitrite is given. Repeat courses of treatment may be necessary.
ETHANOL For: Methanol *(53–426)*	IV ethanol, loading dose in adults of 1 ml of absolute (near 100%) ethanol in 5% dextrose solution per kilogram of body weight over 15 minutes in severe cases or 10% ethanol in 5% dextrose solution, infused the first hour at 6 to 8 ml/kg and maintained at about 1 to 2 ml/kg/hr thereafter; or immediately given oral ethanol (e.g., 40% or 80 proof vodka or whiskey), 1.5 ml/kg and about 0.6 ml/kg every 2 hours until IV alcohol available to achieve near 100 to 125 mg % ethanol blood level. Dialysis may be required.
Ethylene glycol *(53–300)*	Antidote for ethylene glycol (antifreeze) poisoning used in same manner as described for methanol. Dialysis may be required early. Give Ca and HCO_3 prn.
NALOXONE (NARCAN) For: Narcotic drugs *(53–473)* Propoxyphene *(53–581)* Pentazocine *(53–525)* Diphenoxylate *(53–278)*	A specific antagonist of narcotics. Four-tenths mg (1 ml) may be given (IV, IM, SC) and repeated every 2 to 3 minutes for 2 or 3 doses; initial pediatric dosage is 0.01 mg/kg, but may be increased according to clinical response. Larger doses may be needed to reverse effects of overdose with propoxyphene. Duration of naloxone antagonism may be shorter than the narcotic's effect; therefore, repeated doses may be needed. Naloxone does not have central depression narcotic antagonist effects like the older antagonists nalorphine and levallorphan, which were once widely used. Precipitation of narcotic withdrawal syndrome can occur if high doses of naloxone are used in addicted patients.

Table 53–3. NEUTRALIZATION OF POISONS BY SPECIFIC ANTIDOTES (Continued)

Antidote/Poison(s)	Remarks
DEXTROSE For: Insulin *(53–362)*	See Table 32–3. Differential Diagnosis of Hypoglycemia and Hyperinsulinism, 36–6, *Insulin Shock*, and 32–3, *Treatment of Diabetic Coma*
PROTAMINE SULFATE For: Heparin *(53–337)*	*See 45–8, Hemorrhage from Anticoagulant Therapy*
VITAMIN K (AquaMEPHYTON) For: Dicumarol *(53–258)*	*See 45–8, Hemorrhage from Anticoagulant Therapy*
DIMERCAPROL (BAL) For: Arsenic *(53–90)* Gold *(53–328)* Mercury *(53–418)* Antimony *(53–81)* Nickel *(53–476)* Lead *(53–385 to 53–386)*	Antidote for arsenic. Forms a complex that competes with arsenic for enzyme systems. Dose is 3 mg/kg every 4 hours (IM) first 2 days, then 2 mg/kg every 12 hours (IM) for a total of 10 days. When urine arsenic level falls below 50 μg per 24 hours, antidote may be stopped. Dosage varies with the toxic agent.
CALCIUM DISODIUM ETHYLENEDIAMINETETRAACETATE (CaEDTA) (VERSINE) For: Lead *(53–385)* Cadmium *(53–158)* Cobalt *(53–217)* Copper *(53–224)* Nickel *(53–476)*	Given at a total of 50 to 75 mg/kg/day (2% solution IV) in 3 to 6 divided doses for up to 5 days. Lower doses can be given orally if no encephalopathy and lower blood lead level. Stop when urine returns to nontoxic level. BAL is given additionally for lead intoxication.
PENICILLAMINE (CUPRIMINE) For: Mercury *(53–418)*	Antidote of choice for mercury but a highly toxic agent itself and requires close monitoring. Dosage is 100 mg/kg/day to a maximum of 1 g/day (for 1 week) taken orally in 4 divided doses and taken on an empty stomach ½ hr before meals.

DEFEROXAMINE (DESFERAL) For: Iron salts *(53–370)*	Antidote for iron intoxication. If poisoning is severe and patient is in shock, give slowly IV, 15 mg/kg/hr, *after* blood has been drawn for serum iron and iron-binding capacity determination. In less severe cases, give same first hour dose IM then reduce dosage by half for next 2 doses every 4 hours. Maximum dose is 80 mg/kg/day IV, and no more than 6 g total. IM dose is 90 mg/kg q 8 h (maximum single dose: 1 g; maximum total dose: 6 g). Urine will become characteristic red color if iron is chelated with deferoxamine. Fleet's lavage can cause hypernatremia and hyperphosphatemia.
PHYSOSTIGMINE SALICYLATE For: Anticholinergic and atropinic agents Tricyclic antidepressants *(53–723)* Belladonna *(53–115)* Scopolamine *(53–620)*	An antidote of limited value for central nervous system and cardiac toxicity of atropine and anticholinergic-like drugs (tricyclic antidepressants, scopolamine, belladonna). Dose (adult) is 1 mg (usually 0.5 mg first) given IV slowly over 2 to 3 minutes. Wait for changes (3 to 5 minutes) in symptoms (decrease in supraventricular arrhythmias, decreased convulsion, improved mental status) before repeating. Maximum initial dose is 4 mg (adults) or 2 mg (children). The effects are transient (30 to 60 minutes), and lowest effective dose may be repeated when symptoms return. Slow administration of physostigmine helps prevent precipitation of convulsion, bradycardia and asystole caused by physostigmine itself.
N-ACETYLCYSTEINE (MUCOMYST) For: Acetaminophen *(53–19)*	This investigational IV antidote has offered evidence of reducing liver damage from toxic levels of acetaminophen (see Fig. 53–1). To be most effective, acetylcysteine should be started soon and at least within 16 hours. Loading dose is 140 mg/kg orally, and maintenance dose is 70 mg/kg every 4 hours for 17 doses or until toxic levels are reduced to safe range. IV acetylcysteine, given in an initial dose of 150 mg/kg in 200 ml of 5% dextrose over 15 minutes, followed by 50 mg/kg in 500 ml of 5% dextrose over 4 hours, then 100 mg mg/kg in 1 liter of 5% dextrose over the next 16 hours has been shown to be effective in Great Britain, but is still considered investigational in the United States.

Temperature variations: See 62. Exposure to cold environment may complicate mild overdoses, especially in elderly people living alone, and lead to significant hypothermia (low-scale rectal thermometers are necessary). The presence of atropine and other anticholinergics, including phenothiazines and tricyclic antidepressants, impairs the sweating mechanism and may help to bring on heat stress disorders.

Pain: See *12*. The smallest effective dose should be used to avoid complicating the toxic picture; alternatively, nonmedicinal pain relief measures may be used.

Cerebral edema: See 44–7. Cerebral edema may occur not only directly as an effect of the poison but also secondarily as a result of overzealous efforts to achieve forced diuresis—particularly when renal damage is also present.

Fluid and electrolyte administration: See *11* and *46*. Particular caution must be used in the presence of nephrotoxic poisons.

Coma: See 32.

Do not declare a person dead while they still have a treatable poisoning (see *8, Death and Dying Guidelines*).

53–12. METHEMOGLOBINEMIA

When iron in hemoglobin is in its ferric, or oxidized, state in concentrations near or above 2 gm per dl instead of in its normal range of less than half that amount, a cyanotic state unresponsive to oxygen results from the increased methemoglobinemia. Recent onset of cyanosis, particularly with a history of ingestion (or fume exposure) of oxidizing agents—the foremost being nitrites and nitrates—and brownish color of dried blood (when level is over 15%) on a white surface plus normal arterial oxygen saturation, is indicative of an acquired toxic methemoglobinemia. Methemoglobin levels must be ordered as a specific test and cannot be determined from other arterial blood gas determinations. Methemoglobin should not be confused with methalbumin.

The toxic picture may include apathy, dyspnea, convulsions and occasional gastrointestinal upset. Usually cyanosis is disproportionately greater than other symptoms.

Treatment

Treatment consists of lessening the exposure to the oxidizing agent (found in coronary vasodilators, food preservatives, foods such as spinach or beets grown in richly fertilized soil, some water supplies and a number of drugs and chemicals) if the patient is nonsymptomatic. If the patient is grossly symptomatic from the toxic state (this usually occurs with methemoglobin levels of 20–30%), then oxygen administration, removal of remaining enteric chemical, if possible, and slow IV (large vein) infusion of 1% methylene blue solution, 1–2 mg/kg, over 15 to 30 minutes, will usually produce hemoglobin reduction. This can be repeated in 45 to 60 minutes, if needed. In less severe cases, oral intake of methylene blue, 5 mg/kg can be used. If over 40% of the hemoglobin is methemoglobin, then red blood cell (RBC) transfusion should be considered. Treat metabolic acidosis.

53–13. LETHAL OR TOXIC BLOOD LEVELS OF DRUGS *(See also Table on Hematologic Values in Appendix)*

The presence of alcohol and other toxins or medications, extremes of age or prior poor health (especially liver, kidney or heart impairment) of the patient may lower lethal or toxic blood levels of drugs, whereas development of tolerance or tachyphylaxis from prior use in graduated amounts may raise the lethal or toxic blood level several fold from commonly accepted lethal or toxic levels of specific drugs. Blood levels of drugs, nevertheless, can be a guideline for manner and intensity of treatment and a gauge of efficacy of on-going treatment. Often the total blood level is less revealing than the unbound or free drug level in blood. New techniques of measuring blood levels may soon differentiate between carrier-bound, unbound and tissue-bound drug levels.

See Appendix for table giving therapeutic and toxic ranges for some common medications.

53–14. TOXICITY OF HOUSE AND GARDEN PRODUCTS

High-Toxicity Household Products. Though most chemicals commonly in the home are not likely to be highly toxic in the amounts likely to be ingested, the following are notable exceptions.

Drano
Liquid Plumber
Lye
Pesticides
Petroleum distillates (gasoline, kerosene)
Poisons for small animals (rodenticides)

Low-Toxicity Household Products. The following products generally produce insignificant toxicity except when ingested in large doses or when a particular manufacturer's process has combined more toxic chemicals (check with Regional Poison Control Center for current data if in question).

Abrasives
Adhesives
Ballpoint ink
Barium sulfate
Blackboard chalk
Bleaches (<5% Na hypochloride)
Bubblebath soaps (detergents)
Candles (except with insect repellent)
Caps (for toy pistol)
Carboxymethyl cellulose (dehydrating material)
Chalk
Cosmetics
Crayons (modern type)
Detergents (*not* electric dishwasher)
Deodorants
Deodorizers (spray and refrigerator)
Fabric softeners
Fishbowl additives
Incense
Iodoform disinfectants
Lead pencils (graphite)
Linseed oil (raw)
Lipstick
Lubricants
Matches
Mineral Oil (unless aspirated)
Modeling clay
Paint (less than 1% lead, latex)
Pencil (lead, graphite, coloring)
Petrolatum
Polaroid film-coating fluid
Porous-tip ink markers
Putty
Shampoos
Shaving creams
Silica
Soap and soap products
Sweetening agents (saccharin)
Talc
Thermometer (mercury)
Toothpaste

COMMENTS ON SPECIFIC POISONS*†

The numbered and alphabetized listing (*53–15* to *53–765*) on the following pages includes substances that may give toxic signs and symptoms from inhalation of fumes or from skin absorption as well as by ingestion. Unless otherwise specified, ingestion is the mode of entry.

The general index at the end of the book should be referred to for names of substances given by alternate, similar or proprietary names (e.g., Valium is listed in this section only as diazepam).

Whenever the substances listed in this alphabetical list are drugs used medicinally for their therapeutic effect, reference is suggested to a standard pharmacology text, or to the brochures furnished by the manufacturers, for more detailed accounts of recommended dosages, toxicities and side effects. Assistance of a Regional Poison Control Center is encouraged in complex or serious cases or whenever questions regarding treatment arise.

---

*For therapeutic considerations, see also *53–1* to *53–13*.

†TLV (*threshold limit value*) refers to the values established in 1977 by the American Conference of Governmental Industrial Hygienists (ACGIH), based on an 8-hour TWA (*time-weighted average*); a capital letter C following the value cited indicates that it is a ceiling concentration that must not be exceeded.

53–15. ABRUS PRECATORIUS L.

The seeds of this ornamental plant, originally from Africa but now common in the West Indies, Central America and Florida, contain a toxalbumin, abrin. Ingestion of the seeds, called "crab-eyes," jequirity beans, jumbo beans and rosary beads, results in generalized weakness, a rapid weak pulse, extreme and persistent nausea, coarse tremors and severe colicky diarrhea. For signs and symptoms resulting from inhalation of dust from the dried seeds, see *53–376, Jequirity Beans.*

53–16. ABSINTHE (Wormwood)

The dried leaves and flowers of this plant, formerly used as a medicine and liqueur, especially in France, contain a toxic substance, thujone. The signs and symptoms of toxicity are a clammy skin, severe gastric pain, convulsions (tonic and clonic) and cardiac failure.

53–17. ACACIA (Gum Arabic)

Derived from a gum exuded by the stems and branches of an African tree, this substance previously has been utilized in medicine as a colloid in intravenous solutions in the treatment of shock and kidney disease. Occasional severe reactions, with dyspnea, rapid pulse, acute anxiety and terminal circulatory collapse, have been reported, as well as cases of hypersensitivity and anaphylactoid shock *(24, Allergic Reactions).*

53–18. ACETALDEHYDE (CH_3CHO; TLV 100 ppm)

Used in silver plating and industrial chemistry, acetaldehyde fumes in moderate concentration may cause intense mucous membrane irritation, characterized by conjunctivitis, photophobia, corneal injury, rhinitis and anosmia. Removal from exposure usually results in complete clearing of symptoms. High concentrations give a toxic picture similar to that of acute alcoholic intoxication *(53–295, Ethyl Alcohol).*

53–19. ACETAMINOPHEN (Paracetamol, Tylenol, Tempra) ($C_8H_9NO_2$)

Anorexia, nausea, vomiting and diaphoresis occur initially; signs of hepatocellular toxicity with jaundice, coagulation defects, renal failure, myocardiopathy and hypoglycemia usually take several days to develop. Plasma levels must be obtained starting 4 hours after ingestion to help guide therapy (see Fig. *53–1*). Early treatment with *N*-acetylcysteine (Mucomyst) (53–10 and Table 53–3) is mandatory after significant exposures. Use of activated charcoal after emesis is probably not indicated, as it binds *N*-acetylcysteine and decreases its absorption. Early presence of coma is indicative that central nervous system depressant medications have been taken in addition. Death may occur from liver failure.

53–20. ACETANILID (Antifebrin) (C_8H_9NO)

This analgesic is seldom used now. Signs and symptoms include nausea; vomiting; cyanosis (especially of the face); cold, clammy skin; and feeble, rapid pulse with slow respiration. Hemolysis can occur in patients with G6PD deficiency. If acute methemoglobinemia *(53–12)* is present, methylene blue administration may be needed.

53–21. ACETARSONE ($C_8H_{10}AsNO_5$)

This arsenic derivative has been used orally under a great number of trade names for treatment of dysentery (veterinary) and locally for treatment of trichomonal infections. By either route it may cause the toxic effects of arsenicals. For signs and symptoms of toxicity, see *53–90, Arsenic.*

---

*For therapeutic considerations see also *53–1* to *53–13.*

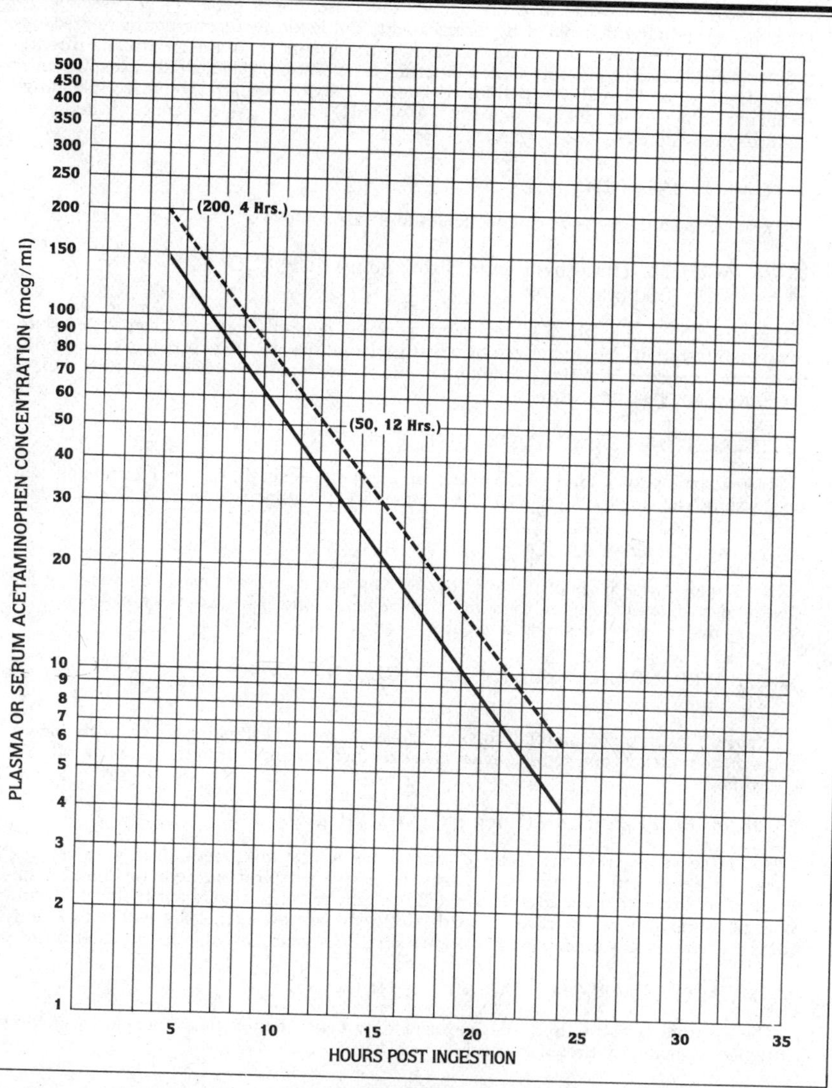

Figure 53–1. •If acetaminophen levels are greater than those depicted by the upper line, hepatotoxicity is likely to occur. •If acetaminophen levels are equal to or greater than lower line (margin of safety calculated), treatment is recommended. •If acetaminophen levels are less than lower line, N-acetylcysteine need not be given or can be discontinued if that approach was used. (From Professional Informational Brochure, Mead Johnson Pharmaceutical Division, 1979.)

53–22. ACETIC ACID (CH_3COOH; TLV 10 ppm)

The most common cause of acute acetic acid poisoning is ingestion of "essence of vinegar," a common household flavoring agent. The toxic picture is characterized by severe pain in the upper alimentary tract; grayish white ulcers in the mouth and throat; profuse vomiting; cold, clammy skin; subnormal temperature; rapid, shallow respiration; acute dyspnea; and sometimes pulmonary edema *(55)* with terminal collapse. Splashing in the eye of household vinegar (4 to 10% CH_3COOH) or on the skin of concentrated acid requires immediate copious flushing.

53–23. ACETOARSENITES

These compounds are powerful pesticides and extremely toxic. See *53–90, Arsenic.*

53–24. ACETONE (Dimethylketone, Propanone) ($[CH_3]_2CO$; TLV 1000 ppm)

Inhalation of fumes, which have a pungent sweet odor or ingestion may cause severe toxic manifestations, characterized by a fruity odor on the breath; severe gastrointestinal symptoms (nausea, vomiting, abdominal pain); and rapid fall in temperature, pulse, respiration and blood pressure.

53–25. ACETONE CYANOHYDRIN ($[CH_3]_2C[OH]CN$)

This extremely toxic liquid used in industry can cause death if a few ml are splashed on the skin. The signs, symptoms and treatment are as outlined under *53–232, Cyanides.*

53–26. ACETOHEXAMIDE (Dymelor)

Excessively large doses of this oral hypoglycemic drug have caused coma lasting for several days in spite of large amounts of intravenous glucose. Patients make complete recovery under energetic supportive care.

53–27. ACETONITRILE (Methylcyanide) (CH_3CN; TLV 40 ppm)

Exposure to this commercial solvent causes severe chest pain, cough with bloody sputum, convulsions and coma. Severe cases require treatment as outlined under *53–232, Cyanides.*

53–28. ACETOPHENETIDIN (Phenacetin) ($C_{10}H_{13}NO_2$)

Too large or too frequent doses of this analgesic and antipyretic drug may cause a weak and feeble pulse, extreme cyanosis, excessive perspiration, hematuria and respiratory and circulatory collapse. Prolonged use may result in severe agranulocytosis and chronic renal failure. In patients with G6PD deficiency, hemolysis will occur. It is metabolized to acetaminophen *(53–19)*, which is less toxic. See also *53–20, Acetanilid.*

53–29. ACETYLCARBROMAL (Abasin) ($C_9H_{15}BrN_2O_3$)

Therapeutic doses of this sedative drug may cause hemorrhagic purpura *(45)* and thrombocytopenia that require treatment.

53–30. ACETYLCHOLINE CHLORIDE ($C_7H_{16}ClNO_2$) *(See Table 53–2, Cholinergics)*

This substance is also a naturally occurring neurotransmitter. Signs and symptoms are sweating, salivation, dyspnea, tightness in chest, excessive micturition and collapse. Specific antidote is atropine; see *53–10.*

---

*For therapeutic considerations see also *53–1* to *53–13.*

53–31. ACETYLENE (Ethine, Narcylene) (HC≡CH)

Inhaled in strong concentrations, this commonly used commercial gas causes rapid onset of deep narcosis. Inhalation of lower concentrations causes dizziness and mental confusion, usually transient. Watch for complications, usually due to impurities, such as hydrogen sulfide *(53–353)* or phosphine *(53–544)*.

53–32. ACETYLSALICYLIC ACID ($C_9H_8O_4$) *(See 53–101, Aspirin; 53–614, Salicylates)*

53–33. ACIDS (Acetic, Acetic Anhydride, Carbonic [Phenol], Hydrochloric [Muriatic], Lactic, Nitric, Sulfuric [Oil of Vitriol], Trichloracetic)

For exceptions to the therapy outlined below, see *53–351, Hydrofluoric Acid; 53–501, Oxalic Acid; 53–587, Pyrogallic Acid;* and *53–671, Tannic Acid.*

Treatment of External Contact

- Repeated flooding with copious amounts of water, followed by treatment as for a burn *(28)*. See also *38–31, Injuries to the Conjunctiva.*

Treatment of Ingestion

- Do not use stomach tube or emetics if concentrated acid has been swallowed. Early endoscopy should be considered.
- Dilute immediately with water and milk or aluminum hydroxide, magnesium oxide or milk of magnesia.
- Treat severe pain *(12)*.
- Perform a tracheostomy *(18–34)* if edema of the glottis is severe.
- Hospitalize if there is any evidence or suspicion of corrosion of the esophagus.

53–34. ACONITE

Known as blue rocket, monkshood, wolfsbane, friar's cowl and mousebane, this flowering plant is common in gardens. Ingestion of the flowers, foliage or stems by children may cause severe toxic symptoms. Fatalities are usually due to respiratory or cardiac abnormalities. Acute poisoning also may result from mistaking the aconite plant for horseradish or from ingestion of medicinal compounds containing aconite. It is characterized by a burning sensation in the mouth and throat, acute dysphagia, impairment of speech, vertigo and eye signs (lacrimation, muscle imbalance and diplopia). Paresthesias, generally starting with the fingers but sometimes involving the whole body, may develop. Nausea, vomiting and diarrhea are common, as are marked hypotension and tonic and clonic convulsions. Fatalities are usually due to respiratory failure. Fatalities have been reported from ingestion of 20 ml of the tincture and from as little as 2 mg of aconitine.

53–35. ACRIDINE (Acrylaldehyde) ($C_{13}H_9N$)

This coal tar derivative causes yellow discoloration of the skin and mucous membranes, tracheobronchitis and asthma, all of which clear when exposure is terminated.

53–36. ACROLEIN ($CH_2 = CHCHO$; TLV 0.1 ppm)

This commercial solvent, used in the resin industry, may cause acute toxic symptoms through inhalation of fumes as well as by ingestion. The usual signs and symptoms consist of a sensation of tightness in the chest, drowsiness, nausea, vomiting and diarrhea. Vertigo, occasionally syncope, may occur.

---

*For therapeutic considerations see also *53–1* to *53–13*.

53–37. **ACRYLONITRILE** (Ventox) ($CH_2 = CHCN$; TLV 20 ppm)

Used as an insecticide and in the rubber industry, this inflammable liquid may give an acute toxic picture following inhalation of the fumes or absorption through the skin. This picture is characterized by acute conjunctivitis, vomiting and diarrhea. Restlessness and irritability are evident at first, then are supplanted by somnolence and coma. Respiratory arrest may occur. Remove contaminated clothing at once. See also 53–232, *Cyanides*. The Occupational Safety and Health Administration (OSHA) has recommended an emergency temporary standard (ETS) of 2 ppm with a ceiling concentration (C) of 10 ppm for any 15-minute period.

53–38. **AGROSTEMMA GITHAGO** (Corn Cockle, Corn Campion, Corn Rose)

Ingestion of cereal grains contaminated by the saponin-containing seeds of this widespread weed can result in nausea, vomiting, diarrhea, severe headache, pain in the spine, impaired locomotion, respiratory collapse, coma and death.

53–39. **AKEE** (Soapberry, Mock Orange)

After apparent recovery from acute gastrointestinal irritation from eating this saponin-containing fruit, convulsions, hypertension, hypoglycemia and coma may develop.

53–40. **ALCOHOL** *(See 53–295, Ethyl Alcohol; 53–372, Isopropyl Alcohol; 53–426, Methanol; 53–41, Alcohols [Higher])*

53–41. **ALCOHOLS** (Higher) (ROH)

The aliphatic liquid alcohols (amyl, butyl, ethylhexyl, isoamyl, etc.) are used extensively in industry as solvents. All are extremely toxic if ingested. For signs and sympoms of toxicity and treatment, see 53–69, *Amyl Alcohol*.

53–42. **ALDEHYDES** (RCHO) *(See 53–315, Formaldehyde)*

53–43. **ALDRIN** (Aldrite) ($C_{12}H_8Cl_6$; TLV 0.25 mg/m^3)

This complex insecticide is similar in actions and toxicity to dieldrin (53–260).

53–44. **ALFALFA**

Decoctions of the seeds of this extensively cultivated fodder have an undeserved reputation as a remedy for arthritis. In some individuals, intense dermatitis results from ingestion. This clears when oral intake is stopped.

53–45. **ALKALIES** (Caustic Alkalies) ([OH^{1-}])

Treatment of External Contact

Flood with copious amounts of water. Consider use of a weak boric acid solution in the eyes after prolonged irrigation with tap water. Also see 35–31, *Injuries to the Conjunctiva*.

Treatment of Ingestion

1. Neutralize or dilute with water immediately.
2. Do not use a stomach tube or give emetics if a concentrated solution has been swallowed or if marked erosion of the mucous membranes of the mouth or throat is apparent or suspected.
3. Give activated charcoal.
4. Sodium bicarbonate and acidic antidotes are not indicated.

---

*For therapeutic considerations see also 53–*1* to 53–*13*.

5. Hospitalize if evidence of erosion or corrosion is present or if ingestion of a large amount of a strong alkali is known or suspected to have occurred.

6. Opiates for control of pain *(12)* as well as for treatment of shock *(53–7)* may be necessary. An emergency tracheostomy may be indicated. Strictures of the esophagus may occur and require prolonged treatment. Early endoscopy is often needed in severe cases.

53–46. ALKALOIDS

A large group of basic organic plant substances that includes atropine *(53–103)*, caffeine *(53–159)*, coniine *(53–223)*, morphine *(53–455)*, nicotine *(53–478)*, quinine *(53–592)* and strychnine *(53–659)*; the term is also applied to synthetic substances with chemical structure similar to plant alkaloids, such as procaine *(53–578)* and other local anesthetics *(53–73)*.

53–47. ALKYL MERCURY COMPOUNDS

These compounds, especially the chlorides and phosphates, are widely used commercially as seed fungicides. Exposure, which may occur by ingestion or fume inhalation, causes fatigue and myalgia, headache and vertigo, sometimes associated with hyperactive reflexes, ataxia and cerebellar signs. There may be some decrease in visual fields, delirium and hallucinations. See *53–418* for further discussion, including treatment.

53–48. ALKYL SODIUM SULFATES

These complex compounds are the active agents in many household detergents. Their toxicity is very slight. Emetics, followed by a saline cathartic, should be given if large amounts have been ingested. See *53–634, Soaps and Detergents.*

53–49. ALLETHRINS (Allyl Cinerin) ($C_{19}H_{26}O_3$)

Allethrins are synthetic analogs of the naturally occurring insecticides cinerin, jasmolin and pyrethrum (see *49–584*).

53–50. ALLIUM SATIVUM L. (Garlic)

The cloves may cause burning and blistering of the skin, with formation of indolent ulcers.

53–51. ALLYL DIBROMIDE ($CH_2 = CHCHBr_2$)

This substance is used in the manufacture of other allyl compounds. Inhalation of fumes results in nausea, bradycardia, conjunctivitis, blurred vision and strabismus—all transient.

53–51A. ALOIN

All species of aloes contain aloin, a strong gastrointestinal irritant and veterinary purgative. Toxic effects are usually more uncomfortable than dangerous. Among the aloin-containing plants are columbine and clematis.

53–52. ALUMINUM AND ITS SALTS (Aluminum Ammonium Sulfate [Alum], Aluminum Acetate, Aluminum Chloride) (Al, Al^{3+})

All of the soluble salts of aluminum may cause gastroenteritis if ingested; the only treatment needed is demulcents. Aluminum oxide and hydroxide are insoluble and harmless.

---

*For therapeutic considerations see also *53–1* to *53–13*.

53–53. AMANITA POISONING *(See 53–462, Mushroom Poisoning)*

53–54. AMERICAN PLUM

The active ingredients are cyanogenic glycosides, which are found in the leaves, stems, bark and seed pits. See 53–232, *Cyanides.*

53–55. AMINOPHYLLINE (Aminophyllin) ($C_{16}H_{24}N_{10}O_4$)

Aminophylline is 85% theophylline and also contains ethylene diamine to improve solubility. See 53–694, *Theophylline,* for symptoms and treatment.

53–56. 2-AMINOPYRIDINE ($NH_2C_5H_4N$; TLV 0.5 ppm)

Inhalation of fumes from melting of this industrial material results in the delayed appearance (after 2 to 4 hours) of headache, dizziness, dyspnea, convulsions and marked elevation of blood pressure. Mild cases clear in a few hours after termination of exposure; severe cases require hospitalization for symptomatic treatment and close observation because of the danger of delayed pulmonary edema *(51).*

53–57. AMINOPYRINE (Amidopyrine, Aminophenazone, Pyramidon, Antipyrine) ($C_{13}H_{17}N_3O$)

Common commercial preparations are Aminophen Pulvules, Cibalgine, Felsol Powder and Tablets, Optalidon and Ray-Pyrine. All are sold without prescription except in Denmark, Sweden and the United States (rarely used in the U.S.). Therapeutic doses recommended by the manufacturer may cause hypersensitivity reactions and agranulocytosis. See 53–20, *Acetanilid.*

53–58. 2-AMINOTHIAZOLE ($C_3H_4N_2S$)

Exposure to this industrial chemical and thyroid inhibitor results in deep brown discoloration of the urine, anorexia, nausea and vomiting, and a serum sickness–like syndrome with large wheals, dependent edema and generalized myalgia and arthralgia.

53–59. AMITRIPTYLINE (Amitril, Elavil, Endep; also in Etrafon, Limbitrol, Triavil) ($C_{20}H_{24}ClN$) *(See 53–723, Tricyclic Antidepressants)*

53–60. AMIZOL (ATA)

The toxicity of this herbicide, used especially for control of poison oak and ivy, is probably low, but following ingestion emetics should be given at once as a precautionary measure.

53–61. AMMONIA (Refrigerants, Household Cleansers, Medications) (NH_3; TLV 25 ppm) *(See also 53–604, Rocket Fuels)*

Treatment of External Contact

- Wash the skin or irrigate the eyes with copious amounts of water.

Treatment of Inhalation

- Intensive pulmonary care may be required because of direct caustic irritation to the respiratory tract.

---

*For therapeutic considerations see also 53–*1* to 53–*13*.

Treatment of Ingestion

- Have the patient drink large quantities of water.
- Start artificial respiration or oxygen inhalations at once if dyspnea or cyanosis is present. Cricothyrotomy or tracheostomy *(18–34)* may be lifesaving and should be done without hesitation if acute edema of the glottis and respiratory distress are present. Coma and convulsions may occur.
- If a stomach tube or emetic is used at all, it is best to protect the airway with cuffed intubation.

53–62. AMMONIATED MERCURY *(See also 53–124, Bichloride of Mercury)*

If ingested, this preparation has about the same toxicity as bichloride of mercury. Systemic effects may occur from absorption through the intact skin.

53–63. AMMONIUM CHLORIDE (Sal Ammoniac) (ClH_4N)

In the presence of even slightly impaired liver or kidney function, the usual therapeutic dose of ammonium chloride, continued for a few days, may cause accumulation of toxic amounts of ammonia. See *32–10, Hepatic Coma.*

Acidosis, hypoproteinemia and coma may develop if long-continued use of ammonium chloride has embarrassed ammonia synthesis in the body. If given at the same time as sulfonamides, the danger of deposit of sulfa crystals in the kidneys is markedly increased.

Treatment

Treatment is primarily preventive and includes:

- Limitation of therapeutic use of ammonium chloride to not more than 3 to 6 g for 4 days in persons with normal renal function.
- Avoidance of administration to persons with impaired liver or kidney function.
- Avoidance of administration at the same time as sulfonamide therapy.

Treatment of Overdosage

- Discontinue medication.
- Monitor blood pH and electrolyte levels. IV administration of 5% solution of sodium bicarbonate according to need. As an alternative, a 1/6 molar solution of sodium lactate, 30 ml/kg, may be used.

53–64. AMMONIUM PICRATE (Carbazotate) ($C_6H_6N_4O_7$)

This substance is used in explosives and fireworks. For treatment, see *53–548, Picric Acid.*

53–65. AMMONIUM SULFITE ($H_8N_2O_3S$)

Widely used in metallurgy and photography and as a "cold wave set," ammonium sulfite is extremely toxic if ingested or absorbed through the skin or scalp. The treatment of toxic symptoms is similar to that outlined in *53–353, Hydrogen Sulfide.*

53–66. AMPHETAMINES (Benzedrine, Dexedrine, Methamphetamine, "Crank," "Speed") ($C_9H_{13}N$) *(See Table 53–2, under Stimulants)*

Medical use of more than 20 mg a day may cause toxic signs and symptoms. Following inhalation, the toxic picture usually develops within 5 to 10 minutes; after ingestion, a time lag of 30 to 45 minutes is common. Approved medical uses today are extremely few.

---

*For therapeutic considerations see also *53–1* to *53–13*.

Signs and Symptoms of toxicity are acute restlessness; inability to relax; flushed face (later becoming pale); mydriasis; dryness of the mucous membranes of the nose, mouth and throat; rapid pulse; elevated blood pressure; shallow respiration; and final collapse. Chronic use—short of acute toxicity—may cause personality changes and increased irritability. Paranoid symptoms, hallucinosis (often prolonged), acute anxiety and exhaustion may develop.

Severe withdrawal symptoms (apathy, psychomotor depression, sleep disturbances, aggravation of previous psychopathology and suicidal tendencies) may require a controlled environment for several weeks.

Treatment

- Empty the stomach by gastric lavage if ingested, followed by activated charcoal.
- Control seizures (see *34, Convulsions/Seizures*).
- Acidify the urine by ammonium chloride to accelerate excretion in severe cases.
- Hospitalize for observation and treatment for at least 24 to 48 hours. Psychiatric evaluation and treatment usually is indicated. Illicit ("street") use of amphetamines may consist of oral ingestion of a large number of Benzedrine or Dexedrine pills or intravenous injection of methamphetamine solutions of varying degrees of purity ("speed-balls"). See *53–647*. Treat elevated body temperatures (see 62–7 and 62–8).
- Consider use of alpha- and beta-adrenergic blocking agents, such as phentolamine (Regitine) and propranolol (Inderal), respectively, for severe cases involving life-threatening degrees of hypertension and/or tachycardia.

53–67. AMYGDALIN ($C_{20}H_{27}NO_{11}$)

Amygdalin is present in the pits of stoned fruit such as peaches and apricots; it also occurs in chokecherries, bitter almonds and berries of the jetberry bush. It is the major component of the alleged anticancer remedy Laetrile. For treatment, see *53–232, Cyanides.*

53–68. AMYL ACETATE ($C_7H_{14}O_2$) (Pear Oil, TLV 100 ppm; Banana Oil, TLV 125 ppm) *(See also 53–554, Plastic Cements and Glues)*

Signs and Symptoms may develop following exposure to fumes (fruit-like odor) as well as ingestion—headache, conjunctivitis, vomiting, muscular incoordination, laryngeal edema with or without dyspnea and cyanosis, pulmonary edema (55) and severe central nervous system depression. If from inhalation, remove from exposure; if from skin contact, remove all clothing (including shoes and socks) and wash contaminated areas thoroughly with soap and water; if from ingestion, institute gastric lavage immediately using copious amounts of water, unless profuse vomiting has occurred.

53–69. AMYL ALCOHOL ($C_5H_{11}OH$)

This alcohol is used extensively as a solvent for lacquer and explosives and is extremely dangerous if ingested or if fumes in high concentrations are inhaled. Both methods of exposure may result in headache, sleepiness, irritation of the throat, nausea, vomiting, anorexia, twitching, coma and death. See also 53–68, *Amyl Acetate,* and 53–295, *Ethyl Alcohol.*

53–70. AMYL NITRITE ($C_5H_{11}NO_2$) *(See also 53–10)*

The first evidence of nitrite toxicity is cyanosis, initially of the lips, later spreading to the fingers, toes and remainder of the body. Because of amyl nitrite's ability to induce methemoglobin, it is used in the early treatment of cyanide poisoning. Hypoxemia from methemoglobinemia then develops, followed in severe cases by coma and death from circulatory failure. Shock (*57*) may be severe. Treat methemoglobinemia (*53–12*) with methylene blue. Room deodorizers with amyl nitrite can be toxic.

---

*For therapeutic considerations see also 53–*1* to 53–*13*.

53–71. ANESTHETICS, INHALATION *(See also 53–196, Chloroform; 53–719, Trichlorethylene)*

Some of the substances used for inhalation anesthesia are halothane, nitrous oxide, divinyl ether, ethyl chloride, ethylene, ether and chloroform. Although there is a marked difference in the margin of safety for each gas, the symptoms of toxicity—deepened unconsciousness, rapid heart beat, loss of reflexes and respiratory and/or cardiac failure—and treatment are approximately the same for all.

Treatment

- Stop or significantly reduce administration of the anesthetic as soon as any of the signs of incipient toxicity or cardiac arrest *(29–8)* develop.
- Start oxygen at once, preferably by means of an endotracheal catheter and resuscitation bag or other means of ventilatory support.
- Treat shock *(57)*.

53–72. ANESTHETICS, INTRAVENOUS *(See also 53–526, Pentothal Sodium)*

Ketamine HCl (Ketaject), a newer, effective, short-acting, anesthetic agent, administered either IV or IM, may cause "emergence reactions" - (controlled usually by a short-acting barbiturate) or reactions similar to those from PCP *(53–532)*. There is increasing "street use."

53–73. ANESTHETICS, LOCAL

Toxicity of Usual Doses. The widespread use of local anesthesia in present-day medicine and dentistry has resulted in the recognition of 3 important types of reactions to usual therapeutic amounts.

ALLERGIC REACTIONS. (See also 24.) This type of toxic reaction occurs in persons who are allergic by heredity (atopic) and fortunately is relatively rare. It may be so overwhelming that death occurs in a few minutes, with rapid development of skin wheals and angioedema. Intubation or cricothyrotomy may be necessary. Acute bronchospasm *(56–4)* may occur.

Treatment

- The best treatment is prevention. Patients should be questioned regarding any family or personal history of allergy before the local anesthetic is used. Intracutaneous tests for sensitivity can be done or else a small amount of the solution to be used should be applied intranasally by means of an applicator. In an atopic patient, itching, burning and congestion will develop within 10 minutes. If the test is negative, injection of the local anesthetic can be considered as relatively safe; if positive, find alternate approaches. It is principally the fillers that are allergenic.
- Maintenance of a clear airway and prevention of hypoxemia by whatever means are necessary.
- Treat with vasopressors, antihistamines and possibly corticosteroids as for anaphylaxis *(24–1)*.

PROGNOSIS. Complete recovery unless the onset has been overwhelming and fatal. The need for avoidance of the offending drug, or of others of similar chemical structure, should be stressed to the patient. Constant wearing of a "dog tag" or wristlet *(24, Allergic Reactions)* specifying the offending substances should be recommended.

Immediate toxic reactions may be caused by accidental injection into a blood vessel, use of too concentrated a solution or very rapid absorption through an extremely vascular area. Acute toxic symptoms develop within a few seconds after injection or topical application. If death occurs, it is usually due to complete circulatory and respiratory collapse, which require immediate resuscitative measures *(5)*.

Delayed toxic reactions are the result of a relatively slow building up of a toxic blood level of a particular agent following injection or topical use. The onset is rarely less than 5 or more than 30 minutes after injection or local application. Somnolence, which may

---

*For therapeutic considerations see also *53–1* to *53–13*.

progress to coma, develops gradually. This sleepy stage in certain persons may be replaced by marked euphoria, excitement and elation. Generally, the patient feels that there is something wrong and will tell the physician so. There is a progressive decrease in rate and quality of pulse and development of facial pallor and a cold, clammy skin. Twitching of the face, hands and feet, with hypotension, syncope and convulsions, may occur. Respiratory and circulatory failure may be irreversible and terminal.

Treatment

- Mental changes require no specific treatment; however, these patients should be watched carefully for at least 30 minutes for evidence of more severe reactions.
- Hypotension—with slow, weak pulse; cold, clammy skin; intermittent apnea; and dyspnea—should be treated as primary shock *(57)*.
- Convulsions must be controlled as quickly as possible by IV/diazepam (Valium), initially 15 to 20 mg in adults and 0.1 to 0.3 mg/kg in children, or by barbiturates.

PROGNOSIS. Good if the early symptoms are recognized and proper treatment is given.

Toxicity of Excessive Amounts. Injection, ingestion or absorption of excessive amounts of any of the local anesthetics may cause extreme excitement, euphoria and laughter or acute depression and apprehension, pallor followed by dyspnea and cyanosis, tachycardia, convulsions, respiratory and/or cardiac collapse—especially cardiac arrest *(29–8)*.

Treatment Considerations Include:

- Vigorous supportive care, particularly for the cardiovascular system.
- Prevent further absorption by emesis or gastric lavage if ingested, or use tourniquet to delay absorption from soft tissues if feasible.
- Convulsions are preferably treated with IV diazepam.
- Treat any shock *(57)* and administer O_2 as needed.
- Methemoglobinemia *(53–12)* though uncommon, can occur—mostly in the young.

53–74. ANGEL'S TRUMPET (Nightshade Family, Locoweed, Moonflower)

This compound contains atropine, hyosyamine and scopolamine. Toxic signs and symptoms from ingestion are due to depression of the parasympathetic mechanism and to stimulation of the central system. For toxic effects and treatment, see *53–103, Atropine Sulfate*.

53–75. ANILINE ($C_6H_5NH_2$; TLV 5 ppm)

Aniline is a powerful and dangerous liquid of wide commercial use, which is also used as a rocket propellant *(53–604)*. It may cause toxic symptoms and signs by ingestion or absorption through the intact skin. Common household preparations containing potentially toxic amounts of aniline are paints, varnishes, marking inks, stove polishes and shoe polishes. Poisoning from the many varieties of aniline dyes is most common in children who have ingested certain types of colored crayons, sucked indelible pencils or drunk or eaten stove or shoe polish. Absorption from colored diapers may cause acute toxic symptoms in infants.

Signs and symptoms include a peculiar grayish pallor, amblyopia and decrease in visual fields, photophobia and scotomata, acute dyspnea, apathy, hypotension, generalized myalgia and occasional gastrointestinal upsets and convulsions. Methemoglobinemia *(53–12)* may be severe and require methylene blue administration.

Immediate removal from contact or exposure to fumes is important. To prevent toxic symptoms from absorption through the skin, immediate and thorough washing with dilute vinegar (acetic acid) followed by soap and water in large amounts is indicated.

53–76. ANT PASTES

These may contain arsenic trioxide *(53–92)*, calcium arsenate *(53–162)*, chlordane *(53–190)*, sodium arsenite *(53–635)* or thallium sulfate *(53–692)*. Occasionally, antimony salts *(53–81)* are substituted.

---

*For therapeutic considerations see also *53–1* to *53–13*.

53–77. ANT POWDERS *(See 53–190, Chlordane; Potassium Cyanide (53–232, Cyanides); Sodium Fluoride (53–311, Fluorides)*

53–78. ANTIBIOTICS

Most adverse reactions to antibiotics are allergic reactions *(24)* or are related to alterations of the general bacterial flora; however, some reactions are toxic, such as bone marrow depression and renal and nerve damage.

For a complete listing of adverse reactions or contraindications, see standard current pharmacology texts or the brochures furnished by the manufacturers. Discontinuance of the antibiotic and supportive therapy are basic to treatment of these cases; if continued antimicrobial therapy is required, administration of another type of antibiotic should be instituted. See *24* for treatment of acute hypersensitivity reaction.

53–79. ANTICOAGULANTS

Of the oral anticoagulant drugs, coumarin derivatives have fewer side effects. All may cause conjunctivitis, paralysis of ocular accommodation, nausea, vomiting, bloody diarrhea, hematuria, steatorrhea, jaundice, liver damage and agranulocytosis. Discontinue administration of the drug and control hemorrhage as outlined in the table in *45–8, Hemorrhage from Anticoagulant Therapy.*

53–80. ANTIHISTAMINICS

Use of these commonly prescribed drugs may cause drowsiness, dizziness, headaches, prolonged insomnia, flushing of the skin, dryness of the mouth, dilation of the pupils, rapid heart rate, gastrointestinal symptoms, and mental confusion—occasionally, visual and olfactory aberrations and hallucinations. If symptomatic with drowsiness, have patient avoid driving. Hypotension followed by collapse and unconsciousness may occur. See *53–10* for antidotal use of physostigmine salicylate, although this is of limited value. Control hyperthermia.

53–81. ANTIMONY (Sb; TLV 0.5 mg/m^3)

With or without arsenic compounds *(53–90)*, antimony is an active constituent of certain brands of commercial sprays, weed killers, ant killers and snail baits. It is also a constituent of many medicines. Antimony oxide is used in glazing cheap "china," and pottery. Poisoning from antimony compounds is usually delayed from ½ to 2 hours after ingestion. Toxicity can occur from inhalation; antimony also is an irritant to skin, eyes and mucous membranes.

Signs and symptoms include nausea and vomiting; dehydration; extreme thirst; weak, rapid pulse; a sensation of choking and tightness in the throat, with difficulty in swallowing; cyanosis; painful, profuse, watery (sometimes bloody) diarrhea; and collapse from severe shock. See *53–108, Dimercaprol (BAL)* for specific antidote. There is a tendency toward development of delayed toxicity.

53–82. ANTU (α-Naphthylthiourea) ($C_{11}H_{10}N_2S$; TLV 0.3 mg/m^3)

This rodenticide is of relatively low toxicity to humans, but ingestion of large doses may cause mild respiratory depression. The prognosis is for complete recovery even after large doses. Inhalation causes pulmonary irritation, and pulmonary edema may result.

53–83. APOMORPHINE HYDROCHLORIDE ($C_{17}H_{17}NO_2 \cdot HCl$)

This powerful emetic acts centrally as an opiate and dopamine agonist when ingested or injected hypodermically. Doses of not more than 5 mg will cause pronounced vomiting followed by depression. Larger doses will result in extreme pallor; violent—sometimes

*For therapeutic considerations see also *53–1* to *53–13*.

projectile—vomiting; irregular, weak respiration; vertigo; sometimes mydriasis; muscle weakness and spasm; and asphyxia. The specific antidote for its opiate effects is naloxone hydrochloride (Narcan), 0.01 mg/kg, to combat depressant effects, repeated as necessary (see *53–10*).

The prognosis is good; even with very large doses, complete recovery usually occurs within a few hours.

53–84. APPLE (SEED)

The active ingredients are cyanogenic glycosides. See 53–232, *Cyanides*. The seeds must be disrupted (i.e., chewed) to release the cyanogenic glycosides.

53–85. APRICOT (PIT)

The active ingredients are cyanogenic glycosides. See 53–232, *Cyanides*.

53–86. ARBOR VITAE (Red Cedar, Thuja, Yellow Cedar)

The twigs and leaves may cause severe toxic symptoms if chewed. Decoctions of the young twigs have been used in attempts to induce abortion. Severe abdominal pain, diarrhea, frothing at the mouth, difficult respiration, pulmonary edema (55), tonic or clonic convulsions and circulatory failure may occur.

53–87. ARECOLINE (Betel Nut) ($C_8H_{13}NO_2$)

Ingestion and intravenous injection of this alkaloid has caused nausea and vomiting, extreme diuresis, clonic convulsions and coma.

53–88. ARGEMONE OIL (Prickly Poppy)

Ingestion of preparations of this complex mixture of alkaloids and fatty acids may cause visual halos and glaucoma, in addition to gastrointestinal and peripheral edema.

53–89. ARNICA (Wolf's bane, Mountain Tobacco)

Extracts of this flower contain an irritating substance that was formerly a common constituent of many "patent medicines." Locally, it may cause erysipeloid dermatitis, cutaneous ulceration and gangrene and formation of profuse pus when applied to open wounds. Removal by thorough irrigation is the only treatment required.

Systemically, following ingestion it may result in severe cephalgia, nausea and vomiting, sometimes associated with severe abdominal pain, extreme pallor, dryness of the skin, rapid weak pulse, irregular (sometime Cheyne-Stokes) respiration, extreme miosis, sleepiness, unconsciousness and death through respiratory and cardiac collapse.

53–90. ARSENIC (As; TLV 0.5 mg/m^3)

Arsenic and its compounds are commonly used in medicinal preparations, Fowler's solution, rodenticides and insecticides; in metallurgy; and in the textile and chemical industries. It has been used many times in criminal poisoning.

Methods of absorption are through the intact skin, by inhalation of dust or fumes, by ingestion and by IV injection. In chronic poisoning, as with other heavy metals, it is detectable in the hair many months after it may have disappeared from feces and urine.

Signs and symptoms of toxicity usually develop in from 15 minutes to 1 hour after ingestion, inhalation of dust or fumes or IV injection; or later, if absorbed through the skin. They are characterized by nausea; vomiting (vomitus may have a garlicky odor); acute dysphagia; *acute abdominal pain* (sometimes severe enough to simulate an acute surgical abdomen); watery diarrhea; cyanosis; weak, rapid pulse; cold clammy skin; encephalitis–like symptoms; and severe shock (57). See 53–*10*, *Dimercapral (BAL)*

***For therapeutic considerations see also *53–1* to *53–13*.**

regarding specific antidote therapy. Follow with oral penicillamine. Hemodialysis may be necessary.

53–91. ARSENIC COLOR PIGMENTS *(See also 53–90, Arsenic)*

Auripigment *(53–93, Arsenic Trisulfide)*, Paris green, Schweinfurt green (copper acetoarsenite) and Scheel's green (copper arsenite) are used in industry and are extremely dangerous.

53–92. ARSENIC TRIOXIDE (As_2O_3) *(See also 53–90, Arsenic)*

This substance is insoluble—hence, has a much lower toxicity than the soluble salts but is still very toxic as compared with the pentoxide. It is the primary material for all arsenic compounds and is used in making of glass, rodenticides, pesticides, sheep dips, enamels, and hide preservatives.

53–93. ARSENIC TRISULFIDE (Auripigment) (As_2S_3) *(See also 53–90, Arsenic)*

Arsenic trisulfide is used in yellow and gold paints and may produce symptoms through absorption or ingestion.

53–94. ARSINE (Arseniuretted Hydrogens) (AsH_3; TLV 0.05 ppm)

This colorless, odorless and dangerous gas may be formed during the burning of lead in industry, from ferosilicon and from the action of impure sulfuric acid on metals.

Signs and symptoms of toxicity usually develop 2 to 6 hours after exposure. Severely exposed patients show acute anoxemia; milder cases are characterized by nausea, vomiting, severe epigastric pain, bronze tinting of the skin due to a combination of jaundice and cyanosis, convulsions, delirium and coma. Hemolysis and hemoglobinemia can occur. Hospitalize for possible dialysis and/or exchange transfusions. Dimercaprol (BAL) is of no value in acute arsine poisoning, as it does not protect against hemolysis.

53–95. ARTANE (Trihexyphenidyl HCl)

Dryness of the mouth, blurred vision, dystonic reactions and hallucinations may follow use of this synthetic antispasmodic antiparkinsonian drug. Symptoms clear when the drug is stopped. See Table 53–2, Anticholinergics.

53–96. ARUM FAMILY

The active principle is calcium oxalate crystals, and the family includes fancy-leaf caladium, elephant's ear, dieffenbachia (dumb cane) and split-leaf philodendron.

53–97. ASARUM EUROPAEUM

Ingestion of a decoction of the roots of this shrub may cause transient vomiting and diarrhea. Symptomatic care is all that is required.

53–98. ASBESTOS (TLV 5 fibers/cc>5 μ in length; OSHA standard: 2 fibers/cc >5 μ in length)

Severe cough and chest pain in a person exposed to the dust of this common insulating material may require emergency care followed by referral for thorough investigation, including x-rays, if there has been chronic, in addition to acute, exposure. Long-range delayed effects (commonly seen 15 to 35 years later) include mesothelioma, bronchogenic carcinoma and cancer of the stomach, colon and rectum.

---

*For therapeutic considerations see also *53–1* to *53–13*.

53–99. ASIMINA TRILOBA (Pawpaw)

Contact with the fruit of this North American shrub causes nausea and vomiting and vesicles with acute pruritus. Symptoms clear slowly when contact is avoided, but a brownish discoloration at the site of the vesicles may be permanent.

53–100. ASPIDUM (Male Fern)

Even small doses of this anthelminthic may give acute toxic symptoms. Among these are cephalgia, vertigo, amblyopia, yellow vision, rapid pulse, dyspnea, vomiting, diarrhea and transient syncope followed by coma, acute myalgia, trismus and occasional toxic psychoses (*54–17*). The prognosis is good even with relatively large doses.

53–101. ASPIRIN (Acetylsalicylic Acid) ($C_9H_8O_4$) *(See also 53–614, Salicylates)*

Three types of toxic reactions to this widely used antipyretic and analgesic are relatively common.

Allergic Sensitivity. This has been reported to occur in as high as 10% of persons with allergic tendencies. For treatment, see *24, Allergic Reactions*. Asthma and nasal polyps may be present.

Gastritis and Gastric Bleeding. This irritative or ulcerative bleeding generally ceases when intake of the drug is stopped. The capacity of aspirin to decrease platelet "stickiness" is an advantage therapeutically in individuals in whom there is a tendency to increased thrombotic episodes; however, it is a disadvantage in the presence of bleeding-clotting problems.

Toxicity from Acute or Chronic Ingestion of Large Doses. The minimal lethal dose is usually considered to be between 0.3 and 0.4 g/kg. For qualitative test for salicylate ingestion, see *19–7*. For estimation of clinical severity of peak serum salicylate levels after a single dose, see Figure 53–3. For signs, symptoms and treatment of acute toxicity, see *53–614, Salicylates*.

53–102. ASTHMA REMEDIES

The active agents contained in these proprietary preparations are usually atropine (*53–103*), belladonna (*53–115*), potassium nitrate (*53–481*) or stramonium (*53–657*), although aminophylline (*53–55*), antihistaminics (*53–80*), barbiturates (*53–110*), bromides (*53–146*), ephedrine (*53–287*), and iodides (*53–364*) may be present. Mixed with beer or soft drinks, some of these proprietary preparations have been used as hallucinogens (*53–332*).

The signs and symptoms of toxicity and appropriate treatment depend upon the active agent.

53–103. ATROPINE ($C_{17}H_{23}NO_3$) *(See also 53–115, Belladonna and Belladonna Alkaloids and Table 49–2, Anticholinergics)*

Acute atropine poisoning may be caused by skin absorption from belladonna plasters, by ingestion of jimson weed berries or by medicinal use (usually as atropine sulfate). The toxic picture is characterized by dryness of the mouth, difficulty in swallowing, widely dilated pupils, red hot and dry skin, tachycardia, increased body temperature, delirium and collapse.

Treatment

- If ingested, immediate emptying of the stomach by gastric lavage with a weak solution of tannic acid followed by activated charcoal in water through the lavage tube.
- Physostigmine salicylate (Antilirium), 0.5 to 2.0 mg SC, IM or IV (See *53–10*), may be used cautiously in severe cases; repeat as necessary to reverse the central nervous system effects of atropine.

---

*For therapeutic considerations see also *53–1* to *53–13*.

- Administration of oxygen as indicated.
- Control of body temperature by ice bags and alcohol sponging.
- Sedation by barbiturates or diazepam in small doses.
- Hospitalization for close observation for at least 48 hours in more severe cases. Relapses may occur after apparent complete recovery. The patient should be in a darkened room because of photophobia.

53–104. AUTUMN CROCUS (Meadow Saffron, Naked Lady)

Postingestion effects are similar to those outlined for colchicine *(53–220)*.

53–105. AZALEA

Andromedotoxin, the poisonous substance contained in these plants, is similar to aconite in many respects; in addition, it has a curare-like effect on voluntary muscles and a depressant action on the heart. See *53–34, Aconite; Curare.*

53–106. BABY POWDERS *(See 53–140, Borates; 53–669, Talc)*

53–107. BACITRACIN *(See also 53–78, Antibiotics)*

Nontoxic if applied locally; intramuscular injection of bacitracin may cause pain at the injection site, skin rashes, petechiae, tinnitus, nausea, vomiting and serious renal damage.

53–108. BAL (British Anti-Lewisite, Dimercaprol, Dithiopropanol ($C_3H_8OS_2$) *(See also 53–10)*

Originally developed to neutralize the effects of lewisite war gas, BAL at the present time is used for its ability to alleviate toxic symptoms caused by certain heavy metals.

Intramuscular (not intravenous) injections of BAL have a definite and effective place in the treatment of poisoning from certain heavy metals (antimony [*53–81*], arsenic [*53–90*], gold [*53–328*], mercury [*53–418, Bichloride of Mercury*], nickel [*53–476*] and lewisite war gas [*53–746*]). In some cases of bismuth (*53–127*), lead (*53–386*) and thallium (*53–692*) poisoning, it may be of some value. It is ineffective or contraindicated in poisoning from cadmium (*53–158*), iron (*53–369*), tellurium (*53–681*), selenium (*53–622*) and zinc (*53–759* to *53–764*). For local effects of lewisite war gas, a 2 to 5% solution or ointment of BAL is recommended.

Toxic effects are almost always caused by excessive dosage (although BAL has a large margin of safety) and develop within 30 minutes of the time of application, injection or ingestion. Most of them can be prevented by premedication with ephedrine sulfate.

SIGNS AND SYMPTOMS OF TOXICITY OF BAL

From local application—urticaria and wheals with intense pruritus, papular eruptions, mottling and increased pigmentation of the skin.

From ingestion or parenteral administration—severe headache, conjunctivitis, lacrimation, blepharospasm, a burning sensation of gums and pharynx, nausea, vomiting, rapid pulse, elevated blood pressure and tetany-like symptoms with positive Chvostek and Trousseau signs *(46–25)*. Prognosis is for complete, rapid recovery.

53–109. BANEBERRY

If ingested, it causes nonlethal gastrointestinal irritation and skin irritation from contact.

53–110. BARBITURATES *(See also 7–2, Addiction; 32, Coma; and Table 53–2, Sedatives)*

All of the numerous derivatives of barbituric acid act in a similar manner, although there is a marked variation in speed and duration of action and in toxicity. Since

*For therapeutic considerations see also *53–1* to *53–13*.

barbiturates are often prescribed in large amounts, cases of acute poisoning from accidental overdosage and suicide attempts are encountered quite frequently. Toxic effects include severe headache, disturbances in sensation (especially of the extremities), slurred speech and general impairment of coordination. The pupils may be any size. In early poisoning, foggy vision, diplopia and color variations may be present. Respirations at first are rapid, then slow and become weak from respiratory center depression. Absence of bowel sounds is indicative of severe poisoning. Pulmonary edema *(55)* from increased capillary permeability may develop. The skin is cold, clammy and cyanotic, and bullous skin lesions may arise. A weak, rapid pulse; extreme hypotension; and anuria may be present. Acute excitement, hallucinations and delirium followed by increasing sleepiness may progress to coma and death from respiratory failure. See 32, *Coma,* for grading of depressed states of consciousness.

Treatment

- Insurance of an adequate airway *(5–10)*. Administer O_2 as indicated.
- Gastric lavage with large quantities of warm water, if the drug has been ingested within 6 hours or if the gag reflex is still present. If suicidal intent *(17)* is suspected, the rectum and vagina should be examined and emptied if indicated. Follow with activated charcoal even if poisoning was by a parenterally administered long-acting barbiturate.
- If hypothermia is present, rewarm with caution depending on circumstances.
- Slow IV infusion of D5W or normal salt solution. Monitor the serum potassium level and supplement appropriately.
- Protection of the eyeballs from drying by taping the eyelids together, if in coma.
- Insertion of a retention catheter with careful measurement of intake and output if need be. Furosemide (Lasix) may aid diuresis as may urine alkalization.
- Support of the circulation by vasopressors such as dopamine if patient is properly hydrated; this may require central hemodynamic monitoring.
- Avoidance of the use of all analeptic drugs, including amphetamine sulfate (Benzedrine), pentylenetetrazol (Metrazol) and picrotoxin.
- Hospitalization in all severe cases, with careful respiratory and hemodynamic monitoring, is indicated. Peritoneal dialysis *(18–24)* or hemodialysis—especially in the case of long-acting barbiturates with hemodynamic instability—may be lifesaving. Painstaking nursing care is an essential part of therapy.

53–111. BARIUM COMPOUNDS ($BaCO_3$, $BaCl_2$, BaS, BaO_2, $BaSO_4$; TLV 0.5 mg/m^3)

Toxic reactions may follow ingestion of barium carbonate, chloride or sulfide or inhalation of dust of barium carbonate or peroxide. Barium salts are the active ingredient in several brands of commercial rodent poisons *(53–595)*. Barium sulfide is used in some depilatories *(53–244)*.

Severe toxic effects have been reported following the use in x-ray studies of barium sulfate contaminated with barium carbonate. Inhalation causes irritation and baritosis.

Signs and Symptoms: Dryness and sense of constriction of the mouth and throat; metallic taste; dilated pupils with loss of accommodation; weak, irregular pulse; rapid, shallow breathing, cyanosis, nausea; vomiting; severe gastritis with acute watery or bloody diarrhea; and gradually increasing sleepiness with mental confusion. Collapse and death from respiratory failure, severe hypokalemia *(46–16)* and cardiac arrest may occur.

Treatment Considerations Include:

- After gastric emptying, oral administration of soluble sulfates (dilute sulfuric acid, alum. magnesium or sodium sulfate) to cause formation of insoluble barium sulfate.
- Gastric lavage with 1 to 3% sodium sulfate in warm water.
- Atropine sulfate, 0.5 to 1.0 mg, to decrease colic. Small doses of morphine may be necessary to control abdominal pain.
- Intravenous potassium if hypokalemia is present.

---

*For therapeutic considerations see also 53–*1* to 53–*13*.

53–112. BARRACUDA *(See also 53–314, Rare Causes of Food Poisoning; 27–3, Barracuda Bites)*

During certain seasons, use of this fish as a food may cause acute toxic symptoms coming on many hours after ingestion. The characteristic picture includes paresthesias around the mouth, metallic taste, acute gastrointestinal irritation, severe myalgia and arthralgia and marked hypotension, which may reach shock levels *(57)*. For treatment, see *53–314, Rare Causes of Food Poisoning.*

53–113. BEECHNUT

Ingestion of beechnuts may cause facial pallor, severe headache, vomiting, abdominal pain, syncope and lassitude lasting for 5 or 6 hours. If seen early, gastric lavage followed by activated charcoal in water and saline cathartics is indicated. Complete recovery is to be expected.

53–114. BEE VENOM *(See 60–1, Bee Stings)*

53–115. BELLADONNA AND BELLADONNA ALKALOIDS

The effects, toxicity and treatment of belladonna are approximately the same as those of atropine sulfate *(53–103)* and other anticholinergics (Table 53–2). In certain individuals, the use of belladonna plasters may result in acute symptoms through absorption. Children may develop acute toxic symptoms from ingestion of any part of the plant, which is common in many household gardens, and also from deadly night shade, jimsonweed, henware and poison black cherry. Extracts of *Atropa belladonna L.* (family Solanaceae) yield atropine hyoscyamine scopolamine, asparagine and choline.

Elderly arteriosclerotic patients are especially prone to hallucinations. Urinary retention may be acute, especially if prostatic hypertrophy is present. Respiratory and circulatory depression may be extreme.

53–116. BENZANTHRONE ($C_{17}H_{10}O$)

Dermatitis, with melanosis of those portions of the skin exposed to light, has been reported following industrial exposure.

53–117. BENZENE (BENZOL) AND ITS DERIVATIVES (Toluene, Xylene, Xylol) (C_6H_6; TLV 10 ppm, OSHA ETS 1 ppm)

Acute benzene poisoning is usually caused by inhalation of fumes in industry, where it is used as a solvent, cleanser and fuel. It may be used by drug abusers for the temporary euphoria that may result with inhalation.

Signs and symptoms after inhalation: Acute conjunctivitis; severe headaches; general malaise and weakness [sometimes preceded by a brief period of exhilaration ("benzene jag")]; nausea; vomiting; facial pallor; cyanosis of the lips and fingertips; weak, rapid pulse; unconsciousness; and convulsions. Death from CNS and respiratory depression may occur. More prolonged exposure causes bone marrow depression and sometimes aplastic anemia or leukemia.

Treatment

- Remove from exposure to fumes.
- Wash the eyes with large amounts of water.
- Protect against injury during convulsions.
- Give oxygen inhalations for dyspnea and cyanosis.
- Support circulation.

Toxic effects appear more rapidly and are much more severe following ingestion than after inhalation. There is increased cardiac sensitivity to catecholamines.

---

*For therapeutic considerations see also *53–1* to *53–13*.

Signs and symptoms after ingestion: Nausea, vomiting, burning sensation in the epigastrium, headache, dizziness, staggering gait, convulsions and sleepiness progressing to stupor and loss of consciousness.

Treatment

- Precautions against aspiration must be taken. Consider emesis if there are toxic signs or if large amounts have been ingested (see 53–323, *Gasoline*). Use a cuffed endotracheal tube prior to any gastric lavage tube placement. If emesis is contraindicated, gastric lavage with warm water or 5% sodium bicarbonate solution should be initiated, followed by activated charcoal.
- Avoid products that increase absorption (alcohol, oils, fats) or ventricular fibrillation (epinephrine).
- Oxygen inhalations.
- Ascorbic acid, 50 to 100 mg IV.
- Control of convulsions by diazepam or rapid-acting barbiturates.
- Correction of fluid-electrolyte imbalance.
- Continuous electrocardiogram (ECG) monitoring because of the danger of ventricular fibrillation. External cardiac compression or defibrillation may be necessary.
- Treatment of pulmonary edema (55).
- Hospitalization after control of the acute symptoms. Delayed development of tracheobronchitis, cardiac irregularities, lung infection and severe blood changes may occur.

53–118. BENZENE HEXACHLORIDE (BHC, Benzahex, ChemHex, Lindane, 662, Gammexane) ($C_6H_6Cl_6$)

Acute toxic symptoms from this common chlorinated cyclic hydrocarbon insecticide usually follow ingestion or absorption through the intact skin, although inhalation of dust or fumes may cause an acute toxic picture. Commercial preparations contain either a mixture of several isomers in varying proportions or the gamma isomer alone (Gammexane, Lindane). The latter preparations are more dangerous because they are usually in the form of oily sprays that adhere to the skin and aid absorption. A fat biopsy may be needed to determine increased cholinesterase inhibitor levels found in chronic poisoning.

Signs and symptoms: Extreme hyperirritability to outside stimuli, with intermittent muscular spasm and convulsions, and cyanosis followed by rapidly developing circulatory and respiratory depression.

Treatment

- Remove all contaminated clothing. Wash the body thoroughly; avoid oily preparations. Protect from external stimuli.
- Empty the stomach (if ingested) by gastric lavage, leaving 30 ml of magnesium sulfate (Epsom salts) in the stomach if desired. Give activated charcoal.
- Sedate by diazepam. Calcium gluconate IV may be beneficial.
- Severe cases with marked hypotension may require levarterenol bitartrate (Levophed) or metaraminol bitartrate (Aramine) for circulatory support. *Do not* use epinephrine (Adrenalin) because of the danger of inducing ventricular fibrillation. Give oxygen prn.
- Hospitalize for close observation. Apparent recovery may be terminated by acute collapse as long as 4 days after initial exposure.
- Cholestyramine (Questran), the chloride salt of a basic anion exchange resin, has reportedly shortened the tissue half-life of other chlorinated hydrocarbons (e.g., Kepone) in patients with chronic exposure, and it may be of benefit in lindane poisoning.

53–119. BENZETHONIUM CHLORIDE (Phemerol, Syntho-San) ($C_{27}H_{42}ClNO_2$)

Ingestion of a 10% solution of this topical anti-infective agent may cause nausea, vomiting, respiratory failure and death.

---

*For therapeutic considerations see also *53–1* to *53–13*.

53–120. BENZIDINE (Diaminodiphenyl) ($NH_2C_6H_4C_6H_4NH_2$)

Used in the chemical industry and as a laboratory reagent, prolonged exposure to benzidine may cause papillomas of the bladder with secondary carcinomatous degeneration. No TLV is assigned because of carcinogenic potential.

53–121. BENZODIAZEPINES (Chlordiazepoxide [Librium], *53–191*; Diazepam [Valium], *53–248*; Flurazepam [Dalmane], *53–313;* Oxazepam [Serax], Lorazepam [Ativan])

The effectiveness and relative safety of the benzodiazepines causes them to be the most commonly prescribed antianxiety (anxiolytic) agents. The benzodiazepines may be categorized as long-acting (e.g., chlordiazepoxide, diazepam) or short-acting (e.g., oxazepam or lorazepam). A nonaccumulating benzodiazepine, such as oxazepam, is more rapidly eliminated (primarily by the kidneys) and is preferred for elderly patients and patients with hepatic impairment.

Cimetadine and alcohol can significantly compound the effect of the benzodiazepines by affecting metabolism.

Drowsiness, ataxia and mental confusion are among the more frequent adverse reactions. Extrapyramidal reactions, edema, altered libido and blood dyscrasias have been reported. Early benzodiazepine withdrawal symptoms (anxiety, tremors, sleeplessness) can be easily confused with the complaints for which the drug was originally prescribed and in rare cases of withdrawal can lead to life-threatening symptoms.

Treatment of overdose is supportive and may require vasopressors for correction of hypotension and ventilatory assistance. Dialysis is of limited value. New benzodiazepine receptor antagonists are being tested and may play a future major role in benzodiazepine overdose cases.

53–122. BENZYLCHLORIDE ($C_6H_5CH_2Cl$, TLV 1 ppm)

Fumes of benzylchloride may cause severe eye and nose irritation that subsides rapidly when exposure is stopped. Pulmonary edema may also result.

53–123. BERYLLIUM (Be; TLV 0.002 mg/m^3)

Beryllium is widely used in industry; and before being banned was used for the inside coating of fluorescent tubes and lamps. The metal itself may be the offending agent, but cases of acute poisoning have also been reported from beryllium carbonate, fluoride, hydroxide, oxide, oxyfluoride, silicate and sulfate. Tremendous variation (from a few hours to several months) in the time lag between exposure and the development of acute symptoms has been noted.

Beryllium disease is of 4 main types. Each type may be acute or chronic. The Be lymphocyte transformation test may help in identification.

Dermatitis contact type, usually from solution of beryllium salts. This condition is characterized by itching papulovesicular lesions on exposed parts.

Treatment

- Removal from exposure.
- Alum and lead acetate compresses (10%).

PROGNOSIS. Good, but re-exposure should be avoided.

Skin Ulcers—caused by minute lacerations from glass particles carrying beryllium into the skin, with formation of nonhealing ulcers.

Treatment

Surgical excision of the ulcers followed by primary closure.

Tracheobronchitis. Rarely seen as an emergency.

---

*For therapeutic considerations see also *53–1* to *53–13*.

Treatment

Treatment consists of removal from contact with beryllium. A baseline chest film should be obtained for later reference.

Chemical Pneumonitis. This condition must be distinguished from acute miliary tuberculosis. If beryllium pneumonitis is suspected from the history or physical findings, immediate hospitalization is indicated, since the reported mortality varies between 18 and 35% Delayed pulmonary interstitial fibrosis may occur.

53–124. BICHLORIDE OF MERCURY (Corrosive Sublimate) ($HgCl_2$)

Signs and Symptoms following ingestion of bichloride of mercury consist of metallic taste, whitish tongue, choking sensation, intense esophageal and gastric pain, vomiting, bloody diarrhea, drowsiness, mental confusion, anuria, convulsions and coma.

Treatment Considerations Include:

- Induction of vomiting or gastric lavage at once.
- Followed with activated charcoal in water through the lavage tube, or if gastric emptying has been achieved by emesis, give by mouth.
- Treat shock *(57)*.
- Obtain urine and blood mercury levels.
- Dimercaprol (BAL) (see *53–108*; penicillamine (cuprimine) is used as a specific antidote; see *53–10)*.
- Hospitalization at once for treatment of shock *(57)* and possible renal insufficiency or failure and for continuation of dimercaprol (BAL) therapy. Follow-up care for possible strictures is essential.

53–125. BIRD OF PARADISE (Strelitzia)

Acute gastrointestinal irritation, vertigo and drowsiness may follow ingestion. After the stomach is emptied, symptomatic treatment should be given.

53–126. BIRTH CONTROL PILLS

The active ingredients of oral contraceptive pills are usually conjugated estrogens, dimethisterone, ethinyl estradiol, mestranol and norethindrone in varying mixtures. The pills, often in attractive containers, are readily available to children in many households.

Toxic effects are mild and consist primarily of gastrointestinal irritation. Emptying the stomach by emetics or gastric lavage followed by saline cathartics is the only treatment required.

53–127. BISMUTH (Bi)

Bismuth is used in the manufacture of electric gases (low conductivity), low melting solders and fusible alloys.

Stomatitis, a purplish line on the gums, albuminuria and collapse characterize bismuth poisoning. For moderate to severe cases, dimercaprol (BAL) *(53–108)* is used.

53–128. BISMUTH SUBNITRATE

The toxicity of this commonly used gastrointestinal remedy is due not to bismuth but to reduction of the nitrate radical to nitrites in the intestinal tract. See *Nitrites, 53–484.*

53–129. BISMUTH SUBSALICYLATE ($C_7H_5BiO_4$)

Used commercially as a fungicide and, more commonly, medicinally by adults as part of an antinauseant and antidiarrheal agent (Pepto-Bismol), this practically insoluble salt

---

***For therapeutic considerations see also *53–1* to *53–13*.**

may give signs and symptoms of bismuth poisoning *(53–127)* and/or salicylate toxicity *(53–614)* in the presence of alkalies.

53–130. BITTER ALMONDS, OIL OF *(See 53–232, Cyanides)*

53–131. BLACK LAUREL

All parts of this shrub contain andromedotoxin (see *53–105, Azalea*).

53–132. BLACK LOCUST

The bark and leaves of this shrub or tree contain a dangerous toxalbumin, phytotoxin. The signs and symptoms of toxicity and treatment are similar to those outlined in *53–180, Castor Beans.*

53–133. BLEACHES (Laundry) *(See 53–356, Hypochlorites, 53–501, Oxalic Acid; 53–140, Sodium Perborate [Borates])*

Contrary to general belief, although nausea and vomiting may be severe, even the most concentrated commercial bleaches do not cause erosion or strictures. In contrast to the effects of caustic alkalies *(53–45)* complete recovery invariably occurs under symptomatic treatment.

53–134. BLEEDING HEART (Dutchman's Breeches)

All parts contain a mixture of alkaloids that may cause respiratory distress, ataxia and convulsions. The treatment is symptomatic and supportive.

53–135. BLIGHIA SAPIDA

The green and incompletely ripened fruit of this West Indian and Canal Zone tree is acutely toxic if ingested, causing nausea, vomiting, stupor, coma and convulsions. Extreme hypoglycemia is usually present, with death in about 12 hours. Children are especially susceptible. Dextrose administration is an important aspect of treatment.

53–136. BLOODROOT

All parts of the plant contain a toxic substance (sanguinarine) that on ingestion causes nausea, vomiting, diarrhea and collapse.

53–137. BLUEBERRY LEAVES

Blueberry leaves contain myrtillin, an antiglycemic agent that may cause severe and permanent liver damage.

53–138. BLUEWEED (Viper's Bugloss)

The stems and leaves contain a toxic alkaloid, pyrrolizidine. Ingestion may cause a picture similar to acute toxic hepatitis.

53–139. BLUING (Laundry)

This contains minute amounts of aniline dyes *(53–75)* and oxalic acid *(53–501).*

53–140. BORATES, BORIC ACID AND BORON ($B_4O_7^{2-}$;BH_3O_3; B) *(See also 35–604, Rocket Fuels)*

Once considered harmless and found in the form of solutions and powder in many household medicine cabinets, boric acid and its salts are now known to be extremely

*For therapeutic considerations see also *53–1* to *53–13.*

dangerous, especially to infants. Several series of severe poisonings, with some fatalities, have been reported following accidental oral administration of boric acid solution to hospital nursery infants.

Signs and symptoms include nausea, vomiting, epigastric pain, diarrhea and collapse. Acute gastroenteritis following skin and mucous membrane absorption, has been reported. In severe cases, particularly in children, cyanosis, tachycardia, metabolic acidosis, hypotension and severe shock (57) may develop. There is generally an erythematous rash extending over the whole body, sometimes involving the pharynx and tympanic membranes. The temperature may be slightly elevated but usually is subnormal.

Delirium and coma, sometimes delayed for as long as a week, may develop, followed by death from central nervous system depression. Chronic and intractable renal damage may occur.

The colorless gas boron trifluoride (BF_3; TLV 1 ppm—C) is severely irritating to the eyes, skin and lungs.

53–141. BORON OXIDE (Diborane) (B_2O_3; TLV 10 mg/m^3)

Exposure to fumes of this substance (used as a metal hardener in alloys and as a neutron absorber) causes an increase in body temperature, shortness of breath, dizziness, double vision and generalized severe myalgia. All symptoms clear when exposure is terminated.

53–142. BOTULISM *(See also 33–8 and 53–314, Food Poisoning)*

In many instances a history of eating home-canned or home-preserved foods can be obtained. A few cases of botulism following puncture wounds have been reported. It is considered to be a factor in the deaths of some infants (*Sudden Infant Death Syndrome*, 52–30).

Toxic signs and symptoms consist of descending motor paralysis and usually are delayed for 12 to 100 hours after ingestion or exposure, with development in the following order:

- Nausea and vomiting.
- Malaise, fatigue, constipation and subnormal temperature.
- Dizziness, headache and blurring of vision.
- Difficulty in swallowing and speech.
- Generalized muscular weakness.
- Coma and death from respiratory paralysis.

Botulism must be distinguished from basilar artery thrombosis, poliomyelitis (33–52) Guillain-Barré syndrome, myasthenia gravis (*49–12*) tick paralysis (27–30) and intoxication such as that due to arsenic (53–90).

Treatment

Hospitalize at once for treatment with trivalent botulinum antitoxin and symptomatic and intensive supportive care. Since 12 to 100 hours have usually elapsed before postingestion toxicity develops, emetics and lavage are of little value, but are advised. Follow with a cathartic, preferably one containing no magnesium. Ventilation assistance and oxygen therapy usually are necessary.

53–143. BOXWOOD

Boxwood contains an alkaloid, buxine—a powerful intestinal irritant and central nervous system depressant. For treatment, see 53–46, *Alkaloids*.

53–144. BRIONIA

Brionia is a strong irritant poison and may cause severe gastrointestinal irritation followed by severe shock. Treatment consists of gastric lavage, activated charcoal by mouth and supportive therapy.

---

*For therapeutic considerations see also 53–*1* to 53–*13*.

53–145. BROMATES (BrO_3^{1-})

Deaths from irreversible kidney damage have been reported following ingestion of popular brands of cold-wave hair preparations containing potassium bromate. The sodium salt, used in the processing of gold ores, is also extremely toxic. CNS depression occurs.

Treatment Considerations Include:

- Emetics and/or gastric lavage with warm water or 1% sodium thiosulfate solution followed by activated charcoal in water by mouth or via the lavage tube.
- Methylene blue tends to enhance bromate toxicity and should not be used.

53–146. BROMIDES (Br^{1-})

Sodium bromide as well as other alkaline salts of this halogen cause toxic symptoms by replacement of the chloride radical in the tissues of the body. The toxic picture is quantitative and varies depending upon the degree of intoxication, which, in turn, varies with the tolerance of the individual. Bromides are contained in a number of nonprescription sedatives. An unexplained increase in serum chloride and low anion gap (measured by an auto-analyzer, which does not distinguish chloride ion from bromide ion) along with mental status changes should lead to consideration of bromide poisoning.

Mild Intoxication (from 100 to 200 mg/dl of blood)—characterized by general listlessness, malaise, insomnia, inability to concentrate and loss of memory. Increasing the urine volume and increasing the daily sodium chloride intake (4 to 6 g) help to displace the bromide ion. Because of synergistic action, all tranquilizers and barbiturates should be stopped.

Moderate Intoxication (more than 200 mg/dl of blood, depending on individual tolerance)—causes restlessness, irritability, insomnia, generalized myalgia and arthralgia. Severe headache, acute depression and paranoia may occur, as may disorientation, retrograde amnesia and hallucinations (usually visual but sometimes auditory), incoordination and tremors. Vision changes (blurring, diplopia, photophobia, disturbances in color vision) are common. Exophthalmos and ptosis of the lids may be present.

Severe Intoxication (300 to 500 mg/dl of blood)—results in dilated, fixed pupils; shallow muddy complexion; acneform skin rashes; fetid breath; and dehydration. Sexual impotence or menstrual irregularities may be present.

Treatment

- All sources of bromide as well as tranquilizers and barbiturates (because of synergistic effect) must be stopped.
- Consider increase of sodium chloride to 6 to 10 g/day plus oral intake of 3500 to 4000 ml of fluid daily, and in severest cases also consider ammonium chloride administration and hemodialysis.

53–147. BROMINE (Br_2; TLV 0.1 ppm)

Bromine gives off brown, heavy, irritant fumes. Inhalation of even low concentrations causes lacrimation, conjunctivitis, rhinitis, pharyngitis, glottal spasm and edema, a feeling of suffocation and pulmonary edema *(55)*. High concentrations are rapidly fatal.

Treatment After Inhalation

- Removal from exposure to fumes.
- Inhalation of nebulized 5% sodium bicarbonate solution and oxygen therapy.
- Sedation.
- Hospitalization of severe cases for symptomatic and supportive therapy because of glottal edema and danger of pulmonary edema *(55)*.

Note: Swallowing of minute amounts of liquid bromine has been reported as causing stomatitis, esophagitis, gastric hemorrhage and bloody diarrhea.

---

*For therapeutic considerations see also *53–1* to *53–13*.

Treatment After Ingestion

- Gastric lavage followed by activated charcoal in water by mouth.
- Saline cathartics.
- Hospitalization according to clinical status.

53–148. BROMOFORM (Tribromethane) ($CHBr_3$; TLV 0.5 ppm)

Small doses of this sedative drug cause transient listlessness, vertigo and headache. Large doses may be fatal. The toxic picture is characterized by a burning sensation in the mouth, somnolence, stupor and coma. Areflexia, trismus, convulsions and death from respiratory failure may occur. Delayed pulmonary edema (55) may also occur.

53–149. BROOM TOP (Scoporius, Scotch Broom)

This plant contains an alkaloid, sparteine, similar in action to coniine (53–223) and nicotine (53–478).

53–150. BRUCINE ($C_{23}H_{26}N_2O_4$)

Ingestion of brucine, commonly used as a denaturant, may cause a toxic picture similar to but less serious than that of strychnine (53–659).

53–151. BUCKEYE

The flowers, seeds and nuts contain toxic glycosides. Treatment consists of emptying the stomach by emetics or gastric lavage, with symptomatic and supportive measures.

53–152. BUCKTHORN (Coyotillo, Tullidora, Wild Cherry)

Ingestion of the drupes of this shrub, indigenous to northern Mexico, Texas and New Mexico causes gradual development of symmetrical polyneuropathy, starting in the legs and progressing to quadriplegia, respiratory involvement and bulbar paralysis. It can be distinguished from Guillain-Barré syndrome by the absence of spinal fluid abnormalities. If the patient survives the initial acute progressive stage, complete recovery without residual permanent disability usually takes place.

53–153. BUPHANINE

Derived from a native herb, this alkaloid is used by African medicine men. Its action is similar to that of scopolamine (53–620).

53–154. BUTANE (C_4H_{10})

Found in natural gas and as a petroleum refinery cracking product, this explosive gas is used in the production of synthetic rubber and motor fuel. Inhalation may cause varying degrees of anesthesia. It is very explosive. For toxic effects, see 53–526, *Pentothal Sodium.*

53–155. BUTANOL (*n*-Butyl Alcohol) (C_4H_9OH; TLV 50 ppm—C)

This solvent alcohol has the same effects as ethyl alcohol (53–295) but is more toxic.

53–156. BUTESIN PICRATE (Butamben Picrate) ($C_{11}H_{15}NO_2$)

Used as an antiseptic ointment, butesin picrate has given rise on many occasions to serious dermatitides. Clearing usually occurs slowly when use of the ointment is discontinued.

---

*For therapeutic considerations see also 53–*1* to 53–*13*.

53–157. *n*-BUTYRALDOXIME

In itself, this substance, used in printing inks, is nontoxic, but inhalation of its vapors causes extreme sensitivity to ingestion of small amounts of alcoholic beverages.

53–158. CADMIUM AND ITS SALTS (Cd, CdO; TLV 0.05 mg/m^3 [dust]; 0.05 mg/m^3—C [fumes])

Acute poisoning occurs in manufacturing and use of cadmium alloys, smelting of ores, coating of bearings and tools with cadmium, electroplating, soldering and welding, process engraving, manufacturing of storage batteries, use of cadmium pigment paints and use of silver polishes containing cadmium carbonate. Small cadmium-containing batteries may leak when ingested and require immediate removal.

Methods of Poisoning

Inhalation of Fumes—usually from silver-cadmium solder. These fumes are odorless and do not produce immediate irritation; hence, dangerous amounts may be inhaled before acute symptoms occur—usually up to 12 hours later. Symptoms are dry throat, cough, headache, nausea, vomiting, a feeling of constriction and pain in the chest, dyspnea and pneumonia. Except for the occasional development of pneumonia, symptoms from inhalation disappear spontaneously in from 12 to 15 hours after onset. Symptomatic treatment only is indicated. Maintain airway and ventilation.

Ingestion. Following ingestion, acute symptoms develop in ½ to 1 hour. Use of cadmium-lined food or drink containers and cadmium-plated eating utensils is banned in some localities because of the tendency of cadmium to dissolve in the acids commonly found in food, thereby producing toxic cadmium chloride. Contamination of the water supply by industrial wastes has been reported from Japan (Itai-itai ["ouch-ouch"] disease). Symptoms consist of salivation, choking, vomiting, abdominal cramps, myalgia and diarrhea. Later symptoms include renal failure and depression.

Treatment Considerations Following Ingestion

- Empty the stomach immediately by producing emesis with syrup of ipecac or by insertion of a gastric tube for lavage. Perform immediate endoscopic or surgical removal of ingested nickel-cadmium–containing batteries if they remain present.
- Follow with activated charcoal via gastric tube or by mouth.
- After the gastrointestinal tract has been emptied, consider calcium disodium edetate administration (see *53–10*) in more severe cases.
- Correct dehydration and acid-base imbalance by intravenous fluids.
- Give supportive therapy for acute renal failure. Use of dimercaprol (BAL) should be avoided. Pulmonary edema *(55)* may be a late complication.

53–159. CAFFEINE

Acute toxic symptoms may be caused by overdoses of medications containing salts of caffeine or by excessive drinking of caffeine-containing beverages (coffee, maté, tea and many "soft drinks"). Infants and small children are peculiarly susceptible to caffeine, and acute toxic symptoms may be caused by ingestion or therapeutic injection of minute amounts. Signs and symptoms include vomiting, epigastric pain, dizziness, ringing in the ears and eye signs (constricted pupils, decreased visual fields, amblyopia, diplopia and photophobia). Headache, occasionally hallucinations and delirium, palpitation, tachycardia and a tight feeling in the chest may occur, as may trismus, opisthotonus and convulsions. Prognosis is for complete recovery without residual ill effects. As a prophylactic measure, many drinks are being "decaffeinated."

53–160. CALABAR BEAN *(See 53–547, Physostigmine [Eserine])*

53–161. CALADIUM

The varicolored leaves and the roots contain calcium oxalate crystals, which can cause severe irritation of the tongue and mucous membranes.

---

*For therapeutic considerations see also *53–1* to *53–13*.

53–162. CALCIUM ARSENATE AND ARSENITE ($Ca_3[AsO_4]_2$; TLV 1 mg/m^3) *(See 53–90, Arsenic)*

53–163. CALLA LILIES

Ingestion causes severe irritation of the mouth and throat, with acute gastroenteritis and ulceration. Large amounts may cause severe shock and death.

53–164. CALOMEL (Mercurous Chloride) (Hg_2Cl_2)

This irritant cathartic is sometimes ingested in relatively large doses, with resultant severe abdominal discomfort and greenish-black diarrhea. Control excessive diarrhea and cramping pain with paregoric, or with atropine sulfate or diphenoxylate HCl with atropine sulfate (Lomotil). Observe for nephrotic syndrome.

53–165. CALTHA PALUSTRIS (Cowslip, Marsh Marigold)

Chewing the leaves of this common plant causes transient burning of the mouth, violent abdominal pain and generalized pemphigus-like skin eruptions. Symptomatic treatment only is needed, with rapid complete recovery.

53–166. CAMBOGIA (Gamboge)

Cambogia is a violent cathartic. Doses of more than 3 g may cause complete collapse and death.

53–167. CAMELLIA

The seeds contain a glucoside that acts like digitalis *(53–265)*.

53–168. CAMPHOR (Camphorated Oil, Spirits of Camphor, Borneol) ($C_{10}H_{16}O$; TLV 2 ppm)

Vicks' VapoRub, Camphor Ice, and other proprietary medical preparations, and some moth repellents, contain camphor as the active ingredient.

Signs and symptoms include headache; sensation of warmth; characteristic odor of the breath; weak, rapid pulse; convulsions (often epileptiform); and terminal circulatory collapse. Control of convulsive seizures *(34)* may be an important aspect of the supportive therapy. Alcohol and oils enhance absorption and should be avoided.

53–169. CANTHARIDES (Spanish Fly, Russian Fly)

This substance has an undeserved reputation as an aphrodisiac, but its most common use is in hair tonics. Ingestion of small amounts may cause nausea, vomiting, abdominal pain, bloody diarrhea, delirium, coma and death from circulatory collapse.

Treatment

- Immediate emptying of stomach by emetics or gastric lavage followed by activated charcoal in water by mouth or through the lavage tube. Avoid giving oils.
- Supportive therapy as required. Shock *(57)* may be severe.

53–170. CARBAMATE PESTICIDES *(See 53–172, Carbaryl)*

53–171. CARBARSONE (p-Carbamylaminophenylarsenic Acid) ($C_7H_9AsN_2O_4$)

Used medically in the treatment of amebiasis and *Trichomonas vaginalis* infection, this substance may cause severe toxic symptoms by absorption through the skin. See *53–90, Arsenic.*

---

*For therapeutic considerations see also 53–*1* to 53–*13*.

53–172. CARBARYL (Arylam, SEVIN, 7744) ($C_{10}H_7OC[O]NHCH_3$; TLV 5 mg/m³)

The carbamate insecticides cause acetylcholine accumulation at synapses because it is a short-acting binding agent that interferes with cholinesterase activity. Signs and symptoms are those of the cholinergics (see Table 53–2) and also include (after a short delay period) abdominal pain, vomiting, diarrhea, lacrimation and cramps. Decontamination, ventilatory support and large doses of atropine (2 to 4 mg IV), as for organophosphates *(53–497)*. Atropinization of at least a slight degree may be necessary for 48 hours in severe poisonings. Use of 2-PAM in these cases is controversial and probably contraindicated.

Dithiocarbamates *(53–280)* do not have a cholinesterase inhibitor effect.

53–173. CARBON DIOXIDE (Carbonic Acid Gas, Carbonic Acid Anhydride) (CO_2; TLV 5000 ppm)

In industry, carbon dioxide, because of its weight, tends to collect in deep enclosures, especially if some fermenting substance is present. Dry ice is the solid state of carbon dioxide. Caution is advised, and even self-contained oxygen breathing apparatus (SCUBA equipment) may be needed by rescuers. Inhalation of concentrations of more than 8% may cause headache, vertigo, apparent inebriation, vomiting, dizziness, paresthesias, malaise, unconsciousness and death from asphyxia. Immediately remove to fresh air and give supportive therapy with ventilation as necessary and oxygen administration.

53–174. CARBON DISULFIDE (CS_2; TLV 20 ppm)

Carbon disulfide is used as a solvent for fats, oils, waxes, resins and rubber; in the manufacture of rayon and nylon fiber; and as an insecticide. In addition, it is a metabolite of disulfiram *(53–279)*. Ingestion or inhalation of concentrated fumes may cause respiratory depression, nausea, vomiting, convulsions and death from respiratory failure. CNS and peripheral nerve injury occur with mental impairment, paresthesias and muscle weakness. Arrhythmias and worsening of coronary heart disease may develop. Milder toxic symptoms can be caused by absorption through the intact skin; immediate washing with soap and water and removal of all contaminants is necessary. Carbon disulfide presence in the body may be confirmed by iodine-azide reaction with the urine.

Treatment Considerations Include:

- Respiratory support by expired air methods *(5–10)* after removal from exposure and insurance of a clear airway. Oxygen therapy should be instituted as soon as possible.
- If ingested, immediate gastric lavage with copious amounts of warm water.
- Circulatory support.
- Control of excitement and convulsions by intravenous diazepam (see *31, Convulsive Seizures*).

PROGNOSIS. Rapid recovery without permanent ill effects if signs and symptoms are mild; in severe cases, the patient may develop severe neuropsychiatric disorders simulating manic-depressive and paranoid states *(54)*. Increased incidence of coronary artery disease is noted.

53–175. CARBON MONOXIDE (CO; TLV 50 ppm)

This colorless, odorless gas, resulting from incomplete combustion, may be inhaled in the presence of improperly functioning or inadequately vented equipment that burns heating or illuminating gas, in the presence of automobile exhaust fumes and during the use of open circuit diving apparatus (26–5). Many deaths credited to smoke inhalation *(25–4)* are in fact due to carbon monoxide poisoning.

DIAGNOSIS. History of exposure, cherry red color to lips (may be absent or transient), peaceful expression, facial twitchings, elevated temperature, pale skin. Progressive throbbing headache, nausea, vomiting, light-headedness, tachypnea, tachycardia and weakness are earlier signs. Brownish-red stippling may be present on the arms or trunk.

---

*For therapeutic considerations see also *53–1* to *53–13*.

Syncope, coma, cardiac ischemia, permanent neurologic consequences, cardiopulmonary failure and death occur with higher carboxyhemoglobin levels. Increasing headache intensity correlates well with rising carboxyhemoglobin levels. Check arterial oxygen saturation also; carboxyhemoglobin levels are determined by a separate test, from ABG's.

Treatment

- Immediate expired air respiration after removal from exposure and determining that the airway is clear, followed by 95 to 100% oxygen inhalations initially under positive pressure using face mask or endotracheal catheter (*5*).
- Dextrose solution (50%), 100 ml. slowly IV.
- Oxygen administration, high flow 100% O_2 initially. Immediate hyperbaric oxygen chamber use with about 2.5 to 3 atmospheres of 100% O_2 for up to 90 minutes is ideal.
- Patients with atherosclerosis and cardiac disease should be hospitalized and monitored (ECG, enzyme levels) if carboxyhemoglobin level is 15% or more.
- Treat seizures (*34*) with IV diazepam and cerebral edema (*44–7*) as necessary.
- Hospitalization for close observation and symptomatic therapy (including consideration of transfusions). The patient should be kept on complete bed rest for at least 48 hours. In severe cases, induction of hypothermia should be considered. Do not give methylene blue.

53–176. CARBON TETRACHLORIDE (CCl_4; TLV:10 ppm)

Commercial uses—fire extinguishers, cleaning fluids, plant-forcing preparations and dry shampoos. Toxic effects may arise from inhalation of fumes or skin absorption as well as from ingestion. Liver necrosis may occur.

Treatment Considerations Include:

1. *Following inhalation:* Fresh air, expired air or mechanical artificial respiration (*5–10*). Administration of air or oxygen may be necessary.
2. *Following ingestion:*
   a. Gastric lavage followed by activated charcoal in water by mouth or through the lavage tube.
   b. Magnesium sulfate (Epsom salts) by mouth as a saline cathartic.
3. Small doses of morphine or meperidine (Demerol) may be necessary, since abdominal pain may be severe enough to simulate an acute surgical condition.
4. Dextrose, 5% IV.
5. Severe cases require hospitalization for peritoneal dialysis or hemodialysis, blood transfusions and measures to prevent liver and kidney damage.

Do Not Do Any of the Following:

1. Give fats or oils—they facilitate absorption.
2. Administer epinephrine hydrochloride (Adrenalin) or ephedrine—these increase the danger of ventricular fibrillation.
3. Prescribe or administer alcohol in any form—it tends to increase hepatic damage.

53–177. CARBROMAL (Adalin, Bromadal, Uradal, Nyctal) ($C_7H_{13}Br\ N_2\ O_2$)

Used as a sedative and hypnotic, carbromal in large doses (0.5 to 1.5 g) produces central nervous system depression, sometimes followed by respiratory arrest. See *53–110, Barbiturates.*

53–178. CASHEW NUTS

The oil from these nuts contains phenols, which resemble in structure and action the irritants in poison oak, poison ivy and poison sumac (*58–13*).

---

*For therapeutic considerations see also 53–*1* to 53–*13*.

53–179. CASTOR BEAN EXTRACT *(See also 53–180)*

Commercial extraction of castor oil, which of itself is a harmless cathartic, results in a residual pomace containing a very potent toxalbumin (ricin) that is notorious for causing severe allergic reactions (24), especially severe asthma and bronchospasm. Ricin causes a serious delayed onset of febrile illness, which can progress to fatal outcome; it has recently been used by assassins for such purposes. No specific antidote is known. Plasmapheresis may be considered.

53–180. CASTOR BEANS (*Ricinus communis*)

The large, varicolored, pleasant-tasting beans of this shrub are very attractive and dangerous to children, since they contain a deadly lectin poison, ricin. Ingestion of 4 or 5 seeds is usually fatal to a child; the mortality in recorded cases of all age groups is about 6%.

Evidences of castor bean poisoning usually do not come on for several hours, but then progress for 1 to 3 days after ingestion and consist of severe headache, nausea, persistent vomiting, and acute gastroenteritis, often with bloody diarrhea. Jaundice from acute hemolysis may be present. Ricin acts to inhibit protein synthesis of the intestinal wall, and severe fluid and electrolyte loss can occur. Convulsions may be followed by death in 6 to 10 days.

Treatment Considerations Include:

- Immediate emptying of the stomach followed as soon as possible after ingestion by activated charcoal in water, even if ingestion is only suspected.
- Close observation for at least 3 days; hospitalize as necessary.
- Correct for fluid and electrolyte loss. Consider parenteral alimentation and plasmapheresis.

For toxic reactions during commercial processing of castor beans, see *53–179.*

53–181. CASTRIX

If ingested, this insecticide may cause severe convulsions. See *53–659, Strychnine.*

53–182. CEDAR OIL

Cedar wood oil has been used as an abortifacient, with development of rapid irregular respiration; cold, clammy skin; convulsions; and coma.

53–183. CHELIDONINE

This substance is the active principle of a common plant, golden celandine. Chewing the leaves causes burning of the mouth and throat, acute gastric pain, somnolence, diarrhea and collapse.

53–184. CHEMOPODIUM (Wormseed, Santonin)

Medicinal use as an anthelmintic may cause acute toxic symptoms even with extremely small doses.

Signs and symptoms include nausea, vomiting, abdominal pain, headache, dizziness, impairment of vision and hearing, acute depression, low back and flank pain from kidney damage, delirium and clonic convulsions. Slow, weak respirations, sometimes Cheyne-Stokes in type, may occur, with death from respiratory paralysis.

The prognosis is fair; sequelae such as polyneuritis, paresis and decreased hearing may persist for a lengthy period.

---

*For therapeutic considerations see also *53–1* to *53–13*.

53–185. CHERRY

The bark, leaves and pits of certain cherry trees, especially the wild black cherry (*Prunus serotina*), are toxic owing to the presence of amygdalin (53–67), which breaks down into hydrocyanic acid. See also *53–205, Chokeberry; 53–307, Finger Cherry; 53–152, Buckthorn (Wild Cherry).*

53–186. CHLORAL HYDRATE ($C_2H_3Cl_3O_2$) *(See also Table 53–2; Sedatives)*

"Knockout drops," sometimes administered in alcoholic beverages, usually contain chloral hydrate.

DIAGNOSIS. History of intake, muscles relaxed, pupils constricted, respiration weak and shallow, pulse barely perceptible, skin cold and clammy, temperature and blood pressure below normal. Cardiac arrhythmias may occur. An abdominal x-ray will reveal this radiopaque substance.

53–187. CHLORAMINE T ($C_7H_7Cl\ N\ NaO_2S$)

Several series of cases have been reported in which severe toxic symptoms have followed accidental ingestion of this commonly used drinking water disinfectant.

Signs and Symptoms: Rapid onset of respiratory embarrassment, cyanosis, marked hypotension, subnormal temperature, abdominal pain and convulsions. Death from respiratory failure usually occurs within a few minutes if a large amount has been ingested; if the patient survives more than 30 minutes, the prognosis is usually good.

53–188. CHLORAMPHENICOL (Chloromycetin) ($C_{11}H_{12}Cl_2N_2O_5$) *(See also 53–78, Antibiotics)*

Usual doses may cause nausea, vomiting, diarrhea, acute skin reactions and vulval and rectal irritation. Prolonged use may result in stomatitis, aplastic anemia and serious liver damage. Children apparently are more susceptible than adults.

53–189. CHLORATES (ClO_3^{-1})

Potassium chlorate ($KClO_3$) is used extensively in industry as an oxidizing agent and is found in explosives, fireworks, matches and medicinally formerly was used as an antiseptic and astringent.

Signs and symptoms include dryness of throat, severe gastric pain, vomiting, diarrhea, yellow sclerae, cyanotic skin due to methemoglobinemia, tendency to hemorrhage (epistaxis, metrorrhagia and purpura hemorrhagica) and respiratory collapse.

Dialysis may be needed in severe cases. Oxygen and whole blood or red blood cell transfusion are used to treat methemoglobinemia *(53–12)* in preference to methylene blue.

53–190. CHLORDANE (Compound 1068, Dowklor, Octa-Klor) ($C_{10}\ H_6\ Cl_8$; TLV 0.5 mg/m^3)

This complex substance has wide commercial use as an insecticide spray and dust. Evidences of toxicity may develop following inhalation of the mist or dust or following skin absorption or ingestion. Convulsions and deep depression, often fatal, may develop. Immediately remove all contaminated clothing using caution also not to contaminate others. The skin should be washed thoroughly with copious amounts of soap and water. The eyes should be irrigated with tap water. Diazepam may be necessary for control of convulsions, but because of the already present respiratory depression, close observation is necessary and ventilatory support may be needed.

---

*For therapeutic considerations see also *53–1* to *53–13*.

53–191. CHLORDIAZEPOXIDE (Librium) ($C_{16}H_{14}ClN_3O$) *(See also 53–121, Benzodiazepines)*

In commonly used dosages this sedative-tranquilizer may cause mental confusion, hypotension, edema (especially pretibial) and decreased libido.

53–192. CHLORINE (Cl_2; TLV 1 ppm)

This irritant gas, when inhaled, causes acute respiratory irritation, which may be followed by pulmonary edema (sometimes delayed) *(55)*, pneumonia and circulatory collapse. Removal from exposure and removal from the skin by use of copious amounts of soap and water is necessary. More severe cases may require hospitalization because of danger of development of pneumonia *(56–16)* or pulmonary edema *(55)*.

53–193. CHLOROACETOPHENONE (Mace or CN) (C_8H_7ClO; TLV:0.05 ppm) *(See also 53–746, War Gases)*

Chloroacetophenone, dissolved in an ether alcohol solution, is the active ingredient in most police "tear gas" guns. It is emitted, together with paper wadding and synthetic packing, under considerable pressure, usually by a freon propellant. An aerosol preparation containing a 1% chloroacetophenone solution, used by law enforcement officers, is known as "Mace."

Chloroacetophenone, a skin and mucosal irritant, is a powerful lacrimator, causing profuse tearing, smarting and burning of the eyes, blurred vision and temporary blindness. Skin irritation, including blistering, and headache occur. The effects are usually transient, owing to high volatility, unless particles have been driven into the tissues by the propellant.

A more toxic, less volatile tear gas, chlorobenzalmalononitrile (CS), has the effects of CN plus greater respiratory tract symptoms. Dibenzoxazepine (CR) is less toxic, but more potent than CN; increase of arterial and intraocular pressure, even with precipitation of acute glaucoma, have been noted.

Treatment

Initial treatment consists of removing victim from exposure, facing victim toward any wind, removing contaminated clothing, general hosing and thorough rinsing of eyes with water if available, restricting rubbing of eyes and assurance that most symptoms subside spontaneously in about 15 minutes. Aeration and vacuuming of particles further prevent secondary affliction of others.

Thorough irrigation of the eyes with 2% sodium bicarbonate, saline or water is indicated, followed by use of sunglasses for comfort. More severe cases require referral of the patient to an ophthalmologist; a few cases of permanent blindness have been reported. The skin may be cleansed with 5 to 10% sodium bicarbonate, then with soap and water shower.

53–194. CHLOROBENZENE (Monochlorobenzene) (C_6H_5Cl; TLV 75 ppm)

This is used in the dry cleaning industry and in the preparation of coal tar pigments and dyes. It may produce toxic symptoms through skin absorption, inhalation of fumes or ingestion. Evidence of poisoning is usually delayed for 2 to 5 hours after exposure and is characterized by headache, sleepiness deepening into coma, pallor, cyanosis from methemoglobinemia *(53–12)*, fibrillary twitching and respiratory and circulatory collapse.

53–195. CHLORODINITROBENZENE

Skin contact with this substance, used in the explosives industry, causes severe dermatitis and acute sensitization. Serious changes (cyanosis, dyspnea, giddiness, stag-

---

*For therapeutic considerations see also *53–1* to *53–13*.

gering gait and liver and spleen enlargement) may follow inhalation of fumes or ingestion. Symptomatic treatment, after stopping exposure, results in a slow clearing of toxic signs and symptoms.

53–196. CHLOROFORM (Trichloromethane) ($CHCl_3$; TLV 25 ppm)

In addition to its use as a general anesthetic, chloroform is used extensively in industry as a solvent for fats and resins. It is not absorbed through the skin but may cause severe erythema and purulent blebs locally.

Three types of acute chloroform poisoning may require emergency treatment.

Inhalation Type. Overdosage during chloroform anesthesia or ingestion of large amounts results in sudden dilation of the pupils (terminally, the corneas become dull and cloudy), sudden disappearance of the pulse, complete respiratory failure and rapid death from circulatory collapse and ventricular fibrillation (29–25).

Treatment Considerations Include:

- Stop anesthesia if from inhalation; start gastric lavage immediately if from ingestion.
- Begin oxygen administration and ventilation at once.
- Support the cardiovascular system. Epinephrine hydrochloride (Adrenalin) is contraindicated; it may cause acute ventricular fibrillation.

Ingestion Type. Signs and symptoms include burning sensation in the mouth, throat, esophagus and stomach; nausea, vomiting; cold, clammy skin, cyanosis of the extremities and face; gasping, irregular respiration; extreme dilation of the pupils; and muscular cramping, especially of the masseters. Progressive hypotension from increasing cardiac weakness, peripheral vasodilation and respiratory failure may occur. The prognosis, however, is much better than that for the inhalation type. Hospitalization for observation and treatment of possible liver damage is usually indicated.

Delayed toxicity type. Delayed toxic reactions to chloroform usually develop 3 to 5 days after administration of an anesthetic to elderly, rundown or cachectic persons and are characterized by severe liver and kidney damage, gradual development of drowsiness and sleepiness, nausea and vomiting and changes in size of the liver—it is usually enlarged and painful but may be contracted. Signs of kidney irritation may be present, and the urine may contain acetone and bile pigments. Delirium and coma may develop.

53–197. CHLORONAPHTHALENE (Halowax)

Signs and symptoms of toxicity follow absorption through the skin and inhalation of the vapors, fumes and dust; these consist of acute gastrointestinal irritation, jaundice, convulsions and coma. Severe liver damage may occur.

53–198. CHLORONITROBENZENE ($C_6H_4ClNO_2$) *(See 53–485, Nitrobenzene)*

53–199. CHLOROPICRIN (Nitrochloroform) (CCl_3NO_2; TLV 0.1 ppm)

Developed originally as a war gas, chloropicrin (trichloronitromethane) is now used as a fumigant. Vomiting is the chief symptom of toxicity. For treatment, see 53–746, *War Gases.*

53–200. CHLOROQUINE PHOSPHATE (Aralen Diphosphate) ($C_{18}H_{32}ClN_3O_8P_2$)

Blindness and retinopathy have been reported following long-term use of this antimalarial drug. Accidental ingestion by children of even small amounts has a high mortality rate. Fatalities have been caused by as little as 1 g.

Signs and symptoms of toxicity develop rapidly, usually within 30 minutes. Very severe

*For therapeutic considerations see also *53–1* to *53–13*.

headaches, visual disturbances and convulsions are common. Respiratory and cardiac arrest *(29–8)* may develop suddenly and without warning. Methemoglobinemia *(53–12)* may occur.

53–201. CHLOROTHIAZIDE (Diuril) ($C_7H_6ClN_3O_4S_2$) *(See 53–696, Thiazide Diuretics)*

53–202. CHLORPHENIRAMINE (Histadyl HCl) ($C_{16}H_{19}ClN_2$)

Usual therapeutic doses of this antihistaminic drug may cause transient nausea, vomiting, headache and nervous tension. Large doses taken by accident or with suicidal intent have caused tetanic jerking, tachycardia, dilated pupils, clonic convulsions, cyanosis, pulmonary edema, anuria and death.

53–203. CHLORPROMAZINE HYDROCHLORIDE (Thorazine) ($C_{17}H_{19}ClN_2S$) *(See also 53–536, Phenothiazines)*

This valuable drug has multiple actions and may give a wide variety of toxic side effects. Primarily, it is a central nervous system depressant, but it has also a mild antispasmodic and antihistaminic action. The amount required to cause undesirable side effects varies markedly in different individuals. These side effects are more uncomfortable than dangerous; they include the following:

Hypotension. Although the decrease in blood pressure is usually mild and transient, in occasional instances it may be severe enough to require therapy for shock *(57)*. With even a small initial dose—particularly by injection—the patient should be lying down when the drug is given and kept under observation for at least 20 minutes. Transient syncope and tachycardia occur, as do allergic reactions *(24)*.

Drowsiness and dizziness. These symptoms are transient but may occur after small oral doses. All patients receiving chlo-promazine hydrochloride (Thorazine) should be warned against driving a motor vehicle.

Parkinsonian syndrome symptoms. These may follow large doses but will often disappear on cessation of therapy. Extrapyramidal side effects are also seen and can be treated with anticholinergics.

Autonomic nervous system symptoms (nasal congestion, dryness of the mucous membranes, constipation, etc.) These are mild and require no treatment.

Secondary symptoms. These may be caused by the tendency of chlorpromazine to accentuate and prolong the effects of sedatives, narcotics, analgesics and anesthetics.

Jaundice. This is usually transient and benign.

PROGNOSIS. Good for rapid complete recovery, unless serious blood changes such as agranulocytosis have occurred. The drug has a wide margin of safety.

53–204. CHLORTETRACYCLINE HYDROCHLORIDE (Aureomycin) ($C_{22}H_{24}Cl_2N_2O_8$) *(See 53–78, Antibiotics)*

53–205. CHOKECHERRY

Sometimes eaten in large quantities by children, campers and tourists, this wild fruit may cause serious and even fatal toxic symptoms. The toxicity is due to the presence of *amygdalin (53–67)*. The treatment is the same as outlined in 53–232, *Cyanides.*

53–206. CHROMATES, CHROMIC ACID (CrO_4^{2-}, CrO_3; TLV 0.05 mg/m^3)

Chromic acid and its salts are used medicinally, in paints and in the chemical and leather industries. Chromates are found in cement.

Modes of Toxicity

Exposure to dust may cause chronic sloughing of the nasal cartilages, with epistaxis and acute macular dermatitis. Acute allergic reactions *(24)*, sometimes severe, may also

---

*For therapeutic considerations see also *53–1* to *53–13*.

occur. The incidence of bronchogenic cancer is higher in workers with chronic exposure to chromates.

Ingestion may cause yellow discoloration of the mouth and pharynx; cold, clammy, cyanotic skin; and dysphagia from corrosion and edema of the posterior pharynx, glottis (at times requiring tracheostomy) and esophagus. Severe gastric burning, with vomiting of yellowish and greenish material, followed by watery, bloody diarrhea, often occurs. Generalized myalgia may be acute. Acute kidney damage may cause coma and death. Methemoglobinemia *(53–12)* may be present. Tracheostomy should be done if swelling of the glottis is progressive and possible interference with breathing is anticipated.

53–207. CHRYSAROBIN

Accidental ingestion of this substance, sometimes used in the treatment of fungous infections, has caused severe nausea, vomiting, gastric pain and diarrhea. It apparently acts only as a simple irritant. Treatment consists of demulcents and emetics by mouth, followed by magnesium sulfate (Epsom salts). Complete recovery without residual ill effects is the rule.

53–208. CICUTA VIROSA (Musquash Root, Spotted Cowbane, Water Hemlock)

The whole plant, but particularly the rhizomes of this plant contain a toxic substance, cicutoxin, which is an unsaturated aliphatic alcohol. Ingestion of any part of the root results, after a lapse of about 1 hour, in lassitude (or excitement), nausea, vomiting and convulsions, with trismus and opisthotonus. Loss of consciousness and death from circulatory failure may occur within a few hours.

There is danger of delayed circulatory collapse after apparent recovery, and close observation is advised.

53–209. CIGARETTES AND CIGARS

Ingestion of cigarette and cigar butts by small children has been fatal. Smoking may result in acute toxic symptoms in nonaccustomed persons; the developing fetus in utero also may be affected adversely. The toxic effects are due to nicotine (53–478). Statistics indicate a direct relationship between chronic smoking and lung cancer, bronchitis and atherosclerotic heart disease. Legislation and organizational policy is increasingly restricting smoking in airplanes, hospitals, work sites and other public places, to diminish the deleterious effects of involuntary smoking.

53–210. CIMETIDINE (Tagamet)

Cimetidine effectively inhibits gastric acid secretion, not as an anticholinergic agent but rather as a new class of medication, by competitively inhibiting the action of histamine at the histamine H_2 receptors. As one of the most frequently prescribed drugs, significant adverse interactions with other medications have surfaced which require caution in its use.

Infrequent mild transient diarrhea or constipation, fatigue, mental status changes, rash, dizziness and (rarely) muscular and joint pain may occur with cimetidine alone. Cimetidine potentiates certain medications, such as warfarin-type anticoagulants, chlordiazepoxide, diazepam, phenytoin, propranolol and theophylline. The mechanism of action of cimetidine-induced drug interactions is either inhibition of hepatic microsomal enzyme systems or decreasing of local hepatic blood flow. Conservative dosage and close monitoring is advised. Reduction in dose is mandatory in patients with renal failure.

In cases of overdosage supportive care is usually all that is needed; occasionally a beta-blocking agent may be used to control tachycardia, and ventilatory support may be required.

---

*For therapeutic considerations see also *53–1* to *53–13*.

53–211. CINCHONINE ($C_{19}H_{22}N_2O$)

Cinchonine is one of the alkaloids of cinchona bark and has been used as a bitter tonic. The toxic picture from ingestion of moderate amounts resembles that from quinine *(53–592)*. The treatment is the same as that for quinine.

53–212. CINEOL ($C_{10}H_{18}O$)

Cineol is one of the chief toxic substances in oil of cajeput and oil of eucalyptus. (See *53–303, Eucalyptol; 53–494, Oil, Essential.)*

53–213. CINNAMON OIL (Oil of Cassia)

Exposure to cinnamon oil in industry may cause acute dermatitis and cheilitis. Hypersensitive persons who use bubble gum, chewing gum, toothpaste or cosmetics containing cinnamon oil may develop similar toxic pictures. Symptoms clear rapidly when exposure is terminated.

53–214. CITRIC ACID ($C_6H_8O_7$)

Small amounts of citric acid are harmless. Ingestion of large amounts may cause acute but transient gastrointestinal irritation. Transfusions of citrated blood may cause serious reactions, with tetany-like symptoms *(18–35)* and serious abnormalities of cardiac function.

53–215. CLEANING FLUIDS AND COMPOUNDS

These preparations—often attractively packaged—are readily available in most households and account for many cases of severe poisoning in children. Common offenders are ammonia *(53–61)*, benzene (benzol) and its derivatives [naphtha, toluene, toluol, xylene; xylol *(53–117)*, carbon tetrachloride *(53–176)*, chlorine *(53–192)*, gasoline *(53–323)*, hypochlorites *(53–356)*, kerosene *(53–379)*, oxalic acid *(53–501)*, sodium hydroxide *(53–639)*, Stoddard solvent *(53–656)* and trichloroethylene *(53–719)*.

Mixtures of household cleaning agents can be dangerous. Sodium hypochloride *(53–636)* and vinegar give off toxic concentrations of chlorine gas *(53–192)*. Sodium hypochlorite and ammonia-containing preparations give off ammonia gas *(53–61)*.

53–216. CLONIDINE (Catapres) ($C_9H_9Cl_2N_3$)

This common, effective antihypertensive medication appears to be a central alpha-adrenergic stimulator and decreases sympathetic outflow from the brain. Oral dryness, drowsiness and sedation are common. Profound rapid hypotension, weakness, bradycardia, somnolence, diminished or absent reflexes, constricted pupils and a picture simulating narcotic overdose may occur with excess ingestion. Cardiac and dermatologic complications present less frequently. In severe massive overdoses, profound hypertension has been noted that has required vasodilator therapy! *Note:* Rapid withdrawal of clonidine can cause marked hypertensive episodes.

Treatment

Treatment with gastric emptying, an analeptic as needed, and a vasopressor usually result in complete recovery in 24 hours or so. Naloxone has been recommended, but its efficacy is as yet unproved. Atropine has been used when bradycardia is present. In the hypotensive patient who has not responded to fluids, alpha-blockers such as tolazoline or phentolamine have been used to raise the blood pressure, but their use is controversial.

---

*For therapeutic considerations see also *53–1* to *53–13*.

53–217. COBALT (Co; TLV 0.1 mg/m³) *(See 53–423, Metal Fumes)*

53–218. COCAINE ("Snow") ($C_{17}H_{21}NO_4$) *(See also 53–73, Anesthetics, Local)*

Cocaine and its salts may cause severe toxic symptoms in a number of ways.

By Absorption. Cocaine may be absorbed through the skin or mucous membranes following topical use. See 53–73, *Anesthetics, Local.* Ischemic ulcerations also can develop in the nose from "snorting" due to recurrent intense vasoconstriction.

By Use in the Eyes. *Signs and symptoms* include acute conjunctivitis sometimes with hemorrhage, chemosis, lacrimation, photophobia, edema of the lids, corneal ulceration, keratitis, glaucoma and acute systemic symptoms as outlined later in this section.

By Self-Administration. Cocaine and its salts in certain individuals cause euphoria, elation and increased mental and physical activity. Sniffing of the powder or solution, ingestion, or hypodermic injection may result in toxic effects that will cause the user to be brought for examination and treatment. Tachyphylaxis occurs allowing tremendous doses to be tolerated, but the remarkable absence of acute withdrawal symptoms results in few, if any, cases of true addiction (7). Continued use, however, results in mental and moral deterioration (including criminal activity, to support the habit), cachexia, insomnia, diplopia, transient paresthesias, hallucinations and mania—sometimes homicidal. Self-administration is reportable at once to the proper authorities.

Signs and symptoms of cocaine intoxication following overdosage by any method, or in hypersensitive persons consist of widely dilated pupils; weak, rapid pulse; severe chills; pale, clammy skin; burning and feeling of constriction in the pharynx; dysphagia; and vomiting. Gastric pain, with tenesmus and diarrhea, may be severe enough to be mistaken for an acute surgical abdomen. Acute dyspnea (occasionally Cheyne-Stokes respiration) may occur. Central nervous system symptoms (headache, dizziness, excitement, confusion, hallucinations and loss of the senses of taste and smell) are fairly common. Slowly developing coma may be followed by death from respiratory failure.

Treatment

If cocaine has been recently injected subcutaneously or intramuscularly, absorption sometimes can be controlled to some extent by application of a compression bandage or judicious cooling. If the drug has been injected intravenously, the onset of toxic effects is so rapid that a tourniquet is of no value. After the stomach is cleared, repeat doses of charcoal are administered, or the patient is placed on NG suction to remove any cocaine that has been secreted into the gastric contents. Diazepam (Valium) may be used to control excitement states if a gentle manner and subdued environment are inadequate. Alpha- and beta-adrenergic blocking agents (phentolamine [Regitine] and propranolol [Inderal], respectively), preferably orally if circumstances permit, can reduce cardiovascular stimulatory effects of cocaine. Information for addicts available by dialing 800-COCAINE.

53–219. CODEINE (Methylmorphine) ($C_{18}H_{21}NO_3$)

This widely used (and overused) narcotic is relatively safe for occasional use (chronic administration is best avoided). Large oral or parenteral doses may cause slowing of the pulse (which usually remains regular and of good quality), flushing of the face, a feeling of tightness in the head (especially in the occipital region), extreme generalized vasodilation, nausea, vomiting, gastric pain, temporary anuria, constipation and fecal impaction. Extreme miosis may occur in early stages, followed by terminal mydriasis. Exophthalmos may be present. Muscle fibrillation, tremors, generalized convulsions and respiratory failure are indicative of severer states of toxicity. Naloxone hydrochloride (Narcan) *(53–10)* is the specific narcotic antagonist.

53–220. COLCHICINE ($C_{22}H_{25}NO_6$)

Colchicine is an active and toxic alkaloid occurring in a common plant, meadow saffron. Ingestion of any part of the plant may cause acute poisoning. If colchicine is

---

*For therapeutic considerations see also *53–1* to *53–13*.

used medicinally as an antigout remedy, overdosage may cause severe toxic signs and symptoms coming on about 2 hours after ingestion.

Signs and symptoms include a sensation of suffocation and tightness in the chest, difficulty in swallowing, nausea, violent vomiting and watery or bloody diarrhea. Severe generalized myalgia and arthralgia with twitching of iolated muscle groups—especially in the calves—are common. Late symptoms are cyanosis and dilated pupils, severe shock, hematuria and oliguria, ascending paralysis, delirium and convulsions. The patient usually remains conscious, but death can occur in from 10 to 36 hours from generalized exhaustion and respiratory failure.

53–221. COLOCYNTH (Bitter Apples)

Signs and symptoms of toxicity following ingestion include visual and auditory disturbances, vertigo, confusion disorientation, severe abdominal pain, watery or bloody diarrhea, kidney irritation (polyuria, oliguria), liver and pancreas damage and circulatory disturbances (weakness, faintness, clammy skin, etc.), followed by collapse.

53–222. COLUMBINE *(See 53–51A, Aloin)*

53–223. CONIINE (Poison Hemlock, Horseradish, California Fern, Blue Lupin)

The whole plant contains coniine, with especially high concentrations in the seeds and roots. The leaves containing this alkaloid may be confused with parsley, celery, carrot and parsnip. Ingestion may cause nausea, vomiting, salivation, acute dysphagia, dilated pupils, diplopia, amblyopia, impaired hearing, convulsions and progressive weakening of skeletal musculature with terminal involvement of the respiratory muscles. Illness is severe, but mortality is low.

53–224. COPPER (Cu; TLV 1 mg/m^3 [dust] or 0.2 mg/m^3 [fume])

Chronic copper poisoning gives a toxic picture similar to that of lead poisoning *(53–386, Lead Salts)*. Certain soluble copper salts may cause vomiting and acute gastroenteritis. Further information on specific copper compounds is as follows:

- Copper acetoarsenite (verdigris, Paris green): See arsenic poisoning symptoms *(53–90)*, which are also caused by this pigment.
- Copper oxides: See *53–423, Metal Fumes.*
- Copper solutions used in the treatment of phosphorus burns: See *28–23.*

Treatment

Hospitalize in severe cases for symptomatic and supportive care and because of the danger of renal and hepatic complications. Consider treatment with calcium EDTA *(53–10)* or penicillamine.

53–225. CORTICOTROPIN (ACTH, ACTHAR)

This potent anterior pituitary hormone is a polypeptide that has many adverse physiologic side effects in addition to its main function of stimulating the adrenal cortex to produce and secrete steroids. Any combination of these side effects may result in symptoms severe enough to cause the patient to seek emergency care. The most common are headache, dizziness, transient blurring of vision, bizarre paresthesias, nervousness, insomnia, fatigue, exhaustion, psychoneurosis, signs of fluid balance disturbance (edema, anasarca, polydipsia, etc.) and alkalosis with lowered potassium levels. Acute sensitivity reactions *(24)* may develop in individuals sensitive to porcine proteins.

---

*For therapeutic considerations see also *53–1* to *53–13*.

53–226. CORTISONE ($C_{21}H_{28}O_5$)

Prolonged use of excess amounts of this crystalline hormonal substance may cause many types of toxic symptoms, especially through sodium retention and metabolic alkalosis *(46–3)*. Hypertension, sleepiness, nervousness, extreme weakness, osteoporosis, hirsutism, psychosis and pain and hemorrhage from the upper gastrointestinal tract may occur. Except for stopping the cortisone and administering sedation, the only treatment required is arrangement for thorough evaluation, preferably under hospital control in severe cases.

53–227. COSMETICS

Although an almost endless variety of substances are used in cosmetics, antimony *(53–81)* and arsenic-containing compounds *(53–90)* are the main offenders in the production of acute toxic symptoms. The use of "indelible" lipsticks may cause soreness of the tongue and throat, coryza, sinusitis, dermatitis and urticaria. Patch tests may be necessary to identify the offending substances. Rapid recovery usually takes place when use of the offending cosmetic is discontinued.

53–228. CRAYONS

Most varieties of children's chalk and wax crayons are required by law to be harmless. In spite of this, ingestion of some types of wax crayons—usually red or orange—may cause toxic symptoms from paranitraniline and/or benzidine *(53–120)*. In addition, toxic symptoms from arsenic salts *(53–90)*, chromium *(53–206)*, copper *(53–224)* and lead *(53–385)* have been reported. Some marking crayons, such as those used by carpenters, contain aniline dyes *(53–75)* and may be dangerous if even small amounts are ingested.

53–229. CREOSOTE (Wood Creosote, Beech Creosote)

The toxic properties of this substance are the result of its phenol and cresol content. Cresol is methylphenol and is obtained from coal tar and toluene. Creolin contains about 15% cresol, and saprol contains about 40% cresol. For toxic picture and treatment, see *53–534, Phenol.*

53–230. CROTON OIL *(See also 53–447)*

Acute and dangerous toxic signs and symptoms caused by this potent irritant cathartic and purgative are sometimes encountered following ingestion in an alcoholic drink [the so-called "Mickey Finn" *(53–447)*, used by bartenders to get rid of offensive or obstreperous customers.] There is a burning sensation in the mouth, severe stomach pain, nausea, vomiting, severe purging (often with bloody diarrhea), collapse and coma.

53–231. CURARE (Intocostrin, Metubine Iodide, *d*-Tubocurarine Chloride)

Curare is obtained mostly from the bark (although the leaves and shoots may also be toxic) of various trees (e.g., strychnos, chondrodendron and crybaby).

Acute toxic signs and symptoms may follow parenteral injection of any derivatives of curare as adjuncts to anesthesia or as muscle relaxants and are characterized by prolonged apnea, bradycardia, vascular collapse and symptoms resulting from histamine release.

Treatment Considerations Include:

- Maintenance of a patent airway, oxygen and ventilation.
- Neostigmine methylsulfate, 1 to 3 mg IV, combined with 0.6 mg to 1.2 mg of atropine sulfate. Edrophonium, 10 mg IV, repeated as necessary, may be helpful.

---

*For therapeutic considerations see also *53–1* to *53–13*.

53–232. CYANIDES ($Ca[CN]_2$, KCN, NaCN HCN; TLV:5 mg/m^3)

Use of cyanide compounds is prevalent in the metal industries and in photography, and calcium cyanide is used as a fumigant. Cyanide is also released from stone fruit seeds (*53–67*). Cyanides inhibit cytochrome oxidase and other metabolic enzymes in the body and cause asphyxia. Criminal contamination of Extra Strength Tylenol in 1982 demonstrated cyanide's high lethality (and also led to greater tamper-proof containerization).

Signs and Symptoms. Victims of acute cyanide poisoning are often either dead or in deep coma when first seen by a physician. Occasionally, recognition of the known exposure and the odor of bitter almonds on the breath may give time for administration of pure oxygen, followed by nitrites and sodium thiosulfate solution. The objective of treatment is to produce methemoglobin (which binds the CN) by nitrate administration; then sodium thiosulfate is given, which causes the CN to be readily eliminated as a thiocyanate. If this therapy can be given while vital signs are still present, there is some chance of recovery. After these measures, the routine treatment measures given in the following outline should be begun and continued in the ambulance en route to the hospital. If the skin or clothing is soaked with liquid cyanide, wash skin and remove clothing. Several kits are produced that include the various medications needed to treat CN poisoning—these kits (e.g., Lilly) should be kept immediately available.

Routine Treatment Considerations Include *(See also Table 53–3, Sodium Nitrite)*

1. Amyl nitrite inhalations for 30 seconds of every minute at 15-second intervals, alternating with 100% oxygen therapy, while a 3% solution of sodium nitrite (30 mg/ml) is being prepared. A syringe containing 1:1000 epinephrine hydrochloride (Adrenalin) or other vasopressor should be ready at all times to combat a sudden drop in blood pressure. Use a fresh pearl every several minutes until 3 to 4 pearls have been administered. Continue oxygen supplements.

2. Discontinue the amyl nitrite inhalations and inject 10 ml of freshly prepared 3% solution of sodium nitrite or 300 mg in adults (10 mg/kg, or 0.33 ml of 3% solution/kg in children with Hb of 12 g/100 ml) slowly IV over 5 minutes, immediately followed by 50 ml of a 25% aqueous solution of sodium thiosulfate (children's dose: 0.7 ml/kg) given over a period of 10 to 15 minutes. Repeat in 30 minutes with sodium nitrite at 50% of initial dose. Do not give a total of more than 12 g of sodium thiosulfate in an adult.

   The dose of 3% sodium nitrite given in children varies according to the Hb level; if the initial Hb level is 7 g%, then 5.8 mg/kg is administered; if the Hb level is 14 g%, 11.6 mg/kg is given; the volume ratio of 3% sodium nitrite given to 25% sodium thiosulfate is 1 ml/5 ml. There is inadequate time for hemoglobin level determination in the acute poisoning state; therefore, unless Hb level has been previously determined, administer sodium nitrite as though the Hb level was 12 g%.

3. Gastric lavage, but steps 1 and 2 have precedence. Administration of activated charcoal is not of value in cyanide poisoning, unless another drug has also been ingested.

4. Parenteral administration of hydroxocobalamin (vitamin B_{12a}) has been found to be of value, as well as cobalt ethylene diamine tetraacetate.

5. Hospitalization for observation and follow-up care, including possible transfusions because of the danger of sudden relapse. Monitor closely. Methemoglobin levels should be kept below 40%. Treat lactic acidosis and monitor ABG's. There is a high incidence of noncardiogenic pulmonary edema (*55–4*) in patients with cyanide poisoning. Venous blood is noted to be bright red.

Prognosis. If the patient is alive 1 hour after severe exposure, there is some chance of recovery, but sudden unexplained fatal relapses may occur 4 to 5 hours after apparent improvement. The sodium nitrite and sodium thiosulfate may be repeated, using half the initial dose, if signs of cyanide intoxication persist or reappear; they may also be repeated prophylactically in 2 to 3 hours if the original poisoning was severe.

---

*For therapeutic considerations see also *53–1* to *53–13*.

53–233. CYCLAMEN

The stalks and leaves contain a saponin that causes intense gastrointestinal symptoms without nausea or vomiting. Ingestion of large amounts may cause convulsions or coma.

53–234. CYCRIMINE HYDROCHLORIDE (Pagitane) ($C_{19}H_{30}ClNO$)

Excessive doses of this antiparkinsonian drug have been reported as causing decreased body temperature; restless, convulsive movements; and impaired speech and vision. Symptoms clear completely after treatment.

53–235. CYTISINE

Chewing or eating the seeds, flowers or roots of common plants containing this toxic alkaloid results in gastrointestinal irritation, dyspnea, vertigo, myalgia, delirium and hallucinations. Death may occur from respiratory failure.

53–236. DAPHNE (Dwarf Bay, Wild Pepper, Dog Parsley)

The attractive red berries and the bark of this shrub are sometimes ingested by children, with a fatality rate of about 20%. Contact of the juice with the skin may cause severe and even fatal symptoms, although recovery following this method of absorption usually occurs.

53–237. DATURA STRAMONIUM (Devil's Apple, Jamestown Weed, Jimsonweed, Stinkweed, Thorn Apple)

Drinking a decoction or chewing the roots, leaves or seeds of this common annual plant results in a toxic picture caused by the alkaloids hyoscyamine and hyoscine, characterized initially by dryness of the mouth, fever, flushed skin, mydriasis and diplopia. Later symptoms are muscle weakness, confusion, delirium and loss of memory. Circulation collapse and coma may develop.

A similar toxic picture has been reported from eating tomatoes grown on plants grafted to *Datura stramonium* roots. See *53–103, Atropine,* and *53–657, Stramonium.*

53–238. DD COMPOUNDS (Chlorinated Propylene Propanes)

All of the chlorinated hydrocarbons are used full strength as fumigants. They are toxic by ingestion, by absorption through the intact skin and by inhalation. Fortunately, they have a garlic-like odor that is offensive and repellent, even to small children. All may cause blistering of the skin on contact, eye and upper respiratory tract irritation, substernal pain, dyspnea, cyanosis, gastroenteritis and pulmonary edema *(55)* from inhalation of the fumes. Gastric pain, acute diarrhea and pulmonary edema develop rapidly after ingestion. Paresthesias, weakness and convulsions occur in more severe cases.

Toxicity may occur by *skin absorption* (blisters require treatment as second-degree chemical burns; see *28–10*), by *inhalation* (aminophylline infusion IV may be needed to combat bronchospasm) or by *ingestion.*

53–239. DDD (Tetrachlorodiphenylethane)

For toxicity and treatment, see *53–240, DDT.*

---

*For therapeutic considerations see also *53–1* to *53–13.*

53–240. DDT (Dichlorodiphenyltrichlorethane, Chlorophenothane) ($C_{14}H_9Cl_5$; TLV 1 mg/m^3)

Used extensively as an insecticide, and now widely banned, DDT has often been credited with the production of serious conditions—especially pulmonary edema (55)—caused in part by the solvents used in the insect sprays, usually petroleum derivatives *(53–531)*. If inhaled in strong concentrations, or if ingested, DDT has a definite toxic action that usually comes on 2 to 4 hours after exposure and is characterized by vomiting from gastric irritation, apprehension, acute depression, incoordination, giddiness, paresthesias of the face and lips, muscular tremors, convulsions (both tonic and clonic), dyspnea and cyanosis followed by respiratory failure. Death may occur from sudden ventricular fibrillation *(29–25)*. Chronic exposure to DDT has been reported as causing blurred speech, loss of coordination and other neurologic signs and symptoms; however, improvement begins when the patient is removed from exposure, (although fat stores last for long periods).

53–241. DELPHINIUM (Larkspur)

The roots and seeds contain several toxic alkaloids. Ingestion may result in burning and dryness of the mucous membranes of the mouth and throat with stiffness of the facial muscles, nausea, vomiting, loss of urinary and rectal sphincter control, extreme hypotension and respiratory depression.

53–242. DEMETON (Systox) ($[C_2H_5O]_2$ $P[S]OC_2H_4SC_2H_5$; TLV 0.01 ppm) *(See 53–497, Organic Phosphates)*

53–243. DEODORANTS AND DEODORIZERS

Preparations used to neutralize body odor usually contain 3 ingredients in varying proportions.

Antiperspirants—Usually aluminum salts *(53–52)* or zinc salts *(53–759)*. Iron salts *(53–370)* and silver salts *(53–630)* are used occasionally but may cause discoloration. Zirconium salts have been reported to cause skin granulomas. The most commonly used anions are chlorides, hydroxychlorides, phenolsulfonates and sulfates.

Deodorants—usually halogenated salicylanides, hexachlorophene, QAC and thiuram disulfide.

Perfumes—often with essential oil bases *(53–494)*.

Deodorizers used in the home may contain formaldehyde *(53–315)*, essential oils *(53–494)*, p-dichlorobenzene *(53–251)*, naphthalene *(53–469)* or isopropyl alcohol *(53–372)*. Although most deodorant and deodorizer preparations contain only small amounts of toxic materials, ingestion of more than a minute quantity calls for emptying the stomach by emetics or gastric lavage followed by activated charcoal in water by mouth and a saline cathartic.

53–244. DEPILATORIES (Hair Removers)

These cosmetics usually contain a mixture of inert ingredients, with a small amount of barium sulfide, calcium sulfide, sodium sulfide or thallium. See *53–111, Barium Compounds; 53–642, Sodium Sulfide; 53–692, Thallium.*

53–245. DERRIS

Powdered derris root contains rotenone *(53–584, Pyrethrum)* and is used as a fish poison and insecticide. Exposure to the powder may cause severe dermatitis, which clears rapidly when exposure is terminated.

Ingestion of the fresh root has been reported as causing vomiting, collapse and CHF.

---

*For therapeutic considerations see also *53–1* to *53–13*.

53–246. DETERGENTS *(See 53–48, Alkyl Sodium Sulfates and 53–642, Sodium Sulfide)*

53–247. DEXTROAMPHETAMINE SULFATE ($C_{18}H_{28}N_2O_4S$) *(See 53–66, Amphetamines, and Table 53–2, Stimulants)*

53–248. DIAZEPAM (Valium) ($C_{16}H_{13}ClN_2O$) *(See also 53–121, Benzodiazepines)*

Diazepam is a benzodiazepine, as is chlordiazepoxide (Librium) *(53–191)* and causes similar effects [central nervous system (CNS) depression]. Toxicity is low and deaths that have occurred are generally in presence of combination with other drugs. Forced diuresis, peritoneal dialysis and hemodialysis are not effective. Treatment is supportive.

53–249. DIAZOMETHANE (CH_2N_2; TLV 0.2 ppm)

This dangerous gas is used in industry as a methylating agent. Inhalation can cause choking, dyspnea and severe chest pain followed by pulmonary edema *(55)* and severe shock *(57)*.

53–250. DICHAPETALUM TOXICARIUM (Ratsbane)

Ingestion of the seeds of this South American and African plant has resulted in a peculiar, often fatal, syndrome called "broke back," characterized by intense gastrointestinal irritation, incoordination and paralysis, areflexia and extreme hyperesthesia.

53–251. DICHLOROBENZENE ($C_6H_4Cl_2$; TLV 0–50 ppm—C)

Both the ortho isomer (used as a wood preservative) and the para isomer (used in mothproofing sprays) are toxic when inhaled or ingested. Signs and symptoms of toxicity and treatment are approximately the same as those for naphthalene *(53–469)*.

53–252. DICHLORODIFLUOROMETHANE (Freon-12, Halon, Isotron) (CCl_2F_2; TLV 1,000 ppm)

This colorless gas, like the monofluoromethane variant, is both a propellant for aerosol bombs and a refrigerant. Sniffing fluorochlorinated hydrocarbons in large doses may lead to CNS dysfunction and cardiac arrhythmias, particularly ventricular fibrillation. Treatment is supportive; avoid epinephrine to reduce risk of ventricular fibrillation.

53–253. DICHLOROETHYLETHER ($C_4H_8Cl_2O$; TLV 5 ppm)

Fumes from this insecticide, soil fumigant and solvent irritate the eyes and upper respiratory tract. A severe persistent cough with a peculiar glassy sputum is characteristic. Sensitization may occur. Eosinophilia is common.

53–254. DICHLOROETHANE ($C_{14}H_{10}Cl_4$)

This liquid is used as a solvent for fats, gums, rubber and resins.

Toxic signs and symptoms may be caused by inhalation or ingestion and consist of nausea, vomiting, diarrhea, somnolence, weakness and respiratory and circulatory collapse.

53–255. DICHLOROHYDRIN

Inhalation of fumes causes symptoms in workers in the nitrocellulose and lacquer industries. The toxic manifestations range from nausea, vomiting and vertigo to somnolence, delirium and death.

---

*For therapeutic considerations see also *53–1* to *53–13*.

By ingestion, the toxicity of dichlorohydrin is even greater; dysphagia, vomiting and severe gastric pain may be followed by conjunctival, scleral and gastric hemorrhage and coma. Toxic hepatitis, nephritis, hemolytic anemia and pulmonary edema *(55)* may develop.

53–256. DICHLOROPHENE ($C_{13}H_{10}Cl_2O_2$)

Used as a mild antiseptic in antiperspirants, deodorants, tooth powders and toilet waters, dichlorophene may cause contact dermatitis, glossitis, stomatitis and cheilitis. Symptoms clear slowly when use of the offending preparation is stopped.

53–257. 2,4-DICHLOROPHENOXYACETIC ACID (2,4-D) ($C_8H_6Cl_2O_3$; TLV 10 mg/m^3)

This acid, used in the preparation of herbicides utilized principally in the control of broad-leafed weeds, is a potentially dangerous substance. Peripheral neuropathy following exposure to the diethylamine salt during manufacture has been reported. CNS excitation and convulsions can occur.

Treatment Considerations Include:

- Support of the circulatory system. Antiarrhythmic medications may be needed. Continuous ECG monitoring is advisable.
- Epinephrine (Adrenalin) may precipitate ventricular fibrillation and should not be used.

53–258. DICUMAROL (Dicoumarin, Melitoxin) ($C_{19}H_{12}O_6$)

Because this anticoagulant causes bleeding that persists for some time after discontinuance of therapeutic use, emergency care may be required for some or all of the toxic effects—especially hemorrhage—in the following list. 4-Hydroxycoumarin *(53–746, Warfarin)*—used as a rodenticide only—is even more toxic, especially to children.

Signs and symptoms: Generalized ecchymoses; hematuria; hemorrhage from the nose, gums or gastrointestinal tract; menorrhagia; and extreme weakness from secondary anemia. Look for retroperitoneal hemorrhage if site of blood loss is not apparent.

Treatment Considerations Include:

- Stop the anticoagulant. If a large amount has been ingested, empty the stomach immediately by gastric lavage followed by activated charcoal through the lavage tube.
- Transfer for hospitalization for vitamin K therapy *(45–8)*, fluid replacement *(11)* and, as necessary, transfusions *(18–35)*.

53–259. DIEFFENBACHIA SEQUINE (Dumb Cane, Elephant's Ear)

Chewing the leaves of this common decorative house plant results in immediate burning of the lips and mouth with difficulty in talking and swallowing and, occasionally, difficulty in breathing. Swelling of the parts with which the juice comes in contact is immediate and intense. If the juice or pulp is swallowed, severe corrosion of the esophagus and stomach may occur. Systemic effects are due to oxalate poisoning *(53–501)* and include bradycardia, hypotension, vomiting, gastric cramping and acute respiratory distress.

53–260. DIELDRIN (Compound 497, Octalox, Isodrin) ($C_{12}H_8Cl_6O$; TLV 0.25 mg/m^3)

Dieldrin is a chlorinated hydrocarbon insecticide and pesticide (and powerful rodenticide—isodrin) used when long-continued action is desirable, usually in combination with kerosene *(53–379)* and xylene *(53–755)*, both of which may complicate the toxic picture.

---

*For therapeutic considerations see also *53–1* to *53–13*.

Central nervous system symptoms may be caused by absorption through the intact skin, by inhalation or by ingestion. Hepatorenal damage may occur (and in mice, hepatocarcinogenicity has been shown).

Signs and symptoms of toxicity (delayed for 1 to 10 hours after ingestion) consist of severe headache, vertigo, nausea, vomiting, muscular twitching, tremors and respiratory failure. Severe epileptiform convulsions may be the first evidence of poisoning.

Treatment

- Removal of contaminated clothing; thorough washing of the skin with soap and water. *The attendant must wear gloves.*
- Prevention or control of convulsions by diazepam or rapid-acting barbiturates.
- Immediate hospitalization with supportive treatment, which may be needed up to 1 week after the last convulsion. Recovery is usually slow but complete.
- Cholestyramine (Questran) may be helpful (see 53–*118*).

53–261. DIETHYLAMINE (Acetylarsen) ($[C_2H_5]_2NH$; TLV 25 ppm)

The principal exposure to this agent comes from contact with resins and dyes and from working in the rubber and petroleum industries. Therapeutic use in the past as an antiluetic drug (Acetylarsen) has resulted in gingival and gastrointestinal bleeding, encephalopathy and agranulocytosis.

53–262. DIETHYL-BETACHLORETHYLAMINE

Fumes of this compound cause severe ophthalmic and respiratory irritation that increase in intensity for 10 to 12 hours after exposure. Delayed pulmonary edema (*55*) may occur.

For treatment, see mustard gas (under *War Gases*, 53–*746*).

53–263. DIETHYLENE GLYCOL (Diethylene Ether) ($C_4H_{10}O_3$)

Used in industry as a solvent, lubricant and hygroscopic agent, this liquid if ingested may have serious immediate and delayed effects including ataxia, nausea, vomiting, abdominal cramping, heartburn, generalized weakness, myalgia (especially of the lumbar muscles), severe kidney damage, convulsions, coma and death from respiratory failure.

53–264. DIETHYLSTILBESTROL ($C_{18}H_{20}O_2$)

Therapeutic doses or overdosage of this estrogenic agent may cause extreme lassitude, nausea, vomiting and abdominal pain, followed by bloody diarrhea and temporary psychoses.

53–265. DIGITALIS (Digitalis Purpurea, Foxglove)

The entire plant is toxic. The plant usually has pink or purple tubular flowers that are spotted on the inside.

For mild toxic signs and symptoms following therapeutic use in cardiac patients, see 29–*11*; difficulty usually occurs because of hypokalemia with or without increased sensitivity due to disease or excess administration, or both.

Ingestion or injection of large amounts of digitalis preparations by accident or with suicidal intent results in headache, depression, muscular weakness, vomiting, drowsiness, slow pulse, bigeminal rhythm, visual disturbances (amblyopia, blurring, diplopia, bizarre color vision changes) and characteristic extreme ECG changes (29–*11*). Prolongation of conduction through the atrioventricular node and increased automaticity of the Purkinje fibers (as with coupled extrasystoles or bidirectional ventricular tachycardia or ventricular fibrillation) are characteristic effects of digitalis.

---

*For therapeutic considerations see also 53–*1* to 53–*13*.

Treatment

- Stop digitalis. In mild cases not associated with serious dysrhythmia, this may be all that is necessary.
- Support ventilation and give oxygen as necessary.
- Start continuous electrocardiographic monitoring if serious dysrhythmia is present.
- If patient is seen early after oral digitalis preparation has been taken, cautiously (so as not to further increase vagal activity) empty the stomach by gastric lavage.
- Administer potassium chloride orally, 1 to 2 g q4h as needed, or give IV, as follows, unless hyperpotassemia is present or ECG's show definite A-V block without atrial tachycardia. Potassium chloride (40 mEq in 500 ml of D5W) may be given IV over a period of 1½ hours, unless the conditions cited in the preceding sentence are present. For children, the dose should be 5 to 10 mEq dissolved in 100 ml of D5W.
- If the patient's condition is degenerating and ventricular arrhythmias are developing (and there is no severe sinus bradycardia, sinoatrial block, or 2nd or 3rd degree A-V block), give 100 mg of diphenylhydantoin (Dilantin) slowly IV every 3 to 5 minutes at a rate not to exceed 50 mg/min up to a maximum of 1000 mg with frequent blood pressure and ECG monitoring. Pediatric dosage is 5mg/kg/day in divided doses up to a maximum of 300 mg. Diphenylhydantoin can be continued as necessary IV or PO until the digitalis is excreted. Lidocaine may also be used (50 mg bolus IV every 3 to 5 minutes up to a total of 300 mg), and propranolol has been used.
- All of the previously mentioned agents may cause hypotension; therefore, a pressor agent such as dopamine hydrochloride (Intropin) should be ready for immediate injection.
- A pervenous temporary demand pacemaker may be advisable for 3rd degree A-V block and sometimes for 2nd degree A-V block or severe sinus bradycardia or sinoatrial block. Because of increased occurrence of ventricular arrhythmia, isoproterenol (Isuprel) is advised against in digitalis toxicity.
- Use of hemoperfusion in severe cases is controversial.
- Successful use of a digoxin antibody has been reported in digoxin overdose, but this experimental substance is not widely available.

53–266. DILAUDID (Hydromorphone Hydrochloride)

The signs and symptoms of acute toxicity, addictive tendencies *(7–4)* and treatment of this powerful narcotic (formerly known as dihydromorphinone hydrochloride) are approximately the same as those for morphine *(53–455)*, for which it may be substituted under certain emergency conditions. Naloxone hydrochloride (Narcan) *(53–10)* is an effective antagonist.

53–267. DIMENHYDRINATE (Dramamine) ($C_{24}H_{28}ClN_5O_3$)

Usual doses prescribed for motion sickness may cause drowsiness, nausea, vomiting and paresthesias. Deaths have been reported from ingestion of large amounts, with preliminary hyperexcitability and convulsions. See *53–10* for possible cautious antidotal treatment with physostigmine salicylate with severe poisonings.

53–268. DIMETAN ($C_{11}H_{17}NO_3$)

Dimetan is a hydrocarbon aphicide that is not absorbed through the skin. It is a cholinesterase inhibitor. Ingestion may cause a toxic picture similar to that caused by physostigmine *(53–547)*.

53–269. DIMETHYL PHTHALATE ($C_{10}H_{10}O_4$; TLV 5 mg/m^3)

Ingestion of this insect repellent may cause an immediate burning sensation of the mucous membranes of the mouth, throat and pharynx and delayed coma coming on 1 to 2 hours after ingestion.

---

*For therapeutic considerations see also *53–1* to *53–13*.

53–270. DIMETHYL SULFOXIDE (DMSO) (C_2H_6OS)*

Dimethyl sulfoxide itself is a substance of low toxicity with a half-life after topical application of approximately 11 to 14 hours.

DMSO increases skin permeability to other substances that may be grossly toxic and may, for instance, be present as contaminants in industrial grade DMSO. Reddening and blistering of the skin are common with application of DMSO concentrations of 70% and over. Medical use other than for interstitial cystitis is experimental.

Ingestion of a water solution containing 1 tsp of pure DMSO crystals in a cup of water generally does not produce ill effect, but nausea, vomiting and diarrhea can occur after taking more concentrated solutions. Large daily oral doses (in the 3 to 5 g/kg range) taken over prolonged periods have produced renal and hepatic toxic changes in rats; short-range IV administration of the same dosage has not revealed renal or hepatic toxicity. Renal and hepatic toxicities at therapeutic DMSO levels, reported by some, have not been substantiated, nor has paresis, paralysis or neuropathy. Patients receiving high doses of 10% IV DMSO (1 g/kg/day) who die from severe trauma may still be successful renal/organ donors.

Forty per cent DMSO given IV causes hemolysis until diluted. DMSO may slightly lengthen blood coagulation time.

DMSO has been reported to cause temporary refractive index changes of the rabbit lens, but these alterations have not been found in man or primates. Hypersensitivity to DMSO is known.

Storage at room temperature in a dark area helps prevent breakdown to dimethyl sulfide, which is a relatively toxic substance.

53–271. DINITROBENZENE ($C_6H_4[NO_2]_2$; TLV 0.15 ppm)

Evidence of acute toxicity may come on suddenly or may develop following several weeks of exposure in industry. Toxic symptoms may be precipitated by prolonged exposure to sunlight or by overindulgence in alcoholic beverages. The toxic picture consists of a bitter almond-like taste in the mouth, headache, vertigo, fatigue, dyspnea, nausea, vomiting with severe gastric pain and a peculiar cyanosis, ranging from pale yellow to a grayish black. Jaundice may be present. Marked blood picture changes may be a late development. See *53–12* concerning methemoglobinemia. For prevention of further skin absorption, cleanse all skin and remove contaminated clothing.

53–272. DINITROCRESOL ($CH_3C_6H_2OH[NO_2]_2$; TLV 0.2 mg/m^3)

For symptoms and signs and treatment of toxic effects of this fungicide and pesticide, see 53–273, *Dinitrophenol.*

53–273. DINITROPHENOL (Capsine, Elgetol, Sinox) ($C_6H_4N_2O_5$)

Prescription or sale of this substance for use as a weight-reducing medication is prohibited by law. It is used extensively in the explosives industry and as a fungicide, insecticide, miticide and herbicide.

Signs and symptoms following inhalation or ingestion consist of temperature elevation, profuse perspiration, extreme thirst, fatigue, flushing of the skin followed by development of a yellow color, rapid deep breathing, restlessness, acute anxiety and sometimes convulsions and coma followed by death from respiratory failure. Temperature elevation may require specific cooling measures (*62, Temperature Variation Emergencies*).

53–274. DINITROTOLUENE ($C_6H_3CH_3[NO_2]_2$; TLV 1.5 mg/m^3)

This drug may cause arthralgia, dyspnea, cyanosis, severe headache, dizziness, nystagmus and severe chest pain, usually in persons handling the material. Ingestion of

---

*For therapeutic considerations see also *53–1* to *53–13*.

alcohol in any form accentuates the toxic picture. See *53–271, Dinitrobenzene,* and *53–12; Methemoglobinemia.*

53–275. DIOXANE ($C_4H_8O_2$; TLV 50 ppm)

Low concentrations of this commercial solvent cause acute mucous membrane irritation of the respiratory tract, including the lungs. Inhalation of high concentrations results in dyspnea, nonreactive pupils, lung congestion, decreased reflexes and serious liver and kidney disease.

53–276. DIOXIN *(See also 53–677, TCDD)*

Dioxin is the family name of about 75 chemical compounds that are becoming increasingly ubiquitous, some of which rank as the most toxic substances produced by man, ranking just below the bacteria-produced botulin, tetanus and diphtheria toxins in potency. Despite this, its degree of toxicity varies enormously from one species to the next, and the minimum toxic dose for man, as well as the exact binding reaction within the mammalian cell, is not known.

The herbicides Silvex, 2–4–5T and Agent Orange contain dioxin. Contamination resulted in abandonment of the entire town of Times Beach, Missouri.

Avoidance, protective clothing and mask, and surface decontamination, if exposed, are the mainstays of treatment.

Chloracne (which may be the only sign) appears a few days to weeks after exposure and can be followed by anorexia and weight loss, liver disorders, peripheral nerve damage and psychological manifestations such as diminished libido, insomnia and irritability. Serum cholesterol and lipids may elevate.

Excretion from the body and breakdown in the environment appear extremely slow. Fat biopsy is necessary to detect levels in the body. Production of birth defects in the offspring of exposed individuals and carcinogenicity are highly suspected, but not confirmed.

53–277. DIPHENHYDRAMINE (Benadryl, Amidryl) *(See 53–80, Antihistaminics)*

53–278. DIPHENOXYLATE *(See 53–399, Lomotil)*

53–279. DISULFIRAM (Antabuse, TTD) ($C_{10}H_{20}N_2S_4$) *(See also 53–702, Thiram; 53–758, Zerlate)*

Toxic effects from disulfiram and disulfiram-like substances (e.g., metronidazole [Flagyl]) are rapidly incurred with patients who have recently ingested alcohol (or alcohol-containing products such as tonics or cough syrups) and paraldehyde. Disulfiram given with phenytoin increases the toxic effects of phenytoin.

Two types of reactions to this drug, which is used in the treatment of chronic alcoholism (and also as a vulcanizer, seed disinfectant and fungicide) may occur.

Side Effects from Administration of Excessive Doses. Although there is marked individual variation in tolerance, one 0.5 g tablet daily usually is adequate for the desired therapeutic effect; larger doses may cause drowsiness (especially in the morning), headache, loss of appetite, fatigue, and psychoses. Optic neuritis and polyneuritis may also occur.

Treatment

Unless a psychosis has developed, nothing is required except reduction of the size of the dose. If psychotic symptoms are present, disulfiram should be discontinued and symptomatic treatment begun. Complete recovery within 1 to 2 weeks almost invariably occurs if the drug is the causative factor.

Antabuse-Alcohol Reactions. These may be brought on by ingestion of alcohol in any form—drinks, foods cooked with wine or medications in alcoholic vehicles. Generally, the amount of alcohol ingested determines the severity of the reactions, but in some individuals even very small amounts may cause severe, even dangerous, toxic manifes-

---

*For therapeutic considerations see also *53–1* to *53–13*.

tations. These usually begin with flushed skin, severe headache, burning of the eyes, salivation and dyspnea, and nausea and vomiting come on within ½ hour after ingestion of the alcohol-containing substances. A feeling of tightness in the chest may be severe enough to be mistaken for a cardiac condition. Hypotension, cyanosis and severe shock (57) may occur. Treat shock. The efficacy of intravenous vitamin C (500 mg to 1 g) has not yet been proved. Oral or IV antihistaminics may be given.

PROGNOSIS. Complete recovery within a short time. Even if untreated, all except the most severe cases in profound shock will make a complete recovery in 8 to 12 hours.

53–280. DITHIOCARBAMATES (Blightox, Blistex, Blue Mold Dust, Corozate, D-14, Dithane, Ferbam, Maneb, Nabam, Zeneb, Zerlate, Ziram)

These substances, usually in an oily base, are used as insecticides. For toxic signs and symptoms, see *53–279, Dilsulfiram; 53–758, Zerlate.* In contrast to the carbonates *(53–169)*, dithiocarbomates and thiocarbomates do *not* have a cholinesterase inhibitor effect.

53–281. DMSO *(See 53–270, Dimethyl Sulfoxide)*

53–282. DJENKOL BEANS

These beans are used as a food by natives of Java and Sumatra and, as a rule, are well tolerated; however, occasionally they may cause acute and very uncomfortable effects, even in persons accustomed to them for years. There is a musty odor to the breath, severe bladder and inguinal pain, milky urine with a very offensive odor, hematuria, anuria and intense colic, with flatulence, vomiting and diarrhea. Alkalinization of the urine with sodium bicarbonate, 2 to 4 g PO 3 to 4 times a day, aids elimination. Complete recovery in 3 to 4 days is the usual course.

53–283. DYES

Aniline Dyes. See *53–75.*

Azo Dyes. The most commonly used azo dyes are alizarine blue S, brilliant vital red, Chicago blue, chlorazol fast pink, indigo carmine, Pyridium (a commonly used urinary antiseptic that may cause methemoglobinemia if given in large doses), scarlet red and toluidine blue. All the members of this group have approximately the same toxicity as scarlet red *(53–619)* and require the same treatment.

Benzidine Dyes. These have been used extensively as trypanocides. The most commonly used members of this group are diamidinostilbene, pentamidine, trypan blue and trypan red. All are toxic if large amounts are ingested, and all have a cumulative toxic action if therapeutic doses are continued over a long period. Fever, acute dermatitis (often generalized, may be exfoliative), acute or chronic kidney irritation and occasional agranulocytosis occur. Symptoms may persist for as long as 6 weeks after withdrawal of the drug. Ingestion of large amounts requires immediate emptying of the stomach by emetics and/or gastric lavage followed by vigorous catharsis.

Coal Tar Dyes. This category comprises all dyes derived from benzene *(53–117)* and includes all of the dyes discussed in the remainder of this section.

FLAVINS (acridine dyes) are derived from a coal tar base and, before the development of sulfa drugs and antibiotics, were frequently used in 1:1000 to 1:10,000 solutions to check surface infection. The two most common preparations are acriflavine and proflavine. Neither is very toxic if applied to raw surfaces or ingested at the above concentrations. Industrial exposure has been reported as causing acute conjunctivitis, lacrimation and acute dermatitis.

GENTIAN VIOLET (methylrosaniline chloride) is a triphenylamine dye. Large amounts of gentian violet, as well as the other common triphenyl dyes (brilliant green, acid fuchsin and basic fuchsin) can be ingested without danger to life, although in some persons nausea, vomiting and diarrhea may occur.

---

*For therapeutic considerations see also *53–1* to *53–13*.

Treatment Considerations Include:

- Removal of large amounts from the stomach by emetics and/or gastric lavage followed by activated charcoal in water by mouth or through the lavage tube.
- Administration of magnesium sulfate (Epsom salts) by mouth to clear the lower gastrointestinal tract.
- Assurance of the patient or family that the color of the skin, sclerae and mucous membranes will slowly return to normal.

HAIR DYES. See *53–331.*

METHYLENE BLUE (tetramethylthionine chloride) is a coal tar dye that has been used medicinally (and usually ineffectively) for its supposed parasiticidal, antiseptic and analgesic action. It has a very low toxicity. A 1% solution is used intravenously in the treatment of acute methemoglobinemia *(53–12)*, such as from nitrite *(53–484)*, acetanilid *(53–20)* and sulfanilamide poisoning *(53–660)*, because of its ability to decrease the methemoglobin and to increase the oxygen-carrying capacity of the red blood corpuscles when the ferric state is reduced to ferrous condition.

Ingestion of large amounts of methylene blue may cause gastrointestinal and bladder irritation, depression of the parasympathetic receptive system similar to that caused by atropine *(53–103)* and temperature elevation by central action. See *53–10* for antidotal treatment with physostigmine salicylate.

PHTHALEIN DYES

Eosin (tetrabromofluorescein) is harmless if ingested, even in large amounts. Use of lipsticks containing eosin may cause acute dermatitis or gastrointestinal symptoms in certain sensitive individuals.

Fluorescein sodium (Uranine) is used locally in a 1 or 2% solution to demonstrate defects in the conjunctiva and cornea. The eye can be anesthetized with a few drops of ½% tetracaine (Pontocaine) before testing, and all fluorescein removed after examination by thorough irrigation with saline.

Fluorescein in a 20% solution has been given PO and IV for diagnosis of intraocular disease and for determination of renal function. If large, potentially dangerous amounts have been ingested, emptying of the stomach by emetics or gastric lavage may be indicated to prevent the characteristic yellowish discoloration of the sclerae and skin, which may be very disturbing to the patient. No other treatment is necessary.

Phenolphthalein. See *53–535.*

Phenoltetrachlorphthalein and phenolsulfonphthalein, used frequently at one time in liver function tests, are harmless. Tetrabromphenolphthalein, used in gallbladder visualizations, is usually nontoxic, although a few serious allergic reactions have been reported.

Shoe dyes. Ingestion may cause severe toxic reactions, as may absorption through the skin from recently dyed shoes. See *53–485, Aniline Dyes; 53–485, Nitrobenzene.*

Triphenyl dyes (acid fuchsin, basic fuchsin, brilliant green, gentian violet) are relatively nontoxic.

53–284. EMETINE ($C_{29}H_{40}N_2O_4$)

This alkaloid occurs in ipecac *(53–367)* and is used medicinally in the treatment of amebic dysentery and, in small doses, as an emetic and expectorant. It may cause nausea, vomiting, difficulty in swallowing, a sensation of tightness in the chest, acute stomach pain, intestinal cramping, diarrhea, cardiac depression and collapse.

53–285. ENDRIN ($C_{12}H_8Cl_6O$; TLV 0.1 mg/m^3)

This is an insecticide similar in action to, but more toxic than, dieldrin *(53–260).*

53–286. ENGLISH IVY

The active ingredient is hederagenin steroidal saponin. Symptoms are excess salivation, thirst, nausea, vomiting, diarrhea.

---

*For therapeutic considerations see also *53–1* to *53–13*.

53–287. EPHEDRINE (Racephedrine, I-sedrin) ($C_{10}H_{15}NO$)

Excessive use of nose drops or nasal sprays containing ephedrine may cause transient symptoms that clear rapidly when the medication is discontinued. Ingestion may cause extreme nervousness with tonic and clonic convulsions; cold, clammy skin; mydriasis; and dysphagia.

53–288. EPINEPHRINE (Adrenalin) ($C_9H_{13}NO_3$) *(See Table 53–2, Stimulants)*

In certain hypersensitive persons, even minimal therapeutic doses may produce great discomfort from tenseness, restlessness, acute anxiety, tremors, dizziness, respiratory distress and palpitation. These symptoms are usually more uncomfortable than serious and in most instances can be cleared up rapidly by sedation with barbiturates. Severe, sometimes fatal, reactions from inadvertent, ill-advised or excessive IV injections of epinephrine hydrochloride have been reported. Persons with hyperthyroidism, cardiovascular disease and angina pectoris are notoriously susceptible. Aggravation of preexistent psychomotor symptoms and activation of psychoses may take place. When epinephrine is given IV, its action as an alpha- and beta-adrenergic agent is extremely rapid. Severe reactions, almost always caused by the accidental injection of a large dose rather than by ingestion, are characterized by cerebrovascular accidents (*63–4*), acute pulmonary edema (*55*), cardiac dilatation and ventricular fibrillation (*29–25*).

Treatment Considerations Include:

- Limitation of absorption by application of a venous tourniquet to an extremity proximal to the site of injection if the error in the amount injected is realized in time.
- If ingested, emptying of the stomach *at once* by gastric lavage or emesis.
- Treatment with alpha- and beta-adrenergic blocking agents (phentolamine [Regitine] and propranolol [Inderal], respectively). *Note:* Epinephrine has a very short half-life.
- Sedation with diazepam or barbiturates, preferably given parenterally, as needed.

53–289. EPN ($C_2H_5O[C_6H_5]P[S]OC_6H_4NO_2$; TLV 0.5 mg/m^3) *(See 53–497, Organic Phosphates)*

53–290. EPOXY RESINS

Used as surface protectants and concrete adhesives, these substances may cause severe contact dermatitis. The catalysts or hardeners used with epoxy compounds may cause erythema, pruritus, periorbital and facial edema and, apparently, permanent hypersensitivity. Inhalation of the fumes may result in severe and persistent bronchospasm.

53–291. ERGOT (Spurred Rye)

Contamination of flour with this fungus may cause acute toxic symptoms, as may ingestion or injection of medicinal preparations. Ergonovine maleate (Ergonovine) or the methyl compound (Methergine) is used for prevention and treatment of postpartum and postabortal hemorrhage. Ergotamine tartrate (Gynergen, Cafergot) is used to prevent or treat migraine headache.

Signs and symptoms of ergotism are mostly related to excess smooth muscle/vasomotor contraction. They include extreme pallor of the face, with cyanosis of the extremities; small, weak rapid pulse; visual, auditory and sensory disturbances; hallucinations; and myocardial infarction. Frequent use of large doses—especially as an abortifacient—results in a tabes-like clinical picture. Gangrene, especially of the fingertips and toes, may develop. Amyl nitrite may be inhaled or papaverine hydrochloride, 30 to 60 mg SC or IV, or sodium nitroprusside IV may be given for their vasodilatory effects, depending on the severity of vasoconstriction.

---

*For therapeutic considerations see also *53–1* to *53–13*.

53–292. ERYTHRITYL TETRANITRATE ($C_4H_6N_4O_{12}$)

This is used commercially in the explosives industry and medicinally as a coronary vasodilator (Cardilate); tablets are nonexplosive. Its toxic signs, symptoms and treatment are similar to those outlined in *53–484, Nitrites.*

53–293. ETHCHLORVYNOL (Placidyl) (C_7H_9ClO)

Signs and symptoms of overdosage are characteristic aromatic odor on the breath; deep coma—often prolonged; respiratory depression and apnea; hypotension; bradycardia; pulmonary edema; and cardiac arrest. In severe cases, consider therapy with resin hemoperfusion.

53–294. ETHIDE (Dichloronitroethane) ($C_2H_3Cl_2NO_2$)

Inhalation of fumes or ingestion of this grain fumigant may cause severe toxic symptoms. The treatment is similar to that outlined in *53–502, Oxides of Nitrogen.*

53–295. ETHYL ALCOHOL (Ethanol) *(See also 7–1, Addiction; 19–1; Alcohol Intoxication Tests; 32, Coma; 37–4, Alcoholism; 37–6, Delirium Tremens; 49–13; Table 53–2, Sedatives/Hypnotics; Alcoholic Neuritis)*

Ethyl alcohol and isopropyl alcohol *(53–372)* vary in some side effects but give practically identical pictures following ingestion. Both are commonly used in rubbing alcohol compounds, and ethyl alcohol is the active agent in intoxicating beverages and the vehicle in many medicinal preparations. The denaturing substances commonly used to make rubbing compounds nonpotable give unpleasant symptoms but, as a rule, are harmless in themselves.

The amounts of ethyl and isopropyl alcohol necessary to produce acute toxic symptoms vary markedly, not only in different individuals but also in the same individual at different times, depending on several modifying factors. Barbiturates, meprobamate, chlorpromazine and other commonly used tranquilizing drugs may potentiate the toxicity of alcohol to a dangerous degree. Metabolic acidosis and increased osmolarity occur (20 mOsm/L for 100 mg%).

Treatment of Acute Alcoholism

- Obtain a blood specimen for determinations of alcohol level *(19–1)* and blood sugar level.
- If the last ingestion of alcohol was within 2 hours, lavage with a large volume of water, taking precautions against aspiration of vomitus or lavage fluid, leaving activated charcoal in water in the stomach. Apomorphine hydrochloride should not be used as an emetic.
- Keep the patient warm.
- Support the respiration by expired air and mechanical means *(5–10)*, with administration of oxygen as required. Circulatory support should be given.
- Treat stomach and bowel complaints symptomatically.
- Give sodium chloride solution IV for dehydration and acidosis. Ringer's lactate may increase lactic acidosis.
- Combat hypoglycemia by IV glucose.
- In the moribund patient, hemodialysis may be lifesaving.
- Hospitalization under strict supervision and control for supportive care and evaluation and treatment of neurologic and psychiatric aspects. Parenteral multivitamin preparations can aid if there is also chronic poor nutrition.

53–296. ETHYL CHLORIDE (CH_3CH_2Cl; TLV 100 ppm) *(See 53–71, Anesthetics, Inhalation)*

---

*For therapeutic considerations see also *53–1* to *53–13*.

53–297. ETHYLENE CHLOROHYDRIN (CH_2OHCH_2Cl; TLV 1 ppm)

Used in the chemical and textile industries, this liquid gives acute toxic symptoms by absorption through the skin, inhalation of fumes and ingestion. The toxic picture is characterized by mucous membrane irritation (especially of eyes and nose), visual disturbances, dizziness, incoordination and paresthesias. Severe thirst, soft weak pulse and extreme hypotension develop, followed in severe cases by shock *(57)* and coma. Death is usually caused by brain congestion or pulmonary edema *(55)*. Because of its tendency to cause ventricular fibrillation, epinephrine should not be used.

53–298. ETHYLENEDIAMINE TETRA-ACETIC ACID (Calcium Disodium Edetate, EDTA, Versene) ($C_{10}H_{12}CaN_2NaO_8$)

This chelating agent in therapeutic dosage may cause internal hemorrhage and symptoms of kidney irritation. Symptoms clear rapidly when use of the drug is discontinued. See *53–10*.

53–299. ETHYLENE DIBROMIDE (EDB) ($[CH_2Br]_2$; TLV 15 ppm; C 500 ppm)

This substance is used as a soil, fruit-grain fumigant, leaded gasoline additive, and in fire extinguishers. It is a colorless, nonflammable liquid with a chloroform-like odor detectable at 10 ppm. The highly toxic metabolites of EDB are potent alkylating agents. In addition to acute symptoms from skin absorption, inhalation or ingestion, there is potential for later problems such as cancer (proved in animals) and genetic and reproductive system damage (abnormal sperm morphology and motility, decreased fertility). Patients on disulfiram (Antabuse) should avoid EDB exposure for at least 30 days after their last dose of disulfiram. On the skin it causes reddening and blisters; inhalation of the fumes results in headache, weakness, excitement, prolonged vomiting and diarrhea that is very resistant to treatment. Heavy concentrations may cause death from cardiac failure. Effects on the central nervous system may be delayed. Remove clothing and wash skin to prevent delayed contact absorption. Treat as under 53–2.

53–300. ETHYLENE GLYCOL (Diethylene Glycol, Antifreeze, Prestone) ($C_2H_6O_2$; TLV 50 ppm [vapor])

This toxic liquid is commonly used in automobile "permanent" antifreeze mixtures; hence, it is often available for ingestion by children. Toxic effects are due to breaking down of these liquids to oxalic acid *(53–501)*. If ingestion is even suspected, do not wait for symptoms to develop, conduct immediate emesis procedures or lavage.

Signs and symptoms of toxicity (usually delayed 1 to 2 hours after ingestion) consist of temporary exhilaration followed by development of progressively deepening coma; rapid, weak pulse; acute respiratory distress; muscular paralysis; and loss of reflexes. A positive Babinski sign may be present. Profound metabolic acidosis and high serum osmolarity result. Oxalate crystals are seen in the urine. Severe hypocalcemia *(46–14)* can occur. If anuria and uremia develop, the condition is generally fatal. Treatment should include immediate IV ethyl alcohol *(53–295)*. Dialysis aids elimination of this nephrotoxic agent and must be considered early.

53–301. ETHYLENE OXIDE (C_2H_4O; TLV 50 ppm)

Used as a food and textile fumigant, ethylene oxide fumes cause a peculiar sweetish taste in the mouth, vomiting, severe cough and vertigo. Bradycardia and extrasystoles are common, as is intense abdominal pain. May cause chromatin exchange mutagen.

53–302. ETHYL GASOLINE

The symptoms and treatment following ingestion are the same as those for gasoline *(53–323)*. Tetraethyl lead apparently is relatively nontoxic in the concentrations com-

---

*For therapeutic considerations see also *53–1* to *53–13*.

monly found in ethyl gasoline, although persons concerned with its manufacture or those who experience prolonged cutaneous contact may develop the clinical picture of acute or chronic lead poisoning *(53–386)* from absorption through the intact skin.

53–303. EUCALYPTOL *(See also 53–494, Oil, Essential)*

Oil of eucalyptus (50% eucalyptol) is an ingredient of many widely used household remedies, especially counterirritant salves and lotions (e.g., Vicks' VapoRub). Ingestion of even small amounts may have serious effects. Vicks' Throat Lozenges, even though the eucalyptol is greatly attenuated, should not be given to children under 3 or to adults for more than 2 days.

Signs and symptoms of toxicity are nausea, vomiting, abdominal pain, diarrhea, miosis, dizziness, mental confusion, dysuria, hematuria, convulsions in children, dyspnea, cyanosis and circulatory collapse, followed by coma. Late development of pulmonary edema *(55)* and severe pneumonitis may occur.

53–304. EUONYMIN

Euonymin is a digitalis-like substance *(53–265, Digitalis)* found in the fruit of many varieties of bushes and trees (arrowwood, bitter ash, burning bush, spindle tree, strawberry tree).

Ingestion may result in vomiting, watery diarrhea, hallucinations and somnolence deepening to coma.

53–305. FAVA BEANS *(See also 45–6, Hemolytic Anemia)*

Favism, characterized by chills, fever, nausea, vomiting, jaundice, red-brown or black urine, gastrointestinal bleeding and hemoglobinemia, may be caused by ingestion of green or incompletely cooked broad (Windsor) beans or horse beans, or by inhalation of the pollen or by dust from grinding. Different individuals show wide variations in susceptibility (most who are affected have glucose-6-phosphate dehydrogenase deficiency); in addition, the same individual may vary in susceptibility at different times. Supportive care is usually all that is needed, but if hemolysis is great, blood transfusion may be required.

53–306. FENFLURAMINE HYDROCHLORIDE (Pondimin)

Overdosage of this sympathomimetic amine anorectic drug may cause agitation or drowsiness, confusion, fever, dry mouth, diarrhea, abdominal pain, malabsorption and hyperventilation. Acidification of the urine aids elimination.

53–307. FINGER CHERRY

The fruit of this Australian flowering shrub may cause sudden onset of complete and permanent blindness from optic nerve damage. If ingested, signs and symptoms of toxicity usually do not develop for 18 to 24 hours; hence, only symptomatic treatment can be given.

53–308. FINGERNAIL POLISH *(See 53–24, Acetone; 53–75, Aniline Dyes)*

53–309. FIRE EXTINGUISHERS

Toxic ingredients depend on the type, as follows:

1. *Dry type*—magnesium stearate, tricalcium phosphate.
2. *Foam type*—aluminum sulfate *(53–52)*, methyl bromide *(53–435)*.
3. *Gas type*—compressed carbon dioxide gas *(53–173)*.
4. *Liquid type*—carbon tetrachloride *(53–176)*, dichloromethane, difluorodibromomethane, chlorobromethane and trichlorethylene *(53–719)*.

---

*For therapeutic considerations see also *53–1* to *53–13*.

For treatment, see the specific toxic constituents and institute general therapeutic principles.

53–310. FIREWORKS

Many acutely toxic substances may be present in fuel, binders, oxidizers and coloring agents of fireworks. In some instances, mild transient toxic signs and symptoms may be caused by inhalation of fumes. Among commonly used toxic constituents are:

Antimony salts *(53–81)*
Arsenates *(53–90)*
Barium salts *(53–111)*
Chlorates *(53–189)*
Copper salts *(53–224)*
Lead salts *(53–386)*
Mercury *(53–418)*
Nitrates *(53–481)*
Perchlorates *(53–189, Chlorates)*
Phosphorus *(53–546)*
Strontium salts
Thiocyanates *(53–698)*

Ingestion of some types of fireworks by children may be fatal if the stomach is not emptied at once and careful symptomatic follow-up care administered.

53–311. FLUORIDES (F^{1-}; TLV 2.5 mg/m³) *(See also 53–312, Fluoroacetates; 53–351, Hydrofluoric acid)*

Sodium, barium and zinc fluorides are often the active toxic ingredients in ant, insect, roach and rodent poisons. Ingestion (especially by children) and inhalation of the dust during manufacture and use have caused many cases of acute and serious poisoning.

Signs and symptoms of acute fluoride poisoning consist of nausea, vomiting, severe abdominal pain, burning, cramps, bluish-gray cyanosis, muscular tremors, myalgia (especially of the calf muscles) and convulsions. Death usually occurs in 2 to 4 hours; the prognosis is good if the patient survives for 24 hours. Hypocalcemia and hyperkalemia can occur.

Treatment Considerations Include:

- If inhaled, removal from exposure followed by oxygen inhalations.
- If ingested, immediate gastric lavage (even if evidence of corrosion is present) with copious amounts of 1% calcium chloride or lime water (0.15% calcium hydroxide) or milk or calcium chloride solution of 5 ml/L of water. Follow with copious amounts of aluminum gel by mouth.
- Oxygen administration; treatment of shock *(57)*.
- Maintain mild diuresis and correct dehydration. If renal output is inadequate or ingestion is severe, consider hemodialysis.
- Calcium gluconate, 10 ml of 10% solution IV, for severe myalgia and as an inactivator of the fluoride ion; as necessary can be repeated in half dose in 30 minutes and every 4 to 6 hours until recovery is complete. Dosage for children is 0.1 ml/kg.
- IV bicarbonate therapy may afford additional protection.

53–312. FLUOROACETATES (Compound 1080)

These compounds, used as rodenticides, are toxic in a different manner from other fluoride derivatives, apparently because of blocking of cellular energy production resulting in the slow development of convulsions. Their toxicity is high, with 5 mg/kg estimated to be the human lethal dose.

Signs and symptoms: Acute apprehension, anxiety, nausea, vomiting, aberrations of special senses [especially auditory, visual (nystagmus) and mental (hallucinations)], paresthesias (usually facial) and muscle twitching. Epileptiform convulsions are often followed by development of cardiac abnormalities [pulsus alternans, ectopic beats, ventricular tachycardia *(29–26)* and fibrillation *(29–25)*].

---

*For therapeutic considerations see also *53–1* to *53–13*.

Treatment Considerations Include:

- Immediate emptying of the stomach by emetics (unless patient is convulsing) or gastric lavage if fluoroacetic poisoning is even suspected. Activated charcoal in water should be left in the stomach. General supportive care.
- Control of convulsions by rapidly acting barbiturates or diazepam IV.
- Glyceryl monoacetate (Monacetin), 0.25 g/kg IM, repeated in ½ to 1 hour if necessary, for effect as an antidote; can also give orally. (*Note:* Although efficacy of this agent is suggested, relatively little clinical experience exists.)
- Hospitalization for close observation, ECG monitoring and symptomatic care.
- Procainamide or lidocaine IV for ventricular arrhythmias.

53–313. FLURAZEPAM (Dalmane) *(See also 53–121, Benzodiazepines)*

Flurazepam is a benzodiazepene hypnotic drug that has similarities to diazepam (Valium) *(53–248)*. Gastrointestinal distress, lethargy, lightheadedness, CNS depression, euphoria, ataxia, sweating, flushing and coma may occur. If a paradoxical reaction, such as hyperactivity or excitement, occurs, avoid use of barbiturates or diazepam. Treatment is supportive.

53–314. FOOD POISONING *(See also Table 40–1, Common Causes of Acute Bacterial Diarrhea)*

Botulism *(53–142)*. Evidence of toxicity from botulism usually does not develop until 12 to 36 hours after eating improperly processed canned foods; in some instances, the time lapse is much longer. The toxic picture is caused by an exotoxin produced under anaerobic conditions by *Clostridium botulinum*. The prognosis depends upon the amount of toxin ingested in relation to body weight. For treatment, see *53–142*.

Bacterial. From enterotoxins in food produced by the growth of staphylococci or by the organisms themselves (*Salmonella, Streptococcus, Clostridium perfringens, Shigella, Bacillus cereus, Vibrio parahaemolyticus*).

Signs and symptoms of toxicity from staphylococcic enterotoxins develop in 2 to 6 hours. Both are characterized by vertigo, weakness, general malaise, salivation, nausea, vomiting, gastric pain, tenesmus, diarrhea, muscular cramps and shock *(57)*—which is usually transient but may be severe and resistant to treatment. Diagnosis is aided when a number of people who have shared common food and drink become acutely ill.

Treatment

- Gastric emptying has usually already occurred spontaneously; use of emetics, lavage or cathartics is not indicated for food-borne bacterial illness (except when due to *C. botulinum*), as the toxins are not eliminated by vomiting and diarrhea.
- Control severe pain *(12)*.
- Decrease tenesmus and diarrhea by 1 g of bismuth subcarbonate or 7.5 g of kaolin by mouth. Camphorated tincture of opium (paregoric), 4 to 8 ml, or diphenoxylate hydrochloride (Lomotil) or bismuth subsalicylate (Pepto Bismol) may be given to reduce diarrhea when appropriate.
- Hospitalize if severe shock *(57)* or dehydration is present; usually it is not necessary.

Chemical. Ingestion of acid foods stored in containers lined with antimony *(53–81)*, cadmium *(53–158)*, lead *(53–386)*, or zinc *(53–759)* may result in nausea, vomiting and diarrhea lasting 2 to 3 days if not treated. Eating unwashed fruit and vegetables that have been sprayed with preparations containing the metal salts may give the same picture. Food preservatives and sugar and salt substitutes may give toxic signs and symptoms. (See *53–484, Nitrites; 53–609, Saccharin.*)

Treatment Considerations Include:

- Emetics followed by gastric lavage if profuse vomiting has not occurred. Activated charcoal in water should be given by mouth.

---

*For therapeutic considerations see also *53–1* to *53–13*.

- Saline cathartics may be administered.
- Atropine sulfate, 0.5 mg SC.
- Bismuth subcarbonate or bismuth subsalicylate (Pepto Bismol) by mouth.
- Specific treatment as outlined under the offending metal.

Radioactive Contamination. See *3–12*.

Rare Causes of Food Poisoning. Poisoning from ingestion of certain plants and animal foods may be due to contaminants or to naturally occurring poisons contained in the foods. Among the foods or food contaminants that have been reported as giving toxic symptoms—usually from nonbacterial poisons—are the following:

Abalone. *See Mytilotoxism* (later in this section); *53–464, Mussel Poisoning.*

Aconite. The roots of this plant, also called Friar's cowl, monkshood and mousebane, may be mistaken for edible horseradish. See *53–223, Coniine.*

Agrostemma githago (corn campion, corn cockle, corn rose). See *53–38.*

Amanita muscaria. This variety of mushroom is very toxic. Toxic symptoms develop in from a few minutes to 3 hours after ingestion. See *53–462, Mushroom Poisoning, 53–460, Muscarine.*

Amanita pantherina. See *53–462, Mushroom Poisoning.*

Amanita phalloides. Delayed, severe, often terminal, toxic symptoms (6 to 24 hours) are characteristic of poisoning from this variety of poisonous mushroom. See *53–462, Mushroom Poisoning.*

Amanita verna. This variety of poisonous mushroom is responsible for many cases of acute toxicity in Europe. See *53–462, Mushroom Poisoning.*

Amberjack. See *Fish poisoning* (later in this section).

Asari. See *Venerupin* (later in this section).

Balloon fish. See *Fish poisoning* (later in this section).

Barracuda. See *Fish poisoning* (later in this section); *53–112*. For barracuda bites, see 27–3.

Black ulna. See *Fish poisoning* (later in this section).

Blaasoportoby. See *Fish poisoning* (later in this section); *53–691, Tetraodontiae.*

Blood (Polish Kiszra) sausage. See *Sausage cyanosis* (later in this section).

Blowfish. See *Fish poisoning* (later in this section); *53–691, Tetraodontiae.*

Botete. See *Fish poisoning* (later in this section); *53–691, Tetraodontiae.*

Bread poisoning. See *Senecio* (later in this section); *53–623, Senecio.*

Bream. See *Haff disease* (later in this section).

Broad beans. See *53–305, Fava Beans.*

Cadmium. See *53–158, Cadmium and Its Salts.*

Chlorinated hydrocarbon pesticides. Contamination of bulk cereal foods has resulted in several series of severe poisoning. Endrin (*53–285*) has been the most common offender.

Ciguatera. This is a gastrointestinal and neurotic disorder (with paresthesias, abnormal sensations of hot and cold, and sensory dysesthesias) caused by ingestion of certain fish. It differs from all other types of fish poisoning because its toxin (cinguatoxin—probably from the dinoflagellate *Gambierdiscus toxicus*) is heat stable and not deactivated by cooking. Treatment is supportive.

Clams. See *Mytilotoxism* (later in this section).

Claviceps purpurea. Ergot fungus as a contaminant of cereal grains (especially rye) can cause acute circulatory symptoms followed by evidence of central nervous system damage. For treatment, see *53–291, Ergot.*

Coprinus atramentarius. This variety of edible mushroom, called "inky caps," gives toxic symptoms usually only in the presence of alcohol. For toxic picture and treatment, see *53–279.*

Corn campion. See *53–38, Agrostemma Githago.*

Corn cockle. See *53–38, Agrostemma Githago.*

Corn rose. See *53–38, Agrostemma Githago.*

Deathfish. See *Fish poisoning* (later in this section); *53–691, Tetraodontiae.*

Eel. See *Fish poisoning* (later in this section); *Haff disease* (later in this section); *53–330, Gymnothorax Flavimarginatus.*

---

*For therapeutic considerations see also *53–1* to *53–13*.

Ergot. See *Claviceps purpurea* (earlier in this section); *53–291, Ergot.*

Fava beans. See *53–305, Fava Beans.*

Favism. See *53–305, Fava Beans.*

Fish poisoning (ichthyosarcotism) is widespread and is usually classified in 3 groups depending on the geographic area in which the fish are found. See also *Ciguatera,* above.

Caribbean Type (amberjack, great barracuda, cavallas, groupers, sierra and fish of related species). Usually not fatal.

Pacific Type (barracuda, black ulna, eels, red snapper, sea bass, trigger fish, mahimahi). Mortality about 5%.

Japanese (Tetraodon) Type (balloon fish, globe fish, puffers). This type is limited to the waters bordering Japan. The mortality is about 70%. For toxic effects and treatment, see *49–691. Tetraodontiae.*

Fugu. See *Fish poisoning* (above); *53–691, Tetraodontiae.*

Fungicides. These preparations are sprayed on grain fields and may give toxic effects when the cereal is used as food. A large series of cases of acquired porphyria *(46–24)* in Turkey was caused by fungus control with hexachlorobenzene.

Galerina venenata. See *53–322.*

Giobe fish. See *Fish poisoning* (earlier in this section).

Groupers. See *Fish poisoning* (earlier in this section).

Gymnothorax flavimarginatus. See *53–330.*

Haff disease. Eating bream, burbot, eels, perch and roach has resulted in an unusual type of food poisoning in countries bordering on the North Sea. The etiology of Haff disease is unknown, but it is characterized by agonizing pain in muscles of the back and extremities coming on about 18 hours after eating the fish. The condition clears spontaneously after 36 to 48 hours. The only treatment required is relief of the severe muscle pain.

Helvella (lorchel, morel, false morel). See *53–462, Mushroom Poisoning.*

Honey. If bees collect the honey from certain plants, it may be very toxic. See *53–347.*

Ichthyosarcotism. See *Fish poisoning* (earlier in this section).

Jatropha curcas. See *53–375, Jatropha Nut Oil.*

Jugfish. See *Fish poisoning* (earlier in this section); *53–691, Tetraodontiae.*

Kiszka. See *Sausage cyanosis* (later in this section).

Lathyrism. The exact etiology of this type of food poisoning, occurring in India, southern Europe and other tropical countries during times of famine, is not known although ingestion of the seeds of *Lathyrus sativa L.* (vetching, green vetch) is suspect. It occurs mainly in middle-aged persons and is characterized by spastic paralysis, paresthesias, hyperreflexia and patellar and Achilles clonus. Symptomatic treatment is all that can be given.

Lead. Food poisoning from lead is usually due to ingestion of unwashed fruits or vegetables that have been sprayed with lead-containing insecticides. See *53–386, Lead Salts.*

Lolium temulentum. See *53–398.*

Mahimahi. See *Fish poisoning* (earlier in this section); *53–691, Tetraodontiae.*

Metals. Arsenic *(53–90)* and lead *(53–386)* may be present on unwashed vegetables and fruits. Antimony *(53–81)*, cadmium *(53–158)*, tin *(53–707)* and zinc *(53–759)* poisoning may be acquired by eating foods stored in containers lined with these metals. Mercury *(53–418)* has contaminated tuna fish. For treatment, see *Chemical poisoning* (discussed earlier).

Milk sickness. See *53–716, Tremetol.*

Mushrooms. See *53–462, Mushroom Poisoning;* see also *Amanita muscaria, Amanita pantherina, Amanita phalloides, Amanita verna* and *Coprinus atramentarius* (earlier in this section).

Mussels. See *53–464, Mussel Poisoning; Mytilotoxism* (following paragraph).

Mytilotoxism. (See also *53–464, Mussel Poisoning)* On the Pacific Coast of North America, abalones, clams, mussels and oysters during certain months of the year (usually June to October) feed on dinoflagellates, which contain a toxic substance that is not destroyed by cooking. Ingestion of the shellfish may cause nausea, vomiting, abdominal

---

*For therapeutic considerations see also *53–1* to *53–13*.

cramps, muscle weakness, peripheral paralysis and death from respiratory failure. Symptoms of toxicity appear within ½ hour of ingestion. The mortality is extremely high.

Treatment

- Immediate emptying of the stomach by emesis (53–7). Alternatively use thorough gastric lavage, leaving activated charcoal in water in the stomach.
- Administration of a saline cathartic.
- Control of pain (*12*).
- Oxygen administration.
- Treatment of shock (*57*).
- Fluid replacement to overcome dehydration and acid-base imbalance (*11*).
- Hospitalization for several days after apparent improvement. Relapses are common.

PROGNOSIS. Good if the toxic material is completely removed from the stomach within ½ hour; poor if the clinical picture of mytilotoxism is full-fledged.

Organic phosphate (organophosphate) pesticides. Contamination of bulk flour and sugar has resulted in several series of organic phosphate poisoning cases with many fatalities. For mode of action and treatment, see 53–497, *Organic Phosphates.*

Oysters. See *Mytilotoxism* (discussed earlier); 53–464, *Mussel Poisoning.*

Panmyelotoxicosis. This disease is well known in Russia and is caused by ingestion of toxic substances elaborated by a fungus growing on cereal grains, especially millet. Toxic effects begin with burning in the mouth and throat followed in a few days by acute gastrointestinal symptoms lasting about 1 week. Four to 8 weeks later, purpura, anemia and thrombocytopenia may develop. Death is usually caused by severe sepsis and bronchopneumonia. Treatment has to be symptomatic and supportive.

Parathion. See 53–497, *Organic Phosphates.*

Perch. See *Haff disease* (earlier in this section).

Phalloidine. See 53–462, *Mushroom Poisoning; Amanita phalloides* (discussed earlier).

Potato. Sprouting or unripened potatoes contain a toxic amount of solanine (*53–644*).

Puffer. See *Fish poisoning* (earlier in this section); 53–691, *Tetraodontiae.*

Red snapper. See *Fish poisoning* (discussed earlier).

Rhubarb. See 53–501, *Oxalic Acid.*

Roach. See *Fish poisoning* (earlier in this section).

Sausage cyanosis. Use of large amounts of nitrate-nitrite to preserve the blood-red color of Polish blood sausage has caused acute toxic effects due to methemoglobinemia (*53–12*). For treatment, see 53–484. *Nitrites.*

Sea bass. See *Fish poisoning* (earlier in this section).

Senecio. Native to South Africa, the seeds of several varieties of this plant as a contaminant of cereal grains have caused many cases of "bread poisoning," a high percentage of which have been fatal. Fatalities are usually the result of irreversible liver damage. See also 53–623.

Shellfish. See *Mytilotoxism* (earlier in this section); 53–464, *Mussel Poisoning.*

Sierra. See *Fish poisoning* (earlier in this section).

Solanine. See *Potato poisoning* (earlier in this section); 53–570).

Tetraodon. See *Fish poisoning* (earlier in this section); 53–691, *Tetraodontiae.*

Tin. See 53–707.

Toadfish. See *Fish poisoning* (earlier in this section); 53–691, *Tetraodontiae.*

Tomato. Several series of cases have been reported, especially from the Middle West area of the United States, in which acute toxic symptoms have developed from eating tomatoes picked from plants grafted on *Datura stramonium* (jimsonweed, stinkweed) roots (*53–237*). The toxic picture and treatment are similar to that outlined under *Atropine* (*53–103*).

Trigger fish. See *Fish poisoning* (earlier in this section).

Venerupin. Limited to Japan, this type of food poisoning follows ingestion of asari and oysters. Acute gastrointestinal symptoms develop in 24 to 36 hours, with evidence of liver damage and increase in blood coagulation time. The mortality is about 30%.

Vitamin A. Poisoning from excessive intake of vitamin A is limited to Arctic regions where animal organs (especially of the polar bear, bearded seal, fox and husky dog) are used as food. Discontinuance of the food and symptomatic care is the only treatment required.

---

*For therapeutic considerations see also 53–*1* to 53–*13*.

Windsor Bean. See *53–305, Fava Beans.*
Zinc. Storage of food in galvanized containers may cause symptoms of zinc poisoning. For treatment, see *Chemical poisoning* (earlier in this section); *53–759, Zinc Chloride.*

53–315. FORMALDEHYDE (HCHO; TLV 2 ppm—C)

A solution of this pungent gas is the active ingredient in many commonly used household antiseptics, deodorizers and fumigants. It is sometimes used in hospitals to sterilize dialysis units. Irritating fumes may emanate for long periods from composition materials and fabricated plastics made with formaldehyde. Formaldehyde solutions are also used to wrinkle-proof clothing. Skin reactions are irritation with pustules, vesicles and tan staining with or without allergic reaction. Inhalation of fumes or ingestion of solutions of the gas may cause an acute toxic picture. The breath has a characteristic odor. If inhaled, acute irritation of the eyes, nose and upper respiratory tract, bronchospasm and/or laryngeal edema may occur. If ingested, there is mucosal erosion and soreness of the mouth and throat with difficulty in swallowing. Nausea, vomiting, hematemesis, severe abdominal pain, diarrhea (often bloody), severe shock, convulsions, coma and death from respiratory failure is the chain of events in terminal cases. In addition to toxic reactions, hypersensitivity to formaldehyde may develop and cause bronchospasm.

Treatment Considerations Include:

- If on the skin, wash off immediately with soap and water. Have the patient change clothes.
- Perform prompt gastric lavage with copious water for ingestion unless severe ulceration is present. Swallowing of water can aid by dilution process. Hospitalize for close observation if esophageal-gastric corrosion is suspected.

53–316. FORMALIN

Formalin is an aqueous solution containing 40% formaldehyde and small amounts of ethyl or methyl alcohol, or both. For treatment of poisoning, see *53–315, Formaldehyde.*

53–317. FORMIC ACID (HCOOH; TLV 5 ppm)

The fumes of formic acid, which is used in the chemical and leather industries, cause acute inflammation of the eyes, nose and throat. Ingestion causes acute stomatitis, glossitis, esophagitis and gastritis with delayed serious kidney damage.

53–318. FOUR-O'CLOCK

The roots and seeds contain a mildly narcotic gastrointestinal irritant that causes immediate nausea and vomiting without permanent ill effects.

53–319. FREONS (*See also 53–252, Dichlorodifluoromethane*)

These chlorinated-fluorinated hydrocarbons are used in refrigerators and as the propelling agents in aerosol containers. Inhalation of fumes may cause respiratory tract irritation from the freezing effect and mental confusion from the narcotizing effect. Another danger lies in contact of the containers with fire in the home. At high temperatures, freons break down into chlorine (*53–192*), fluorine, hydrogen fluoride (*53–311, Fluorides*) and phosgene (*53–543*)—all volatile gases that are dangerous in even low concentrations. Avoid use of isoproterenol (Isuprel) and epinephrine in treatment, because they can cause cardiac excitability. Pulmonary edema (55) and severe ventricular dysrhythmia can occur from freons; patients with these symptoms will require resuscitation (5)

---

*For therapeutic considerations see also *53–1* to *53–13*.

53–320. FURNITURE POLISH

Ingestion of these preparations by children is common and may cause severe illness and even death owing to the toxic effects of the chief ingredient, mineral seal oil, a hydrocarbon distillate. These effects are similar to but more severe than those of gasoline (53–323) and kerosene (53–379), which should be referred to concerning treatment safeguards. There can be delayed development of severe pulmonary involvement. The degree of gastrointestinal absorption is variable.

53–321. GADOLINIUM CHLORIDE (Gd C13)

This lanthanide by-product of the uranium industry has caused cardiovascular collapse in laboratory animals, but no cases of human toxicity have been reported.

53–322. GALERINA VENENATA

Ingestion of this North American fungus has been reported to cause acute gastrointestinal symptoms coming on after about 10 hours, followed by hypotension, convulsions and pulmonary edema (55).

53–323. GASOLINE

Its wide use as a motor fuel and as a cleansing agent makes gasoline one of the main present-day causes of poisoning. Toxic signs and symptoms may follow contact with the skin over large areas of the body, inhalation of fumes or ingestion. The mouth should never be used to initiate suction for siphoning of gasoline. Repeated voluntary inhalation of gasoline fumes has been reported (see 53–332). Coughing and choking following ingestion are presumptive signs of aspiration and pneumonitis.

Skin Contact. Repeated or prolonged washing of the skin with gasoline results in removal of the protective fat layer, with subsequent lowering of resistance to infection. Exposure of large areas of skin to gasoline may cause severe toxic symptoms from absorption similar to those given later in this section for inhalation of high concentrations. Acute symptoms from skin absorption are sometimes encountered following automobile accidents in which the clothing has been saturated with gasoline.

Treatment Considerations Include

- Remove all contaminated clothing at once.
- Wash the skin and hair thoroughly with copious amounts of soap and water.
- Give symptomatic therapy as outlined in the following discussion of inhalation of high concentrations.

Inhalation. Low or medium concentrations of gasoline fumes cause flushing of the skin, staggering gait, confusion, incoherence and disorientation—a clinical picture that may be mistaken for acute alcohol intoxication.

Treatment

- Removal from exposure.
- Fresh air or inhalations of oxygen.

PROGNOSIS. Complete recovery in a short time.

High concentrations may cause muscular twitching, tonic and clonic convulsions, dilated nonreactive pupils, delirium followed by sudden loss of consciousness and death from ventricular fibrillation (29–25) or complete respiratory arrest. Chest x-ray will usually reveal pulmonary involvement within a few hours.

Treatment

- Removal from exposure.
- Oxygen administration.
- *Do not* give epinephrine hydrochloride (Adrenalin) or isoproterenol (Isuprel) because of the danger of inducing ventricular fibrillation. Monitor with ECG if tachycardia or dysrhythmia (usually atrial fibrillation) is present.

---

*For therapeutic considerations see also 53–*1* to 53–*13*.

- Hospitalization as soon as possible. The acute stage may be followed in 2 to 3 hours by peripheral and retrobulbar neuritis, epileptiform seizures, paresthesias and pneumonitis.

PROGNOSIS. Fair if the patient survives the initial exposure. Permanent mental changes as well as serious kidney damage may develop.

Ingestion. Swallowing gasoline causes a burning sensation in the mouth and throat, nausea, vomiting and diarrhea, followed by extreme restlessness, with muscular twitching and incoordination. Aspiration of fumes when gasoline is swallowed may result in a severe chemical pneumonitis. Urinalysis may reveal albuminuria and red cell casts. Blood studies may show leukocytosis, methemoglobinemia and enzyme changes of liver dysfunction.

Treatment Considerations Include:

- If only minor amounts (e.g., less than 1 ml/kg or 30 ml maximum) have been ingested, insufficient to cause CNS, myocardial or other toxicity, emesis should not be induced.
- Toxic amounts should be removed by induction of emesis with syrup of ipecac if the patient has not lost consciousness, the gag reflex is present and he or she is not convulsing. Have the patient upright to minimize aspiration. If emesis is contraindicated and gastric emptying is necessary, insert and inflate a cuffed endotracheal tube before positioning a gastric lavage tube; have the patient lying on his or her side with the head and shoulders dependent before starting lavage.
- Administration of a cathartic and activated charcoal.
- Oxygen administration. Obtain x-ray to look for basilar infiltrates or perihilar changes.
- Hospital for observation and symptomatic and supportive care to minimize the chance of development of respiratory tract, kidney or brain damage. Antibiotics have no value in preventing chemical pneumonitis, but can be used for secondary bacterial infection. Steroids are not indicated except possibly in severest life-threatening situations. If chest x-ray and laboratory studies are normal after 8 hours, and the patient is in good condition, he or she may be released with caution to continue observation for delayed pneumonitis.

53–324. GELSEMIUM (Yellow Jasmine, Carolina Jasmine)

Used medicinally in some localities as an antineuralgic and antispasmodic, gelsemium contains a toxic alkaloid (gelsemine).

Signs and symptoms include great weakness, unsteady gait, vertigo, headache, aphasia, paralysis of the tongue with inability to swallow, lowered body temperature and a pale clammy skin, which later becomes olive green, then flushed and cyanotic. The pupils are dilated and nonreactive. Ptosis of the eyelids is often present. There may also be a weak strychnine action with tetanic contractions and extensor spasms after tendon taps.

53–325. GLORIOSA (Climbing Lily)

Ingestion of the roots, stalks or leaves of this climbing lily results in a toxic picture similar to that caused by colchicine (*53–220*).

53–326. GLUTAMIC ACID

Under the trade names of Accent, Lawry's Seasoned Salt and others, the sodium salt of glutamic acid is used as a food flavoring. Allergic reactions characterized by abdominal discomfort, acute distention, eructations and epigastric fullness have been reported. All disappear when use of the offending preparations is discontinued.

53–327. GLUTETHIMIDE (Doriden)

Overdosage of this nonbarbiturate sedative can result in dryness of the mucous membranes, fever, flushing of the skin, mydriasis, nystagmus, ataxia and coma. Perform gastric emptying followed by administration of activated charcoal. In the comatose

---

*For therapeutic considerations see also *53–1* to *53–13*.

patient, multiple repeat doses of charcoal are indicated. An active metabolite of glutethimide has been identified to be more potent than the parent compound and contributes to the long periods of coma associated with this drug in severe poisonings. Give supportive care; do not overhydrate. Dialysis may be considered in severe cases.

53–328. GOLD SALTS (Au^{3+})

Gold salts used medicinally in the treatment of arthritis and lupus erythematosus are extremely toxic. Sodium aurothiomalate (Myochrysine) is most commonly used now. There may be great variation in personal tolerance of these drugs, not only in different individuals but also in the same person at different times; close medical monitoring and expertise is required.

Signs and symptoms include fever, characteristic facial puffiness, various skin disorders, intense pruritus, nausea, vomiting, abdominal pain and diarrhea. Polyneuritis affecting almost exclusively the motor nerves, liver and kidney damage and blood changes may occur. See *53–108*, dimercaprol (BAL) for antidote administration.

PROGNOSIS. Good unless agranulocytosis has developed, in which case mortality is about 30%.

53–329. GUAIACOL (Methoxyphenol ($C_7H_8O_2$)

Toxic signs, symptoms and treatment of this compound, used as an expectorant, are similar to those listed under *Phenol (53–534)*.

53–330. GYMNOTHORAX FLAVIMARGINATUS

Indigenous to Hawaii, the Philiippines and South Africa, this edible eel for as yet undetermined reasons has been responsible for many cases of acute poisoning. Toxic symptoms, which consist of numbness of the lips, impaired speech, progressive paralysis and convulsions, usually last for several days and are followed by complete recovery without residual ill effects.

53–331. HAIR DYES AND SPRAYS

Many of the preparations used to color, curl, straighten or set hair contain ethyl alcohol (53–295), isopropyl alcohol (53–372), higher alcohols (53–*41*), borates (53–*140*), cadmium salts (53–*158*), caustic hydroxides (53–45 *Alkalies*), copper salts (53–224), dichromates (53–206 *Chromates*). These various substances may cause systemic poisoning through absorption from the scalp and surrounding skin or by ingestion, in addition to localized damage to the hair and scalp.

Among the more complex constituents that may give toxic reactions are:

- Aminodiphenylamines
- Aminonisole
- Chloroaminophenols
- Chlorodiamines
- Diaminophenols
- Henna
- Nitrodiamino compounds
- Phenetols
- Polyvinylpyrrolidones
- Pyrogallol

Treatment

In mild cases the only treatment required is to stop use of the preparation. More severe cases may require extensive supportive therapy. See also 53–587, *Pyrogallol.*

53–332. HALLUCINOGENS (AND OTHER COMMON MIND-AFFECTING CHEMICALS)

Plants containing small amounts of psychotomimetic (sometimes called "consciousness-expanding") drugs have been used for many years as a means of escape from reality in Asia and the Orient [e.g., hashish or marihuana (53–409)] and in religious rites in southwestern United States and Mexico where sliced peyote nuts (53–422, *Mescal*) and certain varieties of mushrooms containing psilocybin (53–462) are chewed by partici-

---

*For therapeutic considerations see also 53–*1* to 53–*13*.

pants. A synthetic, derivative of lysergic acid, the diethylamide (LSD), has a similar but more powerful effect. Illegal sale and use of LSD remains fairly common. The toxic effects (hallucinations, increased perception, personality dissociation, etc.) last for from 6 to 8 hours to 2 to 3 weeks. It is possible that some of the reported unpredictable ill effects may be due to impurities resulting from improper synthesizing. Phencyclidine, which is not a new drug, is being used increasingly (details for treatment of its unique effects are given in *53–532*). True addiction to nonnarcotic hallucinogens does not occur.

In addition to the drugs and plants just mentioned, some of the many substances that have been reported as having hallucinatory effects are as follows:

Acetanilid (*53–20*)
Alkyl mercury compounds (*53–47*)
Amantadine hydrochloride (Symmetrel). This is a recently developed chemical virostat used orally in prevention of influenza. Large doses have a definite hallucinatory effect.
Amyl nitrite (*53–70*)
Arsenic trioxide (*53–92 Arsenic*)
Arsine (*53–94*)
Asthma remedies (*53–102*)
Atropine (*53–103*)
Banana peel scrapings. The dried inner pulp of banana peels has been reported as having some hallucinatory effect ("mellow yellow"). This, however, is very questionable.
Barbiturates (*53–110*)
Belladonna and its alkaloids (*53–115*)
Bromides (*53–146*)
Caffeine (*53–159*)
Camphor (*53–168*)
Carbon monoxide (*53–175*)
Carbon tetrachloride (*53–176*)
Colchicine (*53–220*)
Cortisone (*53–226*)
Dilantin (*53–541*)
DMT (dimethyltryptamine) is a hallucinogen that occurs naturally in certain plants. It can be synthesized very easily. Its action can be obtained only by intramuscular or intravenous injection and is more rapid but less prolonged than LSD.
Epinephrine hydrochloride (Adrenalin) solutions that have turned brown from age or exposure to light.
Ergot (*53–291*)
Euonymin (*53–304*)
Freons (*53–319*)
Gasoline fumes (*53–323*)
Hydrogen sulfide (*53–353*)
Hyoscyamus (*53–355*)
Insulin (Hypoglycemia)
Ketamine (ketaject)—has PCP-like effects
L-dopa (L-dihydroxyphenylalanine)
Meparidine—large doses
Mercury fumes ("Mad Hatter's syndrome") (*53–418*)
Methamphetamine (*53–429, Methedrine*)
Model airplane glue and cement (*53–554*)
Morning glory seeds. Decoctions of the seeds have been used for their alleged hallucinatory effects. The active ingredient is closely related to LSD.
Morphine (*53–455*)
Muscarine (*53–460*)
Nitrous oxide (*53–71, Anesthetics, Inhalation; 53–502, Oxides of Nitrogen*)
Nutmeg (*53–465, Myristicin*)
Oxygen—high concentrations (*53–503*)
Paradichlorobenzene (*53–514*)
Phencyclidine (PCP) (*53–532*)

---

*For therapeutic considerations see also *53–1* to *53–13*.

Prophenpyridamine (53–580)
Quinine (53–592)
Saccharin (53–609)
Salicylic acid (53–614, *Salicylates*)
Scopolamine (53–620)
STP is a more powerful hallucinogen that LSD and is chemically related to amphetamine (53–66) and mescaline (53–422, *Mescal*).
Tetraethyl lead (53–686, *Ethyl Gasoline*; 53–323 *Gasoline*)
Thallium (53–692)
Thiocyanates (53–698)
Trinitrotoluene (53–725)
Tripelennamine hydrochloride (53–727)
Yage. This plant has been used for centuries by Central American witch doctors to promote hallucinations. Its action is similar to that of LSD and mescaline (53–422, *Mescal*).

The following table includes most of the mind-modifying substances usually encountered in drug abuse patients. (Modified from *Medical Economics (Special Edition)*, April 20, 1970.)

Name of Drug	Short-Term Effects	How to Spot Abuser
	Hallucinogens	
DMT	Exhilaration, excitation. Extremely potent when taken intravenously, producing a "blast." Smoking effects are milder.	Same symptoms as LSD.
LSD	Distortion and intensification of sensory perceptions, especially visual hallucinations. Suggestibility.	Dilation of pupils. Exhilaration. Rambling speech, talk of "hearing" or "tasting" colors and "seeing" sounds.
Marijuana and hashish (53–409)	Euphoria, heightened sensory awareness, time/space distortions, increased appetite or lessening of inhibitions. Transient loss of memory and paranoia.	Euphoria with often no physical signs of intoxication, tendency to talk excessively or giggle without provocation, odor of burnt leaves or hemp on breath or clothes, reddened eyes.
Mescaline (53–422)	Same general effects as LSD. High-dose symptoms similar to those after high dose of amphetamine. Acute episode may be mistaken for acute schizophrenia.	Same symptoms as LSD.
Phencyclidine (53–532)	Obtunded consciousness to violent behavior.	Nystagmus, unusual strength, uninhibited behavior.
Psilocybin (53–462)	Initial reactions of nausea, muscular relaxation, headaches, followed by visual and auditory hallucinations.	Same symptoms as LSD.

*For therapeutic considerations see also 53–*1* to 53–*13*.

Name of Drug	Short-Term Effects	How to Spot Abuser
	Depressants	
Barbiturates *(53–110)*	Sedation, relaxation. Relief from anxiety and mental stress. Resultant impaired memory, defective judgment, incoordination.	Drunken behavior with no smell of alcohol. Drowsiness, slowed reflexes, pulse and respiration. Often not diagnosed until onset of acute withdrawal symptoms.
Codeine *(53–219)*	Euphoria obtained only with large amounts, which may also cause excitement and restlessness. Used to "tide over" addict between "fixes" of his usual drug.	Very little evidence of general effect unless taken intravenously.
Heroin *(53–340)*	Rush of euphoria when injected intravenously, but requiring constantly increasing dosage. Drowsiness. Constipation, urinary retention.	Pinpoint pupils (less contraction in seasoned addicts), slow pulse and respiration, needle marks, "nodding."
Methadone *(53–425)*	Analgesia, euphoria. A synthetic narcotic, taken by abusers for its own sake, it is also given to opiate addicts for blockage of craving for and euphoria from their usual drug. Also blocks sickness otherwise produced by withdrawal from opiates.	Heroin-like symptoms.
Morphine *(53–455)*	Similar to heroin except lacking its characteristic euphoric rush.	Same symptoms as heroin.
Plastic or cement glue, toluene, cleaning fluids, aerosols, etc. *(53–554)*	Hazy euphoria. Impaired perceptions, coordination and judgment. Irritation of mucous membranes, slurred speech. Initial excitation is followed by depression, stupor.	See short-term effects.
	Stimulants	
Amphetamines *(53–66)*	Feeling of energy and excitation. Loss of appetite. Insomnia. Feeling of inceased initiative. Euphoric rush when injected.	Extreme restlessness or nervousness. Tremor. Dryness of mouth. Tachycardia. Excessive sweating. Needle marks when injected.
Cocaine *(53–218)*	Flashing, intense euphoria, pleasurable hallucinations. Feeling of great mental and muscular strength.	Garrulity, restlessness, excitement. Hyperactivity of reflexes. Rapid pulse and irregular respiration.

*For therapeutic considerations see also 53–*1* to 53–*13*.

Treatment Considerations Include:

- Close observation under controlled circumstances, with a sympathetic and physically able attendent present at all times. Relapses may occur as long as several weeks after the original exposure.
- Symptomatic and supportive therapy based on the hallucinogen used. Diazepam (Valium) in appropriate doses is a safe sedative. Chlorpromazine hydrochloride (Thorazine) should not be used in the treatment of unidentified hallucinogens. If STP is a component, fatalities may occur.
- Psychiatric evaluation and treatment as needed.

53–333. HEADACHE REMEDIES (Nonprescription)

These proprietary compounds generally contain one or more of the following: acetaminophen (*53–19*), acetanilid (*53–20*) combined with caffeine (*53–159*), bromides (*53–146*) and salicylates (*53–614*).

53–334. HEATHER

Andromedotoxin is the active toxic agent in all varieties of heather. See *53–34, Aconite; 53–231, Curare.*

53–335. HELLEBOREIN

This is one of several glucosides found in the roots and seeds of plants of the Helleborus family (Christmas Rose). Ingestion of even small amounts results in rapid development of nausea, vomiting, abdominal pain, diarrhea, headache, vertigo, tinnitus, dilation of the pupils, photophobia, visual disturbances and myalgia, especially of the calves. More serious cases develop delirium, convulsions, coma and death from respiratory collapse.

Treatment

- Emetics followed by gastric lavage with large amounts of water. Activated charcoal in water should be left in the stomach.
- Artificial respiration by expired air or mechanical methods (*5–1*), followed by administration of oxygen if respiratory depression is acute.
- Administration of 10% calcium gluconate IV for acute myalgia.
- Hospitalization for close observation for at least 24 hours after apparent complete recovery.

53–336. HELVELLA (False Morel, Lorchel, Morel)

Generally considered to be edible, these mushrooms occasionally cause severe toxic symptoms coming on from 6 to 8 hours after ingestion. For signs and symptoms of toxicity and treatment, see *53–462, Mushroom Poisoning.*

53–337. HEPARIN

Purpura, ecchymosis and hematuria from the use of this anticoagulant may be severe enough to require immediate therapy for shock (*57*). Plasma volume expanders should be given for temporary support and the patient hospitalized at once for thorough investigation and possible blood transfusions or protamine administration. (See also *45–8, Hemorrhage After Anticoagulant Therapy,* for specific treatment.)

53–338. HEPTACHLOR ($C_{10}H_5Cl_7$; TLV 0.5 mg/m^3)

Heptachlor is a complex insecticide that by inhalation, skin absorption or ingestion can give a toxic picture similar to that produced by chlordane (*53–190*). In addition, severe and permanent liver damage may develop.

---

*For therapeutic considerations see also *53–1* to *53–13*.

53–339. HERACLEUM LANATUM (Cow Cabbage, Cow Parsnip, Hayweed, Masterwort)

The sap of this perennial meadow plant, indigenous to the northern section of the United States, on contact with the skin causes photosensitization and acute eczematous eruptions, which heal with permanent pigmentation.

53–340. HEROIN (Diacetylmorphine) *(See also 7–4, Addiction)*

This powerful narcotic is more toxic and addictive than any of the other opiates. Prescription or administration of heroin is forbidden in the United States and many other countries. It is common in the illegitimate narcotic market for heroin to be adulterated with substances that in themselves may be toxic, infectious or contain contaminating particles.

Signs and Symptoms of heroin overdosage [usually following IV ("mainline") injection are as follows:

- Marked respiratory depression (apnea or 3 to 4 gasping respirations per minute).
- Cyanotic, clammy pallor.
- Pinpoint pupils (may be dilated if anoxia is extreme).
- Weak pulse, but may be strong and full if extreme hypoxia is present. Arrhythmias and cardiac cessation may occur.
- Evidence of pulmonary edema.
- Areflexia, deep coma and death.

Treatment Considerations Include:

- Establish and maintain an adequate airway.
- Start artificial ventilation by expired air or mechanical methods (5–*1*).
- Begin external cardiac compression (5–*1*) if the heartbeat is ineffective or absent. Monitor cardiac status by ECGs.
- Inject naloxone hydrochloride (Narcan) IV, 0.01 mg/kg (see *53–10*). Repeat doses of naloxone may be needed, because of its short half-life (see *53–10*).
- Give intravenous glucose and electrolytes.
- Treat metabolic acidosis with intravenous glucose and electrolyte administration.
- Treat pulmonary edema (55).

Withdrawal symptoms from heroin are very uncomfortable but rarely life-threatening. Beginning about 10 to 12 hours after the last injection, reaching maximum intensity in about 36 hours and subsiding on about the 5th day, they are characterized by frequent exaggerated yawning and gaping, nausea, vomiting, abdominal cramping and diarrhea, hypersalivation, excessive tearing, photophobia, intense myalgia, jitteriness and insomnia.

Treatment of Withdrawal Symptoms

- Psychologic and physiologic supportive care is best.
- *For pain and myalgia:* Salicylates, acetaminophen or ibuprofen (Motrin) orally.
- *For gastrointestinal symptoms:* Belladonna preparations or dicyclomine hydrochloride (Bentyl) every 4 hours.
- *For nervousness and sleeplessness:* Diazepam (Valium), 5 to 10 mg 4 times a day, or chloral hydrate, 1 g PO at bedtime, may be helpful, but are best avoided to help break up the drug-seeking behavior.
- Recent evidence suggests that clonidine *(53–216)* may be helpful.

53–341. HEXAMETHYLENETETRAMINE (Methenamine, Mandelamine)

In acid urine, this drug, used in treatment of chronic UTI, slowly releases formaldehyde. Excessively large doses may give mild toxic symptoms. See 53–315, *Formaldehyde.*

---

*For therapeutic considerations see also *53–1* to *53–13*.

53–342. HEXYLRESORCINOL

Use of high concentrations or large doses by mouth, in addition to being irritating to tissues, may give a picture suggestive of mild phenol poisoning. See also 53–534, *Phenol.*

53–343. HIPPOMANE MANCINELLA (Mancellier, Manzanillo)

Growing along the seashore of Florida, the Caribbean islands and Central America, this small tree exudes a latex that on contact gives a multiplicity of acute toxic eye symptoms—vesicles, bullae, conjunctivitis, photophobia and corneal ulcers. Ingestion of the fruit causes vomiting, violent gastric pain and bloody diarrhea that may be followed by cardiovascular collapse.

53–344. HISTAMINE ($C_5H_9N_3$)

Medical use of excessive amounts of this potent vasodilator and bronchoconstrictor may cause severe, sometimes fatal, shock and bronchospasm (56–4). It also is present widely in nature as part of the putrefactive process. For treatment, see 24 and 57.

53–345. HOLLY (*Ilex aquifolium*)

Severe gastroenteritis with prolonged vomiting and diarrhea may follow ingestion of any portion of this plant. Eating 20 to 30 berries may be fatal to children.

53–346. HOMATROPINE ($C_{16}H_{21}NO_3$)

Therapeutic use in ophthalmology of this anticholinergic (see Table 53–2, Anticholinergics) may cause a slow pulse, dysphagia, vertigo, weakness, excitement and collapse, as well as the expected mydriasis and cycloplegia. Complete recovery in a short period is the rule. No special treatment is required.

Overdosage has been reported as causing excitement, confusion and coma, with very slow respiration, rapid pulse and hypotension.

53–347. HONEY

Nectar collected by bees from certain flowering plants may yield toxic honey. Among these plants are aconite (53–34), azalea (53–105), foxglove (53–265, *Digitalis*), gelsemium (53–324), laurel (53–384), oleander (53–495), and rhododendron (53–600).

53–348. HYACINTH

The bulb of the hyacinth plant causes severe gastrointestinal symptoms when ingested. Treatment is supportive.

53–349. HYDROCARBONS

See *Gasoline (53–323)* for general treatment measures for toxicity by hydrocarbons, which are highly absorbed gastrointestinally. See also *Benzene (53–117), Furniture Polish (53–320), Kerosene (53–379), Naphthalene (53–469)* and *Turpentine (53–730).*

Benzene and its allied products (toluene, xylene, naphthas) are found in many solvents and thinners. They are highly aromatic and toxic by both inhalation and ingestion. Toxic absorption and indications for selective gastric emptying are similar to those for gasoline.

Furniture polish, lighter fluid, turpentine and kerosene are poorly or not absorbed in the gastrointestinal tract.

53–350. HYDROCHLORIC ACID (HCl; TLV 5 ppm) *(See 53–33, Acids)*

---

*For therapeutic considerations see also 53–*1* to 53–*13*.

53–351. HYDROFLUORIC ACID (HF)

The extremely corrosive solution is used in etching and engraving. It may cause severe toxic symptoms by contact with the skin or nails, contact with the eyes, inhalation of fumes and ingestion. Death may occur.

Skin Contact

Even small amounts of hydrofluoric acid on the skin or nails will cause severe damage. The onset is insidious; after the acid is removed, the skin or nails will appear to be normal for about 1 hour. Erythema, followed by vesication and tissue destruction then develops rapidly, resulting in a nonhealing ulcer that sometimes extends to the bone. Fingernails and nail beds may be completely destroyed.

Treatment Considerations Include:

1. Removal of all contaminated garments.
2. Immediate washing with copious amounts of water for 30 minutes or longer, followed by application of a dressing soaked with a solution of calcium carbonate or chloride (or alternatively a 1:500 solution of quaternary ammonium [e.g., Hibiclens]. An ice pack may add to comfort.
3. After lengthy washing and soaking, 2.5% calcium gluconate gel or a paste made from equal parts of magnesium oxide and magnesium sulfate (Epsom salts) may be applied.
4. Injection of small amounts of calcium gluconate (5 to 10% solution), using a 25-gauge needle, into, under and around the affected area may be done in more severe cases. If the nails are extensively involved, it may be necessary to remove the nail and inject small amounts of the solution into the nail bed. Any infiltration done around the digits, hand, feet or face must be done with much care and knowledge that vascular compromise, tissue irritation and scarring may occur from higher concentrations of calcium. Repeat injection in about 24 hours may be needed if pain persists. Small ulcers can be excised en bloc and the base injected with 5 to 10% calcium gluconate in an area (up to 0.5 ml per sq cm). Relief of pain with calcium gluconate solution can be rapid and an index of adequacy of treatment; concomitant local anesthetic injection would mask this sign, although an anesthetic is acceptable if pain is too severe. Following injection, the areas should be treated as an open wound or third-degree chemical burn.
5. IV injection of 10 ml of 10% calcium gluconate.

Contact with the Eyes

Hydrofluoric acid in the eyes may cause serious and permanent damage.

Treatment

- Immediate and protracted washing with copious amounts of water.
- Instillation of 1% tetracaine hydrochloride (Pontocaine) for examination and initially to control pain, followed by 1% atropine sulfate to dilate the pupil. A dressing of 20% magnesium oxide may be applied.
- Application of an eye patch.
- Immediate referral for ophthalmologic care.

Inhalation of Fumes

Treatment

- Removal from exposure.
- Inhalation of 1% calcium chloride solution sprayed into the respiratory tract with a nebulizer. Consider steroid administration.
- Hospitalization if marked irritation of the respiratory tract is present.

Ingestion. See *53–311, Fluorides,* for treatment.

---

*For therapeutic considerations see also *53–1* to *53–13*.

53–352. HYDROGEN SELENIDE (H_2Se; TLV 0.05 ppm)

Low concentrations of this colorless industrial gas may cause severe eye and throat irritation (cough, hoarseness, dysphagia), rhinitis, anosmia, urticaria, extreme hypotension, dyspnea and cyanosis, followed by pulmonary edema (55).

53–353. HYDROGEN SULFIDE (H_2S; TLV 10 ppm)

Toxic symptoms from this colorless, caustic, foul-smelling ("rotten egg") gas, formed by putrefaction of sulfur-containing material, are common among petroleum and sewer workers. It is extremely important to get away at the first smell, as olfactory fatigue (anosmia) rapidly occurs. Its lethality is comparable to that of hydrocyanic acid.

Low concentrations are irritants only and may cause acute conjunctivitis, photophobia and seeing of colored rings around bright lights, rhinitis with decrease or loss of the sense of smell, tracheitis, bronchitis, pneumonia (56–*16*) and pulmonary edema (55).

Treatment Includes:

- Removal from exposure.
- Installation of bland ointment into the eyes for conjunctivitis.
- Oxygen administration and pain control (*12*).

High concentrations are very depressant and may cause nausea; vomiting; progressively increasing somnolence; amnesia; transient unconsciousness, coming on especially after exertion; dysphagia; rapid pulse; low blood pressure; and eye signs (strabismus, diplopia, exophthalmos, fixed nonreactive pupils). Delirium and hallucinations may be followed by convulsions and death from respiratory failure. Extremely high concentrations are rapidly fatal.

Treatment Includes:

- Removal from exposure. Complete rest.
- Oxygen administration and ventilation (5–*1*) as needed. Treatment of pulmonary edema (55) may be required.
- Treat shock as necessary (57).
- In severe cases, use amyl nitrite therapy and sodium nitrite as outlined in *53–232, Cyanides* (except do not use thiosulfate); the objective is to produce methemoglobin, which binds the sulfide and is renally eliminated as sulfmethemoglobin. Hospitalization for prevention or treatment of delayed sequelae (pneumonia, pulmonary edema, cardiac dilation, severe gastrointestinal symptoms and peripheral polyneuritis) is indicated.

53–354. HYDROQUINONE ($C_6H_4(OH)_2$; TLV 2 mg/m^3)

Most of the cases of acute poisoning from hydroquinone arise from its use as a photographic developer. Signs and symptoms include dizziness, ringing in the ears, rapid respiration, profuse sweating, nausea, vomiting, restlessness, muscular twitching, cyanosis (probably due to methemoglobinemia) (53–*12*) and collapse. Severe hemolytic anemia may occur.

53–355. HYOSCYAMUS (Henbane)

If the foliage or stalks of this flowering garden plant are chewed, severe toxic symptoms similar to those from atropine (53–*103*) may develop. For the toxic picture and treatment, see *53–103, Atropine Sulfate.*

53–356. HYPOCHLORITES (Chlorinated Lime, Clorox, Bleaching Powder, Labarraque's Solution, Dakin's Solution, Emergency Water Sterilizers) (Varying proportions of $Ca[OCl]_2$, $CaCl_2$, $Ca[OH]_2$)

Concentrated solutions have severe caustic alkali actions (53–*45*); dilute solutions cause only mild gastrointestinal symptoms. Although the antiseptic and bleaching actions

---

*For therapeutic considerations see also *53–1* to *53–13*.

depend on the chlorine content, this is too low to give toxic symptoms and can be disregarded in treatment. For treatment, see *53–45, Alkalies.*

53–357. INDELIBLE INKS, PENCILS AND STAINS *(See 53–75, Aniline Dyes; 53–630, Silver Salts)*

53–358. INDIAN POKE

This plant will cause principally gastrointestinal symptoms.

53–359. INDIGO

Ingestion of small amounts of natural or synthetic indigo may cause retching, vomiting, abdominal pain, diarrhea, fever, muscle twitching and renal colic.

53–360. INKY CAPS *(See also 53–462, Mushroom Poisoning)*

This variety of mushroom is considered by some authorities to be edible but in the presence of alcohol can give toxic effects similar to those of disulfiram (53–279).

53–361. INK ERADICATORS *(See 53–356, Hypochlorites; 53–501, Oxalic Acid)*

53–362. INSULIN *(See also 32–3, Diabetes Mellitus)*

Prolonged glucose support may be required if hypoglycemia is due to subcutaneously administered insulin.

53–363. IODATES (IO_3^{1-})

Intravenous use of solutions of sodium and potassium iodate in the treatment of sepsis at one time was common and accounted for a considerable number of fatalities. Iodates are no longer used for this purpose. No recent cases of iodate toxicity have been reported.

53–364. IODIDES (I^{1-})

Iodides are relatively nontoxic, but excessive doses or prolonged use of therapeutic doses can cause iodism (see *53–365, Iodine*), as well as enlargement of the salivary glands, which may be mistaken for mumps (33–43).

53–365. IODINE (I_2; TLV 0.1 ppm—C)

Local application causes mahogany-brown discoloration of the skin, with marked erythema and desquamation, vesication and corrosion of mucous membranes.

Exposure to fumes results in sparkling before the eyes, conjunctivitis, lacrimation, severe cough, headache, somnolence and swelling of the parotid glands (see 53–364, *Iodides*).

Ingestion results in a characteristic metallic iodine taste, with severe pain and burning in the esophagus and stomach, often associated with brownish discoloration of the mucous membranes of the mouth and throat, nausea, vomiting (blue color of vomitus if the patient has been given starch) and extreme thirst. Convulsions may occur if large amounts have been swallowed.

Treatment Considerations Include:

- Give large amounts of 1% to 10% starch solution (or 1 to 4 tablespoons of cornstarch or laundry starch in 1 pint of water) by mouth.
- Unless there is evidence of extensive mucous membrane corrosion, empty the stomach by emesis or gastric lavage and follow with 1% sodium thiosulfate solution (helps transform pure iodine to less harmful iodides); repeat until the returned fluid no longer shows any blue color.
- Support circulation; severe shock requiring energetic management (57) may develop.

---

*For therapeutic considerations see also *53–1* to *53–13*.

53–366. IODOFORM

Absorption from wounds packed extensively with iodoform gauze or ingestion may cause nausea, vomiting, rapid pulse, acute excitement and convulsions.

53–367. IPECAC *(See also 53–7 regarding avoidance of syrup of ipecac)*

Syrup of ipecac orally is an excellent emetic, with a wide margin of safety; however, deaths have occurred when the fluid extract (14 times as toxic as the syrup) has been administered by error in place of the syrup. In addition to being an emetic, ipecac is an efficient sedative. If satisfactory emptying of the stomach does not occur after 2 doses of syrup of ipecac, gastric lavage (*18–11*) should be done at once. Excessive vomiting can be controlled by chlorpromazine (Thorazine) parenterally. Treatment of shock (57) frequently is necessary. Continuous ECG monitoring is advisable because of the cardiotoxic effects—bradycardia, atrial fibrillation, tachycardia and cardiac arrest—of substances such as emetine, which are found in ipecac.

53–368. IRIS

All members of this family contain solanine (*53–644*), mostly in the underground stems. The powdered rhizomes of certain varieties of iris used in cosmetics and tooth powders may cause skin reactions, rhinitis and asthmatic symptoms; these clear rapidly when exposure is terminated.

53–369. IRON OXIDE *(See 53–370, Iron Salts; 53–423, Metal Fumes)* (Fe_2O_3; TLV 5 mg/m^3)

53–370. IRON SALTS Fe, Fe^{++}, Fe^{+++}

Since the common salts of iron oxidize rapidly on exposure to air to form basic ferric sulfate, acute poisoning from this source may occasionally be encountered. The majority of the cases of acute toxicity, however, result from ingestion by children of candy-coated ferrous sulfate tablets, with a mortality rate of up to 30%. Abdominal x-ray may reveal countable radiocontrast iron tablets.

Signs and Symptoms: A metallic taste in the mouth; vomiting of bluish green material; rapid, weak pulse; hypotension; blackish or bloody diarrhea, often persistent enough to cause acute dehydration; and severe shock (57), especially in children.

Treatment Considerations Include:

- Emesis or gastric lavage with copious amounts of tap water through a large-bore tube; then lavage with a 1% bicarbonate solution to promote formation of ferrous carbonate, which is poorly absorbed. *Note:* Any dilute phosphate solution used to precipitate the iron in the GI tract must be used with extreme caution.
- Parenteral deferoxamine (Desferal) (see *53–10*) in symptomatic patients or patients with serum iron levels greater than 300 to 500 μg/dl. Deferoxamine is used until the "vin rosé" color in the urine disappears.
- Treatment of shock (57), which may not appear for 12 hours. Whole blood transfusions may be required. Calcium edetate, oral or IV, is of value.
- Immediate hospitalization for fluid replacement (*11*) and treatment of acidosis. A specimen of gastric washing and a blood specimen taken before starting deferoxamine therapy should be obtained and sent to the laboratory for iron level determinations. Peritoneal dialysis and hemodialysis are of little, if any, value. Dimercaprol (BAL) therapy is ineffective.

53–371. ISONIAZID

Large doses (20–25 mg/kg) of this drug used in the treatment of tuberculosis may be toxic, especially in children.

---

*For therapeutic considerations see also *53–1* to *53–13*.

Signs and symptoms include nausea, vomiting, cyanosis of the extremities, generalized convulsions and coma. Pyridoxine hydrochloride (vitamin B_6) is an important part of therapy and must be given IV in large doses equal to or greater than the amount of isoniazide ingested.

Severe cases may require dialysis.

53–372. ISOPROPYL ALCOHOL (Avantine, Dimethylcarbinol) ($CH_3CHOHCH_3$; TLV 400 ppm)

Isopropyl alcohol has many uses—as a rubbing compound (usually with a denaturant to make it unpotable); as a solvent for waxes and resins; in the production of safety glass, paints and varnishes; and in the manufacture of perfumes and cosmetics.

Signs and symptoms (usually following ingestion but may be caused by inhalation of concentrated fumes) are dizziness, muscular weakness and incoordination (no exhilaration as with ethyl alcohol), severe headache, slow pulse and low blood pressure, acute gastrointestinal irritation with bloody vomitus and diarrhea, anuria and uremia. See also *53–295, Ethyl Alcohol,* for comments and treatment. Acetone is a metabolic product and can be found in blood. Dialysis is rarely necessary.

53–373. ISOPROTERENOL HYDROCHLORIDE (Isuprel, Norisodrine) ($C_{11}H_{17}NO_3 \cdot HCl$)

Used as an inhalant in asthmatic and allergic conditions and IV in the treatment of bradycardia (29–7), Isuprel in certain individuals can cause tachycardia, palpitation, precordial pain and irregularities in blood pressure. Large doses may cause dizziness, mental confusion, hypotension and cardiac arrest.

All symptoms gradually clear when use of the drug is discontinued.

53–374. JACK-IN-THE-PULPIT

All parts contain calcium oxalate, which may cause severe irritation of the mouth, tongue and upper gastrointestinal tract. Treatment consists of aluminum hydroxide by mouth as a demulcent.

53–375. JATROPHA NUT OIL (Physic Nut Tree)

The nuts of this tropical South American and Asiatic shrub (Barbados nut tree, physic nut tree, purging nut tree) contain an oil known as Turkey red oil and "Hell" oil, which is a powerful purgative. It is used in the manufacture of soap. As an adulterant of olive oil, it has been responsible for several series of acute poisonings. Symptoms of toxicity and treatment are similar to those outlined in *53–230, Croton Oil.*

53–376. JEQUIRITY BEANS ("Crab Eyes")

The beans of the plant *Abrus precatorius,* indigenous to Florida and the Caribbean islands, especially Haiti, and some South Pacific Islands, are bright red with a small black spot and are very attractive—and dangerous—to tourists and children. For toxic effects of ingestion of the soft, easily chewed young beans, see *53–15, Abrus precatorius.*

When the beans mature and develop a hard shell, they become even more dangerous. They are used as ornamental beads on rosaries, as strands of beads on blouses and purses, as the eyes of native dolls and as decorations on "voodoo swizzle sticks." The drier they become, the more dust escapes from the hilum. If this powder is ingested or enters the tissues through a break in the skin, it causes serious, often fatal, effects from abrin poisoning. See also *53–15, Abrus precatorius.*

53–377. JERUSALEM CHERRY

This plant contains glycoalkaloids and causes cardiac decompensation.

---

*For therapeutic considerations see also *53–1* to *53–13.*

53–378. JUTE

Processing of jute fibers in the manufacture of bags, mats and rope may cause severe allergic reactions—asthma, bronchitis, bronchospasm, laryngitis and tracheitis.

53–379. KEROSENE (Coal Oil) *(See 53–349, Hydrocarbons)*

This common petroleum distillate mixture has a wide use as a fuel, solvent and cleanser and also as the inert ingredient in many types of household and garden sprays. Although often considered to be of low toxicity, the exact opposite is true; the mortality is close to 10% following ingestion of significant amounts, probably owing in great part to aspiration during ingestion, vomiting and gastric lavage. Inhalation of the fumes may cause transient excitement, headache, hallucinations and delirium, but these signs and symptoms clear rapidly when the concentration of the fumes is lowered by adequate ventilation. It is after these transient and uncomfortable symptoms clear up that the serious pathologic conditions (pneumonitis, pneumonia) become apparent.

Signs and symptoms from ingestion are gastrointestinal irritation, circulatory disturbances, severe respiratory depression, coma, convulsions and pulmonary symptoms, especially aspiration pneumonia. Absorption of kerosene is of low magnitude. Treatment is the same as for *Gasoline* (53–323), except that the need for removal is less imperative.

53–380. KNOCKOUT DROPS *(See 53–186)*

53–381. LABURNUM (Golden Chain)

The flowers, leaves and shoots of this ornamental tree contain the toxic alkaloid cystisine (53–235), which is similar in action to nicotine (53–478).

53–382. LACTIC ACID

Ingestion may cause severe burning of the mouth, pharynx, esophagus and stomach; nausea and vomiting; bloody emesis; rapid, weak pulse; cold perspiration; dyspnea; cyanosis; and death from dehydration and exhaustion secondary to acute gastroenteritis. Ingestion or lavage of lime water followed by activated charcoal aids deactivation.

53–383. LANTANA (Red Sage, Wild Sage)

Fatalities have been reported from ingestion of the berries of this ornamental plant. Acute toxic symptoms resemble those from atropine. For treatment, see 53–*103, Atropine Sulfate; 53–115, Belladonna Alkaloids.*

53–384. LAUREL

All varieties of laurel contain andromedotoxin. Allergic skin reactions are common in hat makers who use laurel oil for "fattening" felts. Termination of exposure results in slow disappearance of symptoms. See 53–*34, Aconite; 53–231, Curare.*

53–385. LEAD ARSENATE ($PbHAsO_4$; TLV 0.15 mg/m^3)

Lead arsenate (and arsenite), both commonly used as insecticides, may cause toxic symptoms through inhalation. See 53–*386, Lead Salts,* and 53–*90, Arsenic.*

53–386. LEAD SALTS (Pb, Pb^{++})

In addition to resulting from exposure in industry, signs and symptoms of toxicity (plumbism) may occur, especially in children, from ingestion of flakes of old-fashioned paints and from use of improperly glazed china and other ceramics. Toxic symptoms also may be caused by inhalation of dust and fumes (particularly lead oxide—see 53–423, *Metal Fumes*), and by absorption through the skin. Several series of cases from

---

*For therapeutic considerations see also 53–*1* to 53–*13*.

illicitly distilled ("bootleg") whisky have been reported. Lead chromate is particularly toxic.

Signs and symptoms of acute plumbism consist of a sweetish metallic taste, with dryness of the throat and extreme thirst, dizziness and severe cramping abdominal pain, with either constipation or bloody diarrhea. Severe arthralgia may occur, with parasthesias, impaired mental status, convulsions and coma. There is often evidence of severe liver and kidney damage.

Following routine gastric emptying for recent ingestion, give specific antidote, IV calcium EDTA (see *53–10*) and dimercaprol (BAL) (see *53–10*) concurrently, guided by serum lead levels. D-Penicillamine (*53–10*) has been found in investigational studies to be effective. Correct conditions that led to toxicity.

53–387. LEMON GRASS OIL

This is a volatile (essential) oil (*53–494*) that not only is toxic if ingested but also causes a dermatitis similar to poison oak (*58–13*) on contact with the skin.

53–388. LETHANE

Lethane is used as a contact insecticide and may give acute toxic signs and symptoms, if ingested. See *53–698, Thiocyanates (Organic derivatives).*

53–389. LIGHTER FLUID *(See also 53–349, Hydrocarbons)*

Lighter fluid is usually a mix of petroleum naphtha (see *53–117, Benzene*) and kerosene (*53–379*). It is poorly absorbed by the gastrointestinal tract, decreasing the need for removal.

53–390. LILY OF THE VALLEY (Pieris Japonica)

The flowers, leaves, stalks and roots contain a glucoside, convallamarin, similar to digitalis (*53–265*) in action and toxicity. Ingestion may cause death in children.

Lily of the valley belongs to the same family (Ericaceae) as other toxic genera: *Rhododendron (53–600), Kalmia* (mountain laurel) and *Lencothe* (fetterbush).

53–391. LIMA BEAN (some varieties, e.g., *Phaseolus lunatus* and *Phaseolus limensis*)

The beans contain cyanoglycosides, which when ingested and metabolized cause signs and symptoms of cyanide poisoning (*53–232*).

53–392. LIME

Quicklime (unslaked lime, calcium oxide) is a powerful caustic that liberates heat when exposed to moisture. It may cause serious damage if ingested or allowed to come in contact with any portion of the eyes. When ingested, the signs, symptoms and treatment are about the same as for any strongly caustic alkali (*53–45*). In the eyes it may cause hyperemia, edema and corneal ulceration, sometimes with resultant permanent opacities and loss of vision (see *35–31*).

53–393. LINDANE *(See 53–118, Benzene Hexachloride)* ($C_6H_6Cl_6$; TLV 0.5 mg/m^3)

53–394. LIPSTICKS *(See 53–227, Cosmetics)*

In general, the more "kiss-proof," the more the chance of toxic reactions (usually of the allergic or contact dermatitis type), which clear rapidly when use of the particular cosmetic is discontinued.

---

*For therapeutic considerations see also *53–1* to *53–13*.

53–395. LITHIUM CARBONATE (CLi_2O)

This is one of the substances that in minute amounts may cause acute toxic signs and symptoms in certain individuals. Apparently, the tolerance of different persons varies tremendously. Since, in addition to its commercial use in fireworks and in soldering aluminum, it is a constituent of some mineral waters and sodium chloride substitutes and is used medically, generally as the lithium carbonate compound, in the treatment of manic episodes of manic-depressive illness, familiarity with its toxic effects is important. Patients with renal or cardiac disease, dehydration or sodium depletion are most prone to serious effects. Severe nephrogenic diabetes insipidus can occur at therapeutic levels. Therapeutic levels (usually 1.0 to 1.5 mEq/L in acute mania, and 0.6 to 1.2 mEq/L for long-range treatment) lie close to toxic levels, which are usually over 1.5 mEq/L; levels over 3.5 mEq/L are life-threatening. Immediately measure blood levels to guide treatment.

Signs and symptoms: Tinnitus; vertigo; ataxia, blurred vision; sleeplessness; vomiting; diarrhea; generalized weakness; tremors of the extremities, often associated with muscular twitching; bizarre shifting disturbances in sensation; acute dysphagia; mental confusion; coma; seizures; and (occasionally) death. Withhold any thiazide diuretics. Restore sodium and water balance. Marked hypersensitivity to stimuli may be controlled by IV short-acting barbiturates or diazepam. Dialysis may be indicated in severe cases. Excretion may be aided by IV mannitol.

PROGNOSIS. Guarded because of the marked variation in reactions and responses to therapy.

53–396. LOBELIA (Indian Tobacco) *(See also 53–478, Nicotine)*

Ingestion of leaves and seeds of this common plant causes serious symptoms due to a toxic alkaloid, lobeline. The characteristic picture consists of throat dryness, vomiting, abdominal pain, diarrhea, anxiety, muscular twitching and somnolence. In fatal cases, severe convulsions precede death. Do not confuse with wild tobacco (53–752).

53–397. LOCUST

The seeds of certain varieties of these common ornamental trees contain a toxic substance similar to that found in castor beans (53–*180*).

Signs and symptoms are usually less severe than in castor bean poisoning and the mortality rate is lower. The treatment is the same.

53–398. LOLIUM TEMULENTUM (Darnel, Ivray, Poison Rye-Grass, Tares)

This widespread weed, as a contaminant of cereal grains and of their derivatives—especially linseed oil—has given rise to numerous cases of poisoning characterized by somnolence, vertigo, staggering and trembling. Eye signs are common, with blurred vision (often greenish) and dilated pupils. Severely affected patients show the symptoms of severe shock (57).

53–399. LOMOTIL

Lomotil contains the opiate diphenoxylate hydrochloride and atropine sulfate. The first effects of overdosage with this popular diarrhea remedy are from atropine (53–*103*) and are often complicated by hypothermia. Later, symptoms resembling those of morphine (53–455) develop. See 53–*10* for use of naloxone hydrochloride (Narcan) as a specific antidote.

53–400. LUPINE

All parts of this flowering plant contain lupinine, an alkaloid that causes respiratory and circulatory depression, paralysis and convulsions if ingested even in small amounts.

---

*For therapeutic considerations see also 53–*1* to 53–*13*.

53–401. LYE (Lixivium)

Lye originally was made by leaching wood ashes, but the term is now used for several of the strong alkalies, especially sodium and potassium hydroxide and carbonate. All act as severe caustics on direct contact with exposed parts of the body, and all may cause severe, often fatal, damage if ingested. Because lye is available in many households (washing powders, drainpipe cleaners, oven cleaners, paint removers, etc.), contact with the eyes or skin or ingestion by accident or with suicidal intent is relatively common.

Treatment

For eyes, see *38–31*; for skin, see *Alkali Burns, 28–5;* for ingestion, see *53–45.*

53–402. MAGNESIUM (Mg)

Metallic magnesium is used in the manufacture of light metal alloys; grinding may cause fine, sharp fragments that perforate the skin and cause marked swelling and crepitus from formation of hydrogen bubbles. Xerography may aid location. Treatment is by surgical excision and primary closure.

Inhalation of finely ground metallic magnesium may cause metal fume fever; for treatment, see *53–423.*

53–403. MAGNESIUM OXIDE (MgO; TLV 10 mg/mv³) *(See 53–423, Metal Fumes)*

53–404. MAGNESIUM SULFATE (Epsom Salts)

Especially in persons with impaired renal function, ingestion of excessive amounts, absorption through the rectum or intravenous injection may result in vomiting, with acute gastric pain, dilation of the pupils, cyanosis, generalized weakness, and collapse from respiratory and cardiac failure. Dialysis against a magnesium-free bath is required for patients with severe overdoses or renal failure.

53–405. MAGNOLIA

The seeds of all of the numerous varieties of magnolias contain a substance similar in action and toxicity to picrotoxin (*53–549*).

53–406. MALATHION ($[CH_3O]_2P[S]S[CHCOOC_2H_5]_2$; TLV 10 mg/m³

This is one of the few organic phosphate insecticides approved for household use. In spite of its extremely low toxicity, treatment may be necessary if exposure has been excessive. Massive area spraying was done, for eradication of the Mediterranean Fruit Fly in California in 1981—including dense population areas—without significant untoward effects. See *53–497.*

53–407. MANGANESE

Although metal fume fever (*53–423*) may be caused by inhalation of finely ground magnesium, more serious toxic symptoms may follow inhalation of manganese dust by workers in the steel and battery industries and among ore handlers.

Signs and symptoms are usually low grade and chronic, but severe acute muscular cramps (especially in the calves), uncontrollable laughter, slurred speech and staggering gait may require emergency therapy. Both the chronic and acute pictures can easily be mistaken for drug addiction (7). Hospitalization for thorough investigation is indicated if the history or symptoms suggest manganese poisoning. The incidence of a subsequent, peculiarly virulent type of pneumonia is relatively high. Calcium edetate may be considered in treatment of acute poisoning and L-dopa for chronic poisoning.

---

*For therapeutic considerations see also *53–1* to *53–13.*

53–408. MANGO

The skin and sap can cause severe dermatitis and gastrointestinal irritation. Treatment is symptomatic.

53–409. MARIJUANA (Bhang, Cannabis sativa, Hashish, Indian hemp, "Pot") *(See also 53–332, Hallucinogens; 53–516, Paraquat)*

Signs and symptoms of marijuana intoxication are the same for ingestion or smoking and consist basically of inebriation, motor excitement, restlessness, euphoria and gaiety (sometimes anxiety) coming on about 1 hour after smoking or ingestion. Extreme thirst may be present as may wide dilation of the pupils with sluggish reaction to light. Aphrodisiac effects are much less marked than usually believed. Vertigo and transient collapse may occur. Spontaneous recovery occurs in a short time on withdrawal, and only supportive treatment is needed. Increasing evidence indicates that chronic use can cause permanent damage. Spraying of the marijuana plant with pesticides (e.g., Paraquat, *53–516*) has added to toxicity.

53–410. MATCHES

Most present day matches contain trisulfurated phosphorus, or phosphorus sesquisulfide, which is almost inert chemically and therefore relatively nontoxic. "Safety matches" have no toxic ingredients in harmful amounts in the head (the phosphorus compound is on the friction surface on the box or book); therefore, children who suck or eat the head need no treatment except disciplining. Ingestion of large numbers of the heads of "strike anywhere" matches requires treatment, because many brands contain potassium chlorate and antimony sulfide in addition to a phosphorus compound. Old-fashioned "sulfur matches" contain yellow phosphorus and are dangerous; ingestion of 16 of these matches has been reported as fatal to an adult.

For toxic signs, symptoms and treatment, see *53–546, Phosphorus*.

53–411. MAYAPPLE (Mandrake)

The leaves, roots and green fruit contain a powerful cathartic, podophyllin. The treatment is symptomatic and supportive.

53–412. MECAMYLAMINE (Inversine) ($C_{11}H_{21}N$)

Used in treatment of hypertension because of its ganglion-blocking effect, mecamylamine may cause constipation and paralytic ileus, muscular weakness, palpitation, anginal pain, acute depressions, profound orthostatic hypotension and bladder atony. If mild toxic symptoms are detected early, gradual reduction in dose helps avoid extreme hypertensive rebound, which may occur following abrupt discontinuance.

53–413. MELIA AZEDARACH (Bead Tree, Chinaberry, White Cedar)

The pulpy fruit (and to a lesser extent the leaves and bark) of the Australian variety of this tree is considered to be acutely toxic, although the North American variety is usually classified as nontoxic. The toxic picture, after ingestion, may consist of mental confusion, dizziness, syncope and stupor.

53–414. METHOL

Ingestion may cause nausea, vomiting, severe abdominal pain, dizziness, staggering gait, slow respiration, flushed face, sluggishness, sleepiness and, in large amounts in children, coma.

---

*For therapeutic considerations see also 53–*1* to 53–*13*.

53–415. MEPERIDINE HYDROCHLORIDE (Demerol) ($C_{15}H_{21}NO_2 \cdot HCl$)

The narcotic affects of Demerol can be neutralized by naloxone (Narcan), 0.01 mg/kg IV, repeated as necessary. See *53–455, Morphine.*

53–416. MEPROBAMATE (Equanil, Miltown)

This once popular non-benzodiazepine tranquilizer now has few medical indications. ***Usual doses*** may cause drowsiness or excitement, generalized diplopia, muscle weakness, acute hypersensitivity reactions, stomach pain, abdominal cramping and diarrhea.

Treatment

- Withdrawal or reduction of dosage of the drug.
- Treatment of hypersensitivity reactions (24).

Excessive doses (over 5 g) may cause shallow respiration with cyanosis, muscular weakness, loss of reflexes, hypotension and acute mental depression.

Treatment

- Oxygen administration and artificial ventilation, as needed.
- Emptying of the stomach by emetics or gastric lavage if meprobamate has been ingested in large amounts, followed by repeated activated charcoal if patient is in coma.
- Support of the circulation and control of hypotension.
- Hospitalization for observation and supportive therapy. Hemodialysis may be helpful in extremely severe cases. Forced osmotic diuresis may also be of aid.

Sudden discontinuance can cause acute life-threatening withdrawal symptoms, often magnified by the fact that many habitual users of tranquilizing drugs have prepsychotic tendencies. These symptoms consist of severe headache, persistent insomnia, excessive salivation and epileptiform convulsions. Activation of psychotic tendencies, especially acute depression states that may be presuicidal, has been reported. Mild cases need only symptomatic care with close supervision and observation at home. Severe cases require hospitalization for symptomatic care and psychiatric evaluation and control.

53–417. MERCAPTANS

Mercaptans are released during the process of petroleum refining. Inhalation of high concentrations of the fumes may cause fever, dyspnea, cyanosis, convulsions and coma. Hospitalize for observation for at least 24 hours; delayed pulmonary edema (55) may occur.

53–418. MERCURY (Hg; TLV 0.05 mg/m^3)

All forms of mercury are toxic if absorbed. This includes metallic mercury, mercurous chloride (calomel), corrosive sublimate, mercurial dyes and mercuric diuretic drugs. About 100 occupations offer definite industrial hazards, usually through inhalation of fumes or dust containing mercury. Fatalities in the home have occurred from fumes from gas heaters and radiators painted with "aluminum" paint. Mercury salts may cause toxic effects by absorption through the intact skin, open wounds, lungs and gastrointestinal tract. Organic mercury compounds are the most toxic forms. Metallic mercury is poorly absorbed from the GI tract.

Toxic signs and symptoms in industry are generally chronic and may be unrecognized until an acute picture develops or is superimposed. For signs, symptoms and treatment of acute toxicity, see *53–124, Bichloride of Mercury,* including use of dimercaprol (BAL), Ca EDTA and penicillamine chelation therapy.

53–419. MERCURY ANTISEPTICS

Numerous commercial compounds intended to utilize the antiseptic action of mercury are available. The most common are mercocresol (Mercresin), merbromin (Mercuro-

---

*For therapeutic considerations see also *53–1* to *53–13*.

chrome) and thimerosal (Merthiolate). All are relatively nontoxic, but if large doses have been ingested, gastric emptying and supportive treatment may be needed. These types of antiseptics have largely been replaced by others that cause less skin injury.

53–420. MERCURY DIURETICS

The effective irritant diuretic action of certain mercury compounds led to the medical use of mersalyl (Salyrgan), mercurophylline (Mercuzanthin) and many others. All may cause acute toxic signs and symptoms if given too frequently or in excessive doses. Their medical use now is practically entirely supplanted by other less toxic drugs. Sodium depletion may require treatment. Treatment is usually discontinuation of the drug and supportive care.

Allergic Reactions. These are characterized by chills, fever, urticaria and, occasionally, bronchospasm and laryngeal edema. For treatment see *Allergic Reactions*.

Immediate Toxicity. Acute symptoms may come on during intravenous injection of the therapeutic dose to which the patient is accustomed. These symptoms consist of apprehension, substernal pain, dyspnea, cyanosis, bradycardia, hypertension, mental confusion, delirium and collapse, probably due to ventricular fibrillation (29–25).

Deferred Toxicity. Coming on from 1 to 3 hours after injection, this type is characterized by chills and fever, dyspnea, cyanosis, asthmatic symptoms, pulmonary edema and evidence of sodium deficiency.

53–421. MERCURY OXYCYANIDE ($C_2Hg_2N_2O$)

Local use as an antiseptic agent can cause severe mucous membrane erosion. If absorbed through mucous membranes or ingested, nausea, vomiting, abdominal pain and collapse may occur. Patients with terminal cases usually die from cyanide poisoning resulting from the action of the gastric hydrochloric acid on the oxycyanide radical.

See also 53–232, *Cyanides; 55–124, Bichloride of Mercury.*

53–422. MESCAL (Peyote)

Intoxication from ingestion of this substance, derived from a certain type of cactus, is sometimes encountered, especially in areas where the cactus grows. Also see 53–332, *Hallucinogens.* A rapid fall in blood pressure and hallucinations similar to those of schizophrenics can occur. Except in severe cases, complete recovery without permanent ill effects occurs in 6 to 8 hours, and only supportive and protective treatment is needed.

53–423. METAL FUMES

Inhalation of high concentrations of freshly formed metallic oxide fumes from smelting, brazing, galvanizing and welding may give rise to a type of poisoning known variously as metal fume fever, brass chills, metal ague, foundry workers' ague, zinc chills, smelter shakes or Monday morning fever. The clinical picture, treatment and prognosis are completely different from those for the toxic symptoms caused by ingestion of the different metals. The following metallic oxides may cause the condition:

Antimony (53–*81*)
Beryllium (53–*123*)
Cadmium (53–*158*)
Cobalt (53–*217*)
Copper (53–*224*)
Lead (53–*386*)
Magnesium (53–*402*)
Manganese (53–*407*)
Nickel (53–*476*)
Zinc (most common) (53–*759* to 53–*764*)

Signs and symptoms (usually coming on from 1 to 3 hours after exposure) consist of profuse perspiration, a peculiar metallic taste in the mouth, dryness of the throat, cough, tightness in the chest, nausea, vomiting, severe general malaise, exhaustion and an elevated temperature [rarely above 39°C (102.2°F)].

Treatment

- Complete bed rest until improved.
- Codeine sulfate and acetylsalicylic acid (aspirin) PO every 4 hours.

---

*For therapeutic considerations see also 53–*1* to 53–*13*.

Complete recovery from the acute phase in 1 to 2 days is usual, and the patient suffers generally more from overtreatment than from undertreatment.

53–424. METALDEHYDE (Metafuel) (C_2H_4O)

This toxic substance is a constituent of many snail baits. In the form of compressed tablets it is used as fuel for small heaters. Signs and symptoms (usually a 1- to 3-hour time lag after ingestion before onset): Salivation, nausea, vomiting, severe abdominal pain, flushed face, high temperature, muscle twitching and incoordination and coma, sometimes fatal in 5 to 8 hours.

53–425. METHADONE HYDROCHLORIDE (Dextrolevomethadone Hydrochloride, Dolophine) ($C_{21}H_{27}NO{\cdot}HCl$)

Methadone is a potent and long-acting, cumulative, synthetic narcotic that has strong addictive tendencies (7–3). The recent increase in treatment of heroin and morphine addiction with oral methadone, often on an ambulatory basis, has resulted in a considerable series of acute methadone poisoning, especially in children who are attracted by the bright orange, clover-leaf shaped tablets and by methadone-containing fruit juices. The usual maintenance dose does not cause any ill effects in a narcotic addict but can cause extreme respiratory depression in nonaddicts.

Treatment Includes:

- Achieve gastric emptying and give activated charcoal.
- Give naloxone hydrochloride (Narcan) (see *53–10*).
- Hospitalize under close observation until all signs of methadone effects have cleared—usually about 2 days. Since naloxone hydrochloride (Narcan) has a short antagonist action (30 to 60 minutes) and the respiratory depressant effects of methadone last for as long as 48 hours, repeated injections of naloxone are necessary to prevent recurring coma, which may be terminal. Large doses of naloxone may be required.
- Analeptic drugs, hemodialysis and peritoneal dialysis are of no value.

53–426. METHANOL (Methyl Alcohol, Methyl Hydrate, Carbinol, Wood Alcohol, Wood Spirit, Wood Naphtha, Columbia Spirit, Colonial Spirit) (CH_3OH; TLV 200 ppm)

Widespread use of this toxic liquid as a solvent in industry, in antifreeze mixtures, in the chemical industry and as a fuel makes accidental ingestion fairly common. In addition, many serious cases have been caused by ingestion, by accident or intent, of methyl alcohol in place of ethyl alcohol. There is a wide variation in susceptibility of different individuals, but as little as 60 ml has been fatal. Inhalation of the fumes also may give an acute toxic picture.

Mild cases are characterized by severe headaches, aching pain in the extremities, nausea, vomiting, gastric pain, dilated sluggish pupils and visual disturbances with temporary (sometimes permanent) blindness. Slow and labored respiration usually is present, often with dyspnea and cyanosis. If marked dyspnea or extreme metabolic acidosis is present, the prognosis is unfavorable.

Severe cases show all the signs and symptoms of mild cases but in greater degree. In addition, there is usually increased reflex hyperexcitability, with trismus; opisthotonos and convulsions; hypotension with a weak, rapid pulse; and hallucinations—sometimes mania. Acute visual disturbances and eye signs usually become acute 18 to 24 hours after ingestion. These consist of dilated fixed pupils, sometimes responsive to convergence tests but rarely to light; sensitivity of the eyeballs to pressure; painful eye motion; ptosis of the lids; and retrobulbar neuritis with partial or complete permanent loss of vision. Acute peripheral neuritis is common.

---

*For therapeutic considerations see also *53–1* to *53–13*.

Treatment Includes:

- Emesis or gastric lavage followed by activated charcoal in water by mouth or through the lavage tube.
- Control of severe pain (*12*).
- Oxygen administration for dyspnea and cyanosis.
- Treatment of severe metabolic acidosis by IV sodium bicarbonate, 1 mEq/kg, repeated according to results of arterial blood gas determination.
- Ethyl alcohol (50% in water) (see 53–*10*) or whiskey, 30 ml to 60 ml every 2 to 3 hours orally pending IV ethanol, until ethyl alcohol blood level of 100 to 125 mg/dl is obtained—continued as necessary for 2 to 3 days. Assay formic acid in the urine.
- In severe cases, hemodialysis may be sight- and lifesaving and should be instituted for methanol levels greater than 50 mg/dl and continued until levels reach 20 mg/dl. "Rebound" rises in methanol level can occur after termination of dialysis.
- Folate should be administered.

PROGNOSIS. Poor; the mortality rate is high even if relatively small amounts of methyl alcohol have been ingested. Death may be due to respiratory or cardiac failure or to severe kidney damage. If recovery occurs, it is a prolonged process. Residual eye, kidney and heart damage is common.

53–427. METHANTHELINE BROMIDE (Banthine) ($C_{21}H_{26}BrNO_3$)

Ordinary doses may cause acute skin reactions, even exfoliative dermatitis, and an increase in intraocular tension. Overdosage may cause extreme weakness, loss of sphincter control, mental confusion and stupor. See Table 53–2, Anticholinergics.

53–428. METHAQUALONE (Quaalude)

This mood-modifying medication is characterized in overdosage by increased deep tendon reflexes, tonic-clonic spasms, coma, hypotension and respiratory depression. A popular drug of abuse, it is no longer manufactured legally in the United States. Repeat doses of charcoal are probably indicated for severe overdoses.

53–429. METHEDRINE (Methamphentamine HCl, Desoxyephedrine HCl, Amphedroxyn, Desoxyn, Estimulex, Isophen, Syndrox) *(See 53–66, Amphetamines; 53–647, "Speedballs")*

53–430. METHENAMINE (Urised) ($C_6H_{12}N_4$)

Toxic signs and symptoms are due to slow decomposition of methenamine into formaldehyde and are characterized by severe diarrhea, pain in the kidney and bladder, painful urination and albumin and blood in the urine. Prognosis is for complete recovery.

53–431. METHIMAZOLE (Tapazole) ($C_4H_6N_2S$)

Skin rash and other allergic manifestations (24), arthralgia, gastrointestinal irritation, toxic hepatitis and neuropathy with footdrop may occur when methimazole is used in the treatment of hyperthyroidism. Loss of the sense of taste has been reported as have serious reactive blood changes (leukopenia, granulocytopenia and agranulocytosis) that mandate immediate discontinuation of the drug.

53–432. METHORPHINAN HYDROBROMIDE (Dromoran)

Overdosage with this synthetic narcotic gives toxic signs and symptoms similar to, but less serious than, those of morphine sulfate (53–455). Response to IV administration of the physiologic antagonist, naloxone hydrochloride (Narcan) (see 53–*10*), may be slow, with frequent injections of naloxone required at short intervals. Not sold in U.S. now.

---

*For therapeutic considerations see also 53–*1* to 53–*13*.

53–433. METHOXYCHLOR ($C_{16}H_{15}Cl_3O_2$)

This insecticide is slightly less toxic than DDT, although signs and symptoms of toxicity are more prolonged. Muscular twitching, tremors and acute depression may require symptomatic care. No fatal cases of poisoning from methoxychlor have been reported. For treatment, see *53–240, DDT.*

53–434. METHYL ACETATE ($CH_3C[O]OCH_3$; TLV 200 ppm)

Through inhalation of fumes or by ingestion, this solvent for nitrocellulose, resins and oils may give toxic signs and symptoms similar to those of methyl alcohol (*53–426*).

53–435. METHYL BROMIDE (CH_3Br; TLV 15 ppm)

Acute toxic signs and symptoms from this dangerous volatile liquid (used in fire extinguishers, as a refrigerant and as an insecticide) may not develop for 30 minutes to 12 hours after inhalation of the fumes. On the skin, ethyl bromide causes itching, prickling and blistering, followed by a sensation of cold and the development of the systemic toxic picture after 4 to 6 hours.

Signs and symptoms: Transient blurred and double vision (sometimes followed by temporary blindness), nausea, vomiting, abdominal pain, sleepiness, loss of memory, profound weakness and slurred speech. Muscular twitching may be present, with incoordination and temporary paralysis. Mental confusion, psychoses, mania and epileptiform convulsions may develop. Pulmonary edema (55) or circulatory and/or respiratory collapse may be terminal.

Treatment Includes:

- Remove from exposure. Remove the victim's clothing and wash contaminated areas of the body with soap and water.
- Hospitalize for observation for at least 48 hours, even if the toxic picture is relatively mild, because of the tendency toward late development of pulmonary edema (55). Although severe metabolic acidosis rarely occurs, the cautious administration of alkalies is to be considered. Unlike methyl alcohol blindness (*53–426*), the impairment of vision from methyl bromide intoxication is temporary and clears spontaneously. Diazepam may be required to control seizures. Observe also for concomitant carbon monoxide poisoning.

53–436. METHYL CELLOSOLVE ($CH_3OCH_2CH_2OH$; TLV 25 ppm)

Methyl cellosolve is used in the leather industry; as a solvent and in stains, paints, enamels, nail polishes and varnishes. Its fumes may cause burning of the eyes, severe headache and signs and symptoms of encephalopathy. Severe reactive blood changes also occur. Hospitalize for supportive care and possible blood transfusions.

53–437. METHYL CHLORIDE (Chlormethane) (CH_3Cl; TLV 100 ppm)

This toxic gas is used in refrigeration systems and in the chemical industry. For signs and symptoms of toxicity and treatment, see *53–435, Methyl Bromide.*

53–438. METHYLENE BLUE ($C_{16}H_{18}ClN_3S$) *(See 53–438, Dyes; 53–12, Methemoglobinemia)*

53–439. METHYLENE DICHLORIDE (CH_2Cl_2; TLV 200 ppm)

Fumes of this common solvent cause intense eye and mucous membrane irritation, with central nervous system depression and pulmonary edema (55) if high concentrations have been inhaled.

---

*For therapeutic considerations see also *53–1* to *53–13*.

53–440. METHYL ETHYL KETONE ($CH_3C[O]CH_2CH_3$; TLV 200 ppm)

This is an industrial solvent that on brief contact can cause extreme thickening of the fingernails, with permanent destruction of the nail beds. Treatment is symptomatic only.

53–441. METHYL FORMATE ($HC[O]OCH_3$; TLV 100 ppm)

Widely used as a solvent in industry, methyl formate may cause severe toxic effects through absorption from the respiratory tract or by ingestion. *Signs and symptoms* include a feeling of suffocation and constriction of the chest, acute dyspnea and visual disturbances (amblyopia and nystagmus). For treatment see *53–426, Methanol.*

53–442. METHYL IODIDE (CH_3I; TLV 5 ppm)

Inhalation of small amounts of the fumes results in acute intoxication with dizziness, sleepiness, irritability and diarrhea. Higher concentrations cause marked nervous system involvement (slurred speech, amblyopia, nystagmus, acute excitement and delirium). Hospitalize for observation, since signs of central nervous system involvement may not appear until after apparent recovery from acute toxic effects. The latency period may be days.

533–443. METHYLROSANILINE CHLORIDE (Methyl Violet)

Methyl violet is used as an antiseptic and in the leads of indelible pencils. Skin contact may cause acute eczematous and acneform eruptions; contact with the lips may cause cheilitis and gingivitis, with a systemic picture of headache, malaise, vomiting, general weakness and low-grade kidney and liver damage.

53–444. METHYL SALICYLATE (Oil of Sweet Birch, Teaberry Oil, Oil of Wintergreen) ($C_8H_8O_3$)

This pleasant-smelling liquid is used as an aromatic flavoring extract, as a rubefacient in rubbing liniments and ointments and as an antirheumatic and antiseptic agent. Because of its attractive smell and taste, it is frequently ingested by infants and children, with a very high mortality rate (about 55%). Absorption through the intact skin also can cause an acute toxic picture. Methyl salicylate is from 10 to 20 times as toxic as acetylsalicylic acid but is much more slowly absorbed from the gastrointestinal tract.

Signs and symptoms: Odor of wintergreen or acetone on the breath; labored, rapid "panting dog" respiration; cyanosis; sleepiness; profuse perspiration; nausea; persistent vomiting; dehydration; thirst; disturbances in sight and hearing; convulsions; and coma. Circulatory and respiratory depression may be terminal. See also *53–614, Salicylates.*

53–445. METHYSERGIDE MALEATE (Sansert)

This congener of ergonovine is used for prevention of migraine attacks; it is a potent serotonin antagonist. Its toxic effects are similar to those caused by ergot (*53–291*), plus acute apprehension, excitement, nightmares, hallucinations and precipitation of psychotic states (*54–17*). See also *53–291, Ergot.*

53–446. MEXICAN JUMPING BEANS

Diarrhea of varying degrees of intensity, probably caused by surface contaminants, may make a child who eats several of these peculiarly acting beans very uncomfortable and the parents very apprehensive. However, larvae in the beans, which cause the "jumping," are harmless. Administration of a saline cathartic and reassurance of the parents are generally all that is required.

---

*For therapeutic considerations see also *53–1* to *53–13*.

53–447. "MICKEY FINN"

Several formulas are occasionally (and illegally) added to alcoholic beverages in some disreputable cocktail lounges and bars to get rid of obstreperous or offensive customers:

Drops: 1 to 2 ml of croton oil *(53–230)*. Powders: A mixture of powdered jalap and milk sugar.

Both are effective, although in different ways, and, in certain instances, dangerous. Neither should be confused with "knockout drops," which contain chloral hydrate *(53–186)* and which usually are administered with a more sinister purpose.

Signs and Symptoms: An acute burning sensation in the mouth; nausea; violent vomiting associated with tenesmus; severe abdominal pain; violent diarrhea; cold, clammy skin; weak pulse; hypotension; and collapse. Death from respiratory and/or circulatory failure may occur if an extremely large dose has been given.

Treatment Includes:

- Empty the stomach (if vomiting has not been profuse) by emetics or lavage. Activated charcoal in water should be given orally or through the lavage tube.
- In extreme cases, support the circulation by means of IV vasopressors after intravascular volume has been restored.
- Hospitalize if respiratory or circulatory depression is profound. Sudden collapse may occur several hours after apparent control of acute signs and symptoms of toxicity.

53–448. MILKWEED

Milkweed contains a resin that is highly irritating to the gastrointestinal tract. Treatment consists of emptying the stomach by emetics or gastric lavage followed by activated charcoal by mouth.

53–449. MIMOSA

This saponin-containing plant has toxic effects similar to those of cyclamen *(53–233)*.

53–450. MISTLETOE

All parts, but especially the berries, contain a potent hypertensive substance, tyramine, that on ingestion may give severe toxic effects, including vasoconstriction, reflex bradycardia and negative inotropism of heart muscle. Fatalities have been reported from use of a decoction of the berries as an abortifacient, as well as from drinking "tea" brewed from the berries. The European variety is more toxic than the American.

Signs and Symptoms of toxicity consist of acute gastroenteritis with vomiting and diarrhea, hypertension, dyspnea, delirium, hallucinations and cardiovascular collapse.

53–451. MONKSHOOD

Aconite *(53–34)* is the toxic principle. It is found only in the root.

53–452. MONOSODIUM L-GLUTAMATE (MSG)

Used to enhance the flavor of Chinese food, this substance may cause paresthesias and a sense of facial pressure, chest pain and (occasionally) severe headache. The amounts necessary to produce symptoms vary markedly in different individuals and in the same individual at different times.

These symptoms, although often extremely uncomfortable, are self-limiting and require no treatment.

53–453. MOONSEED

Ingestion of the roots and fruit may cause acute gastrointestinal symptoms. The sharp-edged pits may cause mechanical intestinal injury.

---

*For therapeutic considerations see also *53–1* to *53–13*.

53–454. MORNING GLORY

The seeds of this climbing plant have a mild hallucinatory effect (53–332).

53–455. MORPHINE (Laudanum, Tincture of Opium) ($C_{17}H_{19}NO_3$) *(See also 7, Addiction; Table 53–2, Narcotics)*

Acute Morphinism. Acute morphinism may follow ingestion; subcutaneous, intramuscular or intravenous injection; or (occasionally) absorption of morphine through mucous membranes. If subcutaneous or intramuscular injections are given to a patient whose circulatory system is extremely depressed (for instance, in severe shock), overwhelmingly cumulative—even lethal—toxic effects may occur when the circulation improves.

Signs and symptoms: Pinpoint nonreactive pupils (during terminal asphyxia the pupils may dilate), subnormal temperature, gradually slowing respiration with slowly increasing cyanosis and increasing somnolence deepening into coma. Convulsions are common in children, rare in adults. Collapse from respiratory failure is the final stage. Noncardiogenic pulmonary edema has been recognized after overdoses.

Treatment Includes:

- If seen during the precoma stage keep the patient awake and moving if possible. Muscular activity such as walking is beneficial in mild cases but can be detrimental if respiratory depression is acute.
- If ingested, perform gastric lavage. Attempts at induction of vomiting by emetics can be unsuccessful and are often dangerous if the airway is not protected.
- If only a short time has elapsed after subcutaneous or intramuscular injection into an extremity, apply a tourniquet proximal to the injection site—tight enough to shut off the venous return but not tight enough to interfere with the arterial pulse. An icebag may delay absorption.
- Combat hypoxemia and cyanosis as necessary by expired air methods (5–*10*) followed by administration of oxygen by face mask or endotracheal catheter and resuscitation bag.
- Inject naloxone hydrochloride (Narcan) (see *53–10*) IV as needed; remember that the half-life of morphine is longer than that of naloxone. If marked improvement in the patient's condition does not occur, look for another cause, or causes, for coma (32). If the patient is an addict who is suffering from overdosage, naloxone may bring on acute withdrawal symptoms requiring immediate treatment as outlined in *53–340, Heroin.*

Chronic Morphinism with Withdrawal Symptoms *(see also 7, Addiction).* This serious condition is a true emergency. Since many states and countries consider prescribing opiates of any type for an addict a crime, except in an extreme emergency or as a lifesaving measure, symptomatic supportive therapy and sedation through diazepam may be indicated until the patient can be transferred for treatment to a properly accredited institution. A generally recognized exception to this rule is that if the patient has been booked and is in police custody, narcotics may be administered for control of acute withdrawal symptoms. Also, it is becoming increasingly recognized in many parts of the world that persons who seek relief from addiction or from withdrawal symptoms should be treated as patients and not as criminals. Use of clonidine *(53–216)* in withdrawal states is gaining favor.

For methadone treatment of morphine addiction and its complications, see *53–425.*

53–456. MOTHER OF PEARL

Although the osteitis caused by inhalation of mother of pearl dust is usually chronic, flare-ups may be acute. These flare-ups consist of sudden acute arthralgia and myalgia with low-grade fever. Symptomatic treatment usually gives relief.

---

*For therapeutic considerations see also *53–1* to *53–13*.

53–457. MOTH REPELLENTS

These may be of several strengths. For slightly toxic repellents, see *53–514, Paradichlorobenzene;* for moderately toxic kinds, *53–168, Camphor;* and for extremely toxic types, *53–469, Naphthalene.*

53–458. MOUNTAIN LAUREL (Kalmia)

All parts of this plant are poisonous and cause principally gastrointestinal and cardiovascular response, with nausea, vomiting, bradycardia and hypotension plus convulsions and paralysis. Treatment is supportive and symptomatic, including use of atropine.

53–459. MUCUNA PRURIENS (Cowhage, Cow-itch, Elephant's Scratchwort, Stinging Bean)

The seed pods of this Central American plant contain a proteolytic enzyme that causes transient extremely severe itching, pain and edema of the skin on contact. Symptoms subside rapidly when exposure is terminated.

53–460. MUSCARINE *(See Table 53–2, Cholinergics)*

This toxic substance occurs in certain varieties of poisonous mushrooms ("fly mushrooms") and toadstools (*53–462*) but not in most fungi.

Signs and symptoms after ingestion: Rapid onset and course with acute symptoms lasting only 1 to 3 hours. Death from cardiac arrest (*29–8*) or complete collapse may occur in a few hours. In nonfatal cases, complete recovery usually occurs in 1 to 2 days. The toxic signs and symptoms are due to parasympathetic stimulation characterized by lacrimation, salivation, miosis, sweating, dyspnea, abdominal pain, vomiting, diarrhea and intense excitement, followed by circulatory and respiratory depression.

Treatment Includes:

- Induction of vomiting or gastric lavage followed by activated charcoal in water.
- SC or IV injection of atropine sulfate (*53–10*), the physiologic antagonist of muscarine. Doses of 1 mg and over may be necessary; repeat until the muscarine effect has been neutralized.
- Administration of magnesium sulfate (Epsom salts), 30 mg by mouth.
- Symptomatic and supportive care.

53–461. MUSCLE RELAXANT DRUGS *(See also 53–231, Curare)*

The toxic effects of average doses of drugs commonly used for muscle relaxation are uncomfortable but rarely serious. Among these drugs are:

Baclofen (Lioresal)
Carisoprodol (Soma, Rela)
Chlormezanone (Trancopal)
Chlorzoxazone (Paraflex)
Cyclobenzaprine (Flexeril)
Diazepam (Valium)
Methocarbamol (Robaxin)
Orphenadrine citrate (Norflex)

Signs and symptoms of toxicity consist of drowsiness, apathy, anorexia, nausea (rarely vomiting), headache, dizziness and dryness of the mouth and throat. All disappear slowly when use of the drug is discontinued.

53–462. MUSHROOM POISONING (Muscarine, Psilocybin)

Rapid Poisoning. Acute toxic signs and symptoms developing from a few minutes to 3 hours after ingestion and occasionally causing death are usually due to the muscarine contained in *Amanita muscaria* and *Amanita pantherina.* Considerable variation in the degree of toxicity in different localities has been noted; for example, in Switzerland *A.*

---

*For therapeutic considerations see also *53–1* to *53–13*.

muscaria ("fly agaric") is considered to be very dangerous, whereas in Alaska it is eaten by Eskimos as a source of pleasurable intoxication. For treatment, see *53–460, Muscarine*. Thioctic acid, an investigational drug, has shown some promise in treatment of toxicity due to *Amanita phalloides* type mushrooms, as has charcoal hemoperfusion, but results are not conclusive. Gastric lavage and activated charcoal administration should be done immediately in cases of unidentified mushroom poisoning.

Delayed Poisoning. Toxic signs and symptoms coming on 6 to 24 hours after ingestion are almost invariably due to *A. phalloides* and allied forms in the United States and to *A. verna* in Europe. These varieties of bulb agarics account for about 90% of all fatalities from mushroom poisoning; ingestion of the "amanita toxins" has a mortality rate of about 50%. A less frequent offender is the *Helvella* (false morel; 53–336), which may cause acute toxic signs and symptoms from 6 to 8 hours after ingestion.

Identification. Members of the amanita family are responsible for practically all cases of serious mushroom poisoning; hence, one simple rule may be lifesaving: *never eat a mushroom that has two swellings on the stalk!* These 2 enlargements—the annulus just below the gills and the volva at or slightly beneath ground level—are characteristic of the deadly amanita family only; other mushrooms may have 1 but no other important variety has both. An even simpler rule: *Never eat uncultivated mushrooms!*

Signs and symptoms (after a latent period of 6 hours or more). Sudden severe abdominal pain, nausea, bloody vomitus, diarrhea with blood and mucus, extreme thirst, dehydration and rapidly developing weakness. Apparent marked improvement, usually lasting a few hours, may occur, followed by sudden development of acute cyanosis with coldness of the skin of the extremities, collapse of the circulatory system and progressive central nervous system involvement. Death usually occurs 48 to 72 hours after ingestion.

See previous discussion in this section and *53–460, Muscarine*, for treatment.

In severe cases, peritoneal dialysis and hemodialysis may assist in the removal of amanita toxins. Thioctic acid is still under evaluation as a specific therapeutic agent.

Hallucinogenic Effects. Psilocybin, an unsaturated indole, is the active toxic agent in certain varieties of mushrooms used in religious rites in Mexico because of their peculiar ability to produce hallucinations (53–332). Recovery in 8 to 10 hours after ingestion is to be expected. No specific treatment is required.

53–463. MUSHROOM "MIASMA"

In certain localities, crews engaged in dumping compost and cleaning the bins used in growing mushrooms have developed dryness of the nose and throat lasting about 8 hours, nausea and restlessness, with a burning sensation in the nose and throat. These symptoms are followed after 24 hours by fever, rapid pulse, dry cough, dermatitis (usually involving the nose, the area below the eyes and the scrotum), sweating, chills and chest pain lasting until about the 8th day after exposure. Gradual abatement of signs and symptoms occurs in about 2 weeks. Symptomatic treatment only is required. No fatalities have been reported.

53–464. MUSSEL POISONING *(See also 53–314. Rare Causes of Food Poisoning [Mytilotoxism])*

Poisonous heat-stable alkaloids are present in certain seafoods during certain months. Mussels, clams, oysters and abalone may be affected.

Signs and symptoms: Acute progressive respiratory paralysis coming on without warning generally causes the patient to be brought for emergency care. The diagnosis depends wholly upon the history—usually several members of the same family or party are affected. After initial treatment, hospitalize for observation and supportive care for at least 24 hours, as relapses are common.

53–465. MYRISTICIN (Nutmeg)

Myristicin is the active ingredient of oil of nutmeg and nutmeg flower oil. Ingestion of these substances or of 2 or 3 ground nutmegs may cause a rapid pulse, clammy skin, tremors, acute excitement, hallucinations and unconsciousness.

---

*For therapeutic considerations see also *53–1* to *53–13*.

53–466. NAIL POLISH *(See 53–75, Aniline; 53–315, Formaldehyde; 53–436, Methyl cellosolve)*

53–467. NAIL POLISH REMOVERS *(See 53–24, Acetone)*

53–468. NAPHTHA (Coal Tar Naphtha: OSHA Standard 100 ppm; Petroleum Distillates: OSHA Standard 500 ppm) *(See also 53–117, Benzene)*

Do not confuse with Naphthol (*53–470*). Petroleum naphtha is an amorphous entity of various hydrocarbons, the average molecular weight of which is higher than that of gasoline.

53–469. NAPHTHALENE (Naphthalin, Tar Camphor)

This is the most toxic of the insect repellents commonly found in moth balls. It is also a constitutent of some brands of deodorant cakes. Toxic signs and symptoms may be caused in children by contact with clothes that have been stored in mothballs as well as by ingestion.

Signs and symptoms following ingestion: Characteristic odor on the breath, nausea, vomiting, gastroenteritis and profound depression, with development after 3 to 7 days of symptoms due to hemolysis from metabolites. Hyperkalemia may follow.

Treatment Includes:

- Fatty substances (including milk) should be avoided.
- Induce vomiting by warm water, ipecac or other emetics. Follow with activated charcoal in water by mouth.
- Hospitalize patients with severer cases; hemolysis may require repeated transfusions. Acute renal failure may occur. Peritoneal dialysis may be beneficial.

53–470. NAPHTHOL ($C_{10}H_8O$)

Both the alpha and beta isomers of naphthol may give severe toxic signs and symptoms after ingestion as well as after absorption through the intact skin. Signs and symptoms include nausea; vomiting; convulsions; coma; severe liver, kidney and spleen damage; jaundice; albuminuria; and anemia.

53–471. NAPHTHYLAMINE ($C_{10}H_9N$; no TLV established)

The beta isomer of naphthylamine may cause fever and severe bladder irritation after ingestion or inhalation of fumes. Hemorrhagic cystitis may be followed by carcinomatous degeneration of polyps of the bladder.

53–472. NARCISSUS (Daffodil, Jonquil, Grape Hyacinth)

Ingestion of the bulbs of these European and North American spring-flowering plants may cause violent vomiting with delayed development of tetanic convulsions

53–473. NARCOTICS *(See 7–3, Narcotics; 13–3, Schedule II and Schedule III Drugs; Table 53–2, Narcotics)*

53–474. NEOSTIGMINE BROMIDE (Prostigmin) ($C_{12}H_{19}BrN_2O_2$) *(See also Table 53–2, Cholinergics)*

Overdosage—especially in the treatment of myasthenia gravis (*49–12*)—may cause difficult respiration, giddiness, anxiety and muscular twitching. In addition to supportive care, atropine sulfate is the physiologic antagonist in more severe cases.

---

*For therapeutic considerations see also *53–1* to *53–13*.

Treatment

- Administration of the physiologic antagonist, atropine sulfate (53–*103*).
- Supportive and symptomatic care.

53–475. NERVE GASES *(See 53–497, Organic Phosphates; 53–746, War Gases)*

53–476. NICKEL *(See also 53–477, Nickel Carbonyl)*

Acute dermatitis, gingivitis and stomatitis may be caused by dust and fumes of nickel and its salts. Removal from contact and symptomatic treatment usually result in rapid recovery. Ingested small nickel-cadmium batteries should be removed from the GI tract immediately, as they can leak and cause a rapid drop in pH.

53–477. NICKEL CARBONYL (C_4NiO_4; TLV 0.05 ppm)

Inhalation of the fumes of this industrial liquid may result in acute poisoning. More than 1 part of fumes to 1 million parts of air may cause severe, even fatal, toxic effects characterized by nausea, vomiting, dizziness and severe cephalgia.

Treatment

Removal of the patient to fresh air usually results in apparent recovery, but observation for 2 to 3 days is necessary. Delayed toxic signs and symptoms (latent period of 12 to 30 hours) may develop, with thoracic pain, a feeling of constriction in the chest, severe cough, slow pulse, rapid respirations, dyspnea, cyanosis and convulsions. Enlargement of the liver may be present after even short exposure. Dimercaprol (BAL) (53–*10*) is the specific antidote. Hospitalize for observation and treatment because of the possibility of delayed development of severe brain, lung and liver damage.

PROGNOSIS. Good in most cases. If convulsions or cyanosis is present, the chances of bronchopneumonia are much increased. Carcinogenicity of this substance is controversial.

53–478. NICOTINE ($C_{10}H_{14}N_2$; TLV 0.5 mg/m^3) *(See also 53–209, Cigarettes and Cigars; 53–711, Tobacco; 53–633, Snuff)*

Nicotine poisoning is characterized by initial stimulation, followed by depression; muscular weakness; prostration; pupils first contracted, then dilated; nausea; vomiting; profuse diarrhea; dyspnea; tachycardia; and muscular tremors, followed by convulsions. Nicotine is readily absorbed orally and from the skin. Nicotine-containing leaves of the tobacco plant are sometimes mistakenly used to make a salad. All plant parts contain nicotine. Treat tachyarrhythmias with propranolol. Atropine use is governed by symptoms.

53–479. NICOTINIC ACID (Niacin)

Used as a preservative in foods and as a medication, nicotinic acid may give toxic signs and symptoms in both therapeutic and excessive doses.

Signs and symptoms are characterized by a sensation of heat that starts in the face and spreads to arms and hands, then to the body, especially the perianal region; flushing of the face; generalized itching; and vague, nonlocalized abdominal discomfort.

Although the effects are uncomfortable, complete recovery in 1 to 1½ hours takes place.

53–480. NIGHT BLOOMING CEREUS

Night blooming cereus contains a toxic active principle with actions similar to those of digitalis (53–265).

---

*For therapeutic considerations see also 53–*1* to 53–*13*.

53–481. NITRATES *(See also 53–484, Nitrites)*

Nitrates are used for many purposes in industry, especially in the processing and pickling of meat products. Nitrates occur naturally in high (although nontoxic) concentrations in certain foods, such as beets, carrots and spinach. Contamination of well water with organic matter may cause sufficient concentration of nitrates to give toxic signs and symptoms. Fatalities have been reported from inhalation of silage gases. Potassium nitrate is a constituent of many asthma remedies (*53–102*).

The breaking down of nitrates to nitrites by bacterial action in the intestine is the causative factor in dietary-induced methemoglobinemia (*53–12*); this is more common in children. For signs and symptoms of nitrite toxicity, see *53–484, Nitrites.*

Large doses may cause nausea and vomiting, with tenesmus, bloody diarrhea and generalized weakness, cardiac irregularities, dysuria and hematuria, convulsions and collapse—sometimes death. Chronic exposure may be associated with increased incidence of cancers.

53–482. NITRIC ACID (HNO_3; TLV 2 ppm) *(See 53–33, Acids)*

53–483. NITRIC OXIDE (NO; TLV 25 ppm) *(See 53–502, Oxides of Nitrogen)*

53–484. NITRITES *(See also 53–481, Nitrates)*

Poisoning from nitrites may occur through inhalation or through ingestion. Both nitrates and nitrites (nitroglycerin, amyl nitrite) cause vasodilation, which results in flushing of the face, throbbing headache, dizziness, syncope, hypotension and tachycardia. Nitrites oxidize hemoglobin to methemoglobin; cyanosis occurs with a 10% level of methemoglobinemia (*53–12*). Metabolic acidosis, ECG evidence of ischemia, convulsions and coma occur with methemoglobin concentrations over 50%.

Treat ingestion cases with emesis or lavage followed by activated charcoal. Hypotension usually responds well to the horizontal or head-down position and administration of saline fluids if necessary. Vasopressors such as dopamine or norepinephrine are usually not needed. Hospitalize in more severe cases, and treat with methylene blue solution (*53–12*). Transfusions with whole blood are indicated if methemoglobinemia is greater than 40%, or plasma expanders may be necessary.

53–485. NITROBENZENE (Oil of Almond, Oil of Mirbane) ($C_6H_5NO_2$; TLV 1 ppm)

Nitrobenzene is a common ingredient in shoe polishes and dyes, often in combination with aniline dyes (*53–75*). Ingestion may cause tinnitus, vertigo, incoordination, nausea, vomiting, dyspnea, cyanosis, convulsions and coma. Methemoglobinemia (*53–12*) may occur.

Hospitalize for supportive care in acute cases; there is a tendency toward delayed development of cardiac, hepatic and renal damage.

53–486. NITROCHLOROBENZENE ($NO_2C_6H_4Cl$; TLV 1 mg/m^3)

Ingestion may cause rapid onset of staggering gait, pallor or cyanosis from the formation of methemoglobinemia, dyspnea, excitement and hallucinations.

Inhalation may cause a similar picture except that the toxic effects usually are less severe and do not become apparent for 1 to 2 hours. See also *53–485, Nitrobenzene.*

53–487. NITROFURAZONE (Furacin, Vabrocid)

Used as a bacteriostatic agent, nitrofurazone on surface application may cause maculopapular and vesicular rashes and occasionally exfoliative dermatitis. Symptoms clear slowly when topical use is discontinued.

---

*For therapeutic considerations see also *53–1* to *53–13*.

53–488. NITROGEN

Short exposure to high concentrations of nitrogen causes dizziness and dyspnea; prolonged exposure may result in unconsciousness and respiratory arrest.

53–489. NITROGEN MUSTARD (Dichloren, Mustine, Mustargen)

Industrial exposure has resulted in acute skin reactions, liver damage and bone marrow depression. Overdosage in the treatment of Hodgkin's disease and lymphosarcoma may result in severe psychoses, leukemia, thrombocytopenia and bone marrow abnormalities.

53–490. NITROPRUSSIDE

Accidental or suicidal ingestion or effects from use in treatment of hypertensive crisis may result in pallor, mydriasis and respiratory paralysis. Prolonged IV use, particularly in renal failure patients, can cause release and accumulation of cyanide. For treatment, see 53–232, *Cyanides*.

53–491. NORTRIPTYLINE HYDROCHLORIDE (Aventyl, Pamelor) *(See 53–723, Tricyclic Antidepressants)*

53–492. NYLON

Certain individuals develop transient skin erythema, hyperhydrosis and whitened erythematous patches on the soles of the feet from contact with nylon.

53–493. OBESITY "CURES" *(See 53–66, Amphetamines; 53–110, Barbiturates; 53–265, Digitalis; 53–696, Thiazide Diuretics; 53–706, Thyroid)*

53–494. OILS†

Essential. Oils of absinthe, apiol, cajeput, cedar, eucalyptus, menthol, nutmeg, pennyroyal, rue, savin and tansy are complex mixtures of alcohols, esters, ketones and hydrocarbons. Ingestion of very small amounts (less than 30 ml) may be fatal. The signs and symptoms of toxicity are similar to those listed under Eucalyptol (53–303) and Turpentine (53–730). Treatment follows the same lines.

Lubricating. In general, the toxicity of lubricating oils varies inversely with the viscosity. Treatment following ingestion of lighter grades should follow that outlined for *Kerosene* (53–379), for heavier grades, all that is required is gastric lavage and administration of saline cathartics.

Mineral. Habitual use may cause fibrosis of the lung or pneumonia. The section of the lung involved depends on the user's position in bed after the nightly dose.

53–495. OLEANDER

Cardioactive glycosides that are released by chewing of the leaves, flowers or bark of this common ornamental shrub may result in fatal poisoning. Cases have been reported from eating food roasted while spitted on oleander sticks, from breathing smoke from burning cuttings and from drinking water in which the flowers have been placed. There is usually a time lag of 2 to 5 hours before the onset of nausea; vomiting; severe abdominal pain; localized cyanosis of the ears, lips and fingertips; and cold perspiration. The respiration becomes shallow and weak and the temperature subnormal; hypotension develops. Pinpoint nonreactive pupils and increasing sleepiness are followed by coma and collapse, with death from acute respiratory paralysis. Intensive supportive care (see

---

*For therapeutic considerations see also 53–*1* to 53–*13*.

†See also specific oils (e.g., *Cedar Oil*) and sources of oil (e.g., *Cashew Nuts*) cited throughout this chapter.

Digitalis, 53–265) is required. Monitor electrolyte levels, digoxin levels (immunologic cross-reactivity with oleander levels) and ECG.

53–496. OPIUM (Laudanum [Tincture of Opium]; Paregoric [Camphorated Tincture of Opium]) *(See also 7, Addiction; 13–3, Narcotics; 53–455, Morphine)*

The milky exudate of the unripe capsules of certain varieties of poppy (Papaver Somniterum and Papaver Album DeC) contains a complex mixture of toxic alkaloids, the most important of which is morphine *(53–455)*. Opium eating and smoking, common in the Orient, give similar pictures to injection of morphine, although withdrawal symptoms may be more severe and more resistant to treatment. For treatment, see *53–455, Morphine.*

53–497. ORGANOPHOSPHATES (Organic Phosphate Esters) *(See also 53–746, War Gases)*

Originally developed for wartime use, organic phosphate esters are now used as insecticides and pesticides by spraying and dusting, often by airplane. Accidental contamination of bulk cereal foods has been responsible for fatalities. The clinical picture may be confused with that of asthma *(56–4)*, encephalitis *(33–20)*, food poisoning (especially botulism [*53–314*] and mushroom poisoning [*53–462*]), pilocarpine intoxication *(53–550)* and heat exhaustion *(62–6)*.

Common Compounds

Azodrin	Dimethoate	Parathion
Bidrin	Dipterix	Paroxon
Bladen	Di-Syston	Phosdrin
Chlorthion	EPN	Phosphamidon
Ciodrin	Fenthion (Baytex)	Ronnel (Korlan)
Co-ral	Gruthion	Schraden
Delnay	HETP	Sulfotepp
Demeton (Systox)	Isolan	TEPP (Bladex, Tetrin)
Dialkylphosphate	Malathion	Thimet
Diazinon	Metacide	Trichlorfon
Dibrom	Mipafox	Trithion
Dicapthon	OMPA	

All of these compounds are available under numerous trade names. Each must bear a label stating the name and amount of each toxic constituent.

Mode of Action. In all of these compounds, the organic phosphorus–containing portion of the molecule is strongly cholinesterase inhibiting; hence, the accumulation of acetylcholine in the body may result in stimulation of the entire parasympathetic nervous system (muscarine effect [*53–460*] and nicotine effect [*53–478*] on the ganglia and skeletal muscle). Acquired sensitivity to or tolerance for these compounds has not been reported, and skin lesions do not occur. There is marked variation in the toxicity of the various compounds and in the amount required to cause toxic effects in different individuals.

Entrance into the Body. Entrance may be through the intact skin, by inhalation or by ingestion. Skin penetration occurs easily with many of these compounds, making them extremely dangerous.

Incidence of Poisoning. Anyone who comes in contact with dust-spraying or dusting apparatus or plants or vegetables to which organic phosphate preparations have been applied within 30 days may develop toxic signs and symptoms. Poisoning has occurred in the following:

- Agricultural, greenhouse and nursery workers; formulators, packagers and distributors.
- Crop dusters (pilots, flagmen and mechanics; persons servicing equipment used in application).

---

*For therapeutic considerations see also *53–1* to *53–13*.

- Occupants of houses in or near treated areas, especially in the leeward; children playing in or near treated areas.
- Persons handling contaminated clothing (housewives, laundry workers, etc.)
- Travelers passing the fields during application; casual trespassers.
- Beekeepers.

Time of Onset of Toxic Effects. This varies from 15 minutes to 24 hours—most commonly within ½ hour of exposure or while in bed at night. Exposure may not take place until a worker changes the contaminated clothing at the end of the day's work. If an individual gives a history of exposure within 24 hours to any of the organic phosphate (phosphate ester) pesticides and presents, even mildly, any of the signs and symptoms in the following list (especially severe headache, fixed contracted pupils, cough, bronchorrhea, diarrhea, and rapid respiration), treatment should be begun at once. Laboratory tests are of no value as an emergency measure, but a specimen of vomitus or of material obtained on gastric lavage should be saved for later analysis. Blood for cholinesterase levels should be sent.

Signs and symptoms of organic phosphate (phosphate ester) poisoning: Premonitory indications are headache, fatigue, giddiness, nausea, salivation, diarrhea, bronchospasm, lacrimation and excessive perspiration. Acute toxic signs and symptoms (½ to 1 hour after the premonitory stage) are dim vision; fixed miosis; dizziness; fainting; severe headache; rapid, difficult breathing; vomiting (with or without diarrhea); and increasing cyanosis. Severe poisoning is indicated by sphincter incontinence, muscular twitching, tonic convulsions, respiratory failure, pulmonary edema (55), total collapse and death. The following mnemonic (DUMBELS) helps recall the salient features of this poisoning: *D*iaphoresis (and defecation), *U*rination, *M*iosis, *B*ronchial secretions, *E*xcitation of muscles (fasciculation or twitching), *L*acrimation, *S*alivation.

Treatment

- Respiratory support by insurance of a patent airway, removal of secretions by suction and administration of oxygen under positive pressure. Intubation may be necessary. Pulmonary edema may occur and require therapy (55).
- Decontamination. All clothing should be removed and the skin, hair and nails washed thoroughly with soap and water. The eyes should be irrigated for 5 to 10 minutes with normal saline or water. *Attendants must wear rubber gloves and protective clothing.*
- Atropine sulfate parenterally in large doses. Individuals with mild cases usually require 1 to 2 mg IV or IM, repeated whenever symptoms reappear. Patients with severe cases should be given 2 to 4 mg IV every 5 to 10 minutes until signs of atropinization (particularly decreased salivation, but also tachycardia and mydriasis) appear, then every 30 to 60 minutes until the toxic effects of the organic phosphate subside—often many hours. Dosages for children should be adjusted by age or weight (9); the usual test dose is 0.05 mg/kg IV. Poisoned persons commonly receive too little, practically never too much, atropine.
- 2-PAM (Protopam chloride). Although this drug is a specific chemical antidote for organic phosphates, it should be used as an adjunct to, not as a substitute for, large doses of atropine. In mild cases, 0.5 g should be given slowly IV. Severe cases require 1 g IV, followed in 30 minutes by 0.5 g (dosage by age or weight in children[9]).
- If the material has been ingested, institute gastric lavage with warm water only, followed soon afterward by activated charcoal.
- Hospitalization as soon as possible if seen during the prodromal or premonitory stage but not until an adequate dose of atropine (No. 3 preceding discussion) has been administered. Since onset of acute toxic symptoms may be terminal if proper symptomatic and supportive treatment is not given at once, the patient should, if possible, be accompanied during transportation to an emergency hospital by a physician, registered nurse or other trained attendant. Close observation in the hospital for at least 48 hours after the disappearance of acute symptoms, or after the last injection of atropine sulfate or 2-PAM, is essential.
- Send for plasma and RBC cholinesterase levels.
- All pesticide-related health problems are reportable by law in some states.

PROGNOSIS. Poor, unless the condition is recognized and given proper emergency treat-

---

*For therapeutic considerations see also *53–1* to *53–13*.

ment at once. Good, if proper immediate treatment is given—complete recovery without residual ill effects usually occurs even after severe exposure. After plasma and red cell cholinesterase levels are at least 50% normal and the patient is symptom free, he or she can usually be allowed to return to regular work with the warning that any exposure to organic phosphates must be avoided for several months.

53–498. ORTHODICHLOROBENZENE

For treatment of toxic effects of this wood preservative, see *53–469, Naphthalene.*

53–499. OSMIUM TETROXIDE (Osmic Acid) (OsO_4; TLV 0.0002 ppm)

The extremely low TLV value is an index of the potency for irritation of this oxidizing agent. Skin contact with osmium preparations causes intense dermatitis with black discoloration. Inhalation of the fumes results in acute eye, nose and throat irritation; bronchitis and pneumonia; and, occasionally, hematuria and other evidence of kidney damage. Close observation is indicated because of the danger of delayed development of pneumonia and nephritis.

53–500. OUABAIN

The toxic effects of this rarely used digitalis-like alkaloid are much greater, faster and less predicatable than those of the more frequently used digitalis preparations. See *53–265, Digitalis.*

53–501. OXALIC ACID (HOOCCOOH; TLV 1 mg/m^3)

This acid is the active agent in many household bleaching and cleansing preparations (see also *49–568, Potassium Oxalate)* and in some ink eradicators. It also occurs in the leaves and blades (not the stalks) of rhubarb plants *(53–602)* and in the leaves of a common household plant, dieffenbachia *(53–259). Note: Treatment of oxalic acid ingestion does not follow the outline given under acids.*

Signs and symptoms include burning of the mouth, throat and esophagus; dysphagia; rapid, weak pulse; cold, clammy skin; bloody vomitus caused by erosion of the gastric mucosa; and violent diarrhea and subsequent acute dehydration.

Treatment Includes:

- Have the patient swallow copious amounts of milk, calcium lactate, lime water (0.15% calcium hydroxide solution), or egg white. *Do not* induce vomiting or pass a stomach tube if concentrated oxalic acid has been swallowed and there is any evidence of mucosal erosion. In mild cases, cautious gastric lavage with a large amount of lime water may be done. *Do not* give the usual alkalies used to neutralize strong acids; they form salts with oxalic acid that may be more corrosive than the acid itself.
- Inject 10 ml of calcium gluconate (10% solution) slowly IV; repeat as necessary to prevent hypocalcemic tetany. Check serum calcium level and ECG for long QT interval.
- Hospitalize. Acute edema of the glottis may require tracheostomy *(18–34)* before transfer. Esophageal strictures may occur, as may serious renal damage.

53–502. OXIDES OF NITROGEN

All of these substances are volatile and all can cause acute toxic symptoms following inhalation of relatively small amounts.

Exposure to Toxic Concentration. This may occur in commercial production of explosives, nitrocellulose and photographic and x-ray films; photoengraving; metal etching; pickling, welding and oxyacetylene operations; use of the carbon arc; and in silo cleaning. Decomposition of nitrates in silage may result in a fatal concentration of nitrogen oxides.

Modes of Toxic Action

---

*For therapeutic considerations see also *53–1* to *53–13*.

Anesthetic Action. See 53–71, Anesthetics, Inhalation. This is unimportant in industry since nitrous oxide is never present in high enough concentration to cause anesthetic symptoms.

Nitrite Action. Results from breaking down of NO, NO_2 and N_2O_4 in the lungs. See *53–484, Nitrites.*

Local Irritative and Corrosive Action in the Lungs. This is due to NO_2 and N_2O_4.

Clinical Types of Toxic Reactions

Shock Type. Immediate death from asphyxia may occur. There is generally no time for treatment of any kind.

Irritant Gas Type. This type is characterized by an immediate burning sensation in the mouth and throat, with violent nonproductive cough. A latent period of up to 24 hours may follow, with secondary development of severe, frequently fatal, pulmonary edema (55). If the patient survives the initial acute symptoms, pneumonia or pulmonary fibrosis is a frequent complication.

Reversible Type. This type is characterized by mild respiratory irritation, with nausea, vomiting, vertigo, severe dyspnea, cyanosis and syncope. These persons generally recover spontaneously and completely.

Combined Type. Various combinations of the types just outlined.

Exposure should be terminated immediately. Remove frothy, foamy exudate from the respiratory tract by suctioning, postural drainage and sodium bicarbonate–sodium chloride aerosols.

53–503. OXYGEN (O_2) *(See also 53–604, Rocket Fuels)*

In addition to retrolental fibroplasia in premature infants, protracted inhalations of high concentrations of oxygen can cause pulmonary oxygen toxicity (respiratory distress, pulmonary exudation and later bronchopulmonary fibrodysplasia, initial roentgenographic signs of edema with opacity and subsequently mixed appearance of areas of overexpansion and consolidation or fibrosis). Prolonged administration of concentrations of 60% or more can cause severe cough and acute chest pain associated with decreased vital capacity; inhalation of pure oxygen can bring on symptoms and signs as early as 6 hours and irreversible changes can occur in several days. Breathing of high concentration oxygen over a period of long duration is one of the aggravating factors of shock lung. These factors should not dissuade use of pure or high concentration oxygen for short periods up to a few hours in emergency resuscitation of hypoxemic states. In persons with chronic pulmonary disease, oxygen may cause a decrease in respiration. Inhalation of oxygen at high pressures may cause severe poisoning and mechanical injury in flyers and in professional and sport divers (26–5).

Prophylactic Treatment. If cyanosis and low arterial oxygenation are present, give the lowest concentration of oxygen that will restore normal oxygenation—50% is generally adequately tolerated initially. Monitor arterial blood gases.

Signs and Symptoms. Restlessness; nervousness; extreme hilarity; impaired cerebration, judgment and sensation; and muscle fibrillation and spasm, followed by severe convulsions.

Treatment

- Artificial ventilation *(5–10) at once* by expired air or mechanical methods if ventilatory failure is present. Keep oxygen content for inspiration at normal air level or lowest supplement level consistent with adequate arterial oxygen saturation.
- Immediate transfer to a pressure chamber for recompression if the patient has become unconscious while diving with any type of gas-filled apparatus (26–5). Artificial ventilation must be continued en route.

53–504. OXYQUINOLINE DERIVATIVES

Overdosage of these amebicides may result in acute symptoms that are practically never fatal provided proper treatment is obtained.

Signs and symptoms include nausea, vomiting, upper abdominal pain (sometimes

---

*For therapeutic considerations see also *53–1* to *53–13*.

severe enough to be mistaken for an acute surgical condition) and hepatitis (with or without jaundice).

53–505. OZONE (O_3)

Consumable electrode welding has resulted in an increase in the number of cases of acute ozone poisoning. In addition, ozone-producing equipment, allegedly of therapeutic benefit, may give toxic concentrations of ozone (more than 0.1 part per million of air).

Signs and symptoms: Headache, lethargy, generalized malaise, persistent (usually nonproductive) cough, and chest pain—sometimes severe enough to be mistaken for the pain caused by a myocardial or pulmonary infarct. There are usually only minimal clinical and x-ray findings in spite of the acute clinical picture.

Treatment Includes:

- Remove from exposure.
- Control restlessness and pain by administration of sedatives and analgesics.
- Administer oxygen.
- Keep under observation until acute symptoms have subsided. Delayed pulmonary edema *(55)* may occur.

53–506. PAINT *(See 53–90, Arsenic; 53–206, Chromates, Chromic Acid, Chromium Trioxide; 53–323, Gasoline; 53–379, Kerosene; 53–386, Lead Salts; 53–426, Methyl Alcohol; 53–436, Methyl Cellosolve; 53–708, Titanium Tetrachloride; 53–730, Turpentine)*

White lead (a basic carbonate) and red lead (the tetroxide) are the bases of many paints. Petroleum solvents give toxic signs and symptoms similar to those of gasoline and kerosene. Harmless titanium salts are the base of many modern inside house paints.

53–507. PAINT REMOVERS *(See 53–24, Acetone; 53–117, Benzene (Benzol) and Its Derivatives; 53–176, Carbon Tetrachloride; 53–254, Dichloroethane; 53–401, Lye; 53–426, Methyl Alcohol; 53–440, Methylethylketone; 53–730, Turpentine)*

53–508. PAMAQUINE NAPHTHOATE ($C_{42}H_{45}N_3O_7$)

Under the trade name of Plasmochin, this drug is used for specific antimalaria therapy. Excessive or prolonged dosage may cause dizziness, drowsiness, cyanosis and jaundice. Methemoglobinemia *(53–12)* also may occur. (*Note*: Not sold in U.S. now.)

Hospitalize severe cases for symptomatic care. Permanent ill effects are rare.

53–509. PANSY

The roots contain a mildly toxic alkaloid, violine. For treatment, see 53–46, *Alkaloids.*

53–510. PANTOPON

Containing about 50% morphine, Pantopon is a mixture of opium alkaloids and is used as an analgesic and narcotic. For treatment, see 53–455, *Morphine.*

53–511. PAPER PRODUCTS

Ornamental paper products, such as colored crepe, are often sucked or chewed by children. They are not toxic.

---

*For therapeutic considerations see also *53–1* to *53–13.*

53–512. PARACHLOROMETACRESOL (PCMC)

Although ordinary commercial concentrations do not cause skin irritation, ingestion gives a toxic picture similar to that from ingestion of phenol (53–534).

53–513. PARACHLOROMETAXYLENOL (PCMX)

This complex insecticide can give an acute picture by penetration of the skin as well as by ingestion. For toxic signs, symptoms and treatment, see 53–534, *Phenol.*

53–514. PARADICHLOROBENZENE (PDB)

This is the least toxic of the active agents used in moth repellent balls and flakes. Ingestion rarely causes acute toxicity, but prolonged exposure to fumes may be serious.

See also 53–469, *Naphthalene.*

53–515. PARALDEHYDE ($C_6H_{12}O_3$)

Although this effective sedative has a large margin of safety, some hypersensitive patients react unfavorably to even small doses. Paraldehyde solutions deteriorate rapidly in the presence of light, with formation of toxic products. Rectal administration causes considerable local irritation. A characteristic profound odor from exhaled clearance is present regardless of route of administration.

Signs and symptoms include sudden onset of rapid pulse, accelerated respiration, cyanosis, coma and cardiac and respiratory failure.

53–516. PARAQUAT (Methylviologen) ($C_{12}H_{14}N_2$; TLV 0.5 mg/m^3)

Paraquat is a common herbicide that is used alone or, often, in conjunction with diquat, which is related. Toxicity can occur via skin absorption, inhalation and ingestion. *Signs and symptoms* include skin and mucosal irritation, fingernail abnormality with ridging and transverse white markings, severe eye injury, epistaxis, a wide range of respiratory tract pathology following inhalation (such as pulmonary edema and hemorrhage) and gastrointestinal plus multiorgan destruction after ingestion. Sometimes toxicity attributed to marijuana (53–409) in some cases is actually due to paraquat.

Treatment

Treatment includes removal from exposure, with cautions in handling as listed under organic phosphates (53–497). If paraquat has been ingested, induce emesis or lavage followed by administration of activated charcoal or Fuller's Earth (Bentonite) and magnesium sulfate. Avoid oxygen unless arterial saturation is inadequate. Lowered oxygen concentrations (FIO_2 = 18%) are advised, but this requires arterial and possibly central (mixed venous) PO_2 monitoring. Hemoperfusion and/or dialysis is probably indicated. Hospitalization, monitoring and intensive supportive treatment are needed in serious exposure cases.

53–517. PARATHION (Alkron, E605, Niran, Paraphos, Thiophos) ($[C_2H_5O]_2$ $P[S]OC_6H_4NO_2$; TLV 0.1 mg/m^3)

This anticholinesterase compound is one of the most toxic of the organic phosphate insecticides. See 53–497, *Organic Phosphates.*

53–518. PAREGORIC (Camphorated Tincture of Opium) *(See 13–3, Narcotics; 53–455, Morphine; 53–727, Tripelennamine Hydrochloride ["Blue Velvet"])*

---

*For therapeutic considerations see also *53–1* to *53–13*.

53–519. **PARIS GREEN** (Copper Acetoarsenate, Schweinfurth Green) *(See 53–90, Arsenic)*

53–520. **PARTHENOCISSUS QUINQUEFOLIA** (Virginia Creeper, American Woodbine, False Grape, Wild Wood Vine)

Although this North American climbing vine is usually considered to be nontoxic, chewing the leaves and eating the berries has caused violent vomiting, diarrhea, stupor, and collapse.

53–521. **PCB** (Polychlorinated biphenyls, Arochlor 1242 [$C_{12}H_7Cl_3$; 42% Cl; TLV 1 mg/m^3], Arochlor 1254 [$C_{12}H_5Cl_5$; 54% Cl; TLV 0.5 mg/m^3])

This prevalent straw-colored fluid is found in heat exchange and hydraulic fluids, is a dielectric in old capacitors and transformers and is used in casting processes. Toxicity generally occurs from inhalation of fumes or skin absorption, but there was mass poisoning in Japan from ingestion of PCB-contaminated rice bran oil. Acneform dermatitis (chloracne), paresthesias and liver damage occur, and there is a possible link to malignancy change with chronic exposure. Blood plasma PCB tests are not highly reliable; PCB's accumulate in human fat. Decontaminate skin and remove clothing immediately if exposed. Check liver function tests (LFT) for hepatic damage. Transient exposure to small amounts of PCB is not of consequence.

53–522. **PEACH (PIT)**

The pit contains amygdalin *(53–67)*. For treatment, see *53–232, Cyanides.*

53–523. **PELLETIERINE** (Punicine)

This toxic alkaloid is found in the bark (especially in the root bark) of the pomegranate tree. Ingestion of moderate amounts may cause mydriasis, partial blindness, severe headache, vertigo, vomiting, diarrhea and convulsions.

53–524. **PENNYROYAL** (Squaw Mint, *Hedeoma*) *(See 53–494, Oil, Essential)*

The leaves and flowers of this plant contain substances that are powerful stimulants, carminatives and emmenagogues. Ingestion has been reported to cause symptoms of shock, confusion, delirium, twitching and respiratory depression.

53–525. **PENTAZOCINE HYDROCHLORIDE** (Talwin) ($C_{19}H_{27}NO$)

The toxicity of pentazocine is similar to that of narcotics but generally less intense. Addiction is somewhat less likely to occur. Treatment includes induced emesis, activated charcoal, supportive care and use of naloxone *(53–10)*, which is often needed in much larger doses than with other opiates.

53–526. **PENTOTHAL SODIUM**

This relatively safe and effective intravenous anesthetic (thiopental sodium) may cause myocardial depression and cardiac arrest in certain hypersensitive persons, or if administered improperly or carelessly in addition to respiratory and CNS depression. Artificial ventilation is often required, and reduction or discontinuance of the drug may be necessary. Laryngospasm with light thiopental sodium anesthesia may be relieved with skeletal muscle relaxants, and hypersecretion may be reduced with atropine. Shivering,

---

*For therapeutic considerations see also *53–1* to *53–13*.

extremity tremors and facial twitching are relieved with warming, time and, if necessary, chlorpromazine. It is shorter acting than pentobarbital.

53–527. PENTYLENETETRAZOLE

Pentylenetetrazól has been used in the past as a potent analeptic and is occasionally used in EEG studies. In hypersensitive individuals, use of pentylenetetrazol (Metrazol) even in small "therapeutic" doses has resulted in brief but extremely violent convulsions and in auricular fibrillation. Seizure precautions are indicated to prevent fractures, dislocations, tongue biting, etc. The auricular fibrillation is usually transient and not dangerous. Airway protection should be provided. The benzodiazepines are excellent and safe in preventing or terminating phenylenetetrazole seizures.

53–528. PERFUMES

The exact constituents of most perfumes are the closely guarded professional secrets of the various manufacturers, but, basically, ambergris, volatile hydrocarbons, alcohols and natural or synthetic scents are used. If more than 4 ml has been ingested, gastric emptying followed by activated charcoal in water and by symptomatic and supportive therapy is indicated.

53–529. PERU BALSAM (China Oil)

A mixture of resins and aromatic esters, balsam of Peru is used topically in the treatment of indolent ulcers and pediculosis. Absorption may cause a rapid pulse, convulsions and nephritis, with slow recovery when use is discontinued.

53–530. PESTICIDES

Pesticides include a wide range of potent chemicals used commercially and domestically to abate and eliminate pests (bugs, insects, rodents) that interfere with the growth and harvesting of vegetable kingdom products. Some pesticides such as DDT *(53–240)* have proved so persistent and lethal that their production is banned. Mass leakage of methyl isocyanate gas, used in pesticide production, killed over 2000 people and injured approximately 100,000 in India in 1984; this was history's worst industrial accident.

Among the groups of pesticides used are:

- Organophosphate cholinesterase inhibitors. See *53–497, Organic Phosphates.*
- Carbamate cholinesterase inhibitors. See *53–170.*
- Solid organocholine pesticides. See *53–117, Benzene Hexachloride and pentachlorophenol.*
- Nitrophenolic and nitrocresolic herbicides.
- Chlorophenoxy compounds (e.g., *53–257, 2,4 Dichlorophenoxyacetic Acid)*
- Paraquat and Diquat. See *53–516, Paraquat.*
- Dithiocarbamates and Thiocarbamates. See *53–280; 53–702, Thiram.*
- Pyrethrum, Pyrethrius, Pyrethroids and Pyronyl Butoxide. See *53–584, Pyrethrum.*
- Arsenicals. See *53–90.*
- Rodenticides. (e.g., *53–747, Warfarin; 53–597, Red Squill)*
- Fumigants:
  - —Halocarbons (e.g., *53–176, Carbon Tetrachloride; 53–196, Chloroform; 53–299, Ethylene Dibromide)*
  - —Oxides and aldehydes (e.g., *53–301, Ethylene Oxide; 53–315, Formaldehyde; 53–36, Acrolein)*
  - —Sulphur and phosphorous compounds (e.g., *53–663, Sulfur Dioxide; 53–232, Cyanides* (e.g., *53–37,* Acrylonitrile)

Treatment

For therapeutic considerations, see *53–1* to *53–13* and specific poisons. In moderate to severe poisonings, contacting the Poison Control Center is advisable; product ingredients and concentrations may vary. Prompt reporting to the Public Health Department *in addition to* reporting injured workers to the Division of Industrial Accidents may be mandatory, as in California. An excellent overview, *Recognition and Management of Pesticide Poisonings,* by Donald P. Morgan, M.D., Ph.D., is available (EPA-

---

*For therapeutic considerations see also *53–1* to *53–13.*

540/9–80–005, Third Edition, 1982, Supt. of Documents, U.S. Govt. Printing Office, Washington, D.C. 20402).

53–531. PETROLEUM DISTILLATES *(See 53–117, Benzene (Benzol) and Its Derivatives; 53–323, Gasoline; 53–379, Kerosene; 53–468, Naphtha; 53–656, Stoddard Solvent)*

53–532. PHENCYCLIDINE (PCP, Angel Dust)

Use of phencyclidine by smoking or insufflation (less often by ingestion or injection) presents a complex clinical picture of physical signs and symptoms (Fig. 53–2) and behavior (ranging from an obtunded consciousness "zombie" state to violent, unusually strong, release of physical power, not infrequently accompanied by loud uninhibited snarling, growling or other animal sounds). Coma with the eyes open is often diagnostic. Ketamine is often sold as PCP and is similar in nature.

Consciousness and pain response are used to classify toxicity into the following three stages: Stage I, both present; Stage II, unconscious but pain response present; Stage III, neither present. Stage I psychologic changes include thought pattern and body image derangement, apathy, drowsiness and occasional hostility and amnesia. The electroencephalograph (EEG) shows slowed delta rhythm in all stages and dysrhythmic theta activity in Stage III.

Usual absence of chromatographic analysis equipment in the emergency setting makes history and clinical evaluation paramount in establishing the diagnosis and managing treatment of intoxication by this potent psychedelic, sympathomimetic street drug. The only other common drug besides PCP that causes horizontal and vertical nystagmus is phenytoin. Attenuation and prophylactic prevention of adrenergic "storms," supportive care with gentle handling and efforts to speed elimination of the drug are basic to treatment. As pointed out by Done and Aronow (JACEP, 7:56, 1978), ion trapping of this weakly basic compound by continuous gastric suction and acidification of urine or blood, or both, speeds elimination of PCP. Administration of repeated doses of activated charcoal is considered by some to achieve the same goal.

Treatment

- See Table 53–4 for basic elements of treatment.
- Stage I patients require a quiet environment and gentle handling; the reassuring "talk down" approach is of benefit. Gastric emptying is not attempted unless there is some indication the patient has just taken additional PCP.
- If a Stage II case is deepening, prepare to proceed with gastric lavage, with a standby expert for airway intubation; otherwise avoid unnecessary instrumentation and suctioning.
- In Stage II and Stage III patients, obtain blood studies and send any specimens for analysis as described in *Coma (32).* Monitor closely. Start IV fluids with 5% dextrose in lactated Ringer's solution.
- Consider propranolol (Inderal) if signs of impending hypertensive crisis; if occurring also give IV propranolol, 1 mg every minute as needed to a maximum of 10 mg in 10 minutes. Monitor ECG and blood pressure. If response inadequate, consider use of diazoxide or nitroprusside with appropriate arterial blood pressure monitoring.
- Even in patients who are clearing from confusion, particularly those in Stage II and Stage III, continue medications orally for 1 week to avoid postingestion adrenergic crisis as follows: 0.5 g ascorbic acid qid, 40 mg propranolol (Inderal) tid, 40 mg furosemide (Lasix) qid, plus 10 mg diazepam (Valium) tid [with 5 mg haloperidol (Haldol) qid and 25 mg diphenhydramine (Benadryl) if patient had severe violent episode].

53–533. PHENOBARBITAL (Barbenyl, Dormiral, Gardenal, Luminal, Somonal, etc.)

In some persons, even small doses of this long-acting sedative may cause headache, dizziness, acute skin changes (including exfoliative dermatitis) and personality changes. For treatment, see *53–110, Barbiturates.*

---

*For therapeutic considerations see also *53–1* to *53–13*.

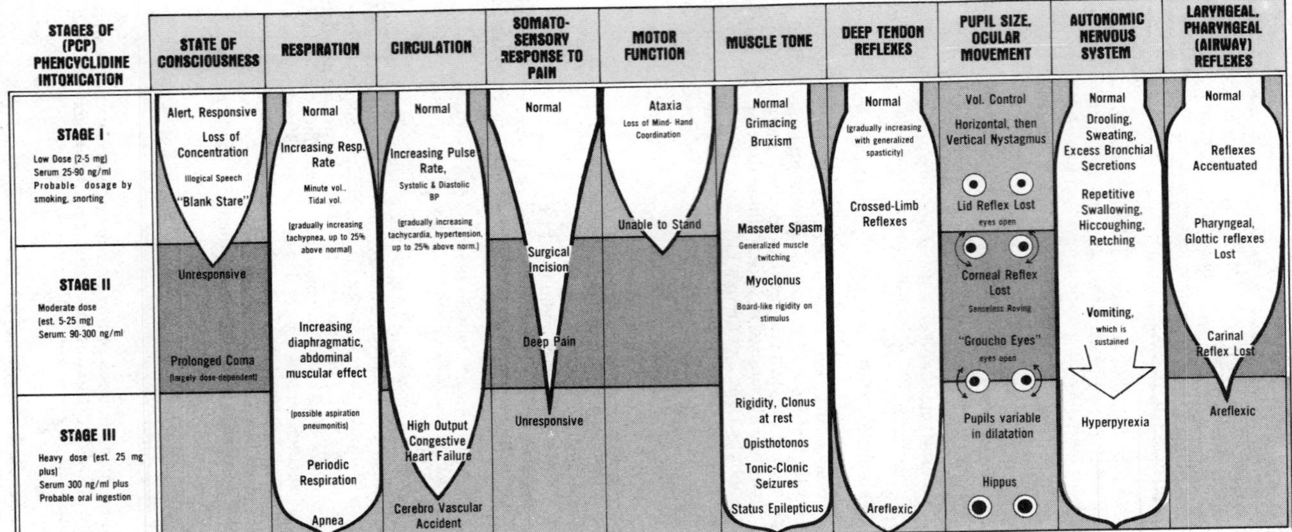

Figure 53–2. Signs and symptoms of phencyclidine (PCP) intoxication. (From Rappolt, R. T., and Gat, G. T.: JACEP, 8:68, 1979.)

Table 53–4. TREATMENT OF PCP INGESTION

	Quiet & reduced handling	Emetics	Gastric lavage & steady suction or activated charcoal	Cooling measures	Diazepam	Ascorbic acid	Propranolol	Furosemide	Nitroprusside or Diazoxide
Stage I (conscious, pain response)	Yes	No	No	±	10 to 30 mg orally	0.5 to 1.5 g orally	40 to 80 mg orally	±	±
Stage II (unconscious but pain response)	Yes	No	±	Yes, prn	2.5 mg IV to total of 5 to 15 mg prn	1 to 1.5 g IV solution (slowly) every 6 hours	1 mg IV every 30 minutes while stable for hypertensive crisis: 1 mg IV every 1 to 5 minutes to maximum of 10 mg	40 mg IV every 6 hours	Use IV if hypertensive crisis isn't controlled by sedatives, diuretics, or propranolol; do arterial BP monitoring
Stage III (coma and no pain response)	±	No	Yes	Yes, prn	Same as Stage II, prn	1 to 1.5 g IV solution (slowly) 4 to 6 hours		40 mg IV every 4 to 6 hours	

53–534. PHENOL (Carbolic Acid) (C_6H_5OH; TLV 5 ppm)

Acute toxic signs and symptoms may occur from absorption through the skin, absorption through the mucous membrane of the rectum or vagina and ingestion by accident or with suicidal intent.

Signs and symptoms following ingestion are acute and consist of the odor of phenol on the breath; burning in the mouth and throat, with whitish discoloration of the tongue and mucous membrane of the throat; nausea; vomiting; severe abdominal pain; slow, weak pulse; faintness; hypotension; and coma. Renal insufficiency may develop. Esophageal strictures are a rare complication.

Treatment Includes:

- Removal as soon as possible by washing the skin or eyes with copious amounts of water or by giving warm water enemas or douches, depending upon portal of entry. If ingested, the stomach should be washed with large quantities of warm water until the odor of phenol has disappeared. This should be followed by activated charcoal in water by mouth or through the lavage tube. Mineral oil should not be used. Alcohol increases absorption of phenol and is contraindicated.
- Artificial respiration (*5–10*) and oxygen therapy as required.
- Morphine sulfate or meperidine (Demerol) in small doses for control of pain.
- Sodium bicarbonate IV for correction of severe metabolic acidosis.
- Treatment of incipient or actual pulmonary edema (*55*).

53–535. PHENOLPHTHALEIN ($C_{20}H_{14}O_4$)

This cathartic is the active ingredient in several popular "candy laxatives." Although phenolphthalein is relatively nontoxic, large doses, especially in children, may cause severe enteritis and colitis lasting for 3 to 4 days. Aside from treatment of dehydration, no specific therapy is required.

53–536. PHENOTHIAZINES

Used in the treatment of gastrointestinal and psychiatric complaints, phenothiazines may cause characteristic side effects following average as well as excessive doses.

Common Preparations

Acetophenazine (Tindal)
Carphenazine (Proketazine)
Chlorpromazine (Thorazine)
Fluphenazine (Permitil)
Perphenazine (Trilafon)
Prochlorperazine (Compazine)
Promazine (Sparine)
Thioridazine (Mellaril)
Trifluoperazine (Stelazine)
Triflupromazine (Vesprin)

Extrapyramidal Reactions. Dyskinesia, dystonia, cervical muscle spasm, facial muscle spasm (trismus, sardonic grin, etc.), lack of control of movements of the tongue, bizarre involuntary movements of the extremities and embarrassment of respiration.

Parkinsonian Symptoms. Drooling, tremor, rigidity, abnormal posture and gait, restlessness and profuse speech.

Treatment Includes:

- Discontinue or decrease the dose of the medication. Use gastric lavage rather than attempting to induce emesis if stomach must be emptied.
- Give diphenhydramine (Benadryl), 25 mg IV or 50 mg IM (children, 5 mg/kg every 24 hours); in milder cases, oral administration may be substituted for dystonic reactions only.
- Support respiration as needed.
- If continuation of phenothiazine therapy is necessary, decrease the dosage and give antiparkinsonian agents.

Hypotension and Shock. For treatment, see 57. Prolonged QT may appear on the ECG.

Jaundice, Dermatitis and Agranulocytosis. These may persist for lengthy periods after the drug has been stopped.

---

*For therapeutic considerations see also *53–1* to *53–13*.

Somnolence. This usually clears rapidly when use of phenothiazine is discontinued. Avoid use with alcohol or other CNS depressants.

53–537. PHENYLBUTAZONE (Butazolidin) and OXYPHENBUTAZONE (Tandearil)

Both of these drugs have important toxic side effects.

Signs and symptoms: Acute gastrointestinal symptoms, including activation of healed ulcers, fluid retention, acute skin changes, sometimes severe exfoliative dermatitis *(58–8A, Toxic Epidermal Necrolysis)*, stomatitis, sore throat and serious progressive blood changes that may develop rapidly and may be irreversible.

Prevention and Early Recognition of Toxic Reactions

- Limitation of dosage to 600 mg daily for no more than several days, then 300 mg daily. A baseline complete blood count should be established.
- Discontinuance at the end of 1 week usually if no clinical improvement.
- Hematologic examinations every week for the first 6 weeks of treatment, then every 6 to 8 weeks for as long as therapy is continued—repeat sooner if signs or symptoms occur.

Treatment Includes:

- Stop administration at once.
- Symptomatic care, local and general. Mild cases as a rule do well under home care; severe cases require hospitalization including possible transfusions, etc.

53–538. PHENYLENEDIAMINE ($C_6H_4[NH_2]_2$; TLV 0.1 mg/m³)

Used in eyelash dyes, this substance may give severe toxic reactions *(24)* in hypersensitive individuals.

Local Reactions. Severe smarting and pain in the eyes, edema, lacrimation and acute conjunctivitis with photophobia and corneal ulcerations.

Systemic Reactions. Headache; sleepiness; bizarre paresthesias; nausea; epigastric pain; edema of the face, neck and glottis; asthmatic attacks (probably allergic); and severe liver damage. All cases should be checked by an ophthalmologist, since permanent eye damage may result if prompt treatment is not given.

53–539. PHENYLHYDRAZINE ($C_6H_5NHNH_2$; TLV 5 ppm)

Accidental ingestion or therapeutic use in the treatment of polycythemia vera may cause severe toxic manifestations. Skin absorption and sensitization occurs easily.

Signs and symptoms include fatigue, headache, vertigo, edema of the eyelids and upper extremities, acute gastritis with or without diarrhea, cyanosis secondary to blood destruction and toxic hepatitis with severe anemia. Blood transfusions may be required.

53–540. PHENYL SALICYLATE (Salol)

Mild toxicity is due to phenol *(53–534)*—not to salicylates.

53–541. PHENYTOIN (Dilantin, Diphenylhydantoin)

Usual doses or overdosage of this drug, used for prevention of epileptic attacks and in the treatment of digitalis toxicity *(53–265)* may cause apprehension, tension, tremulousness, dizziness, ataxia, nausea, vomiting, blurring of vision, diplopia, nystagmus, generalized lymphadenopathy and hepatosplenomegaly. Allergic reactions, including liver damage, blood dyscrasias and dermatitis, can occur.

Treatment Considerations Include:

- Discontinue therapeutic use and find satisfactory alternative medications or decrease the size of the dose of the drug. In severe cases, emesis or lavage and activated charcoal are indicated.

---

*For therapeutic considerations see also *53–1* to *53–13*.

- Impress on the patient or patient's family the need for further medical treatment. The patient should be made to understand that stopping the drug completely for continuing periods may cause an increase in the number and severity of convulsive seizures.
- Blood serum levels may help to guide therapy.

53–542. PHILODENDRON

The leaves and stalks of this common household plant contain clusters of small needle-sharp crystals of calcium oxalate that may cause an acute inflammatory process in the mouth or throat; swelling of the throat may be severe enough to interfere with breathing. Systemic reactions to the oxalate are rare.

53–543. PHOSGENE (Carbonyl Chloride) ($COCl_2$; TLV 0.1 ppm)

Although phosgene originally was used as a war gas (see 53–746, *War Gases*), toxic signs and symptoms from respiratory tract irritation occur occasionally in the chemical industry.

Signs and symptoms: A foul taste in the mouth, with a "scratchy" feeling in the throat. Anosmia develops after the first few whiffs, so that large quantities of the gas may be inhaled without knowledge of its presence. Dyspnea, severe cyanosis, bronchitis, emphysema, pulmonary edema (*55*), bronchospasm and acute cardiac failure may occur. Pulmonary edema and cardiac failure may occur even after apparent recovery.

53–544. PHOSPHINE (Phosphoretted Hydrogen) (PH_3; TLV 0.3 ppm)

Formed by the decomposition of phosphides in industrial processes, this foul-smelling gas in low concentrations may cause headache, dizziness, restlessness, tremors, general fatigue, burning substernal pain, nausea, vomiting and diarrhea. Bronchitis with fluorescent green sputum, acute dyspnea and pulmonary edema (*55*) may develop. Death is usually preceded by tonic convulsions, which may occur suddenly after the patient has apparently recovered. The garlic odor threshold of this substance is about 7 times higher (2.0 ppm) than the toxic level, so smelling it offers no protection.

53–545. PHOSPHORIC ACID (H_3PO_4; TLV 1 mg/m³)

For systemic effects, see 28–23, *Phosphorus Burns*; 53–33, *Acids*; 53–546, *Phosphorus*. Locally, phosphoric acid burns require special emergency therapy (28–23).

53–546. PHOSPHORUS (P; TLV 0.1 mg/m³) *(See also 28–23, Phosphorus Burns)*

Yellow and white phosphorus are extremely toxic; red phosphorus is insoluble and hence nontoxic. Acute poisoning may arise from ingestion of rat or roach poisons, certain types of fireworks, imported matches (especially from China and Japan) and old-fashioned "sulfur" matches. Severe, even terminal, effects have been caused by the ingestion of the heads of "strike anywhere" kitchen matches or of the friction striking areas of "safety" book or box matches (*53–410, Matches*).

Signs and symptoms of phosphorus poisoning after ingestion are a garlicky taste in the mouth and odor on the breath, a burning sensation in the mouth and throat, nausea, vomiting (the vomitus may be luminous in the dark), abdominal pain, slow weak pulse, faintness and collapse. Severe systemic damage may be evident 2 to 3 days after apparently complete recovery. Fatty enlargement of the liver, intense icterus, severe hemorrhage and serious blood dyscrasias may occur.

Treatment Includes:

- Immediate gastric lavage with 30 to 60 ml of 1% copper sulfate solution diluted to 200 ml; follow with copious gastric lavage with tap water or half normal saline. The

---

*For therapeutic considerations see also 53–*1* to 53–*13*.

patient and attendants must be protected from contact with vomitus and gastric washings.

- Treatment of severe shock. Corticosteroid therapy may be of value.
- Control of convulsions by rapid-acting barbiturates or diazepam.
- Vitamin K_1 IV to combat hypoprothrombinemia. Fresh blood transfusions may be necessary.
- Hospitalize for observation to ascertain possible liver and kidney damage. Mortality is high.

For local and systemic effects of burns from phosphorus-containing bombs, rockets and flares in wartime, see *28–23, Phosphorus Burns.*

53–547. PHYSOSTIGMINE SALICYLATE (Eserine)

This is a powerful parasympathetic stimulator that may cause bradycardia, intense salivation, miosis, twitching of skeletal muscles, coma, heart block, convulsions and collapse. In therapeutic doses, it is the antidote for atropine and similar compounds (see *53–10* and Table 53–2, Cholinergics).

Treatment

Administration of the physiologic antagonist, atropine sulfate *(53–10)* or propantheline bromide (Pro-Banthine). Gastric lavage, followed by activated charcoal in water, is indicated if large amounts have been ingested.

53–548. PICRIC ACID ($HOC_6H_2[NO_2]_3$; TLV 0.1 mg/m^3)

Used industrially in the manufacture of explosives and dyes and medicinally (usually as the picrate) as an antiseptic ointment, picric acid may cause bright yellow discoloration of the skin. Intense bitter taste, nausea, vomiting, abdominal pain, epigastric tenderness, bladder tenesmus and severe liver and kidney damage. After gastric emptying, 5% sodium bicarbonate solution is satisfactory for lavage.

53–549. PICROTOXIN ($C_{30}H_{34}O_{13}$)

Picrotoxin, a GABA antagonist, is the toxic ingredient of the bright red berries of an East Indian plant, commonly known as "fish eggs." Medicinally it was formerly used as an analeptic, especially in barbiturate poisoning, but its use for this purpose is not indicated. Ill-advised injection of picrotoxin in the treatment of coma has caused uncontrollable convulsions and death.

Signs and symptoms after ingestion: A burning sensation in the mouth, pallor, cold perspiration, nausea, vomiting and shallow respiration. After ½ to 3 hours, confusion, stupor, unconsciousness and clonic or tonic convulsions may occur, especially in children. Treatment includes seizure precautions *(34)* and benzodiazepines.

PROGNOSIS. The mortality from ingestion is very low.

53–550. PILOCARPINE

This medication is used for pupil constriction in the treatment of glaucoma. Toxic manifestations and treatment are approximately the same as those given for *Physostigmine (53–547).*

53–551. PINE OIL

Ingestion of small amounts of this complex mixture of terpene alcohols may cause acute toxic effects, especially gastritis (sometimes hemorrhagic), decreased body temperature, central nervous system depression and respiratory failure. See also *53–682, Terpineol; 53–730, Turpentine.*

---

*For therapeutic considerations see also *53–1* to *53–13.*

53–552. PINKS

The seeds are the only toxic part of the plant. Ingestion may cause intense gastrointestinal irritation—never fatal because of the emetic action. Treatment is symptomatic only.

53–553. PLASTER OF PARIS (Anhydrous Calcium Sulfate or Dihydrate)

Plaster of Paris has no intrinsic toxicity but if swallowed may harden and cause obstruction requiring surgical relief. *Immediate* ingestion of large amounts of water, gelatin or glycerin will sometimes delay setting long enough to allow removal by emesis or gastric lavage.

53–554. PLASTIC CEMENTS AND GLUES (Model Airplane Cement)

Sniffing the fumes from model airplane adhesive materials has become fairly common. Transient exhilaration, euphoria and increased tolerance to pain result—probably due to the solvents employed (often toluene and amyl acetate [53–68]). Habitual glue-sniffing may result in intoxication, anoxia and coma. Similar effects have been reported from sniffing paint thinner, lacquer and marking pencil fumes. Treatment is symptomatic and supportive.

53–555. PLASTICS

Ever-widening uses of plastic materials have focused attention on 3 main types of toxic reactions:

1. Irritation of the skin and mucous membranes during manufacture. This is often due to solvents, plasticizers and dyes and is rarely serious.
2. Polymer fume fever. The exact cause of this condition is unknown. The toxic picture and treatment are similar to those for metal fume fever (*53–423*).
3. Acute toxic signs and symptoms may be caused by decomposition products resulting from heating plastic materials used in industry and medical and surgical, therapy i.e., fluorocarbons such as Teflon. Under certain conditions, extremely toxic substances, including hydrocyanic acid (*53–232, Cyanides*), oxides of nitrogen (*53–488*) and tetrafluoroethylene, may result from exposure of plastics to intense heat. The smoke from burning plastics is highly irritating and dangerous (see also 25–4).

53–556. PMA (Phenyl Mercuric Acetate)

This fungicide is more toxic than mercuric chloride. For treatment, see *53–124, Bichloride of Mercury*.

53–557. POKEWEED (Inkberry, Phytolacca; American Nightshade, Pigeonberry, Scoke)

All parts of this common plant (especially the unripe berries) contain a saponin and resin that are intense gastrointestinal irritants. Toxic effects (burning in the mouth, severe gastroenteritis, drowsiness, impaired vision and respiratory depression) develop about 2 hours after ingestion.

53–558. POINSETTIA

The sap from this plant can cause severe contact dermatitis and temporary blindness. Chewing the leaves results in irritation and swelling of oropharyngeal mucosa, gastroenteritis, vomiting, and diarrhea.

---

*For therapeutic considerations see also *53–1* to *53–13*.

53–559. POISON HEMLOCK

The active poison factor is lambdaconiceine. See *53–223, Coniine.*

53–560. POISON IVY, OAK, SUMAC *(See 58–13* and *58–18, Urushiol Contact Dermatitis)*

53–561. POLYCHLORINATED BIPHENYL *(See 53–521, PCB)*

53–562. POLYMER FUME FEVER *(See 53–554, Plastics)*

53–563. POMEGRANATE

The bark and stems contain toxic alkaloids. *See 53–523, Pelletierine.*

53–564. POPPIES

California poppies contain a mixture of alkaloids with a depressant action on heart muscle. Oriental poppies have a high content of opium alkaloids. For treatment, see *53–46, Alkaloids; 53–455, Morphine.*

53–565. POSTERIOR PITUITARY EXTRACTS

The most commonly used extracts are posterior pituitary (Pituitrin), oxytocin (Pitocin) and vasopressin (Pitressin). All are oxytocic agents and may cause nausea, vomiting, intestinal cramping, extreme facial pallor and cramping similar to menstrual cramps in women.

Treatment

No physiologic antagonist to posterior pituitary extracts is known; therefore, symptomatic treatment is all that is indicated.

PROGNOSIS. Complete and rapid disappearance of symptoms, provided use of the offending extract has been discontinued.

53–566. POTASSIUM CHLORATE ($KClO_3$)

Formerly present in many household toilet articles and medications (cough mixtures, gargles, mouthwashes and toothpastes). Ingestion of large amounts may cause nausea, vomiting, epigastric pain, dyspnea, cyanosis and methemoglobinemia *(53–12)*, acute delirium, anuria and jaundice. Perform gastric emptying and administration of activated charcoal for ingestion of large amounts.

53–567. POTASSIUM ION *(See 46–12, Hyperpotassemia)*

53–568. POTASSIUM OXALATE ($K_2C_2O_4$) *(See also 53–501, Oxalic Acid)*

Potassium oxalate is the active constituent of many popular household cleansing and bleaching agents. Acute toxic, even fatal, effects may be caused by ingestion (accidental or with suicidal intent), by injection in the vagina or uterus in an attempt to produce an abortion or by inhalation of fumes or steam from cleansing or bleaching solutions.

Signs and symptoms of oxalate toxicity consist of a burning sensation in the mouth and throat with difficulty in swallowing; edema of the glottis; nausea; vomiting, often bloody and associated with severe epigastric pain; weak pulse; low blood pressure; muscular fibrillation and twitching; exaggerated reflexes with patellar clonus; uremic convulsions; coma; and death from circulatory collapse.

Treatment is based in part on the formation of insoluble calcium oxalate. For details, see *53–501, Oxalic Acid.*

---

*For therapeutic considerations see also *53–1* to *53–13.*

53–569. POTASSIUM PERMANGANATE ($KMnO_4$)

Crystals or solutions of potassium permanganate are common in many household medical cabinets and often are available to children. Ingestion of a few crystals usually does no harm, but larger amounts may be dangerous. Severe mucous membrane burns, even perforation and peritonitis, have occurred following attempts at induction of an abortion by insertion of large amounts of the crystals into the vagina. Ingestion causes a film in the mouth or on other mucous membranes that may be violet or dark brown, stomatitis, nausea, vomiting, acute gastroenteritis with abdominal tenderness and shock from circulatory collapse (*57*), which may be severe and resistant to therapy.

Treatment

- Local treatment of mucous membrane burns (*28–19*).
- Gastric lavage with large quantities of saline solution followed by activated charcoal in water and saline cathartics.
- Control of pain by small doses of narcotics.
- Treatment of shock (*57*).
- Hospitalization if there is evidence of deep erosion or penetration of any mucous membrane.

PROGNOSIS. Good unless a concentrated solution (more than 3%) or a large amount of crystals have been swallowed or perforation of a body cavity or viscus has occurred.

53–570. POTATOES

Seeds, sprouts, leaves and berries contain toxic glucosides. *See 53–644, Solanine.*

53–571. PRECATORY BEAN (Rosary Pea)

Ingestion may result in delayed severe gastrointestinal distress, seizures, hemolytic anemia and death. *See 53–15, Abrus Precatorius; 53–376, Jequirity Beans.*

53–572. PREDNISOLONE (Delta-Cortef, Hydeltra, Meticortelone)

This synthetic steroid is used in the treatment of arthritis and may give a toxic picture similar to that of cortisone (53–226).

53–573. PREDNISONE (Deltasone, Deltra, Meticorten) *(See 53–226, Cortisone)*

53–574. PRIMIDONE (Mysoline)

Used as an antiepileptic drug, primidone in large doses may cause drowsiness, ataxia, vertigo and psychotic episodes. Toxic symptoms subside when use is stopped or reduced. Primidone is metabolized to PEMA and phenobarbital; thus its toxic effects can be very prolonged in cases of overdose. After initial measures, repeat doses of activated charcoal may be advisable in severe cases. *See 53–110, Barbiturates.*

53–575. PRIMROSE (Primula)

Hypersensitivity to this common garden plant is common and is characterized by acute skin reactions and swelling, burning and itching of the fingertips. Symptoms clear slowly when contact is avoided.

53–576. PRIVET (Ligustrum vulgare)

The leaves and berries of this hedge shrub have a toxic effect similar to those of aloes and adromedotoxin. *See 53–34, Aconite; 53–231, Curare.*

---

*For therapeutic considerations see also *53–1* to *53–13*.

53–577. PRIVINE (Naphazoline Hydrochloride)

Ingestion, as well as local use, of this powerful vasoconstrictor may result in disturbing and uncomfortable (but rarely dangerous) toxic effects. Many persons are hypersensitive to Privine and show extreme reactions after relatively small doses *(24, Allergic Reactions)*.

Signs and symptoms include severe headache, acute anxiety and excitement, cold perspiration and cyanosis, especially of lips and fingertips, followed by respiratory failure.

53–578. PROCAINAMIDE HYDROCHLORIDE (Pronestyl)

In hypersensitive persons or after administration of large doses, Pronestyl may produce bradycardia *(29–7)* and cardiac arrest *(29–8)*, sometimes preceded by extreme hypotension. Sore throat, fever, dysphagia, lupus-like syndrome and bone marrow depression have also been reported.

Prolonged QT intervals are seen.

53–579. PROLAN

Readily absorbable through the intact skin, this chlorinated hydrocarbon insecticide gives a toxic picture similar to that of chlordane *(53–190)*.

53–580. PROPHENPYRIDAMINE (Trimeton) AND CHLORPHENIRAMINE (Chlor-Trimeton) *(See also 53–202 and Table 53–2, Anticholinergics)*

Overdosage of these complex drugs, which are used in the treatment of allergic conditions, may cause facial flushing, mydriasis, muscle stiffness, dizziness, ataxia, confusion, delirium and hallucinations.

53–581. PROPOXYPHENE HYDROCHLORIDE (Darvon) ($C_{22}H_{30}ClNO_2$)

Either convulsions or coma may result from an overdose of this popular analgesic agent. Both may be preceded by deep respiratory depression, cardiac arrhythmias and signs and symptoms of cerebral and pulmonary edema.

Treatment Includes:

- Gastric lavage followed by activated charcoal in water by mouth or through the lavage tube.
- Assisted ventilations by expired air or mechanical methods *(5–1)*.
- Perform cardiac monitoring. Conduction abnormalities, bigeminy, lengthening of the QRS complex with ST wave modifications may be noted among findings.
- Control of convulsive seizures by rapid-acting barbiturates or diazepam.
- Naloxone hydrochloride (Narcan) *(53–10)* administration; large doses of naloxone may be required to reverse action of propoxyphene.
- Correct any severe metabolic acidosis.
- Treatment of pulmonary edema *(55)*, which must be differentiated from aspiration pneumonitis.

53–582. PROPRANOLOL (Inderal)

The benefits of this valuable beta-adrenergic blocking medication, which is used as an adjunct in the treatment of hypertension, angina pectoris, cardiac arrhythmias (particularly supraventricular), pheochromocytoma and migraine, must always be monitored to guard against excessive decreases in heart rate, blood pressure and cardiac output. Other medications of this group with similar effects are atenolol (Tenormin) and metoprolol (Lopressor).

---

*For therapeutic considerations see also *53–1* to *53–13*.

Because it competes with beta-adrenergic receptor stimulating agents for available beta receptor sites, propranolol is contraindicated when sympathetic stimulation is vital, as in: (1) cardiogenic shock, (2) bronchial asthma, (3) sinus bradycardia with greater than first-degree block, (4) right ventricular failure secondary to pulmonary hypertension, (5) congestive heart failure (unless due to a tachyarrhythmia treatable by propranolol, as with thyrotoxicosis), (6) patients receiving MAO inhibitors and other adrenergic-augmenting psychotropic drugs.

Treatment

Treatment of excess beta blockade consists of judicious withdrawal of propranolol (too rapid withdrawal may excite angina pectoris and myocardial infarction in susceptible patients) and administration of atropine for bradycardia, plus supportive care, with use of a Pacemaker if needed to relieve severe bradycardia or heart block. IV Levophed is indicated for hypotension not responding to pacing or blood volume replacement.

Cardiac failure (*29–8*) is treated with diuretics and digitalization. Epinephrine or levarterenol can be used for hypotension (see 57, *Shock*). Treat bronchospasm (see *56–4*) with aminophylline and a selective β_2 agonist (e.g., metaproterenol [Alupent]).

53–583. PYRACANTHA (Fire Bush, Firethorn)

Ingestion of the berries causes a toxic picture similar to that caused by belladonna. (*See 53–103, Atropine Sulfate; Belladonna and Belladonna Alkaloids.*

53–584. PYRETHRUM (Persian Insect Powder) (TLV 5 mg/m³)

Many household and garden insecticides contain this relatively nontoxic compound, often combined with other more toxic insecticides, especially organophosphates (*53–497*). Pyrethrum sprays often have a kerosene or xylene (*53–755*) base.

Signs and symptoms after inhalation or ingestion of large amounts consist of nausea, vomiting, acute gastrointestinal pain followed by diarrhea and a burning and stinging sensation around the anus.

Treatment is symptomatic and symptomatic only unless pyrethrum is combined with more dangerous insecticides or suspended in harmful vehicles (distillate, kerosene, xylene, etc.). Pyrethrum alone rarely causes dangerous toxic effects.

53–585. PYRIDINE (NC_5H_5; TLV 5 ppm)

Used commercially as a solvent and medicinally as an antiseptic and antispasmodic, pyridine may cause acute but transient toxic reactions following inhalation of the fumes or ingestion.

Signs and symptoms include headache, restlessness, insomnia, vertigo, muscular incoordination, disturbances in hearing and severe peripheral neuritis.

53–586. PYROCATECHOL (Catechol) ($C_6H_6O_2$)

This substance has, in general, the same actions as phenol but is more toxic, especially in its tendency to cause convulsions. For treatment, see *53–534, Phenol.*

53–587. PYROGALLOL (Pyrogallic Acid) ($C_6H_6O_3$)

Pyrogallol is used commercially in hair dyes and proprietary ringworm "cures." Severe toxic signs and symptoms similar to those caused by phenol (*53–534*) may occur from absorption through the intact skin as well as by ingestion. In addition, renal damage, methemoglobinemia (*53–12*) and red blood cell destruction similar to the effects of aniline (*53–75*) have been noted after prolonged use. Toxicity is usually manifested by the sudden onset of collapse, convulsions and albuminuria due to severe toxic nephritis.

---

*For therapeutic considerations see also *53–1* to *53–13*.

This characteristically sudden onset may occur after use of a preparation containing pyrogallol for a long period without apparent previous ill effects. Dyspnea, cyanosis and acute respiratory depression may occur.

53–588. PYROLAN

This is a phosphate ester pesticide, similar in action and toxicity to parathion. For treatment, see *53–497, Organic Phosphates.*

53–589. QUATERNARY AMMONIUM SALTS (QAC)

In 0.01 to 1% concentrations, many complex combinations of quaternary ammonium salts are used as antiseptics, deodorants and fungicides. Lauryl benzyl dimethyl ammonium chloride is used commonly in medicine under the USP name of benzalkonium chloride and the proprietary name of Zephiran.

Ingestion of large amounts of concentrated solutions or absorption from a mucous membrane-lined cavity such as the vagina may cause severe toxic effects. A few fatalities coming on 1 to 2 hours after ingestion have been reported. The extreme muscle weakness is not relieved by curare antagonists such as neostigmine *(53–474)* and edrophonium (Tensilon).

Signs and symptoms, A severe burning sensation in the mouth, throat and stomach if a concentrated solution has been ingested; restlessness; apprehension; dyspnea; cyanosis; generalized muscle weakness; and death from respiratory failure, sometimes preceded by convulsions.

53–590. QUINACRINE HYDROCHLORIDE (Atabrine)

Effective therapeutic doses used in the treatment of malaria may cause severe toxic effects, as may overdosage. Individual tolerance varies markedly. Signs and symptoms of toxicity following excessive doses are similar to those given in *53–200, Chloroquine Phosphate.*

53–591. QUINIDINE

Quinidine is used in the treatment of auricular fibrillation and other cardiac arrhythmias *(29)*. Overdosage (or therapeutic doses in hypersensitive persons) may produce nausea, vomiting, diarrhea, bizarre behavior, cardiac abnormalities (including extrasystoles, paroxysmal tachycardia, variable AV heart block, ventricular fibrillation *(29–25)* and cardiac arrest *(29–8)*. In addition, respiratory paralysis and pulmonary infarction may occur.

For treatment, see *53–592, Quinine.* Cardiac irregularities are less likely to occur if the patient is digitalized; they usually subside rapidly when quinidine therapy is discontinued. Prolonged QT, wide PR and QRS segment are noted.

53–592. QUININE

The most important alkaloid of cinchona bark, quinine is used in the treatment of malaria *(33–38)* as a tonic and as a hair dressing and is an ingredient of many common proprietary preparations. Allergic hypersensitivity reactions *(24)* are common. Acute quinine poisoning is characterized by nausea, vomiting, abdominal pain, diarrhea, generalized edema and hypotension. The patient may have decreased vision and hearing, severe headache, tinnitus and auditory hallucinations. Jaundice and evidence of renal damage may develop. Fatalities are the result of excessive dosage and are due to respiratory arrest. Constant ECG monitoring should be conducted during the acute toxic state because of danger of cardiac irritability and arrest *(29–8)*. Acidosis may require correction. The clinical picture of acute quinine poisoning may resemble in many ways that of acute malaria *(33–38)*, the disease for which the drug is often prescribed. Prevent further absorption with emesis or lavage and activated charcoal.

---

*For therapeutic considerations see also *53–1* to *53–13*.

53–593. RAGWORT

If ingested, ragwort causes severe liver damage without other toxic effects.

53–594. RANUNCULUS SCLERATUS (Buttercup, Crowfoot)

Chewing or swallowing flowers or leaves of this common flowering meadow plant results in acute salivation, peeling of the surface of the tongue, loss of taste and colicky gastric pain. All symptoms are of short duration and leave no permanent ill effects.

53–595. RAT KILLERS (Rodenticides) *(See 53–90, Arsenic; 53–111, Barium Compounds; 53–232, Cyanides; 53–311, Fluorides; 53–597, Red Squill; 53–638, Sodium Fluoroacetate; 53–659, Strychnine; 53–692, Thallium; 53–747, Warfarin; 53–762, Zinc Phosphide)*

53–596. RAUWOLFIA ALKALOIDS (Reserpine, Serpasil) ($C_{33}H_{40}N_2O_{10}$)

Rauwolfia and its alkaloids in therapeutic doses may cause nasal congestion and epistaxis, acute gastrointestinal symptoms, flare-ups of healed ulcers, acute colitis simulating an acute surgical abdomen, acute mental depression and parkinsonism. Cardiac irritability may occur with increased incidence in conjunction with use of digitalis preparations and quinidine.

Treatment

Decrease in dosage or stopping administration of the drug usually results in spontaneous and complete clearing of symptoms. In severe cases, treatment includes:

- Even if several hours have passed since ingestion, gastric emptying with copious amounts of water, followed by activated charcoal via the lavage tube and a saline cathartic.
- Conservative therapy if coma and hypotension are present. Analeptic and vasopressor drugs should be avoided, as should rapid intravenous infusions.
- Give small doses of atropine for control of parasympathomimetic side effects.
- Local antacid therapy for gastric pain.
- Antiparkinsonian drugs for control of stiffness and tremors.
- Frequent ECG monitoring regarding cardiac abnormalities.

53–597. RED SQUILL

Ingestion of even small amounts of this commonly used rat poison causes a toxic picture similar to that caused by digitalis *(53–265)*.

53–598. REFRIGERATING AGENTS *(See 53–61, Ammonia; 53–435, Methyl Bromide; 53–437, Methyl Chloride; 53–663, Sulfur Dioxide; 53–741, Vinyl Chloride)*

53–599. RESORCINOL

Similar in many respects to phenol in its toxicity, resorcinol may give acute signs and symptoms from skin absorption as well as from ingestion. The toxic picture is generally not as severe as that caused by phenol, although the tendency toward convulsions is greater.

Hexylresorcinol *(53–342)* is slightly less toxic than resorcinol.

For treatment, see *53–534, Phenol.*

---

*For therapeutic considerations see also *53–1* to *53–13*.

53–600. RHODODENDRON

The foliage and shoots of the numerous flowering plants in this genus contain andromedotoxin (or grayanotoxin). Poisoning usually occurs from children chewing on leaves (which causes oral burning) or people eating honey produced by bees taking the flower nectar. The signs and symptoms of toxicity and treatment after ingestion are similar to those for aconite *(53–34)* and curare *(53–231)*. Recovery is usually complete in 24 hours, but fatalities do occur. Atropine may correct the bradycardia.

53–601. RHODOTYPOS KERRIODES (Jet Bead Tree)

A native of Japan, this flowering tree produces drupes called "jet beads." Ingestion by children of 2 or 3 of these attractive drupes has caused dilated pupils, tonic-clonic convulsions and glucosuria—all transient.

53–602. RHUBARB

Ingestion of large amounts of rhubarb greens (leaves or blades) may be dangerous. For signs and symptoms of toxicity and treatment, see *53–501, Oxalic Acid.*

53–602A. RICIN *(See 53–179, Castor Bean Extract)*

53–603. ROACH PASTE *(See 53–90, Arsenic; 53–311, Fluorides)*

53–604. ROCKET FUELS

None of the chemical substances now in use as rocket propellants are new; their properties and toxicities have been well known to chemists, laboratory workers and toxicologists for many years. What is new is the utilization of their peculiar physical and chemical properties in rocketry. Elaborate methods for protection from toxic effects of persons working with tremendous amounts of these dangerous substances have been put in effect, so far successfully. Protection of the general public from transportation accidents, wind-blown fumes, explosions, etc., so far has been effective.

The following list contains some of the chemicals in use at the present time, with a notation regarding toxicity or other dangerous characteristics.

Rocket Fuel	Characteristics and Toxicity
Ammonia	Fumes acutely toxic (53–*61*)
Anhydrous hydrazine	Explosive; fumes toxic
Aniline	Acutely toxic (53–*75*)
Boron derivatives	Flammable; fumes acutely toxic; all exposed personnel required to wear special masks and protective clothing.
Chlorine trifluoride	Reacts violently; toxic effects of both chlorine (53–*192*) and fluorides (53–*311*)
Decaborane	See *Boron derivatives* (earlier in table). In addition, borates break into flame on contact with the atmosphere; therefore, special containers are necessary for transportation. Boron fires cannot be controlled by the usual methods.
Diborane	See *Decaborane* (earlier in table).
Ethyl nitrate	Will explode when exposed to slight shock or temperature variations; fumes acutely toxic.
Fluorine (liquid)	Will ignite spontaneously in the presence of another chemical (hypergolic); fumes toxic.
Fuming nitric acid	Hypergolic; fumes toxic (53–482); severe burns on contact.
Hydrazine	See *Anhydrous hydrazine* (earlier in table).

Table continued on following page

*For therapeutic considerations see also 53–*1* to 53–*13*.

Rocket Fuel	Characteristics and Toxicity
Hydrogen (liquid)	Explosive. Exposure to air may result in severe burns before the presence of a fire is recognized, since hydrogen burns with a completely nonluminous flame.
Hydrogen peroxide (90%)	Explosive; causes severe burns on contact; fumes toxic.
Isocyanates	Toxic; see 53–232 *Cyanides*.
LOX	See *Oxygen (liquid)* (later in table).
Mixed amines	Ignite spontaneously on contact with nitric acid (hypergolic).
Nitrogen tetraoxide	Must be kept absolutely dry; in presence of moisture forms nitric acid. See 53–502, *Oxides of Nitrogen*.
Nitroglycerin	Extremely sensitive to percussion; see 53–484, *Nitrites*.
Oxygen (liquid)	Acutely flammable; reacts violently with hydrocarbons and other combustible materials.
Pentaborane	See *Decaborane* (earlier in table)
Perchlorates	Break down into hydrochloric acid and corrosive substances.
UDMH (unsymmetrical dimethylhydrazine)	Highly explosive, flammable; fumes toxic. Based on experimental evidence, injection of pyridoxine hydrochloride, 25 mg/kg, has been recommended.

53–605. ROSEMARY

Oil of rosemary is used medicinally as a rubefacient but is extremely toxic if ingested. Signs and symptoms include nausea; vomiting; severe gastric pain; rapid, weak pulse; hyperactive reflexes; pulmonary edema *(55)*; marked albuminuria; collapse; and coma.

53–606. ROTENONE ($C_{23}H_{22}O_6$; TLV 5 mg/m^3) *(See 53–245, Derris; 53–584, Pyrethrum)*

Rotenone is widely used as an insecticide, often in combination with DDT *(53–240)* and pyrethrum *(53–584)*, because it has a low toxicity for plants and animals. No human fatalities have been reported.

53–607. RUBBING ALCOHOL *(See 53–295, Ethyl Alcohol; 53–372, Isopropyl Alcohol)*

Contrary to common belief, rubbing alcohol never contains methanol.

53–608. RUMEX ACETOSA L. (Sorrel)

In some localities sorrel is sometimes used as a salad green. Ingestion of large amounts gives a toxic picture similar to that caused by rhubarb *(53–602)*, owing to the oxalate content. (See *53–501, Oxalic Acid.*)

53–609. SACCHARIN (Glucide, Saccharinol) ($C_7H_5NO_3S$)

Commonly used as a sugar substitute in diabetic or reducing diets, this benzoic acid derivative may give toxic reactions in hypersensitive persons or if excessively large doses are ingested. *Signs and symptoms* include loss of appetite, nausea, vomiting, gastric cramps and pain, diarrhea, acute myalgia with muscular fibrillation and twitching, delirium and hallucinations (especially auditory).

53–610. SAFFRON

The stigmas of the crocus plant contain saffron. Although oil of saffron is occasionally used as a flavoring and coloring agent, most of the cases of acute toxicity that have been

---

*For therapeutic considerations see also *53–1* to *53–13*.

reported have been caused by drinking extremely strong teas or concentrated decoctions in attempts to induce abortions.

Signs and symptoms of saffron poisoning consist of vomiting of blood-tinged material; severe gastric pain; bloody diarrhea; rapid, weak pulse; hypotension; hematuria; convulsions; and coma. The prognosis is good with general treatment although irritative symptoms referable to the stomach, intestines and kidneys may persist for several weeks.

53–611. SAFROLE ($C_{10}H_{10}O_2$)

Safrole, the active ingredient in oil of sassafras and Macassar oil, is extremely toxic. Ingestion of a few milliliters has caused vomiting, hallucinations, vascular collapse and coma. Local application of oil of sassafras to the scalp has caused vertigo, stupor, aphasia and circulatory collapse. Psychic disturbances may persist for weeks after other symptoms have cleared.

53–612. SAGE

Oil of sage if ingested in small amounts may cause marked dyspnea; weak, rapid pulse; lowered blood pressure; shock *(57)*; and epileptiform convulsions.

53–613. SALICYLANILIDE (Ansadol, Shirlan) ($C_{13}H_{11}NO_2$)

Used for mildew control and as a fungicide, salicylanilide can cause both aniline and salicylate poisoning by inhalation or by ingestion. For treatment, see *53–75, Aniline; 53–614, Salicylates.*

53–614. SALICYLATES ($C_7H_5O_3^{1-}$) *(See also 53–101, Aspirin; 53–444, Methyl Salicylate)*

Salicylic acid and all of the soluble salicylates may cause additive severe toxic signs and symptoms, grouped under the heading of "salicylism"; toxicity occurs through skin absorption as well as by ingestion. The widespread use of oil of wintergreen *(53–444, Methyl Salicylate)* and candy-coated "baby aspirin" tablets makes therapeutic and accidental poisoning relatively common in children; the highest mortality is in the 1 to 4 age group. Any dosage over 65 mg per year of age every 4 hours will produce acute toxic signs and symptoms in a child less than 8 years old in a short time; if renal function is impaired even smaller doses may be dangerous. The minimal lethal dose of acetylsalicylic acid (aspirin) is usually considered to be between 0.3 and 0.4 g/kg. Peak serum salicylate levels are usually reached about 2 hours after ingestion and may be roughly estimated by the following equation:

$$\frac{\text{Amount ingested in milligrams}}{\text{Total body water (70\% of body wt. in grams)}} \times 100 = \begin{array}{c}\text{Mg of salicylate per}\\ \text{dl of serum}\end{array}$$

For assistance in clinical evaluation of the severity of peak serum salicylate levels after a single dose, see Figure 53–3 (this nomogram does not apply to chronic exposures to salicylates). For qualitative test for salicylates, see *19–7, Salicylate Ingestion Test.* Adjust interpretation of the serum salicylate level in association with concomitantly determined arterial pH.

The clinical picture of salicylate intoxication consists of faintness, tinnitus, loss of hearing, disturbed vision, nausea, vomiting, gastrointestinal hemorrhage and dehydration; it may suggest a viral infection syndrome in the young. There may be an acetone odor on the breath (for methyl salicylate only). Salicylism and diabetes *(32–3)* may give practically the same clinical picture of acidosis and increased glucose levels. However, grossly depressed glucose levels may also be noted. Rapid hyperpneic ("panting dog") respiration if most common in children. Cyanosis is usually present. Edema of the larynx may be serious. Convulsions (especially in children), delirium, coma and hemorrhage secondary to hypoprothrombinemia may occur. Ingestion of massive doses can cause death through acidosis, electrolyte imbalance, irreversible respiratory collapse and pulmonary edema. See also effect of salicylates in Reye's syndrome (33–55).

---

*For therapeutic considerations see also *53–1* to *53–13*.

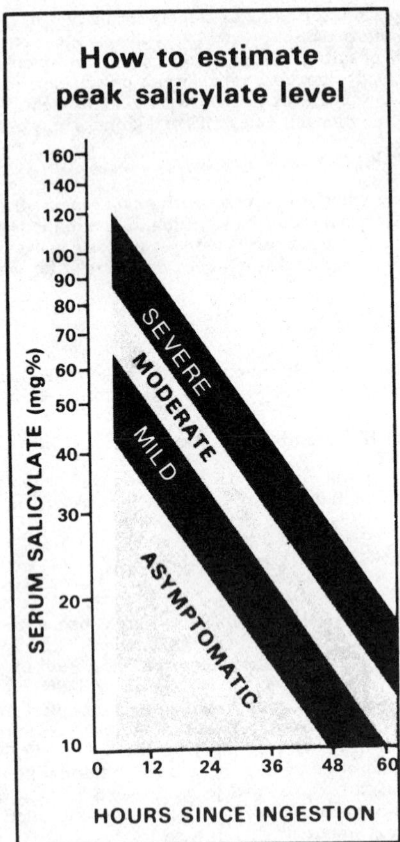

Figure 53–3. Hours after a single aspirin overdose it is possible to estimate peak salicylate level and severity of intoxication by using this nomogram. (From Done, A. K.: Pediatrics, 26:800, 1960.)

Treatment

Therapy for salicylate overdosage should be monitored by frequent tests of serum salicylate level and acid-base and electrolyte studies; higher acidity is more toxic.

If the peak serum salicylate level [24 hours after single ingestion for aspirin *(53–101)*; much longer for oil of wintergreen *(53–444)*] is below 30 mg/dl, little further treatment (after preventing further absorption) is required—spontaneous recovery will take place. Clinical status, however, must be the guide if there has been multiple or chronic ingestion of salicylates.

From 40 to 70 mg/dl: Mild symptoms require emptying of the stomach and supportive care. Hospitalization may not be needed if patient is diuresing well and serum salicylate level drops below 40 mg/dl, although the patient should be kept under close observation for several hours.

---

*For therapeutic considerations see also *53–1* to *53–13*.

From 70 to 100 mg/dl: Moderate to severe toxic symptoms are to be expected. The patient should be hospitalized and aggressively treated; treatment should include repeat doses of charcoal and diuresis.

From 100 to 140 mg/dl or more: Severe, critical symptoms (hyperventilation, acute dehydration, severe metabolic acidosis, convulsions, coma) require treatment as indicated below, including possible dialysis. Noncardiogenic pulmonary edema can occur.

Treatment of Severe Salicylate Intoxication

- Immediate emptying of the stomach by emetics or gastric lavage with water, followed by activated charcoal in water orally or through the lavage tube. Since spontaneous stomach emptying is often delayed after ingestion of salicylates, it is infrequent that emesis or gastric lavage is not indicated.
- Copious amounts of fluids intravenously and orally to increase renal excretion. IV isotonic solutions (lactated Ringer's solution, normal saline, D5W or 1.25% sodium bicarbonate depending on the status of the acidosis), can be started with an initial infusion rate of 1 to 2 L/hr, then dropped to 500 ml/hr and repeated as necessary according to arterial pH level and electrolyte and serum salicylate levels. Discontinue rapid fluid infusion after salicylate level is less than 40 mg/dl, or if monitoring indicates beginning fluid overload or a decrease in renal status is noted.
- Sodium bicarbonate solution IV to combat severe metabolic acidosis and to alkalinize the urine. Monitor with ABG's. Avoid use of acetazolamide (Diamox) in alkalinizing the urine.
- Potassium chloride IV or PO in large doses, provided urine output is adequate.
- If oliguria persists, give a trial of 20% solution of mannitol (1 g/kg) IV, at a rate of 1 ml/min, or furosemide), 20–40 mg, to increase renal clearance.
- If large fluid volumes are needed, and oxygenation, blood pressure or urine output are abnormal, monitor CVP.
- Control of hyperpyrexia by cooling blankets or other means.
- If treatment as outlined above has not resulted in definite clinical and serum level improvement, then hemodialysis or hemoperfusion should be done. If not available, peritoneal dialysis should be done and repeated 2 to 3 times if necessary. The dialysis fluid should consist of 5% human albumin in an electrolyte solution (Albumisol), to which 5 mEq/L of potassium has been added.
- Patients with moderate to severe salicylate intoxication should receive parenteral vitamin K therapy. Treat any hypoglycemia.

53–615. SALT *(See also 53–636, Sodium Chloride)*

Several series of accidental severe poisoning in nursery infants have been reported. Severe toxic symptoms have followed the use of a strong solution of table salt as a household emetic.

53–616. SALTPETER (Potassium Nitrate)

Potassium nitrate is used in the manufacture of gunpowder and fireworks, as a fertilizer, in the chemical industry and as a constituent of some proprietary asthma remedies *(53–102)*. Use as a food preservative and medicinally for suppression of sexual excitement is no longer common. Chile saltpeter is sodium nitrate. See also *53–481, Nitrates; 53–484, Nitrites.*

53–617. SAMARIUM CHLORIDE

This is a by-product of the uranium industry. Like gadolinium chloride *(53–321)*, it is toxic to laboratory animals, but there have been no reports of human toxicity.

53–618. SAPONIN

Saponin occurs in many common plants and has the ability to produce foam with water. Ingestion of the seeds may result in acute toxic symptoms. For the toxic picture, see *53–38, Agrostemma Githago.*

---

*For therapeutic considerations see also *53–1* to *53–13.*

53–619. SCARLET RED (Aminoazotoluene) ($C_{24}H_{20}N_4O$)

In ointment form, scarlet red is used medicinally to promote epithelization. Its attractive color may result in ingestion by children, producing a toxic picture similar to that resulting from absorption from wound surfaces.

Signs and symptoms include nausea, vomiting, abdominal pain, diarrhea, fever, general malaise and hypotension.

53–620. SCOPOLAMINE

An alkaloid occurring naturally in *Datura stramonium* and *Hyoscyamus niger*, scopolamine on ingestion gives a toxic picture resembling that of atropine sulfate. For treatment, see *53–103, Atropine*, and antidote, physostigmine salicylate (*53–10*).

53–621. SCORPION VENOM *(See 60–12, Scorpion Stings)*

53–622. SELENIUM AND ITS SALTS (Se, Se^+)

This nonmetallic element is most dangerous if vaporized; however, its salts are acutely toxic by inhalation of dust or fumes, skin absorption or ingestion. The treatment is the same as that given for arsenic (*53–90*), except that BAL is ineffective and not indicated.

53–623. SENECIO (Golden Ragwort, Squaw Weed)

Several varieties of this South African plant as a contaminant of cereal grains have caused numerous cases of food poisoning, with many fatalities.

Senecio glicifolicus and burchelli seeds cause bloody vomiting, epigastric pain, enlargement of the liver with ascites, pleural effusion and collapse. The mortality rate from this type of poisoning is very high.

Senecio vulgaris (groundsel) seeds cause "bread poisoning" characterized by nausea, vomiting, epigastric pain, bloody diarrhea and evidence of acute liver damage. The presence of ascites makes the prognosis very poor.

Senecio canicida. The toxic principles of this variety are contained in the roots and resemble picrotoxin (*53–549*).

53–624. SESAME OIL (Benne, Teel, Gingilli Oil)

Large doses of this complex mixture of glycerides produce extreme catharsis. Acute dehydration may require oral or intravenous fluid replacement.

53–625. SHEEP DIP *(See 53–90, Arsenic; 53–534, Phenol; 53–715, Toxaphene)*

53–626. SHELLAC

White shellac contains rosin; other colors contain arsenic trisulfide. All varieties are dissolved in ethyl or methyl alcohol to which various aliphatic hydrocarbons and ketones in small amounts have been added. For treatment, see *53–90, Arsenic; 53–426, Methyl Alcohol.*

53–627. SHOE CLEANERS

Usually shoe cleaners contain a small amount of trisodium phosphate with isopropyl alcohol (*53–372*).

53–628. SHOE DYES AND POLISHES *(See 53–75, Aniline Dyes; 53–372, Isopropyl Alcohol; 53–485, Nitrobenzene)*

---

*For therapeutic considerations see also *53–1* to *53–13*.

53–629. SILVER POLISH *(See 53–232)*

53–630. SILVER SALTS AND COMPOUNDS (Ag, $AgNO_3$; TLV 0.01 mg/m^3)

Silver acetate and nitrate are available in many households and are acutely toxic if ingested. Halogen salts of silver are of little or no toxicity. Silver nitrate caustic pencils may be broken up and eaten by children. Less than 2 g is generally harmless; larger amounts may cause burning of the throat and epigastrium, black vomitus, violent abdominal pain and convulsions and coma that may be terminal. After gastric emptying, lavage with saline solution to precipitate the silver ion is advised.

Prognosis is good with small amounts. Ingestion of 2 to 10 mg of silver nitrate may be fatal; more than 10 g almost always causes death.

53–631. SNAIL BAITS *(See 53–424, Metaldehyde)*

Some older proprietary products may contain arsenic *(53–90)*.

53–632. SNAKE VENOM *(See 27–27, Snake Bites)*

53–633. SNUFF *(See 53–478)*

53–634. SOAPS AND DETERGENTS ("Non-Soap" Cleaners)

White, unperfumed household soaps are harmless even if ingested in large quantities; addition of antiseptics, disinfectants, deodorants, coloring or perfume may cause nausea, vomiting and mild gastrointestinal irritation but no life-threatening symptoms. Some laundry soaps contain enough caustic alkalies to cause severe mucous membrane damage and require treatment as with other alkalies *(53–45)*, together with fluid replacement if vomiting has been prolonged.

Household detergents are divided into 3 classes, depending on the purpose for which they are intended.

Class 1. Light-duty, high sudsing: for dishes, baby clothes, etc.—these are slightly toxic.

Class 2. All-purpose, high sudsing: for laundry and general use—moderately toxic.

Class 3. Washday, low sudsing: Made for use in automatic washers—relatively high toxicity.

Deaths from ingestion have been reported.

Treatment for Classes 1 and 2

- Immediate dilution with copious amounts of water.
- Induction of vomiting if large amounts have been swallowed and vomiting has not already occurred. After the stomach has been emptied, activated charcoal in water should be given by mouth.
- Evaluate for presence of hypocalcemia and treat accordingly.

Treatment for Class 3

- Dilution; administration of activated charcoal.
- Gastric lavage (if mucous membrane erosion is not extreme), followed by a saline cathartic.
- Control of pain. Small doses of a narcotic may be required.
- Administration of air or oxygen by face mask and rebreathing bag.
- Endotracheal tube or tracheostomy *(18–34)* for advancing laryngeal edema.
- Recognition and treatment of pulmonary edema *(55)*.
- Hospitalization for prolonged observation, supportive and symptomatic treatment. Permanent strictures of the esophagus may occur.

Treatment of cationic detergent poisoning may require management of seizures *(34)* but otherwise is supportive and symptomatic, as is also the case for anionic and nonionic detergent poisoning.

---

*For therapeutic considerations see also *53–1* to *53–13*.

53–635. SODIUM ARSENATE AND ARSENITE

These contain about 50 and 75% arsenic respectively and, because they are very soluble, are extremely toxic. See 53–90, *Arsenic*.

53–636. SODIUM CHLORIDE (Salt) (NaCl) *(See also 46–10, Hypernatremia)*

Common table salt in excess can cause severe toxic effects in infants and small children, characterized by nausea, vomiting, excitement, hypertonicity, extensor spasticity, convulsions and eventual coma. *Table salt and water should never be used as an emetic.*

Treatment

- Control of hypertonicity and convulsions by sedatives and rehydration.
- Prevention of dehydration and potassium depletion *(11, Fluid Replacement)*.
- Removal of salt as by repeated peritoneal dialyses *(18–24)*, using 5% dextrose plus potassium in water as the dialysate, may be necessary in severe cases.

53–637. SODIUM CYANIDE (NaCN)

Inhalation or ingestion of even minute amounts may be fatal. See 53–232, *Cyanides*.

53–638. SODIUM FLUOROACETATE *(See also 53–312, Fluoracetates)*

Sodium fluoroacetate is a tremendously toxic substance that occurs naturally in a South African plant *(Dichapetalum cymosum)* that has caused many fatalities. The synthetic commercial preparation (Compound 1080) is used as a rodenticide. Accidental ingestion of a few crystals has caused tingling around the mouth and nose, severe vomiting, blurred vision from loss of focusing ability, epileptiform convulsions, stupor and coma. Gastric lavage followed by magnesium sulfate solution in the stomach is advised. Hospitalization for supportive therapy and close observation for several days is often needed. Delayed hypertension and cardiac dilation may occur. Lidocaine or procainamide (Pronestyl) can be given IV to control ventricular arrhythmia.

53–639. SODIUM HYDROXIDE (Caustic Soda) (NaOH) *(See 53–45, Alkalies)*

53–640. SODIUM ION (Na^{1+}) *(See 46–18, Hypernatremia)*

53–641. SODIUM NITRITE ($NaNO_2$) *(See 53–484, Nitrites)*

53–642. SODIUM SULFIDE (Na_2S)

Usually mixed with barium sulfide or thallium salts, sodium sulfide is the main active agent in many depilatories (hair removers). Toxic effects following ingestion are due partly to local corrosive action on the mucous membranes and partly to formation of hydrogen sulfide *(53–353)* and consist of foul breath from the odor of hydrogen sulfide; a burning sensation in the mouth, throat and stomach; rapid onset of pulmonary irritation and pulmonary edema *(55)*. Convulsions and coma followed by death from respiratory paralysis may occur. Hospitalize for observation for at least 24 hours after control of the acute signs and symptoms. Pulmonary edema *(55)* may also be a late complication.

53–643. SOIL FUMIGANTS *(See 53–238, DD Compounds; 53–736, Vapam)*

---

*For therapeutic considerations see also 53–*1* to 53–*13*.

53–644. SOLANINE

A mixture of very toxic glucosides, including solanine, is present in several species of plants. Among these are the following:

Bittersweet (Dulcamara). The toxic alkaloid occurs in the leaves, berries and seeds of this common North American and European plant. Green berries contain large amounts of solanine and dulcamerin; ripe berries, very little.

Jerusalem Cherry. The fruit contains a large amount of solanine and is extremely poisonous.

Nightshade. The green, unripened berries and the leaves of several varieties (deadly nightshade, black cherry, blue nightshade, climbing nightshade, woody nightshade) of this plant are toxic; the ripe berries are relatively nontoxic.

Potato. In the sprouts, leaves, berries and seeds.

Tomato. In the leaves and stems. The green fruit of wild tomato (horse nettle, sand briar) also contains solanine.

Signs and symptoms: Poisoning is usually delayed for 1 to 3 hours after ingestion; symptoms consist of a cold, clammy skin; nausea; vomiting; multiple soft stools; mental confusion; delirium; muscular twitching; mydriasis; and acute respiratory and cardiac depression. Since delayed toxic effects may occur, have patient observed for at least 6 hours after ingestion.

53–645. SOMINEX

This proprietary preparation, extensively advertised as a safe somnifacient, has caused numerous cases of acute toxicity due to its scopolamine content. See *53–103, Atropine; 53–620, Scopolamine.*

53–646. SPANISH BAYONET (Yucca)

Plants of this family contain toxic saponins, which on ingestion produce irritation of the gastrointestinal tract. See *53–233, Cyclamen.*

53–647. "SPEEDBALLS"

A "speedball" is generally a combination of cocaine and heroin. Euphoria and stimulation are the objective, but psychoses and hyperthermia are among the adverse effects. Two well-known preparations have been substituted by ingeniously minded individuals—often narcotic addicts—for the more difficult to obtain drugs, cocaine and heroin. These are Percodan, a proprietary preparation containing dehydrocodeinone, homatropine, acetylsalicylic acid, acetophenetidin and caffeine in a nonsterile tablet for oral use, and methamphetamine hydrochloride (Methedrine). These and other combinations may be used intravenously, and neither quality nor quantity of medications can be predicted from a given street name.

53–648. SPIDER LILY

The bulbs contain a toxic alkaloid (lycocine). Fatalities are rare because of its rapid irritant action on the stomach.

53–649. SPIDER VENOM *(See 27–28, Spider Bites)*

53–650. SQUILL (Sea Onion)

White squill is used medicinally as a diuretic and cardiac agent; red squill is used as a rat poison. The toxicity and treatment are practically the same as outlined in *53–265, Digitalis.*

53–651. SQUIRREL POISONS

These preparations usually contain sodium fluoroacetate *(53–638)*, thallium *(53–692)* or strychnine *(53–659)*.

---

*For therapeutic considerations see also *53–1* to *53–13*.

53–652. STAGGERBUSH

Staggerbush contains andromedotoxin, which may cause toxic effects that may be mistaken for acute alcoholic intoxication. The action is primarily a peripheral paralysis of the vagus and depression of the brain associated with a voluntary muscle effect similar to that caused by curare *(53–231)*.

53–653. STANNIC AND STANNOUS SALTS *(See 53–707, Tin)*

53–654. STAR ANISE

This plant belongs to the magnolia family. Ingestion of its seeds may result in toxic symptoms similar to those caused by picrotoxin *(53–549)*.

53–655. STAR OF BETHLEHEM (Snowdrop)

Star of Bethlehem contains a toxic resin similar to that described under milkweed *(53–448)*.

53–656. STODDARD SOLVENT (TLV 100 ppm)

This is a petroleum distillate composed of approximately 20% aromatic hydrocarbons and 80% paraffin and naphthenic hydrocarbons; it has about the same toxicity as kerosene. For treatment, see 53–379, *Kerosene*.

53–657. STRAMONIUM

Stramonium is found in common plants (jimsonweed, stinkweed, thorn apple, etc.) in many localities. The toxicity and treatment are similar to that outlined for *Atropine Sulfate (53–103)*. It has a mild hallucinogenic effect *(53–332)*. Stramonium poisoning has been reported following ingestion by immature persons of Asthamaclor, a stramonium-belladonna mixture.

53–658. STREPTOKINASE (Kabikinase, Streptase)

Streptokinase is being used more frequently now for clot lysis in acute MI and massive pulmonary embolism.

Allergic reactions to this mixture of proteolytic enzymes have been reported. These include chills, restlessness, apprehension, profuse perspiration, chest pain, dyspnea and anaphylactic shock. Bleeding is another major complication. For treatment, see 24, *Allergic Reactions*. There is no known specific treatment other than supportive care and blood replacement.

53–659. STRYCHNINE *(Nux Vomica)* ($C_{21}H_{22}N_2O_2$; TLV 0.15 mg/m^3)

Strychnine is an alkaloid contained in the seeds of the nux vomica plant. It is a powerful glycine antagonist poison that formerly had wide use medicinally as a tonic and respiratory stimulant and commercially as a glycine antagonist rodenticide. Its presence in old patent medicines (usually laxatives and tonics), which may contain appreciable quantities, constitutes a household hazard for children. Strychnine acts by increasing the reflex excitement of the spinal cord and the medullary center. The toxic picture can be confused with acute tetanus *(33–68)* and is characterized by dyspnea, cyanosis, a feeling of suffocation, profuse perspiration, opisthotonos and tetanic convulsions. No matter how acute the poisoning, the patient is fully conscious.

Treatment Includes:

- Absolute rest in a quiet room to prevent initiation of tetanic convulsions by external stimuli.

---

*For therapeutic considerations see also *53–1* to *53–13*.

- Activated charcoal in water by mouth. Unless the patient is seen within a few minutes of ingestion or is asymptomatic regarding hypertonicity, *do not give emetics or attempt gastric lavage unless the airway is controlled and IV medication for relaxation is ready.*
- IV diazepam or phenobarbital for control of convulsions or severe muscle spasms, repeated as necessary.
- Assistance with ventilation by mechanical methods *(5–10)* if necessary. Muscle paralyzation and intubation may be indicated in severe cases.
- Hospitalization for close observation and symptomatic treatment. Relapses after several hours are common.

DO NOT USE

Emetics of any type. Once the patient is symptomatic, choking, strangling and aspiration of vomitus may result, and emetics should be avoided.

Gastric Lavage. If the patient is not seen within 10 minutes and is asymptomatic, attempts to empty the stomach should be postponed until reflex irritability, convulsions and the airway have been completely controlled.

Caffeine. It increases the strychnine effect.

Bromides. Their action is too slow to be beneficial.

Opiates of synthetic narcotics. Acute respiratory depression may result.

Cathartics, purgatives or diuretics. They are of no value.

PROGNOSIS. Good if the patient can be kept alive for 5 to 6 hours.

53–660. SULFONAMIDES

Some of the sulfonamides are oral, including salicylazosulfapyridine (Azulfidine), sulfadiazine (Suladyne), sulfamethizole (Thiosulfil), sulfamethoxazole (Gantanol), sulfisoxazole (Gantrisin), and others are administered IV, such as Septra, a combination of sulfamethoxazole and trimethoprim.

All may give toxic reactions following overdose or accidental ingestion of large amounts. Some persons may demonstrate hypersensitivity to small doses. Toxic manifestations of greater or lesser degree occur in about 50% of adults and 20% of children. Although the symptoms may be alarming, few fatalities have been reported.

Minor toxic effects consist of fever, usually accompanied by skin rashes suggestive of measles; pruritus, cyanosis, gastrointestinal irritation; precordial and abdominal pain; acidosis; central nervous system disturbances; confusion; restlessness; headache; vertigo; nausea; vomiting; depression (or elation); and lassitude. The medication should be discontinued and, if necessary, another type of antimicrobial substituted.

Dangerous toxic effects are characterized by the following:

Skin Rashes. Generalized serious exfoliative dermatitis (see *58–8A, Toxic Epidermal Necrolysis)* may occur, sometimes associated with hepatitis.

Jaundice. Acute hemolysis apparently has no relationship to the level of sulfonamides in the blood. There is usually an associated hemoglobinuria.

Toxic nephrosis.

Acute hemolytic anemia with hemoglobinuria, severe leukopenia and agranulocytosis.

Crystalluria.

Renal calculi with resultant suppression of kidney function.

53–661. SULFUR (S)

Sulfur has a relatively low toxicity. Toxic signs and symptoms may develop after ingestion of large amounts that break down in the large intestine to hydrogen sulfide *(53–353).*

53–662. SULFUR CHLORIDE (S_2Cl_2)

Sulfur chloride is a commonly used insecticide that in the presence of moisture breaks down into hydrochloric acid and sulfur dioxide. For treatment, see *53–33, Acids; 53–663, Sulfur Dioxide.*

---

*For therapeutic considerations see also *53–1* to *53–13.*

53–663. SULFUR DIOXIDE (SO_2; TLV 5 ppm)

Sulfur dioxide is used as an insecticide and as a food preservative. It is one of the toxic components of the "smog" common in highly industrialized areas. Even moderate concentrations cause irritation of the upper respiratory tract (choking, coughing, sneezing, dyspnea, cyanosis), asthma *(54–6)* and pulmonary edema *(55)*. Acidosis *(46–1)* may develop. Convulsions and reflex respiratory arrest may be terminal.

53–664. SULFURIC ACID (Oil of Vitriol) (H_2SO_4; TLV 1 mg/m^3) *(See 53–33, Acids)*

53–665. SULFURYL CHLORIDE (SO_2Cl_2)

Inhalation of the fumes of this solvent, used in the chemical and rubber industries, causes severe mucous membrane and skin irritation with conjunctivitis, palpebral edema, rhinitis, tracheitis, bronchitis and pneumonitis. The patient should be removed from exposure and given inhalations.

53–666. SULINDAC (Clinoril)

This antiarthritic medication is a nonsteroidal, anti-inflammatory agent. Adverse reactions that can occur include nausea, vomiting, peptic ulcer, gastrointestinal bleeding, liver function abnormalities and edema; increased prothrombin time in patients on oral anticoagulants; and some hypersensitivity and dermatologic problems. There is no specific antidote; see general measures *(53–2, 53–4)*. Other drugs in the same category include ibuprofen (Motrin), indomethacin (Indocin), tolmetin (Tolectin) and Naproxen (Naprosyn).

53–667. SUN TAN CREAMS AND LOTIONS

These cosmetic preparations are used as "sun screens" to absorb ultraviolet rays and to prevent sunburn and usually contain dicumarol and amyl salicylate. Toxic effects from skin absorption usually do not develop except in allergic individuals. If ingested, severe toxic effects may develop due to the dicumarol *(53–258)* and the salicylate content.

53–668. SWEET PEAS

The stalks and stems of sweet peas contain active toxic alkaloids and beta-amino proprionitrite. Ingestion of large amounts has been known to cause cerebral motor paralysis and acute cardiac depression. The clinical syndrome from ingestion resembles that of curare ingestion 53–231 and is known as lathyrism *(53–314, Rare causes of food poisoning)*.

53–669. TALC (French Chalk) ($Mg_3Si_4O_{10}[OH]_2$; TLV 6 mg/m^3)

Talc (magnesium silicate) is harmless unless large amounts are aspirated, but some popular brands of talcum powder contain a considerable amount of boric acid *(53–140)* and zinc stearate *(53–763)*.

53–670. TANACETUM VULGARE (Tansy)

The stems and leaves of this perennial plant contain a mixture of toxic terpenes and volatile oils. "Therapeutic" doses given as abortifacients and anthelminthics have been fatal.

53–671. TANNIC ACID (Tannin) ($C_{27}H_{24}O_{18}$[Corilagin])

If ingested, this powerful astringent will cause uncomfortable but never fatal signs and symptoms, including nausea, vomiting, gastritis and lower bowel disturbances.

---

*For therapeutic considerations see also *53–1* to *53–13*.

In contrast, by injection it is a deadly poison and may cause severe convulsions, circulatory or respiratory collapse, or both, and death from hepatic necrosis.

53–672. TAR

All types and derivatives of tar are toxic if ingested, because of their cresol content. Tar is found in many medicinal scalp shampoos. For signs and symptoms of toxicity and treatment, see *53–534, Phenol.*

53–673. TARTARIC ACID ($C_4H_6O_6$)

Although relatively nontoxic, large doses of tartaric acid may cause severe signs and symptoms. Fatalities have been reported.

Signs and symptoms include nausea, vomiting, severe abdominal cramping, diarrhea and circulatory collapse. Tartar emetic is antimony *(53–81)* and potassium tartrate.

53–674. TAXUS BACCATA L. (English Yew)

The leaves, the stems and, to a lesser extent, the fruit of this ornamental evergreen tree contain taxines, toxic substances that, if ingested, cause dry mouth, mydriasis, vomiting, gastric and abdominal pain, pallor, dizziness, hypotension and respiratory and cardiac conduction blockade (which may require a temporary pacemaker) with secondary arrhythmia. Onset of symptoms is usually within 1 to 3 hours. Anaphylactoid reactions have been reported from chewing the needles.

53–675. TCA (Trichloracetic Acid)

This is a powerful local caustic but has no systemic toxic actions. See *53–33, Acids.*

53–676. TCE (Tetrachlorethane)

TCE is similar in action to, but more dangerous than, carbon tetrachloride. For treatment, see *53–176, Carbon Tetrachloride.*

53–677. TCDD *(See also 53–276, Dioxin)*

TCDD is the most toxic of the 75 or so compounds in the dioxin family of chemicals. It is 2,3,7,8-tetrachlorodibenzo-p-dioxin. It breaks down slowly in the body, persists in the environment and is the most prevalent source of dioxin.

53–678. TDE (Tetrachlorodiphenylethane)

Used as an insecticide, TDE is much safer than most of the other preparations used for the same purpose. Signs and symptoms of toxicity following inhalation or ingestion (general malaise, prostration and collapse) are usually relatively mild, with recovery in 2 to 4 days without residual ill effects. Treatment is similar to that outlined for DDT *(53–240).*

53–679. TEETHING POWDERS

These usually contain calomel *(53–164)* with talc *(53–669)* or chalk. Some brands contain small amounts of boric acid or borates *(53–140)* and bromides *(53–146).*

53–680. TEFLON *(See 53–555, Plastics)*

Fine Teflon dust causes a condition similar to metal fume fever *(53–423).* Inhalation of fumes has been reported to cause pulmonary edema *(55).* Though nontoxic when in contact with the skin, recent casting of bullets with Teflon can greatly increase bodily injury from deeper penetration in gunshot wounds.

---

*For therapeutic considerations see also *53–1* to *53–13.*

53–681. TELLURIUM (Te; TLV 0.1 mg/m^3)

Most of the cases of toxicity from tellurium are caused by inhalation of the fumes of the oxide. A garlicky odor to the breath is characteristic, with gastric pain, fatigue and severe headache. Accidental ingestion of potassium tellurite has resulted in a similar picture, followed by cyanosis, dyspnea, hepatic involvement and death.

53–682. TERPINEOL (Lilacin) ($C_{10}H_{18}O$)

This toxic substance occurs in pine oil and because of its attractive lilac odor is a constituent of many perfumes and cosmetics. Ingestion of preparations containing terpineol in even small amounts may cause acute gastritis (sometimes hemorrhagic), general malaise, weakness, decreased body temperature, vertigo, excitement, drowsiness, convulsions and other signs of central nervous system disturbances and respiratory depression. See also 53–730, *Turpentine.*

53–683. TERPIN HYDRATE ($C_{10}H_{20}O_2$)

This commonly used expectorant in large doses can give a toxic picture similar to that of turpentine. See also 53–730, *Turpentine.*

53–684. TETRACHLORODIPHENYLETHANE (DDD)

This insecticide has the same action as, but less toxicity than, DDT (53–240).

53–685. TETRACHLOROETHYLENE ($Cl_2C{=}CCl_2$; TLV 100 ppm) *(See 53–176, Carbon Tetrachloride)*

53–686. TETRAETHYL LEAD ($Pb[C_2H_5]_4$; TLV 0.1 mg/m^3) *(See 53–302, Ethyl Gasoline; 53–323, Gasoline)*

Used as an antiknock component of gasoline, tetraethyl lead may cause toxic symptoms by absorption through the intact skin or by inhalation of the fumes. It is not added to so-called "unleaded" gasoline. Acute poisoning is characterized by sleeplessness, restlessness, mental confusion, hallucinations, delirium and maniacal outbursts. Later developments are tremors, fibrillary twitching, myoclonus and spasticity.

53–687. TETRAETHYLPYROPHOSPHATE (TEPP, Nifos, Tetrin) ($[C_2H_5]_4P_2O_7$; TLV 0.004 ppm) *(See 53–497, Organic Phosphates)*

53–688. TETRAFLUOROETHYLENE *(See 53–555, Plastics)*

53–689. TETRAHYDRONAPHTHALENE (Tetralin)

Inhalation of the fumes of this commercial solvent for fats, oils and waxes causes severe headache, acute conjunctivitis, nasotracheobronchitis and nephritic irritation, with grass-green urine. If toxic nephritis develops, it usually clears in 7 to 10 days without permanent ill effects.

53–690. TETRAMETHYLTHIURAM DISULFIDE *(See 53–702, Thiram)*

53–691. TETRAODONTIAE *(See also 53–314, Rare causes of food poisoning)*

The viscera, especially the ovaries, of this world-wide variety of edible fish contain an extremely toxic substance, tetradotoxin, that is heat resistant and not destroyed by usual

---

*For therapeutic considerations see also *53–1* to *53–13.*

cooking methods and that varies in amount in different species in different seasons. Local names for the fish vary in different countries—in Australia they are called toadfish, in Great Britain puffers, in the Hawaiian Islands death fish or mahimahi, in Japan fugus, in the Philippines botete, in South Africa blaasoportoby and in the United States blowfish, jugfish or puffers.

The clinical picture of poisoning from all types develops at any time up to 36 hours after ingestion and is characterized by facial tingling, numbness of the extremities, intense pruritus, vomiting, abdominal pain, arthralgia, myalgia, paralysis and prostration. Hypotension may reach shock levels.

53–692. THALLIUM (Tl; TLV 0.1 mg/m^3)

Thallium is handled by the cells in a manner similar to potassium. With or without the sulfides of barium *(53–111)* and sodium, thallium acetate was formerly used in depilatories (hair removers) in spite of the fact that it is only slightly less toxic than arsenic *(53–90)*. Alopecia occurs. Thallium sulfate is the active toxic ingredient in some brands of pesticides, ant poisons *(53–76)* and rodenticides *(53–651, Squirrel Poisons)*.

Toxic signs and symptoms usually develop 1 to 2 hours after ingestion but may be delayed for as long as 36 hours if thallium has been administered medicinally.

Signs and symptoms of thallium poisoning consist of nausea, vomiting, severe abdominal pain, bloody diarrhea, ulcerative stomatitis, bizarre paresthesias, ptosis, strabismus, mydriasis, facial palsies, superficial ecchymoses and petechiae, convulsions, delirium and delayed respiratory failure. Potassium chloride, 1.5 g 2 to 3 times per day for 5 days, helps to reduce intracellular distribution of thallium. Careful observation of a patient undergoing potassium therapy should be done because of transient increases of blood thallium and potassium levels.

53–693. THEOBROMINE

Occurring naturally in cacao beans, tea and cola nuts, theobromine was used medicinally in the past as a myocardial stimulant and diuretic. Large doses (2 to 5 g) may cause severe headaches, nausea, vomiting, gastric pain, diarrhea, acute excitement and tremors. See *53–159, Caffeine*, for treatment.

53–694. THEOPHYLLINE (Aminophylline) ($C_7H_8N_4O_2$)

Theophylline, the active ingredient of aminophylline, acts as a bronchodilator, pulmonary vasodilator and smooth muscle relaxant, as well as having the properties of other xanthine derivatives (diuretic, coronary vasodilator and cerebral and cardiac stimulant). The toxic effects of theophylline—tachypnea, tachycardia, dysrhythmia, irritability and restlessness—may mimic some signs of exacerbation of chronic asthma or obstructive pulmonary emphysema, the conditions for which theophylline is most often prescribed. Immediate blood serum theophylline concentration delineates the status; adverse reactions most often occur when serum levels exceed 20 mg/L (or μg/ml). The smallest size suppositories commercially available (0.25 g) can cause an acute toxic state in children under 3 years of age; therefore use of theophylline in children under the age of 12 is best avoided.

Treatment

- If potential overdose is established and the patient has not had a seizure: Induce vomiting, administer a cathartic (particularly to propel sustained-release preparations) and administer activated charcoal. (Doses of GI charcoal have been shown to even reduce the half-life of IV-administered theophylline.)
- If the patient is having a seizure: Control seizure *(34)* and maintain airway *(5–10)*. Empty stomach with lavage and proceed otherwise as above, plus supportive measures and repeat doses of charcoal every 6 hours. Rapid metabolism/clearance often obviates the need for hemoperfusion or hemodialysis, although these are indicated in patients with severe toxicity.

---

*For therapeutic considerations see also *53–1* to *53–13*.

53–695. THIAMINE HYDROCHLORIDE (Vitamin B_1 Hydrochloride)

Hypersensitivity reactions are common not only in patients receiving thiamine to correct B_1 deficiency but also in pharmaceutical workers. In addition to pruritus, urticaria, angioneurotic edema and respiratory distress may occur. For treatment, see 24, *Allergic Reactions*.

53–696. THIAZIDE DIURETICS

Note: The furosemide (Lasix) type diuretics are not members of this group. Among available preparations are the following:

Benzthiazide (Aquatag, ExNa)
Bendroflumethiazide (Naturetin)
Chlorothiazide (Diuril)
Cyclothiazide (Anhydron)
Flumethiazide
Hydrochlorothiazide (Esidrix, Hydro-Diuril, Oretic)
Hydroflumethiazide (Saluron)
Methyclothiazide (Enduron)
Polythiazide (Renese)
Trichlormethiazide (Metahydrin, Naqua)

Usual therapeutic doses of any of these may cause many side effects, including aggravation of preexistent systemic conditions, such as diabetes and gout, and accentuation of the effects of drugs such as digitalis. Potassium depletion often requires replacement therapy. Other side effects are muscular weakness, gastroenteritis, pancreatitis, jaundice, hepatic cirrhosis, glomerulonephritis, photosensitization and (rarely) blood dyscrasias.

53–697. THINNER INTOXICATION

Use of paint thinner as an intoxicating agent and hallucinogen has been reported among teenagers. Ordinary paint thinner made up of benzene, butyl acetate, butyl alcohol, ethyl acetate, ethyl alcohol and toluene is used to saturate a handkerchief that is held over the nose. Another method is to spray the thinner into the nose with an ordinary atomizer. Sniffing is further augmented at times by "bagging" (putting the head and intoxicant within a plastic bag)—this adds the further danger of asphyxiation. All degrees of intoxication can be obtained.

Treatment

Treatment is similar to that outlined for acute alcoholic intoxication (53–295). See also 53–323, *Gasoline* and 53–554, *Plastic Glues and Cements*.

53–698. THIOCYANATES (Sulfocyanates, Rhodanates) (SCN^{1-})

Inorganic Salts (ammonium, potassium, sodium, etc.). These present a completely different toxic picture from that given by the more complex organic (aliphatic) thiocyanates.

Average therapeutic doses in certain individuals may cause nausea, vomiting, acute gastric pain, diarrhea, acute depression, exhaustion, edema of the glottis or larynx and signs of hypothyroidism.

Larger doses (with a thiocyanate level greater than 12 mg/100 ml) may cause high fever, angina, gastric hemorrhage, purpura, enlargement of the thyroid, hyperactive reflexes, muscular twitching, convulsions, hallucinations, motor paralysis of the lower extremities, toxic hepatitis, coma and collapse.

Organic (Aliphatic) Derivatives. These substances are used almost exclusively as contact insecticides, usually in kerosene or toluene bases. Not only does their toxicity differ from that of inorganic thiocyanates, but the various members of the aliphatic groups also have different toxic characteristics.

---

*For therapeutic considerations see also 53–*1* to 53–*13*.

Ethyl, Isopropyl and Methyl Thiocyanates. Treat as outlined under 53–232, *Cyanides.*

All Other Derivatives (lauryl, lethane, thanite, etc.) Follow gastric emptying by lavage with at least 100 ml of mineral oil, leaving a small amount of oil, together with 30 g of magnesium sulfate (Epsom salts), in the stomach.

53–699. THIOGLYCOLATES ($C_2H_3NaO_2S$)

These salts are the active ingredients of several "cold-wave" hair setting preparations. On the skin and scalp they may cause acute dermatitis with extreme edema and, occasionally, bleeding. If ingested they have a mild caustic action. Treatment consists of stopping use of the cold-wave preparation.

53–700. THIONYL CHLORIDE (Cl_2OS)

Skin contact may cause first and second degree burns. Inhalation of the fumes results in intense upper respiratory irritation.

Treatment Includes:

- *Do not wash the skin with water unless copious amounts are used;* alternatively, cleanse thoroughly with petroleum solvents.
- Inhalations of 5% sodium bicarbonate mist.
- Symptomatic and supportive therapy.

53–701. THIOURACIL ($C_4H_4N_2OS$)

Used in the treatment of hyperthyroidism, thiouracil and its more modern prototype, propylthiouracil, may cause severe hypersensitivity reactions, parotitis, liver dysfunction, hypothyroidism and agranulocytosis. Exophthalmos from the primary disease may be increased. Blood dyscrasias occur frequently. Discontinue the drug and give supportive treatment. Serious secondary infection may occur, requiring further treatment.

53–702. THIRAM (Tetramethylthiuram Disulfide) ($[(CH_3)_2NCS]_2S_2$; TLV 5 mg/m^3)

This substance is used extensively as a fungicide and in the rubber industry. It is the methyl analogue of disulfiram (Antabuse) and has approximately the same toxic action. For signs and symptoms of toxicity following ingestion of small amounts, see 53–279, *Disulfiram.* If large amounts have been ingested, gastric lavage with copious amounts of water should be done. Ingestion of fats, oils and ethyl alcohol should be avoided for at least 1 week.

53–703. THOMAS SLAG

A by-product of the Thomas steel process, quadribasic calcium phosphate is used in a finely ground state as a fertilizer. Inhalation of the dust causes severe pneumonia.

53–704. THORIUM OXIDE (O_2Th)

Insoluble thorium oxide is a by-product of the uranium industry. Inhalation of dust causes deposits of radioactive particles in the lungs and pulmonary lymph nodes, that are, for practical purposes, permanent.

No serious toxic effects from inhalation of thorium oxide particles have been reported as yet, although a preparation of thorium dioxide (Thorotrast) that was used by IV injection as a roentgenographic contrast medium in the past was related to several radiation-induced malignant tumors of the liver.

53–705. THYMOL ($C_{10}H_{14}O$)

Thymol has been used as an oral antiseptic and mouthwash; as a deodorant in dirty, draining wounds; and as a specific antihookworm agent.

---

*For therapeutic considerations see also *53–1* to *53–13*.

Signs and symptoms of thymol poisoning consist of a sensation of warmth in the stomach, followed by nausea, vomiting and severe epigastric pain. There may be dizziness; ataxia; acute excitement; subnormal temperature; rapid, soft pulse; marked generalized weakness; and collapse with cyanosis.

53–706. THYROID (Crude Thyroid Extract, Synthroid, T_3 or T_4)

Overdosage with thyroid or drugs of similar action (Sodium levothyroxine [Synthroid sodium], sodium liothyronine [Cytomel], thyroglobulin [Proloid]) may result in palpitation, excessive sweating, tremors, nervousness, fever, intolerance to heat, tachycardia, increased pulse pressure, diarrhea and hyperglycemia.

Treatment
- Discontinue or decrease drug dosage.
- In severe acute overdoses, clear stomach by emesis or lavage. Charcoal should be given. Use of propranalol should be considered if severe tachycardia and hypertension are present (see *36–11*).

53–707. TIN (Sn)

Acute tin poisoning is rare but does occur occasionally following ingestion of stannous salts. Usually 5 to 6 hours elapse before vomiting, chest pain, a metallic taste in the mouth and diarrhea develop. Symptoms are usually more uncomfortable than serious and subside after a few hours in response to symptomatic therapy. Organic tin compounds can lead to neurologic emergencies.

53–708. TITANIUM TETRACHLORIDE ($TiCl_4$)

This substance is highly corrosive to soft tissues on contact and its fumes are extremely irritating if inhaled. Severe chemical bronchitis and pneumonia, followed by pulmonary edema (*55*), may be caused by inhalation of a high concentration of fumes. Titanium salts used in paints are harmless. Wash the skin with copious amounts of water to counteract the exothermic reaction.

53–709. TNT *(See 53–725, Trinitrotoluene)*

53–710. TOADSTOOLS *(See 53–322, Galerina Venenata; 53–460, Muscarine; 53–462, Mushroom Poisoning)*

53–711. TOBACCO *(See also 53–209, Cigarettes and Cigars; 53–478, Nicotine)*

Commercial tobacco contains 1 to 2.5% nicotine. A cigarette contains about 15 to 25 mg of nicotine. Except for the fact that tobacco causes vomiting, ingestion of 2 or 3 cigarettes could well be fatal to an adult unaccustomed to tobacco. Fatalities have been reported in small children from ingestion of one half of a cigarette. For treatment of acute toxic effects, see *53–478, Nicotine*. The serious effects from chronic poisoning with tobacco smoke and use are legion. Legislation and organizational policy are increasingly restricting smoking in airlines, hospitals, work sites and other public places to diminish the potential effects of "involuntary smoking."

53–712. TOLUENE (Toluol) ($C_6H_5CH_3$; TLV 100 ppm) *(See 53–117, Benzene [Benzol] and Its Derivatives)*

53–713. TOLUIDINE ($CH_3C_6H_4NH_2$; TLV 5 ppm

Toluidine is similar in action to, but more toxic than, aniline and causes more renal damage. For treatment, see 53–75, *Aniline*.

---

*For therapeutic considerations see also *53–1* to *53–13*.

53–714. TOOTHPASTES AND POWDERS *(See 53–566)*

53–715. TOXAPHENE (Compound 3956, Octochlorocamphene, Chlorinated Camphene) ($C_{10}H_{10}Cl_8$; TLV 0.5 mg/m^3)

Toxaphene is a moderately toxic chlorinated hydrocarbon insecticide and pesticide that is not destroyed by heat; therefore, cases of poisoning from eating cooked vegetables have been reported.

Signs and symptoms from inhalation and ingestion are of about equal intensity. Toxaphene has only a slight irritant effect on the skin and mucous membranes, but inhalation or ingestion may cause dizziness, involuntary muscle tremors and epileptiform convulsions. Treatment is similar to that for other chlorinated hydrocarbons or for benzene hexachloride *(53–118).*

53–716. TREMETOL

A toxic unsaturated alcohol called tremetol is present in many native uncultivated plants in many parts of the United States. It is the cause of "trembles" in cattle and of "milk sickness" in humans resulting from ingestion of milk of animals that have eaten the leaves or shoots. Plants that contain tremetol include deerwort, rayless goldenrod, witchweed, squaw seed, white snakeroot, white sanicle and richweed, all of which are related to *Eupatorium urticaefolium.*

Tremetol intoxication is manifested by the slow onset of toxic effects, beginning with weakness, fatigue, anorexia, subnormal temperature, acetone-like odor on the breath and constipation. Severe vomiting and abdominal pain may develop 24 to 36 hours after ingestion, followed by coma and collapse. The mortality from tremetol poisoning is high (about 50%). If the patient survives the acute stage, it is usually many months before he or she regains full strength and endurance.

53–717. TRIALKYLTHIOPHOSPHATE (Parathion) *(See 53–497, Organic Phosphates)*

53–718. TRICHLOROBENZENE ($C_6H_3Cl_3$)

The fumes of trichlorobenzene, which is used in termite control, may cause mild irritation of the eyes, nose and throat. For treatment, see *53–469, Naphthalene.*

53–719. TRICHLOROETHYLENE (Ethylene Trichloride, Trilene) ($Cl_2C{=}CHCl$.; TLV 100 ppm)

As a solvent for fats and greases in industry, trichloroethylene is used in preference to carbon tetrachloride because inhalation of its fumes does not cause hepatic and renal damage as readily. It is a CNS depressant and is also used medicinally as an anesthetic.

Signs and symptoms following ingestion: Severe burning in mouth, throat, esophagus and stomach; nausea; vomiting; acute excitement followed by depression; hyperactive reflexes; muscular tremors; in severe cases, respiratory or cardiac collapse, or both, with serious liver damage.

Following inhalation of excessive or narcotic concentrations, pallor, profuse perspiration, dyspnea, cyanosis, bradycardia, hypotension and unconsciousness may develop, with death from respiratory or cardiac failure, or a combination of the two.

53–720. TRICHLORONITROMETHANE (Chloropicrin) *(See 53–746, War Gases)*

53–721. 2,4,5-TRICHLOROPHENOXY ACETIC ACID (2-4-5-T)

Used as a weed and shrub killer, 2-4-5-T has toxic effects similar to those of 2-4-D *(53–731).* Of particular concern are cardiac arrhythmias. Dioxin, produced along with 2-

*For therapeutic considerations see also *53–1* to *53–13.*

4-5-T (or Agent Orange), causes severe toxic effects on the nervous system, liver and bone marrow. Some carcinogenic properties have been suggested in the results of some animal/bacterial investigational models.

53–722. TRICRESOL *(See 53–534, Phenol)*

53–723. TRICYCLIC ANTIDEPRESSANTS (TCA; e.g., Amitriptyline Hydrochloride [Elavil], Desipramine Hydrochloride [Norpramin], Imipramine Hydrochloride [Tofranil], Nortriptyline Hydrochloride [Aventyl], Protriptyline [Vivactil])

Overdosage of any of these drugs may cause extreme restlessness, twitching, hyperreflexia, hypo- or hyperpyrexia, persistent tachycardia and coma. Hallucinations may occur. Convulsions and cardiac arrhythmias are additional complications. On ECG the widened QRS duration may be more than 100 msec. The three C's of toxicity are coma, convulsions, cardiac. The newer tetracyclics, such as maprotiline HCl (Ludiomil), tend to have less cardiac toxicity but a higher incidence of seizures.

Treatment

- Gastric emptying by emesis or tube followed by activated charcoal. Repeated doses of charcoal are indicated in severe cases.
- Respiratory assistance by expired air or mechanical methods *(5–1)*.
- Alkalization should be done immediately, to change the relative tissue binding of the TCA. This can be done with hyperventilation, if the patient is on a respirator, or with bicarbonate drip. The goal is to keep the serum pH >7.45 and <7.5.
- Frequent ECG monitoring with appropriate treatment of ventricular ectopy, particularly IV sodium diphenylhydantoin, lidocaine and sodium bicarbonate; use physostigmine if cardiovascular response is not changed by other means. Wide PR, QRS and long QT interval, plus various cardiac arrhythmias (e.g., variable AV block) and cardiac arrest can occur. A temporary pacemaker is sometimes needed.
- Convulsions are usually responsive to treatment with diazepam, sodium diphenylhydantoin (phenytoin) or phenobarbital.
- Neutralization of atropine-like symptoms by physostigmine is rarely needed.
- IV sodium bicarbonate is also important in relief of arrhythmias and hypotension. Levophed can be used if further treatment of hypotension is needed.
- Dialysis is not valuable, since the medication rapidly fixed to the tissues.

Therapeutic doses of tricyclic antidepressants given in conjunction with monamine oxidase (MAO) inhibitor drugs (isocarboxid [Marplan], nialamide [Niamid], phenelzine sulfate [Nardil], tranylcypromine sulfate [Parnate], etc.) can cause serious toxic symptoms, including hypotension or hypertension, hyperpyrexia and convulsions. These symptoms clear rapidly under symptomatic care when concomitant use of MAO inhibitors and tricyclic antidepressant drugs is discontinued.

53–724. TRINITROBENZENE ($C_6H_3N_3O_6$)

The signs and symptoms of toxicity are approximately the same as those for dinitrobenzene *(53–271)*.

53–725. TRINITROTOLUENE (TNT) ($CH_3C_6H_2[NO_2]_3$; TLV 1.5 mg/m^3)

Inhalation of the fumes and dust from TNT may cause a serious toxic picture characterized by loss of appetite; nausea; vomiting; acute diarrhea; cyanosis of the fingertips, ears and lips; delirium; hallucinations; convulsions; hepatitis; jaundice; and aplastic anemia. Treatment consists of removal from exposure and supportive care.

---

*For therapeutic considerations see also 53–*1* to 53–*13*.

53–726. TRIORTHOCRESYL PHOSPHATE (Tri-*o*-cresyl Phosphate, TOCP) ($[CH_3C_6H_4]_3PO_4$; TLV 0.1 mg/m³)

This substance is the toxic agent in so-called "jake poisoning," caused by drinking extract of Jamaica ginger ("Jake") or ingestion of parsley extract (apiol).

Signs and symptoms: Nausea, vomiting and gastrointestinal irritation lasting for 2 to 3 days. After an interval of 5 days to 3 weeks (usually about 10 days), footdrop and wristdrop may develop. Other muscle groups may be involved. The muscle weakness and paralysis may be permanent because of damage to anterior horn cells. Death may occur in severe cases.

53–727. TRIPELENNAMINE HYDROCHLORIDE (Pyribenzamine Hydrochloride)

See *53–80, Antihistaminics,* for signs and symptoms of toxicity following therapeutic or excessive doses.

"Blue velvet" is the name for a peculiarly vicious mixture of tripelennamine and paregoric used by opiate addicts as a substitute for morphine or heroin. Both of the ingredients can be obtained cheaply without a prescription in many localities. One ounce of paregoric is boiled to get rid of the camphor and other volatile ingredients, and a 50-mg tripelennamine oral tablet is crushed into the liquid. This mixture is then injected intravenously, giving a euphoric effect lasting 2 to 3 hours. Since the oral antihistaminic tablets contain talc, veins are rapidly occluded. Pulmonary hypertension, severe bacterial infections and hepatitis may occur. In addition to treatment for acute addiction to opiates (see *53–455, Morphine*), symptomatic care of the serious complications resulting from IV injection of an irritative, nonsterile substance often is necessary.

53–728. TULIPS

A toxic alkaloid, tulipine, contained in the bulbs may cause a severe reaction if ingested in even small amounts. The action and treatment are similar to those for colchicine *(53–220)*.

53–729. TUNG OIL (Chinawood Oil) AND NUTS

Tung oil is nontoxic, but ingestion of the Brazil nut–like nuts may cause severe gastric pain with vomiting and profuse diarrhea, painful muscle cramping and complete prostration from shock and respiratory depression. After prompt gastric emptying and supportive care, complete recovery without residual ill effects is usual.

53–730. TURPENTINE (Gum Turpentine, Oil of Turpentine, Spirits of Turpentine) ($C_{10}H_{16}$; TLV 100 ppm)

Varying combinations of terpenes, especially *o*-pinene, are responsible for the toxicity of this common solvent and medication. Although ingestion is more common, inhalation of high concentrations of fumes as well as absorption through the skin can cause acute toxicity. Absorption from the gastrointestinal tract is of low degree.

Signs and symptoms: Characteristic odor on the breath; a sensation of burning in the mouth, throat, esophagus and stomach; nausea; vomiting; diarrhea; severe abdominal pain; ataxia; delirium; and acute excitement, often followed by convulsions and painful urination with a violet-like odor of the urine. Later, hematuria and albuminuria may be present. Death usually occurs from respiratory failure, often secondary to aspiration pneumonitis.

Treatment is the same as that given for gasoline *(53–323)*.

53–731. TWO-FOUR-D (2-4-D) ($C_8H_6Cl_2O_3$)*(See 53–257)*

---

*For therapeutic considerations see also *53–1* to *53–13*.

53–732. ULTRAMARINE (Lapis Lazuli) ($Na_7Al_6S_6O_{24}S_3$)

In the presence of acid, this mineral decomposes to hydrogen sulfide. It is used in the painting of fabrics and as a bluing agent. Ingestion causes a toxic picture similar to that of hydrogen sulfide (53–353).

53–733. URANIUM DIOXIDE (UO_2; TLV 0.2 mg/m³)

Inhalation of dust of the insoluble radioactive oxide results in accumulation in the lungs and pulmonary lymph nodes; it is slowly, but never completely, eliminated after termination of exposure. The soluble uranium compounds (e.g., uranyl nitrate and fluoride) are toxic to the kidney, but chronic toxicity has not been reported. Avoidance of protracted skin contact is advised to prevent skin radiation damage.

53–734. VACCINIUM ULIGINOSUM L. (Bilberry, Whortleberry)

This berry-producing shrub, which grows in America, Asia and Europe, differs from true blueberry (*Vaccinium myrtillis L.*) in that its juice is colorless instead of purple. Ingestion of the berries has caused a feeling of inebriation, euphoria, headache, bradycardia, dyspnea and aberrations of vision (white appears to be blue and green appears yellow).

53–735. VANADIUM PENTOXIDE (V_2O_5; TLV 0.5 mg/m³—C [dust]; 0.05 mg/m³ [fume])

Vanadium poisoning is usually caused by the pentoxide and occurs in persons working around oil-burning furnaces and oil refineries, in the manufacture of vanadium steel and in the dyeing industry.

Signs and symptoms: Greenish-black discoloration of the tongue, dry nonproductive cough, severe headaches resistant to all therapy, disturbances in vision, hemoptysis, nervousness, psychic derangement and gastrointestinal and urinary disturbances, all of which may persist for 2 to 3 weeks.

Treatment includes ascorbic acid by mouth in large doses. Prognosis is good in acute cases; chronic exposure may result in permanent renal damage.

53–736. VAPAM

This soil fumigant acts much like disulfiram (Antabuse) if ingested. For signs of toxicity and treatment, see 53–279, *Disulfiram.*

53–737. VARNISH AND VARNISH REMOVERS *(See 53–24, Acetone; 53–45, Alkalies [Sodium Hydroxide]; 53–117, Benzene [Benzol] and Its Derivatives; 53–176, Carbon Tetrachloride; 53–295, Ethyl Alcohol; 53–323, Gasoline; 53–386, Lead Salts; 53–426, Methyl Alcohol; 53–437, Methyl Chloride; 53–440, Methylethylketone; 53–468, Naphtha; 53–712, Toluene [Toluol]; 53–729, Tung Oil; 53–730, Turpentine)*

53–738. VENEZUELA (Coco de Mono) NUTS

Ingestion of these nuts has been reported to cause nausea, vomiting, chills, malaise and prostration followed in 7 to 10 days by complete loss of hair from the scalp and body. Gastric emptying, activated charcoal and supportive care are indicated. No treatment seems to affect the loss of body hair, which grows back slowly. No fatalities have been reported.

---

*For therapeutic considerations see also 53–*1* to 53–*13*.

53–739. VERATRINE (Cevadine)

Veratrine is a complicated mixture of alkaloids sometimes used in the treatment of pediculosis capitis and certain types of neuralgia. It (or an allied substance of similar action) is also found in the "death camas" (*Zygadenus*) plant (*53–765*) common in the grazing lands of the northwestern United States. Ingestion may cause burning in the mouth and stomach, salivation, nausea, vomiting, acute abdominal pain, diarrhea, acute anxiety, headache, vertigo, slow and feeble pulse, extreme hypotension, dilated pupils and muscular twitching. Respiratory and circulatory collapse may occur. In spite of the severity of the symptoms, most patients are conscious at all times.

Gastric emptying with emetics or gastric lavage followed by activated charcoal and magnesium sulfate are indicated. Hospitalization is indicated for supportive care; since the toxic substances are excreted very slowly (probably through the kidneys), a relapse may occur after apparent improvement.

53–740. VERATRUM VIRIDE (Green Hellebore, False Hellebore, White Hellebore; *Veratrum californicum* [Corn Lily, Skunk Cabbage])

Acute toxic signs and symptoms may occur following ingestion of the roots (or other parts) or drinking of "herb teas" or through confusion with certain other tinctures used medicinally, especially tincture of valeriana. The toxic action is due mainly to the alkaloid protoveratrine, which should not be confused with cevadine, the toxic agent in veratrine (*53–739*).

Although veratrum was once used medicinally, it is a reflex cardiac depressant, and use of it now is unusual. Most cases of poisoning occur from accidental ingestion of the powder, which is used as an insecticide. The toxic picture is characterized by burning in the throat and stomach, pain on swallowing, vomiting, diarrhea, bradycardia, hypotension, muscular cramping and convulsions, with or without loss of sphincter control.

PROGNOSIS. Most patients with veratrum viride poisoning recover in a short time because its immediate violent emetic action causes early gastric emptying. Bradycardia will respond to atropine.

53–741. VINYL CHLORIDE ($H_2C{=}CCl\ H$; OSHA Standard 1 ppm)

Similar in action to, but weaker than, ethyl chloride (*53–71, Anesthetics, Inhalation*), this substance is used as a refrigerant and in the plastics industry. Its acute toxic effects from high concentration exposure, such as nausea, dizziness and CNS depression, are transient and require only symptomatic treatment. Chronic exposure has been associated with noncirrhotic portal fibrosis and angiosarcoma of the liver. Raynaud's syndrome and degeneration of terminal phalanges of the digits has also been noted.

53–742. VIOLETS

The rhizomes contain violine, a toxic alkaloid. See *53–46, Alkaloids*.

53–743. VIOSTEROL (Vitamin D)

Although commonly and once indiscriminately used medicinally in the treatment of many conditions (rickets, osteomalacia, arthritis, etc.) viosterol is a dangerous substance. Large doses (150,000 to 600,000 units/day) may result in serious, sometimes fatal, toxic reactions from hypercalcemia.

Signs and symptoms are nausea and vomiting associated with abdominal cramping and pain, with or without diarrhea. The abdominal pain may be severe enough to be mistaken for an acute surgical abdomen. Headache, general lassitude, dyspnea, neuralgia, myalgia and signs of urinary tract irritation (polyuria, nocturia, albuminuria) may be present, as may urticaria, asthma (*56–4*) and congestive heart failure (*29–10*).

---

*For therapeutic considerations see also *53–1* to *53–13*.

Treatment includes cessation of the drug, gastric emptying if just taken and supportive care. Hospitalization may be needed for treatment of hypercalcemia (46–6)

53–744. VITAMIN A

Acute hypervitaminosis A in infants causes vomiting and bulging of the fontanelles. In adults it is associated with nausea, vomiting, headache, papilledema (pseudotumor cerebri), mental irritability, sleepiness and localized peeling of the skin. Although excessive intake is the most common cause, hypervitaminosis A may be due to ingestion of food containing large amounts of the vitamin. See *53–314, Food Poisoning, Rare Causes.*

In acute cases, signs and symptoms of toxicity subside rapidly when excessive intake of the vitamin is stopped; in chronic cases, lengthy supportive and symptomatic care usually is required.

53–745. VITAMIN K_1

Therapeutic doses may cause flushing, sweating and a sense of constriction of the chest. Acute sensitivity reactions (24) are fairly common. In certain susceptible persons, usual therapeutic doses may result in hypotension; rapid, irregular pulse; severe chest pain; cyanosis; and coma.

Recovery occurs rapidly under symptomatic and supportive therapy after use of the drug has been discontinued.

53–746. WAR GASES

Lacrimators (brombenzylcyanide and chloroacetophenone; "tear gas"). *Signs and symptoms* are profuse lacrimation, smarting and burning of eyes, blurred vision and temporary blindness. The effects are panic-inducing but transient and usually not dangerous. See *53–193, Chloroacetophenone.*

Treatment for Lacrimators

- Irrigate the eyes thoroughly with water or 2% sodium bicarbonate solution.
- Protect the eye with dark glasses. Do not bandage.

Pulmonary Irritants (chlorine, chloropicrin, palite, phosgene). All of these gases produce symptoms with an insidious onset and are very dangerous.

Signs and symptoms include bronchospasm, dyspnea, pulmonary edema (55), intense cyanosis, nausea, vomiting, coma and collapse.

Treatment for Pulmonary Irritants

- Bed rest; prevention of chilling.
- Insurance of an adequate airway.
- Oxygen therapy. An endotracheal catheter may be necessary.
- Treatment for acute bronchospasm (56–4).

Irritant Smokes (diphenylaminechlorarsine and diphenylchlorarsine). *Signs and symptoms* are violent sneezing, nausea, vomiting, coughing, dyspnea and pulmonary edema (55–4). Dangerous only if very severe.

Treatment for Smoke Irritants

- Wash the nose and mouth with water or 2% sodium bicarbonate solution.
- Prescribe absolute rest.
- Give oxygen therapy.

Vesicants (mustard gas [dichloroethylsulfide] and lewisite [chlorvinyldichlorarsine]). *Signs and symptoms* include itching, blistering, blurred vision, sneezing, blindness, collapse from severe shock (57) and delayed arsenic poisoning (53–90).

Treatment for Mustard Gas in the Eyes

- Wash the eyes with copious amounts of water for examination or 2% sodium bicarbonate solution.

---

*For therapeutic considerations see also 53–*1* to 53–*13*.

- Instill tetracaine (Pontocaine) into the eyes to relieve pain initially.

Treatment for Mustard Gas on the Skin

- Wash the contaminated areas with 2% sodium bicarbonate solution followed by soap and water.
- Spot sponge with alcohol or gasoline; avoid spreading.
- Rub in a paste of chlorinated lime or wipe with sodium hypochlorite solution.

Treatment for Lewisite on the Skin

- Wipe with sodium hypochlorite solution and alcohol; then wash with soap and water.
- Neutralize with BAL by local and systemic administration *(53–10)*.
- Treat the blisters as second degree burns *(28–3)*.
- Treat for collapse and shock *(57)*.

53–747. WARFARIN (Compound 42, Coumachlor [Coumadin Sodium], Deathmore, Decon, Fumarin, Pival, Tomarin, Warficide) ($C_{19}H_{16}O_4$; TLV 0.1 mg/m^3)

This powerful anticoagulant is used in powder form as a rodenticide. It is toxic if ingested but is not absorbed through the skin. For signs and symptoms of toxicity and treatment, see *45–8*.

53–748. WATER GLASS

Used as an egg preservative, as an adhesive, for fireproofing fabrics and as a detergent, water glass contains about 40% sodium silicate, which has a definite caustic alkali effect *(53–45)* on the skin and mucous membranes. Ingestion causes a burning sensation in the mouth and throat, inability to swallow, vomiting and gastric pain.

Treatment

- Thorough washing of the mouth with copious amounts of water.
- Gastric emptying by emetics or gastric lavage followed by activated charcoal in water by mouth or through the lavage tube. A saline cathartic should be given.
- Symptomatic and supportive therapy.

53–749. WATERPROOFING AGENTS (e.g., Scotchguard, Allguard, Shoeguard)

Failure to use these aerosolized products (containing 1,1,1-trichloroethane) in a well-ventilated area—preferably outdoors—can result in dyspnea, cough, pharyngeal irritation, nausea, weakness, generalized aching, headache and chills. Onset varies from immediate to a few hours after exposure. Ingestion causes even greater mucosal irritation, and large doses can result in coma, shock and death. For treatment, see *53–2, Initial Treatment Axioms*. Oral ingestion requires gastric emptying, charcoal and a cathartic.

53–750. WATER PURIFIERS *(See 53–356)*

53–751. "WATERFRONT COCKTAILS"

For a small amount of money, persons who cannot afford the usual alcoholic beverages can obtain about 50 ml of rubbing alcohol *(53–40)* and 100 ml of white (nonethyl-containing) gasoline *(53–323)*. This mixture, when ingested, results in acute intoxication, terminated in 2 to 3 hours by vomiting, triggered by the substances added to the alcohol to make it unpotable. Treatment is symptomatic and supportive, as outlined in *53–295, Ethyl Alcohol.*

53–752. WILD TOBACCO

All parts of this plant contain nicotine *(53–478)*.

---

*For therapeutic considerations see also *53–1* to *53–13*.

53–753. WISTERIA

The active principles are resin and glycoside. If ingested, the pods cause severe gastrointestinal symptoms, sometimes followed by collapse. Treatment consists of emptying the stomach by emetics or gastric lavage followed by activated charcoal in water. Supportive therapy may be necessary.

53–754. WOOD

In addition to skin reactions commonly caused by many different types of wood, several tropical woods used in cabinetmaking may give rise to acute toxic symptoms, apparently resulting from absorption of toxic substances through the intact skin or from inhalation of dust or fumes.

Signs and Symptoms: Swelling and stiffness of the hands and fingers associated with a heavy feeling in the arms, severe headaches, visual disturbances, dyspnea, rapid pulse, dysphagia and watery diarrhea with dehydration.

Treatment is supportive. Complete recovery is the rule upon removal from exposure, although some fatalities have been reported. Desensitization to certain tropical woods has been successful.

53–755. XYLENE (Xylol) ($C_6 H_4[CH_3]_2$; TLV 100 ppm) *(See 53–117, Benzene [Benzol] and Its Derivatives*

53–756. YAUPON, YAUPON HOLLY

Nausea, vomiting, abdominal pain and diarrhea can occur with ingestion.

53–757. YEW

The leaves, shoots and berries of the American, English, Irish and Japanese varieties contain a toxic alkaloid, taxine. For treatment, see 53–674, *Taxus Baccata L.*

53–758. ZERLATE (Zinc Dimethyldithiocarbamate, Ziram)

Combined with an oily base, this substance is an effective insecticide. It also has toxic properties similar to those of disulfiram (Antabuse). See 53–279, *Disulfiram.*

53–759. ZINC CHLORIDE ($ZnCl_2$; TLV [fume] 1 mg/m^3)

Zinc chloride is used medicinally as an escharotic, astringent, deodorant and disinfectant and commercially in zinc plating and in alloys. Inhalation of fumes (common) and ingestion (rare) may cause acute toxic signs and symptoms; a high percentage of ingestion cases are fatal. Inhalation cases generally recover, although there is a tendency toward delayed development of severe pneumonia. Substantial exposure justifies several days of hospital observation.

Signs and symptoms following inhalation of fumes: Hoarseness, loss of voice, chest pain, rapid pulse and respiration, tracheobronchitis and sometimes severe and even fatal pneumonia. Treatment is removal from exposure and supportive care.

Signs and symptoms following ingestion: Severe gastric and substernal pain, swollen lips, edema of the glottis, severe vomiting, bloody diarrhea, cold skin, low blood pressure, dyspnea and collapse with the picture of acute shock and hypocalcemia. Perforation of a viscus may occur.

Treatment includes gastric emptying followed by activated charcoal and supportive therapy. If acute edema of the glottis is present, an endotracheal tube or tracheostomy may be necessary. Chelation therapy with either Ca EDTA or BAL has been shown to be effective in severe cases.

53–760. ZINC CYANIDE ($Zn[CN]_2$)

This zinc salt is a powerful insecticide. For signs and symptoms of toxicity and treatment, see 53–232, *Cyanides.*

---

*For therapeutic considerations see also 53–*1* to 53–*13*.

53–761. ZINC OXIDE (ZnO; TLV[fume] 5 mg/m^3)

Inhalation may cause metal fume fever (*53–423, Metal Fumes*). Ingestion causes toxic signs and symptoms from formation of zinc chloride in the stomach. The treatment is the same as that outlined in *53–759, Zinc Chloride.*

53–762. ZINC PHOSPHIDE (Zn_3P_2)

Decomposition of this zinc salt by water and acids results in the formation of phosphine. If it is inhaled, the treatment given in *53–544, Phosphine*, should be followed; if this zinc salt is ingested, this treatment should be preceded by stomach emptying with emetics or gastric tube with gastric lavage using 1:5000 potassium permanganate solution.

53–763. ZINC STEARATE ($Zn[C_{18}H_{35}O_2]_2$)

Inhalation of the fine dust from zinc stearate talcum powder by infants may result in pneumonia, with a mortality of more than 20%.

53–764. ZINC SULFATE (White Vitriol, Zinc Vitriol) ($ZnSO_4$)

Signs and symptoms following ingestion: Violent vomiting with severe abdominal pain, bloody diarrhea and sudden collapse. Signs of severe kidney injury (albuminuria, acetonuria, glycosuria) may develop after apparent complete recovery.

53–765. ZYGADENUS VENENOSUS (Death Camas)

A native of northwestern America from British Columbia to northern California, this perennial plant contains a very toxic alkaloid, zygadenzine, that is similar in action to veratrine. The toxic principle is found in all parts of the plant, including the flowers, and is not destroye by drying. The species have the appearance of wild onions, but do not have the characteristic odor. For treatment, see *53–739, Veratrine.*

54. Psychiatric Emergencies

Emergency psychiatric care is usually sought by the patient (or for the patient by family members or others closely associated with the patient) for one or more of the following reasons: gross disruption of functional capacity in at least one major activity area, psychic distress, behavior widely deviant from the patient's norm or society's acceptable limits, or indications of homicidal or suicidal intent, or a combination of these. Some aspect of unbearable change usually precipitates an immediate need for control and treatment, with the change generally being organic, functional intrapsychic or interpersonal in nature.

Management and treatment is dependent on ascertainment of the following:

- Has the patient been physically ill? If so, what are the suspected contributing factors?
- What is the apparent underlying and *immediate* precipitating cause(s) for seeking help *now*?
- What is the category and severity of the psychiatric problem?
- Did the patient present of his or her own volition or was he or she accompanied? (Determine by whom and why.)
- Is the patient mentally competent and able to give an informed and free choice consent (see *54–14, Involuntary Treatment and Commitment Process*)?

- At least in part what are the immediate and long-range solutions desired by the person(s) seeking help?

In contrast to the quick action programs of most other emergency situations, the responder to a psychiatric emergency usually needs to Stop/Look/Listen/Listen/Listen. Psychiatric problems require more time involvement, interrelating with the patient's close associates, and continuous patient attendance.

54–1. ESSENTIALS OF THE PSYCHIATRIC EVALUATION

- Ensure decorum by all emergency responders in dealing with the patient and close associates. Establish trust, uninhibited communication channels, and adequate control with a minimum of physical action.
- Obtain details of the presenting complaint and precipitating event(s).
- Obtain medical history and perform a physical examination to determine if any underlying disease or disorder is responsible for the patient's condition. Check TPR, fundi, neurologic features, etc.
- Check mental status; use Table 54–1 for assistance. Estimate intelligence.
- Review psychiatric history: Check for medication, use of illicit drugs and prior psychotherapy. Review jobs, education, military service, socioeconomic status, family history (especially mental illness), any crimes and deviant behavior. Note any changes in ADL (especially food, sex, sleep).
- Record findings and communicate essentials to those on therapeutic team.

54–2. PSYCHIATRIC HOSPITALIZATION INDICATIONS

Inpatient care for patients presenting to the ED with psychiatric crises is sometimes required; the common conditions requiring emergency treatment have been described as the 7 D's:*

- **Destructiveness:** Suicide (*17* and *54–8*), homicide threats (*54–10*) and violent behavior (*54–21*) are indications for admission and control (see *54–14*).
- **Disorganization:** Massive mental disruption as occurs with acute intoxication, disarray of thought processes in schizophrenia and severe anxiety reactions.
- **Deep Depression:** To extent that cessation of competent functioning has occurred.
- **Disorientation:** Diagnostic evaluation and control needed for severe organic mental disorders.
- **Detoxification:** Control and management of withdrawal or overdose (see *53, Poisoning*).
- **Doctor:** The managing psychotherapist advises that outpatient care no longer suffices, and hospital admission is needed for further diagnostic procedures, control and therapy. Inadequate support from family and friends, and inability of the patient to function effectively on his own, are major factors.
- **Deviancy:** Severe psychiatric crisis in some special cases may lead to isolated petty crime with intent to be caught and gain help; merits of hospitalization can exceed those of incarceration.

---

*Modified from Soreff, S.M.: *Management of the Psychiatric Emergency.* New York, John Wiley & Sons, 1981.

Table 54–1. GUIDE TO PSYCHIATRIC EVALUATION AND CEREBRAL FUNCTION

Clinical Aspect	Normal		Neurosis		Psychosis*
Appearance	Appropriate to activity and image being portrayed; usually clean and orderly		Generally socially appropriate; may be increase in "eccentric attire"		Variable; may be total breakdown in self-care and grooming
Behavior	Consistent with affect, activity and situation		Inappropriate (excessive or restrained) when dealing in the neurotic focus		Abnormally variable; exhibited energy ranges from immobile (involutional) to violent (manic)
Content of thought	Communication indicative of logical chain of thought, reflecting direction, associations and reasonable abstract relationships		Select areas of "abnormal content" but often consistent with altered objectivity; watch for "Freudian slips" that clue underlying problems		Gross areas of confused thinking when decompensated; disintegration and aberrant ideation; hallucinations and delusions
Discourse (speech)	Even delivery, reasonably distinct; pitch, tone, intensity appropriate to content and circumstances	Gray Zone	Often interrupted cadence; pitch/tone/volume variably altered by increased emotional energy that alters bodily and vasomotor activity	Gray Zone	Abnormally variable when decompensated, ranging from mute to raving
Elaboration on sensorium	Oriented as to time, place, person. Memory intact. Digit recall, simple math (7's) OK		Usually orientation and memory intact except for highly charged areas		Often impaired as to time, place, person; with multiple disorientation, suspect acute complicating medical problems
Functional capacity	Appropriate to circumstances, usual objectives and past performance level		Variable; average functioning to substantial interference		Variable; often substantial interference to gross disintegration

*See *54–17* for discussion of causes requiring prompt medical intervention in addition to psychiatric evaluation.

54–3. ACUTE SITUATIONAL REACTION (Transient Situational Disorder)

(See also 37–10, Hyperventilation)

Regardless of how well adjusted any person may be, there is a limit beyond which either an event of overwhelming magnitude or the presence of one more even seemingly insignificant problem may cause a precipitous decline in the person's performance and adaptive capacity. To paraphrase an adage it is "the stressor that snapped the subject's sense of sanity and proportion." Often, the greater the number of problems the individual has been dealing with, the more precipitous and complex will be the disruption of adequate functioning.

Types of precipitating problems are often grief reactions, impediment to or destruction of life goals or victimization by assault and battery or other crime.

Treatment

- Situational counseling to aid the person through an appropriate temporary period of mourning for the injury incurred (reasonable mourning that is squelched has a propensity to magnify and require even greater treatment at a later, more inappropriate time).
- Removal of problems or guidance for the resolution of problems. Alternatively recommendation of complete relief from problems for a few days or longer, with enlistment of sufficient resources to keep problems from further accumulating in the interim, can be valuable.
- Appropriate rest (see *54–13, Insomnia*), exercise and a nutritional diet should be prescribed.
- Excessive amounts of caffeine, alcohol, nicotine, illicit drugs, medications, salt and sugar taken while trying to adjust and cope with the acute situation can contribute greatly to the subsequent collapse (a case of the "cure" being worse than the "disease").
- Formal psychotherapy and psychotherapeutic drugs are usually not necessary except in more severe grief reactions; small doses of diazepam, 2 to 5 mg 3 to 4 times daily for several days, may be helpful.
- Enlist further aid of relatives, friends and clergy as necessary and available. Self-help groups centered on peer support (with professional guidance) aid the working through of problems and readaptation; information is available through local mental health association or county mental health service.

54–4. ADDICTION *(See 7)*

54–5. COMMITMENT PROCESS *(See 54–14, Involuntary Treatment and Commitment Process)*

54–6. DEATH AND DYING *(See 8–9)*

54–7. DELIRIUM

Delirium is a state of fluctuating consciousness or advanced acute brain syndrome *(54–17)*, that is short of coma *(32)*. Treatment is aimed at the specific cause; bodily protection and supportive care are necessary in the interim.

One prototype of this disorder is delirium tremens, which may be precipitated in heavy drinkers by sudden withdrawal from alcohol. There is usually a prodromal period of 1 to 2 days, characterized by depression, uneasiness and insomnia, followed by development of a coarse tremor and hallucinations (especially visual). See also *53–295, Ethyl Alcohol,* regarding acute intoxication.

Treatment

- Treatment of underlying problems.
- Thiamine, 100 to 500 mg IV, is effective in the alcoholic patient.
- Chlordiazepoxide (Librium), 10 to 25 mg tid to qid, chlorpromazine hydrochloride (Thorazine), 50 to 100 mg, or prochlorperazine maleate (Compazine), 10 to 15 mg IM, is usually safe and effective.
- Paraldehyde, 10 to 15 ml by mouth or 5 to 10 ml IM, is an adequate drug for sedation, but unpopular because of the smell. It may be given with safety 3 or 4 times a day. Chloral hydrate by mouth may be given as necessary for long-continued sedation.
- Hydration and electrolyte correction by IV route.
- Provide adequate nutrition and vitamins, especially B complex, which includes thiamine.
- Restraint may be necessary but should be avoided if possible. As a rule, if restraint is required, sedation is inadequate.
- Opiates, synthetic narcotics, caffeine and alcohol should not be used.
- Hospitalization in an institution equipped for the care of such patients.

54–8. DEPRESSION AND SUICIDAL IDEATION *(See also 17, Suicide and Suicide Attempts)*

The commonest neurosis of this era is depression. Often its presentation will be a symptom complaint made by the fatigued person who makes a wan smile to show brave defiance against the perceived or actual overwhelming odds. As the inner stress increases, a spiraling set of perpetuating negative events occur, as the patient often drinks more alcohol; sleeps erratically, develops altered appetite patterns; feels constantly sad, guilty and fatigued; seeks more medication; exercises less; and functions increasingly inadequately at work and elsewhere, all leading to less gratification, more stress and more depression. The depression must be more than a grief reaction and longer than a week in duration to meet the diagnostic requirements of DMS III*; it may be single or bipolar with periods of mania. The tendency to depression may be inherited.

The person must be asked forthright questions. Is he or she considering or has he or she considered suicide? If so, what level of specific preparation has occurred? What plans or thoughts does the patient have for getting out of this state? If a suicide attempt has been made, to help determine the severity of intent, ask the patient why he or she is still here—that is, what went wrong with the intention. If the person is in a state of hopelessness and emotional contact cannot be made to establish a positive program, it is wise to obtain an immediate consultation from a psychiatrist, or, if one is not available, from another physician. Handling should be tactful and *an able-bodied attendant present at all times* when activation of suicide threats is imminent. Voluntary hospital admission for evaluation of any contributory illness (such as tumor or endocrine or collagen disorders) and psychiatric treatment may be necessary. Involuntary treatment *(54–14)* may be necessary. Another measure that may help is tricyclic antidepressant therapy, such as amitriptyline hydrochloride (Elavil), 50 to 75 mg at bedtime or larger doses if the depression is more

---

*Diagnostic and Statistical Manual of Mental Disorders, 3rd ed.

severe and the patient is hospitalized; imipramine hydrochloride (Tofranil) is also effective for the nonagitated patient who is depressed. Cardiac effects of tricyclic antidepressants (53–723) must be monitored periodically; doxepin HCl (Sinequan) has fewer such effects. (Note: A week or more delay for onset of therapeutic effect is common; a premedication evaluation of affect by a psychiatrist is advisable in severer cases.) An acceptable resolution must be found to handle psychic management of the precipitating event. Follow-up care is essential, and arrangements should be made for psychiatric consultation (if not previously obtained) unless the depression is of minor proportions. A graduated exercise program can be a key element to recovery; treatment with L-tryptophan, good nutrition, and supplemental vitamins may also aid. Enlistment of family support is extremely important; lack of family support can constitute an indication for hospitalization in conjunction with patients' inability to plan for themselves.

54–9. FAINTING (Vasodepressor Syncope) *(See 49–20, Differential Diagnosis of Episodic Unconsciousness; 63–7, Syncope)*

54–10. HOMICIDAL THREATS

Patients usually have the privilege of excluding disclosure by a physician with whom there has been a confidential communication in a physician-patient relationship. Gradually, however, this is being recognized as a qualified privilege that does not apply to explicit homicidal threats to specific individuals made by the patient. The physician not only *may* disclose this information to the potential victim and proper law enforcement authorities, and obtain an involuntary temporary commitment if danger is imminent, but it is also increasingly recognized that it is the physician's specified *duty* to report, and there is a possibility that the physician will be liable for injury to named victims if a report is not made. Gray zone or nonexplicit threats create a serious dilemma for the physician or psychologist or other emergency responder (RN, EMT, MSW), and in such cases, in addition to getting a psychiatrist's consultation and opinion, it may be advisable to seek legal counsel or a judicial opinion. In general, if in doubt, it is best to report.

54–11. HYPERVENTILATION *(See 37–10)*

54–12. HYSTERIA (Conversion Hysteria) *(See also 49–19, Unconsciousness, Episodic; 49–20, Differential Diagnosis)*

Emotional or physical strain in certain individuals may cause panic states or bizarre hysterical symptoms severe enough to require emergency care. Hysteria is more than a diagnosis by exclusion. Not only is the patient usually in normal condition on examination, but there are also manifestations or symptoms inconsistent with known patterns of physiology and anatomy. Manifestations may subside under hypnosis. Referral for more comprehensive evaluation is usually necessary.

Common manifestations of conversion hysteria are as follows:

- *Blindness.* Usually monocular or tunnel vision—the cone of the vision area outlined does not vary (e.g., between 3 and 6 feet). See *38–41, Sudden Vision Loss.*
- *"Coma."* See *49–19, Unconsciousness, Episodic; 49–20, Differential Diagnosis.*
- *Globus.* A subjective sensation of a lump in the throat, sometimes so severe

that the patient is convinced that he or she is unable to swallow. The gag reflex may be absent.

- *Hyperventilation*. See 37–10.
- *Paralysis*. Transient, partial or complete; usually not corresponding to any motor nerve distribution. The patient is inconsistent in tests that alternatively check muscles for active motion and active resistance, especially when done bilaterally simultaneously or ipsilaterally while contralateral stabilization with the "paralyzed muscles" is being checked.
- *Sensory abnormalities*. Usually hypesthesias or paresthesias, often of stocking or glove distribution. The hypesthesia is often precise midline including the perineal-genital area instead of in conformity with known sensory overlap. Gag and corneal reflexes may be absent.
- *Symptom presentation*. The severity of the problem being presented may not be accompanied by appropriate effect (la belle indifférence). Many symptoms concerning diverse organ systems can be elicited, and if these are absent, the diagnosis of hysteria is suspect.

Treatment

- Reassure the patient that improvement will occur, but further treatment and evaluation are necessary. Challenging the patient with reality is usually ineffective or counterproductive in the emergency setting. Do not tell these patients that there is nothing wrong with them.
- Enlist the aid of responsible family members who may be further helped by working with a mental health evaluator and treatment team.
- Avoid complicating the problem with excessive medication. If considerable agitation is present, treatment with diazepam or IV sodium pentothal may be temporarily helpful.
- Hypnosis relieves the acute panic state.
- Refer for necessary additional neurologic evaluation and psychiatric care.

54–13. INSOMNIA

Persons who request emergency care for sleeplessness usually complain of difficulty in getting to sleep, inability to stay asleep long enough to become rested or to sleep soundly enough to become rested, or early morning awakening pattern. Except in those instances in which severe emotional trauma is a factor, most cases of insomnia are chronic and require emergency therapy only because previous medical and psychiatric care have not yet been effective and lack of rest has resulted in complete exhaustion. After emphasizing to the patient or members of the family that only emergency treatment is being given, one of the following drugs may be administered orally: chloral hydrate, 0.5 to 1.0 g (repeat in 1 to 2 hours if necessary); flurazepam HCl (Dalmane) or temazepam (Restoril), 15 to 30 mg. or L-tryptophan (a nonprescription amino acid), 0.5 to 1 g.

All patients should be advised to make arrangements for further care so that treatment on an urgent basis will not be required again. Large quantities of barbiturates, bromides, "tranquilizers" or sedatives should not be prescribed for home use. Under no circumstances should opiates or synthetic narcotics be administered or prescribed. If the patient is deeply disturbed, all medications should be in the possession of a responsible family member. Since insomnia is often one symptom of anxiety or significant depression, psychiatric referral may be helpful.

Orientation to the benefits of an adequate daily exercise program followed by a warm tub bath or shower, which will relieve mental and muscular tension and lead to natural sleep, is advisable.

54–14. INVOLUNTARY TREATMENT AND THE COMMITMENT PROCESS *(See also 69, Permits and Authorizations in Relation to Emergency Cases)*

In the law there are two opposing views concerning prompt physical restraint and confinement of a mentally troubled patient.

On the nonintervention side is the Fifth Constitutional Amendment, restricting deprivation of life, liberty or property *without due process.* This means that neither federal nor state personnel may aid private citizens in their acts without restriction. Restraint without due cause may subject the restrainer(s) and any superior(s) to charges of false imprisonment, kidnap, assault and battery. There is also the medical consideration that any affirmative patient-physician relationship, if the patient is able to recognize one, will be disrupted.

The issues that promote prompt restraint and involuntary medical treatment of one who refuses voluntary treatment and is gravely disabled or likely to harm him- or herself or others are abandonment *(64)*, negligence *(68–1)* and potential liability for subsequent harm that may occur to the patient or others because of nonrestraint. State legislation regarding "temporary hold" outlines the civil circumstances under which people may be restrained involuntarily, who will make the decision to hold, where the holding will take place and for how long before other due process measures must be enacted. Crisis clinics and local mental health departments can provide specific guidelines. Another important aspect is the medical ethical responsibility to act in such situations. Also, there is frequently a statutory obligation to report situations of potential homicide *(15)*.

The resolution of this conflict is probably best achieved in the following manner:

1. Give due consideration to the previously discussed factors as applicable to the situation at hand and proceed in the most reasonable manner for the best interests of the patient and others. Protection of the patient and others from obvious physical danger should prevail over consideration of the patient's liberty.
2. Obtain immediate discussion or consultation with another capable physician or person whenever possible prior to action. Preferably, paramedical personnel should receive pre-arranged training and orders for functioning when they are not in immediate communication with the responsible physician.
3. Record promptly and thoroughly the salient features of the situation that led to the actions being taken.
4. Documented action taken to the best of one's ability under the circumstances presented minimizes any medicolegal second-guessing that may later occur. A curious situation exists in which the patient may sue if given involuntary treatment, and others may sue if the patient is *not* treated.

Further guidelines that aid are as follows:

1. Knowledge of applicable local statutes and their judicial interpretation. Since it is unlikely that all possible situations will have been covered, documentation of the reasonableness of action under the circumstances presented should prevail.
2. Whenever possible, have the patient voluntarily submit to immediate outpatient psychiatric consultation and care and to any necessary subsequent

hospitalization. Enlist encouragement from relatives who have rapport with the patient as necessary.

3. Obtain emergency judicial review and temporary holding order if feasible for involuntary hold and treatment or proceed under temporary hold and treatment statutes.

4. Promptly report any involuntary restraint and treatment for subsequent judicial review regarding due process and continuance.

54–15. NEUROSES *(See specific type and Table 54–1)*

54–16. PHOBIAS *(See 37–14)*

54–17. PSYCHOSES *(See also Table 54–1)*

Signs and symptoms vary but in general consist of personality changes and progressively poorer functioning. This impairment is manifested by loss of calculating ability and specialized knowledge, poor judgment and memory, faulty orientation, delirium, acute excitement states *(37)*, confusion, anxiety, feelings of persecution and hallucinations. Impairment is sometimes accompanied by neurologic signs, such as ataxia, tremors and slurred speech.

Acute brain syndrome psychoses are most often caused by organic abnormalities in circulation, metabolism or nutrition, infection, injury, intoxication (alcohol, drugs, and so forth) or neoplasms. Guides to the cause and the urgent treatment of this problem are: rapid or sudden onset; fever; toxic appearance; evidence of injury or drug use; neurologic deficit; abnormal laboratory studies, including electroencephalograph (EEG), computerized tomography (CT) scan and lumbar puncture; and age of the patient (more often over 40). Electrolyte imbalance (especially low levels of sodium, potassium, calcium) may be a precipitating factor, as may withdrawal from alcohol or other drugs. The latter is not uncommonly noted after surgery in patients who sequestered information about drug use.

Increasingly, physicians are finding that some organic psychoses are induced by mixed drug usage (narcotics, amphetamines, psychotropic agents, alcohol); therefore, systematic investigation may be required as under *53–4, Poisoning*. In these situations, use caution to avoid further complicating the situation with more psychotropic medication (see *54–19, Prudent Use of Psychotherapeutic Agents*).

Treatment

- Prevent self-injury and injury to others by gentle physical restraint as necessary.
- Maintain an open airway and adequate ventilation if impairment or delirium is present.
- Obtain psychiatric consultation.
- Hospitalize the patient for diagnosis and treatment of the underlying cause.

Subacute Psychoses

Having eliminated the causes just described, particularly subdural hematomas, neoplasm and smoldering infections of the central nervous system, one is confronted with psychoses from poorly defined or less common causes such as Cushing's syndrome, myxedema, collagen diseases or variants of drug use. As more is learned of the biochemistry of psychoses, the term "functional" (a euphemism for ignorance of cause) will probably be dropped, and the issue will be more the urgency and type of treatment. Neuropsychiatric evaluation and treatment beyond the capacity of the time available to most emergency physicians or departments is necessary.

Manic-Depressive Psychoses

Persons suffering from these conditions show marked changes in behavior and personality, with fluctuation between acute excitement and depression, and may demonstrate complete lack of comprehension of their condition. Either mania or depression may be present without a history of the other (unipolar) or one phase may alternate with the other (bipolar). The depressive phase requires close observation. Chlorpromazine (Thorazine) is helpful for acute mania.

Paranoia

This condition is characterized by intense feelings of guilt, failure and persecutory delusions; patients are potentially homicidal and suicidal *(17)*.

Schizophrenia

Inability to distinguish between actual environment and a fantasy world, often with disturbance in thinking (thought disorder), feeling and acting and confusion regarding identity.

Treatment

- Withdraw any associated chemical agent or toxin—particularly alcohol and psychotropic drugs.
- Obtain neuropsychiatric care and as feasible voluntary consent for any treatment or admission.
- Acute evaluatory treatment may be started with fluphenazine hydrochloride (Prolixin), 5 mg IM, or trifluoperazine (Stelazine), 1.0 mg IM, with continuous observation in a quiet area. Chlorpromazine (Thorazine) and haloperidol (Haldol) are also effective. If necessary, doses may be repeated hourly, with dosage appropriately revised until patient is controlled. If patient is not controlled in 6 hours, admit for hospital care. Benztropine mesylate (Cogentin), 1 mg PO bid, may reduce extrapyramidal reactions.
- If patient is violent, see *54–21*. Also see *54–14, Involuntary Treatment and Commitment*.

54–18. PSYCHOPHYSIOLOGIC ILLNESS (Psychosomatic Illness)

Numerous patients present for emergency evaluation multiple complex symptoms that are accompanied by no or minimal objective signs. Though one would prefer that these patients presented for evaluation outside the emergency situation, it should be recognized that they usually are sincerely concerned that what they feel and perceive constitutes an urgent condition requiring help.

The following factors may be related to the psychophysiologic illness presented:

- Negative conditioning by misinformed relatives and friends (e.g., "you'll always have ____________________ as a problem"). The body may begin to conform to what the mind believes.
- Positive conditioning by the medical profession to have problems checked early before they turn into bigger problems and possible recrimination

earlier by a physician for not having reported a problem immediately for evaluation and treatment.

- Depression *(54–8)*.
- Hysterical conversion reactions or panic states *(54–12)* may present similar symptoms also lacking a physiologic component.

Treatment

- Perform sufficient evaluation to assure all concerned that there is, in fact, *not* a primary physical problem needing urgent treatment; this is an important first step in reassurance.
- Acknowledge first, with empathy, that the situation is very difficult for the patient. Then explain that in spite of the intensity of the patient's subjective experience, it is not a dangerous problem, will not be chronic, does not require immediate intense treatment and will improve with subsequent planned follow-up.
- The patient does have a problem that needs correction and that may require anything from plain education in lay person's terms to treatment as under *54–8* or *54–12*. Arrange for follow-up evaluation and treatment.

54–19. PRUDENT USE OF PSYCHOTHERAPEUTIC AGENTS

The guidelines prepared by the AMA Committee on Alcoholism and Drug Dependence and approved by the AMA Council on Mental Health and AMA Department of Drugs are as follows:

AMA Prescribing Guidelines

- Use barbiturates and other sedative-hypnotics for relief of severe symptoms, but avoid them for minor complaints of distress or discomfort.
- Attempt to diagnose and treat underlying disorders before relying on drugs of this class for symptomatic relief.
- Assess susceptibility of the patient to drug abuse before prescribing barbiturates or any other psychoactive drugs. Weigh benefits against hazards.
- Use dosages that will not lower sensory perception, responsiveness to the environment or alertness below safe levels.*
- Know how to administer barbiturates when clinically indicated for withdrawal in cases of drug dependence of the barbiturate type.
- Using periodic checkups and family consultations, monitor possible development of dependence in patients who are on an extended sedative-hypnotic regimen.
- Prescribe no greater quantity of a drug than is needed until the next checkup.
- Warn patients to avoid possible adverse effects because of interaction with other drugs, including alcohol.
- Counsel patients as to the proper use of medication—follow directions on the label, dispose of old medicine no longer needed, keep medicine out of reach of children, do not "share" prescription drugs with others.
- Convey to patients through your own attitude and manner that drugs, no matter how helpful, are only one part of an overall plan of treatment and management.

Though the emergency physician ordinarily should order only several days' supply of such medication, at times he or she also will be the follow-up care physician; also sometimes the request may come from a patient from out of town who has lost or run out of medication and wants several weeks' supply until returning home (beware of a ploy—call the original physician if feasible); in such instances these guidelines should be kept in mind.

---

*Write warning on prescription if substance will cause drowsiness.

54–20. RUNAWAYS AND CHRONIC HOMELESS PATIENTS

Members of these two groups of patients may present themselves for emergency attention in a disheveled, bewildered, depressed, fatigued, moneyless state, suffering from illness due to poor hygiene, unsheltered environment, accident, mugging, or the effects of drugs or alcohol. Their plight requires treatment with dignity.

In addition to the treatment of the principal medical problem, assistance is needed in their socioeconomic status, evaluation of how they got into this predicament and determination as to whether they are receptive to follow-up counseling to change their current situation. Runaways are most receptive to such counseling, and reunification with their families should be attempted (confidential toll-free phone line for messages: 800-621-4000). Homeless patients may be helped to obtain food and shelter through such agencies as Goodwill, the county welfare service, the Salvation Army, etc.; consult the community service list or Social Service for local information.

54–21. VIOLENT BEHAVIOR

Overt, uncontrolled, physically aggressive behavior by a patient is potentially dangerous to all proximately situated. That zone of danger depends upon the endurance and strength (suspect the most) of the patient and what type of weapons are available.

Preservation of the safety of others and oneself is foremost. Isolate the patient as possible, warn others and move them to safety, call for the assistance of security personnel and/or police, with equipment as necessary to control the situation; avoid further action until their arrival, except to assure the patient intermittently that you want to help and not to harm.

If the patient is unarmed, preferably six able-bodied people should be present to exert control—one to each limb, on pre-arranged basis if possible, one to control the head from behind by grabbing the hair with both hands to minimize biting and head-butting and one to give predrawn benzodiazepine, such as diazepam (Valium), preferably IV, 5 mg per minute up to 10 to 20 mg, or IM. Parenteral haloperidol (Haldol); 2.5 to 5 mg IM, repeated every 30 to 60 minutes as needed, may be given in severely agitated patients, with increases as indicated by response under close monitoring. If the patient is armed in any manner, his or her capacity must be neutralized by trained security personnel, preferably by the least injurious method available.

Talking to the uncontrolled violent patient is generally ineffective, but if it is attempted—particularly when other recourses are not available—use a strong authoritarian voice and indicate clearly and briefly, without threats, what the patient must do to enlist your aid (e.g., I can't help you unless you sit down over there; all right, now drop the stick by your left foot).

To help in analyzing the problem and decreasing recurrence, it is advisable to determine what circumstances were present just prior to the violence.

Potential violent behavior can erupt unexpectedly, but often there are forewarnings. Besides using extreme caution with patients who have expressed paranoid ideation or who are using potentially psychic energizing drugs (such as PCP; see 53–532) beware of the patient who grimaces or shifts position away when approached (under these circumstances, do not approach further but in deference move back a step or two), move to the side if blocking easy egress to the door and sit rather than stand above the patient.

If cautious discussion still intensely increases irritability, drop the subject. With increasing agitation or likelihood of violence, advise immediate (rather than elective) psychiatric consultation and follow-up care; if none is available, get evaluation from any other physician. Inform responsible relatives of the situation. Start immediate fast-acting psychotrophic drugs, preferably a phenothiazine, by oral route if it will be taken. Physical restraint or involuntary treatment and confinement *(54–14)* in the absence of an overt threat or act with imminent danger to self or others is best avoided.

55. Pulmonary Edema

55–1. GENERAL CONSIDERATIONS IN PULMONARY EDEMA

Pulmonary edema is a life-threatening complex of clinical conditions in which the patient has increased interstitial and alveolar fluid, symptoms of dyspnea, and acute apprehension ("air hunger"). Signs of impaired blood-alveolar gas exchange due to multiple causes (see Table 55–1) lead to labored respirations, tachypnea, tachycardia, hypoxemia and at least secondary hypoxic cardiac dysrhythmias and acidosis, which lead ultimately to death if untreated. Treatment varies according to the underlying cause.

Pulmonary edema is broadly classified etiologically into cardiogenic and noncardiogenic, as discussed below.

Cardiogenic (CHF). Pathogenesis is ↑ hemostatic pressure from LV pump failure (cause #5, Table 5–2) due to: decompensated LVH from hypertension, mitral and aortic valve disease, acute MI, serious dysrhythmia, vascular compartment overload; pulmonary embolism may be a precipitating factor. RV pump failure may precede.

Noncardiogenic (usually from ARDS). Pathogenesis is most often the "capillary-leak syndrome" from increased permeability of the alveolar-capillary barrier (see also cause #4, Table 5–2, and *56–2, ARDS*). Other less common pathogenic causes—which generally do not present as emergencies—are vascular obstruction (venous/lymphatic) due to trauma, disease or malignancy, and a drop in serum osmotic pressure, as occurs in liver disease with hypoalbuminemia. Noncardiogenic pulmonary edema from ARDS may result from a variety of causes, including:

- Acute poisoning from absorption, ingestion, injection, inhalation or aspiration of many drugs, gases and other toxic substances, such as the following:

  Aconite *(53–34)*
  Acrolein *(53–36)*
  Barbiturates *(53–110)*
  Cadmium salts *(53–158)*
  Carbon monoxide *(53–175)*
  Chlorates *(53–189)*
  Cyanides *(53–232)*
  Dinitrophenol *(53–273)*
  Epinephrine hydrochloride *(53–288)*
  Ethylene *(53–71, Anesthetics, Inhalation)*
  Hydrogen sulfide *(53–353)*
  Iodine *(53–365)*
  Kerosene *(53–379)*
  Methyl bromide *(53–435)*
  Morphine *(53–455)*
  Oxygen *(53–503)*
  Organophosphates *(53–497)*
  Phosgene *(53–543)*
  Salicylates *(53–614)*
  Thallium *(53–692)*
  Thuja *(53–86, Arbor Vitae)*

- Barotrauma, including effects of high altitude *(26–1, AMS* and *HAPE)* and submersion *(26–4, Decompression Sickness)*.
- Acute trauma with massive thoracic concussion *(31, Chest Injuries)*.
- Infection, interstitial pneumonia *(33–51)*—diffuse, due to acute viral infections, particularly *Varicella (33–76)* and Eaton agent.
- Embolus (fat, pulmonary).

Table 55–1. DISTINGUISHING FEATURES OF NONCARDIOGENIC AND CARDIOGENIC PULMONARY EDEMA

Distinguishing Features: Clinical (Hx, Sx, Px, Dx, Rx) Laboratory (Lx)	Noncardiogenic Pulmonary Edema (ARDS)	Cardiogenic Pulmonary Edema (CHF)
Hx (History of Prior Events)		
• ASHD and other heart disease or risk factors	Variable; not dominant factor	Usually present; often prior Rx
• Exposure to primary ARDS events	Usually noted; see 55–*1*	Variable; can precipitate CHF
Sx (Symptoms and Signs, Current)		
• Dyspnea, DOE, orthopnea	Present (usually recent)	Present (± long prodrome)
• PND	Absent	Present often
• Sx from primary ARDS event	Usually noted; see 55–*1*	Variable; can precipitate CHF
Px (Physical Exam)		
• ↑ HR, ↑ R/R	Present	Present; PVC's common
• Hypotension	Occurs as event progresses	Common
• Hypoxemic dysrhythmia	May occur early	May occur anytime
• Cyanosis, mental confusion	May occur early	Later finding usually
• Pitting edema (legs), NVD, tender hepatomegaly, HJR	Absent usually	Present usually
• Moist rales; cough; sputum with or without blood tinge	Variable; severe with toxic fumes; dry crackles most common	Present usually; ± Cheyne-Stokes respiration
Lx (Laboratory Exam)		
Chest x-ray:		
• Enlarged heart; enlarged pulmonary artery "knob"	No, unless secondary problem present	Present; ± calcifications
• Diffuse pulmonary findings	Asymmetrical infiltrate often; nonvascular	↑ ↑ vascularity; ± Kerley A or B lines; hilar "batwing"/"butterfly"
ECG		
• Primary QRS abnormality	Absent usually	Yes: LVH/MI (see Fig. 29–1, *R, O, P*)
• Dysrhythmia	Hypoxic dysrhythmia common	Dysrhythmias common
ABG's		
• PaO_2 (n ≐ 91 ± 17 mm Hg)	↓ ↓ PaO_2 (e.g., < 40 mm Hg)	↓ PaO_2
• $PaCO_2$ (n = 39 ± 7 mm Hg)	↓ $PaCO_2$ often	↓ $PaCO_2$ or n range
• pH (n = 7.41 ± 0.04)	n or ↑; will decrease if not treated	n or ↓; will decrease if not treated
Swan-Ganz		
• Pulmonary wedge pressure	n to slight ↑	↑ ↑; > 30 torr/mm Hg
Dx (Diagnosis)	ARDS; may lead to hypoxic CHF/MI	CHF; may or may not precipitate ARDS
Rx (Treatment)		
• Furosemide, morphine sulfate; *optional*: phlebotomy, digitalis	Not indicated for ARDS	Lifesaving measures; see 29–*10* and 55–3
• Oxygen	High % O_2; see 55–4	Start O_2; do ABG's; see 55–3
• Mechanical ventilation	↑ flow with PEEP; see 55–4	No, unless severe abnormality of ABG's; see 55–3

- Airway obstruction, smoke inhalation, near drowning.
- Ketoacidosis, uremia, pancreatitis, hypoglycemia.
- Shock

55–2. COMPARISONS BETWEEN CARDIOGENIC (CHF) AND NONCARDIOGENIC (ARDS) PULMONARY EDEMA

- As noted in *55–1*, pulmonary edema of both types may be clinically similar and may stay so, being distinguished with certainty only by pulmonary wedge pressure; mixed conditions also can occur, in which case the dominant one must be treated, but not to the exclusion of the other.
- It is crucial to differentiate these primary types of pulmonary edema before initiating treatment, as patients with ARDS are not helped by digitalis, diuretics, morphine, or phlebotomy, whereas their absence in CHF may be critical and even fatal.
- See Table 55–1 for assistance in distinguishing CHF from ARDS.

55–3. TREATMENT OF ACUTE CARDIOGENIC PULMONARY EDEMA *(See 29–10, Congestive Heart Failure)*

Insertion of a cuffed endotracheal tube with positive pressure ventilation (see fourth treatment measure under *55–4*, below) may be lifesaving if the patient is unconscious or cyanotic, or if other methods are not adequately effective as demonstrated by ABG revelation of acute respiratory acidosis and increasing wedge pressure.

55–4. TREATMENT OF ACUTE NONCARDIOGENIC PULMONARY EDEMA—ARDS *(See also 55–1, 55–2)*

- Removal from exposure to exciting toxin or event (see *55–1*).
- Complete rest with patient in position of maximum comfort. Encourage patient to try pursed lip expiratory breathing.
- Close observation (vital signs, cardiac monitoring) for changes in condition.
- Oxygen by mask or intranasal cannula (100% at 6 to 8 L/min initially, but reduce as soon as possible and do not use for more than 1½ to 2 hours); adjust volume according to history and response. Volume-controlled ventilation with positive end-expiratory pressure (PEEP) of 10 cm H_2O can be beneficial. Intubation is often necessary. Increased tidal volumes within the range of 10 to 20 ml/kg may produce response. Monitor response with ABG's and in more severe cases with pulmonary wedge pressures. Adjust therapy to achieve a PaO_2 of 65 to 80 mm Hg. If response is inadequate even with high settings of tidal volume, high FIO_2 (> 60%), PEEP in high range (> 20 cm H_2O) and high-driving pressures (> 40 cm H_2O), then avulsion of the bronchial tree *(56–17)* and inadvertent iatrogenic pneumothorax are hazards with continued similar efforts. Under these circumstances, consider use of high-frequency jet ventilation (HFJV; high flow, rapid rate, small volume), which is emerging as a possible solution (although this is still experimental, and carries the risk of possible tracheal necrosis), or consider HBO.
- Correct acidosis *(46–1)*.
- Sedate with caution (if at all), using agents that have a minimal depressant effect on the respiratory center (e.g., chloral hydrate, 0.5 g PO or 1.5 g by rectal route, q 4 to 6 h), unless the patient is safely on ventilatory assistance, in which case sedatives may be given as often as indicated for comfort and compliance. Excessive narcotic effects may be reversed with naloxone.

- Bronchial dilatation by intermittent use of an aerosol if bronchial spasm is present—e.g., 5 ml of 0.25% isoetharine hydrochloride (Bronkosol) (adult). Observe closely for cardiac arrhythmia, particularly in the presence of tachycardia, although it is probably best not to use an aerosol in the presence of very rapid tachycardia (i.e., greater than 140 beats/min) unless the tachycardia is just secondary to the bronchospasm effect, rather than symptomatic of cardiac disease. (See also *Measures for Acute Severe Bronchospasm*, under 56–4.)
- Treatment of any specific bacterial infection (see 33–83, *Antimicrobial Drugs of Choice*).
- Steroid therapy (controversial). Dexamethasone, 10 to 15 mg in a single loading dose by oral or parenteral route, or prednisone, 100 mg orally, with the same amount repeated in divided doses during the ensuing 24 hours, may be associated with dramatic improvement in severe, life-threatening interstitial pulmonary edema and inflammation. Dexamethasone may also be aerosolized and administered via IPPB for topical respiratory system application.

56. Respiratory Tract/Lung Conditions

56–1. GENERAL CONSIDERATIONS

Many persons who request emergency care have respiratory tract signs and symptoms that appear more discomforting than life-threatening. Considering, however, that worsening of some respiratory problems follows an exponential curve rather than an arithmetic line, careful early evaluation of the cause (see Table 5–2) of respiratory distress and the level of any airway obstruction (see Table 5–3) is always imperative. Some of the acute respiratory tract conditions that may warrant emergency care are listed below.

Infants and young children have a much smaller zone of tolerance to worsening of respiratory conditions than do adults, and pediatric consultation or referral is often advisable.

Clinical Evaluation of Respiratory Tract

Emergency treatment of respiratory tract problems is aided by careful early assessment of airway patency, including ventilation power/airway/gas exchange (Steps 2/3/4 respectively of Table 5–2, Respiratory Distress Evaluation). Since involvement at any level in the respiratory chain ultimately affects all other levels, recovery is most rapidly achieved if the weak link or aggravating factor is identified early.

Laboratory Tests in Respiratory Conditions

Tests that are of value in evaluating and monitoring more extensive respiratory tract involvement are determinations of arterial blood gas levels, chest x-ray, ECG, pulmonary function tests (particularly tidal air, FEV_1 or PEFR, and vital capacity), sputum culture and Gram stain. Special techniques are required for making acid-fast bacillus, anaerobe and fungus cultures when needed. Hematocrit, blood urea nitrogen (BUN) and urine specific gravity values are indices to state of hydration, and CBC and differential cell counts—including total eosinophil counts when allergy is suspected—can give an indication of type and severity of infection. These tests can be initiated and/or performed in the ED. Pulmonary angiogram and pulmonary isotope scan require special arrangement.

56–2. ACUTE RESPIRATORY DISTRESS SYNDROME (ARDS)

(See 55–4)

56–3. ACUTE RESPIRATORY FAILURE

The major causes and corrections of acute respiratory failure (defined as impaired exchange of respiratory gases between ambient proximate environmental atmosphere and the circulating blood) are outlined in Steps 2, 3 and 4 of Table 5–2, Respiratory Distress Evaluation. Important points are as follows:

- Effective mechanical ventilation gas flow techniques, usually with endotracheal intubation, are required for treating each type of cause in its severe stage, with severity generally signaled by: (1) apnea or severe drop in respiratory rate; (2) FVC < 10 to 15 ml/kg; (3) fatigue, decreased inspiratory force and failing effective aeration despite a respiratory rate above 35 to 40/min; (4) $PaCO_2 > 50$ mm Hg; (5) $PaO_2 < 50$ mm Hg.
- The gas flow techniques that appear to be most effective for each type vary. Pressure and/or volume ventilation support with or without PEEP is used when neuromuscular aspects of ventilation are impaired but lung is normal; for moderate ARDS; and for COPD (except when ratio of inspiratory to expiratory time is decreased, in which case consider use of expiratory retard valve to smooth and prolong exhalation—equivalent of pursed lip exhalation). Include *PEEP* for ARDS of greater severity.
- Oxygenation is indicated in all cases (even for COPD when $PaO_2 < 50$, but it must be used with great caution—e.g., 1 to 2 L/min), with close monitoring of voluntary ventilatory capacity and ABG's.

56–4. ASTHMA AND BRONCHOSPASM *(See also 39–6, Foreign Bodies in the Airway [especially in children])*

Asthma is a condition of acute partial (but reversible) airway obstruction marked by recurrent attacks of paroxysmal dyspnea with mucosal edema, excess tenacious mucus production, and wheezing due to spasmodic contraction of the peribronchial smooth muscles. Once stimulated, these smooth muscles physiologically always have prolonged contractile periods before they very slowly relax.

Of great importance before, during and after the asthmatic attack are prevention and avoidance of the numerous precipitating or aggravating factors. Among these are: dehydration, allergens (pollens, house dust, animal danders, molds and certain foods), cold dry air, upper respiratory infections, dust, cigarette smoke and other noxious effluvia, extremes of physical activity in susceptible individuals—including competitive athletes without heart disease—and emotional stress (certain asthmatics can throw themselves into even cyanotic episodes at will; hypnosis helps to relieve these attacks). Treatment measures for both nonallergenic (intrinsic) and allergenic (extrinsic) asthma are the same, except that no specific avoidance or desensitization is required with the intrinsic type. Foreign bodies in the respiratory tract (39–6), infections and left heart failure (see 55, *Pulmonary Edema)* may also cause asthmatic wheezing.

The physical signs of asthma are signs of partial airway obstruction (Table 5–3), bronchial wheezing (inspiratory and expiratory with prolonged expiratory phase), and clinical signs of pulsus paradoxus, hypoxemia and early respiratory alkalosis or later acidosis (confirmed by ABG's) as the problem progresses from mild to one of moderate severity. The rapid ventilation studies performable in the office or ED—PEFR ($\cong FEV_1$), VC (FVC)—show breathing capacity decreased to 50 to 75% of normal in mild cases, to <25% of normal in severe cases and to ≤10% of normal in cases of profound respiratory failure. The demonstrated correlation that patients in one series (Martin et al.*) with a PEFR ≥ 25% did not have ABG findings of pH < 7.35 or $PaCO_2$ > 45 mm helps serve as a guideline to defer ABG's in moderately severe asthma pending the results of early therapy. Tests should be repeated after use of bronchodilators. Chest x-rays may be normal early or may later show overinflation, atelectasis and pneumonia.

Treatment

Initial Measures—All Cases

- Check vital signs and clinically categorize as mild, moderate or severe.
- Eliminate any foreign body (*39–4* and Table 5–3) as a causative factor (history and examination).
- Evaluate for infection, pulmonary embolus, CHF or precipitating/aggravating factors, and pulsus paradoxus.
- Obtain serum level of theophylline if there is history of recent administration.
- Obtain sputum Gram stain culture and sensitivity plus CBC if there are signs of infection; prescribe antibiotics accordingly.
- Measure ventilation performance before and after use of bronchodilators. Obtain ABG's if condition is severe or not improving with treatment.
- Chest x-ray is ordered on specific indication and in all patients whose condition is severe enough to warrant admission.
- Hydrate by oral or IV route (D5NS or D5½NS) according to degree and type dehydration (see *11*). Urine specific gravity is an aid in evaluating.
- Administer humidified O_2 100% at 5 L/min by face mask or cannula, unless involvement is only slight or COPD is present.
- DO NOT
  —Administer opiates, synthetic narcotics, antihistamines or sedatives. (Instead, consider alternative nonmedicinal approaches to management [*12–5, 12–6*].)
  —Administer cromolyn sodium; it is not of value in acute attack.
  —Encourage coughing until tenacious mucus is well liquified.

Measures for Mild to Moderate Asthma

- Review initial measures for application as appropriate.
- Bronchodilation by β-adrenergic medications, e.g.:
  —Epinephrine hydrochloride (Adrenalin), 0.25 to 0.5 ml of 1:1000 solution SC in adults, repeated in 15 to 20 minutes if bronchospasm has not decreased. Give a total of three injections before proceeding to theophylline. (The pediatric SC dose of epinephrine is 0.01 ml/kg [maximum total for 1 dose: 0.3 ml] and of Sus-Phrine is 0.005 ml/kg [maximum total for 1 dose: 0.15 ml].) Epinephrine is also α-adrenergic.
  —Terbutaline sulfate (Brethine), 0.01 mg/kg SC up to 0.25 mg may be used instead; may repeat in 15 to 30 minutes, but not more than 0.5 mg in 4 hours. Like all adrenergics, terbutaline must be used with great caution in the presence of, or when there is the potential for, cardiac dysrhythmia. Use in adults only.

*Ann. Emerg. Med., *11*:2, February 1982, p. 70.

—Aerosol of 0.25 ml of 5% inhalant solution of metaproterenol (Alupent) or of a 0.5-ml dose of isoetharine hydrochloride (Bronkosol), plus 2.5 ml of distilled water by mask; do not repeat for 4 hours generally.

- Theophylline orally or (less preferably) by rectal solution enema is generally effective only in early or milder attacks. Therapeutic serum levels are in the 10 to 20 μg/ml range and should be measured to achieve and maintain this level. If the patient has been taking theophylline recently, have blood sample taken immediately, and give IV theophylline at only maintenance level pending results of blood level. In patients who have not been recently treated, a loading dose of 5.6 mg/kg given slowly IV over 20 minutes will often be helpful if the above hasn't been effective. Maintenance dose is usually 0.8 to 0.9 mg/kg/hr; in presence of CHF or impaired liver function, loading and maintenance dose should be from one-quarter to one-half this amount and must be monitored frequently.
- IV corticosteroids are still controversial and are indicated at this level of severity only if the patient has been taking corticosteroids within the past 6 weeks. (IV corticosteroids require from 2 to 4 hours to take effect.) Some start a 10-day course of oral prednisone in cases of moderate asthma to prevent recurrence of visits to the ED.
- Observe till stabilized. PEFR or FEV_1 should be at least 50 to 60% of predicted normal and PEFR improved to at least 60 L/min or more than 17% improvement with use of bronchodilators before discharge can be considered.
- Generally, order oral maintenance doses of a theophylline preparation without ephedrine and sedative combinations. Sustained release forms of theophylline result in better patient compliance and more even blood levels. Separate doses of oral theophylline (Theo-Dur, Theolair, Quibron) and adrenergics (Alupent, terbutaline, Proventil) are preferable to ease dose adjustment.
- Arrange for detailed follow-up medical supervision with a physician experienced in asthma care. The need for further care should be stressed most emphatically, since after relief from an acute attack, many patients will postpone medical care until another acute episode occurs.

Measures for Acute Severe Bronchospasm

Diagnosis of acute severe bronchospasm is based on findings of ventilation under 25% of normal, acidosis, PaO_2 <50, and $PaCO_2$ >40. Correction of hypoxemia and hypercapnia requires control of asthma; if ABG's are not rapidly improved, ventilatory assistance may be required.

- Review all of the preceding measures cited under *Treatment* for application, as appropriate.
- Hospitalize as soon as possible.
- Correct any severe metabolic acidosis *(46–1)* by rapid IV administration of 25 to 100 ml of sodium bicarbonate (44.6 mEq per 50 ml—prefilled syringe).
- Give corticosteroids by IV route: hydrocortisone sodium succinate (Solu-Cortef), 250 to 1000 mg, or methyl prednisolone sodium succinate (Solu-Medrol), usually 1 to 3 mg/kg, to a maximum of 5 mg/kg initially, followed by 1 mg/kg q 6 h in life-threatening situations or if previously described measures do not initiate rapid relief. Steroids given by aerosol are not indicated until the acute attack is resolved (as with cromolyn sodium).
- Intubation and mechanical ventilation using a cuffed endotracheal tube may be required in the most severe cases (as occur with tetanus—see *33–68*). Bronchial lavage with 30 to 60 ml of 0.25% to 0.50% lidocaine in normal saline gradually instilled over ½ hour along with periodic suctioning may be lifesaving, as when ischemic multifocal ventricular arrhythmia is

developing from associated hypoxemia. Lidocaine can be administered in an aerosol. Efforts at effective mechanical ventilation may be impossible in the most severe cases until relief of smooth muscle spasm of the bronchi has occurred.

- Institute monitoring of serial PEFR, theophylline levels and ABG's, which are important in guiding therapy.

56–5. BRONCHITIS AND BRONCHIOLITIS

Fever, chills, productive cough, pleuritic pain and dyspnea are frequent with general inflammation of the tracheobronchial system. Bronchitis is generally caused by either a bacteria (particularly *Pneumococcus* and *H. influenzae*), a virus, or, in industry especially, numerous chemically irritating fumes. Bacterial infection is often a secondary complication.

Bronchiolitis is a viral respiratory disease seen frequently in children under 1 year of age, generally in the winter and early spring, and characterized by rapid respirations with wheezing, fine inspiratory rales and absence of response to bronchodilators. X-rays usually reveal small diffuse infiltrates and signs of hyperinflation.

Treatment

- Supportive measures, as under 56–6, *"Coryza,"* and 56–4, *Asthma.* Noncardiac pulmonary edema (55–4) can develop.
- Administer antibiotics on evidence of specific infection.
- Hospitalize for administration of IV fluids and monitoring in more severe cases and when there is extensive chronic pulmonary disease.

56–6. "CORYZA" ("COMMON COLD") *(See 33–13)*

56–7. CROUP (Subglottic Laryngeal Obstruction and Laryngotracheobronchitis) *(See also 56–8, Epiglottitis; Table 5–3)*

Croup is more than a viral disease; it is a complex inflammatory disorder with swelling that results in subglottic laryngeal and lower respiratory tract obstruction. It is important to rule out the presence of foreign bodies (39–6, *Esophagus*) and epiglottitis (56–8), which can give similar initial clinical appearances. Croup is characterized by stridulous cough, usually preceded by or associated with mild respiratory infection, and has a notorious tendency to develop without warning during sleep and to become worse rapidly. Usually there is little temperature rise. Children are the most often affected and the worst affected, because of their smaller-diameter laryngotracheobronchial airway. As the patient coughs, the voice becomes progressively hoarse.

Home treatment, as in the following outlines, may be tried if the condition is mild and not progressing rapidly and if there is responsible home supervision with adequate guidelines for care.

Treatment

- Position of comfort; most patients are more comfortable sitting up.
- Increase moisture content of the air by one of the following:
  —Cold vaporizers (preferred).
  —Running a hot shower in a closed bathroom.
  —Use of a hot steam device if other means are not available. (*Note:* Every precaution must be taken to prevent burning the patient if such a device must be used.) Heat may increase edema.

- Sedation should be avoided.
- Acetaminophen, 1 grain per year of age up to 10 grains every 3 to 4 hours orally as necessary for fever control.
- Antibiotics are not indicated for illnesses that are only viral in origin. Culture and stain sputum specimen. Steroids are not indicated. Hospital treatment is definitely indicated if these measures do not result in a decrease in the mild signs and symptoms, or if there is any suspicion of significant or progressing loss of airway patency or evidence of hypoxemia even without cyanosis. If in doubt, hospitalize.
- Obtain arterial blood gases and chest and lateral neck x-rays (see note on *Caution* while taking x-rays, second paragraph under 56–8).
- Start oral or IV hydration.
- Humidified 40% O_2 may be given by face mask if PaO_2 is dropping and under 60 to 70 mm Hg. Smaller water particle size for loosening of bronchial secretions may be produced with an ultrasonic nebulizer. Masks and nasal cannulas deliver better concentrations, but tents are better accepted by some children.
- If nebulized racemic epinephrine (see *56–8*) is needed and leads to rapid improvement in the ED, hospital admission is still indicated because of the possibility of rebound.
- If laryngotracheobronchial (LTB) airway appears compromised clinically or by ABG determinations, prepare early for nasotracheal intubation, e.g., if PaO_2 <60 mm Hg and $PaCO_2$ >45 mm Hg despite above therapeutic measures.

56–8. EPIGLOTTITIS (Supraglottic Laryngitis) *(See also Table 5–3, Guide to Localization of Airway Obstruction)*

Acute fulminant swelling of the epiglottis due to severe focal infection is often overlooked as a cause of respiratory obstruction in children; fatalities due to epiglottitis are notorious. Any toxic, febrile child with rapid onset (within hours) of stridor, difficulty in swallowing, drooling, neck jutting forward and dyspnea has epiglottitis until proved otherwise—particularly when these symptoms are accompanied by nasal flare and neck-thorax inspiratory retractions—and must be admitted for immediate treatment and constant observation.

Diagnosis is based on the above clinical picture. A swollen epiglottis may be seen directly or be revealed by x-ray demonstration of swelling. *Caution:* Pulling on the tongue and vigorous attempts to observe the cherry-red epiglottis have precipitated acute airway closure. If having the patient open the mouth does not provide for adequate observation, wait for immediate standby assistance of someone well trained in airway management and equipped to help if there are complications from any further attempts at direct observation. If direct observation is not possible, take the patient to the x-ray department accompanied by physician and airway management equipment; a single lateral inspiratory x-ray may show characteristic changes (ballooned hypopharynx, thickening of the epiglottis, widening of the aryepiglottic fold).

Treatment

- In established cases, hospitalize the patient and perform endotracheal intubation in the operating room (OR) with tracheotomy set at hand; follow with nasotracheal care in ICU and close observation. Attempts at intubation should be avoided outside the OR or area set up for emergency cricothyrotomy *(5–19)* and tracheostomy *(18–34)*. Sometimes in borderline critical situations, use of IPPB with racemic epinephrine aerosol (below) by mask (or transtracheal jet ventilation temporarily) will improve the situation sufficiently to permit less precipitous procedures.

- IPPB with aerosol of 0.5 ml in children (up to 2.5 in adults) of racemic epinephrine (Vaponefrin) may reduce airway obstruction rapidly by vasoconstrictive action; some object to use of this agent because of side effects—e.g., tachycardia, arrhythmia, hypertension, irritability—which must be watched for. Administer in the ED or hospital. Do not release from the ED just because there is improvement, as rebound is common and thus hospitalization is still necessary.
- Treatment of the causative infection, which is generally due to *H. influenzae*. Owing to increasing incidence of ampicillin-resistant bacteria and even chloramphenicol-resistant bacteria (though uncommon), chloramphenicol may be started concomitantly with ampicillin in more severe cases; discontinue the chloramphenicol if the bacteria is demonstrated to be ampicillin sensitive (or vice versa if the converse situation is present). Alternatively, chloramphenicol can be started alone, with a switch to ampicillin later if the organism is found to be sensitive to ampicillin.

56–9. HICCUPS (Singultus)

Episodic diaphragmatic spasms (hiccups) are caused by an irritative chain of events occurring anywhere along the phrenic nerve (neck/mediastinum/diaphragm), the vagal nerve (and all its associations in the abdominal and thoracic organs up to the throat, ear and meninges) and the CNS (e.g., lesions, ischemia, toxins such as alcohol, uremia). Onset may be related to identified events such as overdistention of the stomach from food or swallowed air (most prominent in infants and relieved by "burping"), general anesthesia or posterior myocardial infarction; most cases are idiopathic, however.

- Attention should first be directed toward identifying any primary events that need treatment (e.g., MI, uremia).
- Most cases of hiccups will stop spontaneously within an hour ("intractable" cases are considered to be those lasting beyond 48 hours), but a number of "remedies" (household and otherwise) may hasten the recovery process. Some of these are as follows:
  —Swallowing finely cracked ice or tsp. granulated sugar.
  —Temporarily increasing $PaCO_2$ by rebreathing using a paper bag, breath holding with neck held in extension—may or may not abort hiccups.
  —Stimulating hard to soft palate with a cotton-tipped applicator.
  —Gastric emptying by NG tube followed by lavage with iced water or saline or by stimulation of the posterior pharyngeal wall at C_2-C_3 level.
- Vigorous medicinal or surgical management should be considered only if deemed absolutely necessary in light of the fact that the condition is usually self-limiting and nonhazardous (albeit annoying and occasionally fatiguing). Measures for intractable cases include the following:
  —Sedation by chlorpromazine, 25 to 50 mg PO tid to qid. If more intensive intervention is indicated, slowly infuse a solution of 50 mg chlorpromazine diluted in 1000 ml D5NS and monitor.
  —Comprehensive evaluation should be done before advancing to such measures as phrenic nerve block.

56–10. HYALINE MEMBRANE DISEASE *(See 56–3; 52–24)*

56–11. HYPERVENTILATION *(See 37–10)*

56–12. LARYNGITIS

The emergency assessment and management is the same as outlined for croup *(56–7)* and epiglottitis *(56–8)*.

56–13. MECONIUM ASPIRATION *(See 52–4)*

56–14. METAL FLUME FEVER *(See 53–423)*

56–15. PLEURITIS (PLEURISY) AND PLEURAL EFFUSION

Even in the absence of traumatic injury to the parietal pleura, the inflammation and dermatomal thoracic pain (along with referred pain—e.g., to the upper abdomen or shoulder and neck) is generally of abrupt onset. Most commonly trauma (with or without rib fracture), infection (viral pleuritis or extension from bacterial pneumonia) or pulmonary embolism *(56–20)* underlies the problem when seen on an emergency basis.

Thoracic excursion or inspiration increases the steady pain in the involved area; a characteristic crackling friction rub is heard, underlying breath sounds are decreased and there is dullness on percussion. Problems with effusion (e.g., due to tumor, collagen disease, tuberculosis, multiple myeloma) are less likely to present in an emergency situation unless ventilation is compromised, because pain diminishes with the fluid buffer between the moving parietal and visceral pleura. Calcifications of the pleura—as with asbestosis—indicate longstanding inflammation and often are an incidental finding.

The chest x-ray may identify the primary pathologic process (e.g., rib fracture, pulmonary embolus, pneumonia), but definitive signs of the pleural pathology are unlikely to be seen on chest x-ray unless only a small amount of effusion is present. Obtain an ECG if there is a pleuropericardial rub or if associated cardiac events have occurred. If thoracentesis *(18–33)* is necessary to remove pleural effusion for diagnostic or therapeutic reasons, perform slowly and monitor pressures if more than 1 liter is being taken. Note color, volume, odor and turbidity of effusion. Send sample for cell count, stains, culture, pathologist cell block exam, pH, total protein, LDH and amylase as indicated.

Treatment

- Treat the underlying problem. Perform thoracentesis *(18–33)* for diagnosis if effusion is present.
- Give analgesics for pain. Codeine-containing medications are usually adequate. TNS units may give significant relief.
- Rib belts may help limit excursion and give partial relief. Avoid tight constriction with tape.
- Hospitalize if the primary problem requires further diagnostic measures or if therapeutic measures (e.g., thoracentesis for large effusion) are required.

56–16. PNEUMONIA *(See 56–1, Laboratory Tests; 33–51, Interstitial Pneumonia)*

Bacterial Pneumonia

Pneumonia, particularly of the bacterial type, is heralded by chest pain with rapid respiration, fever, dyspnea, cough (often producing mucopurulent sputum with or without blood tinging) and cyanosis; these symptoms, together with the physical findings of abnormal breath sounds (rales, decreased breath sounds), percussion dullness with consolidation, friction rub and toxic appearance, help to establish the diagnosis of acute infection of interstitial and alveolar portions of the lungs. Chest x-ray, Gram stain and sputum culture, and ABG's (in the presence of signs of hypoxemia) may be needed to determine the extent of involvement and the causative organism and to aid management of the case. (*Note:* In infants and children, tracheal cultures have been shown to be more definitive than cultures of expectorated sputum.) Hospitalization is required almost invariably with lobar pneumonia and legionnaire's disease (33–35), often with bronchopneumonia, and sometimes with viral pneumonia.

The patient's current general condition and prior medical state should be the deciding factors in the management of cases of suspected or proved pneumonia. Many patients with extensive lung involvement can be treated satisfactorily at home with bed rest, use of a vaporizer, antibiotics, analgesics and good nursing care. Penicillin or ampicillin in adequate doses is often sufficient to achieve control, but other antibiotics (see 33–83, *Antimicrobial Drugs of Choice)* may be more effective if a mixed infection or a penicillin-resistant organism is present. Results of Gram stain and subsequent culture results should guide drug choice. Hospitalization and intensive treatment is required for patients who show advancing signs of ARDS (55–4).

Viral Pneumonia

The auscultatory findings of the lungs in interstitial pneumonia may be normal or consist only of faint, dry crackles; at the same time, the chest x-ray can reveal a "snow blizzard" appearance. These patients may be extremely ill; see ARDS (55–4). Antibiotics are not required in treatment or prophylaxis.

All patients, particularly those who appear to have been recovering satisfactorily from a viral respiratory infection and become precipitously seriously worse, should be suspected of having a secondary staphylococcal infection; they should be immediately hospitalized for vigorous treatment, including parenteral antibiotics such as oxacillin, methicillin or a cephalosporin. Steroids may be required for treatment of septic shock.

Aspiration Pneumonia

Aspiration of more than minimal amounts of gastric contents or of severe toxins such as hydrocarbons and other chemical irritants presents a severe emergency. Immediate bronchoscopy for removal of *particulate matter in the laryngotracheobronchial airway* is indicated. Lavage with saline/steroid or neutralizing solution is not helpful and may be detrimental. Correction of bronchospasm and acidosis is soon needed. Start vigorous supportive care (see 55–4, *ARDS*). *Note:* Prevention is the best treatment—e.g., preliminary placement of cuffed endotracheal tube or esophageal obturator airway (EOA [5–16] or EGTA [Fig. 5–4]), avoidance of initiating gastric reflux till prepared, positioning of unconscious patients in the "coma position" (Fig. 4–5).

56–17. PNEUMOTHORAX *(See also 31–12, Tension Pneumothorax; 31–13, Traumatic Pneumothorax)*

Pneumothorax indicates the presence of free air in the normally occluded space between the parietal and visceral pleurae; it may be of several types:

- *Spontaneous (non-tension) pneumothorax.* This type is usually a benign process caused by spontaneous rupture of an air-containing vesicle or of an alveolus, resulting in the passage of air into the pleural cavity or mediastinum. The onset is usually sudden and accompanied by pain, apprehension and dyspnea. Cough, decreased breath sounds and percussion tympany are usually present unless the volume of air involved is small. X-rays are useful not only in establishing the diagnosis, magnitude of involvement and mediastinal shift but also in disclosing any underlying causative disease. Symptomatic treatment with sedation and bed rest (preferably in a hospital) for a few days is generally all that is required for most patients, but if the patient has borderline respiratory reserve as a result of prior diffuse disease, then the onset of hypoxemia, hypercarbia and acidosis can be rapid and intense. These are indications for chest tube and decompression *(18–33)* plus ABG's to guide oxygen administration and acidosis correction. Underlying disease processes should be recognized and arrangements made for proper care. Patients with emphysema, high-pressure IPPB, and pulmonary blebs (especially during exertion and Valsalva maneuver) are more prone to spontaneous pneumothorax.

- *Tension pneumothorax*. See *31–12*.
- *Traumatic pneumothorax*. See *31–13*.
- *Therapeutic pneumothorax*. Emergency care may be needed for bleeding following therapeutic injection of air. Only supportive care is usually necessary.

56–18. PULMONARY ABSCESS *(See 23–25)*

56–19. PULMONARY EDEMA *(See 55)*

56–20. PULMONARY ARTERY EMBOLISM

Complete Occlusion

Lodging of a clot large enough to completely occlude the bifurcation of the common pulmonary artery ("saddle embolus") results in sudden obstruction of blood flow to the entire distal pulmonary parenchyma, causing collapse and death within minutes. Resuscitative measures are ineffective.

Embolization of Medium-Sized and Small Branches of the Pulmonary Artery

Signs and Symptoms vary with the size and number of the occluded arteries; most frequently recognized are those cases with sudden onset of severe chest pain, dyspnea, tachypnea, tachycardia (sinus or atrial), cyanosis, extreme anxiety and apprehension. Hemoptysis may occur. Signs of shock *(57)*, pulmonary hypertension, secondary cor pulmonale, pulmonary infarction and arterial hypoxemia often develop with larger or multiple emboli.

Physical findings vary; there may be none or those previously mentioned—a pleuritic friction rub, increased pulmonary second sound (due to pulmonary hypertension) and pleural effusion. Pulmonary infarction doesn't always occur but is most likely present with the combination of hemoptysis, fever, pleural pain/friction rub/effusion, and chest x-ray evidence of consolidation and effusion.

Further diagnostic measures may include enzyme studies (LDH, AST/SGOT, and bilirubin), roentgenographic studies (posteroanterior and lateral of chest, pulmonary arteriography), radioisotope lung scan combined with ventilation studies (ventilation–perfusion lung scan), ABG's and electrocardiograms taken immediately and at 6 and 12 hours. (Transient atrial arrhythmias, prominent P waves, S_1Q_3 pattern, right bundle branch block, nonspecific ST-T changes or no electrocardiographic abnormality may be present.) Differential diagnosis from other cardiac and pulmonary disease (myocardial infarction *[29–15]*, pneumonia *[56–16]*, pericarditis *[29–19]* and septic shock *[57]*) may be difficult, but diagnosis is greatly aided with lung scan, with the greatest accuracy achieved by pulmonary angiography as needed.

Phlebothrombosis or deep vein thrombosis (DVT) is the most common underlying cause of pulmonary embolism (see *63–12*). Emboli from the right heart, fractures (fat emboli) and amniotic fluid are much less common.

Treatment *(See also 63–12, DVT; 55, Pulmonary Edema;* and *55–4, ARDS)*

Therapy varies with the severity of the clinical condition and with the medicosurgical resources available. Treatment measures include:

- Position of comfort (see General Prophylactic Measures, below).
- Oxygen by cannula, face mask, or IPPB with PEEP (see *55–4, ARDS*).
- Heparin, 10,000 units IV, to help prevent further thromboembolism (unless contraindicated by evidence of current or recent bleeding, hemorrhagic disorder, septic embolism or planned use of streptokinase or surgery).
- Morphine sulfate, 10 mg IV, for pain. Segmental pain may be relieved by intercostal nerve blocks.
- Treatment of shock (*57*) initially by IV drip infusion of dopamine, starting with 2 to 5 μg/kg/min and increasing dosage as necessary, by increments of 5 to 10 μg/kg/min, to 20 to 50 μg/kg/min, with continuous monitoring of ECG and BP and appropriate adjustment of the drip to keep systolic pressure at least over 90 mm Hg.
- Referral for pulmonary embolectomy is indicated pending the following:
  —Availability of an experienced surgical team and cardiopulmonary bypass unit.
  —Clinical and preliminary supportive evidence of a major embolism.
- Evidence by x-rays, ECG or direct measurement of rapidly increasing pulmonary artery pressure.
  —Pulmonary arteriographic or radioactive isotope evidence of gross vascular bed involvement, or evidence of pending cardiac arrest.
  —Femoral venoarterial bypass is a possible interim emergency procedure pending embolectomy or thrombolytic medication procedure.
  —Thrombolysis with IV streptokinase is a readily available alternative to embolectomy in selected cases (see *63–12* regarding use and contraindications).

General Prophylactic Measures for Prevention of Occurrence or Recurrence of Pulmonary Emboli

The following measures help to decrease the thromboembolic process:

- Maintenance of proper fluid balance and prevention of dehydration (*11*).
- Activity and frequent changes in position (as soon as not contraindicated in postoperative or debilitated patients).
- Encouragement of active and passive leg exercises. Especially helpful are repeated periodic 5- to 7-second isometric contractions of all muscles of the lower extremities (caution patient not to hold breath).
- Positioning with no pillows under the knees; foot of the bed or leg supports of wheel chair slightly elevated.
- Firm, even application of compression bandages or elastic stockings from toes to infrapatellar level or upper thighs in patients with lower extremity deep vein thrombosis (*63–12*) and subsequent necessary prolonged bed rest.
- Administration of anticoagulant therapy (unless contraindicated) under careful control and observation for those with a high likelihood of developing thromboembolism. Heparin is the drug of choice initially. Avoid aspirin.
- Reduction of weight to within a normal range.

56–21. PULMONARY HEMORRHAGE (Massive Hemoptysis)

Massive pulmonary hemorrhage is life-threatening and identified by hemoptysis of from 200 ml to 600 ml per 24 hours or more. Once started, sudden rapid increases can occur and should be planned for. Bronchiectasis, lung abscess, pulmonary tuberculosis and trauma are the most common causes, but malignancy and, in children, cystic fibrosis, rheumatic heart disease and congenital heart disease also should be considered. Prevention of asphyxiation from blood occlusion of the airway (see *5–1*) is of primary concern. Obtain chest x-rays, lung scan and thoracic surgical/medical consultation for assistance in locating bleeding site and possible emergency lung resection. (*Note:* Patients with coagulation disorders, bleeding from diffuse pulmonary disease and bleeding entirely (see *5–1*) due to mitral valve stenosis, congenital heart disease or diffuse malignancy are not generally candidates for lung resection.)

Treatment

- If the probable focus of bleeding is known, place the patient with the involved lung in the dependent position and the uninvolved lung in superior position. Encourage periodic effective coughing. Periodic postural drainage may also be beneficial.
- Maintain a clear airway and give ventilatory assistance as needed. Perform endotracheal intubation if necessary for suctioning or have it at hand. Use an 8-mm or larger tube if possible.
- Obtain immediate specialist assistance for emergency bronchoscopy to localize the bleeding; remove clots from major bronchi, which may be causing atelectasis, and possibly insert a tamponade balloon (e.g., Fogarty, Swan-Ganz) or perform other measures for temporary bleeding control and protection of the uninvolved lung. With special tubes it is possible to differentially ventilate, suction and/or occlude each main-stem bronchus. Arteriography may also help to localize.
- Obtain chest x-rays and draw blood for typing and crossmatching, complete blood count (CBC), differential blood count and coagulation studies *(45)*.
- Treat shock *(57)*.
- Correct any coagulation disorders *(45)*.
- Prepare surgical candidate patients with identified focal bleeding for focal resection.
- Patients who are not surgical candidates and whose bleeding is not controlled with balloon tamponade should be considered for bronchial arteriography and guided catheter injection of 1-mm absorbable gelatin sponge segments to occlude the particular bleeding bronchial artery.
- Avoid use of narcotics.

56–22. RHINORRHEA

Drainage of spinal fluid, usually mixed with blood, from the nose indicates a fracture of the skull *(44–12)*, whether or not x-rays show bony injury. See *44–18, Middle Fossa Fractures*.

56–23. SINUSITIS *(See also 48–1, Aerosinusitis)*

Sinusitis is an inflammatory condition of the respiratory or paranasal sinuses. Bacterial inflammation is the most common severe condition requiring attention and is many times a secondary complication following stasis due to viral or allergic inflammation. Fungal infection (check for diabetes mellitus) and mechanical obstruction from trauma or growths also occur, but not commonly.

Frontal headache, toothache (maxillary sinusitis), focal tenderness to pressure over the sinuses, reddened nasal mucosa, purulent discharge, fever and malaise are common. In fulminant cases the patient may be obtunded, and sinusitis as a cause of FUO (fever of unknown origin) can be a diagnostic challenge. Failure of the sinuses to transilluminate and x-rays of the sinuses (look also for fluid level) confirm the diagnosis.

Treatment

- Obtain culture.
- Penicillin V, 250 mg PO q 6 h for 10 days (or erythromycin if patient is allergic to penicillin). Septra, ampicillin or tetracycline is better for repeat attacks.
- Phenylephrine hydrochloride (Neo-Synephrine) nose drops (⅛% to ¼% for children or ½% to occasionally 1% for adults) or oxymetazoline hydrochloride (Afrin) shrink the engorged mucous membranes and promote drainage. Use <5 days. Postural drainage may be effective.
- Application of local moist heat over the sinuses.
- Bed rest; copious fluids.
- Aspirin and codeine phosphate by mouth for pain and headache.
- Ultrasound therapy over the frontal and maxillary sinuses for 7 to 10 minutes daily may be of great value in promoting drainage.
- Referral to an otolaryngologist for further treatment if symptoms persist. Fluid levels in maxillary sinuses may necessitate needle aspiration.

56–24. SHOCK LUNG *(See 55–4, ARDS)*

56–25. SMOKE INHALATION *(See 25–4 and 55–4, ARDS)*

56–26. TONSILLITIS *(See 61–16)*

56–27. VIRUS INFECTIONS *(See 33)*

57. Shock

57–1. DEFINITION

Shock is "a rude unhinging of the machinery of life" (Samuel D. Gross, 1872) that is still incompletely understood, although it is recognized that its dramatic and various clinical pictures are based more on impairment of cellular function than on specific anatomic changes. This condition of acute peripheral circulatory failure due to derangement of circulatory control or loss of circulatory fluid may be induced by a multitude of causes, many times in combination, including injury, blood loss, fright, dehydration, cardiac inadequacy, hypersensitivity reactions, endotoxins from gram-negative organisms, impairment of nervous function, blockage of blood flow in major vessels, impaired function of certain endocrine glands and poisons. Any of these conditions may cause hypotension with reduction of effective tissue perfusion to a level that is too low to sustain general cellular metabolism. This, in turn, further impairs tissue perfusion. Thus, shock begets shock. Restoration and maintenance of normal circulating vascular fluid volume is imperative.

The following tables in this chapter give a quick review of data for assessing, stopping and correcting the otherwise frequently lethal cyclic process of shock:

Table 57–1. Initial General Measures in Shock Management

Table 57–2. Rapid Physical Review for Patients in Shock

Table 57–3. Methods for Rapid Clinical Monitoring of Cellular Metabolism and Organ Perfusion

Table 57–4. Guidelines for Determining Degree of Severity of Shock

Table 57–5. Common Physical Findings by Type of Shock

Table 57–6. Treatment of Shock by Type

This chapter should also be used in conjunction with other relevant chapters to treat any significant problems underlying the shock (e.g., *Burns, 28; Pulmonary Edema, 55; Poisoning, 53*); see also Respiratory Distress Evaluation, Table 5–2.

57–2. SIGNS AND SYMPTOMS

The clinical manifestations of shock depend to a great extent upon the cause, magnitude and duration as well as upon the patient's prior general health. An individual showing the characteristic picture of shock is prostrated but usually conscious, restless and apprehensive, with moist, cool, clammy skin; circumoral pallor; and sunken eyeballs ("Hippocratic facies"). Cyanosis may occur except when profound anemia is present. The pulse is rapid, feeble and of small volume. Measured urine output is scanty or absent. The blood pressure becomes progressively (and sometimes rapidly) lower, with the systolic pressure usually falling more rapidly than the diastolic. Increasing acidosis *(46–1)* due to progressive hypoxemia of the tissues develops.

Duration of the acute shock state is a reliable index of prognosis—the longer the duration the worse the prognosis. Therefore, treatment of shock takes precedence over all other emergency measures except control of gross hemorrhage and insurance of adequate oxygenation. Any adult patient with a systolic blood pressure of 40 to 55 mm Hg below his or her usual resting level or below 80 to 90 mm Hg, should be checked thoroughly for other manifestations of shock (see Tables 57–2 to 57–5), and treatment should be instituted accordingly.

57–3. PHYSIOLOGIC EVALUATION OF SHOCK SEVERITY

An important contribution to the understanding of the pathophysiology of shock and of the effects of treatment (including use of vasodilator and vasoconstrictor drugs) has been the recognition of the role of pre– and post–capillary vasoconstriction mechanism. If effective treatment is started in the earlier or ischemic stage, reversal of the process with improvement of tissue perfusion occurs more readily than if treatment is delayed until the stagnant phase has become established.

Peripheral arterial blood pressure measurement as a single test is not the only efficient means of assessing the degree or severity of shock or of evaluating response to treatment, but rather represents one of the valuable methods for minute-by-minute monitoring of essential organ tissue perfusion and function outlined in Tables 57–3 and 57–4.

57–4. TYPES OF SHOCK

Importance of Patient History

Details of events leading to development of shock and a detailed history of prior health are usually of assistance in determination of the cause, type and

Table 57–1. INITIAL GENERAL MEASURES IN SHOCK MANAGEMENT*

Initial Measures

- Check vital ABBCS rapidly (Airway, Breathing, Bleeding, Circulation, Sensorium; [5–*1*]). Proceed with rapid physical survey (57–3) if condition permits; otherwise perform rest of these initial measures and return.
- Clear the airway and institute resuscitation (5) if necessary, continuing until the condition has stabilized. Oxygen is administered on clinical grounds.
- Control gross bleeding; splint major fractures [apply pneumatic splints/trousers (MAST) as indicated and available (*18–25*)]. Keep the patient warm. Keep the head level, and keep the legs level or slightly elevated.
- Explain to the patient what is happening in positive clear terms, and convey assurance (this is very important even if it is thought that the patient cannot hear).
- Insert two IV catheters (preferably) or a No. 15 needle. A blood pressure cuff may be used first to take a blood pressure reading and then as a precision temporary tourniquet. Keep a sample of blood for testing of blood sugar and electrolytes. Do a saphenous or other vein cutdown if necessary (two or more lines are advisable).
- Start rapid infusion of D5RL or D5NS, unless an unusual situation (such as hypernatremia) is suspected. Particularly if shock is associated with coma (see 32), give 50 ml of 50% dextrose in water IV plus 100 mg of thiamine IM at once (also consider use of naloxone). If there is obvious hypovolemic shock from severe blood loss, start colloids or whole blood IV as soon as available. Treat acidosis (*46–1*) vigorously as needed: start with 0.5 to 1.0 mEq $NaHCO_3$/kg initially. Monitor therapy results.
- Reassess and complete the rapid physical examination of entire exposed body (see Table 57–2). It is important that normal body temperature be obtained.
- Obtain any further available information concerning onset and past history.

Further Measures

- Reassess status, including rectal temperature.
- Draw blood specimens for the following:
  - —Hgb, Hmct, WBC and diff (one tube of citrated blood).
  - —Serum sugar/amylase, creatinine, BUN, Na, K, Cl, CO_2 content (one tube of clotted blood).
  - —Sample for type and crossmatch for blood transfusion (1 tube).
  - —Obtain 1 extra tube of clotted blood for special tests as needed (e.g., levels of serum acetone, barbiturates, bromide, bilirubin, enzymes).
  - —If there is gross hemorrhage—particularly if disproportionate to trauma, if prolonged, or if patient is known to be on anticoagulants—take a blood specimen for PT, PTT, fibrinogen content and platelet count.
  - —Note the gross clotting time and put aside a sample for evaluation of clot retraction. If a patient with hemorrhage has been taking anticoagulation drugs (*45–8*), start indicated IV therapy at once after drawing blood for PT.
  - —Arterial blood sample for pH and blood gas determination.

Table 57–1. INITIAL GENERAL MEASURES IN SHOCK MANAGEMENT *(Continued)*

Further Measures *(Continued)*

- Insert a urinary bladder catheter (*18–6*) in moderate/severe shock and check output every few minutes until the output becomes adequate. Obtain immediate evaluations of urinary specific gravity, sugar, acetone and pH and send specimen to the lab for culture and micro exam.
- Test responses to sitting (tilt test) if not in severe shock and to the capillary blanching test (Table 57–3).
- Obtain a standard 12 lead electrocardiogram—evaluate particularly for myocardial infarction (*29–15*), cardiac arrhythmias and electrolyte imbalance; establish ongoing monitoring accordingly.
- Recheck vital signs and urine output (Table 57–3).
- Insert a nasogastric tube (unless contraindicated—e.g., by ingestion of corrosives/hydrocarbons); observe the aspirate for volume, color and blood. Save specimen for possible later examination if poisoning suspected. Lavage with 500 ml of 1/6 molar sodium lactate or saline or water. Maintain suction if gastric distention or blood is present.
- Insert a central venous pressure catheter, or a Swan-Ganz catheter, and possibly an arterial line, if the patient is in severe shock. Pulmonary wedge pressures are especially important in severe shock associated with pulmonary edema, acute myocardial infarction, respiratory failure and sepsis, to determine fluid load and to guide therapy, including use of diuretics and digitalis. Label all lines.
- If the patient is febrile and toxic, obtain at least three blood cultures in rapid succession. Culture any wounds or drainage. Perform a lumbar puncture (*18–29*) if meningeal irritation, coma or focal central nervous system deficit is present. Culture throat, any petechiae, and—in females—the cervix. Consider culdocentesis (*18–9*) for women with possible pelvic intra-abdominal pathology. Make Gram stains of any probable sources of infection and start immediate appropriate massive antibiotic therapy (*33–29, Antimicrobial Drugs of Choice*).
- If urinary output is scanty (4 to 6 ml in 10 minutes) or absent, inject 100 ml of a 25% solution of mannitol IV, or consider fluid challenge with saline or Ringer's solution. If the urine volume doubles in the next 10 minutes, continue to force appropriate fluids (blood or saline); if there is no increase, fluids must be given very cautiously.
- Obtain additional laboratory tests (such as blood volume, radioisotope organ scans) as required and retest based on current condition and response to therapy (such as serial arterial pH, $PaCO_2$, PaO_2) and proceed with therapy for the type and degree of shock (Tables 57–4 and 57–6) and with treatment of underlying causes.
- Consider heparin administration if pulmonary embolism (*63–6*) is present.

*Use of a slide rule nomogram giving calculated IV bolus and IV infusion dose rates of medications for shock and resuscitation management for varying pediatric and adult weights is of great assistance. A device available from EMERG-DOSE Inc., 152 Highland St., Holden, MA 01520) accomplishes this.

Table 57–2. RAPID PHYSICAL REVIEW FOR PATIENTS IN SHOCK*

Skin (Expose entire body surface for examination as soon as feasible.)
*Gross bleeding seen at or beneath the skin surface
Burns—surface area, degree, depth (see 28)
Turgor
*Color
*Temperature (by tactile perception of examiner first; obtain rectal recording later)
*Rash, petechiae or purpura
Capillary filling
Infections or wounds
Otoscopic inspection

Central Nervous System
*Sensorium
*Pupils—size and reactivity
Papilledema
Gross focal pathologic neurologic signs (motor or sensory loss, reflexes, rectal sphincter tone, pathologic toe signs); cranial nerve deficit
Meningeal irritation (*33–40, Meningitis*)

Cardiopulmonary Vascular System
*Pulse rate and rhythm
*Respiratory volumes: estimate TV first (*19–9*); later measure TV, PEFR, FVC prn
*Blood pressure
Jugular vein size, angle of collapse
Lungs—breath sounds, dullness, tympany
Heart—gross size, thrills, quality of heart tones, murmurs

Enteric System and Abdomen
Odor of breath and oral cavity
Presence of oral blood, blood in the stool (*40–5, Gastrointestinal Hemorrhage*) or foreign substances (*39–7, Foreign Bodies in Gastrointestinal Tract*)
Abdominal distention, tenderness, guarding or masses; rectal examination
Organomegaly, including area of splenic dullness
Widening of the abdominal aorta and presence of femoral pulses

Genitourinary System
See *41, Genitourinary Tract Emergencies*. A bimanual pelvic examination should be done in women, followed later by a speculum examination, with rectal examination if posterior cul-de-sac pathology is suspected. In evaluation of toxic shock syndrome (*33–70*), culture the vagina, cervix and any tampon present, plus remove the tampon and send to Pathology lab.

Musculoskeletal System (*See also 47, Musculoskeletal Conditions*)
A thorough visual inspection should be made followed by rapid but careful checking for evidence of injury to the neck, thorax, back, pelvis and extremities. Massive soft tissue trauma should be evaluated carefully. In the prevention and treatment of shock, splinting of long bone fractures has a high order of priority (see *2, Triage*).

*Examinations preceded by an asterisk (*) should be done at once.

Table 57–3. METHODS FOR RAPID CLINICAL MONITORING OF CELLULAR METABOLISM AND ORGAN PERFUSION

Parameter	Primary Organ or System
Respiratory rate, tidal volume (estimated) skin color, temperature, capillary blanching and filling; measured TV, PEFR, FVC prn	Pulmonary and ventilatory system. Peripheral cellular metabolism and perfusion
Pupillary size; sensorium	Central nervous system
Pulse and heart rate; stethoscope; oscilloscope with electrocardiograph (cardiac rate and rhythm; ventricular depolarization and repolarization)	Heart (If stethoscope not available, placing the ear directly against the thorax permits a good index of heart and breath sounds)
Urinary output determined by indwelling bladder catheter	Kidney
Tilt test, jugular vein filling, capillary blanching test, venous and pulse pressure	Extracellular and intravascular fluid volume

Other periodic measurements (cardiac output, blood pH, expired air and arterial blood gas determinations and blood volume) may be necessary in some cases but are not as simple or immediately available as those listed above

prognosis of shock. A history of trauma, operative procedures, exposure to poisonous substances (including drugs and medications), infection, fever and focal pain may be significant. In addition, estimates of prior blood loss, duration of vomiting and diarrhea and comparison with normal body weight can be of great importance in planning an effective therapeutic regimen. Inability of the patient to give a coherent history is an indication of impaired brain cell function, possibly secondary to perfusion.

Classification of Shock Types

The following classification of the types of shock is not satisfactory in some ways, but it does furnish a basis for rapid evaluation and emergency therapy. A combination of the types listed may be present in the same patient at a given time and may, by a common mode or an interrelated action, cause disruption of tissue perfusion and cellular metabolism. Common physical findings by type of shock are listed in Table 57–5.

1. ***Hypovolemic shock*** is the result of gross loss of one or more of the following: blood, plasma, water, saline and electrolytes, either from the body and intravascular compartments or into a relatively inaccessible "third compartment" (peritoneal and pleural cavities, massive soft tissue effusion).

2. ***Cardiogenic shock*** results from electrical or mechanical failure of the heart or peripheral vascular collapse, or both. Acute myocardial infarction, serious cardiac dysrhythmias and acute cor pulmonale—particularly from pulmonary embolus—are the most common causes.

3. ***Septic shock*** is caused by bacterial toxins or by endotoxins from gram-negative organisms. Septic shock may result in severe effective fluid volume loss (hypovolemia).

Table 57–4. GUIDELINES FOR DETERMINING DEGREE OF SEVERITY OF SHOCK

Test or Sign		Normal or Average	Degree of Shock (Class)		
			Preshock State to Mild Shock (I)	*Moderate (II)*	*Moderately Severe (III) to Severe (IV)*
Sensorium	Orientation	Well-oriented Time Place Person	Oriented	Fairly well-oriented	May be confused and disoriented to uncommunicative
	Enunciation	Distinct	Normal—slurred words	Possibly slowed, with slurred words	Slow and slurred to not speaking
	Content	Appropriate; structured sentences	Sentences normal; concerned	Apprehensive; slow sentences or phrases	Apprehensive; confused to incoherent
Pupils	Size	Equal (2 to 4 mm)	Normal	Normal	Normal to dilating or dilated
	Constriction with light	Rapid	Rapid	Rapid	Slow or nonreactive
Pulse	Rate	60 to 80/min	80 to 100/min	100 to 120/min	120 to 140/min (III) >140 (IV)
	Amplitude	Full	Full amplitude to slight decrease	Variable—mild decrease	Thready or absent
Blood pressure (mm Hg)	Systolic	110 to 145	Normal or slightly low	Decreased—often 40 to 50 mm of Hg below usual B.P.	Less than 80 to unobtainable
	Diastolic	60 to 90	Normal or slightly low	Decreased, but less so than systolic	40 to 50 to unobtainable
	Pulse pressure	40 to 60	35 to 40	30	20 or less
Jugular vein filling*	Patient flat	Fills to anterior border of sternocleidomastoid	Normal to trace of filling	Trace to no filling	No filling

Urinary output via catheter	ml/min	0.6 to 1.0	0.5 to 0.6	0.4 to 0.5	0.1 to 0.3 or less
	ml/10 min	6 to 10	5 to 6	4 to 5	1 to 3 or less
Tilt test— Rapid lying to sitting position	Pulse	Transient increase	Increased	Rapid	Already maximal
	Blood pressure	Less than 10 min decrease	10 to 25 mm decrease	25 to 50 mm decrease	Marked decrease to unobtainable
	Symptoms	No "lightheadedness"	No lightheadedness	Lightheadedness	Unable to sit up
	Therapeutic, if whole blood loss	—	Crystalloids	Crystalloids; usually no blood transfusion	Crystalloids plus blood transfusion
	Est. blood loss (average adult male)	—	To 750 ml	1000 to 1250 ml	1500 to 1800 ml (III) 2000 to 2500 ml or more (IV)
	Est. % blood volume loss	—	15%	20 to 25%	30 to 35% (III) 40 to 50% (IV)
Capillary blanching test	Blanching of forehead skin or nailbed with thumb pressure	Return of circulation in 1.25 to 1.5 sec.	1.25 to 1.5 sec.	More than 1.5 sec.	Pallor before and after test
			Note: With hypercapnia, there may be almost instantaneous return		
Central venous pressure (CVP)		Normal (3 to 12 cm) of saline)	Normal	Low	Extremely low
			May be normal (unusual) or elevated (common) in cardiogenic shock		
			May be elevated (unusual) in hypovolemia with secondary congestive heart failure; give monitored fluid challenge		
Pulmonary wedge pressure	Normal (4 to 12 torr)		Same as CVP		

*May be grossly distended in cardiogenic shock and pericardial tamponade.

Table 57–5. COMMON PHYSICAL FINDINGS BY TYPE OF SHOCK

Hypovolemic	Cardiogenic	Septic
Whole Blood Loss History of prior focal bleeding, blood dyscrasia or anticoagulant therapy (*45–10*) Acute trauma Observed gross bleeding Extreme pallor, including the conjunctivae and palmar creases Palpation, percussion and needle aspiration of large blood masses	Signs and symptoms of myocardial infarction (*29–15*) or congestive heart failure (*55–3*)	Feverishness Malaise Symptoms often of genitourinary or enteric disease or disorder or prior treatment and instrumentation thereof
Water, Saline and/or Plasma Loss Rapid body weight loss Poor tissue turgor Inadequate input or abnormally increased output via skin, stomach, rectum or kidneys Demonstration of fluid loss into "third space"	Serious arrhythmias and abnormal rates (increased or decreased) Gallop rhythm and murmurs Poor heart tones Cardiac enlargement	Toxic appearance Focus of infection Fever (can be minimal or absent if septic shock is overwhelming, occurs in a person already in a debilitated condition [e.g., due to myxedema] or is masked by subsequent hypothermia as is prone to occur in the elderly, in people living alone, or in those debilitated by alcohol, drugs or disease)

57–5. SPECIFIC MEASURES IN SHOCK TREATMENT

No protocol, regardless of its length or structure, can take the place of frequent close observation of the patient and appropriate individual adjustments of treatment. Evaluation of a person who is in shock begins the moment that the physician first sees the patient. Therapy must take into consideration not only correction of immediate deficits and replacement of current losses but also normal physiologic requirements.

Moderate and severe shock must be treated energetically and corrected as soon as possible using periodic monitoring to evaluate progress. On the other hand, persons in mild shock who are making satisfactory progress toward normalcy should be treated more conservatively and cautiously—especially the very young, the very old and persons with underlying chronic organic diseases so as to minimize the likelihood of problems that may be caused by overtreatment. Therapy must take into consideration not only correction of immediate deficits and replacement of current losses but also normal daily physiologic requirements (see *11*).

General measures in shock treatment are started as outlined in Table 57–1. The severity and type of shock are evaluated according to the guidelines in Tables 57–2 through 57–5; once these are determined, specific treatment measures are instituted as suggested in the guidelines of Table 57–6. The major specific treatment measures for shock are outlined on page 652 and described more fully in the following paragraphs. (Again, reference should also be made to sections dealing with specific underlying problems.) *The goal is restoration of normal fluid compartment volumes and composition plus normal tissue perfusion pressures.*

Table 57–6. TREATMENT OF SHOCK BY TYPE

KEY:
++ Prime factor
\+ Generally indicated
± Variable—based on clinical state
0 Not indicated or not necessary

Treatment	Hypovolemic Shock	Cardiogenic Shock	Septic Shock
Insurance of an adequate airway and ventilation	++	++	++
Control of hemorrhage if present (gross/occult)	++	0	0
Control of pain and apprehension	++	++	++
Oxygen	++	++	++
Preservation of normal body temperature	++	++	++
Restoration and maintenance of normal circulating vascular volume	++	++	++
Correction of acidosis; avoidance of alkalosis	++	++	++
Saline and electrolytes	++	±	+
Plasma volume expanders	±	±	±
Whole blood	++ (Severe blood loss type)	0	±
Vasopressors; cardiotonic drugs	±	++	+
Vasodilators	±	±	±
Antibiotics	±	±	++
Steroids	±	±	±

Outline of Specific Measures

A. Maintenance or Restoration of Blood and Tissue Fluid Volume
B. Metabolic Correction
C. Vasopressor and Cardiotonic Medications
D. Vasodilators
E. Ventilation Assistance and Oxygen Administration
F. Corticosteroid Therapy
G. Antibiotic Therapy
H. Control of Pain
I. Transportation

A. Restoration and Maintenance of Blood and Tissue Fluid Volume

- Volume and type of crystalloids and/or colloids, and rate of fluid administration are key issues in correction of shock.
- Volume and type must be adequate to replenish prior, current and future losses (see *11–1* to *11–3*).
- Data from a fluid balance sheet (*11–1*) initially estimating prior and current losses of crystalloids and colloids, along with the data provided in Table 57–4, Guidelines for Determining Degree of Severity of Shock, should be used to determine the volume and type of fluids needed. The composition of common crystalloids and colloids is given in *11–4*.
- The rate of administration must be adequate to restore effective blood flow rapidly for vital organ function; this is measured on a minute-by-minute basis (Tables 57–3 and 57–4), with the rate adjusted until restoration and stabilization is occurring and at appropriate frequent intervals thereafter.
- Crystalloids are the principal fluid given generally unless blood or a colloid is indicated on the basis of one or more of the following:
  —Acute blood loss of 30% or more.
  —Prior severe anemia.
  —Preexistence of a disease state that places the patient at a higher-than-average risk to relative ischemia.
  —Need for greater osmotic pressure of colloids (e.g., peripheral edema exists, but blood volume is still low).
- Crystalloids are usually still given at a 3:1 volume ratio to blood/colloids even when blood/colloids are indicated.
- Set up multiple large-bore IV cannulae for administration and monitoring as noted in Table 57–1.
- A guideline for fluid administration in one type of complex situation—burns—is given in Table 28–2.

Crystalloid Solution Administration

- D5RL or D5NS is usually given IV initially unless special electrolyte problems exist.
- An IV fluid challenge of 20 ml/kg/hr of D5RL given in 10-minute aliquots in adults (and up to twice that rate in the younger pediatric age group) may be given for therapeutic response.
- Usually give adults up to 200 to 250 ml increments every 10 minutes and check CVP (or use Swan-Ganz catheter in patients with cardiovascular disease); continue to administer at 10-minute intervals if general response is favorable and if CVP increase is not more than 2 cm H_2O or more than a total of 10 to 11 cm H_2O. If CVP increments or total is greater than the

aforementioned, or if urine output rises to over 17 ml/10 min in an adult (or over 2 ml/kg/hr in pediatric age group), reduce or stop the challenge for 5 to 10 minutes to permit readjustment and reevaluation.

- Gradually reduce fluid administration rates to maintenance levels while continuing monitored responses (Table 57–4) and assuring adequate urine output (50 to 60 ml/hr in the adult; 2 ml/kg/hr for children under 1 year, and 1 ml/kg/hr if older).

Colloid Administration Other Than Blood

Among the colloid substances other than blood that may be used to increase plasma volume are: dextran-70 (best to avoid administration of over 1000 ml; generally creates fewer problems than dextran-40); serum albumin (5% or 25%: both are effective plasma expanders but are expensive and can cause salt and fluid retention and coagulation problems); plasma protein fraction (hypotension can result); and plasma (hepatitis virus a problem). Newer preparations for which protocols are being evaluated are: Hetastarch, HALF-D, and blood substitutes such as Fluosol DA (approved under special circumstances; see *18–35*).

Blood Administration

- Before any plasma volume expander is given, collect 7 ml of venous blood (serum) in a plain red top tube for each 1 to 3 units of blood to be typed and crossmatched. The need to increase hemoglobin—particularly if there is acute blood loss of 30% or more as determined by guidelines above—will determine further procedure.
- Starting from the time of drawing the sample, the need for accurate labeling and patient identification is paramount.
- Current preference is to give crystalloids for support until complete ABO-Rh type and antibody screening crossmatch of packed RBC's is available—this takes about 45 to 60 minutes or more, depending on difficulty (particularly presence of positive recipient antibody screen) and on whether more than one technician is available.
- If unique circumstances permit consideration of autotransfusion (see *18–35*), that procedure can be begun immediately. Some religious sects (e.g., Jehovah's Witnesses) do not permit autotransfusion; blood substitutes such as Fluosol may be used in these cases. See also *69–16*.
- Urgent need for rapid replacement of the blood oxygen transport system may justify the physician's subjecting the patient to increased risk of using blood that is less than completely typed and crossmatched.
- ABO-Rh typing takes about 10 minutes, and type-specific blood is preferred over O-negative blood. Saline–immediate spin crossmatch takes approximately another 10 minutes and helps eliminate severe reactions that may occur with ABO mismatch and potent minor blood group antibodies (albumin crossmatch, screening for antibodies in the recipient's blood and Coombs test are done additionally in a complete T & C).
- Acquisition of O-negative blood (the universal donor) takes practically no more time than transport from the blood bank. Particularly in females of potential childbearing status, it is best to use low-titer O-negative blood or packed O-negative RBC's plus fresh frozen plasma or normal saline if there is insufficient time to obtain type-specific blood.
- The following considerations should also be taken into account:
  —Normal saline is the most compatible solution in IV lines carrying blood.
  —Macrofilters are generally used instead of microfilters, which may also screen out platelets.

—A unit of RBC/blood should be preferably transfused in less than 2 hours. Monitor the patient closely for reactions (*18–35*) during initial administration.
—With massive transfusion requirements, 3 or 4 large-bore IV catheter lines may be needed in conjunction with frequent CVP monitoring.
—Warming of the blood to 37°C (98.6°F) is desirable, especially during multiple transfusions; if warmth of blood is inadequate, then warm the patient (*62–3*).
—Use blood as fresh as available for multiple transfusions.
—Coagulation deficiencies (*45*) may occur with multiple transfusions. Massive hemorrhage may be defined as blood loss requiring 6 to 10 units transfused in less than 2 hours. Monitor platelets, fibrinogen, PTT and serum calcium (e.g., after each 5 to 10 units of RBC/blood). With each 6 to 10 units of bank blood transfused, 5 to 10 platelet packs and 1 to 2 units or more of frozen plasma may be needed; most patients do not require calcium administration separately.

B. Metabolic Correction

Control severe metabolic acidosis by initial IV injection of 0.5 to 1.0 mEq/kgbw of sodium bicarbonate solution (contains 44.6 mEq in 50 ml of solution) and repeat as required or according to specific schedules, as in cardiac arrest (*5–2*) or diabetic coma). Correct any electrolyte imbalance (*46*). Include periodic ABG determinations as a guide to therapy. Avoid alkaline pH state.

C. Vasopressor and Cardiotonic Medications

In noncardiogenic shock, vasopressors must not be employed until after the restoration of adequate intravascular volume. The vasopressor drugs can be valuable adjuncts in treatment of shock, particularly shock in which the skin is warm (rather than cold and clammy). In cardiogenic shock due to myocardial infarction, use vasopressors cautiously to help avoid extending the infarct size. As a rule, they should be given slowly in 500 to 1000 ml of intravenous fluids. Evaluation of therapeutic response to vasopressors can be more easily monitored with an arterial line and Swan-Ganz catheter. The most effective vasoconstrictors are as follows:*

1. Levarterenol bitartrate (Levophed) or *l*-norepinephrine, 4 mg, given slowly IV in 250 ml of D5W or saline continued for as long as necessary. The speed of IV injection should be controlled by blood pressure readings every 2 minutes until a plateau at which the systolic pressure is slightly below normal has been reached. A plastic catheter inserted into a large vein—by cutdown if necessary—is preferable to a needle because extravasation of levarterenol bitartrate into soft tissues will cause sloughing. If long-continued use is necessary and blanching along the course of the vein develops, the site of injection should be changed at once. If extravasation into the soft tissues does occur, infiltration of the area through multiple punctures, using a fine (No. 26) needle, with 5 to 10 mg of phentolamine methanesulfonate (Regitine) and 150 turbidity reducing units (TRU) of hyaluronidase dissolved in 15 ml of normal salt solution may prevent extensive necrosis.

**Note*: Although levarterenol is the most potent, use of dopamine or dobutamine is usually preferred.

2. Dopamine hydrochloride (Intropin) has both alpha- and beta-adrenergic actions plus unique dopaminergic properties and, like norepinephrine and metaraminol, is inotropic and chronotropic but may exhibit vasodilatory effect under some circumstances and may be noted to particularly improve splanchnic and renal blood flow. Dopamine may be preferable for patients in cardiogenic shock or for patients with known cardiac problems; administer with monitored continuous IV infusion beginning at 2 to 5 μg/kg/min. Increase by increments of 5 to 10 μg/kg/min up to 20 to 50 μg/kg/min as necessary. Administer with same type of precautions as used for norepinephrine. If there is no response to dopamine, a 4-mg bolus of IV glucagon may be given, followed by an infusion of 10 mg/hr if response is favorable.

3. Dobutamine HCl (Dobutrex) has more beta-adrenergic activity and is inotropic and chronotropic with vasodilatory action. It does not cause release of norepinephrine as does dopamine. Its onset of action is rapid, occurring within 1 to 2 minutes with IV infusion of 2.5 to 10 μg/kg/min, with peak effect reached within 10 minutes. It is effective in cardiogenic shock, but should not be given with IHSS (idiopathic hypertrophic subaortic stenosis).

4. Metaraminol bitartrate (Aramine) given intravenously is now rarely used. This drug in small doses has a beta-adrenergic effect and decreases blood pressure, increases the heart rate and decreases venous pooling. In large doses it acts as an alphamimetic, with a rise in blood pressure, a decrease in pulse rate and an increase in venous pooling.

5. Phenylephrine hydrochloride (Neo-Synephrine), 0.1 to 0.5 mg IV directly or 3 to 5 mg added to 500 to 1000 ml of IV solution. This drug is a potent alphamimetic and raises blood pressure, slows the heart (no direct cardiac stimulatory effect; effect is reflex) and increases venous pooling. Methoxamine hydrochloride (Vasoxyl) has a similar effect.

Note: Digitalization *(29–11)* with digoxin should be considered if there are signs of pulmonary congestion or failure of response in the presence of adequate fluid volume. See also *29–15, Treatment of Acute Myocardial Infarction.*

D. Vasodilators

Cardiogenic shock with severely decreased cardiac output is the single most important indicator for the use of vasodilators in shock management. If pulmonary wedge pressure (PWP) and peripheral resistance are both increased, as measured by an arterial line, IV sodium nitroprusside or IV nitroglycerine may be used to decrease the resistance and thus obtain an increase in the cardiac output. Using an infusion pump and close monitoring, IV sodium nitroprusside may be started at a rate of 0.5 to 1.0 μg/kg/min. The usual adult starting dose of IV nitroglycerine is 5 μg per minute; special non–polyvinyl chloride (non-PVC) IV infusion sets are required. Dopamine may also be indicated in dopaminergic dose levels (2 to 5 μg/kg/min) to increase renal blood flow and perfusion as determined by frequent urinary output measurement.

E. Ventilation Assistance and Oxygen Administration

Assisted ventilation of moisturized oxygen supplement may be necessary rather than just administration of oxygen by mask or cannula if the minute volume is low, the tidal volume is less than 5 ml/kg, the vital capacity is less than 12 ml/kg, the PaO_2 is less than 80 or the $PaCO_2$ is more than 50. Acute respiratory distress syndrome (ARDS; see 55–4) is often a leading component in death due to shock; monitored oxygen therapy is beneficial.

F. Corticosteroid Therapy

The use of steroids for types of shock other than anaphylaxis and adrenal endocrine deficiency shock is generally considered controversial. In cases of severe hypersensitivity (*24–1, Anaphylactic Shock*) or endocrine failure shock (*36–1, Acute Adrenal Cortical Insufficiency; 36–8, Acute Parathyroid Intoxication; 36–11, Hyperthyroid Emergencies*) that do not respond readily to general measures, including use of epinephrine and restoration of fluid volume, corticosteroids may be indicated. Corticosteroids are generally considered not to be indicated for cardiogenic shock. The sooner corticosteroids are given, the more likely they are to provide a beneficial response, if they provide one at all. Draw a blood sample for cortisol level first, if prior deficiency may be an issue. In severe septic or refractory shock, methylprednisolone sodium succinate (Solu-Medrol), 30 mg/kg in a single dose and half that dose repeated in 4 to 6 hours, may be considered. If there is no response after two doses, this approach can be discontinued. In children, the IV dose should be not less than 0.5 mg/kg/day. Provided corticosteroid therapy has not been in use for more than 3 days, administration can be discontinued abruptly without ill effects; if it has been used for longer periods, it should be gradually decreased.

G. Antibiotic Therapy

In cases of infection, as specific treatment as possible must be started as soon as cultures have been obtained. This is of critical importance in septic and toxic shock. Selection of antibiotic is aided by Gram stain, patient age, febrile course, history of exposures, and characteristics of any wounds (see especially *59–42, Soft Tissue Infections, Deep and Anaerobic*). For further guidelines, see *33–83, Antimicrobial Drugs of Choice*. Prophylactic use of antibiotics is not generally recommended. Females of childbearing age should be checked for the presence of a tampon or diaphragm, which may predispose to toxic shock.

H. Control of Pain *(See also 12)*

Restoration of perfusion and blood pressure should be commenced before morphine sulfate administration. Morphine sulfate given slowly IV may be used in small doses (e.g., 1 mg every 30 to 60 seconds up to a 5-mg dose or until pain has stopped; repeat in 10 minutes if no adverse effects but pain persists) if the patient is acutely apprehensive and in severe pain, provided chest injuries *(31)* or head injuries *(44)* are not present. Pentazocine lactate (Talwin), 30 mg IV or IM, does not cause significant respiratory depression and is an effective anodyne. Control of pain *(12)* is an important factor in management, as pain can contribute significantly to the severity of shock.

I. Transportation *(See also 4, Transportation)*

Transportation for hospitalization and definitive treatment should be arranged as soon as feasible. Speed of transportation is not as important as care during transportation, which should be in full compliance with speed and traffic regulations. Intravenous fluids, respiratory assistance and supportive therapy should be continued during transportation as necessary, preferably under protocol and/or supervision of a physician.

58. Skin and Mucous Membrane Conditions

The skin surface area of an average-sized adult (70 kg or 154 lb) is about 1.73 square meters (18½ square feet) and is exposed to multiple infections, irritants, trauma and allergenic factors; the response to these is readily visible and can rapidly cause physical and psychological distress. These factors cause numerous patients with dermatologic conditions to come to the emergency department for evaluation and treatment, though few are life threatening. The skin, with its complex interrelationship with the nervous system (both develop embryologically from the ectoderm), has important thermoregulatory, fluid and electrolyte functions in addition to being an impressive buffer organ against the environment. Although the eyes may be the "window to the soul," the skin is the mirror of the psyche (e.g., vasomotor manifestations, acute and chronic, and dermatitis factitia).

The skin, in contrast to internal organs and structures, lends itself easily to direct examination. The skilled observer can usually differentiate causes of tissue reaction, e.g., allergic, vascular, infectious, degenerative and neoplastic; and appropriate therapy can be initiated. Burns *(28)* and soft tissue injuries *(59)* are considered in separate sections.

58–1. ALLERGIC REACTIONS *(See 24)*

58–2. ANGIOEDEMA *(See 24–2)*

58–3. BITES *(See 27)*

58–4. BLISTERS *(See also 12, Edema Reduction)*

Blisters from abrasive activity cause pain that may detract from physical performance during sports or work and present the potential for secondary infections. Avoidance of further activity and circumferential padding are ordinarily all that is required.

Temporary relief (and sometimes lasting relief) of sufficient degree to usually permit continuance of competition or urgent work can be obtained with the following approach:

1. Cleanse the skin.
2. Drain the fluid from the blister with a syringe via a needle inserted into adjacent normal skin and undermined up into the blister—topical Fluori-methane spray is an adequate anesthetic.
3. Coat the blister and a generous surrounding area with tincture of benzoin followed by 4 to 5 layers of 1-inch or 2-inch Micropore paper tape. Application of a broad covering, such as Second Skin or Moleskin, is also of value.

58–5. BURNS *(See 28; see also 3–6, Thermal Effects of a Nuclear Blast)*

58–6. CONTAGIOUS AND COMMUNICABLE DISEASES *(See also 33–82, Common Exanthems; 49–13, Neuritis)*

General treatment of the following conditions requires care of any associated wounds (See *59, Soft Tissue Injuries; 20, Tetanus Immunization*). Communicable disease control of the patient's person and belongings to protect the family and others is of paramount importance. (See *33–1, Infectious Disease Control Techniques.*)

Erysipelas (St. Anthony's Fire). Erysipelas is an acute infectious disease due to *Streptococcus pyogenes* and its toxin or *Staphylococcus aureus*. It is ushered in rapidly with a prodromal systemic toxemia, then characterized by an indurated crimson or erythematous raised and sharply demarcated skin border.

Specific treatment consists of immediate oral or intramuscular penicillin (if allergic, then erythromycin), depending on severity. Topical antibacterials are of limited value. Initially the exact inciting organism will be unknown, but often the condition is due to a penicillinase-producing *Staphylococcus* species. Therefore it may be safer to give a cephalosporin, vancomycin, dicloxacillin, nafcillin or cloxacillin rather than penicillin G or Pen Vee K.

Impetigo Contagiosa. This acute, highly contagious skin disease may occur at any age and is caused by pyogenic cocci, either streptococcus, staphylococcus or both. The skin lesions are characterized by onset with an erythematous macule that rapidly changes to a vesicle then a pustule with subsequent irregular crusting. Bullae may occur. Deeper skin involvement causing circinate ulcerations with adjacent skin induration and reddening is called ecthyma. Lesions should be cultured and testing done for antibacterial sensitivity; a Gram stain may aid immediate diagnosis and treatment selection.

Treatment

1. See *33–83*. The antimicrobial of choice for oral or parenteral administration is usually erythromycin, cloxacillin or dicloxacillin in the presence of a penicillinase-producing *Staphylococcus* species and penicillin in the presence of streptococci.
2. Warm, moist compresses several times daily with gentle opening of pustules and removal of crusts. Cleanse adjacent skin and then infected sites with Hibiclens or Phisohex.
3. Topical antibacterials such as bacitracin or polymyxin B combination (Polysporin) aid infection control. Lesions may be left open and exposed to the air periodically if patient is at home in bed but should be covered with protective dressing if up and about.
4. Disease control against autoinoculation and spread to close contacts (and even community epidemics) is of paramount importance.

Toxic Epidermal Necrolysis (TEN, Scalded Skin Syndrome). Acute toxemia, early skin tenderness and redness, bullae and easy desquamation with pressure on skin that appears scalded are characteristic. This potentially lethal dermatologic emergency is caused most often by an infectious process (*Staphylococcus* organisms) or a drug reaction. Differentiation as to exact cause is essential, as treatment approaches vary greatly. Toxic shock syndrome (*33–70*) should be considered in the differential diagnosis.

Evaluate with the following measures:

1. Get history of *all* drug ingestions and chemical exposures.
2. Perform Gram stain and obtain culture of skin lesion exudates. Culture the pharynx, blood and urine.
3. Age is not an absolute indicator, though more infants and young children have staphylococcal infection and more adults have drug reaction.
4. Frozen section examination of the border of a fresh reddened piece of a peeled or denuded skin lesion shows a deep split (full thickness) in drug reactions, whereas denuding of only the outermost layers (*S. corneum*) typifies staphylococcus infections with toxin release.
5. Cytologic examination of the sample described under measure 4 or of a smear made from gentle scrapings at the base of a fresh lesion, in addition to

showing cells characteristic of the level of skin splitting, will show a paucity of inflammatory cells in the intradermal split if the lesion is due to staphylococcus infection with toxin release.

Treatment of Drug Reaction TEN *(See also 58–8, Treatment of Infection-Induced TEN)*

1. Start IV infusion of sodium methicillin (Staphcillin) 50 mg per kilogram per day. If penicillin allergy is known, give erythromycin or clindamycin in high doses.
2. Hospitalize at once for continued treatment, including those measures performed for burn patients to treat and preserve skin.
3. If differentiation between the two major causes of TEN cannot be made initially, in addition to withdrawing all prior possibly culpable drugs, start intravenous (IV) antibiotics then add steroids.

Scabies (Mites) and Pediculosis (Lice). The principal urgency in these pruritic dermatoses is to make the diagnosis and start management to stop their epidemic proportions.

SCABIES. Scabies is distinguished by the eruptive skin lesions produced by the burrowing of the female parasitic mite *(Sarcoptes scabiei)* while laying eggs. Characteristics are grayish-brown, dotted, slightly raised, straight or twisting tracts 5 to 6 mm in length; noninflammatory vesicles on the interdigital webs and sides of fingers; erythematous urticarial papules; and excoriations from scratching. They may appear anywhere on the body but are generally below the neck, particularly in friction areas. Urticaria *(58–19)* may occur. Diagnosis is confirmed by finding the mite in a burrow using a hypodermic needle for unroofing and a hand lens.

Treatment

1. Take a hot shower and clean with soap and a soft brush.
2. Apply a scabicide such as gamma benzene hexachloride (Kwell) all over the body from the neck down for 8 to 12 hours (overnight) followed by thorough washing; use according to manufacturer's instructions in adults and older children (do not use in pregnant women). Prescribe enough (1 to 2 ounces per adult) for one treatment course only for all family members and close personal contacts. The scabicide crotamiton (Eurax Lotion) can be used safely for infants and young children (and adults), as it is less toxic; massage into skin of whole body from chin down, particularly all folds and creases; repeat in 24 hours, and shower 48 hours after that. Wash furred family pets, particularly dogs, which may harbor the mites, according to veterinarian's instructions.
3. Use freshly laundered (hot wash and dry) underclothing and bedding after the general cleansing off of lotion at 8 to 12 hours. Mites are obligate parasites that do not survive away from animal-human hosts, so general cleaning is not required.
4. Either wash all clothes and bedding used in the past 2 days on hot wash/dry cycle, dry clean nonwashable items or seal items in a plastic container for 2 full days before reuse.
5. Diphenhydramine hydrochloride (Benadryl) and hydroxyzine hydrochloride (Atarax) for relief of pruritus or other antipruritic measures, as under *58–12*. Itching may continue for several days despite successful scabicide treatment.
6. Antibacterial treatment, topical or systemic, for any secondary infection.

PEDICULOSIS. Pediculosis is an infestation with obligate lice parasites (head louse, *Pediculus humanus capitis;* body louse, *Pediculus humanus* var.

corporis—"cooties"; or crab louse, *Phthirus pubic*—"crabs") that, with the exception of the body louse, propagate in the hairy regions of the body and irritate the skin. Identification of the louse (about ⅛" long) and its eggs (nits), seen with the naked eye or magnifying glass, establishes the diagnosis. Nits are opaque, pear-shaped bodies of white to dark brown color (about 1/16" long) that fasten to clothing (particularly in seams) and hair shafts (mostly at the hair-skin junction) by a glue-like substance. Lice that fall onto inorganic material die in 2 to 3 days. Nits take approximately 10 days to hatch, so they may survive during that period without nourishment.

Principles of therapy are similar to those for scabies, namely, to destroy the parasite and its eggs and to treat the irritated skin. If prescription pesticides such as gamma benzene hexachloride (e.g., Kwell lotion or shampoo) are unobtainable, nits may be destroyed or loosened from hair shafts for easier removal by soaking with equal parts of alcohol and vinegar solution. Over-the-counter products, such as RID, BARC and TRIPLEX, used as directed, can also be effective. Nits may be removed from the scalp with a very fine comb or tweezers. Shirts, underclothing, sheets and pillowcases used within the past 7 days should be washed and dried at hot cycle; boiling is not necessary; alternatively these items can be sealed in a plastic bag for 10 days and then used. Also, nits may be removed with a tweezers. Turn outer clothing inside out and shake and vacuum. Press inseams with a hot iron after moistening; dry cleaning is also effective. Clean all personal effects, particularly combs, brushes and hats. Mattresses, rugs and furniture should be vacuumed; spraying is not necessary.

Infestation of the scalp by *Pediculus humanus* var. *capitis* or *Phthirus pubis* is treated by a 4- to 6-minute shampoo with 2 to 3 teaspoons of gamma benzene hexachloride—1% lindane—followed by thorough rinsing and rewashing with nonmedicated shampoo (Kwell shampoo). If any nits survive, repeat in 10 days may be necessary. (*Note:* Kwell should not be used on children under 8 or pregnant women.)

Check close contacts every 2 to 3 days for 10 days; close contacts need not be treated unless the person sleeps in the same bed or room as the patient or evidence of nits is found.

58–7. DERMATITIS

Irritant Contact. Primary irritant contact dermatitis is the response of the skin to irritant exposure—the concentration and duration required varying from individual to individual. Many are caused by occupational chemicals (for reporting see *75, Worker's Compensation Cases*).

For primary antipruritic and corticosteroid treatment, see *58–12*. Prophylactic treatment with use of tools, proper protective gloves and/or protective substances (e.g., Arretil or Kerodex) is advisable; recurrence despite these may necessitate a change in occupation or work site.

Allergic Contact. This type of dermatitis is due to an individual's hypersensitivity reaction to allergens contacted. For example, see *58–13, Poison Oak, Ivy and Sumac; 58–18, Urushiol Contact Dermatitis.*

Treatment

- Identify and remove from exposure to the causative agent. Proper identification may require extensive testing in some cases.
- See *58–12, Pruritus,* for antipruritic measures.

58–8. DRUG AND CHEMICAL REACTIONS

Practically every drug in therapeutic use can cause pruritus, skin rashes, urticaria, angioedema and serum sickness severe enough to activate an urgent patient problem.

Toxic Epidermal Necrolysis (TEN) *(See 58–6)*. Severe cases may cause an exfoliative reaction of the skin and mucous membranes; for example, arsenic preparations (*53–90, Arsphenamine*) and phenylbutazone (*53–537*) are notorious offenders. Salicylates (*53–614*), penicillins (*53–78*), barbiturates (*53–110*) and sulfonamides (*53–660*) are other leading causes.

Erythema Multiforme. Drug and chemical reactions are among the multiple causes (e.g., viral, fungal, bacterial, collagen disease) of this acute skin and mucous membrane disorder. Iris or target lesions are most characteristic, but red macules, blisters and mucous membrane ulcerations also occur.

Stevens-Johnson Syndrome. This serious, acute and occasionally fatal dermal problem may begin as erythema multiforme, then extend to a toxic condition with severe ulcerations of mucous membranes, especially in the nose, oropharynx, lips, conjunctivae and genitalia. Bleeding, purpura, pneumonia and manifestations of TEN are further complications.

Treatment consists of removal of the offending drug or chemical plus steroid administration. Hospitalization, intravenous steroids (100 mg hydrocortisone every 6 to 8 hours) or oral prednisone, initial loading and daily dose of 60 mg, and treatment similar to that of a burn victim (28) are necessary for severe cases. Oral lidocaine (Xylocaine viscous) before meals, 1 to 3 teaspoonsful swirled around in the mouth for 5 minutes and then expectorated. This will reduce oropharyngeal pain and permit drinking and eating of soft foods; impairment of pharyngeal phase of swallowing can occur with swallowing of lidocaine so caution and discretion are necessary. Alternatively, lesions may be swabbed. This avoids anesthetizing the tongue and decreases the likelihood of impairment of the swallowing reflex and is preferable for children and older adults. See also *24, Allergic Reactions; 53, Poisoning.*

58–9. ECZEMA

Many individuals suffer from atopic eczema in infancy. Others acquire the condition later, and such cases often are manifestations of the close relationship between the skin, nervous system and psychic stress. Inherited, allergic, systemic, infectious and psychologic factors influence the degree of adverse skin response and require consideration in modifying treatment. This type of dermatologic reaction is subject to exacerbations and avoidance of or protection from irritants is necessary. Scratching secondary to pruritus leads to breaks in the skin that serve as portals for alien organisms, particularly streptococci and staphylococci, and may cause infection. Treat infections, including use of oral and/or topical antibacterial therapy. Reduce stress and anxiety; tranquilizers and antidepressants can be important adjuncts. See *58–13* for antipruritic measures and use of corticosteroids.

58–10. HIVES *(See 58–19, Urticaria)*

58–11. PARESTHESIAS

Variations in normal sensation of the skin without evident surface pathology or stimulation (in contrast to dysesthesias) are disturbing and, fortunately, often result in an emergency visit early enough in a cerebrovascular or other potentially serious condition so that neurologic and medical evaluation can be done and preventive therapy begun. Tranquilizers aid in symptomatic relief.

58–12. PRURITUS

Pruritus is one of the most common and annoying of skin symptoms. It results principally from inflammation and edema in the skin and has a plethora of causes, including insect bites, contact and atopic dermatitis, pediculosis, scabies, urticaria and dermatitis factitia (neurotic self-induced lesions).

Treatment

- Treatment of the primary cause.
- Avoidance of scratching, which causes a cyclic irritation problem and protective skin breakdown and introduces bacteria leading to infection. Keep fingernails cut short. Avoid contact with irritating substances and materials, such as wool.
- Application of crushed ice in a thin plastic bag for 5 to 10 minutes and reapplication as needed. Heat aggravates the problem in many instances.
- Topical wet cool compresses [of colloidal oatmeal preparation (Aveeno) or modified Burow's solution or baking soda—about 2 teaspoons per liter of water], or sitz baths with 1 cup of Aveeno, baking soda or vinegar in ⅓ bathtub of tepid water.
- Diphenhydramine hydrochloride (Benadryl), 25 to 50 mg PO every 4 hours, or hydroxyzine hydrochloride (Atarax), 10 to 25 mg PO every 4 to 6 hours, helps to promote relaxation and sleep. Caution regarding drowsiness. Aspirin in usual doses may also be helpful.
- Topical cream or ointment according to cause. A corticosteroid cream such as 0.25% to 1.0% hydrocortisone cream or 0.025% to 0.1% triamcinolone cream applied 3 to 4 times daily to affected areas will relieve corticosteroid-responsive dermatoses. Use corticosteroids cautiously, if at all, in the presence or the likelihood of bacterial and fungal infections. A thin layer of vegetable cooking oil or white petrolatum (Vaseline) may be helpful.
- Oral or parenteral corticosteroids or parenteral adrenocorticosteroid hormone (ACTH) may be needed for short courses in severe cases that are corticosteroid-responsive (such as allergy-, toxin-, or chemical-induced pruritus). Adults may be given prednisone in an initial dose of 40 to 80 mg, followed by tapered doses over the next 7 to 10 days.

58–13. POISON OAK, IVY AND SUMAC *(See also 58–18, Urushiols)*

The skin lesions caused by these plants are due to a fixed nonvolatile oil, toxicodendrol, and contrary to general belief, are not contagious. The contact dermatitis resulting from contact with these plants is due to a delayed allergic reaction; the lesions may not appear for 2 to 7 days after contact and often do not disappear for 2 to 4 weeks.

Treatment

- Washing of exposed parts with nonmedicated soap (e.g., Lava soap) and hot water as soon as possible after exposure.
- Local application of soothing lotions, wet compresses or sodium bicarbonate

paste (see also *58–12, Pruritus*). Preparations containing phenol (carbolic acid) and topical anesthetics should not be used.

- Antihistaminics, aspirin and hydroxyzine hydrochloride (Atarax) are helpful in controlling pruritus and discomfort.
- Hospitalization if there is severe generalized skin involvement, especially of the face or genitals, or if secondary infection is present.
- Topical and oral corticosteroids are excellent therapeutic agents. Use 0.1 to 0.5% triamcinolone (Aristocort) or 1% hydrocortisone cream topically. In severe cases, start with divided daily doses of 60 to 80 mg prednisone for several days and taper over the next 10 to 14 days.
- Poison oak or ivy antigens should not be administered, since their use during the acute state may cause serious aggravation of symptoms; in addition, their use has not yet been perfected.

58–14. PRURITUS ANI

Itching in and around the anus and rectum may be so persistent and severe that it is practically unbearable. Persons suffering from this condition may scratch so forcibly that they tear off strips of skin, subcutaneous tissue and mucous membrane with their fingernails, further aggravating the problem. Pruritus may be relieved with the measures indicated in *58–12*.

COMMON CAUSES OF PRURITUS ANI

Fissure-in-Ano *(See 40–7, Anorectal Conditions)*

Food Allergy

Treatment

- Give sedatives and antihistaminics by mouth.
- Treat secondary infection from scratching by sitz baths and application of bacitracin or polymyxin ointment.
- Give a topical hydrocortisone or triamcinolone (e.g., 0.1% Aristocort) cream or lotion.
- Arrange for further medical care, preferably by an allergist.

Fungus Infection

Treatment

- Topical miconazole nitrate (Micatin), tolnaftate (Tinactin) clotrimazole (Lotrimin), haloprogin (Halotex), Loprox or Spectazole creams or solution.
- For proven severe and very pruritic cases, prescribe oral griseofulvin—consultation by a dermatologist may be needed.
- Iodochlorhydroxyquin and hydrocortisone (Vioform) cream is effective in mixed infections or infected eczematoid dermatitis sites.
- General treatment of pruritus as outlined previously.

Hemorrhoids *(See 40–19)*

Medications

The wide use of antibiotics, especially the tetracyclines and birth control pills, has resulted in a very stubborn type of pruritus ani resulting from suppression of the normal intestinal organisms, with increased monilial *(Candida albicans)* growth and infection.

Treatment

- Discontinuance of the offending medication.
- If *Candida albicans* or fungus infection is present or suspected, start with miconazole, Loprox or Spectazole cream.
- If diagnosis is indefinite, use iodochlorhydroxyquin and hydrocortisone cream.

Pinworms (Oxyuriasis) *(See also 40–18)*

Pinworms are frequently the cause of anal itching in children and occasionally adults, as well as vulvar itching in females.

Treatment

- Pyrvinium pamoate (Povan) orally, 5 mg/kg, should be given to the patient and all members of the family or other close contacts. Tablets should be swallowed whole to avoid staining the teeth.
- Personal care to prevent contamination and reinfection through hands, fingernails, etc.
- Sanitary measures, as follows:
  —Boil all bed linen, underclothes, washcloths and towels daily.
  —Scrub toilet seats daily.
  —Sterilize metallic objects used by the patient by baking in a hot oven for at least 10 minutes.

58–15. PRURITUS VULVAE

The usual causes and treatment are the same as outlined in 58–14, *Pruritus Ani*, especially under Fungus Infection.

58–16. STINGS *(See 60)*

58–17. SUNBURN *(See 28–29)*

For systemic effects, see 62–8, *Sunstroke*.

58–18. URUSHIOL CONTACT DERMATITIS *(See also 58–13, Poison Oak, Ivy and Sumac)*

Many plants of the urushiol category (Anacardiaceae family) may cause acute contact dermatitis, as outlined in the table on page 665.

For treatment, see 58–13, *Poison Oak, Ivy and Sumac*. Antihistaminics are of no value in treatment.

58–19. URTICARIA *(See also 24, Allergic Reactions)*

Urticaria (hives), like angioedema and serum sickness, results in part from the release of histamine from mast cells following an antigen-antibody reaction. Acute urticaria is most often caused by drugs, insect bites and foods and is characterized by the appearance on the skin and mucous membranes of pruritic reddened or whitish swellings of various sizes and shapes called wheals. Acute urticaria may have many causes including the following:

Animal dander
Animal serums used in injections
Commercial chemicals such as DDT (53–240)
Drugs (often penicillin, aspirin)
Feathers

Common Names	Distribution	Modes of Contact
Cashew nut shell oil *(53–178)* (Cashew oil)	Africa, Central America, East Indies, India	Electrical insulation, glues, printer's ink, resins, swizzle sticks
Ginkgo tree (maidenhair tree)	China, Europe, Japan, U.S.A. (southeast),	Cosmetics, lacquerware, soaps
Indian marking nut (washerman itch)	India, Malaya	Laundry marking ink
Lacquer tree (Japanese lacquer tree)	China, India, Japan	Bar rails, bracelets, ornamental wooden novelties
Mango ("apple of the tropics," "king of fruits")	California, Central America, Hawaii, Mediterranean	Direct—plant or fruit to skin; indirect—particles in air, contaminated insects or animals
Oakleaf poison ivy *(58–13)* (eastern oakleaf, poison ivy)	U.S.A. (southeast)	Same as mango (above)
Poison ivy *(58–13)* (poison creeper, markweed)	Canada, China, Mexico, Taiwan, U.S.A. (except southwest)	Same as mango (above)
Poison oak *(58–13)* (Western poison oak, yeara)	U.S.A. (Pacific coast)	Same as mango (above)
Poison sumac *(58–13)* (Poison dogwood, poison elder, swamp sumac)	U.S.A. (southeast)	Same as mango (above)
Rengas tree (black varnish tree)	Malaya	Furniture, wood carvings

Food—especially berries, chocolate, fish (particularly shellfish) tomato, pork, nuts, spices, additives
Microorganisms
Parasites
Perfumes and cosmetics
Physical factors—heat, cold, light
Products of metabolism (complement factor)
Psychogenic stimuli
Secretion from endocrine glands

Treatment

1. Removal from or elimination of causative source and administration of epinephrine hydrochloride (Adrenalin), 0.3 to 0.5 ml of 1:1000 solution IM or, in severe cases, diluted to 10 ml with normal saline and given slowly IV.
2. Immediate endotracheal intubation *(18–10)* or tracheostomy *(18–34)* if there is serious airway obstruction. See *24–1, Anaphylactic Shock.*
3. Consider use of the following:

- Antihistaminics orally or intramuscularly.
- Corticosteroid therapy orally or parenterally (acute cases).

- Hydroxyzine hydrochloride (Atarax), 25 mg PO every 6 hours is helpful in recurrent chronic cases.

Note: For treatment of pruritus, also see *58–12*.

4. Observation for several hours after initiation of therapy may be necessary. If response to the measures described here is not satisfactory, patients with severe cases may require hospitalization.

58–20. VARICOSE ECZEMA AND ULCERS *(See 58–9)*

58–21. VINCENT'S ANGINA *(See 61–15)*

58–22. "WELDED SKIN" (Bonding by "Superglue Adhesives")

New cyanoacrylate adhesives ("superglues") may cause accidental firm skin-to-skin bonding, but surgery should not be necessary to separate with immediate use of appropriate measures. *In all instances, avoid trying to pull bonded surfaces directly apart.* Nail polish remover helps to release bonding at all external locations, but of course its use around the eye must be limited; if not available, the following alternative measures should be taken:

Skin Bonds

1. Immerse involved parts in soapy water and gently peel or roll the surfaces apart by using a blunt edge such as a tongue blade or spoon handle.
2. Wash off the adhesive with soap and water.

Lip Bonds

1. Apply a stream of warm water to the lips. The edge of a tiny bar of soap may be used to peel or roll the lips gently apart.

Eyelid-to-Eyelid or Eyeball Bonds

1. Do not try to open the eyes by manipulation.
2. Wash thoroughly with warm water and apply a gauze patch if bonding has occurred. The eye should open in 1 to 4 days without further action.
3. Refer to an ophthalmologist.

Adhesive on the Eyeball

1. Wash with warm water if lid open.
2. Cover the eye with a patch (38).
3. Cyanoacrylate will attach itself to the superficial eye protein and will dissociate from the eye in several hours even with gross contamination.
4. Refer to an ophthalmologist.

Oral Ingestion

Cyanoacrylate is almost impossible to swallow; the adhesive adheres to the mucosa and solidifies. Saliva will separate the adhesive within 1 to 2 days. Have the patient lie in the prone position to avoid swallowing or gagging on the solidified lump.

58–23. X-RAY (RADIATION) BURNS *(See 28–34)*

59. Soft Tissue Injuries

Soft tissue injuries of varying degrees of severity make up the bulk of cases treated on any emergency service.

59–1. SOFT TISSUE TRAUMA AND ASSOCIATED INFECTIONS—INITIAL GENERAL MEASURES *(See also 44–1, Hand Trauma and Infection; 59–42, Soft Tissue Infections (Life Threatening); 23, Abscesses; 27, Bites; 57, Shock; 69–9, Operative and Treatment Permit)*

Remove Potentially Constrictive Materials from Affected Parts. Remove all jewelry and other materials from affected parts. Remove clothing, using scissors if necessary, from involved areas.

Preliminary Cleaning

1. Cleanse the area around the wound for at least several inches. Clip any hair that may protrude into the wound (do not shave eyebrows; although they will grow back, they will not always grow back the same way). Remove any clothing or dressings adherent with coagulated blood by soaking in sterile saline or half-strength hydrogen peroxide.
2. Cover the wound with sterile gauze. Cleanse the surrounding uninvolved skin with a water-soluble iodophor (Betadine) or chlorhexidine gluconate (Hibiclens) or with soap and water. Substances such as petrolatum, mineral oil, bacitracin or polysporin ointment, and even mayonnaise may be used to clean off oily substances. Irrigate thoroughly with saline. Ethyl chloride in spray form (caution: explosive) is another good degreasing agent. See *28–6* for tar removal.
3. Remove the gauze and mechanically clean the wound with bland, nonmedicated soap and water, loosening and removing superficial foreign bodies and following with copious sterile saline irrigation. Three to 4 liters of saline may be used for large or contaminated wounds. Irrigation can be done initially with a syringe (with a 25-gauge needle) or WaterPic, then a gravity apparatus. Deep cleaning need not be done now. Cover wound with sterile gauze during subsequent steps as applicable (this amount of cleaning is adequate for superficial wounds; proceed to section *59–2*).
4. Tetanus immunization *(20)* can be given before or after specific procedures.

History. Obtain a detailed account of the type of injury, the duration of injury and exposure to any substance that may require special management. Record dominant hand and upper extremity injuries and occupation (functional needs may affect therapeutic approach).

Brief Examination for Other Injuries. Before attention becomes focused on the affected area, rapidly check for any other bodily areas that may be involved.

X-ray. Unless the involvement is superficial and slight, preliminary soft tissue x-ray films of the area are advisable; this includes views of amputated parts prior to reimplantation.

Examination for Nerve and Tendon Injury. Motor and sensory function should be tested before any anesthetic use. See *44–1* for hand function testing.

Anesthesia. See *12, Anesthesia and Analgesia.* Operative and humane interests dictate that one or more of these methods be in effect before deep cleaning and debridement are done or repair procedures are started.

Tourniquet (TK) Control. If an extremity is involved and control of anticipated bleeding will be required at the time of surgical cleaning and repair, elevate it for 1 to 2 minutes and clear it of as much blood as possible before tightening or inflating the proximate tourniquet to exert 200 to 250 mm Hg extrinsic pressure. A broad thigh blood pressure cuff should be used in the lower extremity (or in obese upper extremity) to improve the hemostatic effectiveness and to decrease the likelihood of compression neuronapraxia ("tourniquet paralysis"). Maximum period of TK application is 1½ to 2 hours, after which 15 to 20 minutes of recirculation should be permitted before any further shortened period of reapplication (preferably by a specialist) is begun. (*Note:* A tourniquet can be used for approximately 15 to 20 minutes without undue pain, but longer periods require the use of anesthetics.)

Final Cleaning for More Complex Surgery and Repair

1. Sterile operating room technique is essential for all cases. All persons in the operating room *including the patient* should be capped (with hair confined) and masked, and operating personnel should wear sterile gloves after preliminary scrubbing. A sterile operating gown should be worn and full operating room technique in effect if a lengthy or an extensive repair is needed.

2. The affected part is rewashed with soap and water and again copiously lavaged with sterile saline, then wrapped in a sterile towel while the operator changes gloves. The skin is again cleaned with a water-soluble iodine (Betadine) and draped for surgery.

Examination of the Wound. After final cleaning, the wound is thoroughly examined, the operator looking for severance of large blood vessels, muscles, nerves or tendons; fractures; dislocations, epiphyseal displacements; foreign bodies; hematomas; and openings into or contamination of joints, tendon sheaths or fascial spaces. Except in the hands or fingers, tag gently any lacerated tendons or nerves with long suture material. If unexpectedly severe damage is encountered that is beyond the skill of the operator, the tourniquet should be removed and a sterile pressure bandage applied and the patient transferred at once to an adequately equipped hospital. Administration of a sedative may be advisable. A summary of findings and treatment to date should be sent with the patient.

Debridement. The object of debridement is to convert an area of traumatized and potentially infected tissue into a surgically clean wound. With a small-toothed forceps, sharp scalpel and small curved scissors, sharp dissection should be used to remove any damaged structures to a depth of 1 to 2 mm, starting with the skin and working toward the depths of the wound. If exposure is inadequate with use of nontraumatic retractors, the surface laceration should be extended, bearing in mind the areas of safe incisions, particularly in the hand (see Fig. 43–1). Excise grossly nonviable, dark noncontractile muscle. Nerves, tendons, blood vessels and articular surfaces should be preserved, as should bone fragments with periosteal and soft tissue attachments.

All dead spaces should be eliminated by closure in layers or application of mattress sutures after careful evacuation of blood clots except from the flexor crease of the wrist distally, where only skin sutures should be used; any dead space that cannot be closed should either be drained (using an exit site separate from the laceration site) or left open and covered with moist sterile saline dressing for later closure. Bleeding not controllable by pressure should be stopped by cautery, by vessel-twisting technique or by clamping and tying with No. 000 catgut or polyglactin 910 (Vicryl) or Dexon. Buried suture material, however, should be kept to an absolute minimum and the knots inverted and buried deep.

Completely severed small sections of soft tissue (for instance, fingertips) that are not badly macerated, in some instances (especially in small children), can be carefully cleaned and debrided for suturing back in place as full-thickness grafts. Pieces of skin should be thoroughly defatted. The quicker this suturing is done, the better the chance of a "take." Intact skin from amputated parts that are to be discarded can be used for grafting denuded areas.

Debridement should be limited in certain areas; little, if any, tissue should be removed from these regions unless nonviable, gross contamination or maceration is present. The most important of these areas are the following:

- *Eyelids*. Superficial linear lacerations in this region should be thoroughly cleansed and closed with fine, nonabsorbable suture material to prevent ectropion *(38–8)* or entropion *(38–11);* sutures should be removed after 3 to 4 days, to lessen the chance of cysts forming along suture lines. Deep, nonlinear and marginal lacerations should be covered after cleaning and referred to an ophthalmologist or plastic surgeon for repair (Fig. 38–3).
- *Hands and fingers (44–1).*
- *Face*. Simple lacerations may be cosmetically closed after cleansing, but complex lacerations are better treated by sterile dressing coverage after cleaning and referral to a plastic surgeon for primary plastic repair. Align the eyebrows, when involved, before further area repair.
- *Lips*, especially in the region of the vermilion border.
- *Penis (41–4).*

No antibiotics, antiseptics, disinfectants, sulfonamides or other substances of any type should be painted, sprayed, insufflated or sprinkled into the wound, which is now ready for any repair or closure procedures (see 59–2).

59–2. SPECIFIC PROCEDURES (CLOSURE, REPAIR, INCISION AND DRAINAGE *(See also 43–2, Hand Injuries, Procedures; 23, Abscesses; 27, Bites)*

Repair by primary closure is generally considered safe within 6 hours of injury except where indicated otherwise. This time may be extended at the discretion of the physician if the wound is not grossly contaminated or obviously infected (get C & S if it is infected).

Closures and Repairs

Simple Closures

SKIN SURFACE. Even tension sufficient to just cause physiologic and cosmetic skin line approximation of opposing wound edges in simple lacerations can be obtained with one of the following methods:

- Adhesive butterflies (Fig. 59–1)
- Steri-strips (Fig. 59–2)
- Long body hair (as in the scalp) of sufficient length (make a twisted strand from several hairs on each side of the laceration) tied in a surgical knot across the wound like suture material. Hair must usually be wiped with tincture of benzoin (keep it out of wound) prior to tying—the stickiness will help prevent slippage of the knot, as will a drop of collodion on the knot after tying.
- Skin clips
- Running or interrupted (used most often) subcuticular stitch (Fig. 59–3)
- Interrupted sutures of Dermalon or Prolene (see Figs. 59–4 and 59–5); generally use 6–0 on the face, 5–0 on the hands, and 4–0 on other skin surfaces. All external knots should be placed away from the approximated

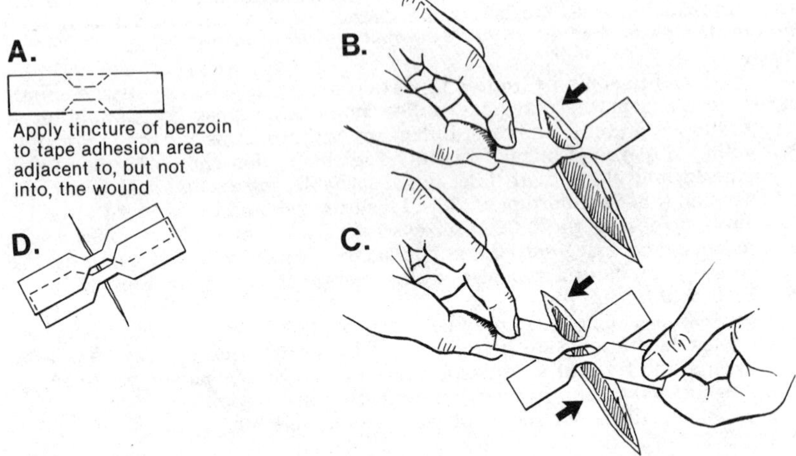

Figure 59–1. Counter-opposing interlocking butterflies. Multiple pairs can be used for longer wounds.

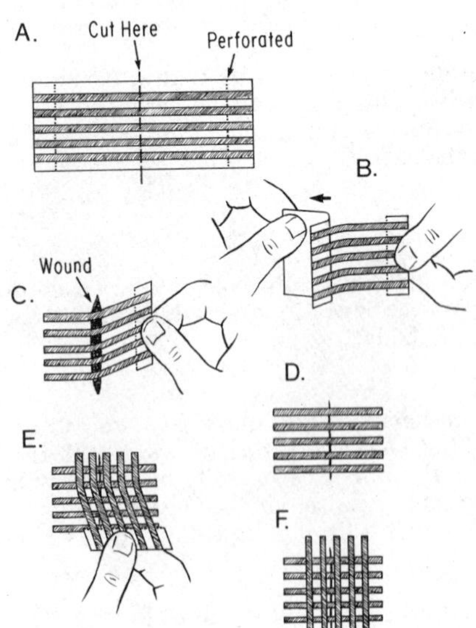

Figure 59–2. Technique for maximum closure and adhesion by Steri-Strips (3M). *A,* A 3″ long packet is first cut in half (for smaller wounds). *B,* The protective covering is removed from one part, and after tincture of benzoin has been applied to area adjacent to, but not into, the wound, the wound is closed with Steri-Strips *(C* and *D).* The process is then repeated, but second strips are placed perpendicular to the first *(E* and *F).*

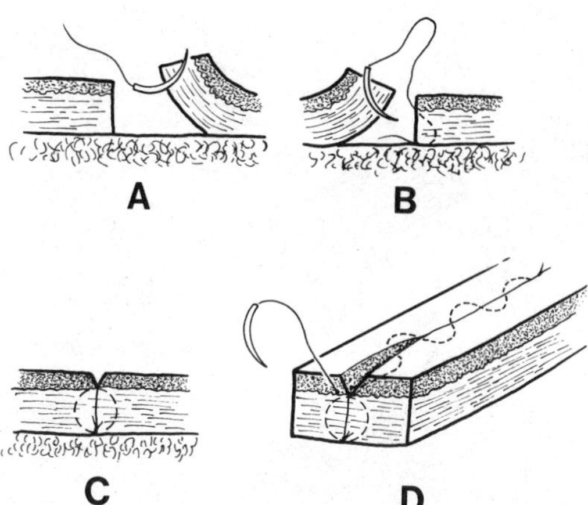

Figure 59–3. *A, B* and *C,* Insertion of a deep suture with the knot buried. *D,* Insertion of a subcuticular suture. For easier removal of a long subcuticular suture, at the midpoint, the suture may be brought up through the skin and a small identifiable loop made, after which the subcuticular stitch may be continued. When the stitch is removed, the knot is cut off at each end and pulled from the center.

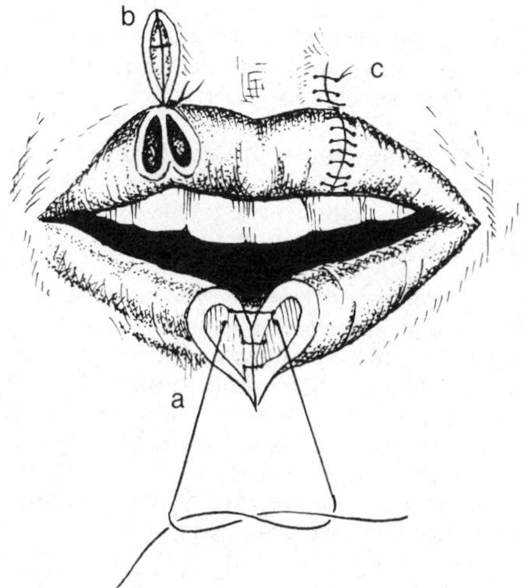

Figure 59–4. Suturing of the lip. Deep sutures are placed first in the muscle (a). Then the vermilion border is aligned (b) followed by completion of the sutures (c).

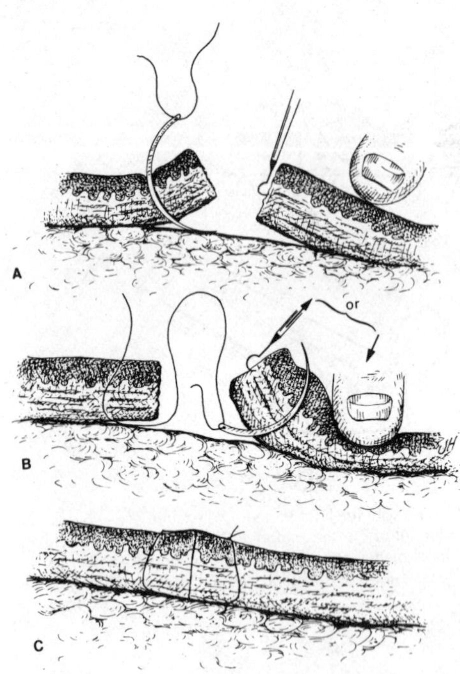

Figure 59–5. Technique for insertion of an interrupted suture. The base is wider than the top; and eversion by thumb pressure or skin hook helps accomplish this.

skin edges (Fig. 59–6). Sutures are the most common enduring closures used in areas where moisture and continuing motion around the wound will be present. A corner stitch may be required in wounds with pointed flaps (Fig. 59–7).

DEEP SPACES. Obliteration of dead spaces should be achieved by closure in layers (see Fig. 59–8) using mattress sutures of No. 000 catgut. Buried sutures should be kept to a minimum; avoid these in the digits, hand and foot.

Complex Closures. For wounds that require complex closures that are beyond the usual experience of the operator, it is best to cover the wound with a sterile saline-soaked dressing and transfer the patient promptly to a center with adequate facilities and appropriate specialists if circumstances permit. Closures may be complex because of the site of the wound (intricate structures involved or need for cosmetic repair), the nature of the injury (ragged or mutilating laceration) or the extent of area and structures to be covered.

COVERAGE OF LARGE AREAS AND ESSENTIAL STRUCTURES. Essential structures (tendons, nerves, blood vessels, joints, bone) must be covered; keep these structures moist with sterile saline-soaked gauze while awaiting any transportation or delayed primary coverage. See also 28–3 for comments on broad area coverage. Attempt to keep suture lines away from tendons, nerves, blood vessels, joints and bone.

Repair of Small, Avulsed and Amputated Parts *(See also 59–44, Reattachment of Amputated Parts).* Completely severed soft tissue, if of small quantity and not macerated (e.g., fingertips, portions of nose and ear), may be thoroughly cleansed, defatted and sutured in place as a full-thickness graft. If replace-

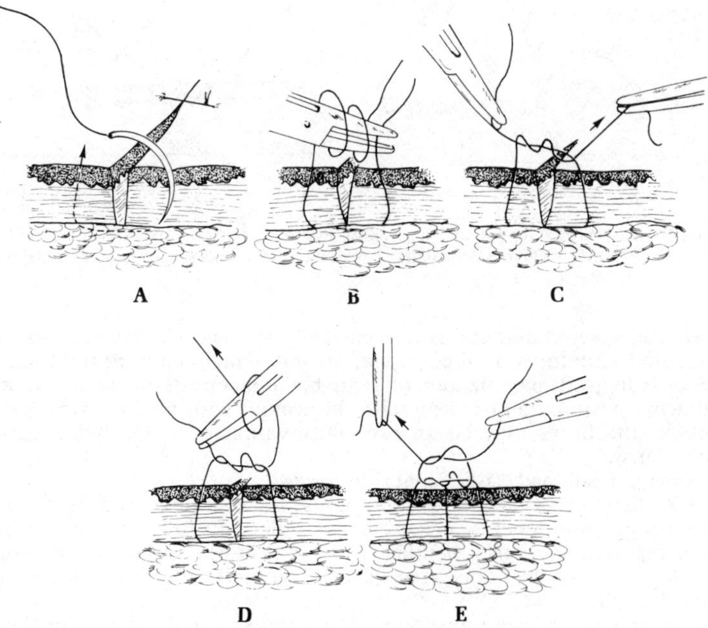

Figure 59–6. Steps in use of two instruments to perform a square knot tie of a suture. The double looping shown in *B* is not essential but provides some resistance of the suture line to keep the wound from gaping while the tie is being made.

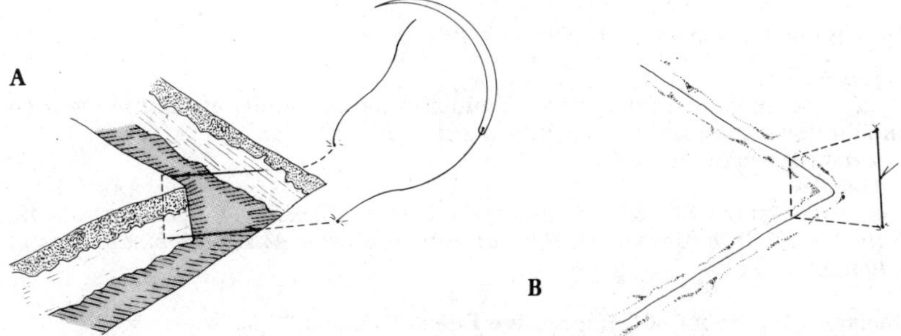

Figure 59–7. Corner stitch. This should be used to suture any pointed flaps so that the blood supply to the point is not strangulated.

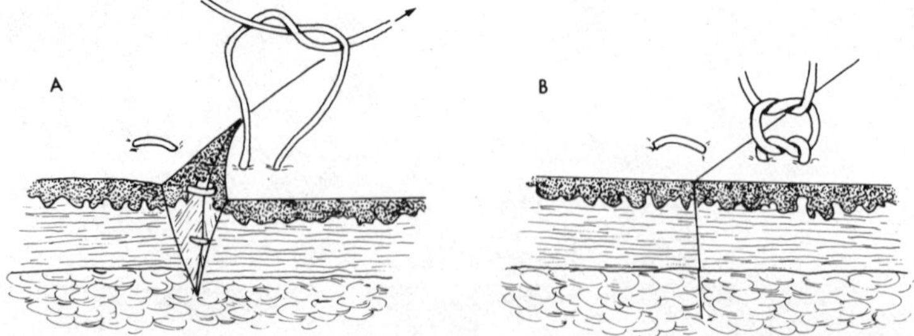

Figure 59–8. Technique for performing a vertical mattress suture—the medial suturing next to the wound is done last. This suture is helpful in compressing tissue for hemostasis, such as in the scalp.

ment of the severed material is not feasible, the choices available (assuming no essential structures need coverage) are subsequent split- or full-thickness graft, pedicle graft, mobilization of available adjacent tissue by undercutting or allowing granulation of tissue into the wound with healing by secondary intention (the latter may be an especially valuable approach for fingertip amputations).

Common Cosmetic and Plastic Surgical Techniques

- The Z-plasty converts a laceration across or transverse to a flexor crease into a horizontal laceration more compatible with fuller range of motion. After repair, the central member of the Z-plasty is parallel to the normal creases of the body. This procedure is generally not done as an initial procedure, however.
- Repair of jagged lacerations depends on the size and viability of the flap areas. Larger viable flaps can be sutured directly. Nonviable flaps can be trimmed to make a linear laceration and surrounding tissue mobilized (Fig. 59–9). Grafts *(28–3)* may be required.
- Curvilinear lacerations with avulsed tissue can be managed with a "dog ear" repair (Fig. 59–10).

Arterial Repair. See Figure 59–11.

Nerve Repair. See *43–10;* Figure 59–12.

Tendon Repair. See *43–12;* Figure 59–13.

Infections *(See also 43–2, Hand Injuries, Procedures)*

Simple

CELLULITIS. Specific antibacterial administration is usually all that is required in addition to applicable measures described in *59–1* and *59–3.*

SUPERFICIAL ABSCESS. See 23.

Complex

MASSIVE INFECTIONS. See *23, Abscesses; 43–2, Hand Injuries,* Procedures; *59–42, Soft Tissue Infections (Life Threatening); 33–83, Antimicrobial Drugs of Choice.*

Incisions for Relief of Compressive Edema *(See also 28–3, Burns; 47–60, Compartment Syndromes; 59–40, Wringer-Type Injuries)*

Fasciotomy or escharotomy may be required within 24 hours of onset of serious injury or infection to relieve circulatory compromise caused by massive

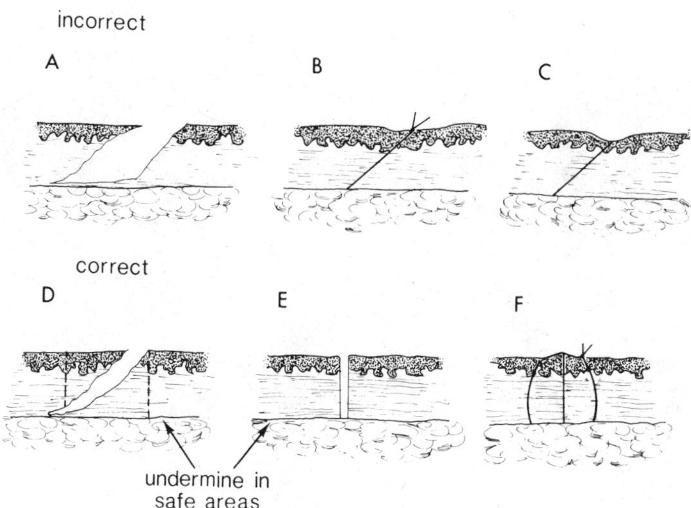

Figure 59–9. To align laceration edges of a slicing wound properly, the avulsed or sliced area may be blocked off with a scalpel *(D)* and the skin undermined in safe areas *(E)* and then sutured *(F)*.

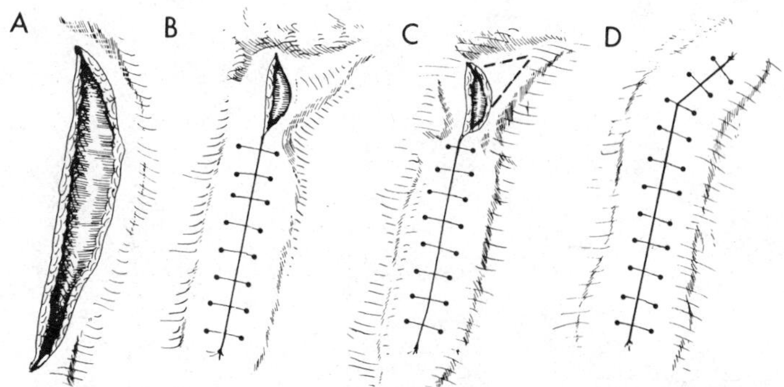

Figure 59–10. Suturing of an elliptical wound results in a terminal bunching of skin ("dog ear"). To remove the excess tissue, an incision is first made along the distal dotted line area *(C)*. Then the flap is smoothed out and, using the underneath incision line as a guide, a second wedged incision is made proximally to remove just the excess tissue. Then the angled area is sutured *(D)*.

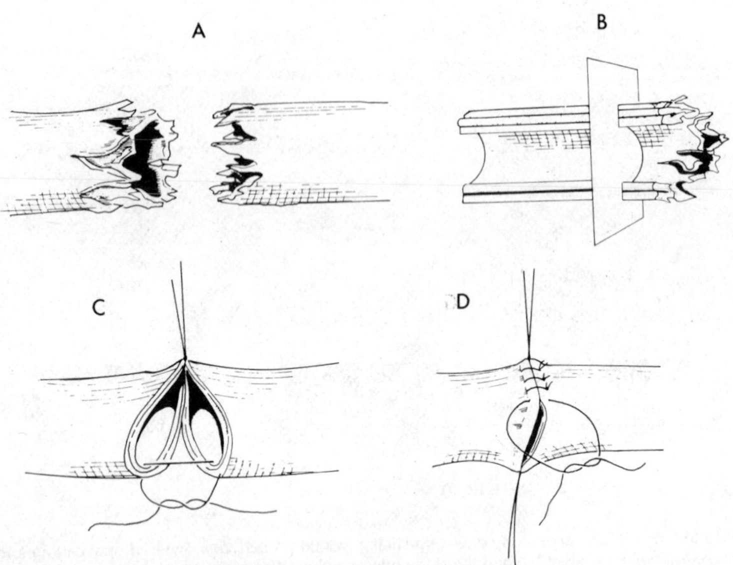

Figure 59–11. Repair of a lacerated blood vessel *(A)*. The injured vessel is debrided back to normal intima *(B)* after proximal and distal blood flow are controlled. Accurate approximation of the intimal surfaces is important—everting the edges as possible *(C)*. Circumferential suturing follows *(D)*. (Modified from Grabb, W. C., Kleinert, H. E., and Puckett, C. L.: Technics in Surgery: Facial and Hand Injuries. Ethicon, Inc., 1976.)

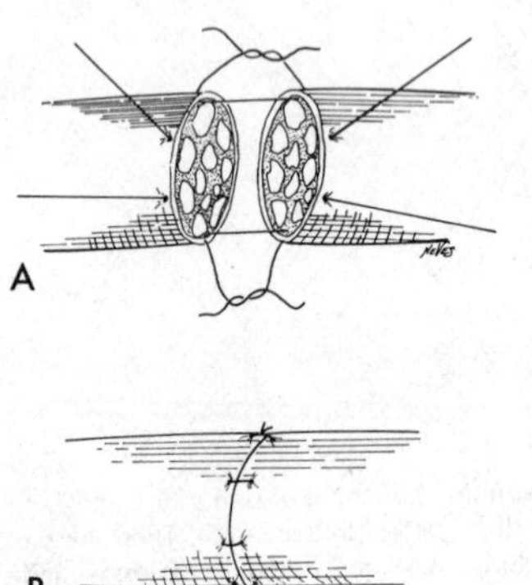

Figure 59–12. Repair of a lacerated nerve. Magnification is necessary for nerve repair and should be done by a skilled surgeon. Size 10–0 nylon sutures are placed through the epineurium. Splinting should follow repair. (Modified from Grabb, W. C., Kleinert, H. E., and Puckett, C. L.: Technics in Surgery: Facial and Hand Injuries. Ethicon, Inc., 1976.)

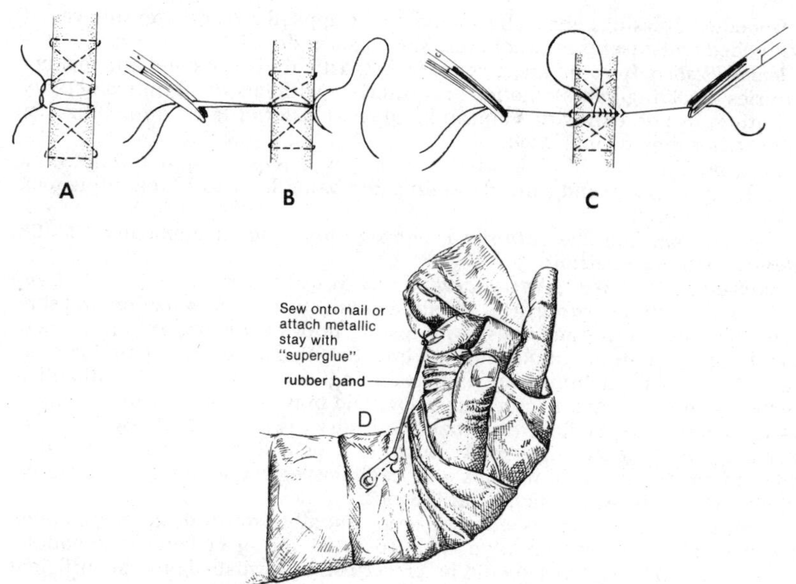

Figure 59–13. Tendon repair. The stepwise repair of a flexor tendon and subsequent proper splinting is depicted in *A* through *D*. It is particularly important that all repairs of tendons in the zone from the midinterphalangeal area to the metacarpal heads be done by an expert because of presence of the intricate multiple pulley system in this region. The Kessler suture (not shown) is also popular; instead of making ×'s, the suture is placed internally directly parallel to the tendon sheath and run perpendicularly at the same sites as shown above. (Modified from Grabb, W. C., Kleinert, H. E., and Puckett, C. L.: Technics in Surgery: Facial and Hand Injuries. Ethicon, Inc., 1976.)

edema. In general, incisional lines are longitudinal on the trunk and extremities, approximately in the coronal plane and deep enough to relieve constrictive planes of tissue while avoiding major nerves and blood vessels; arced transverse incisions are also made across the pectoral, suprapubic and umbilical levels.

59–3. POSTPROCEDURE MEASURES

Dressings. A nonadherent dressing (Adaptic, Telfa) should be applied over the wound and sutures and covered with sterile gauze (the surrounding area can be painted with compound tincture of benzoin). When this has dried enough to be "tacky," an elastic pressure bandage can be applied. Zinc oxide can be copiously applied over wounds that would otherwise require soaking. On any portion of an extremity, care should be taken to allow for postoperative edema. Tight circular bandages completely around an extremity should never be applied.

Facial wounds may be left open and Bacitracin ointment applied tid to keep the wound free of clots. The wound also may be washed gently with soap and water.

Bismuth tribromophenate (Xeroform) gauze may be used for the original dressing in clean wounds or in wounds in which evidence of gross infection has been noted.

Collodion dressings generally should not be applied directly over the wound, but collodion is useful for anchoring the edges of dressings.

Immobilization. In some areas of the body (particularly the hand and foot and injuries involving joints), motion may interfere with healing. Limited activity, splinting, use of a sling or Velpeau bandage, plaster of Paris immobilization or crutches may be indicated.

Elevation. Elevation of an injured extremity will help to improve venous and lymphatic drainage and control swelling and pain. See also *12* regarding focal edema control.

Immunization. See *20, Tetanus Immunization*, and, if applicable, *33–28, Hepatitis Immunization.*

Antibiotics. See *33–83, Antimicrobial Drugs of Choice; 59–42, Soft Tissue Infections (Life Threatening).* Obtain a Gram stain to aid selection and send specimen for culture and sensitivity testing prior to starting antibiotic treatment. Gross contamination, current infection and delay of repair for more than 6 hours from injury are important indications for use of antibiotics. Severely contused and necrotizing soft tissue may become a focus for anaerobic bacteria growth following massive injury *even in the absence of skin perforation.* An excellent initial antibiotic is penicillin; for mixed organism contamination of fresh wounds use cephalosporin and for gram-negative infected wounds, gentamicin (Garamycin).

Analgesics. *(See also 12, Pain Management).* Usually aspirin or acetaminophen given singly or in combination with 16 to 64 mg of codeine is adequate. Analgesics and sedatives should be prescribed or furnished only in sufficient number to last until the next scheduled recheck.

Follow-up Care. Specific instructions must be given to the patient regarding care at home (see Table 59–1, Laceration Care) and regarding follow-up care (64–2). All grossly contaminated or severely crushed or contused injuries must be rechecked in 24 hours; so should injuries in which debridement only, without closure, has been done. All finger, hand, wrist or elbow injuries should be seen by a physician on the day following surgical repair. Status of minor lacerations should be inspected in not more than 3 days. Compromise in circulation, rising or spiking fever, gross bleeding and uncontrolled pain are indications for immediate recheck. Sutures are generally removed in 7 to 10 days except for facial (4 days) and skin areas under stress, as in the distal lower extremities (14 days). See Table 59–1 for patient instructions on laceration care.

SOFT TISSUE INJURIES NEEDING SPECIAL MANAGEMENT*

59–4. ABDOMINAL INJURIES *(See also 22, Abdominal Pain)*

Nonpenetrating Injuries. Nonpenetrating injuries caused by direct blunt trauma to the abdominal wall are far more common than penetrating or perforating injuries and may be so severe that hemorrhage and shock (57) cause death before any treatment can be given, or so slight that no treatment is required. Between these two extremes lies the intermediate field in which accurate diagnosis and prompt and proper treatment can influence the chance of recovery.

The severity of the trauma inflicted on an underlying viscus by a blunt object depends upon the force exerted, the size and shape of the striking

*For general therapeutic considerations, see *59–1* to *59–3.*

Table 59–1. LACERATION CARE

- Keep wound clean and dry.
- Remove our dressing in ______day(s).
- Keep a dry, sterile dressing on wound until sutures are removed. Change dressing daily. If steri-strips have been applied, remove them in ______days. Change dressing over the strips daily.
- Watch for signs of wound infection; report to physician if any of the following are present:
    - Redness and swelling
    - Heat and increasing tenderness
    - Drainage of pus
    - Fever
- The following instructions apply especially to FACIAL INJURIES.
    - You may have mild pain after the anesthetic wears off. Usually two (2) aspirin tablets will alleviate it. (Use Tylenol if you are allergic to aspirin.)
    - You may have swelling and/or discoloration around the wound. This is normal. The swelling will decrease more rapidly if you stay upright during the day and if you use three or four pillows when you sleep.
    - There may be a small amount of bloody crust on or around the sutures for one or two days. This is normal.
    - STARTING THE DAY AFTER THE REPAIR OF THE WOUND: Wash area gently with soap and water two or three times daily. Do not wash the wound if steri-strips have been applied.
    - Do not apply any so-called "antiseptics" such as alcohol, iodine, merthiolate, etc. These fluids will harm the tissues, slow healing, increase scarring, and may cause unwanted reactions.
    - Do not cover the wound other than as instructed. The moisture and warmth produced by covering slows and interferes with the healthy process and may cause infection.

object, the location of impact, the ability of the person struck to give way with the blow or to tighten the muscles in preparation for it, the strength of the abdominal musculature and status of filling of any hollow viscus.

Spleen and kidney injuries, followed by intestine and liver injuries, are the most common nonpenetrating abdominal injuries with retroperitoneal hemorrhage. Mesentery, pancreas and diaphragm injuries are among others occurring less frequently.

More than 80% of abdominal injuries from blunt trauma are the result of automobile accidents; industrial accidents (75) account for another 10%. The mortality from nonpenetrating abdominal injuries is about three and one-half times that for penetrating injuries, probably owing in great part to the difficulty in making an accurate diagnosis.

Treatment

For treatment, see under the organ involved.

Clear indications for laparotomy or laparoscopy no matter what viscus is suspected are as follows:

- Pneumoperitoneum demonstrable by x-rays.
- Abdominal paracentesis (see *18–23, Peritoneal Aspiration*) or culdocentesis (*18–9*) that yields blood [must be associated with clinical signs of active bleeding or evidence of contamination from contents of a hollow viscus (stomach contents, bile, feces, urine)].
- Secondary collapse following recovery from primary posttraumatic shock, with localized evidence of abdominal injury.

Perforating Abdominal Injuries. These are usually bullet wounds (*59–9*) or stab wounds (*59–33*).

Treatment

- Application of sterile dressings to entrance and exit wounds.
- Hospitalization for definitive care and laparoscopy or laparotomy if perforation is through the peritoneum. Any observations that might be of value to law enforcement agencies (powder marks on clothing, powder burns on skin, course of wound tract) should be recorded on the emergency chart and permanent evidence marked to be submitted to them (see *14–5, Medicolegal Documentation*).

59–5. ABRASIONS *(For corneal abrasions, see 38–32)*

If removal of all embedded foreign bodies and devitalized tissue from the skin or subcutaneous structures cannot be accomplished with a knife and scrub brush under topical or local anesthetic, hospitalization for administration of general anesthesia may be necessary to prevent permanent and disfiguring tattooing. All foreign material must be removed. Extensive abrasions may be dressed with petrolatum gauze.

59–6. BITES *(See 27)*

59–7. BLADDER INJURIES *(See 41–1)*

59–8. BRAIN INJURIES *(See 44)*

59–9. BULLET WOUNDS *(See also 45–1, Control of Bleeding)*

The amount of injury and treatment required varies with the velocity, caliber and type of bullet (hard or soft) used and the tract of the projectile into or through the body. Whenever possible, the exact site of entry, the course of the bullet and the point of exit should be described in detail in the patient's record. If there is no exit site, obtain sufficient x-ray views or fluoroscope to locate; if final location is far from entry area, suspect and observe for vascular injury and delayed bleeding. Removal of a bullet may be contraindicated. The presence or absence of powder burns or marks on the skin and clothing should be noted. If the bullet is recovered, it should be turned over to the proper law enforcement officers; see *14–5* for discussion of proper collection and handling of medicolegal evidence. For treatment, see *59–1* to *59–4* and the discussion of the specific body area involved (see *57, Shock,* for treatment of hypovolemia). A penetrating bullet wound of the abdomen and peritoneum is usually considered a mandatory indication for laparotomy. In some abdominal injuries from high velocity shells, exploration may be advisable even if the peritoneum is intact. All bullet wound patients require protection against tetanus (*20*).

59–10. BURNS *(See 28)*

59–11. CARDIAC INJURIES *(See 31–4)*

59–12. CHEST INJURIES *(See 31)*

59–13. CONTUSIONS *(See also 59–1, Initial Measures, and 59–3, Postprocedure Measures)*

Mild Contusions. Ordinary contusions (provided fracture has been ruled out) need only symptomatic treatment to reduce pain and swelling. The patient should be instructed to limit use of an extremity, given crutches or a splint if indicated and instructed regarding application of hot or cold compresses at home. As a general rule, cold is more effective for the first 24 to 48 hours; on about the 4th to 5th day warm compresses or contrast baths may be used (see also 7). Marked relief, especially of throbbing fingers and toes, may be obtained by gentle inunction of the injured part for 10 to 15 minutes every 3 to 4 hours with a 2.5% ointment of hydrocortisone acetate in neomycin sulfate (Neo-Cortef).

Severe Contusions. These injuries, especially of the extremities, may require elevation and snug elastic bandages to prevent and control intramuscular bleeding. Severely contused and necrotizing soft tissue following massive injury may become a focus for anaerobic bacteria growth, even in the absence of skin perforation.

59–14. CRUSHING INJURIES

Crushing Injuries to the Chest. These may cause serious damage without external evidence of trauma. The following types of injury may be present:

- Pulmonary contusion with alveolar rupture and hemorrhage, especially in children *(31–5)*.
- Cardiac contusion with or without severe symptoms such as myocardial infarction *(29–15)*, hemopericardium *(31–4)* and cardiac arrest *(29–8)*. Milder contusions may result in electrocardiogram (ECG) changes (ST segment variations and T-wave flattening) that persist for lengthy periods.
- Diaphragmatic damage *(31–7)*.
- Fractured ribs and sternum *(31–8)*.
- Mediastinal hemorrhage *(31–2)*.
- Tension pneumothorax *(31–12)*.

Crushing Injuries to the Extremities. These injuries may cause severe damage not apparent on initial examination. X-rays are indicated in all cases. See also *59–40, Wringer-Type Injuries*.

Crushing Injuries to the Low Back or Flanks may cause severe kidney damage *41–2*). Hematuria, gross or microscopic, is present in 75 to 80% of cases.

59–15. DIAPHRAGMATIC INJURIES *(See 31–7)*

59–16. EAR INJURIES *(See 35–8)*

59–17. EYE INJURIES *(See 38–29 to 38–37)*

59–18. FOREIGN BODIES *(See also 39–1 and 39–7)*

For removal of fishhooks in soft tissue, see Figure 59–14. Use Fluorimethane spray, lidocaine injection or nitrous oxide inhalation to reduce pain during the procedure.

59–19. GALLBLADDER AND BILE DUCT INJURIES

Because of its sheltered location, the gallbladder and its duct system are rarely injured by blunt trauma unless there is also extensive liver damage

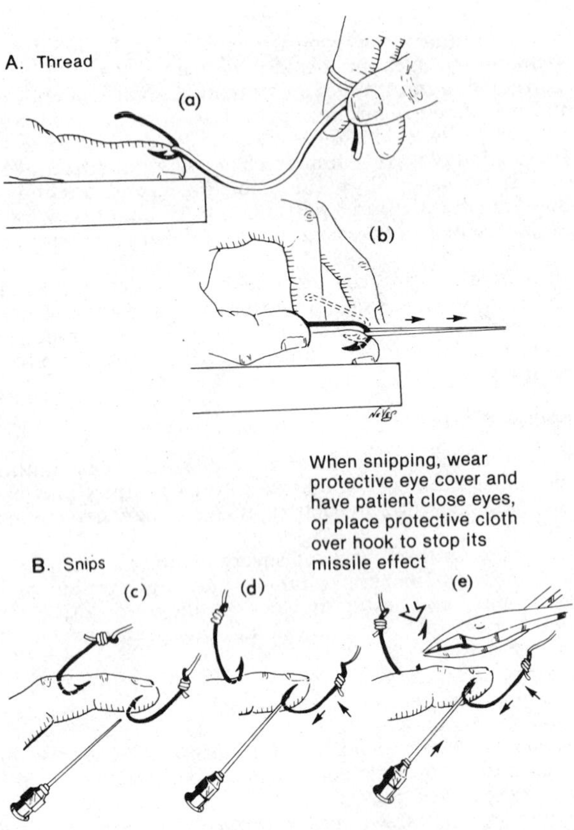
A. Thread
(a)
(b)
When snipping, wear protective eye cover and have patient close eyes, or place protective cloth over hook to stop its missile effect
B. Snips
(c)
(d)
(e)
C. Needle

Figure 59–14. Three methods for removal of a hook from the body. *A,* Thread. To fish for fishhooks, you'll need about one foot of line. Loop the line around the curve of the hook and wrap the ends several times around your forefinger *(a)*. Then take the hook's eye and shank in the thumb and forefinger of your free hand and push down, disengaging the barb. Finally, align the string with the shank's long axis—and pull *(b)*. *B,* Snips. Advance the hook through the skin *(c)* in the arc of the hook until the barb is exposed *(d)*. Then snip off the barb *(e)* and back the hook out in an arced manner. *C,* Needle. To remove a hook without using a string or snips, all you need is an 18-gauge disposable needle *(f)*. Introduce the needle along the barbed side of the hook, with the bevel toward the inside of the hook curve. Apply slight pressure upward on the hook shank, so that the barb is disengaged from the flesh. Then push the needle gently upward and rotate until the lumen locks firmly over the barb. Keeping the needle locked over the barb with gentle upward pressure, rotate the hook shank slightly upward and the hook curve downward until needle and hook are removed through the original wound. (Modified from Longmire, W. T., Jr., Emergency Medicine, Vol. 3, No. 7, p. 98, July 1971.)

(59–23). It may, however, be injured by penetration or perforation. Suspicion or evidence (usually by abdominal paracentesis) of gallbladder or duct damage calls for immediate evaluation for exploratory laparotomy.

59–20. GASTROINTESTINAL INJURIES

Rupture by severe, blunt, nonpenetrating trauma or perforation of any portion of the bowel calls for immediate surgical exploration and repair. Blows to either the upper abdomen or the back can cause retroperitoneal rupture of the duodenum. A history of possible trauma, with some immediate severe abdominal pain followed by a brief pain-free period, is typical. Demonstration by x-ray of free air on lateral decubitus or under the diaphragm in an upright film is conclusive, but absence of air does not rule out perforation (if possible, have the patient sit up for 5 minutes before taking the upright film). Penetrating wounds from the back or flank may give no immediate symptoms even if the retroperitoneal portion of the ascending or descending colon is injured; if injuries in this area are not operated upon, they must be watched closely and possibly a barium enema performed.

59–21. GREASE AND PAINT HIGH-PRESSURE GUN INJURIES

Severe injuries, usually to the hand, may result from injection through a small puncture wound in the skin of lubricating grease or paint under as much as 600 pounds per square inch pressure. Although these injuries may appear innocent, open exploration should be performed in most cases, particularly in the digits. Following the tracts of least resistance (fascial compartments, intermuscular septa, tendon and nerve sheaths), the grease or paint may dissect for considerable distance in the brief moment of contact. Even with extensive damage, immediate pain is unusual but becomes agonizing within a few hours due to tissue ischemia. Since the grease is not radiopaque, x-rays are of little, if any, value in determining the extent of damage, but radiopaque paint is identifiable.

Treatment

- Release of tension and removal of the contaminant as an immediate emergency procedure. Wide surgical exposure with extremely diligent debridement, usually under regional nerve block, must be done to minimize permanent disability. Consider use of short-term steroids with tapering doses; continuous saline irrigations may also be beneficial.
- Intensive and prolonged antibiotic therapy for infection control.

59–22. LACERATIONS *(See 59–1 to 59–3)*

59–23. LIVER INJURIES

If severe blunt trauma to the right lower ribs or abdomen (usually the result of vehicular or industrial injury) without external evidence of injury has occurred and severe shock (57) not explainable by other injuries is present, damage to the liver should always be suspected. Usually, however, hepatic damage is associated with other injuries (fractured ribs, fractured pelvis, ruptured diaphragm, mediastinal hemorrhage) and is signaled by upper abdominal pain, tenderness and spasm. Right shoulder pain may be present, often only on deep inspiration. Treat shock (57) before and during transfer for evaluation for laparoscopy or laparotomy or both.

59–24. NASAL INJURIES *(See 48–5; see also 59–22, Lacerations)*

59–25. NERVE INJURIES *(See 43–10, Nerve Injuries in the Hand; see also 49–15 and Fig. 49–1, Anatomical Location of Peripheral Nerve Injuries)*

59–26. PANCREATIC INJURIES

Blunt trauma to the abdomen, usually from automobile accidents and usually associated with other serious injuries, is a common cause of traumatic pancreatitis. Injury limited to the gland is usually the result of bullet or stab wounds. Elevated serum and urine amylase levels are of value in diagnosis.

Treatment

Wide exposure at laparotomy, with opening of the lesser omental sac to allow inspection of the complete gland for ecchymoses, edema, fat necrosis, tears of the capsule and parenchyma and retroperitoneal hematomas, and for surgical procedures as indicated.

59–27. PENETRATING AND PUNCTURE WOUNDS *(See also 31–4, Hemopericardium; 31–11, Penetrating Chest Wounds; 38–29 to 38–37, Eye Injuries; 59–1 to 59–3)*

This general category covers all types of injuries, usually but not necessarily caused by small pointed objects, in which there is a wound of entrance but none of exit. Diagnosis is usually apparent and treatment [exploration, debridement, closure, protection against tetanus *(20)*] well-standardized; therefore, the mortality rate is lower than that of injuries resulting from blunt force without external evidence of injury. If there is contamination of the puncture wound with foreign human blood products or feces, also protect against hepatitis with 0.02 ml per lb. of body weight of gamma globulin intramuscularly (IM).

Power lawn mowers propel small objects with nearly the same velocity as a bullet and leave a deceptively benign entry site but deep, injurious penetration. On the other hand, chain saw injuries, usually caused by faulty handling and improper clothing measures, cause wide mutilating wounds, often requiring a plastic surgeon's assistance. Explosions from bottles containing carbonated beverages can cause both deep, penetrating and wide, avulsing wounds.

Soft tissue penetrating wounds to the neck must all be meticulously explored; surgery is performed in selective cases following careful guidelines (Shuck) and combined with close ongoing observation. Indications for immediate surgery are:

- Active bleeding not readily controlled by topical pressure.
- Hematoma that is pulsating or enlarging.
- Bruit or thrill.
- Carotid pulse deficit.
- Crepitation or dysphagia (evaluate larynx, trachea, esophagus).

Even in the absence of any of the above, arteriogram or barium swallow are appropriate if the wound tract is close to the carotid sheath or esophagus respectively. Platysma penetration is a strong, but not absolute, indication for exploratory surgery.

59–28. PERFORATING WOUNDS

Through-and-through wounds with unmistakable skin defects at the points of entrance and exit are most often caused by bullets. The mortality rate is lower than that of contusions caused by blunt force or of penetrating wounds because surgical exploration without delay is more frequently and promptly carried out. See *59–27.*

59–29. SCALP WOUNDS *(See 44–22)*

59–30. SPINAL CORD INJURIES *(See 47–17)*

59–31. SPLENIC INJURIES

Injuries to the spleen represent the largest group (approximately 26%) in most statistical series concerned with the effects of blunt trauma. Automobile accidents represent the chief cause of such injuries. Rupture of the spleen is often associated with rib fractures and other chest and abdominal traumatic pathology.

Signs and Symptoms. Upper abdominal pain that may vary markedly in intensity and tenderness and muscle spasm or guarding in the left upper quadrant, sometimes extending below the umbilicus. An enlarging spleen and percussible dullness above the 10th rib laterally will occur if the capsule is intact. Left shoulder pain, elicited by pressure over the left upper quadrant and by deep inspiration, is present in about 50% of cases. Bleeding may be temporarily tamponaded by perisplenic hematomas, with irreversible circulatory collapse *(57, Shock)* when capsular rupture occurs—sometimes several weeks after injury. A spleen scan aids diagnosis.

Treatment

Immediate surgery for repair of the spleen, if possible, or splenectomy as soon as the condition is recognized. If the diagnosis is in doubt, or conservative measures are used for any reason, cross matched blood should be available for immediate use.

59–32. SPRAINS AND STRAINS *(See 47–3)*

59–33. STAB WOUNDS

The treatment of stab wounds depends upon the injury tract, the structures involved and the length of time since injury. Close observation for several hours, followed by surgical exploration, may be required to determine the true extent of injury, particularly if the weapon used has produced a very small entrance wound with deep penetration (hatpins, ice picks, thin knife blades). See also *59–27.*

59–34. STINGS *(See 60)*

59–35. STUD AND STAPLE GUN INJURIES

A modern stud-driving device used in the construction industry utilizes small explosive powder charges for propulsion of rivets and studs. As a result, it offers two sets of hazards:

- The bullet-like effect of the stud or rivet. Large industrial staple guns, spring propelled, may cause severe soft tissue and bone injuries.
- The gunpowder danger from the charge. Any break in the skin is an indication for protection against tetanus *(20).*

59–36. TEAR GAS PEN AND GUN INJURIES

The increasing use of small tear gas pistols for self-defense has resulted in permanent impairment of sensation and mobility when the gun has exploded in the user's hand—apparently from imbedding of particles of the lacrimating agent, alpha-chloracetophenone, in nerve and muscle tissue. Serious eye injuries have been reported.

Treatment

- Thorough debridement with removal of imbedded foreign bodies, followed by thorough irrigation. Hospitalization may be required because of need for repeated debridement.
- Application of a sterile dressing, leaving the wound open.
- Reference for follow-up care in 1 or 2 days. Reexploration of the wound in 3 to 4 weeks may be necessary.
- For treatment of chemical eye injuries, see *53–193, Chloracetophenone (Mace).*

59–37. TRACHEOBRONCHIAL INJURIES

Rupture of the trachea or of the bronchi can be caused by direct trauma such as steering wheel impact, by heavy glancing blows to the chest and by falls. Increased intraluminal pressure with a closed glottis may be a factor. Tremendous cervical and facial emphysema ("puffball like") may be rapidly fatal. Tension pneumothorax *(31–12)* may require treatment. In some cases, immediate intubation *(5–18)* or tracheostomy *(18–34)* followed by thoracotomy may have a successful outcome; in all cases, immediate hospitalization for close observation and possible emergency surgical intervention is indicated.

59–38. "WHIPLASH INJURIES" *(See 47–10)*

59–39. WINDSHIELD GLASS INJURIES

In 1966, safety regulations made the use of shatter-proof glass mandatory. Since this type of glass breaks into many small shards on impact, the facial injuries it causes usually consist of small puncture wounds and elliptical lacerations. Accompanying head injury *(41)* can be a serious problem.

Treatment

- Thorough irrigation and inspection and palpation for possible foreign bodies, which may be numerous.
- Debridement with conversion of elliptical lacerations into straight lines, corresponding whenever possible to the normal skin lines of the face. Revision of disfiguring scars should be postponed until at least 12 to 18 months after injury to allow the scars to mature.

59–40. WRINGER-TYPE INJURIES ("Degloving Injuries")

The advent of the household spin-dry washer has, fortunately, resulted in a great decrease in this serious type of injury. Classic wringer injuries, which are confined almost exclusively to children old enough to run about and a rare industrial occurrence, can result in extensive, permanent disability and deformity. The same type of injury occurs most frequently now when an upper or lower extremity is severely impinged during motion between any two or more hard surfaces. Severe crushing and avulsion of soft tissues, abrasions, lacerations, friction burns and nerve and blood vessel damage may occur.

DANGER SIGNS WITH WRINGER-TYPE INJURIES

Massive edema	Skin pallor or poor color return on pressure and release. Pulse may be obscured. Digital or radial pulse absent or difficult to palpate
Discolored abrasions	Deep red to purple color with no blanching on digital pressure
Avulsion of skin with a distally based flap	Skin rolled distally Flap discoloration (cyanosis or pallor)
Pain	Ischemic variety, unrelieved by splinting, aggravated by repeatedly opening and closing hand Crying, fretfulness
Anesthetic skin	Possible nerve severance or contusion or loss of arterial supply Absence of sweating Diminished or absent pinprick and discriminatory sensations
Absent pulses in fingers or major arterial trunks	Possible diminished or absent blood flow due to internal pressure

Fractures and epiphyseal damage may be demonstrated by x-ray films. See also 47–60, *Compartment Syndrome.*

Treatment *(See also 59–1, Initial Measures; 59–2, Specific Procedures; 59–3, Postprocedure Measures)*

- Cleansing of abrasions and superficial lacerations; application of petrolatum or bacitracin gauze dressings. Debridement; evacuation of hematomas; obliteration of dead spaces; and suturing of gaping, deep or extensive lacerations under general anesthesia are usually necessary.
- Reduction of any fractures, followed by application of a removable splint or plaster shell.
- Arrangement for immediate hospitalization and close observation, particularly for circulatory impairment. Extreme edema, common following crushing injuries, may require fasciotomy. No circumferential dressings should be applied, especially around the digits and elbow.
- Explanation to the parents or legal guardian of the injured child of the potential seriousness of the injury, including possible loss of the extremity, and of the possible need for secondary skin grafting, tendon suture or nerve repair at a later date.
- Consider use of hyperbaric oxygen.

59–41. ZIPPER INJURIES

Although other redundant, loose, soft tissues may occasionally be involved, zipper injuries to the penis—especially the prepuce—are by far the most common, particularly when the individual is intoxicated or in an agitated hurry. Sedation and topical anesthetic may be required. If the zipper cannot be backed off, remove the zipper intact from the clothing, and then see if the zipper tab can be advanced without involving more tissue and disengaged from the top. Do not attempt to use sharp tissue dissection, as a wide skin defect may result. See 59–3, *Postprocedure Measures.*

59–42. SOFT TISSUE INFECTIONS (LIFE THREATENING; DEEP AND ANAEROBIC) *(See Table 59–2; see also 58–6, Contagious and Communicable Skin Diseases; 59–1 to 59–3)*

These serious, rapidly destructive and not infrequently fatal infections require prompt recognition and intervention.

Occurrence

Most of these infections occur as a complication of soft tissue trauma (see *59–1* to *59–3*), intra-abdominal surgery or ischemic necrosis. Patients with the following conditions are more often susceptible hosts: diabetes mellitus, malnutrition, decreased immune reaction system and debilitated states of any cause.

Gas Formation in Wounds

- The classic cause of this finding is infection (gas gangrene) from histotoxic clostridia, particularly *Clostridium perfringens*. However, other organisms may cause gas to be present in tissues (anaerobic streptococci, *Bacteroides*, coliform bacteria), but crepitant cellulitis from these latter causes is usually more superficially located, slower in onset and associated usually with less toxicity.
- If air ambulance transfer is necessary, it should be noted that gas expansion occurs at higher elevation, with great increase in pain. Measures in addition to medication that can assist are flying at a lower altitude, a well-pressurized cabin and possibly a relaxing fasciotomy prior to flight.
- Wounds washed extensively with hydrogen peroxide may temporarily show subcutaneous gas bubbles on x-ray film but should not cause diagnostic problems.

Bacterial Identification

- Gram stain of a smear of wound fluids is the most important initial guide to detection of the responsible microbial pathogen and to selection of an effective antimicrobial *(33–83)*.
- Source of contamination and body site affected are indices to microbial type.
- Wound exudate should be cultured under both aerobic and anaerobic conditions in addition to being subjected to antimicrobial sensitivity studies.

Treatment—General Measures

- See principles set forth in *59–1* to *59–3*.
- Prompt wide and deep surgical incision and drainage, plus debridement of necrotic tissue is of paramount importance in these problems. Urgency is the watchword, and undue procrastination can be fatal.
- Hyperbaric oxygen is of value in suppression of anaerobic infections, particularly clostridial infections.
- Antimicrobial therapy must be vigorous and prompt and initially should be parenterally given—preferably intravenously. See *33–83* for antimicrobial agents and doses in specific anaerobic infections. Clindamycin (Cleocin) and gentamicin (Garamycin) are valuable for mixed anaerobic infections.
- Treatment of shock (57) and general supportive care. Treatment of ketoacidosis *(46–1)*, hypocalcemia *(46–14)*, renal failure and anemia may be necessary.

Table 59–2. DIFFERENTIAL DIAGNOSIS OF LIFE THREATENING SOFT TISSUE INFECTIONS*

	Clostridial Myonecrosis	Streptococcal Myositis	Synergistic Necrotizing Cellulitis	Necrotizing Fascitis	Progressive Synergistic Gangrene
Incubation	18 hours to 3 days	3 to 4 days	3 to 14 days	1 to 4 days	10 to 14 days
Onset	Sudden	Gradual	Sudden	Sudden	Gradual
Toxemia	Severe	Progressively severe	Severe	Moderate to severe	Slight
Pain	Severe	Usually severe	Severe	Minimal; especially hypesthesia	Severe
Exudate	Usually profuse, serosanguinous, "stench"	Abundant, seropurulent, foul smelling	"Dishwater pus," foul smelling	Serosanguinous	Nil or slight
Gas	Rarely pronounced, except terminally	Present, not pronounced	Not pronounced, present in 25% of cases	Usually not present	Usually not present
Muscle	Edema, pallor to blackish color, nonviable	Little change but edema, viable	Moderate change, viable	Viable	No change
Skin	Tense, often white blebs later	Tense, often with coppery tinge	Discrete bluish-gray necrosis with areas of normal skin	Tense, pale red cellulitis, little demarcation	Fiery red cellulitis often purplish zone, ulceration later
Mortality	15 to 30%	5 to 10%	75%	30%	High

*Modified from Finegold, S. M., Bartlett, J. G., Chow, A. W., et al.: Ann. Intern. Med., *83*:375, 1975; and Oill, P. A., Roser, S. M., Galpin, J. E., et al.: West. J. Med., *126*:196, 1977.

Clostridial Myonecrosis *(See Table 59–1)*

This rapidly toxic and often fatal anaerobic infection may complicate wounds of all types. The toxin generated causes gross tissue destruction and can cause hemolysis.

Treatment *(See also General Measures, above)*

- Hyperbaric oxygen whenever available (see 26–6).
- Prompt surgical excision of all involved tissue. If hyperbaric oxygen is used, surgical delay for better demarcation is tenable.
- Penicillin G intravenously in divided doses of 10 to 20 million units per day or chloramphenicol (Chloromycetin), 4 gm per day in divided doses.
- Polyvalent antitoxin is of equivocal value, but its benefit is most likely if given early (75,000 units IV), after checking for sensitivity *(16)*.

Necrotizing Fasciitis *(See Table 59–1)*

This uncommon infection, which causes diffuse fascial and subcutaneous necrosis, undermining the skin in a plane that permits easy extensive movement of a probe, most often occurs following trauma and intraabdominal surgery. It is caused by a mixed flora of anaerobes and aerobes. Subcutaneous gangrene can be extensive, with skin necrosis, bullae and ecchymoses occurring later.

Treatment

- See General Measures, above.
- Clindamycin (Cleocin) and gentamicin (Garamycin) often form an effective initial combination.

Progressive Synergistic Gangrene *(See Table 59–1)*

Anaerobic cocci and aerobic gram-negative rods or gram-positive cocci synergistically cause an infection that most often occurs along the suture line of an intra-abdominal surgical wound. The area around the suture line becomes very tender, red and edematous, with a purplish center that ulcerates. A slowly advancing greyish-white undermining subcutaneous slough follows.

Aerobic streptococci and staphylococci (gram-positive) are treated with penicillin and methicillin in large parenteral doses. If gram-negative rods are also present, a combination of gentamicin and clindamycin or chloramphenicol should be used initially, or consider metronidazole.

Streptococcal Myositis

Combined anaerobic and aerobic streptococci, with or without concomitant staphylococci, cause this infection, most often as a complication of traumatic wounds. Differentiation from clostridial myonecrosis is usually made before cultures are returned on the basis of Gram stain and observation of the muscle at surgery. In streptococcal myositis, though the muscle is discolored, it usually remains viable and contractile in contrast to findings with clostridial (toxin) muscle involvement (muscle is noncontractile; friable; gangrenous; purple, black or greenish color). Abundance of anaerobic staphylococci may cause abscess in the skeletal muscle; with severe contusions, abscess may occur even when there is no skin perforation.

Streptococcal infection is best treated with 10 to 20 million units of penicillin G daily in divided doses in patients who are not sensitive. If *Staphylococcus* organisms are prominent, nafcillin or a cephalosporin may be used.

Synergistic Necrotizing Cellulitis *(See Table 59–1)*

This type of infection is characterized by distinct areas of bluish-grey necrotic skin separated by normal skin areas, which belies the extensive necrosis of muscle compartments beneath.

Synergistic action of both aerobic gram-negative bacteria (one or more of the following: *Escherichia coli, Proteus mirabilis, Klebsiella* spp., Enterobacteriaceae organisms) and anaerobic bacteria (either anaerobic streptococci or *Bacteroides*, or both) must occur to cause this rapid, extensive destruction.

For specific treatment, a combination of clindamycin (Cleocin) and gentamicin (Garamycin) is usually effective.

59–43. TISSUE COVERING OF WOUNDS (GRAFTS) *(See 28–3, Burns, Principles of Treatment)*

59–44. WOUND REPAIR WITH REATTACHMENT OF SEVERED PARTS

The severed, amputated, or avulsed part should be:

- Promptly and gently rinsed with nonirritating substances (water, saline) if time and skill permits; ok to do no cleaning.
- Wrapped in sterile gauze, if available, or in gauze moistened with saline or water.
- Sealed in a dry plastic bag of appropriate size. Do not put amputated part in direct contact with the ice slurry.
- Kept cool by placing plastic bag in an ice slurry within an ice chest or thermal vacuum container during transportation.

Properly cooled and stored parts have been successfully reapplied up to 24 hours after severance, though the earliest time feasible is best; the more complex the severance, the shorter the period for successful replantation. Prime indications for reattachment in the hand are thumb amputation and amputation of multiple digits proximal to the distal interphalangeal joint or single digits distal to the distal interphalangeal joint in young children.

Reattachment should be done by the most skilled individual reasonably available, using indicated microsurgical techniques.

Relative contraindications to replantation are:

- Massive crushing injury of the entire part.
- Major "degloving injuries" (see *59–40*).
- Tissue necrosis associated with freezing.
- Massive contamination.
- Normothermia of amputated part for more than 6 hours.

Even if reattachment is not conceivable, the part should be cleaned and sent with the patient, as parts of the skin may be used for autografts.

60. Stings*

Approximately 50% of deaths from venomous stings are due to insects of the order Hymenoptera (bees, fire ants, hornets, wasps, yellow jackets); 80% of these deaths occur within 2 hours of the sting.

60–1. BEE STINGS

These are common and may be dangerous. Large numbers of multiple stings (e.g., 500 to 2000) at a single event may be lethal in the absence of hypersensitivity, but this is rare. Extremely great sensitivity (natural or acquired) to

*See also *24, Allergic Reactions; 27, Bites; 53, Acute Poisoning; 59, Soft Tissue Injury.*

hymenopteran venom may be encountered, and a single repeat sting can constitute an acute emergency.

Treatment

These patients present with the clinical picture of severe anaphylactic shock and require immediate energetic handling as a lifesaving measure (24). Epinephrine hydrochloride (Adrenalin), 0.3 to 0.5 ml in adults and 0.2 to 0.3 ml in children (0.01 ml/kg) of 1:1000 solution, should be given SC or 1:10,000 solution slowly IV, followed by therapy for shock (57) and hospitalization.

Persons known to be sensitive to hymenopteran venom, especially those over 40 years of age with known heart disease, should have available an emergency kit for immediate treatment of insect bites and stings. This kit (see also 24 regarding Anakit) should contain the following:

- Needle or pin for lifting out the stinger without compression (which can cause additional injection of venom). This may also be accomplished by gentle teasing out with a fingernail. Avoid squeezing or compression with tweezers.
- A tourniquet to use as a compression band for lymphatics.
- A disposable hypodermic syringe (with needle) containing 1 ml of 1:1000 epinephrine hydrochloride (Adrenalin). These should be replaced if solution turns brown (can occur within about 1 year or sooner in warmer climates—is then ineffective).
- An aerosol inhalator containing epinephrine hydrochloride (Adrenalin) or isoproterenol solution. Isoproterenol infusion may be necessary to neutralize the epinephrine-resistant effect of propranolol in patients who are taking propranolol (Inderal).
- Antihistamine tablets (oral).

Symptomatic Local Treatment

- Cold compresses or an ice cube; application of tincture of iodine, ammonia or baking soda, or magnesium sulfate (Epsom salts) soaks will usually give relief.
- The "stinger" should be identified and removed if present. Afterwards, papain (Adolph's meat tenderizer—a paste of ¼ teaspoonful in a teaspoon of water) immediately applied topically may help destroy and neutralize the hymenopteran venom.

Desensitization

Desensitization to hymenopteran venom sometimes is practical but should always be supervised by an allergist. Pure venom preparations are available for desensitization.

60–2. CADDIS FLY STINGS

Acute allergic reactions have been reported, especially in the Great Lakes area of the United States, from stings from this fly. For treatment, see 24, *Allergic Reactions; 60–1, Bee Stings.*

60–3. CATERPILLAR STINGS

Among the larvae that can cause severe reactions from venom carried in the hair are those of the brown-tail moth, buck moth, flannel moth, Io moth, range caterpillar, saddleback caterpillar, tussock moth and white moth. The venom may cause local edema, swelling and acute pain. Vomiting, convulsions and shock are rare occurrences.

Treatment

- Thorough washing of the site of the sting, followed by application of ammonia, baking soda, papain (Adolph's meat tenderizer) or alcohol solutions.
- Control of pain by aspirin or codeine. Intravenous injection of 10 ml of 10% calcium gluconate may be effective.
- Supportive and symptomatic care *(53)*.

60–4. CONE SHELL STINGS

Conus californicus is the only cone shell (a mollusc) present on North American shores that will give a toxic sting (slight) when handled. *Conus geographus* and other *Conus* species are inhabitants of more tropical Pacific areas; these are dangerous and have caused fatalities through paralytic muscular action; treatment is vigorous supportive assistance, including ventilatory assistance.

60–5. CORAL STINGS

The toxicity of venom from coral varies with the species.

60–6. FIRE ANT STINGS *(See also 24, Allergic Reactions)*

Although these ants (found principally in southern states in the United States) also bite, toxic effects are caused by venom injected through a spine on the ant's abdomen. Since the ants move and sting quickly (each ant 3 or 4 times), 3000 to 5000 stings have been reported on one person following disturbance of an ant mound. Severe reactions, including allergic reactions *(24)*, that are potentially life threatening can occur.

Signs and Symptoms. Immediate development of a characteristic umbilicated papule surrounded by a reddened, acutely painful halo, with severe, burning, stinging pain at, and for some distance around, the site of the sting. The skin temperature is usually elevated. Dyspnea, cyanosis and acute respiratory depression may develop rapidly.

Treatment

- Artificial ventilation *(5–21)* in severe cases.
- Treatment of allergic reactions *(24)* and supportive care *(57)*.
- Protective sterile dressing over involved areas. (See also *60–1, Bee Stings, Treatment*).
- *Control of pain (12)*. Narcotics may be necessary for 12 to 24 hours.

Prognosis. Although rare fatalities from respiratory collapse have been reported owing to multiple stings and hypersensitivity, complete recovery in 3 to 5 days usually occurs.

60–7. HYMENOPTERA STINGS *(See 60–1, Bee Stings)*

60–8. LARVAL STINGS *(See 60–3, Caterpillar Stings)*

60–9. MARINE ANIMAL STINGS *(See 60–5, Coral Stings; 60–10, Portuguese Man-of-War Stings; 60–13, Sea Anemone Stings; 60–15, Stingray; 60–16, Tropical Jellyfish Stings)*

60–10. PORTUGUESE MAN-OF-WAR (Blue Bottle) STINGS

Stings from these marine creatures are relatively common in persons participating in water sports. Severe pain, gross muscle tetany, local tissue changes and anaphylactic shock *(24)* may occur.

Treatment

- Remove any adherent tentacles (which contain nematocysts) at once, with the hands wrapped in cloth or protected by gloves.
- Treat shock *(57)*.
- Wash with cool salt water followed by methyl alcohol or dilute household ammonia or vinegar; dust with sodium bicarbonate paste or flour. When this is dry, scrape off with a noncutting, narrow-edged instrument, Rewash with salt water.
- Give tripelennamine hydrochloride (PBZ), 50 mg PO q 4 h prn.
- Inject 10 ml of 10% calcium gluconate IV over about 5 minutes for muscle spasm relief, if needed.
- A corticosteroid-analgesic-antihistamine ointment (such as Sea Balm*) is beneficial.

60–11. PUSS CATERPILLAR STINGS *(See also 60–3, Caterpillar Stings)*

Of the more than 50 species of larvae that may produce toxic effects from venoms contained in the hair, the larval stage of the flannel moth is the most common. It is known in different localities by various names—el perrito ("little dog"), Italian asp, possum bug, puss caterpillar, wooly slug and wooly worm. In appearance, it is a blob of neatly combed brown fur, shaped like a Brazil nut and 20 to 30 mm long. The venom is contained in hidden clusters of specialized hair on the back; it is not found in all hairs.

For treatment, see *60–3, Caterpillar Stings.*

60–12. SCORPION STINGS

The seriousness of toxic reactions to scorpion stings varies with the species, with the site of the sting and with the age of the victim. In North America, the species are relatively harmless except for *Centruroides exilicauda.* Infants and small children generally become more seriously ill and should be hospitalized.

The victim may have local pain, dizziness, circulatory and respiratory depression, hypersensitivity to touch, weakness or paralysis and hypertensive crisis. Transverse myelopathy has been reported.

Treatment

- Compress the sting site with ice.
- Control pain *(12)*.
- Administer scorpion antivenin after evenomation from *C. sculpturatus* or other toxic species after testing for sensitivity. (See *16, Serum Sensitivity and Desensitization*).
- Hospitalize for close observation and symptomatic and supportive care *(53–11)*.

60–13. SEA ANEMONE ("Sea Nettle") STINGS

Sea anemones can cause severe burning stings from their nematocysts,

*Sea Balm is available from Marine Tech, 3115 E. 40th Ave., Denver, Colorado 80205.

similar to other coelenterates, including the Portuguese Man-of-War.

For treatment, see *60–10, Portuguese Man-of-War Stings.*

60–14. SEA URCHINS

Long- and short-spined sea urchins are fairly common causes of marine injury. Injury mainly involves tissue penetration *(59)*, and treatment requires removal of any of the remaining friable, purplish spines (these rarely are visible on x-ray). Weak acid soaks (e.g., household vinegar) may help to dissolve small fragments. Symptoms from venom are usually minimal except in rare cases of *Tripneustes* pedicellarial envenomation.

60–15. STINGRAY (Stingaree) STINGS

Wounds caused by the stingray are common in the South Pacific and have been reported from Gulf of Mexico and California resorts where water sports are popular. Both the fresh water and the salt water varieties are dangerous. Stingray injuries are characterized by jagged, irregular wounds that may in themselves be fatal and by severe localized pain or, in some instances, numbness of the whole affected extremity, caused by venom carried in the integumentary sheath of the ray's serrated stinger. Nausea, vomiting, headache, hypotension and dizziness, and painful, shallow respiration with pallor and cyanosis, are sometimes present. Symptoms reach maximum severity within 1 to 1½ hours after the sting. Swelling and induration are common.

Treatment

- Thorough irrigation of the wound (see *59–1, Soft Tissue Injuries*).
- Control of severe pain and neutralization of toxin by immersion in hot tub of water (as hot as tolerated). Injection of morphine sulfate or meperidine SC or IV may be necessary.
- Surgical removal of the serrated stinger or sheath, followed by thorough debridement. Elevate the affected part.
- Hospitalization is advised when there are systemic ill effects. Unless thorough debridement is done, large, slow-healing ulcers may develop at the site of the sting.

60–16. TROPICAL JELLYFISH STINGS *(See also 60–10, Portuguese Man-of-War Stings; 60–13, Sea Anemone Stings)*

These cause local pain and generalized myalgia. Severe systemic reactions are variable according to species. The order Cubomedusae—the box jellies or "sea wasps"—are highly toxic, and rapid fatalities have been recorded. Anaphylactic allergic reactions to jellyfish stings also occur (see 24). The muscle pain usually yields readily to intravenous administration of 5 to 10 ml of 10% calcium gluconate solution, but in some cases codeine or morphine sulfate may be necessary. Cool soaks of vinegar or alcohol are helpful. Local treatment as given under *Portuguese Man-of-War Stings (60–10)* should be used. Systemic reactions may require intensive supportive care.

60–17. WASP (Hornet, Yellow Jacket) STINGS

Wasp stings may cause reactions similar to but more severe than those caused by bee stings *(60–1)*. Acute anaphylactic reactions *(24)* may be terminal. The treatment is the same as for bee stings except that there is no buried stinger to be removed. For emergency kit and desensitization, see *60–1, Bee Stings.*

61. Teeth and Orofacial Conditions

61–1. TOOTH PAIN (Toothache)

Tooth pain in the emergency setting is usually due to direct trauma *(61–2)* or to trauma or dysfunction of surrounding structures—e.g., maxilla, mandible *(61–5)*, TMJ *(61–13)*, neuralgia (trigeminal/glossopharyngeal; see *49–13*) or infection of surrounding structures (parotid gland [*61–17*]; maxillary sinus [56–23]) or the tooth itself.

Pain with hot and cold substances usually is present with tooth decay or pulp involvement, although the latter is of a more intense throbbing quality compared with the dull aching of tooth decay. Periapical and alveolar abscesses *(23–1)* cause the teeth to be tender with percussion, palpation or chewing, with the latter producing much swelling.

Fever, observable infection, a history or visible evidence of trauma and results of percussion usually focus the diagnosis. Radiographic evaluation is usually necessary before definitive diagnosis and treatment.

Treatment

- Treat pain *(12)*.
- Antibiotics (usually penicillin or erythromycin) are indicated in the presence of tooth mobility, percussion pain, periodontal swelling or other specific infections.
- Refer to a dentist or oral surgeon for continuing care.

61–2. FRACTURE OF TEETH

Isolated injury to a tooth or teeth may occur, but many times such injuries are associated with lip contusion or laceration *(59–2)* and occasionally with mandibular or maxillary *(61–5)* or cervical *(47–10; 47–11)* fractures or with various degrees of intracranial injury *(44)*. History and examination must include evaluation and checking for abnormal position and motion plus pain and crepitus with motion (see also Fig. 61–2).

Tooth injury is determined by visual inspection, mobility to touch, pain with pressure or tapping with finger on the incisal edge and x-ray (tooth fragments may also be detected in soft tissue wounds by x-ray). The magnitude of injury can be determined by visual inspection or x-ray, or both, and graded into eight classes of fracture for treatment (see Table 61–1 and Fig. 61–1).

A dentist should examine the patient in almost all cases of trauma to the teeth, as early referral can provide for salvaging of teeth and/or their roots. Even a slight hit that leaves a tooth asymptomatic and immobile can cause eventual unesthetic darkening of the tooth, necrosis of the pulp and apical abscess. On the positive side, there have been thousands of teeth replanted successfully from a totally avulsed state.

Treatment of the Traumatically Luxated Tooth

After very gentle washing off of foreign material, the traumatically luxated tooth is to be kept moist by *immediate* placement either in the mouth or in a cup of milk, weak saline or water. Do not scrape or scrub the root surface, as its minute attachment fibers are to be kept. If sufficient alveolar bone exists to allow for splinting with adjacent teeth, the dentist may even perform root

The tooth and its fractures

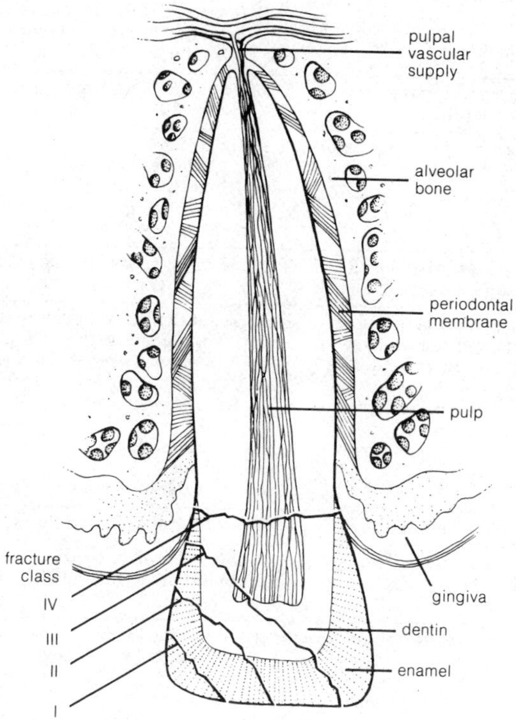

Injuries to the teeth

Class I.	Simple fracture of the enamel of the crown
Class II.	Extensive fracture of the crown involving dentine
Class III.	Extensive fracture of the crown involving dentine and dental pulp
Class IV.	Extensive involvement and exposure of the entire pulp
Class V.	Totally avulsed or luxated teeth
Class VI.	Fracture of the root with or without loss of crown structure
Class VII.	Displacement of tooth without fracture of crown or root
Class VIII.	Fracture of the crown in its entirety

Figure 61–1. Determination of the magnitude of injury to the tooth. (From Emergency Medicine, June 1978.)

Table 61–1. CLASSIFICATION OF TOOTH FRACTURES

Class of Injury	Description	**Treatment** (save all parts for possible reattachment; dental films advisable to evaluate for root fracture)
Class I	Simple fracture of crown enamel	1. Cover fracture site with copal ether varnish for thermal protection. 2. Refer to dentist next day. 3. Send any found fragment for possible bonding.
Class II	Fracture of crown, including dentine	Same as for Class I fractures
Class III	Fracture of crown, including dentine and part of pulp	1. Immediate referral to dentist, endodontist or oral surgeon to prevent infection. Give analgesics as indicated. 2. Immediate application of calcium hydroxide over pulp.
Class IV	Like Class III, but all of pulp revealed	Same as for Class III fractures
Class V	Entire tooth avulsed or luxated from socket Note: immediate dental referral advisable for Classes V to VIII for repositioning and possible root canal treatment.	1. Tepid tap water or saline rinse of tooth without scrubbing. Keep tooth moist. 2. Anatomically reposition tooth in socket prn if out for less than 2 hours. 3. Reduce edema with focal ice pack. 4. Splint (wire, acrylic or bonding) to adjacent teeth and/or immediate dental referral. 5. Consider broad-spectrum antibiotics.
Class VI	Root fracture ± crown	Refer to dentist immediately.
Class VII	Tooth displacement but no root/crown fracture	1. Slowly realign tooth. 2. Splint as needed and/or prompt dental referral.
Class VIII	Entire crown fractured/lost	1. Analgesics/sedation. 2. Prompt referral to dentist or oral surgeon.

canal therapy on the tooth before inserting and splinting it. Once the field is dry, excellent splinting is achieved with the acid etch–epoxy resin (bonding) or acrylic or wiring techniques for almost any mobilized tooth.

If a dentist is not reachable, the physician will need to replant the tooth as soon as possible for the best results to be achieved. X-rays are most helpful in assessing the area for extent of destruction, foreign material, and so on. Injecting 1.8 ml of 2% lidocaine with 1:100,000 epinephrine into the labial vestibule at the apical area of the socket will anesthetize the area. Without scraping the socket, the blood clot is removed. The tooth is inserted to proper alignment by holding the crown. Placing the forefinger and thumb of the opposite hand on the lingual and labial alveolar plates will allow tactile aid in implanting the tooth properly. Ideally, the tooth needs to be immobilized (with gentle finger pressure if no other means are available), to prevent extrusion until the dentist is seen.

In all cases of luxation injuries with mobilized teeth, an antibiotic should be given (penicillin V or erythromycin, 500 mg stat, followed by 250 mg q 6 h for 3 days; 2 to 4 times this dose should be given if the patient is at increased risk of infection because of cardiac valvulopathy, artificial implants, etc). The patient should be advised of a guarded to poor prognosis for permanent retention of the tooth.

61–3. FACIAL NERVE LACERATION

Laceration of one or more of the five branches of the facial nerve must be suspected and tested for whenever lacerations occur anterior to the auditory canal. Use only compressive pressure to control bleeding on the face, as facial nerves may be injured by hemostats. If immediate paralysis occurs with a laceration posterior to an imaginary line dropped from the lateral canthus of the eye to the oral commissure, then refer for nerve repair under the microscope; lacerations anterior to this imaginary line may be repaired even though there is slight paralysis.

61–4. PAROTID DUCT LACERATION

Parotid duct lacerations must be referred for repair promptly and should be suspected if a laceration crosses an imaginary line from the tragus of the ear to the middle of the upper lip. Inspect the inside of the mouth for drainage and bleeding; if necessary, the duct may be cannulated from inside the mouth.

61–5. MAXILLOFACIAL FRACTURES/INJURIES

True maxillofacial emergencies that must be treated are airway obstruction *(5–10)*, hemorrhage (use broad compression bandages whenever possible) and ocular injuries *(38)*. Severe lacerations with tissue displacement needing extensive plastic repair may be approximated temporarily with tacking sutures, dressed and referred for definitive repair.

Assessing the extent and location of maxillofacial injuries (Fig. 61–2) is generally not nearly as critical in regard to time as is performance of lateral cervical x-rays to determine that there was not concomitant cervical vertebral fracture.

Supraorbital fractures may reveal a flattened brow, displaced orbital contents, anesthesia of the forehead, periorbital ecchymoses and lacerations. Patients with fractures of the upper third of the facial skeleton are the most likely to also have neurologic damage from direct trauma to the brain. Ophthalmologic and neurosurgical consultation are generally necessary.

Le Fort classification of maxillary fractures is shown in Figure 61–3. Mandibular-condylar fractures are most easily detected by placement of the examiner's index fingers in the patient's external auditory meatus as the patient opens and closes the mouth; absence of motion to palpation on one side indicates ipsilateral condylar fracture. Malocclusions from maxillary and mandibular fracture must be treated with fracture reduction and interdental fixation. Fractures of the maxilla from the skull need to be immobilized either by wires from an intact zygomatic arch or by external fixation and should be performed by surgeons skilled in maxillofacial trauma.

61–6. NASAL BONE FRACTURES *(See 48–5)*

61–7. EYE AND PERIORBITAL TRAUMA *(See 38–29 to 38–37)*

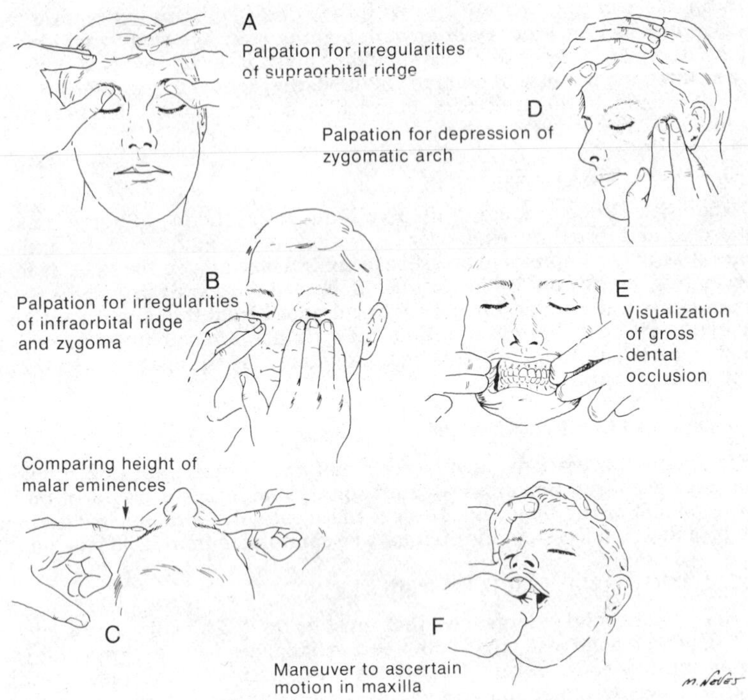

Figure 61–2. *A–C,* Techniques for bilateral palpation about the orbits. *D,* Palpation for irregularities of the zygomatic arch. *E,* Visualization of interdental occlusion. *F,* Maneuver to ascertain maxillary motion. (Modified from Schultz, R. C., and Wood, J. R.: Primary Care, 3:641, 1976.)

61–8. EAR TRAUMA *(See 35–3, Bleeding from Ears; 35–8, Contusions; 35–13, Hematoma)*

Avulsed parts should be cleaned with saline and saved for possible replantation (see *59–44*).

61–9. CONCOMITANT CERVICAL INJURY *(See 47–10 and 47–11, Injuries)*

61–10. CONCOMITANT INTRACRANIAL INJURY *See 44, Head Injuries)*

61–11. POSTEXTRACTION BLEEDING AND PAIN

Postextraction bleeding can result in loss of a large amount of blood.

Treatment

- Have the patient bite firmly on a small pad of gauze or moistened tea bag (tannic acid). Evaluation for contributory causes of hemorrhage *(45)* should be considered in such cases.

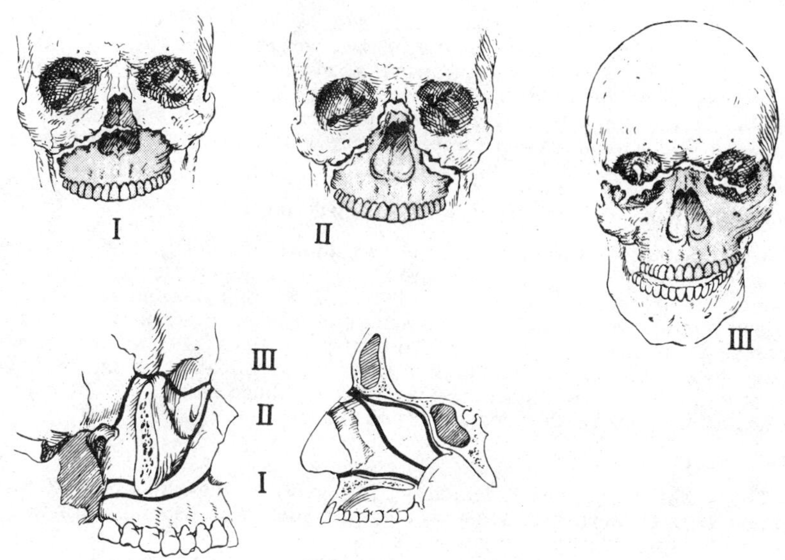

Figure 61–3. Le Fort Classification of Maxillary Fractures. I, Transverse fracture of maxilla; II, Pyramidal fracture of maxilla; III, Craniofacial dysjunction. (Modified from Schultz, R. C., and Oldham, R. J.: Surg. Clin. North Am., *57*:1000, 1977.)

- Pack the area with sterile cotton moistened with aluminum chloride solution (Hemodent). A solution of 1:1000 epinephrine hydrochloride (Adrenalin) can also be used, but sparingly, as systemic reaction with tachycardia may occur.
- Place a small piece of oxidized cellulose (Gelfoam or Oxycel) or topical thrombin on a gelatin sponge in the bleeding socket and hold firmly in place with a pad of gauze held between the teeth. Often the gums may be sutured over the implant.
- Instruct the patient not to eat solid foods of any kind until further dental care is received (this should be done immediately). Also caution the patient not to suck on a straw, as negative air pressure in the mouth can cause the clot to be "sucked out."
- Treat contributory causes of hemorrhage *(45)*.
- If the patient is in pain, give acetaminophen with or without codeine sulfate. Debridement of a "dry socket" often reveals denuded bone. Packing with iodoform and eugenol gauze under local anesthesia is often needed and should be repeated every 2 days. This most often occurs at the mandibular third molar extraction sites.
- If possible, refer the patient back to the original performing dentist.

61–12. POST-TONSILLECTOMY BLEEDING

Post-tonsillectomy bleeding may be delayed, profuse and difficult to control. It may be the first harbinger of a hematologic bleeding and clotting problem (see *45–2*) and should be evaluated accordingly. Hospitalization for suturing under general anesthesia is occasionally required. To prevent the swallowing of blood, the patient should sit up during transportation unless signs of shock *(57)* are present, in which case transportation in the semi-prone position is preferable. Sedation to allay anxiety and to quiet the patient may be necessary. Usually, removing a blood clot in the tonsillar fossa and applying direct pressure or electrocautery in the emergency department, using local anesthesia, will correct the bleeding.

61–13. TEMPOROMANDIBULAR JOINT SYNDROME (TMJS)

In addition to pain surrounding the temporomandibular joint, TMJS involves limitation and deviation of the mandible, a popping sound on opening the mouth, failure of the teeth to make a good chomping sound on closure (malocclusion), tenderness of the masseter muscles and, in some cases, rather intense headaches in the occipital and temporal regions. The patient is most likely to present for treatment after excessive mastication of chewy substances, a stressful jaw-clenching day, or a night of bad dreams and intensive bruxism. X-rays may show degenerative changes.

Treatment

- Mild cases are relieved by analgesics *(12)*, reduced chewing effort, relaxation training, and physical therapy measures such as ultrasound, diathermy, cryotherapy and isometric jaw exercises.
- More severe cases may require corticoid injection or joint operation.
- Referral to dentist for biteplate and correction of malocclusion.

61–14. LUDWIG'S ANGINA (MORBUS STRANGULATORIUS)

This is a life-threatening form of oropharyngeal soft tissue infection, deep and anaerobic *(59–42)*, that additionally requires immediate tracheostomy for signs of airway obstruction. The safeguards used in epiglottitis *(56–8)* are also applicable here. Otherwise, treatment is as described under 59–42. This disease generally follows fractures or infection in or around the mouth (comparable to a human bite from oneself in a vulnerable area—the acquired resistance to one's own organisms having been overcome).

61–15. VINCENT'S ANGINA (Acute Necrotizing Ulcerative Gingivitis [ANUG], Ulcerative Fetid Stomatitis, Trench Mouth, Vincent's Disease)

This ulcer-forming inflammation beginning on the interdental papillae is caused by a fusiform bacillus and a coarsely coiled spirochete, both of which can usually be identified in smears. The marginal and attached gingiva may be involved by direct extension. Laboratory studies should be done, but clinical exam usually differentiates adequately from diphtheria, infectious mononucleosis, tuberculosis, streptococcal gingivitis and fungal infection. Poor oral hygiene, stress, inadequate nutrition, blood dyscrasias, debilitating illnesses and heavy smoking precipitate this disease. Vincent's disease in rare instances may involve areas other than just the gums and oropharyngeal membranes (e.g., external ear, internal nares, genitalia).

Signs and Symptoms. Painful, inflamed marginal gingiva with characteristic ulcerative destruction of the interdental papillae, which are often covered with a grayish-white adherent membrane that on removal or irritation leaves punctate bleeding areas. Occasionally general malaise, fetid odor, chills and fever may be present. There may be pain on swallowing if the oral cavity is involved. A leukopenia is usually present. Incidence is highest in the 16- to 30-year age group.

Treatment

- Referral for dental care. Permanent damage to the gums and mucous membranes may occur without proper and prolonged treatment.
- Gentle debridement of crusts and cleansing of sloughs with 2% hydrogen peroxide rinse or warm saline, with a later appointment made for thorough curettage and lavage.
- Close attention to oral and other personal hygiene, including gentle flossing and brushing immediately after eating.
- In the unusual case of fever and/or lymphadenopathy, penicillin V, 250 mg q 6 h for 7 to 10 days, or a tetracycline or erythromycin at the same dosage, may be added to the above regimen.

61–16. TONSILLITIS-PHARYNGITIS *(See also 33–18, Diphtheria; 33–31, Infectious Mononucleosis)*

Acute (Including Follicular and Abscess Forms)

Acutely inflamed and swollen tonsils, with purulent material filling crypts usually sufficient to cause dysphagia and sometimes dyspnea, are common in childhood. Usually cultures, which should be routinely taken often, reveal group A beta-hemolytic streptococci or occasional staphylococci in children; with delayed treatment, these infections are prone to progress to peritonsillar abscess (quinsy; see 23–22). Adults may have the same organisms, but because of venereal *(33–78)* and oral-anal-genital contact, microbes found in any of these locations may also be cultured. A WBC and diff. is advised.

Treatment

- Aspirin or acetaminophen prn, with or without codeine, for pain relief.
- Gram stain, cultures and sensitivity tests of samples from throat as soon as possible.
- Soft or liquid diet.
- Icebags or cold compresses to the throat.
- Warm (not hot) saline lavages dripped by bulb syringe or nozzle on forming abscesses can help diminish discomfort in some cases. Place affected side down so fluid can drain out the mouth.
- Aqueous penicillin G, 75,000 units/kg/day, is the initial drug of choice (unless allergy is present); other antibiotics can be used based on the results of the Gram stain, cultures and sensitivity tests.
- Acute cases with extreme toxicity or edema require hospitalization and pediatric or otolaryngologic supervision. Controlled surgical drainage of all abscesses is necessary.

Exudative Forms

Usually there is a grayish ulcerative involvement of the tonsil with little distinguishable involvement of the crypts. Conditions affecting the immune mechanism more commonly present this way (leukemia, granulocytopenia and agranulocytosis), as may infectious mononucleosis. The most urgent situation is to discontinue immediately any causative drugs or exposures.

61–17. PAROTITIS *(See also 33–43, Epidemic Parotitis [Mumps])*

Painful tender swelling of the parotid gland can arise rapidly from bacterial infection, usually by *Staphylococcus*. It usually is seen in postsurgical patients and in persons who are on anticholinergic drugs, dehydrated and debilitated, uremic, or who have a parotid duct stone (often palpable and strippable). Serum amylase is often elevated. Gland massage is both diagnostic and therapeutic when purulent material exudes into the mouth; obtain Gram stain and culture. Additional treatment includes hydration, cessation of oral drying agents, and administration of appropriate antibiotics (usually a penicillin). Warm compresses and sucking on a lemon can be beneficial. Surgery and x-ray radiation are rarely indicated.

61–18. PERITONSILLAR ABSCESS *(See 23–22)*

61–19. RETROPHARYNGEAL ABSCESS *(See 23–27)*

61–20. ALVEOLAR ABSCESS *(See 23–1)*

62. Temperature Variation Emergencies

COLD STRESS DISORDERS

62–1. GENERAL CONSIDERATIONS

All the mechanisms of injury from exposure to low temperatures are not completely known, but metabolic and vascular changes with sludging of the blood and later thrombosis are important factors. There is a wide variation in the ability of different individuals to tolerate cold. The chances of injury by exposure to low temperature are increased by a darkly pigmented skin, advanced age, poor general physical condition, hypoxia (as in high altitude climbing or flying) and previous trauma, especially cold injury. For the detrimental effects of high wind velocity, see Figure 62–1.

Avoidance of cold injury is aided foremost by wind protection and by wearing multiple layers of dry, loose clothing (combine newer synthetics/wool/down), outside face protection as needed, with head/ear gear, and mittens with glove liners). *Note:* When wet, natural materials such as wool, and particularly down, lose their effectiveness; rapid-drying synthetics are therefore better under wet conditions. Materials that incorporate a vapor barrier and that decrease radiant heat loss (e.g., reflective space blankets) are essential in cold weather; in an emergency, covering the body surface with layers of dry newspapers that are then covered with plastic bags can help. Avoid vasoconstrictors (e.g., nicotine) and vasodilators (e.g., nitrites/alcohol) in large amounts.

62–2. FOCAL COLD INJURIES (Chilblain, Frostbite, Frostnip, Immersion Foot, Pernio, Trench Foot)

The hands, feet and face—especially the nose and ears—are the most susceptible focal cold injury areas; perform periodic checks in prevention.

Wind chill factor chart

Estimated wind speed (in mph)	Actual Thermometer Reading (° F)											
	50	40	30	20	10	0	-10	-20	-30	-40	-50	-60
	EQUIVALENT TEMPERATURE (° F.)											
calm	50	40	30	20	10	0	-10	-20	-30	-40	-50	-60
5	48	37	27	16	6	-5	-15	-26	-36	-47	-57	-68
10	40	28	16	4	-9	-24	-33	-46	-58	-70	-83	-95
15	36	22	9	-5	-18	-32	-45	-58	-72	-85	-99	-112
20	32	18	4	-10	-25	-39	-53	-67	-82	-96	-110	-124
25	30	16	0	-15	-29	-44	-59	-74	-88	-104	-118	-133
30	28	13	-2	-18	-33	-48	-63	-79	-94	-109	-125	-140
35	27	11	-4	-20	-35	-51	-67	-82	-98	-113	-129	-145
40	26	10	-6	-21	-37	-53	-69	-85	-100	-116	-132	-148
(Wind speeds greater than 40 mph have little additional effect.)	LITTLE DANGER (for properly clothed person). Maximum danger of false sense of security.				INCREASING DANGER Danger from freezing of exposed flesh.				GREAT DANGER			

Trenchfoot and immersion foot may occur at any point on this chart.

Figure 62–1

Accurate determination of the extent of tissue damage at the time of the original examination is impossible. The affected tissues are usually white, very cold to the touch, have lost their pliability and become hard and anesthetic with further cooling.

Treament (For focal cold injuries with no or only minimal core hypothermia)

- Rest in a recumbent position in the warmest, driest, most wind-sheltered area available. Exchange wet for dry clothing. Implement the heat conservation measures mentioned above. If transportation is not imminent, do *not* attempt to thaw tissues if there is danger that refreezing may occur. If warming frozen hands and feet beneath axillae and between thighs, use caution to avoid direct tissue trauma.
- Rapidly rewarm by moist heat—as in a warm tub or with compresses—after the injured person has reached a safe place where there will be no chance of refreezing. It is better to postpone rapid rewarming for a few hours than to be forced to repeat the process; once a safe place has been reached and rapid rewarming has been performed, no further rapid rewarming should be done even if a temporary drop occurs again. The solution should be kept between 37.8°C (100°F) and a maximum of 43.3°C (110°F). Regulated dry heat is also acceptable, but not preferred. Discontinue active rewarming when the skin reddens (becomes blotchy red and painful).
- After active rewarming, exposure to air at room temperature (about 21°C [69.4°F]) is most satisfactory. Elevate the extremity for edema reduction. The four degrees of tissue involvement and grading are similar to those in

burn injuries (see Fig. 28–2). Protect the skin with use of a cradle as necessary.
- Administer analgesics for severe pain (*12*). Aspirin, in addition to having an analgesic effect, reduces platelet stickiness, which may aid in relieving thrombosis formation. Narcotics are often needed.
- Give warm oral fluids, as desired.
- Administer human tetanus immune globulin (TIG) or toxoid (see *20*) if it is possible that there is a break in the integument.
- Evaluate for and treat any contributory diseases.
- Give antibiotic therapy if infection is present or imminent.
- Keep under observation until the extent of damage can be determined.
- Topical use of dilute dimethylsulfoxide is still experimental, as is intra-arterial reserpine injection proximal to the frozen area. Sympathetectomy has not produced consistent results.

Detrimental Measures

Do Not:
- Rub or compress the affected part with ice, snow or cold water. Massage or friction of any type is harmful to the injured skin.
- Attempt to evacuate blebs or blisters.
- Allow use of affected extremities (especially if use involves weight bearing) unless absolutely necessary (as in evacuation from disaster areas, etc.).
- Apply pressure dressings or ointments of any type.
- Allow excessive use of tobacco or snuff.
- Administer anticoagulants, corticosteroids or vasodilators; they are of unproven value and complications can occur.
- Perform early surgery; frequently the tissue loss, if any, is only superficial. A 3- to 6-month delay is often appropriate.

62–3. CORE HYPOTHERMIA (Generalized Hypothermia, "Accidental Hypothermia," Severe Cold Exposure)

Severe chilling of the whole body resulting in a rectal temperature of 35°C (95°F) or lower, either from exposure to natural elements or during therapeutic procedures (e.g., cardiac and vascular surgery, treatment of certain poisonings) leads to a progressive decrease of physiologic processes that eventually becomes irreversible. The ability to survive hypothermia depends on the length of exposure and rapidity of cooling, inherent constitutional factors (some persons tolerate low temperatures better than others), environmental factors (altitude, barometric pressure, humidity) and physical condition (nutritional status, pre-existent disease). Cases in which persons survived after rectal temperatures had reached as low as 16°C (60.8°F) have been reported. Favorable pre-existent physical condition, close monitoring and supportive treatment appear generally to be more important factors in recovery than the particular mode of rewarming.

Unless there is conclusive evidence that a person was dead before becoming hypothermic, do not consider anyone with severe core hypothermia to be "dead" until rewarming measures (e.g., to 30°C [86°F] or greater) fail to produce any signs of life. Whether rewarming and resuscitative efforts without progress should continue beyond 1 or 2 hours is a matter of clinical judgment. It should also be mentioned that it is not possible to effectively rewarm a truly dead person.

Magnitude of Core Hypothermia

- Slight (35 to 32.22°C [95–90°F]): Skin pale, hard, numb; patient shivering.
- Moderate (32.21 to 30°C [89.9–86°F]): Poor mentation, hallucinations; slow physical responses; pupils dilate; bradycardia.
- Severe (less than 30°C [86°F]): Patient obtunded or comatose; slowing or cessation of respiration; heart rate slows with later dysrhythmia, VT or cardiac arrest; oliguria.

Treatment *(See also precautions above listed under Detrimental Measures)*

Initial Procedures (Resuscitation measures [5] continue as necessary)

- Gentle handling is important, to prevent cardiac dysrhythmias and skin injury. Keep patient still; do not give warmed fluids, stimulants or alcohol. Take off wet clothing and protect patient from drafts, wind and further heat loss. *Note:* Rewarming measures should be avoided until the patient has been moved to a controlled environment.
- Hyperoxygenate before all procedures (particularly airway).
- Insert nasotracheal tube *(18–20)*, unless the patient has no ventilation deficit and is fully conscious.
- Monitor vital signs, including extremity pulses (use Doppler prn); rectal thermometer readings (low scale to 10°C [50°F], 2" into rectum; telethermometer preferable); use CVP line prn; establish ECG monitoring.
- Do blood and x-ray studies as listed in Table 57–1. Perform steps in treatment of shock. Adjust ABG results for temperature correction. Watch especially for alterations in Na, K, pH, glucose and elevated alcohol/amylase. *Note:* Treatment with any bicarbonate must be cautious, to avoid overcorrection.
- IV infusion with D5NS initially. IV fluids must be cautiously administered (after possibly a 300-ml initial bolus, which has improved survival in some cases) until kidney function is established (often 12 to 18 hours after starting treatment). Fluids may be warmed, but this is of limited value.
- Careful search for and treatment of underlying disease processes. Alcohol and drugs may have initiated the process. Hypothermia may mask the usual signs and symptoms of trauma, infection and disease and blunt the effect of administered medications.
- Take ECG, using standard 12 lead ECG. An abnormality commonly found in all degrees of hypothermia is the J wave (Osborne wave), best seen on the R downslope of the QRS in precordial leads (subsides with rewarming and is of no prognostic value). Sinus bradycardia occurs in slight hypothermia. Common abnormalities in moderate to severe hypothermia are prolonged QT interval, A-V block, nodal tachycardia and ventricular fibrillation. (Rewarm actively, preferably to over 28 to 30° C [82.4 to 86°F]; consider bretyllium IV; defibrillate.)

Passive and active rewarming methods are not proven protocols, but some guidelines are as follows:

Slow Rewarming

- Slow rewarming is safest and generally preferred, particularly for older individuals, or those with mild hypothermia (>32°C[90°F]) of gradual onset, to help prevent "rewarming shock." The maximum rate of core temperature increase usually should not exceed 0.6°C (1.1°F) per hour in older people; in healthy younger patients, increases of 1.2 to 1.8°C (2.2 to 3.3°F) per hour are permissible.

- Application of blankets for insulation (passive warming). (*Note:* Not effective if core temperature <30°C[86°F].)
- Administration of nebulized air with 40% oxygen (or % O_2 adjusted according to ABG results) heated to 40 to 42°C (104 to 107.6°F) via mask or ETT (improves airway management and oxygenation) helps to relieve moderately severe hypothermia and hypoxemia.

Rapid Rewarming

- *Cautions:* Accelerated external rewarming may increase the risk of ventricular fibrillation, rewarming shock, secondary drop in core temperature, rapid lactic acid rise and possibility of thermal burns. However, unresponsive serious dysrhythmia, deteriorating condition and failure to warm despite institution of other measures—as occurs with some underlying severe endocrine deficiencies and intractable vasodilatation problems (alcohol/drugs)—are relative indications for rapid rewarming measures.
- External measures (e.g., electric thermal blankets, warm water bottles, radiant heaters, immersion in warm water tubs) have been effective but are not generally preferred, because of the problems noted in the preceding paragraph. Avoid direct contact with skin and preferably heat only the trunk, leaving the extremities vasoconstricted for more gradual rewarming.
- Core rewarming measures—warmed air inhalation as described above; peritoneal, gastric, possibly pleural cavity, bladder or colonic lavage with warmed physiologic solutions; warmed IV solutions; hemodialysis—and coronary bypass, as may be required in the most severe cases, are preferable to the external measures but still have risks. Heated nebulized air with oxygen supplementation appears the safest and most effective active measure, even though it is less dramatically invasive and does not raise focal tissue temperature as rapidly. It is important to note that rectal administration of fluids impairs accurate readings of core temperature by rectal thermometer. Warmed fluids administered IV in usual physiologic volumes provide only limited heat increase.

HEAT STRESS DISORDERS

62–4. GENERAL CONSIDERATIONS

The following factors commonly predispose to disruption of the body's ability to adapt to heat stress; hot, humid, windless environment; hard physical activity when unacclimatized; improper clothing (including lack of an adequate hat); debilitated condition; extremes of age and obesity; inadequate fluid and salt replacement; and presence of certain drugs (such as anticholinergics, major tranquilizers and antipsychotic agents).

Graduated (in strenuousness and duration) periodic activity, frequent weight measurements (do not exceed 3 to 5% body weight loss), availability of abundant cool water and cool (25°C[75°F]), shaded rest areas, generous salting of food (or addition of 0.1% NaCl to drinking water) and light-weight clothing help avoidance of heat stress disorders and aid successful acclimatization.

62–5. HEAT CRAMPS

Depletion of body fluid and sodium chloride by prolonged excessive sweating may result in a pale skin, extreme thirst, nausea, dizziness, rapid, strong pulse and normal or slightly elevated temperature. Muscular twitching (sometimes generalized, as in epilepsy) and severe painful muscle cramps of rapid onset may be present if the salt depletion is extreme; calf and abdominal muscular spasms and pain may predominate.

Treatment

- Complete rest in a cool place for remainder of day; oral intake of large volumes of water and generous salting of food are all that are necessary in most cases.
- In severe cases, normal salt solution, 1000 ml IV to correct dehydration and salt depletion; patients with less severe cramps will respond rapidly to oral intake of crushed salt tablets (0.5 to 1 g) with copious water, generous food salting or hypotonic salt solution (1 to 2 level teaspoonsful of table salt in 1 gallon of water); take periodically 8 to 12 ounces (240 to 360 ml) of solution and follow with oral intake of water to satiation or beyond (the thirst mechanism usually lags behind physiologic needs).
- During warm or hot weather oral water intake should take place regularly every 20 to 30 minutes (or more often with strenuous exercise [e.g., 250 ml every 10 to 15 minutes]) without depending on the relatively insensitive thirst mechanism. Also generous salting of food should take place on a prophylactic basis.
- Commercial electrolyte replacement solutions (such as ERG or Gatorade) are generally better tolerated at ½ to ⅓ strength.
- Complete and rapid recovery practically always occurs. Hospitalization generally is not required.

62–6. HEAT EXHAUSTION (Heat Prostration)

This relatively common condition is caused by prolonged exposure to heat, often with high humidity. Fatalities are rare; when they do occur there is generally underlying cardiac or other pathology. The clinical picture is the result of peripheral vasomotor collapse and low blood volume. See Table 62–1 for clinical features and differentiation from other heat stress disorders. High urine specific gravity is present. If water loss has exceeded salt loss, serum sodium value will be elevated *(46–10)* as will chloride level.

Treatment

- Move to cooler and less humid surroundings.
- Allow fluids and salt (as with heat cramps, 62–5) if able to swallow; if not, give normal saline intravenously. Obtain serum electrolyte levels, perform hematocrit and urinalysis.
- Treat as for hypovolemic shock *(57)* and hospitalize in more severe cases.
- If recovery is slow, look for and treat any underlying pathology.

62–7. HEATSTROKE (Heat Hyperpyrexia) *(See also 62–8, Iatrogenic Heat Stress)*

Failure of the body to adequately eliminate body heat as a result of a breakdown of the normal sweating and thermoregulatory apparatus leads to mental confusion, hypohidrosis (or anhidrosis) and core temperatures of over 41°C (105.8°F). This hyperthermic condition is invariably fatal unless recognized early and treated energetically. All untreated patients will die.

Even with rapid and energetic treatment, the mortality may be above 50%, particularly with preexistent pathology. The clinical picture is startling (see Table 62–1) and is heralded by stoppage of sweating. Prior to vigorous treatment, there is a rapidly increasing rectal temperature that may reach as

Table 62–1. DIFFERENTIAL DIAGNOSIS OF HEAT STRESS DISORDERS

	Heat Cramps (See 62–5)	**Heat Exhaustion** (See 62–6)	**Heatstroke** (See 62–6 and 62–7)
Skin	Pale—excessive perspiration	Pale, cool, clammy, sweaty	Hot, ↓ sweat; later dry/gray
Body temperature (rectal)	Normal or slightly elevated	Often ↑ to 40° C (104° F); may be subnormal	Rapidly increasing rise—to over 41° C (105.8° F)
Pulse	Rapid, strong	Rapid (120–200); weak	Early rapid and full; later thready
Respiration	Normal	Normal	Slow/deep; later Cheyne-Stokes
Blood pressure	Normal	Normal to decreased later	Increased early; later decreased
Pupils	Normal	Dilated	Dilated
Body odor	Normal perspiration	Normal	Offensive
Muscle cramps	Severe	Variable	No—except see 62–8
Convulsions	Generalized twitching	Rare	Epileptiform type—early
Nausea and vomiting	Mild nausea—rarely vomiting	May be prolonged	Usually does not occur
State of consciousness	Normal	Lethargy; may progress	Early loss of consciousness
Pain	Severe (from muscle cramping)	Headaches	Only at onset
Treatment	Rest in a cool place. Administer salt and correct any dehydration.	Removal from excessive heat and humidity. Correction of dehydration and salt depletion. Supportive care	*Immediate* reduction of body temperature (apply wet/cold). Control of convulsions. Cardiac and respiratory support
Hospitalization	Not necessary	Rarely necessary unless underlying cardiac or other pathology is present	Essential, with cooling measures during transportation
Prognosis	Complete recovery without residual ill effects	Good in absence of severe preexistent underlying pathology	Hopeless in untreated cases; poor (50% mortality) in treated cases. Possible permanent mental damage

high as 46.5°C (115.7°F). Quality survival requires superb, meticulous care and good fortune; irreversible cell death usually begins near 42°C (108°F).

Treatment

- Immediate reduction of body temperature, starting usually in the field, by means of repeated application of wet compresses (with removal and fanning until the skin has dried between applications); this is followed by wrapping the patient in wet sheets and covering with bags of ice, if available, during transport to the hospital; other alternatives are immersion in an ice cube bath or application of hypothermia blankets. The rectal temperature must be reduced to 38.9°C (102°F) as rapidly as possible by whatever means are available; active chilling below this level is generally not advised. Cold, isotonic saline peritoneal lavage may help. Chilled saline enemas, while effective, prevent effective monitoring of rectal temperature, which should be carried out every 4 to 5 minutes using a rectal telethermometer.
- Maintain ventilation; generally intubate/oxygenate.
- Evaluate with baseline studies and treat as for hypovolemic (fluid and electrolyte) shock *(57)* and coma *(32)*; start IV administration of 5% dextrose in normal saline; check response with venous pressure readings and urine output via catheter. Avoid use of alpha-adrenergic vasoconstrictors.
- Establish cardiac monitoring and perform standard ECG.
- Perform repeated electrolyte and ABG's to combat acidosis *(46–1)* and hypokalemia *(46–16)*.
- Start preventive treatment for cerebral edema *(44–7)*. Mannitol also aids in the treatment of heat-induced rhabdomyolysis (monitor with CPK/urine myoglobin), as does alkalinization of urine with IV acetazolomide.
- Prevention or control of convulsions by IV phenytoin/diazepam (see *34*, Convulsions/Seizures)
- Massage of iced extremities promotes circulation of superficial cooled blood and peripheral return of warm blood.
- Chlorpromazine, 25 mg IV or IM, reduces severe shivering.
- Effect of heat on the hematopoietic system may result in bleeding disorders and hemolysis (see *45–1, Control of Bleeding* for Analysis and Management). Whole blood, plasma, packed RBC's or platelet transfusion may be required.
- Evaluate and treat any problems and eliminate any drugs that may have contributed to heat stroke.

62–8. IATROGENIC HEAT STRESS *(See also 62–7)*

During periods of excessively hot weather with high humidity, hospitalized persons with impaired sweat secretion are especially susceptible to heat stress. The significance of the clinical picture of impending heat stress may be overlooked or misinterpreted in persons under anesthesia if drapes and covering prevent adequate heat loss; in quadriplegics, hemiplegics and paraplegics in whom the perspiration-control mechanism is impaired; in persons on medications that inhibit sweating, especially atropine and phenothiazines; and in psychiatric patients whose mental symptoms are dramatic enough to divert attention from the signs and symptoms of impending heatstroke *(62–7)*. Treat with cessation of contributory medications and as under *Heat Cramps (62–5)* or *Heat Exhaustion (62–6)*.

Malignant hyperthermia is particularly prone to occur in genetically predisposed individuals who are given major general anesthetic agents and succinylcholine chloride (Anectine); in these instances an idiosyncratic reaction can quickly follow the succinylcholine. Rapid onset of severe hypermetabolism can occur with tachycardia, tachypnea, metabolic and respiratory acidosis, and calcium shift through the cell membranes with rigidity and seriously rising body temperature. The death rate is high in untreated individuals.

Treatment consists of immediate cessation of any anesthetic agents, hyperventilation with 100% oxygen administration, and treatment of metabolic acidosis (*46–1*) and heat hyperpyrexia (*62–7*). Dantrolene sodium (Dantrium) should be given immediately and rapidly in a continuous IV push infusion in increments of 1 mg/kg until the process, particularly the muscle rigidity, begins to subside or a maximum of 10 mg/kg is reached; results often are evident after injection of 2.5 mg/kg over a minute or two. Procainamide may be needed for controlling ventricular tachycardia.

62–9. SUNSTROKE

Although "sunstroke" properly applies only to heat hyperpyrexia (*62–7*) developing following direct exposure to hot sun, the term is often used loosely for cases of heat exhaustion (*62–6*) in which there has been disturbance in the state of consciousness, provided there is a history of exposure to sunlight. In many instances, a mixed picture may be present; however, a rapidly rising body temperature associated with a hot, dry skin makes immediate energetic treatment as outlined under *Heat Hyperpyrexia* (*62–7*) mandatory.

Infants and small children are particularly susceptible to the effects of sun and hot weather, which may be confused with other serious conditions, such as brain concussion, or febrile infectious illness. Children left in a poorly ventilated car parked in the sun may be victims, even on a day that is not very hot, as the car condenses heat even with the windows slightly opened.

63. Vascular Disorders

63–1. GENERAL CONSIDERATIONS

Various types of catastrophes can occur from acute pathologic processes involving the vascular system (arteries, veins and lymphatics). Detection is aided clinically by noting the following: skin color, temperature, sensation; edema (including sequential circumferential measurements); hematomas (hardness indicates brisk bleeding); proximity of trauma site to major vessels (see Figs. 47–5 to 47–8). Check also for pulsatile masses, peripheral pulses and bruit. When defects are suspected, compare not only left and right extremities (blood pressure of left upper extremity [LUE] is usually a few mm Hg less than that of right upper extremity; blood pressures of left and right lower extremities are equal) but also UE and LE on each side (BP at ankle is usually 10% less than that of UE; if 10–30% less, there is mild obstruction; a difference of 50% or more indicates severe obstruction). Clinical evaluation of arterial pressure, flow rate and location is abetted by use of the Doppler ultrasound device (*19–3*). See *47–60* for details concerning compartment syndromes. Angiography may be required to visualize site and magnitude of lesions, particularly in preparation for surgery.

63–2. ARTERIAL INJURIES *(See also 47–60, Compartment Syndromes, Acute; 59–2, Arterial Repair)*

Immediate recognition of severe injuries to major arteries, followed by prompt and proper surgical treatment, may be lifesaving or may eliminate the necessity for amputation. Surgical techniques are available for repair of defects in major arteries by direct suturing, venous grafts or prosthetic grafts; even extremely small arteries can at times be repaired successfully using a microscopic lens device for better visualization.

Types of Arterial Injury

1. Contusion. Vasospasm resulting from damage to the intima may give a clinical picture suggestive of complete vessel transection.

2. Compression against a bony prominence, usually near the elbow, wrist, knee or ankle, or in a swollen fascial compartment, causing a compartment syndrome (see Fig. 49–1 and Table 49–1).

3. Laceration may result in fatal external or internal hemorrhage. Partial lacerations may cause more prolonged bleeding than complete severance, because the injured vessel cannot adequately constrict.

4. Severance—complete.

Severe arterial damage results in the appearance of bright red blood, often spurting, if a channel to the surface is available; in the development of a rapidly increasing hematoma that becomes hard and tense when anatomic limits are reached or by bleeding into actual or potential body cavities. Exsanguination from major arteries may occur unless control is accomplished (*45–1*). Pulsations in the arteries distal to the injury may be decreased or absent, and the patient may be in shock. There may be intense pain from ischemia or pressure on surrounding structures, or increased, disturbed or decreased sensation.

Treatment

- Control of major hemorrhage (*45–1*) by the least injurious means possible—preferably by using broad compression bandages, air splints or MAST. This is a lifesaving measure and takes precedence over all other therapeutic measures except CPR, which should be done concomitantly if required.
- Treatment of any shock (57).
- Release of compression by reduction of displaced fractures or dislocations as soon as evidence of arterial compression is recognized or whenever the possibility of compression of a major artery is suspected from the position of displaced bone fragments or joint surfaces. Immediate surgical attention is necessary.
- Hospitalization for definitive surgical care *as soon as possible* in all cases of known or suspected major arterial damage. The time lag between injury and repair must be kept to a minimum (not more than 6 or 7 hours at the most) for a successful result.

63–3. ARTERITIS, TEMPORAL (CRANIAL)

In this condition, the artery is palpably tender in its course. In addition to the temporal artery, the vertebral and internal carotid arteries may be affected, and involvement of the ophthalmic and retinal arteries may cause sudden vision loss—particularly in patients over 50 years of age. Headache, lassitude, myalgia, low-grade fever and highly elevated erythrocyte sedimentation rate (ESR) are common.

Treatment

The patient should be started on large doses of prednisone immediately and referred to a neurologist. Biopsy of the superficial temporal artery confirms the diagnosis.

63–4. INTRACRANIAL HEMORRHAGE

Bleeding within the cranium is one of the common forms of catastrophic events known as cerebrovascular accidents (CVAs) or "strokes," which we define as *the rapid onset of neurologic signs and symptoms due to disturbançe of normal blood supply to or from the brain.* See also 63–6, *Cerebral Embolism; 63–9, Cerebral Thrombosis; 63–10, Transient Ischemia Attacks.* Table 63–1 indicates features in the differential diagnosis of strokes; the need for accurate diagnosis to assure appropriate treatment is evident (see Table 63–2). Note precautions to be taken with subarachnoid puncture (*18–29*).

Epidural Hemorrhage *(See 44–20)*

Intracerebral Hemorrhage

Common Causes

- Congenital weakness of blood vessel walls (saccular aneurysms, berry aneurysms, arteriovenous malformation).
- Hypertension.
- Platelet disorders—either primary (e.g., in myeloproliferative diseases) or secondary to drug-induced thrombocytopenia, ITP, DIC or consumption coagulopathy.
- Excessive anticoagulation.
- Trauma.
- Atherosclerotic degeneration of cerebral arteries.
- Damage of arterial walls secondary to arteritis, congenital malformations, infections and toxins.

SIGNS AND SYMPTOMS are highlighted by the sudden onset of intense headache, nausea, vomiting and (frequently) impairment of consciousness. Focal neurologic signs, such as cranial nerve deficit, weakness or sensory loss, depend upon the location and extent of the hemorrhage. There may be evidence of blood in the spinal fluid and of secondary meningeal irritation.

Treatment

1. General Supportive Measures. The measures outlined in Table 63–1 are applicable to patients with completed strokes resulting in similar deficits, no matter what the cause. Early active exercise is restricted in patients with extensive intracranial bleeding, particularly subarachnoid hemorrhage (discussed later in this section).

2. Specific Measures. Treat any contributing blood coagulation disorders such as hemophilia (*45–7*), thrombocytopenia (*45–12*) or hypoprothrombinemia resulting from medication with heparin or warfarin-like drugs (*45–8*).

Reduce moderate to severe hypertension cautiously. Rapid reduction of the blood pressure to "normal" may cause the clinical condition to deteriorate because of inadequate perfusion levels. See also *Hypertensive Crisis* (*29–14*).

Computerized tomography (CT) scans are valuable in determining the size and location of hematomas or other lesions that would benefit from neurosurgical evacuation.

Cerebellar Hemorrhage

Cerebellar hemorrhage is characterized initially by sudden severe vertigo, nystagmus, ataxia, headache, nausea, vomiting, bloody cerebrospinal fluid (CSF) and later coma. Gaze palsy with ocular deviation to the side opposite the lesion, ipsilateral facial palsy and dysarthria may occur. Swelling may cause critical secondary problems of irregular breath and "long tract signs" (of hemiplegia or quadriplegia with sensory deficit) that require urgent neurosurgical intervention for evaluation for acute surgical decompression. An angiogram or CAT scan may aid in the evaluation if time and accessibility permit. Start medical measures to reduce edema (44–7) and give supportive therapy in the interim.

Subarachnoid Hemorrhage

This type is most frequently the result of a ruptured intracranial aneurysm or arteriovenous malformation. If conscious, the patient often will describe a sudden, severe, generalized headache unlike any experienced previously. Initial lateralization of the pain may be an important clue as to the location of the bleeding source. Focal neurologic signs may be absent. Physical findings are often limited to some alteration in mental state, a stiff neck, presence of Babinski signs and severe occipital pain after a few hours, often followed by frank unconsciousness. Progressive involvement of the vital centers through elevated intracranial pressure and vasospasm can lead to a fatal outcome. Subhyaloid hemorrhage in the eyegrounds is virtually diagnostic in this context. The diagnosis is confirmed by examination of the spinal fluid, which is bloody and under increased pressure. A significant hemorrhage is proved by spinning down the CSF to show that the supernatant is xanthochromic.

Treatment and Prognosis

Treatment is similar to that outlined for intracerebral hemorrhage, and immediate intracranial surgery may be lifesaving. If the only signs are meningeal irritation from blood or mild neurologic deficits, *immediate* arteriograms, followed by neurosurgery if indicated, give the best statistical chance of survival. Hypothermia may be of value in some cases. Dexamethasone (Decadron), 15 to 25 mg IV and/or IV mannitol (Osmitrol) may help to relieve cerebral edema.

Subdural Hemorrhage *(See 44–20; for supportive treatment see Table 63–2; for goals in preventing and treating cerebrovascular accidents, see Table 63–3)*

63–5. DISSECTING AORTIC ANEURYSM

The defect that leads to weakening of the aortic wall is usually cystic central necrosis. Increased stress on the aortic wall from increased intracranial pressure, hypertension or trauma may precipitate acute signs and symptoms consisting of abdominal or thoracic pain (which may be minimal or excruciating, sudden or progressive), pallor, sweating and shock (57). There may be pathologic discrepancies in the blood pressure and pulses between the two arms or between the arms and legs and signs of ischemia or infarction of the brain, kidney, myocardium or spinal cord (with rapid onset of paraplegia). Widening of the aorta may be demonstrable by palpation or radiologic studies.

Treatment

- Immediate hospitalization and surgical evaluation. Type and crossmatch blood for current or potential use.
- Absolute rest.
- Barbiturates and opiates as necessary for control of restlessness, pain and apprehension.

Table 63–1. DIFFERENTIAL DIAGNOSIS OF COMMON CAUSES OF STROKES

	Subarachnoid Hemorrhage	Subdural Hemorrhage	Extradural Hemorrhage	Brain Tumor
Onset	Sudden; variable progression	Insidious, occasionally acute	Rapid; usually minutes to hours	Usually very slow; rapid with hemorrhage
Duration of signs and symptoms	Variable; clearing may occur over days/weeks	Hours to months	Initial fluctuating course common, then steady ↑	Gradually progressive; permanent
Activity	More frequent during activity	Usually but not always related to head trauma	Almost always related to trauma	Unrelated to activity
Contributing or associated diseases	Intracerebral aneurysms, trauma, tumor	Chronic alcoholism	Any condition that predisposes to trauma	If metastatic, primary focus
Sensorium	Coma common	Generally clouded	Rapidly advanced coma	Slow, progressive loss
Nuchal rigidity	Present, but not immediately	Absent	Absent	Absent
Location of cerebral damage	Diffuse; aneurysm may give focal sign before and after hemorrhage	Frontal lobe signs common, ipsilateral pupil may dilate	Temporal lobe signs, dilatation of ipsilateral pupil and IIP	Focal—area of tumor
Convulsions	Common	Infrequent	Common	Variable; Jacksonian type most common
Cerebrospinal fluid	Grossly bloody; increased pressure	Normal to slight elevation of protein	↑ pressure, usually normal color/cells	Increased protein and pressure
Skull x-rays	Usually normal; may show calcified aneurysm	Frequently contralateral shift of pineal	Often fracture across middle meningeal artery groove	May show pineal shift; calcification
Angiography	One or more aneurysms (unless filled with clot)	Avascular subdural mass	May show site of bleeding, avascular mass	Identification of mass, vascularity
CAT scan	Usually prompt positive location	Immediate positive location	Immediate positive location	Positive location
RIS of brain	Usually negative	Often positive location	May be positive	Usually positive location
Recurrence	Common	Can recur after surgery	None with early surgery	Varies with type of tumor

Table 63–2. GOALS AND METHODS OF SUPPORTIVE TREATMENT IN ACUTE PHASE OF CVAs AND COMPARABLE DISABILITIES*

Organ System	Goals	Methods of Treatment
Skin	Prevent pressure ulcers	• Change position q 2 h; antidecubitus boots • Keep all pressure off reddened or blanched skin • Keep skin dry and clean
Respiratory tract	Maintain a clear airway	• Suctioning; tracheostomy if necessary • Postural drainage of secretions • Periodic deep breathing and coughing; incentive spirometer; use of ancillary chemical/mechanical agents prn • Liquefy secretions by adequate hydration and use of aerosols • Antibiotics if clinical x-ray evidence of pulmonary infection
Cardiovascular (CV)	Maintain adequate BP for perfusion of vital organs	• See *Shock* (57) • Preservation of vasomotor tone by early mobilization: sitting, use of standing table, walking
	Reduce peripheral thrombophlebitis	• Lower extremity elastic wraps • Early mobilization • Low-dose heparin, SC
GI	Maintain hydration/electrolyte balance/anabolism	Adequate fluids, minerals, calories and vitamins: PO/NGT/parenterally
	Promote normal bowel function	Proper bowel-training program
GU	Assure complete urinary elimination	Catheter drainage if necessary
	Reduce infection, protect and preserve upper urinary tract	• Adequate hydration and removal of catheter ASAP • Antibacterial medications
CNS	Avoid further depression of CNS	• Restriction of sedatives • Avoidance of narcotics
	Control convulsive seizures	Phenytoin as needed
	Counteract usual depression	Proper attitude and counseling; antidepressant drugs prn
Musculoskeletal	Maintain normal range of joint motion	• Daily exercise, passive then active • Proper positioning with pillows, removable splints • Avoid excessive passive stretching against spastic muscles
	Maintain tone of uninvolved as well as affected muscles	• Early mobilization: standing table, sitting, walking • Supervised resistive exercises

*Modified from Cain, H. D., and Smith, E.: *Hosp. Med.*, Oct., 1965.

Table 63–3. GOALS IN PREVENTION AND TREATMENT OF CEREBROVASCULAR ACCIDENTS*

Type of Stroke	Goals	Methods Used to Achieve Goals
Arterial Occlusion	Remove occlusion	Thrombectomy or embolectomy
	Prevent formation of new thrombi	Anticoagulant therapy, antiplatelet agents, endarterectomy
	Prevent formation of new emboli	Conversion of AF to sinus mechanism; antibiotic treatment of bacterial endocarditis; mitral commissurotomy, ablation of left atrial appendage in mitral stenosis; endarterectomy; anticoagulant therapy
	Improve blood flow to cerebrum (a) Enlarge arterial channels arising from aortic arch and carotid vessels	Endarterectomy; arterial bypass; vasodilation
	(b) Correct decreased cardiac output and oxygen carrying capacity of blood	Treatment of congestive heart failure and serious arrhythmias; blood transfusion for severe anemia
	Reduction of cerebral edema	Dexamethasone IV if herniation; hypertonic agents IV (e.g., urea, hypertonic glucose) prior to surgery; DMSO (still experimental)
Intracranial Hemorrhage	Establishment of normal blood coagulability	Correction of congenital or acquired coagulation defects; avoidance of anticoagulation if hemorrhage may occur or has occurred
	Reduction of cerebral intra-arterial pressure	Hypotensive drugs; postural position (tilt table); ligation of, or Salibi clamp on, common carotid artery; ligation of intracranial artery
	Control of ruptured aneurysm	Surgical reinforcement or isolation (depending on anatomic location and accessibility)
	Elimination of hematoma	Surgical evacuation and control of bleeding
	Reduction of oxygen need of brain	Hypothermia; barbiturate coma (still experimental)

*Modified from Cain, H. D., and Smith, E.: *Hosp. Med.*, Oct., 1965.

- Treatment of shock (57). The blood pressure should be kept at the minimal level to maintain adequate perfusion of vital organs. Cautious reduction of moderate or severe hypertension is indicated.

Prognosis. The mortality from dissecting aortic aneurysms is in the 75 to 80% range; a much better prognosis is offered if the aneurysm can be repaired prior to dissection.

63–6. EMBOLISM

An embolus of either cardiac or noncardiac origin may cause infarction of any organ of the body. The diagnosis is usually made by evidence of sudden infarction and/or malfunction of the involved organ plus determination of the presence of a probable source of the embolus. In general, emergency therapy is designed to be supportive, to reduce the source or likelihood of other emboli and to allow performance of a surgical embolectomy if indicated and possible. See *56–20, Pulmonary Embolism,* for discussion of measures to prevent pulmonary emboli.

Cerebral Emboli

Cerebral emboli usually arise from a cardiac source and may be due to myocardial infarction (*29–15*), chronic atrial fibrillation (*29–3*) or endocarditis (*29–6*). Another source may be atherosclerotic plaques from major arteries of the neck (see *63–10*). Signs and symptoms, which generally correspond to the neurologic areas supplied by the occluded artery, have a sudden onset.

Treatment

- Supportive. (See under *63–4* for general supportive treatment.)
- Surgical attack of thromboembolic occlusions in completed strokes generally has not given favorable results. Surgical approach to remove the source of past and future emboli may be considered (e.g., prosthetic replacement of diseased and defective cardiac valves; endarterectomy of grossly atherosclerotic major neck vessels).
- Anticoagulation may be considered for reduction of thrombotic emboli if evidences of infection and secondary hemorrhage are *not* present (as confirmed by lumbar puncture and CAT scan). It is generally preferable to wait at least 2 days (but no more than 2 weeks) post CVA and start with heparin.

Embolus in Peripheral Arteries

Whether the blocking of a peripheral artery is due to embolism or arteriosclerotic thrombus, the emergency treatment for the artery is similar. Recognition of the condition and proper handling may be the deciding factors in saving a limb or a life.

Signs and Symptoms. Acute pain, usually severe, pallor, coldness and numbness of the affected extremity, absence or gross diminution of pulsation in the arteries distal to the lesion and puffiness and pitting edema if there is concomitant venous involvement. Doppler studies can help grade decreased arterial pulsation.

Treatment

- Protect the extremity from mechanical injury and place in a level or slightly dependent position.
- Relieve pain and vasospasm by administering morphine sulfate, 10 to 15

mg SC or IV; papaverine hydrochloride, 0.2 g PO or 30 to 60 mg intra-arterially proximal to the occlusion (if the embolism is in a small distal artery); and atropine sulfate, 0.6 mg SC or IV.

- Transfer to a hospital as soon as possible. Immediate embolectomy (frequently removal with a Fogarty catheter) or paravertebral sympathetic nerve blocks may be indicated.
- After obtaining control specimens, begin anticoagulation therapy, preferably with heparin, 10,000 units IV, initially if indicated.

Air Embolism (Arterial Embolism) *(See also 26–5, Diving Hazards; 63–11, Venous Air Embolism)*

In an adult of average weight, 60 to 80 ml of air in the vascular tree may be a lethal amount, although the speed of entry, pressure and position of the patient may cause marked variations in the amount that can be tolerated.

Causes

- Intrinsic air in the alveoli, pulmonary cavity or pleural cavity (pneumothorax).
- Extrinsic air accidentally injected during diagnostic procedures, open operations and traumatic incidents.

Signs and Symptoms. Dizziness, cold clammy skin, thready pulse, extreme hypotension, dyspnea and cyanosis often followed by Cheyne-Stokes respiration. Convulsions, coma and localized neurologic signs (hemiplegia, blindness) may be present. Confirmatory findings are detection of air in the retinal vessels by ophthalmoscopic examination, appearance of sharply defined areas of pallor in the tongue (Liebermeister's sign), "marbling" of the skin and bubbling of air mixed with blood from a skin incision. X-ray demonstration of air in the cerebral vessels is sometimes possible. Coronary artery involvement can give the characteristic electrocardiographic changes of myocardial injury or infarction (29–15).

Treatment

- Keep the patient's head down; place on left side.
- Give symptomatic supportive therapy (artificial respiration, oxygen under positive pressure, support of circulation, etc.).
- Treat pneumothorax (31–12).
- Hyperbaric oxygen chamber therapy (26–6).
- Hospitalize immediately for further treatment.

63–7. SYNCOPE (Fainting, Vasodepressor Syncope) *(See also 34, Convulsive Seizures, and 49–20, Episodic Unconsciousness)*

Transient loss of consciousness is not a serious condition unless the patient is injured in falling. Various mechanisms may lead to collapse of arterial vasomotor tone and temporary insufficiency of cerebral circulation; thorough investigation should be made to determine the underlying cause. Distinguishing between simple syncope and other causes of "collapse" or "blackout" is easier if the event is witnessed and there is a description of preceding comments, actions and circumstances as well as one of events during unconsciousness (e.g., no tongue biting, clonic or tonic muscle contractions or involuntary defecation or urination). If episodic cardiac arrhythmia is suspected as a cause, a Holter monitor may aid detection. See 29–23, *Stokes-Adams Attacks*, and 49–20 for differential diagnosis.

Treatment

- Recumbent position until recovered.
- Monitor the pulse, which is usually within normal limits in simple syncope but often slow, weak or irregular in Stokes-Adams attacks.
- Inhalations of aromatic spirits of ammonia.
- Treatment of any injuries sustained in falling.
- Prevention of repeated falling; instructions for mild preliminary exercises and gradual arising when orthostatic hypotension is present.
- Prohibit operation of motor vehicles or exposure to potentially hazardous situations (height, moving machinery) if recurrence is likely until effective preventative treatment is established. If susceptibility to repeat occurrence is likely, official reporting (*15*) of case is obligatory.

63–8. THROMBOANGIITIS OBLITERANS (Buerger's Disease)

The extremely severe pain caused by this progressive condition may bring the patient for emergency relief.

Treatment of Acute Episodes

- Advise against tobacco use and exposure to cold.
- If tissue viability not impaired, encourage exercise to near tolerance; rest and repeat till slow, long distance activities obtained. Use simple analgesics, including aspirin (minimum 10 grains/day).
- Bed rest with positioning of the involved extremity for most comfort and least blanching. Do not elevate the extremity.
- Peripheral vasodilators are of equivocal value.
- Consider trial with temporary preganglionic lumbar sympathectomy with local or spinal anesthetics or autonomic blocking agents.
- For severe pain, codeine sulfate or morphine sulfate may be required. Check for possible addiction to narcotics (*7–3*).
- Hospitalization may be indicated if the acute pain cannot be controlled by the measures just described or if the patient shows signs of impaired circulation threatening tissue viability. Obtain vascular surgical consultation regarding possible angiography and segmental resection with synthetic vessel replacement or bypass procedure.

63–9. THROMBOSIS

Cerebral and Major Arteries of Neck. Signs, symptoms and treatment are similar to those for emboli (*63–6*) occurring in the same arteries, except that the onset is frequently slower. In the early hours after cerebral thrombosis, it is desirable to keep the head down, eliminating any element of postural hypotension. Thrombolysins have not proved their value in treatment. For treatment of completed stroke due to cerebral thrombosis, statistics favor non-use of anticoagulants. Acute surgery for thrombectomy is usually too late for preservation or restoration of cerebral function, and sudden restoration of blood flow in the acute postinfarction period may be further injurious to the softened, swollen brain tissue.

Peripheral Artery Thrombosis. See *63–6, Embolism of Peripheral Arteries*, and *63–12, Phlebothrombosis*.

63–10. TRANSIENT ISCHEMIA ATTACKS ("TIA's")

Recurrent episodes of cerebral ischemia lasting from seconds to a few minutes—or up to 24 hours on occasion—may give any of the signs and symptoms of a "stroke," but the patient reverts spontaneously to his or her prior normal or near normal state. Patients who have *reversible ischemic neurologic deficit* ("RIND") are those with apparent brain infarction who improve substantially or completely after 24 hours (or sometimes after days or weeks).

Treatment

- Obtain and record an accurate history of events.
- Auscultate for bruit over major neck arteries, palpate carotid and temporal arteries and record blood pressure in both arms. Abnormal findings in these areas indicate more surgically accessible vascular pathology.
- Refer the patient to a vascular surgeon or neurosurgeon for diagnostic evaluation, which may include lumbar subarachnoid puncture, arteriography and electroencephalography. Surgical removal of large atherosclerotic lesions in major branches of the aortic arch and arteries of neck may prevent recurrence of ischemia and development of completed strokes.
- Anticoagulation therapy or preferably antiplatelet therapy (which is safer) is effective in reducing the number of recurrences in some patients. Aspirin (5 to 10 grains daily) appears to reduce the adhesiveness and embolization of platelet material. So far other antiplatelet drugs, such as sulfinpyrazone (100 mg PO daily) and dipyridamole (50 mg/day) have not demonstrated clear superiority to aspirin.
- Evaluate for any associated hypertensive or cardiac problems.

63–11. VENOUS AIR EMBOLISM

This condition may follow diagnostic injection of air (peritoneum, pleura, subarachnoid space); retroperitoneal trauma; operation on the head, neck and genitourinary tract; administration of fluids into, or removal of blood from, any vein; or extreme changes in atmospheric pressure (26, *Barotrauma*).

Signs and Symptoms. Deep inspiration followed by coughing exhalation, then a few attempts at breathing followed by apnea. The blood pressure drops and the pulse becomes weak or imperceptible.

Treatment

- Immediate left lateral position, with the head down below shoulder level (unless the patient has the rare condition of dextrocardia, in which case place on right side).
- Artificial respiration followed by administration of oxygen under positive pressure by endotracheal catheter and rebreathing bag.
- Immediate hospitalization for aspiration of air from the right atrium, preferably by open operation.

63–12. PHLEBOTHROMBOSIS *(See also 63–6, Pulmonary Artery Embolism)*

Few clinical signs may be produced even in the presence of extensive thrombotic involvement of the deep veins of the lower extremities and the pelvic veins. These thrombi may dislodge and migrate; phlebothrombosis or deep vein thrombosis (DVT) is the most common cause of pulmonary embolism (63–6). Confirm presence of embolism with venogram. Occurrence is most common in inactive or debilitated patients, but it may also be post-traumatic.

Signs and Symptoms. Moderate elevation of temperature, unilateral leg edema with enlargement of thigh and calf and positive Homan's sign (pain in the calf of the involved leg on forced dorsiflexion of the foot).

Treatment

- Complete rest; 10° to 15° elevation of the extended extremity.
- Application of moist heat.
- Treatment of pain and vasospasm.
- Anticoagulation with sodium heparin, 10,000 units IV, followed by maintenance dosage after obtaining a preliminary coagulation time (if streptokinase therapy is not planned).
- Referral to a hospital for observation and care.
- Surgical consultation regarding thrombectomy or removal of thrombus with a Fogarty catheter is indicated if there is gross edema and secondary arterial circulation compromise. Recurrent emboli may require inferior vena cava ligation.
- Streptokinase may be used when risks of thrombolytic treatment are outweighed by the benefits to be achieved.

Contraindications to use are: active internal bleeding, CVA, intracranial or intraspinal surgery within 2 months, intracranial neoplasm.

Risks of thrombolytic therapy include allergic reactions, bleeding and fever. The manufacturer's listing of conditions with increased risk should be thoroughly reviewed; the major risks include major surgery, serious GI bleeding, organ biopsy, obstetrical delivery within the past 10 days, cerebrovascular disease, pregnancy and left heart thrombus.

Use: The usual initial dose is 250,000 IU streptokinase (Streptase) infused over 30 minutes into a peripheral vein, following the manufacturer's instructions, followed by a maintenance dose of 100,000 IU/hr. Special precautions are necessary before instituting anticoagulation after discontinuance of streptokinase.

63–13. THROMBOPHLEBITIS

Thrombophlebitis is usually an inflammation of a superficial vein, with infection and varicosities being contributing factors. The most common sites are the veins of the lower extremities, although veins in any portion of the body may be involved.

Signs and Symptoms. Severe pain with redness and induration over the course of the vein, fever (sometimes chills) and swelling of the extremity. Embolization may occur and cause pulmonary artery occlusion, but it is much less common in such cases than it is with phlebothrombosis (*63–12*).

Treatment

- Bed rest.
- Heat (hot, moist compresses are best) at about body temperature.
- Elevation of the extremity about 6 inches above the heart level to allow lymphatic-venous drainage.
- Avoidance of dehydration by oral and IV administration of fluids (*11*).
- Compressive wrapping or elastic stockings from toes to above the knee when upright or ambulatory.
- Hospitalization if the condition persists, if deep vein involvement occurs or if any signs of emboli appear (treat as for phlebothrombosis [*63–12*]).

63–14. VARICOSE VEINS

Esophageal Varices *(See 40–5)*

Hemorrhoids *(See 40–7)*

Postinjection Thrombophlebitis

Inflammation of a vein wall of varying degrees of severity may follow local injection of varicose veins with sclerosing solutions. For treatment, see *63–13*.

Postligation Hemorrhage

Bleeding may occur several days after surgical procedures for ligation of varicose veins of the lower extremities.

Treatment

- Sedation.
- Application of local pressure.
- Hospitalization if bleeding is persistent or if blood loss has been extreme.

Pruritus due to Varicose Eczema

The itching caused by chronic eczema, especially that secondary to degenerative changes in the vessels of the lower legs, may be severe enough to bring the patient for emergency care.

Treatment

- Sedation.
- Application of local anesthetic preparations such as calamine lotion with 1% phenol (*do not bandage or compress*) or dibucaine (Nupercaine) ointment.
- Referral to a dermatologist for definitive care.

Rupture of a Varicose Vein of an Extremity

Rupture of a varicosity may be spontaneous or traumatic and may cause stubborn and persistent bleeding severe enough to result in secondary anemia. The bleeding is usually not enough to cause symptoms of shock.

Treatment

- Elevate the extremity; restrict activity initially.
- Apply direct pressure by an elastic bandage or gauze fluffs held in place by a roller elastic bandage; then allow patient to walk.
- Administer sedation as needed.
- Place mattress sutures, under local anesthesia, if necessary.
- Refer for further surgical care, preferably within 24 hours.

Varicose Ulcers with Secondary Infection and Cellulitis

Treatment

- Give oral ampicillin, 250 to 500 mg qid.
- Wash ulcer daily with antibacterial solution. Apply sterile gauze dressing and fluffs covered by a heavyweight elastic wrap/stocking, or apply an Unna boot.
- With effective external compression in place (Unna boot or elastic wrap), encourage walking to tolerance at least tid (fluid is pumped out of the extremity by active muscle contractions, thereby lowering venous pressure.
- Elevate lower extremity at night and when sitting.
- Hospitalize if cellulitis is extensive or spreading despite conservative treatment.

63–15. LYMPHATIC SYSTEM EMERGENCIES

Lymphangitis

Uncontrolled infection in an extremity, frequently of streptococcal origin, will cause involvement of the lymphatics and adjacent blood vessels. The condition is identified by pain, tenderness, swelling and characteristic superficial red streaks in the involved extremity.

Treatment

- Antibiotics, broad-spectrum or penicillin.
- Moist heat and hypertonic solutions, such as magnesium sulfate, locally.
- Rest and elevation of the extremity.
- Analgesics.

Obstruction

Enlargement of lymph nodes secondary to various types of pathology may cause acute obstruction of the superior vena cava or extrahepatic bile ducts. Treatment is primarily surgical. Lymph fluid may clot if stagnant for long periods.

63–16. RAYNAUD'S PHENOMENA AND REFLEX NEUROVASCULAR SYNDROME

In this condition, severe vascular spasm—usually in the distal upper extremities—is associated with uncomfortable paresthesias, pain, pallor of the fingers during the arteriospasm phase, cyanosis during the venospasm phases then rubor and residual edema of the digits (probably due to venospasm, diapedesis of proteins through capillary walls during the ischemic phase and clotting of lymph fluids in lymphatic channels). Trophic ulcers in edematous fingers and small areas of gangrene—usually at the tips of the fingers—may occur.

Precipitation of events by exposure to cold is characteristic. The idiopathic type (Raynaud's disease) occurs almost entirely in women. Numerous other causes of the reflex neurovascular syndrome (shoulder-hand syndrome) are associated with Raynaud's phenomenon (e.g., occlusive arterial disease, neurogenic lesions, trauma, collagen diseases).

Patients with these conditions may present themselves for emergency evaluation and treatment because of acute discomfort in hand and/or shoulder or because of presence of tender pregangrenous or gangrenous lesions.

Treatment

- Mild sedation with phenobarbital, 15 to 30 mg PO 4 times a day, or diazepam (Valium), 5 mg PO 3 or 4 times a day.
- Mild analgesics. Avoid narcotics.
- Evaluate and treat any underlying contributing cause; particularly eliminate tobacco use.
- Avoid exposure to cold and improve body and extremity warmth with clothing.
- Whirling the affected extremity in a circle, like a softball pitcher, 20 times, appears to push increased blood flow by centrifugal force into the digits with therapeutic benefit.
- Mild vasodilatation with tolazoline hydrochloride (Priscoline), 25 to 50 mg PO 4 times a day.
- Encourage full use of extremity—otherwise dystrophic changes and disability will ensue.

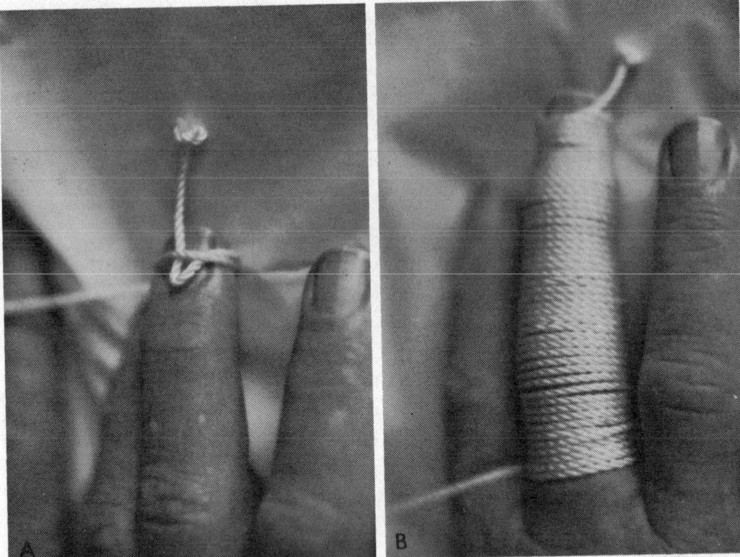

Figure 63–1. Technique of compressive centripetal wrapping. *A*, A small loop of string is placed over the fingernail before the first coil of the helix is turned. *B*, Firm, contiguous, centripetal wrapping is rapidly performed. Immediately upon completion of helix of desired length, the protruding distal tip of string is pulled and the total wrapping is removed centripetally. (From Cain H. D., and Liebgold, H. B.: Arch. Phys. Med., Vol. 48, 1967.)

- Reduction of discomfort, improved range of motion, healing of trophic ulcers and improved circulation occur with rapid reduction of edema in the digits by use of centripetal concentric compression. Ordinary string is wrapped *firmly* and rapidly from the distal to proximal portion of the edematous digit (Fig. 63–1), then removed *immediately*, in a manner similar to removing a ring from a swollen finger. Place thin sterile gauze over any ulceration. Rewrap periodically until the edema is completely gone (removal of a ring from a swollen finger can be achieved by the same technique, except slip the proximal end of the string under the ring, then exert distal pressure while pulling on the string).
- Stellate ganglion blocks may be of value.
- Severe recurrent vasospastic events warrant referral for surgical consultation regarding sympathectomy.

Administrative, Clerical and Medicolegal Principles and Procedures

DEFINITIONS

"Emergency Care"

- The examination, treatment and disposition of a person who has developed or sustained an unforeseen condition which is believed to call for prompt action.

—*Thomas Flint, Jr., M.D., Preface to the First Edition of* Emergency Treatment and Management, *1954*

"Emergency Medicine"

- The immediate recognition, evaluation, care and disposition of patients in response to acute illness and injury;
- The administration, research, and teaching of all aspects of emergency medical care;
- The direction of the patient to sources of follow-up care, in or out of the hospital as may be required;
- The provision, when requested, of emergency, but not continuing, care to in-hospital patients; and
- The management of emergency medical system for the provision of prehospital emergency care.

—*Definition Adopted by the American Medical Association House of Delegates, 1975*

"Emergency Services"

. . . those services required for alleviation of severe pain, or immediate diagnosis and treatment of unforeseen medical conditions, which, if not immediately diagnosed and treated, would lead to disability or death."

—*Section 51056(a) of Medi-Cal Regulations (1975)*

64. Abandonment

64–1. ESTABLISHMENT OF THE PHYSICIAN-PATIENT RELATIONSHIP *(See also 69–8, Consent)*

The legal duty (aside from ethical and moral considerations) to offer and give aid in emergency situations varies greatly:

- In common law and in most states there is no such general requirement.
- In a few states (e.g., Vermont), in Maritime law and in many European countries, it is required that aid be offered and given if consented to (if the patient is unconscious, the request for aid and consent are implied). Failure of a Vermont physician to provide aid in the emergency setting may result in the physician's being fined.
- Duty of emergency personnel is also established if under contract to a hospital or clinic with an emergency room that has a "duty to treat all." Even if there is no contract with obligation to the emergency patient, there is an "ostensible agency" or apparent contractual relationship between the hospital and physician.
- After the physician has given any therapeutic advice (however seemingly trivial—even advising aspirin use over the telephone) or has examined or treated the patient, the physician-patient relationship has been established.

Abandonment is legally "the termination by the physician of a doctor-patient relationship without the consent of the patient and without giving the patient adequate notice and opportunity to find another physician." Paramedical personnel are generally considered the agents of the directing physician or employer and their abandonment of a patient may also be attributed to the physician or employer. The physician is responsible for the patient's care until responsibility has been properly shifted to another physician either by the original attendant or by the patient or the patient's agents. (See also 4, *Transportation and Transfer of Care.*)

Ethically, certain situations may arise in which refusal to establish the physician-patient relationship might result in social and professional criticism in spite of the generally accepted precept incorporated in the Principles of Medical Ethics—"a physician may choose whom he [or she] will serve." The three most commonly encountered situations in which it is unethical to refuse treatment are:

1. **If No Other Medical Help is Available.** This situation occurs most often in traffic accident cases and has been clarified in many localities by "Good Samaritan" laws that specify that a physician giving on-site emergency treatment (which must be given in good faith and not be grossly negligent) need not continue with the ongoing care of the patient after treatment at the scene, unless the physician so desires. Once treatment has been begun, the physician does have the responsibility, however, of seeing that the injured person's care is continued until the person is turned over to a law enforcement officer, ambulance attendant or other responsible person with provision of further physician attendance being established. If the physician or other individual giving aid transfers care to an irresponsible person (one whose irresponsibility is known or clearly evident), there may be liability under "negligent entrustment."

2. **If Assistance in an Emergency Is Requested.** Unfortunately, no universally accepted precise definition of what constitutes an "emergency" has ever been established. The concept that an emergency consists of an unforeseen condition requiring immediate medical care to save life or preserve function has been modified and expanded by judicial interpretation in different areas in different and conflicting ways. In addition, there is often a considerable discrepancy between the view of lay persons (including patients) and physicians as to what constitutes an "emergency" case.

No person who reports to an emergency department should be refused advice or treatment when life and function are threatened—the act of coming to the emergency department constitutes a request for treatment.

Requests for emergency care may be made by the injured or ill individual in person or by telephone or by someone else on his or her behalf. If any questions regarding the patient's complaints or condition are asked by the physician (or by his nurse or other representative) and any recommendations given, or treatment prescribed, a physician-patient relationship has been established that can be terminated only by specific notification. This notification, which should be documented in writing, should give adequate time for finding other professional help. In an emergency, care should continue to be provided until means for satisfactory ongoing alternative care are established.

3. **If Refusal of Treatment Constitutes Abandonment.** Social censure, criticism and condemnation and civil lawsuit can follow refusal of a physician to give further advice or treatment to a person with whom a physician-patient relationship is in effect, provided the patient has a genuine need for the attention requested and advance notice of the intent not to treat is insufficient.

64–2. ADVICE FOR FOLLOW–UP CARE
(and avoidance of abandonment)

Failure of the attending physician to take reasonable steps to complete specific arrangements for follow-up care after emergency treatment and to stress the possible ill-effects of lack of such care may constitute a basis for legal action by the patient (or his natural or legal guardians) on the grounds of abandonment. A practical method of prevention of this type of claim consists of giving or sending (if unable to personally give or in situations in which reinforcement is advisable) the patient (or patient's legal guardian) a brief notation explaining the need for further medical care and outlining the possible consequences of lack of care. This notation should be sent by registered mail, if not personally given, with return receipt requested. A copy of this letter and the return receipt (or the undelivered original letter) should be made a part of the patient's permanent record. The following form (Instructions for Follow-Up Care) has been found to be of value, especially in clinics, offices and stations where large numbers of emergency patients are treated. This form should be completed in duplicate if the information does not appear elsewhere in the record. The original should be given to the patient when emergency care is completed and the copy placed in the patient's record.

INSTRUCTIONS FOR FOLLOW-UP CARE

The examination and treatment that you have received has been on an emergency basis and has not been intended to be a substitute or replacement for complete medical care. For your protection, I hereby suggest that in order to prevent possible complications you follow the recommendations checked below:

☐ Telephone your private physician for an appointment

on ______________________________
(Date)

☐ Report at once to your private physician.

☐ Report at once to ______________________________ Hospital.

☐ Telephone for an appointment in the ______________________________

Clinic at ______________________________ on ______________________________
(location) (date)

☐ Report back to this Emergency Department on ______________________________

______________________________ at A.M.
(date) P.M.

☐ Other (specify) ______________________________

Date ______________________________ Signed ______________________________ M.D.

65. Certificates

65–1. BIRTH CERTIFICATES

The signature of the person delivering the infant (this is usually the attending physician but in some localities may be a licensed midwife or a lay person if there are no medical attendants) in black permanent ink is required on all certificates covering live births and stillbirths.

For uniformity in reporting to public agencies, the following criteria are in general use:

65–2. LIVE BIRTH

Any infant born at any gestational age that after birth shows any sign of life, even momentarily (heart beat, impulse in cord or respiratory activity). Use of EEG to show "brain life" status may become a standard required test in the future.

65–3. PREMATURE BIRTH

Any infant less than 2500 g (5½ lb) in weight, regardless of length or age.

65–4. STILLBIRTH

Any infant born dead (no heart beat, impulse in cord or respiratory activity) and weighing 1000 g (2 lb, 3 oz) or more, regardless of length or age.

65–5. ABORTION

Any infant born dead and weighing less than 500 g (1.1 lb), regardless of length or age, or any infant born dead after a gestation period of less than 20 weeks if weight not known.

65–6. DEATH CERTIFICATES

Whenever an infant weighing 2500 g or more shows signs of life (65–2), even momentarily, both a birth certificate (65–*1*) and a death certificate must be completed and signed by the attending physician or coroner. Abortions (65–5) do not require completion of any certificate; however, a notation must be made in the emergency record and signed by the attending physician.

A death certificate must be completed within a given time (usually 15 or 24 hours), on every death case, no matter what the cause. For detailed information regarding coroner's (medical examiner's) responsibility, see *8–8*.

66. Emergency Case Records*

In many instances, legal actions against physicians and hospitals are based upon incidents alleged to have occurred at the time of initial emergency treatment (68, *Malpractice*). Therefore, to protect the physician and hospital as well as the patient, meticulous care should be used in the completion, filing, and safeguarding of detailed, accurate, legible records on all emergency cases.

66–1. EXAMINATION DATA FOR EMERGENCY REPORT *(See 75–2)*

66–2. EMERGENCY CASE LOG

In those offices, admitting departments, stations or wards that handle emergency cases, a current and chronologic emergency log should be kept by clerical or nursing personnel in addition to the records or charts completed by the attending physician. This log should be a permanent record, typed or written in ink, and should contain the following information:

Classification code (private, industrial, insurance coverage).
Date and time registered.
Name in full, including middle initial (if no middle initial, indicate as N.M.I.). If the patient is a minor, the legal guardian's name, address and telephone number should be given.
Address and telephone number.
Date of birth (if not known, indicate apparent age).
Sex.
Brought for emergency care by (self, family, guardian, friends, police, ambulance).
Brought from (home, address, site of accident, name of hospital).
Type of case (pediatric, surgical, medical, obstetric, undetermined).
Diagnosis. If a specific diagnosis has not been given on the medical record by the examining physician, the working or symptom diagnosis should be entered. "Deferred" *should never be used* as an entry on its own; rather, give a statement containing some

---

*See also 69, *Permits and Authorizations;* 75, *Worker's Compensation (Industrial) Cases;* 67, *Subrogation cases.*

kind of information, e.g., "Headache of undetermined origin; possible causes to be evaluated include: (etc.)."
Treatment, in brief.
Disposition—home, to work, hospitalized, referred (to whom?).
Condition—good, fair, poor, critical, deceased.
Time discharged from emergency care.
Out by (self, friends, ambulance).
Follow-up care—specific instructions.
Name (not initials) of the attending physician.

66–3. RELEASE FROM RESPONSIBILITY

Occasionally a patient, or a patient's guardian, will refuse to follow the recommendations for treatment or disposition made by the examining physician. In cases of this type a "Release from Responsibility" form (below) should be signed by the patient (or patient's natural or legal guardian) in the presence of two witnesses. This signed and witnessed release should be made a permanent part of the emergency record.

RELEASE FROM RESPONSIBILITY
(Cross out portions which do not apply)

Date ____________________ Time ____________________ m.

I hereby certify that of my own free will I am removing my

____ from the
(self, son, daughter, husband, wife, ward)

____
(Office, Clinic, Hospital)

against the recommendation and advice of ____________________ M.D., and that I am hereby refusing further examination, tests, and treatment. I hereby acknowledge that I have been informed of, and understand, the possible consequences of such removal and/or refusal. Having full knowledge of the risks involved, and realization of the dangers that may result from removal of the patient and/or refusal of recommended examination, tests, and treatment, I hereby agree to hold the ____
(Office, Clinic, Hospital)

and ____, M.D.

and all others concerned blameless and free from any and all liability for any direct or indirect injuries or ill-effects which may result by reason of removal of the patient, and/or refusal of examination, tests, and treatment.

Witness ____________________ Signed ____________________

Witness ____________________ Relationship to Patient ____________________
(self, mother, father, husband, wife, guardian)

66–4. UNUSUAL OCCURRENCE REPORTS

Emergency practice is prone to unusual occurrences because of the types of cases that are handled. Any incidents that fall into any of the following categories should be covered by a detailed note made in the patient's record and by an entry in the emergency log (66–2).

- Omission, incorrect administration or improper dosage of any drug or medication ordered or prescribed by the attending physician.

- Incidents that cause, or that might be construed as causing, bodily injury to a patient or other persons.
- Serious reactions caused by drugs or other substances administered or prescribed in the treatment of emergency conditions.
- See *15, Reportable Conditions*, which details conditions that the physician is under a legal duty to report.
- Accidents, breaks in technique or unusual incidences during examination and/or treatment.
- Incidents occurring in the entrance to, or on the property or grounds of, the emergency station, office, clinic, ward or hospital that might be construed as causing or contributing to mental or physical suffering or injury—direct or indirect—to a patient or visitor. (Injuries to emergency personnel or police officers are covered under the compensation acts and require the usual industrial form [75–2.])
- Loss or alleged loss of clothing, money, jewelry or other personal effects.

67. Liability and Subrogation Cases

Many of the cases treated as emergencies result from direct or indirect trauma (assault, auto accidents, railroad wrecks, industrial accidents) that may be the basis for future litigation of considerable complexity; therefore, it is the responsibility of the attending physician to see that *on first examination* all evidences of injury are noted in detail on the patient's chart. These include superficial contusions, abrasions and lacerations, as well as more serious injuries. The exact location and severity (slight, moderate, severe) should be noted in detail on the emergency record. (See also comments in *14–5* regarding preservation of evidence.)

X-rays should be taken whenever necessary to establish, confirm or rule out traumatic, pre-existent or other relevant conditions (*21*).

Any evidence of or tests for any degree of intoxication from alcohol, narcotics or other drugs should be entered on the clinical record with enough detail to refresh the physician's memory in case he or she should be required to testify in court at a later date.

68. Malpractice (Errors and Omissions)

68–1. NEGLIGENCE

Malpractice actions against physicians are usually based on allegations of negligence concerning the physician's performance within the place and course of usual practice or employment. "Good Samaritan" statutes, to encourage trained medical personnel to render emergency care at the scene, require only that the personnel act in "good faith" and without "gross negligence" (intentional failure to perform duty in manifest disregard of the consequences). (See *69–8* for comments on consent.)

In order to prove negligence, the complainant must, as a rule, present evidence concerning the following points (sometimes referred to as the *Four D's*):

Duty. The existence of a physician-patient relationship (*64–1*) assumes the physician's duty toward the patient.

Dereliction of Duty. See *68–3*.

Direct Causation and Proximate Causation. An unbroken chain of causation with foreseeable results from the derelict act, or acts, or omission of acts, to the condition of which the patient complains must be proved by a preponderance of the evidence.

Damage. Proof of general damages (pain, suffering, physical dysfunction or disfigurement) and/or special damages (loss of earnings, medical and hospital expenses, necessary travel and other indirect costs) must be presented.

Negligence may consist of either or both of the following:

- Omission of proper and recognized methods of examination and treatment.
- Commission of improper, unauthorized, experimental or nonrecognized methods of examination or treatment. Application of the legal doctrine of *res ipsa loquitur* may result in inference of actionable negligence from the fact of injury itself, with corroborating medical evidence. Malpractice action for assault and technical battery may be based on alleged lack of informed consent (69–8) on the part of the patient.

68–2. STATUTES OF LIMITATION

This rule varies in different jurisdictions, but generally statutes of limitation run from the time that the patient becomes aware of the damaging incident, not from the date of the procedure.

68–3. STANDARDS OF CARE IN EMERGENCY CASES

The criteria by which proper and recognized methods of examination and treatment are determined have changed markedly during the last few years. Formerly the general ("Locality") rule was usually stated as follows: "A physician is required to exercise or use such reasonable and ordinary care, skill and diligence as a physician in good standing in the same area in the same general line of practice, ordinarily used in like cases." At the present time, the same standards of knowledge, skill and experience are applied to a general practitioner in a remote rural area as to a specialist in a sophisticated urban medical center.

It is sometimes written by statute ("Good Samaritan" laws) that a lower standard of care is required in the management and treatment of emergency cases at the scene than in nonurgent situations and that the ordinary criteria for determining negligence do not apply in these circumstances and, instead, a requirement of good faith and absence of gross negligence exists. In California, a new law establishes that if a physician is sued for emergency treatment given, only a physician with 5 years of emergency department experience can qualify as an expert witness.

The available time or degree of urgency (2, *Urgency Evaluation [Triage]*) does not in any way modify a physician's duty to use reasonable care; this duty remains the same at all times. However, the degree of skill required of the physician may vary according to the skill that good physicians exercise in like cases and circumstances. A correct test is whether or not the physician took such action as a skillful and experienced physician would have taken under similar circumstances.

68–4. MALPRACTICE INSURANCE

All professional medical personnel, especially those who handle a great volume of emergency cases, should be covered adequately by malpractice insurance with a reliable company. The insurance policy should contain the specific provision that no claim can be paid or settled by the company without the approval of the insured.

68–5. ROUTINE SAFEGUARDS AGAINST MALPRACTICE ACTIONS

To avoid malpractice suits, it is helpful to adhere to the following precautions:

- Completion and careful preservation of accurate, detailed and legible records on every patient. The length of time that these records are required by law to be preserved varies in different localities, but records on children must be kept until they reach their majority. Make recommendations for follow-up care (64–2).
- Utilization of maximum skill, knowledge and judgment in examination, treatment and disposition.
- Insistence on competent consultation in problem cases.
- Avoidance of quasi-experimental, controversial or nonaccepted procedures.
- Explanation to the patient (or patient's legal guardian) *in advance* of the purpose, extent, expected results, possible complications and estimated expense of any proce-

dure (see *69–8, Informed Consent*). Under no circumstances should any express, specific or implied guarantee or warranty be suggested, given or endorsed.

- Notation in the patient's record, in detail and in a noncritical fashion, of any complications or unusual situations related directly or indirectly to the management of the case.
- Avoidance of informal direct, indirect or implied criticism of the work of, or the results obtained by, others even under extreme provocation, since the complete accurate facts or circumstances are usually not known (an acceptable alternative is initiation of formal peer review).
- Use of courtesy, kindness, sympathy and tact in all relationships with the patient, family, relatives, friends or other interested parties.

69. Permits and Authorizations in Relation to Emergency Cases*

Some of the following permits and authorizations have been referred to in the preceding text. All have been found useful in the management of emergency cases. (See *69–8* regarding informed and free choice consent.)

69–1. DISCLOSURE OF INFORMATION TO OR FROM PATIENT'S PHYSICIAN

1. I hereby authorize ______________________ M.D. to disclose complete information to ______________________ concerning medical findings and treatment of ______________________ (name or "myself") from ______________________ 19______ until the date of conclusion of such treatment, including psychiatric, alcohol or drug abuse treatment.

2. I hereby waive on behalf of myself and any persons who may have an interest in the matter, all provisions of law relating to the disclosure of confidential medical information.

Witness ______________ Signed ______________________

Date ______________ Date ______________________

69–2. BLOOD ALCOHOL TEST *(See also 19–2)*

Witnesses should be disinterested adults, not the attending physician, the attending nurse or a law enforcement officer.

---

*Some of the forms in this section are modified from "Medicolegal Forms with Legal Analysis" published by the Law Department of the American Medical Association, from "Reference Manual of Permits, Consents and/or Releases; Hospital Administrative Procedure No. 1–10" prepared by the office of the Area Administrator, Kaiser Foundation Hospitals, Oakland, California and from the California Hospital Association Consent Manual. The "Consent to Medical Examination Following Sexual Assault" (69–7) is modified from a form in use at the Michael Reese Hospital, Chicago.)

BLOOD TEST REQUEST BY PEACE OFFICER
AT

_______________Hospital, _______________
City

The undersigned, a duly authorized peace officer of _______________
(name of law enforcement body)
hereby requests that a physician, registered nurse, licensed clinical laboratory technologist or clinical laboratory technician obtain a blood sample from _______________. (name of patient)
This is to certify that said person from whom the blood sample is to be obtained has been lawfully arrested for an offense allegedly committed by said person while driving a motor vehicle under the influence of intoxicating liquor and that the undersigned peace officer has reasonable cause to believe such person was driving a motor vehicle upon the highway while under the influence of intoxicating liquor. The person referred to above has been advised that his or her failure to submit to such a chemical test will result in the suspension of his or her privilege to operate a motor vehicle for a period of six months and that said person has been granted the choice of whether the test shall be of his or her blood, breath, or urine.

____
(signature of peace officer)

Date: _______________ Time: _______________ Witness: _______________

CONSENT TO BLOOD TEST

I, the undersigned, do hereby consent to the withdrawal of a blood sample from my body and do hereby further acknowledge that I have been advised that I have my choice of submitting to a test of either my blood, breath or urine and that I have selected the blood test. I further certify that I am not a person who is afflicted with hemophilia (a bleeder) or a person who is afflicted with a heart condition using an anticoagulant (blood thinner) under the direction of a physician.

____
(patient)

Date: _______________ Time: _______________ Witness: _______________

PERSON WITHDRAWING BLOOD

Upon the request of _______________, I have withdrawn
(name of peace officer requesting test)
a blood sample from the above-named patient on _______________ at _______________.
(date) (time)

The patient was unable to sign the consent. ☐

The patient refused to sign the consent, but willingly submitted to the test. ☐

____
(physician, registered nurse, licensed clinical laboratory technologist or laboratory technician)

69–3. DIAGNOSTIC AND THERAPEUTIC PROCEDURES *(e.g., Arteriograms, Arthograms, Bronchograms, Cisternal Puncture, Myelograms, Paracentesis, Spinal Puncture, Sternal Puncture, Other Procedures Requiring Injection of a Radiopaque Material)*

PATIENT ______________________________ AGE __________

DATE ______________________________ TIME __________ A.M.

I hereby request and authorize ______________________________ M.D.

to perform upon ______________________________ the following
("myself" or name of patient)

procedure : ______________________________ .
I have been fully informed of the risks and possible consequences involved and understand that unforeseen results and complications may occur; among these are: ______________________________

Signed ______________________________

Relationship to patient ______________________________

The foregoing consent was read, discussed and signed in my presence, and in my opinion the person so signing did so freely and with full knowledge and understanding.

Date __________________ Witness ______________________________

69–4. DISPOSAL OF A SEVERED OR AMPUTATED PART OR ORGAN*

Date ______________________________

I hereby authorize the ______________________________ Hospital to preserve for scientific purposes, or to use in grafts upon living persons, or to otherwise dispose of in a proper and suitable manner, the tissues, parts, or

organs of ______________________________ specified below.
(Name of patient or "myself")

____
(Parts or organs)

Witness __________________ Signed ______________________________

Witness __________________ Relationship to patient
(Self, parent, legal guardian) ______________________________

69–5. EMERGENCY CARE WITHOUT A SURGERY PERMIT

The degree of emergency as evaluated by the examining physician is the deciding factor in the handling of patients who are unable to sign their own treatment permits

*The physician may also need to save the amputated part temporarily for skin donor grafting for the patient's own wound sites, even if replantation is not feasible.

because of minority, mental condition or grave disability or whose natural or legal guardians are not available.

When Immediate Treatment Is Required (Gross Hemorrhage, Acute Poisoning, Cardiac Emergencies, Respiratory Embarrassment [2, *Urgency Evaluation—Triage*])

In these cases there is a definitive *positive* obligation for treatment without delay and consent is legally implied. While the patient is being prepared for and undergoing treatment, every effort should be made to locate the natural or legal guardian by telephone, telegraph or other means. The cooperation of law enforcement and social service agencies of the community can often be obtained.

Before emergency surgery or procedures beyond basic life support are undertaken, the Immediate Treatment Form (below) should be signed by a licensed physician and made a part of the patient's permanent record. If another physician is in attendance, it is a wise precaution to have that physician's concurring signature also.

In addition, a standard informed consent treatment permit (*69–8*) signed by the natural or legal guardian or telegraph or telephone permission (*69–15*) should be obtained at the earliest opportunity and before any surgery that can be safely postponed.

Immediate Treatment Permit

(Used when patient is an unemancipated minor or mentally incompetent or unable to sign because of condition; natural or legal guardian not available)

Date ____________Time ____________m.

We, the undersigned physicians,* licensed to practice in the State of ____________

______________________________, hereby certify that it is our considered opinion that

____________________, ______________, is in need of immediate treatment to save
(Name of patient) (Age)
life and/or to prevent serious disability and/or deformity.

We further certify that unsuccessful attempts have been made for a reasonable time to communicate with the parents, spouse, or legal guardian of the patient named above, and that in our professional judgment further delay in rendering treatment will seriously increase the danger to the patient's life and health.

Witness ______________________________Signed ______________________, M.D.

Witness ______________________________Signed ______________________, M.D.

*Some states require the signature of only 1 physician; however, if available, signatures of 2 physicians may add value.

Miscellaneous Provisions Concerning Emergency Permits

- The signer must be clearly aware of the nature of his or her consent.
- Persons witnessing signatures must be mentally competent and 18 years of age or older in most states.
- When emergency procedures are performed without the signature of the patient or patient's natural or legal guardian, a properly signed and witnessed permit should be obtained at the earliest possible opportunity and incorported in the emergency record.
- Permits signed with an "X" should be witnessed by 2 adults able to write their names.
- Surgery or other treatment necessary to prevent a cosmetic or functional defect requires a validly signed operative or treatment permit based on informed consent (*69–8*). This requirement also applies to elective surgery of any type. These procedures cannot be performed under an immediate treatment permit.
- No person who has only temporary custody of a minor has any legal right to authorize treatment of any kind.
- The authority of a duly appointed legal guardian supersedes that of a parent or spouse.

Table 69–1. LEGAL CONSENT REQUIREMENTS FOR MEDICAL TREATMENT OF MINORS IN VARIOUS CIRCUMSTANCES*

Patient's Status	Is Parental Consent Required?	Are Parents Responsible for Cost?	Is Minor's Consent Sufficient?	May M.D. Inform Parents of Treatment?
Under 18, unmarried, no special circumstances	Yes	Yes	No	Yes
Under 18, married or previously married	No	No	Yes	No
Under 18, emergency and parents not available	No	Yes	Yes (if capable)	Yes
Emancipated (over 15, not living at home, manages own financial affairs)	No	No	Yes	Yes
Not married, pregnant, under 18 (care related to pregnancy) (including consent to an abortion)	No	No	Yes	No
Not married, pregnant, under 18 (care not related to pregnancy and no other special circumstances)	Yes	Yes	No	Yes
Not married, under 18, determination if pregnant, no other special circumstances	Probably not	Probably not	Probably yes	Probably not
Under 18, on active duty with Armed Services	No	No	Yes	No
Under 18, over 12, care for contagious reportable disease	No	No	Yes	No
Under 18, birth control	No	No	Yes	No
Under 18, over 12, care for rape	No	No	Yes	Yes
Under 18, care for sexual assault	No	No	Yes	Yes, usually
Under 18, over 12, care for alcohol or drug abuse	No	No	Yes	Yes, usually

*From California Hospital Association Consent Manual, 1978.

- Grandparents, adult brothers or sisters, close relatives, etc. *cannot sign a permit for a minor* [except *in loco parentis*].
- Permits should be signed *before any preoperative medication is given to the patient.*
- If a patient qualified to give permission specifically prohibits any procedure verbally or in writing before becoming incompetent or irresponsible, the procedure cannot be performed under any circumstances, even as a lifesaving measure, in many localities (*69–8*).
- Because the father and mother are charged equally with the control and custody of a child, express prohibition by 1 parent prevents any treatment even though the other has given permission. This applies even if the parents are separated and can be overruled only if the laws in the particular locality provide for the issuance of treatment orders by juvenile or other courts.
- When marriage of a minor, divorce, annulment, legal guardianship, or *in loco parentis* relationship is claimed as a basis for exceptions to the usual rules regarding treatment permits, adequate evidence to substantiate the claim should be required.
- A summary of the legal consent requirements for minors in one jurisdiction (California) is shown in Table 69–1.

69–6. ENTRUSTMENT OF CARE OF MINORS*

Parents or legal guardians who wish to leave their children or wards under the care of another adult during working hours, overnight, while on vacation trips, etc., can ensure prompt emergency care by completing and signing a document of the type shown on page 740. The signed and witnessed document should be kept in the possession of the adult designated to authorize care during the parents' or guardian's absence, to be presented to the attending physician in the case of an emergency involving the persons specified thereon.

69–7. EXAMINATION FOR CRIMINAL SEXUAL ASSAULT† *(For detailed outline of required history and examination, see 14, Rape; see also consent form on p. 741)*

69–8. INFORMED AND FREE CHOICE CONSENT *(See also 69–15)*

No longer is a blanket authorization covering any and all medical, surgical and laboratory procedures considered adequate for emergency or other medical care. It is generally accepted that, if time permits, before giving consent, the patient is entitled to accurate and detailed information not only regarding the projected operation, diagnostic procedure or therapy but also concerning recognized risks, possible complications and their effects and available alternative methods of treatment.

Informed consent and free choice consent are best viewed in a relative sense, since the art of communication is often imperfect despite intentions. The gestalt of word meaning is individually widely varied, and absolute freedom is a rarity. Free choice may be considered to be present under circumstances devoid of obvious or likely duress or coercion. Informed consent means the consenter and the consentee reasonably understand the major issues before them and are in substantial agreement except as expressed otherwise. The consent may be implied through the patient's voluntary submission to a procedure or may be expressed verbally or in writing. Written consent (with the general areas of information communicated and agreed upon as outlined later in this section, unless the patient has written a consent indicating that he or she did not wish to be informed—see page 743) is by far the best policy for avoidance of any later misunderstanding.

To protect the attending physician and his or her assistants, the anesthesiologist and the clinic or hospital and its personnel against subsequent allegations by the patients,

---

*Any person under 18 years of age.

†In some states, a minor who is a victim of a sexual attack can legally sign a consent for examination without requirement of parenteral consent (see *69–15*).

TO WHOM IT MAY CONCERN: Date of Signing ____________

(Cross out words that do not apply)

This is to certify that I/we, ______________________________

______________________ the ______________________

(names in full) (mother, father, legal guardian)

of the persons listed below, do hereby constitute and appoint

____

(name in full) (address)

my/our true and lawful attorney, solely, and with the power to authorize and consent to the administration of any anesthetic or medical treatment to, and the performance of whatever operations or removal of tissue decided to be necessary by the attending physician, on the below named minor(s) for the period from ____________ to ____________, inclusive.

(date) (date)

NAME	AGE OR DATE OF BIRTH
______________	______________
______________	______________
______________	______________
______________	______________

WITNESSED BY:

Name	Date	Name	Relationship
Name	Date	Name	Relationship

Note: A photocopy supply of this form is helpful to have for quick completion in any home in which there are minors. (Permission for photocopy granted.)

CONSENT TO MEDICAL EXAMINATION FOLLOWING SEXUAL ASSAULT

I, ______________________________, voluntarily request ______________________________ M.D., his or her medical and nursing assistants and associates, to conduct an examination to determine the medical implications of an alleged sexual assault made upon me. I fully understand this examination will include tests for presence of sperm and venereal disease, as well as clinical observations for physical evidence of penetration of and/or injury to my reproductive organs.

I fully understand the nature of the examination and the fact that medical information gathered by this means may be used as evidence in a court of law or in connection with the enforcement of public health rules and laws.

I hereby grant permission to ______________________________ Hospital and its agents for the release of this and related information to authorized officials when deemed necessary or advisable and I herewith save and hold harmless said ______________________________ Hospital and its agents from any and all claims of injury, whatsoever, which may in any manner result from the release of such information.

This will certify that I am of legal age and capacity to consent to this examination and that I fully understand all of its implications.

______________________________ ______________________________
Witness Signature of Patient

TO BE SIGNED BY PARENTS OR GUARDIANS
OF MINOR PATIENT

This will certify that while I am not of legal age to consent to this examination, I fully understand all of its implications.

____
Signature of Patient

I, ______________________________, in my capacity as ______________________________ of the patient,
(father, mother, guardian, etc.)

______________________________, do hereby grant permission to ______________________________ Hospital and its agents, as specified above, to conduction this examination on my ______________________________.
(son, daughter, ward)

______________________________ ______________________________
Witness Signed

Date of signing ______________________________

patient's legal guardian or heirs (usually triggered by a result below the expectations of the patient or family or by a dispute concerning charges) that the patient (or patient's legal guardian) was not informed of, or did not have full understanding of, possible risks and/or complications at the time that permission was given, the authorization should whenever possible incorporate the following points:

- *Date.* If a long period elapses between signature of the authorization and the time that the procedure is begun, the claim may be made that the patient had changed his or her mind during the interim and that, therefore, the procedure was done without legal authorization. This should not be a problem in the emergency setting.
- *Time of consent.* The exact time at which permission is given should be indicated and should be before administration of any drug or medication that might be construed as interfering with the patient's complete comprehension and sound judgment.
- *The scheduled procedure*—in lay terms if possible—with the name of the physician who will personally perform it (unless otherwise specified).
- *A general statement* in nontechnical language of recognized risks and complications of the procedure and possible adverse consequences.
- *A specific statement* that no guarantee of the results of the procedure has been made or implied and that alternative methods of treatment have been discussed.
- *A properly executed and witnessed signature of the patient or of the patient's legal guardian.* A patient who is physically unable to sign his or her name should make a mark with a pen held by or against any portion of his or her body. The patient's full name should then be written or printed after the mark, with the notation "________, his (or her) mark" and properly witnessed.
- *Witnesses* to the patient's signature must be disinterested adults—not the attending physician.

The following General Information About Surgery form covers all the points previously outlined and should be used to supplement the Operative and Treatment Permit (69–9).

General Information About Surgery

You and your doctor have decided that for the further diagnosis or treatment of your illness or condition, an operation is necessary. Surgical procedures of any type involve the taking of risks, ranging from minor to serious (including the risk of death) but today are generally safe, helpful and often lifesaving. It is important to be aware of the following possible risks before you give your consent to the operation that you and your physician are planning.

A surgical procedure, whether minor or serious, involves cutting skin, tissue or organs. The following may be the reactions of your body to an operation.

- *Infection*—invasion of tissue by bacteria or other germs occurs to some degree whenever a cut or incision is made. In most instances, the natural defense mechanisms of the body heal the affected area without difficulty. In some instances antibiotic medicines are prescribed and at times additional surgical measures may be necessary.
- *Hemorrhage*—cutting of blood vessels and accompanying bleeding occurs in every incision. This is usually easily controlled. At times blood transfusions are required to replace excessive blood loss. If blood transfusions are given there is a small additional risk of liver inflammation. There is no way to completely predict this undesired reaction. In simple operations there is usually less blood loss than in major ones, but not always. There are instances when excessive bleeding occurs after the original operation (major or minor) is completed, and additional action must be taken to control delayed bleeding.
- *Drug reactions*—unexpected allergies, lack of proper response or illness caused by the drugs can occur. It is important for you to inform your physician of any problems you have had with drugs and to let him or her know which medications you now take regularly.
- *Anesthesia reactions*—there may be unusual or expected responses to the gases, drugs or methods used that can lead to difficulties with lung, heart or nerve function. Except in unusual situations or emergencies you are not allowed to eat or drink for several hours prior to surgery in order to prevent the effects of vomiting. Your reactions to surgery continue to be observed in the recovery room during the period immediately after the operation.
- *Blood vessel inflammation and clotting*—when they happen together, thrombophlebitis results; blood clots may separate and move into other organs and cause more damage.
- *Injury to other organs*—because of closeness of other organs to the area being operated on, it may be unavoidable that other organ functions are affected. The stress of surgery

may also harm other organ systems. Required adjustments in the treatment will be made by your physician in response to these conditions.

- *Other concerns*—it is not possible to list here all the possible risks and complications and their variations that may arise in any surgical operation or procedure. Each situation depends upon the condition of health and the purpose and nature of the operation. Your physician is willing to discuss any further details with you.
- *Alternatives to surgery:* Other ways of managing your illness, which may range from doing nothing to taking different measures, have been considered. Since you and your doctor have decided upon surgery as the treatment indicated, do not hesitate to discuss the reasons and the alternatives. Because there are risks involved in any operation, with no guarantee or assurance of a successful result, it is important that you clearly understand and agree to it as the decision of your choice.

I have read the above information and am satisfied and I understand it. I have discussed with my physician any particular doubts, problems or concerns I may have regarding the intended surgery or procedure. I have no further questions regarding possible risks, complications and alternatives to the intended treatment.

The patient who does not wish to be informed should sign the following form in lieu of the General Information about Surgery form.

> Following the discussion I have had with my doctor regarding my condition, I prefer not to know in any detail the common risks of any surgical procedure.
>
> Date ______________________ Name ______________________
>
> Witness ____

69–9. OPERATIVE AND TREATMENT PERMIT (General) *(See also 69–8, Informed Consent)*

General Considerations. Whenever possible, an informed consent treatment permit, including permission for operative procedures (69–8) should be signed by the patient (or the patient's natural or legal guardian), properly witnessed and made a permanent part of the medical record before any treatment is given. Legally, treatment against the explicit or implied wish of the patient or of the patient's natural or legal guardian may constitute actionable assault. Practically, it is generally considered that the following types of treatment can be given without written authorization; verbal or nonverbal consent is adequate.

- Cleansing and irrigation of a wound (not debridement) with coaptation of the edges by adhesive straps or "butterflies" and application of protective sterile bandages.
- Application of temporary splints (not casts) to prevent aggravation of an injury by motion.
- Oral or rectal administration of medications.
- Diagnostic withdrawal of blood (e.g., by phlebotomy).
- Artificial respiration or assistance to respiration by any unexpired air, manual or mechanical means, including inhalation by tent, catheter or mask, of air, oxygen or other nonanesthetic gases.

In contrast, the following procedures should not be done without a properly signed permit unless an immediate threat to life or health is present:*

- Surgical procedures, major or minor, emergency or elective.
- Administration of local or general anesthesia.
- Insertion of a needle for any therapeutic or diagnostic injection. This includes intracutaneous, subcutaneous, intramuscular, intravenous or intraspinal injections of all types, as well as the withdrawal of spinal fluid, etc., for diagnosis or treatment.

---

*May come under a general consent—although special consent is advisable for riskier procedures.

CONSENT TO OPERATION, ADMINISTRATION OF ANESTHETICS AND THE RENDERING OF OTHER MEDICAL SERVICES

1. I authorize ______________________________ M.D., and/or his or her associates, assistants of his or her choice and personnel assigned by the Hospital, to perform the following operation or procedure upon me ______________________________
____
and/or to do any other procedures that in (his) (her) (their) judgment may be advisable for the patient's well-being, including such procedures as are considered medically advisable to remedy conditions discovered during the procedure or operation. I am satisfied with my understanding of the nature of the operation or procedure, the more common risks associated with it, including the potential for serious harm, and alternative methods of treatment, which have been explained to me by ______________________________
No warranty or guarantee has been made as to the result or cure.
2. I hereby authorize and direct the above named Hospital, Medical Group, physician and/or his or her associates and assistants, to provide such additional services for me as he or she or they may deem medically advisable, including, but not limited to, the selection and administration of anesthesia and the performance of pathology and radiology services.
3. I hereby authorize the Hospital to dispose of any severed tissue or member in accordance with accustomed hospital practice.
4. (Other) ______________________________
____
____

Date ____________________ Signed: ____________________

Hour: ____________________ Witness: ____________________
(If patient is a minor or is unable to sign, complete the following:)

Patient is a minor ____________________ or is unable to sign

because ______________________________
Signed: ____________________

Witness: ____________________ Relationship: ____________________

- Gastric lavage or gavage.
- Catheterization.
- Application or changing of corrective splints or casts.

The best definition of a danger or threat to life or health that would warrant proceeding without proper authorization is as follows: *It must involve a threat which carries danger of major incapacities, permanent or irreversible, through impairment or loss of a function, organ or structural unit of the body.* A satisfactory form of general operative and treatment permit is shown above.

69–10. PERSONS WHO MAY SIGN THEIR OWN EMERGENCY TREATMENT PERMITS *(See also 69–5 and 69–8)*

Any mentally competent person over 18 years of age. The decision regarding mental competency must be made by the attending physician, provided it has not been established by court action.

Any mentally competent male over 16 or female over 15 who is married or divorced or whose marrige has been annulled. Such persons are considered to be emancipated from parental control; hence, they can sign their own permits in many states.

"Mature" Minors. In some states (there is considerable variation) unmarried minors less than 18 may, under certain circumstances sign emergency permits. These circumstances are as follows:

- When the consent of the natural or legal guardian cannot be obtained within the time limit available to save life or prevent suffering or permanent disability.
- The minor is living separately and managing personal finances. The status of being pregnant in and of itself does not give qualification for a "mature minor." In California, however, any minor can consent to her pregnancy treatment (including abortion) without parental involvement.
- When the natural or legal guardians are not available, but the minor has presented himself or herself for treatment accompanied by older relatives and with a parent's knowledge, provided there is no reason to suspect that 1 or both of the parents' consent would not have been given had they been available.

See also special laws concerning minors age 12 and over who seek treatment for venereal diseases (33–78).

69–11. PERSONS WHO MAY SIGN PERMITS FOR MINORS*

A Natural Parent. If the parents have been legally divorced, the parent to whom the court has awarded custody of the child must sign the permit. The signatures of both parents are desirable, although not essential, in cases of this type.

In the rare instances in which there is a difference of opinion between undivorced parents, emergency treatment of any type *cannot be given* if specifically prohibited by 1 of the parents, unless there is a provision in the law of the specific locality for the issuance of a treatment order by juvenile or other court order.

A Legal Guardian (duly appointed by court order).

The husband of a married female over 15 or the wife of a married male over 16, if the patient is mentally incompetent, and provided the patient has not expressly prohibited the procedure verbally or in writing before the onset of mental incompetence.

In Loco Parentis. Any person who, in the *permanent* absence of the parents, has assumed parental obligations without the formalities of legal adoption is *in loco parentis*. For example, if any uncle or grandparent receives a niece, nephew or grandchild into his or her household as a member of his or her family, he or she assumes the rights and duties of the lawful parent. Since permanent, not temporary, custody is required, the important factor to determine in each case is whether the child has actually been deserted or abandoned by the parents. To constitute abandonment there must be actual desertion, accompanied by the intention to sever completely, or as completely as possible, the parental relationship.

69–12. PERSONS WHO MAY SIGN PERMITS FOR LEGALLY ADJUDGED MENTALLY INCOMPETENT ADULTS

A legally appointed guardian, usually a parent, spouse or close relative but in some instances a nonrelated person. In this case, the legal guardian alone can sign permits, and the guardian's decision takes precedence over that of a parent or spouse.

69–13. PERSONS WHO MAY SIGN PERMITS FOR ADULTS WHO ARE TEMPORARILY MENTALLY INCOMPETENT FROM SERIOUS DISEASE OR INJURY

A Spouse—provided that the patient has not expressly prohibited the procedure verbally or in writing before becoming mentally irresponsible.

A Legal Guardian. If a mentally irresponsible patient is brought for emergency care without accompanying identification (transients, auto accident cases, alcoholics, attempted suicides, etc.), handling must be in accordance with the rules outlined under 69–5, *Emergency Care without a Surgery Permit*.

69–14. PHOTOGRAPHING OF PATIENTS

Photographing of injured or ill persons undergoing emergency care should never be allowed without written permission of the patient or, if a minor, of a parent or legal

---

*A minor, in most states, is any person under 18 years of age.

CONSENT TO TAKING AND PUBLICATION OF PHOTOGRAPHS

Patient ______________________________

Place ______________________________

Date ______________________________

In connection with the medical services that I am receiving from my physician, ______________________________M.D., I consent that photographs may be taken of me, or of parts of my body, under the following conditions:

1. The photographs may be taken only with the consent of the physician designated above and under such conditions and at such times as he or she may approve.

2. The photographs shall be taken by my physician or by a photographer approved and designated by him or her.

3. Any and all photographs taken as specified above shall be used for medical purposes only.

4. If, in the judgment of my physician, medical research, education, or science will be benefited by their use, such photographs and information relating to my case may be published and republished, either separately or in connection with each other, in professional journals or medical books, or used for any other purpose that my physician may deem proper in the interest of medical education, knowledge, or research; provided, however, that it is specifically understood that in any such publications or use I shall not be identified by name.

5. The aforementioned photographs may be modified or retouched in any way that my physician, in his or her discretion, may considerable desirable.

Signed ______________________________
(patient)

Witness ______________________________

guardian. Under no circumstances should photographs of unconscious, dazed or mentally irresponsible adult patients be allowed, even if permission has been given by the spouse, unless such photographs are needed by law enforcement agencies.

69–15. TYPES OF VALID EMERGENCY TREATMENT PERMITS

Written. Authorizations should always be signed if possible. If the patient is illiterate or physically unable to write, but is mentally competent, he or she should make an X, with assistance if necessary. The certification by 2 witnesses should be as follows:

"John Doe (his mark)" Witness______________________________
Witness______________________________

Telegraph. A copy of the telegraph authorization must be made a permanent part of the record.

Telephone. This is valid provided 2 persons listen in on the line and both record the time and circumstances in the patient's record. A substantiating written authorization should be obtained as soon as possible.

Verbal. Verbal permission or silent (tacit) acquiescence of a mentally competent adult is a valid consent but is often difficult or impossible to prove at a later date. Therefore, a properly witnessed written consent (69–8) should be obtained at the earliest possible opportunity.

69–16. REFUSAL OF BLOOD OR BLOOD DERIVATIVES

At least one religious group (Jehovah's Witnesses) will not allow administration of blood or blood derivatives, even as a lifesaving measure.* In circumstances of this type, to protect the attending physician and the hospital, the following form should be signed by the patient and spouse, by parents of a minor or by the legal guardian of a mentally incompetent person.

> Because of religious beliefs, I hereby expressly forbid the administration of human blood or any of its derivatives to ______________________________ during this hospitalization. I hereby release the hospital, its personnel and the attending physician from any responsibility whatsoever for any unfavorable reactions or untoward results due to my refusal to permit the use of blood or its derivatives. It has been clearly explained and I fully understand the possible consequences of such refusal.
>
> Date ______________________________ Signed ______________________________
>
> Witness ______________________________ Spouse ______________________________
>
> Parents ______________________________
>
> Legal Guardian ______________________________

69–17. UNIFORM DONOR CARDS (to be signed and carried with you)†

(Face)

> UNIFORM DONOR CARD
>
> OF ______________________________
>
> Print or type name of donor
>
> In the hope that I may help others, I hereby make this anatomic gift, if medically acceptable, to take effect upon my death. The words and marks below indicate my desires.
>
> I give: (a) ______any needed organs or parts
>
> (b) ______only the following organs or parts
>
> ______________________________
>
> Specify the organ(s) or part(s)
>
> for the purposes of transplantation, therapy, medical research or education;
>
> (c) ______my body for anatomical study if needed.
>
> Limitations or special wishes, if any: ______________________________

---

*Blood substitutes ("artificial blood"; see *18–35*) may become an adequate compromise in these situations. An alternative solution in extreme, life-threatening cases concerning a patient who is a minor is to make the minor a ward of the court.

†In at least two states this type of donor card is on the back of the driver's license. In some states, Highway Patrol officers are authorized to check the wallets of dead victims for such donor cards and to consider the need for expedient management.

(Reverse)

Signed by the donor and the following two witnesses in the presence of each other:

______________________	______________________
Signature of Donor	Date of Birth of Donor
______________	______________________
Date signed	City & State
______________________	______________________
Witness	Witness

This is a legal document under the Uniform Anatomical Gift or similar laws.

69–18. IN VIVO CONTRIBUTION OF ANATOMICAL GIFT*

Donor ______________________________ Date __________

Recipient (if known) ______________________ Time __________

1. In the hope and with the expectation that this contribution will inure to the advancement of medical science and education and/or will benefit the above-shown recipient by preservation or prolongation of his or her life and well being, I, a person authorized by the California Anatomical Gift Act to make this contribution, do hereby authorize the retention, preservation, donation and/or transplantation of the following anatomical gifts: ______________________

____

____

2. I hereby acknowledge that this authorization is volunteered without obligation of any kind on the part of the recipient, this hospital, or any individual or organization authorized by law to receive this contribution and that this authorization is motivated exclusively by humanitarian instincts without hope or expectation of reward or compensation of any kind. I therefore release and surrender any and all claims which I may now have or which may be acquired by my legal representatives or me against my physician, his associates, this hospital, its agents or employees, any recipient or authorized individual or organization.

3. This contribution and authorization is subject to and expressely conditional upon the following conditions:

____

____

Witness: ______________________ Signed: ______________________
date

Witness: ______________________ Relationship, if signed for or on behalf of donor:
date

____

*This form is reprinted from the California Hospital Association Consent Manual.

69–19. NATURAL DEATH ACT

In certain instances, individuals (who are at least 18 years of age and of sound mind) with pending or present terminal illness may wish to avoid last-minute emergency efforts to prolong life—in a sense, they wish to "consent to not being treated."

The following form, in accordance with California's Natural Death Act, helps to fulfill that desire:

DIRECTIVE TO PHYSICIANS*

Directive made this ________day of ____________________(month, year).

I ______________________________, being of sound mind, willfully, and voluntarily make known my desire that my life shall not be artificially prolonged under the circumstances set forth below, do hereby declare:

1. If at any time I should have an incurable injury, disease, or illness certified to be a terminal condition by two physicians, and where the application of life-sustaining procedures would serve only to artificially prolong the moment of my death and where my physician determines that my death is imminent whether or not life-sustaining procedures are utilized, I direct that such procedures be withheld or withdrawn, and that I be permitted to die naturally.
2. In the absence of my ability to give directions regarding the use of such life-sustaining procedures, it is my intention that this directive shall be honored by my family and physician(s) as the final expression of my legal right to refuse medical or surgical treatment and accept the consequences from such refusal.
3. If I have been diagnosed as pregnant and that diagnosis is known to my physician, this directive shall have no force or effect during the course of my pregnancy.
4. I have been diagnosed and notified at least 14 days ago as having a terminal condition by ____, M.D., whose address is ____________________________, and whose telephone number is ________________. I understand that if I have not filled in the physician's name and address, it shall be presumed that I did not have a terminal condition when I made out this directive.
5. This directive shall have no force or effect five years from the date filled in above.
6. I understand the full import of this directive and I am emotionally and mentally competent to make this directive.

Signed ______________________

City, County and State of Residence ______________________________

The declarant has been personally known to me and I believe him or her to be of sound mind.

Witness ______________________

Witness ______________________

*This form is reprinted from Mills, D. H., J. Leg. Med., 5(1):23, 1977.

The physician attempting to comply with this type of directive should know that certain conditions also have been met:

- Two examining physicians, one of whom is the regular attending physician, must have certified in writing that the patient has a terminal illness.
- The patient must not be pregnant at the time the directive is to be carried out.
- The two witnesses must *not*: be related to the patient by blood or marriage, be mentioned in the will, be potential claimants to the estate or be involved in the patient's medical care. If the patient was in a skilled nursing home at the time of the signing

of the will, one witness *must* be a "patient advocate" designated by the State Department of Aging.

- If the physician is unwilling to act according to the directive, he *must* transfer the patient to a physician who will.

In California, patients may also choose an alternative route by selecting a durable power of attorney who will act in their behalf according to prior instructions in these situations.

70. Release of Information*

The physician who treats a patient on an emergency basis and all emergency personnel working under his or her supervision, direction or control should always keep in mind that medical information obtained during the physician-patient relationship is confidential and privileged and cannot be divulged without proper authorization (69–1) from the patient (or patient's legal guardian) except by due process of law (see *15, Reportable Conditions*). Therefore, only limited information can be given to friends, attorneys, claim adjustors, investigators, reporters or other interested persons, unless a proper authorization has been signed by the patient or the patient's legal guardian. It is preferable, when a public relations specialist is affiliated with the medical facility, for that individual to be the principal spokesperson for all information released to the public. Release of information to family members varies according to the patient's wishes; special care must be taken in this regard when sensitive issues such as abortion and sterility are involved. If an accident requires investigation and report by a law enforcement agency, is covered by the provisions of city, county or state emergency contracts or concerns a member of the merchant marine or armed services, a brief report, preferably in lay terms, covering the diagnosis, prognosis and disposition may be given to the investigating officer or to the proper law enforcement authorities subject to the following restrictions (which also apply to inquiries by any other members of the public).

Public Release of Information

The following items of public information may be given *without* the patient's consent, unless the patient specifically requests and signs a document indicating otherwise.

- ***Identity:*** (a) Name, (b) sex, (c) age, (d) address (release policy varies), and (e) general description of reason for treatment, general nature of injury or general condition.†
- ***Nature of the Accident:*** (a) Injured by automobile, explosion, shooting; (b) if there is a fracture, it is not to be described in any way except to state the member involved; and (c) more than a statement that it is simple or open (compound) may not be made.
- ***Injuries of the Head:*** (a) A simple statement that the injuries involve the head may be made, (b) it may not be stated that the skull is fractured, (c) no opinion as to the severity of the injury or prognosis should be given.
- ***Internal Injuries:*** (a) It may be stated that there are internal injuries but nothing more specific as to the location or specific condition of the injuries and (b) a statement that the general condition is good, fair, serious or critical† may be made.

---

*State laws vary; check jurisdictional requirements and individual hospital policies.

†Definitions of General Conditions:

- *Good:* Vital signs are stable and within normal limits; patient is conscious and comfortable; indicators are excellent.
- *Fair:* Same as good, but patient may be uncomfortable.
- *Serious:* Patient is acutely ill; vital signs may be unstable and outside normal limits; questionable indicators.
- *Critical:* Unstable vital signs; patient may be unconscious; unfavorable indicators.
- *Deceased:* Announcement of death is not routinely made by the hospital. However, news of a patient's death is public information after all reasonable efforts have been made to notify the family. The hospital may release information that will appear on the death certificate but should not give the cause of death unless it has been entered on the death certificate by the last attending physician or the coroner.

- ***Unconsciousness:*** (a) If the patient is unconscious when he or she is brought to the hospital, a statement of this fact may be made; (b) the cause of unconsciousness, however, should not be given.
- ***Cases of Poisoning:*** (a) A statement may be made that the patient is being treated for suspected poisoning, (b) if patient has ingested a poisonous compound, do not identify it by trade name but only by a general name, i.e., caustic, cleaning compound, etc., (c) no statement concerning the possibility of accident or suicide may be made, (d) make no prognosis.
- ***Suicide Attempts:*** No statement may be made that there was a suicide or attempted suicide.
- ***Sexual Assaults:*** (a) Names should not be released; (b) no statement may be made concerning the nature of the incident or injuries.
- ***Battered Children:*** (a) No statement may be made that a child's injuries appear to be the result of child abuse, even if an official report has been filed; (b) however, the nature and extent of injuries may be released in accordance with the other guidelines in this section.
- ***Psychiatric Emergencies or Drug and Alcohol Abuse:*** Federal regulation (and some state laws) strictly prohibit the giving of any information about psychiatric or drug and alcohol abuse patients, including information as to whether they are in the hospital or not. While reporters may have information from the police concerning persons who subsequently become psychiatric or drug and alcohol abuse patients, it is recommended that all such inquiries be answered, "We cannot, under Federal regulations, comment on this case."
- ***Births:*** No information is given until the mother signs a form for "release of birth information for birth announcement."
- ***Shooting:*** (a) A statement may be made that there is a penetrating wound and the general location given, (b) no statement may be made as to how the wound occurred, i.e., accidental, suicidal, homicidal or in a brawl, and the environment in which the shooting occurred may not be mentioned.
- ***Stabbing:*** The same general statements may be made for stabbing as for shooting incidents (previous paragraph).
- ***Intoxication:*** No statement may be made as to whether or not the patient is intoxicated or whether the ingested material is alcohol or other drugs.
- ***Burns:*** (a) A statement may be made that the patient is burned, also of the general location on the body, (b) a statement may be made also as to whether the patient has first, second or third degree burns, but only after diagnosis by a physician, (c) a statement as to how the accident occurred may be made only when the absolute facts are known, and (d) no prognosis may be given.
- ***Attending Physician:*** If the physician agrees, the hospital may state to the representatives of newspapers, radio stations or television stations the name of the attending physician of private patients and refer such representatives to the physician for information about the case.

Conditions Requiring Reporting *(See also 15 and 52–29)*

Since the reports completed by law enforcement officers become public documents, medical information thereon is not privileged and can be divulged without specific authorization from the patient or the patient's legal guardian.

Written reports concerning diagnosis, treatment and prognosis may be drawn up at the request of insurance adjustors, attorneys or other interested parties, provided a properly witnessed written authorization (*69–1*) signed by the patient (or the parent or legal guardian if the patient is a minor or has been legally declared incompetent) has been completed and made a part of the file, and provided the permission of the emergency physician who treated the case (or his or her superior in a hospital or plant emergency department) has been obtained.

Specific authorization is not a requirement for release of information concerning an industrial case (75). By requesting medical care under the provisions of any of the several worker's compensation acts, the patient waives the physician-patient relationship.

The oral or written request or permission of a patient's spouse to release medical information is not adequate if the patient is mentally competent to make the decision regarding release of information and the spouse is not the legal guardian.

Special Release Requirements *(See also 69–1).*

As required by federal law and some state laws, special specific consent by the patient must be given (or in its absence, a court order requiring divulgence to the judge) for medical information concerning remedial treatment for alcoholism or drug abuse or, for psychiatric treatment.

71. Responsibilities of Physicians Examining and Treating Emergency Cases

- To be available at all times if assigned to an emergency department, room, station or ward.
- To examine, evaluate and give prompt and proper treatment to all persons requiring emergency care in accordance with accepted medical standards.
- To decide whether or not persons requesting examination and treatment do, in fact, require emergency care. This very important decision is the responsibility solely of the emergency physician. Under no circumstances should it be made by a nurse, orderly, aide or clerk, though they may initiate specific emergency treatment under designated circumstances in accord with standing written orders by a physician for such occasions.
- To treat patients in approximate order of urgency (2, *Urgency Evaluation—Triage*).
- To supervise, instruct, direct and assume responsibility for professional assistants, nurses, orderlies, clerks, attendants and other emergency department personnel.
- To be familiar with the location of, indications for and adjustment and application of the various types of mechanical diagnostic and therapeutic equipment available in the emergency and critical care units.
- To be familiar with the application to emergency situations of rites of various religious denominations and sects (*8–11*).
- To be aware of the laws and ordinances relating to emergency situations of the political subdivision in which he or she is practicing.
- To be familiar with and abide by staff association constitution and by-laws and the hospital's rules, regulations and standing orders, including details of any formally outlined disaster plan, if on duty in an emergency department, room or ward.
- To be familiar with accepted actions, doses, side effects and toxicity of commonly used drugs.
- To arrange for future medical management of all persons with whom he or she has established a physician-patient relationship through examination, treatment or advice, with full knowledge of his or her responsibility until another physician takes over active supervision (64, *Abandonment*).
- To evaluate the condition of each patient before transfer or referral to be certain that such transportation or referral will not decrease the patient's chances of recovery or survival. In borderline cases, if, in the considered judgment of the emergency physician, transportation is indicated and feasible, supportive measures (oxygen, plasma volume expanders, vasopressor drugs, etc.) should be continued in the ambulance, preferably under the supervision of a physician, registered nurse or trained ambulance attendant. The résumé sent with the patient should indicate the attending physician's reasons for transfer.
- To complete and send with any referred or transferred patient a medical résumé giving diagnosis and treatment. This résumé should be enclosed in a sealed envelope and a copy made a permanent part of the emergency record.
- To determine and certify the cause and time of death (8–5), or to certify to dead on arrival (DOA) cases (8–7).
- To cooperate with family members, clergy, members of law enforcement agencies, press, photographers and other interested persons within the limits established by the

physician-patient relationship, applicable legal restrictions and staff and hospital regulations.

- To use courtesy, consideration, tact and kindness in relations not only with patients but also with designated spokespersons for the family and significant others.
- To complete a detailed, concise, accurate *and legible* record on each patient, specifying not only *what* was done but also *why* it was done, if the reasons are not self-evident.

72. Service Personnel and Dependents

Only supportive emergency care and measures to prevent aggravation of a condition should be given to active members of any of the branches of the Armed Services and their dependents—enough to insure arrival at the closest Armed Services or Government hospital or clinic in satisfactory condition. Obvious or suspected fractures and dislocations should not be x-rayed unless, in the opinion of the attending emergency physician, films are necessary for adequate interim care. The injured parts should be splinted and pain, shock, etc. controlled by the usual measures. Transportation, by government ambulance if necessary, usually can be arranged by telephone communication with the proper government facility and medical admissions officer of the day in the vicinity.

If medical personnel must be in attendance during transportation (4), establish and document who will provide this care.

The opinion of the present treating physician regarding transportability of the patient should prevail until, when circumstances indicate, there has been personal medical evaluation by an individual from the entity that will be responsible for ongoing care.

Some private health insurance plans (such as Ross Loos Health Plan, Kaiser Foundation Health Plan) with specified physician and facility designation have similar restrictions, except for immediate emergency conditions; notification to these facilities regarding treatment of their members should also be made as soon as possible.

73. Subpoenas

73–1. APPEARANCE IN RESPONSE TO SUBPOENA

Any attending emergency personnel can be subpoenaed to appear in person before any court, administrative agency or investigative board by any party to a related medicolegal action. Attendance at the specified time and place is mandatory provided a legal subpoena (73–4) has been properly served and accepted (73–5). Noncompliance constitutes contempt of court and can be punished accordingly.

73–2. RELIEF FROM UNREASONABLY SHORT NOTICE

If a physician is served with a subpoena that specifies appearance before an administrative agency, investigative board or court on unreasonably or unusually short notice (for example, service at 5 P.M. to appear the next day at 9:30 A.M.), the physician or physician's attorney usually can obtain relief by informing the clerk of the agency, board or court of other pressing medical duties, with the request that attendance be continued to a later time so that arrangements can be made in advance for attendance. Seven days is usually considered reasonable notice.

73–3. DUCES TECUM

A subpoena duces tectum is a court, administrative board or law enforcement investigative agency order that requires production of certain specified documents at a specified place at a given time. This material may include original x-rays and business office records in addition to the medical chart.

73–4. REQUIREMENTS FOR A LEGAL SUBPOENA

- Specification of the date, time and place of appearance.
- Signature of the proper official of the issuing court, board or administrative agency.
- Impress of the official seal of the issuing agency, board or court on the original document.

73–5. PROPER SERVICE

This, as a rule, is considered to mean presentation of the original subpoena (with its impressed official seal) to the subpoenee for inspection, and, upon request at time of service, payment in advance of the appropriate witness fee plus mileage at the established rate per mile from the place at which the subpoena is served to the location of the court or agency at which the subpoenee is ordered to appear.

74. Testimony in Court

Any physician or other emergency personnel is required by law to appear before an investigative agency, administrative agency or in court in response to a properly completed and served subpoena (*73–4; 74–5*). He or she may be required to appear as a factual (nonmedical) witness (*74–1*), as a medical witness (*74–2*) or as an expert medical witness (*74–3*).

74–1. NONMEDICAL TESTIMONY

In some instances, physicians may be called upon to testify regarding an incident concerning which they have firsthand (not hearsay) knowledge. As witnesses they have the same rights, privileges and obligations as any other witness and are entitled to the nominal witness fee (plus mileage). This fee and mileage allowance must be paid in advance by the server at the time that the subpoena is served.

74–2. MEDICAL TESTIMONY

Any physician may be required to testify regarding findings on medical examination or treatment of any patient under his or her care, subject to the privileged communication rule. This means that confidential information obtained during examination or treatment or at any other time when the patient-physician relationship is in effect cannot be divulged except under certain circumstances. These circumstances vary in details in different localities but in general are as follows:

- With the permission of the patient (or patient's legal guardian).
- In criminal cases.
- In civil cases in which there is a question of the mental competency of a deceased person.
- In personal injury or wrongful death cases.
- In certain will contests.

The usual medical witness fees apply unless prior arrangements have been made with the attorney. However, if the line between medical testimony and testimony as an expert witness (*74–3*) is crossed by the request of legal counsel for either side for interpretation of the factual medical testimony or for a medical opinion of any type, the physician may request that the presiding officer of the agency, board or court classify him or her as an expert witness (*74–3*).

74–3. EXPERT WITNESS

Generally speaking, any person who possesses specialized knowledge or can aid the trier of fact about the subject involved significantly beyond those with common experience may be classified as an "expert witness." Therefore, in most medical matters any physician may be qualified as an expert witness (except see *68–3*) even if he or she is not particularly trained or experienced in a given specialty, and even if he or she has not actually examined or treated the patient. Other credentials affect the weight given to the expert's testimony.

An expert medical witness may be required to answer hypothetical questions under oath and to give an opinion concerning diagnosis, disability, further treatment and prognosis. Whenever possible, questions should be answered by "Yes" or "No," but if qualifications are required, they will usually be allowed by the presiding judge or hearing officer. If sufficient facts to permit an accurate and fair answer have not been incorporated in the hypothetical question, the physician may so state and defer the answer until the presiding officer has given a ruling regarding the need for further information.

74–4. PREPARATION OF A COURT CASE

- Careful review of the written records made at the time of prior examinations.
- Pretrial conferences with the attorney.
- Arrangements regarding expert witness fees—including presentation of the billing—should be made with the attorney in advance of court appearance. These fees vary in different localities but are usually based on the time spent in preparation, pretrial conferences and anticipated time in court (the billing should state "for appearance" rather than for "for testimony" in court). *Under no circumstances* should this fee be on a contingent basis. It should always apply in full, regardless of the outcome of the case—won, lost, dismissed or settled out of court.

74–5. OBLIGATIONS OF A PHYSICIAN AS A WITNESS

- To dress and act in a respectful, conservative and dignified manner. To give testimony distinctly with candor, sincerity and accuracy, avoiding medical terminology as much as possible and explaining those medical terms that are used. Above all, "talking down" to the jury in a condescending manner should be avoided. The original medical record can often be used for reference but if so used is admissible as evidence.
- To avoid taking sides, especially by coloring testimony or acting as a medical advocate in other ways.
- To remain calm, even-tempered and alert under cross-examination and to avoid trying to appear clever in debate.
- To keep differences of opinion with other physicians on an impersonal professional level.
- To abide scrupulously by any and all rulings made by the trial judge or presiding officer. Questions concerning privileged information or other similar matters can be asked directly of, and decided by, the judge or hearing officers.

75. Worker's Compensation (Industrial or Occupational) Cases

75–1. MANAGEMENT ON INITIAL VISIT

Special forms for reporting industrial cases (injuries or illnesses caused by or arising out of employment) are used almost universally. All medical information for these forms must be completed by the emergency physician (aided by the staff if desired) at the first examination. Written permission of the patient is not necessary to send an industrial injury report; by requesting treatment as an industrial case, the patient creates a limited waiver of rights to a confidential patient-physician relationship concerning care of the claimed industrial problem with respect to the employer and the industrial insurance-carrier.

Reports to employers, insurance carriers and governmental agencies must be completed and submitted as soon as possible after the first examination. Therefore, for adequate reporting, it is essential that all spaces on the industrial form be filled in. The following is an explanation of the subheadings found on many industrial injury and illness forms.

75–2. EXAMINATION DATA FOR EMERGENCY REPORT

A detailed record of each emergency patient interviewed, examined and/or treated should be written and signed (not initialed) by the attending physician as soon as possible after the patient is seen. The record on each patient should be written legibly in ink and should contain the following information:

Occupation: This gives a perspective on the physical and mental stresses of the job and is helpful in both industrial and nonindustrial problems. Get a brief report on supplemental data as needed (e.g., part-time jobs, non–employment-related and recreational activities).

Chief Complaint(s): What problem caused the patient to seek aid?

History of Onset

- *Illness*: Duration, type of onset, chronological development of symptoms (i.e., when and where signs and symptoms were noted), previous attacks.
- *Injuries*: What? When? Where? How?

Physical Findings: Temperature, respiration, pulse and blood pressure should be recorded. The physical examination (and recording thereof) should be sufficiently complete to give a word picture of the problem at hand. Significant negative as well as positive findings should be recorded. See *1, ABC's of Emergency Problem Analysis*, for assistance in physical exam as needed.

X-rays: The attending physician's interpretation of any films should be recorded (*21*). Careful examination of the films generally will disclose the presence of any pathologic process. A confirmatory reading by a roentgenologist should be obtained as soon as necessary.

Laboratory Results: The results of any laboratory tests performed by, under the direction of or by order of the attending physician should be recorded and appropriate action indicated for significantly abnormal results.

Diagnosis

- Whenever possible, the diagnosis should be specific and descriptive and must indicate the severity of the condition. "Bruised finger" is inadequate for industrial reporting purposes; "mild contusion volar surface distal phalanx left index finger" gives a clear picture of the location, type and severity of the injury. If a definitive diagnosis cannot be established, a symptom diagnosis and probable cause may be given, indicating the relationship (or lack thereof) of the injury to the work history. "Diagnosis deferred" and other disclaimers of any medical opinion are worthless and should not be used as isolated statements or for want of an absolute diagnosis. Citing probable cause is adequate.
- Descriptive names for the digits of the hand should always be given—i.e., thumb, index finger, middle (or long) finger, ring finger and little finger (the terms "first," "second," etc., should never be used). Finger joints should be specified—i.e., "metacarpophalangeal," "proximal interphalangeal," and "distal interphalangeal" (not "first," "second" and "third").
- Negative findings or words of quantitative description are of value in diagnosis and prognosis. *Examples*: "Concussion of the brain—mild; neurologic exam negative." "Laceration volar surface middle phalanx left ring finger—tendons, vascular and nerve supply not injured." "Severe contusion right supraorbital ridge. No evidence of damage to eye." (Record visual acuity.)
- If there is any question as to whether the medical problem is truly job-related, this should be entered in the report.
- Symptoms with or without an anatomic location do not constitute an adequate diagnosis (e.g., metatarsalgia, back pain, cephalgia; pain, left wrist). If the probable cause is not known, then so state (e.g., "cephalgia of unknown cause, type to be determined") or list the diagnostic possibilities.

Accident Sole Cause or Previous Impairment?

- In the majority of accident cases, the event is the sole cause. Certain unusual circumstances, such as syncope causing a fall with resultant injury, or incarceration developing in a previously asymptomatic hernia, do occur. These should be specified under "Contributing Causes." In general, granting of industrially related temporary disability is not reduced because of pre-existent factors; however, such factors may become important in apportionment of later permanent disability ratings.

- Pre-existent condition such as arthritis, limited function from old trauma or disease, previous operative procedures, etc., should be listed. Aggravation of a pre-existent condition by an industrial injury is a frequent and legitimate cause of compensable disability.

Treatment

Include under this heading:

- Medications administered or prescribed; include immunizing injections, antibiotics, analgesics, etc.
- Therapy for shock—time, type, amount.
- Supportive measures—artificial ventilation, parenteral fluids, O_2.
- Splints and casts—type, time applied.
- Gastric lavage—with what? Results?
- Tourniquets—time applied and removed.
- Surgical repair—anesthesia, length of laceration, number and type of sutures.
- Instructions on home treatment.

Disposition

- Sent home? At what time? How and with whom (if impaired capacity)?
- Hospitalized? Where? At what time? Sent by private car or ambulance?
- Referred? To whom? Specify time, name and address of physician.
- Follow-up care arrangements should be in writing, with a copy given to patient before leaving.

Further Treatment (Duration): This is important information for insurance companies or employers because a reserve to meet all expenses of the case usually is set up as soon as the First Report of Injury is received. It is better for all concerned to slightly overestimate than to underestimate the treatment period.

Temporary Disability (How Long). If no time loss from regular work is anticipated, indicate as "N.T.L." (No Time Lost) or "None." If in the opinion of the examining physician the patient is unable to work at all, the expected duration of disability should be given in days, weeks or months. Avoid medically certifying time off prior to initial exam.

Medical recovery and minimal disruption of socioeconomic status are enhanced by the earliest safe return to work. If the patient can't do regular work, presume the availability (or potential availability) of limited duty and write the work prescription accordingly with permitted and prescribed activities; the patient should return to this modified work as soon as possible. The employer can then determine if a suitable position exists or can be created—usually every effort is made to provide one.

Permanent Disability (P.D.). On the initial visit, frequently only an estimate regarding ultimate permanent disability can be made unless the injury is mild or clearly delineated. Answer "yes" or "no." If "yes," specify:

- Amputation—exact level.
- Expected loss of function from limited motion, weakness or deformity—slight, moderate or marked.
- Cosmetic disfigurement sometimes constitutes a ratable permanent disability. For instance, an extensive disfiguring scar on the face might be a handicap in the labor market, whereas a scar on any portion of the body that is usually covered would not be.

Clinic Return: The patient should be told to return to the medical clinic at a specific time on a specified date, with the date entered on the form. An instruction sheet given to the patient indicating possible complications and to whom to report is preferable to general instructions such as "Return if doesn't feel better" or "P.R.N." If discharged from care, so state.

Referred To: If "Clinic Return" has been filled out, this space can be left blank. Otherwise, specify the physician to whom the patient is being referred, the hospital to which he or she has been instructed to report and/or the special examination or procedure the patient is to have.

Appendix

COMMONLY USED ABBREVIATIONS AND SYMBOLS*

ā ante, before
a acute
A auscultation
AAP or **APAP** acetaminophen
Ab antibody
AB abortion
ABB airway/breathing/bleeding
ABBCS airway/breathing/bleeding/circulation/sensorium
ABC airway/breathing/circulation
ABC's outline of material
abd abdomen
ABG's arterial blood gases
ABR alternate birthing room
AC alternating current
A-C acromioclavicular joint
ac before meals
ACEP American College of Emergency Physicians
ACGIH American Conference of Governmental Industrial Hygienists
ACLS advanced cardiac life support
ACTH adrenocorticotropin hormone
AD right ear
ADL activities of daily living
ad lib as desired
A-E above elbow
af afebrile
AF atrial fibrillation
AFB acid-fast bacillus
Ag antigen
A/G albumin/globin ratio
AGA appropriate for gestational age
$AgNO_3$ silver nitrate
AHA American Heart Association
AI aortic insufficiency
ALS advanced life support
AK above knee
AP apical pulse
A-P anterior-posterior
A+P auscultation and percussion
$A_2 > P_2$ aortic 2nd heart sound > pulmonic 2nd heart sound
alb albumin
ALT alanine transferase (=SGPT)
AM morning, after midnight
ama against medical advice
AMA American Medical Association
amb ambulate
amp ampule
ant anterior
APAP acetaminophen
APC aspirin with phenacetin/caffeine
approx approximately
appt appointment
ARC American Red Cross
ARD acute respiratory distress
ARDS acute respiratory distress syndrome
ARF acute renal failure
ARM artificial rupture of membranes
AS left ear
AS Ⓜ aortic stenosis murmur
ASA aspirin
ASAP as soon as possible
ASCVD arteriosclerotic cardiovascular disease
ASD atrial septal defect

*The abbreviations and symbols listed here are among those more commonly used in medicine, with special emphasis on terms used in emergency and occupational medicine. To avoid confusion, none should be used in a medical center unless they are agreed upon by all who will use them; as the JCAH (Joint Commission of Accreditation of Hospitals) notes: "Each abbreviation or symbol should have only one meaning."

Note: If the reader has additional abbreviation(s) of value in the above categories or other relevant data, please direct to Flint's Emergency Treatment and Management c/o W. B. Saunders Co., West Washington Square, Philadelphia, PA 19105.

ASH asymmetrical septal hypertrophy
ASHD arteriosclerotic heart disease
AST aspartate transferase (= SGOT)
ATC around the clock
ATLS advanced trauma life support
ATRO atropine
AU both ears
AUB abnormal uterine bleeding
AV arteriovenous
A-V atrioventricular
AVM arteriovenous malformation
ax axillary

Ba barium
BBB bundle branch block (L or R)
B/E base excess
BE barium enema
bid twice daily
Bili (t/d) bilirubin (total/direct)
BK below knee
BKA below knee amputation
BLS basic life support
BM bowel movement
BMR basal metabolic rate
BOW bag of waters (amniotic sac)
BP blood pressure
BPD biparietal diameter
BPH benign prostatic hypertrophy
BR bathroom
BRET bretylium tosylate
BRP bathroom privileges
BS bowel sounds
bs breath sounds
BSA body surface area
BSC bedside commode
BSP Bromosulphalein
BSO bilateral salpingo-oophorectomy
BTL bilateral tubal ligation
BUN blood urea nitrogen
BUS Bartholin's, urethral and Skene's glands
BW body weight

C ceiling (toxic limit)
°C centigrade
$\bar{c}$ with
C_1C_2 first and second cervical vertebrae (etc., to C_7)
Ca calcium
CA cancer
CAD coronary artery disease
cap capsule
CAT computerized axial tomography (scan)
cath catheter
CBC complete blood count
CBF cerebral blood flow
CC chief complaint
cc cubic centimeter
CCM critical care medicine
CCPR cerebrocardiopulmonary resuscitation
CCU coronary care unit
CD communicable disease
CHF congestive heart failure
CHO carbohydrate (or in context: blood sugar)
chol cholesterol
CICU cardiac intensive care unit
cl clear
Cl chlorine
c/o complains of
co cardiac output
CO carbon monoxide
cm centimeter
CMI cell-mediated immunodeficiency
cmpd compound
CMV cytomegalic virus
CNS central nervous system
CO_2 carbon dioxide
COAD chronic obstructive airway disease
COHb carboxyhemoglobin
COLD chronic obstructive lung disease
conc concentration
cont continue
COPD chronic obstructive pulmonary disease
cor heart
CP cerebral palsy
CPAP continuous positive airway pressure
CPD cephalopelvic disproportion
CPR cardiopulmonary resuscitation
CPK creatinine phosphokinase
Cr creatinine

CRF chronic renal failure
C&S culture and sensitivity
C/S cesarean section
CSM carotid sinus massage
CS continue same
CSF cerebrospinal fluid
CT computerized tomography
cu cubic
CV cardiovascular
cva costovertebral angle
CVA cerebrovascular accident
CVD cerebrovascular disease
CVP central venous pressure
Cx cervix
CXR chest x-ray

d or **D** day
D_1D_2 first and second dorsal (etc., to D_{12})
D5RL dextrose 5% with Ringer's lactate
D5¼NS dextrose 5% with ¼% normal saline
D5W dextrose 5% in water
D50W dextrose 50% in water
DB deep breath
D&C dilatation and curettage
D/C discharge
dc discontinue
DC direct current
DDAVP desamino-D arginine vasopressin
DDP Doctors for Disaster Preparedness
defib defibrillation
DEXA dexamethasone
DI diabetes insipidus
diag or **Dx** diagnosis
diff differential blood count
DIP distal interphalangeal joint
DM diabetes mellitus
DMSO dimethylsulfoxide
DNA deoxyribonucleic acid
DNPA do not publish, adopted
DNPK do not publish, keeping
DNR do not resuscitate
DNS dextrose in normal saline
DOA dead on arrival
DOE dyspnea on exertion
DOP dopamine
DPT diphtheria, pertussis, tetanus
Dr. doctor
DSA digital subtraction angiography
dsg dressing
DSM III Diagnostic and Statistical Manual of Mental Disorders, 3rd ed.
DTR deep tendon reflex
DT's delirium tremens
DVT deep vein thrombosis
Dx see diag

EBS Emergency Broadcast System
EBV Epstein-Barr virus
ECC endocervical curettage
ECF extended care facility
ECG or **EKG** electrocardiogram
ECHO echocardiogram
ED emergency department
EDC estimated date of confinement
EEG electroencephalogram
EENT ears, eyes, nose, throat
EFW estimated fetal weight
e.g. for example
EGTA esophageal gastric tube airway
EHC external heart compression
EKG see ECG
EL or **exp lap** exploratory laparotomy
EMG electromyogram
EMD electromechanical dissociation
EMS emergency medical services
EMT emergency medical technician
ENT ear, nose, throat
EOA esophageal obturator airway
EOM extraocular movements
EPI epinephrine
epis episiotomy
ER emergency room (*note:* ED more common now)
esp especially
ESR erythrocyte sedimentation rate
ETOH ethyl alcohol
ETS emergency temporary standard
ETT endotracheal tube

EUA examination under anesthesia
exam examination
exp expired
exp lap see EL
ext extremities

F Fahrenheit
fb fingerbreadth
FB foreign body
FBS fasting blood sugar
Fe iron
FEC freestanding emergency center
FEV_1 forced expiratory volume in 1 second
FH family history
FHR fetal heart rate
FHT fetal heart tone
FHS fetal heart sounds
fib. fibrillation
FIO_2 fractional inspired O_2 concentration
flex. flexion
FSH follicle-stimulating hormone
FTI free thyroxin index
FTND full-term normal delivery
FTT fingers to toes
f/u follow-up
FUO fever of unknown origin
FVC forced vital capacity
Fx fracture

G gravida
g or **gm** gram
G+ gram-positive
gav gavage
GB gallbladder
GC gonorrhea
GE gastroenteritis
GG gamma globulin
GI gastrointestinal
gm see **g**
Gr grain
GSW gunshot wound
gtt drops
GU genitourinary
gyn gynecology

h or **hr** hour
H_2O water
HA headache
HACE high-altitude cerebral edema
HAPE high-altitude pulmonary edema
HAV hepatitis A virus
HBIG hepatitis B immune globulin
HBO hyperbaric oxygen
HBP high blood pressure
HBV hepatitis B virus
HC hydrocortisone
HCl hydrochloric acid
HCO_3 bicarbonate
Hct hematocrit
HCVD hypertensive cardiovascular disease
HDCV human diploid cell vaccine
HEENT head, eyes, ears, nose, throat
Hg mercury
Hgb hemoglobin
HJR hepatojugular reflex
HM Heimlich maneuver
HMD hyaline membrane disease
H&P history and physical
HP Harvard pump
HPF high-power field
HPI history of present illness
hr see **h**
HR heart rate
hs at hour of sleep
HS heart sounds
HSV herpes simplex virus (types I and II)
ht height
HT heart tone
Hx history

I iodine
^{131}I radioactive iodine
IC icteric
ICC incident control center
ICCE intracapsular cataract extraction
ICH intracranial hemorrhage
ICS intercostal space
ICU intensive care unit
I&D incision and drainage

i.e. that is
IgA immune globulin type A (also types D, E, G, M)
IHSS idiopathic hypertropic subaortic stenosis
IIP increased intracranial pressure
IKD internal knee derangement
IM intramuscular
Imp impression
I&O intake and output
IOP intraocular pressure
IP interphalangeal
IPPB intermittent positive pressure breathing
ISG immune serum globulin
Iso isoproterenol
ITP idiopathic thrombocytopenic purpura
IUD intrauterine device (contraceptive)
IUP intrauterine pregnancy
IV intravenous
IVH intravenous hyperalimentation
IVP intravenous pyelogram

jct junction
jt joint
JVD jugular venous distension

K potassium
kg kilogram
kgbw kilogram of body weight
KUB kidney, ureter, bladder

L or l liter
L or Ⓛ left
L_1L_2 first and second lumbar
LAC long arm cast
lac laceration
lat lateral
lb pound
LBP low back pain
LBW low birth weight
LC_{50} lethal concentration, atmosphere, to 50%
LD_{50} lethal dose, by stated route, to 50%
L+D labor and delivery
LDH lactodehydrogenase
LE lupus erythematosus
LFD low forceps delivery
LFT liver function tests
LGA large for gestational age
LIDO lidocaine
liq liquids
LMP last menstrual period
LLC long leg cast
LLD long leg discrepancy
LLE left lower extremity
LLL left lower lung
LLQ left lower quadrant
LOA left occiput anterior
LOC loss of consciousness
LOP left occiput posterior
LP lumbar puncture
LPF low-power field
LR labor room
L-S lumbosacral
L/S lecithin/sphingomyelin ratio
L+S liver and spleen
LSK liver, spleen, kidney
LTB laryngotracheobronchial(itis)
LTC low transverse cesarean
LUE left upper extremity
LUL left upper lobe
LUQ left upper quadrant
LVH left ventricular hypertrophy
L+W living and well
LYMPH lymphocytes
Lx laboratory examination(s)

m or ⓜ murmur
M.A. metatarsus adductus
MAST military anti-shock trousers
MC metacarpal
mcg or μg microgram
MCH mean corpuscular hemoglobin
MCHC mean corpuscular hemoglobin concentration
MCI mass casualty incident
MCL midclavicular line
MCP metacarpophalangeal
MCV mean corpuscular volume
mec meconium

med medication
MEDEM medical emergency; laboratory report needed stat
mEq milliequivalent
Mg magnesium
mg milligram
mg/m³ milligram of substance per cubic meter of air
MH marital history
MHb methemoglobin(emia)
MI myocardial infarction
MICU medical intensive care unit
min minute
ml milliliter
mm Hg millimeters of mercury
MMK Marshall-Marchetti procedure
Mn manganese
MOM milk of magnesia
mono monocyte
M-P metacarpophalangeal
mppcf millions of particles per cubic foot air
MS morphine sulfate
MS Ⓜ mitral stenosis murmur
MSA medical short appointment
MSW medical social worker
M-T-A mouth-to-airway (mask, tube, etc.)
M-T-M mouth-to-mouth (resuscitation)
Muscle abbreviations see separate listing on page 768
MVA motor vehicle accident
MVL mitral valve leaflet
MVP mitral valve prolapse

ⓝ normal
N nitrogen
Na sodium
NaBi sodium bicarbonate ("bicarb")
NAD no apparent (acute) distress
NAR Narcan (naloxone)
NB newborn
NBP needle biopsy of prostate
neg negative
neuro neurological
NG nasogastric
NIOSH National Institute of Occupational Safety and Health
NKA no known allergies
no. number
noct or **noc** nocturnal (night)
NPO nothing by mouth
N or **V** nausea or vomiting
NS normal saline
NSAID/NSAIA nonsteroidal anti-inflammatory drug or agent
NSILA nonsuppressible insulin-like activity
NSR normal sinus rhythm
NSVD normal spontaneous vaginal delivery
NTG nitroglycerine
NV neurovascular
NVD neck vein distention
NWB non–weight-bearing

ō none
O_2 oxygen
OB obstetrics
OBS organic brain syndrome
occ occasional
OCT oxytocin challenge test
OD overdose
OD right eye
OFC occipital frontal circumference
oint or **ung** ointment
OJ orange juice
OOB out of bed
OP operation
OPD outpatient department
ophthal or **ophth** ophthalmology
OR operating room
ORIF open reduction with internal fixation
Ortho orthopedics
OS left eye
osm osmole, osmolarity
OSHA Occupational Safety and Health Administration
OTC over-the-counter (nonprescription medication)
OU both eyes
oz ounce

p pulse
P phosphorus
p̄ after
P_2 pulmonic second heart sound

P-A posterior-anterior
P&A percussion and auscultation
PA pulmonary artery
$PaCO_2$ arterial partial pressure of carbon dioxide
palp palpable, palpation
PaO_2 arterial partial pressure of oxygen
PAR postanesthesia room
PARA number of deliveries
PAT paroxysmal atrial tachycardia
path pathology
PB phenobarbital
PBS phenobarbital sulphate
pc or **Pc** after meals
PCN penicillin
PCO_2 or **Pco_2** partial pressure of carbon dioxide
PCP phenocyclidine
PCS patient collecting station
PDA patent ductus arteriosus
PE pulmonary embolus
ped pediatrics
PEEP positive end expiratory pressure
PEFR peak expiratory flow rate
PERL pupils equal and react to light
PERRLA pupils equal, round, reactive to light and accommodation
pH hydrogen ion concentration
PH past history
PHN public health nurse
PHS Public Health Service
PI present illness
PICU pediatric intensive care unit
PID pelvic inflammatory disease
PIP proximal interphalangeal joint
PKU phenylketonuria
PM afternoon
PMB postmenopausal bleeding
PMI point of maximal impulse
PML prolapse mitral leaflet
PMN polymorphonuclear cells
PMP previous menstrual period
PND paroxysmal nocturnal dyspnea
PO by mouth
PO_2 or **Po_2** partial pressure of oxygen
POD postoperative day
POF position of function
pos positive
post posterior
pp postpartum
PPD positive protein derivative
ppb parts per billion
ppm parts per million
PR pulse rate
prep preparation
pre-op preoperative
PRN or **prn** as needed
PRO procainamide
prog prognosis
PROM premature rupture of membranes
pro time or **PT** prothrombin time
pt patient
PT see **pro time**
P.T. physical therapy
PTT partial thromboplastin time
PUD peptic ulcer disease
PVC premature ventricular contractions
PVR pulmonary vascular resistance
PVS percussion, vibration, suction
PZI protamine zinc insulin
PWB partial weight-bearing
Px physical examination

q every
qh every hour
q 2 d every 2 days
q 4 h every 4 hours
qd every day
qid four times per day
qn or **qnoc** every night
qns quantity not sufficient
qod every other day
qs quantity sufficient

r respirations
R or **Ⓡ** or **rt** right
RA rheumatoid arthritis
RBC red blood count
rbc red blood cell
RDS respiratory distress syndrome

resp respiratory, respiration
RF rheumatic fever
RHD rheumatic heart disease
RHF right heart failure
RIA radioimmunoassay
RIS radioisotope scan
rks retrograde kidney study
RKS renal kidney stone
RL Ringer's lactate
RLE right lower extremity
RLL right lower lobe
RLQ right lower quadrant
RML right middle lobe
RNA ribonucleic acid
RND radical neck dissection
R/O rule out
ROAD reversible obstructive airway disease
ROM range of motion
ROS review of systems
ROT right occiput transverse
RR regular rhythm
R/R respiratory rate
RS Reye's syndrome
RSR regular sinus rhythm
rt right
RT respiratory therapy
RTA renal tubular acidosis
RTC return to clinic
RTW return to work
RUE right upper extremity
RUL right upper lobe
RUQ right upper quadrant
RV right ventricle
RVH right ventricular hypertrophy
Rx therapy or treatment

$\bar{s}$ without
S_4 fourth heart sound
SAC short arm cast
SAH subarachnoid hemorrhage
SB sternal border
SBE subacute bacterial endocarditis
SC or **SQ, subcu, sub q** subcutaneous
SCA sickle cell anemia
SCI spinal cord injury
sed rate sedimentation rate
SFB surgical foreign body
SG or **sp gr** specific gravity
SGA small for gestational age
SGOT serum glutamic oxaloacetic transaminase (=AST)
SGPT serum glutamic pyruvic transaminase (=ALT)
SH social history
SI stress incontinence
SIADH syndrome of inappropriate antidiuretic hormone
SICU surgical intensive care unit
sl slight
SL sublingual
SLC short leg cast
SLE systemic lupus erythematosus
SLNWBC short leg non–weight-bearing cast
SLNWC Short leg non-walking cast
SLR straight leg raising
SMR submucous resection
SOAP subjective objective assessment plan
SOB shortness of breath
sod bicarb sodium bicarbonate ($NaHCO_3$)
sol solution
S/P status post
spec specimen
sp fl spinal fluid
sp gr see SG
SR system review
SRM or **SROM** spontaneous rupture of membranes
SQ see **SC**
sq squamous
SS soap suds
ss one half
Staph staphylococcus
stat immediately, at once
STEL short-term exposure limit (15 min. continuous max.)
Strep streptococcus
Subcu or **sub q** see **SC**
SVC superior vena cava
SVT supraventricular tachycardia
Sx symptoms and signs

T or **t** temperature
T_3 tri-iodothyronine
T_4 tetraiodothyronine (thyroxine)

T_4; T_8 T-cell helper (inducer); T-cell suppressor
T&A tonsillectomy and adenoidectomy
tab tablet
TAB therapeutic abortion
TAH total abdominal hysterectomy
TAHBSO total abdominal hysterectomy bilateral salpingo-oophorectomy
TAT tetanus antitoxin
TB or **TBC** tuberculosis
tbsp or **tbl** tablespoon
T&C type and crossmatch
TCN tetracycline
$TCPO_2$ transcutaneous partial pressure of oxygen
TC&NP throat culture and nasopharyngeal culture
TCA tricyclic antidepressant
TD temporary disability
TDG touch-down gait
TEN toxic epidermal necrolysis
TEV talipes equino varus
TG triglycerides
THR total hip replacement
TIA transient ischemic attack
tib-fib tibia and fibula
tid three times per day
TIG tetanus immune globulin
tinct or **tr** tincture
TK tourniquet
TKO to keep open
TKR total knee replacement
TL tubal ligation
TLC total lung capacity
tlv total lung volume
TLV—C Threshold Limit Value—ceiling (absolute)
TM tympanic membrane
TMJ temporomandibular joint
TNS transcutaneous nerve stimulator
t.o. telephone order
TOA tubo-ovarian abscess
TPN total parenteral nutrition
TPR or **tpr** temperature, pulse, respiration
tr see tinct
trach trachea, tracheostomy
TSH thyroid-stimulating hormone
tsp teaspoon
TUR transurethral resection
TURB transurethral resection of the bladder
TURP transurethral resection of prostate
TV tidal volume
TWA time-weighted average
Tx traction

U unit
UA urinalysis
UAC umbilical artery catheter
UC uterine contractions
UGI upper gastrointestinal (series)
ung or **oint** ointment
UPJ ureteropelvic junction
URI upper respiratory infection
urol urology
US ultrasound
UTI urinary tract infection

VA visual acuity
vag vagina, vaginal
VC or **vit cap** vital capacity
VD venereal disease
VE vaginal exam/efficiency
vf visual fields
V-fib or **VF** ventricular fibrillation
VDRL Venereal Disease Research Laboratory (serology syphilis test)
VH vaginal hysterectomy
VI volume index
vit or **Vit** vitamin
vit cap see VC
v.o. verbal orders
vol volume
v-p shunt ventriculoperitoneal shunt
Verp verapamil
VS vital signs
VSD ventricular septal defect
VSS vital signs stable
V-tach or **VT** ventricular tachycardia

WBC white blood count
WC wheelchair

WD well-developed
WDWN well-developed and well-nourished
WF white female
WM white male
WNL within normal units
WPW Wolf-Parkinson-White syndrome
w-sec watt-second (=joule)
wt weight

X "times" (e.g., 4 × 6 = 24) or "for" (e.g., × 3 days)

y/o or **Y/O** Years old
yr year

Zn Zinc

Muscle/Anatomy Abbreviations*

Movement	±	Anatomic Location	±	Length/Depth Size/Position
AB abductor		**B** brachial (arm)		**Ant** anterior
Ad adductor		**C** carpi (wrist)		**Br** brevis (short)
E extensor		**D** digitorum (digits)		**I** interosseus
ER external rotation		**H** hallucis (great toe)		**L** longus (long)
F flexor		**P** pollicis (thumb)		**Max** maximum
IR internal rotation		**R** radial (lateral forearm)		**Mini** minimus
Pro pronator		**T** or **Tib** tibial (leg)		**Post** posterior
Sup supinator		**U** ulnar (medial forearm)		**Pr** profundus (deep)
				S superficialis

Some Common Abbreviations

AbPBr abductor pollicis brevis
AbPL abductor pollicis longus
AdL adductor longus
AdP adductor pollicis
ECRL extensor carpi radialis longus
ECRBr extensor carpi radialis brevis
ECU extensor carpi ulnaris
ED extensor digitorum
EHL extensor hallucis longus
EPBr extensor pollicis brevis
EPL extensor pollicis longus
FDPr flexor digitorum profundus
FDS flexor digitorum superficialis
FHL flexor hallucis longus
FPL flexor pollicis longus
FCR flexor carpi radialis
FCU flexor carpi ulnaris

Miscellaneous (Common Usage and Slang)

Achilles tendon of the triceps surae muscle (gastrocnemius-soleus group)
Adductors adductor magnus, longus, minimus (thigh)
Ant Tib tibialis anterior muscle
Delt's deltoideus (shoulder)
Gastroc gastrocnemius-soleus group (calf)
Glut's gluteus maximus, medius and minimus (buttocks)
Hamstrings *inner*: sartorius, gracilis, semimembranosus, semitendinosus; *outer*: biceps femoris (posterior thigh)
Lat's latissimus dorsi (posterior shoulder girdle)
Pec's pectoralis major and minor (anterior shoulder girdle)
Quad's quadriceps femoris: rectus femoris, vastus intermedius, vastus lateralis, vastus medialis (anterior thigh)

---

*Partial listing.

SYMBOLS

↑ increase (d)
↓ decrease (d)
= equal
≅ equivalent to
≠ Is not equal to
> greater than
≥ greater than or equal to
< less than
≤ less than or equal to
~ approximately
\+ positive, plus
− negative, minus
± plus or minus; variable equivocal; varies with circumstances
♂ male
♀ female

→ yields or produces
△ change; trimester of pregnancy (e.g., 1st △, 2nd△, 3rd △)
∴ therefore
∠ angle
ⓜ murmur
ⓝ normal
1° primary
2° secondary
Ⓡ right
Ⓛ left
c̄ With
s̄ Without
÷ divided by
% per cent
× multiply by, "times" or "for"

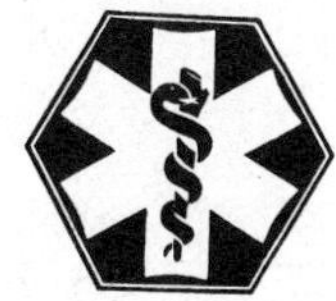

EMERGENCY MEDICAL IDENTIFICATION SYMBOL (designates special medical problem of bearer)

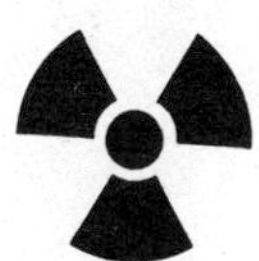

RADIATION HAZARD

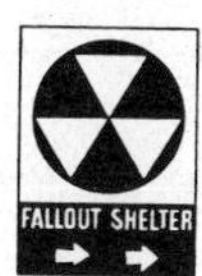

FALLOUT SHELTER

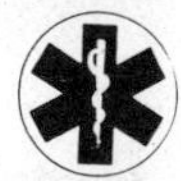

EMERGENCY MEDICAL TECHNICIAN (EMT)
EMT 1, EMT 2 (PARAMEDIC)

CIVIL DEFENSE;
FEDERAL EMERGENCY MANAGEMENT AGENCY

MEDICAL VEHICLE; ARC

APPROXIMATE EQUIVALENTS FOR U.S. AND METRIC MEASUREMENTS

VOLUME

U.S. Customary Unit	U.S. Equivalents		Metric Equivalents	
Liquid Measurement				
Fluid ounce	8.00	fluid drams	29.57	ml
	1.80	cubic inches		
Pint	16.00	fluid ounces	0.473	liter
	28.88	cubic inches		
Quart	2.00	pints	0.946	liter
	57.75	cubic inches		
Gallon	4.00	quarts	3.785	liter
	231.00	cubic inches		
	1⁄31 to 1⁄42 barrel			
Dry Measurement				
Pint	0.5	quart	0.551	liter
	33.6	cubic inches		
Quart	2.0	pints	1.101	liters
	67.2	cubic inches		
	1⁄8 peck or 1⁄32 bushel			

British Imperial Liquid and Dry Measurement	U.S. Equivalents		Metric Equivalents	
Fluid ounce	0.96	U.S. fluid ounce	28.41	ml
	1.73	cubic inches		
Pint	1.03	U.S. dry pints	568.26	ml
	1.20	U.S. liquid pints		
	34.68	cubic inches		
Quart	1.03	U.S. dry quarts	1.14	liters
	1.20	U.S. liquid quarts		
	69.35	cubic inches		
Gallon	1.20	U.S. gallons	4.55	liters
	277.42	cubic inches		

Apothecary Fluid Unit	U.S. Equivalents		Metric Equivalents	
1 minim	0.0167	fluid dram	0.0616	ml
1 fluidrachm or fluidram	0.125	fluid ounce	3.7	ml
1 fluid ounce	8.0	fluid drams	29.57	ml

WEIGHT

U.S. Customary Unit (Avoirdupois)	U.S. Equivalents		Metric Equivalents	
Grain	0.036	dram	64.80	mg
Dram	27.34	grain	1.77	g
	0.063	ounce		
Ounce	16.0	drams	28.35	g
	437.5	grains		
Pound	16.0	ounces	453.59	g
	7000.0	grains	0.45	kg
			(1 kg = 2.2 lb)	

WEIGHT *(Continued)*

Apothecary Weight Unit	U.S. Customary Equivalents		Metric Equivalents	
Scruple	20.0	grains	1.30	g
Dram	60.0	grains	3.89	g
Ounce	480.0	grains	31.10	g
	1.097	avoirdupois ounces		
Pound	12.0	ounces	373.24	g
	0.82	avoirdupois pound	0.37	kg

APPROXIMATE LIQUID MEASURES

(1 ml is approximately equal to 1 cc)

Household Measure (U.S.)	Metric	Apothecary
1 to 2 drops equal (varies with viscosity, specific gravity, type and fullness of container, etc.)	0.6 ml or	1 minim
1 teaspoonful equals about	4.00 ml or	1 fluidram
1 dessertspoonful equals about	8.00 ml or	2 fluidram
1 tablespoonful equals about	15.00 ml or	4 fluidram
1 teacupful equals about	120.00 ml or	4 fluidounces
1 glassful equals about	250.00 ml or	8 fluidounces
one lb of water* or 1 pint equals about	550.00 ml or	16 fluidounces
1 quart equals about	1100.00 ml or	32 fluidounces
1 gallon equals about	4400.00 ml or	128 fluidounces

*"A pint's a pound the world around."

LENGTH

(Approximate equivalents)

1 inch = 2.54 cm	1 cm = 0.3937 inch
1 foot = 0.3048 meter	1 meter = 1.09 yard
1 yard = 0.9144 meter	1 km = 0.6214 land mile
1 mile (land) = 1609 meters (1.6 km) 1760 yd 5280 feet	
1 mile (sea) = 1852 meters (1.8 km)	

To convert

Milliliters into grams

$$\text{Sp. gr.} \times \text{ml} = \text{g}$$

Milliliters into ounces

$$\frac{\text{ml} \times \text{sp gr}}{28.35} = \text{oz}$$

Grams into milliliters

$$\frac{\text{g}}{\text{sp gr}} = \text{ml}$$

Ounces into milliliters

$$\frac{\text{oz} \times 28.35}{\text{sp gr}} = \text{ml}$$

Grains into grams

$$\frac{\text{gr}}{15} = \text{g}$$

Pounds into kilograms

$$\frac{\text{lb}}{2.2} = \text{kg}$$

TABLE OF COMMON DOSE CONVERSIONS

(GRAINS TO GRAMS, APPROXIMATE)

1/200 gr	= 0.3 mg	1/30 gr	= 2 mg	5 gr	= 300 mg (0.3 g)
1/150 gr	= 0.4 mg	1/4 gr	= 15 mg	7½ gr	= 500 mg (0.5 g)
1/120 gr	= 0.5 mg	1/2 gr	= 30 mg	10 gr	= 600 mg (0.6 g)
1/100 gr	= 0.6 mg	1 gr	= 60 mg	15 gr	= 1000 mg (1 g)
1/60 gr	= 1 mg	1½ gr	= 100 mg (0.1 g)		

COMPARATIVE THERMOMETER READINGS

Fahrenheit	Centigrade	Fahrenheit	Centigrade	Fahrenheit	Centigrade
91.0	32.8	96.2	35.6	101.4	38.5
91.2	32.9	96.4	35.7	101.6	38.6
91.4	33.0	96.6	35.8	101.8	38.7
91.6	33.1	96.8	36.0	102.0	38.8
91.8	33.2	97.0	36.1	102.2	39.0
92.0	33.3	97.2	36.2	102.4	39.1
92.2	33.4	97.4	36.3	102.6	39.2
92.4	33.6	97.6	36.4	102.8	39.3
92.6	33.7	97.8	36.6	103.0	39.4
92.8	33.8	98.0	36.7	103.2	39.6
93.0	33.9	98.2	36.8	103.4	39.7
93.2	34.0	98.4	36.9	103.6	39.8
93.4	34.1	98.6	37.0	103.8	39.9
93.6	34.2	98.8	37.1	104.0	40.0
93.8	34.3	99.0	37.2	104.2	40.1
94.0	34.4	99.2	37.3	104.4	40.2
94.2	34.6	99.4	37.4	104.6	40.3
94.4	34.7	99.6	37.6	104.8	40.4
94.6	34.8	99.8	37.7	105.0	40.6
94.8	34.9	100.0	37.8	105.2	40.7
95.0	35.0	100.2	37.9	105.4	40.8
95.2	35.1	100.4	38.0	105.6	40.9
95.4	35.2	100.6	38.1	105.8	41.0
95.6	35.3	100.8	38.2	106.0	41.1
95.8	35.4	101.0	38.3	108.0	42.2
96.0	35.5	101.2	38.4	110.0	43.3

To Convert Centigrade Into Fahrenheit:

Multiply by 9, divide by 5, and add 32 $\left(°F = \frac{°C \times 9}{5} + 32 \right)$

To Convert Fahrenheit Into Centigrade:

Subtract 32, multiply by 5, divide by 9 $\left(°C = \frac{°F - 32 \times 5}{9} \right)$

Clinical Ranges, °F and °C

°F	95	96	96.8	97.7	98.6	99.5	100.4	101.4	102.2	103.1	104
°C	35		36		37		38		39		40

Stages of Human Hypothermia

Slight: 35–32.22°C (95–90°F)
Moderate: 32.21–30°C (89.9–86°F)
Severe: less than 30°C (<86°F)

ADULT NORMAL LABORATORY VALUES*

HEMATOLOGIC VALUES

Determination	Normal Values	Material Analyzed
CBC	WBC 4000–11,000/mm^3† RBC Female = 3.6–5.1 mil/mm^3 Male = 4.1–5.7 mil/mm^3 HGB Female = 11–15 gm/dl Male = 13–17 gm/dl HCT Female = 34–46% Male = 39–51% MCV 80–100 μ^3 MCH 26–34 pg MCHC 31–37%	EDTA (purple top) Whole blood Differential - mean %: Polys 56 Bands 3 Eos 2.7 Baso 0.3 Lymphs 34 Monos 4
Total direct eosinophil count (unopette method)	Newborn 20–850/mm^3 1 yr. old 50–700/mm^3 Adult 0–450/mm^3	EDTA (purple top) Whole blood
Kleihauer test	Reported as fetal/adult RBC ratio; normal = <2.4%	EDTA (purple top) Whole blood
Leukocyte alkaline phosphate	Score = 13–130	Call Hematology Dept.
Mucin test (synovial fluid)	Reported as good, fair, poor, very poor	Heparin (green top)
Osmotic fragility (RBC)	%NaCl — % Hemolysis 0.30 — 97–100 0.40 — 50–90 0.50 — 0–5 0.85 — 0	Heparin (green top) Whole blood
Platelet count	150,000–450,000 per mm^3	EDTA (purple top) Whole blood
Presumptive test for P.N.H. (paroxysmal nocturnal hemoglobinuria)	Little or no hemolysis	Na Citrate (blue top) Whole blood
Retic. count Absolute retic. count	0.5–1.5% 25,000–80,000/mm^3	EDTA (purple top) Whole blood
Sedimentation rate	Westergren: Female = 0–20 mm/hr Male = 0–15 mm/hr Wintrobe: Female = 0–20 mm/hr Male = 0–9 mm/hr	Citrate (blue top) Whole blood EDTA (purple top) Whole blood
Serum hemoglobin	0–15 mg/dl	Serum (red top)
Sickle cell test (Mod. Itano)	Negative (Positive may indicate abnormal Hgb such as S, C, etc. or abnormal protein)	EDTA (purple top) Whole blood
CSF (spinal fluid) (see also *18–29*)	RBC—none seen WBC—0–8/mm^3	Spinal fluid

*Based on normal values from the Sacramento Kaiser-Permanente Medical Center, January 1984. John Rice, M.D., Laboratory Director; Helmut W. Schroeder, Laboratory Manager; and Robert V. Coyne, Ph.D., Assistant Laboratory Manager.

†In pregnancy, normal WBC range increases up to 14,000, with increases in PMN's and stabs (band cells).

COAGULATION VALUES

Determination	Normal Values	Material Analyzed
Aspirin tolerance	Refer to template bleeding time	Call Hematology Dept.*
Bleeding time	Duke—1–5 minutes Template—3.0–7.5 minutes	Call Hematology Dept.
Clot retraction	40–94%	Call Hematology Dept.
Fibrinogen	150–385 mg/dl	Na Citrate (blue top)
Fibrinolysis test	No clot lysis within 72 hrs.	Clot (red top)
Fibrin split products (Thrombin-Wellco test)	Call Hematology laboratory	Call Hematology laboratory
Partial thromboplastin time (activated PTT)	1. "Coagamate" Normal = Less than 38 seconds, routine method. 2. "Fibrometer" Normal = Less than 38 seconds 3. Heparin Therapy = Times should be maintained between 1½ and 2½ times the control.	Na Citrate (blue top)
Protamine sulfate test	Positive = Test shows clot formation or fibrin strands. Negative = Test shows no clot formation or fibrin strands.	Na Citrate (blue top)
Prothrombin time	Normal = Patient value should equal the control range of 10–12 seconds. Coumadin therapy = Times should be 2–2½ times the control.	Na Citrate (blue top)
Thrombin time	Patient time should equal the control or not exceed the control time by a ratio of 1.3	Na Citrate (blue top)
Tourniquet test (Rumpel-Leede)	Normal = 0–20 tiny petechiae may appear.	Call Hematology Dept.

*Call Hematology Department: Special instructions may be necessary.

CHEMISTRY VALUES

Determination	Normal Values	Material Analyzed
Ammonia	20–50 μmol/L	Heparinized* whole blood kept on ice.
Amylase	23–85 IU/L	Serum
Bilirubin	Direct 0–0.4 mg/dl Total 0.2–1.5 mg/dl	Serum
BUN	7–22 mg/dl	Serum
Calcium	8.7–10.2 mg/dl	Serum
CO_2 content (or bicarbonate)	24–32 mEq/L	Plasma (green top)
Chloride	98–108 mEq/L	Serum
CSF Chloride	120–130 mEq/L	Spinal fluid
Cholesterol	120–280 mg/dl	Serum
Creatinine (blood)	Male: 0.8–1.3 mg/dl Female: 0.6–1.0 mg/dl	Serum or plasma
Creatinine (amniotic fluid)	Ratio 3:1 fetal to maternal Abnormal 2:1 at term	Amniotic fluid plus maternal plasma or serum
Creatine phosphokinase (CPK)	17–224 IU/L (Du Pont)	Serum
CPK isoenzymes	0–3% CK-2 (MB)	Serum
Creatinine clearance	Male: 95–135 ml/min Female: 85–125 ml/min	Serum or plasma plus urine
Gamma-GT	Male: 0–83 IU/L (Du Pont) Female: 0–64 IU/L	Serum
Glucose	70–110 mg/dl	Fluoride plasma (gray top)

Table continued on following page

*Universal color key for blood-drawing tube stoppers and anticoagulants: Green, heparin; red, no anticoagulant = serum; gray, fluoride; purple, EDTA; blue, Na citrate.

CHEMISTRY VALUES *(Continued)*

Determination	Normal Values	Material Analyzed
CSF glucose	30–70 mg/dl	Spinal fluid
Glucose-6 phosphate	Normal	1 EDTA tube, whole blood
Glucose tolerance:		
Fasting	70–110 mg/dl	Fluoride plasma (gray tops) for all samples
½ hour	30–60 mg/dl above fasting level	
1 hour	20–50 mg/dl above fasting level	
2 hours	5–15 mg/dl above fasting level	
3 hours	fasting level or below	
Haptoglobin	25–200 mg/dl	Serum
Iron, serum (total)	41–132 μg/dl	Serum
Lactic dehydrogenase (LDH)	100–190 IU/L (Du Pont)	Serum
Lactic acid	Venous 0.5–2.2 mEq/L (Du Pont) Arterial 0.5–1.6 mEq/L	Equal volume EDTA, blood and 7% perchloric acid (call Lab)
Lipase	4–24 IU/dl	Serum
Magnesium	1.8–2.4 mg/dl	Serum
Osmolality	278–305 mOsm/kg serum H_2O	Serum
Osmolality-urine/serum ratio	1.0–3.0 mOsm/kg H_2O	
Phosphatase (alkaline)	Adults 55–151 IU/L (Du Pont)	Serum
Phosphatase (acid)	0–0.8 IU/L (Du Pont)	Serum
Phosphorus	2.5–4.9 mg/dl	Serum
Potassium (K)	3.8–5.1 mEq/L	Serum
Protein total albumin	6.4–8.2 g/dl 3.8–4.8 g/dl	Serum
CSF Protein	15–45 mg/dl	Spinal fluid
Salicylates	Therapeutic 2–29 mg/dl Toxic 30–70 mg/dl Lethal >70 mg/dl	Serum or plasma
Sodium (Na)	135–145 mEq/L	Serum
Transaminase SGOT (AST)	22–47 IU/L (Du Pont)	Serum
Transaminase SGPT (ALT)	3–36 IU/L (Du Pont)	Serum
Turbidity	Negative	Serum
Uric acid	Male 3.8–7.1 mg/dl Female 2.6–5.6 mg/dl	Serum Serum

THERAPEUTIC (Rx) DRUG MONITORING—TOXICOLOGY

(See also specific drugs in 53, *Poisoning*)

Drug Name		Normal/Toxic Values		Units	Specimen Requirements*
		Low	*High*		
Acetaminophen (Tylenol)	Rx range:	2	13	μg/ml†	1.5 ml serum
	Toxic range:	30	300		
Acetone (with alcohol screen)	Toxic level:	20		mg/dl	5 ml whole blood
Amobarbital (Amytal)	Rx range:	3	12	μg/ml†	10 ml whole blood
	Toxic range:	30	60		
Barbiturates Screen (Amobarbital, butalbital, butabarbital, phenobarbital, pentobarbital, secobarbital)		See individual drug			10 ml whole blood
Butalbital	Rx and toxic range:	Not available			5 ml whole blood
Butabarbital (Butisol)	Rx range:	8	17	μg/ml†	5 ml whole blood
	Toxic range:	30	60		
Carbamazepine (Tegretol)	Rx range:	2	10	μg/ml†	1 ml serum
Chlordiazepoxide (Librium)	Rx range:	0.5	3	μg/ml†	10 ml whole blood
	Toxic range:	3	20		
Diazepam (Valium)	Toxic range:	2	30	μg/ml	10 ml whole blood
Digoxin (Lanoxin)		See Table 29–1		ng/ml *or* μg%	1 ml serum
Ethanol	Toxic level:	See 19–1		mg%	5 ml whole blood
Ethchlorvynol (Placidyl)	Rx range:	5	20	μg/ml†	10 ml whole blood
	Toxic range:	20	200		
Ethosuximide (Zarontin)	Rx range:	40	100	μg/ml†	1 ml serum

*All specimens should be refrigerated unless otherwise indicated.
†Therapeutic ranges are guidelines only, since effective levels vary among patients.

Table continued on following page

THERAPEUTIC (Rx) DRUG MONITORING—TOXICOLOGY *(Continued)*
(See also specific drugs in *53, Poisoning*)

Drug Name		Normal/Toxic Values *Low*	Normal/Toxic Values *High*	Units	Specimen Requirements*
Gentamicin	Trough level:	Less than 2		μg/ml†	1 ml serum
	Peak level:	5	10		
Glutethimide (Doriden)	Rx range:	5	12	μg/ml†	10 ml whole blood
	Toxic range:	5	120		
Isopropanol (Acetone metabolite must be present)	Toxic level:	340		mg/dl	5 ml whole blood
Lithium	Rx range:	0.5	1.5	mEq/L†	1.5 ml serum
	Toxic level:	2.0			
Magnesium		1.8	2.4	mEq/L	0.5 ml serum
Meprobamate (Equanil)	Rx range:	10	20	μg/ml†	10 ml whole blood
	Toxic level:	35			
Methanol	Toxic level:	20		mg/dl	5 ml whole blood
Methyprylon (Noludar)	Rx range:	8	10	μg/ml†	10 ml whole blood
	Toxic range:	30	60		
Pentobarbital (Nembutal)	Rx range:	1	5	μg/ml†	10 ml whole blood
	Toxic range:	8	30		
Phenobarbital	Rx range:	10	30	μg/ml†	1 ml serum

Phenytoin (Dilantin)	Rx range:	10	20	µg/ml†	1 ml serum
Primidone (Mysoline)	Rx range:	5	15	µg/ml†	1 ml serum
Procainamide (Pronestyl)	Rx range:	4	8	µg/ml†	1.5 ml serum
	Toxic level:	12			
Metabolite: N-Acetyl Procainamide (NAPA)	Rx range:	2	8	µg/ml†	
	Toxic level:	30			
Quinidine	Rx range:	2	5	µg/ml†	1 ml serum
Salicylate	Toxic level:	30		mg/dl	1.5 ml serum
Secobarbital (Seconal)	Rx range:	2	5	µg/ml†	10 ml whole blood
	Toxic range:	8	30		
Sedative Toxicology Panel I Screen‡		See individual drug			15 ml whole blood
Sedative Toxicology Panel II Screen§					
Theophylline (Aminophylline)	Rx range:				
	Adults:	10	20	µg/ml†	1 ml serum
	Newborns:	5	15		
Tobramycin	Trough level:	Less than 2		µg/ml†	1 ml serum
	Peak level:	5	10		
Valproic Acid (Depakene)	Rx range:	50	100	µg/ml†	0.5 ml serum

*All specimens should be refrigerated unless otherwise indicated.

†Therapeutic ranges are guidelines only, since effective levels vary among patients.

‡Includes drugs listed in Barbiturates Screen (above) plus acetone, ethanol, ethchlorvynol, glutethimide, isopropanol, meprobamate, methanol, methyprylon.

§Includes drugs listed in Panel I Screen plus chlordiazepoxide, diazepam, methaqualone (methaqualone toxic level: 10 µg/ml).

ARTERIAL BLOOD GAS (ABG) VALUES

Determination		Normal Values*	Material Analyzed†
pH	A	7.42 ± 0.4	Arterial whole blood heparinized with buffered porcine intestinal heparin coating barrel of Luer-Lok glass syringe (plunger also glass or Teflon-tipped plastic)
	P	7.35 – 7.50 (48 hr)	
	N	7.27 – 7.47	
	I	7.33 – 7.43	
$PaCO_2$	A	39 ± 7 mm Hg	
	N	27 – 40 mm Hg	
PaO_2‡	A	91 ± 17 mm Hg	
	N	65 – 80 mm Hg	
Bicarbonate	A	25 ± 4 mmol/L	
BE (base excess)	A	0 ± 2 mmol/L	
	N	(−10)–(−2) mmol/L	
	I	(−7)–(−1) mmol/L	
	C	(−4)–(+2) mmol/L	
O_2 saturation	A	94 ± 2%	
	N	40–90%	
	I	95–98%	
O_2 CT	A	20 ± 2 ml/dl	

*A = adult; P = premature; N = newborn; I = infant; C = child

†The same sample is used for measuring all of these parameters. Adjust values for temperature variations.

‡PaO_2 normally decreases with increasing age; a guideline rule of thumb is: PaO_2 = 105 − one-half the patient's age.

CEREBROSPINAL FLUID VALUES: See *18–29*.

URINE VALUES

Determination	Normal Values	Material Analyzed
Acetone	Negative	Random specimen
Addis count	WBC 1,000,000	12-hour specimen
	RBC 0–500,000	
	Casts (hyaline) 0–5000	
	In children, the values are slightly higher for casts; the WBC and RBC counts are slightly lower	
Albumin (quantitative)	Up to 100 mg/24 hr	24-hour specimen
Amylase	Less than 37 IU/hr	2-hour specimen
Bence Jones protein	Negative	Random specimen
Bilirubin (bile)	Negative	Random specimen
Calcium (quantitative)	50–300 mg/24 hr	24-hour specimen
Chloride	110–250 mEq/24 hr	24-hour specimen

URINE VALUES *(Continued)*

Determination	Normal Values	Material Analyzed
Concentration test	Specific gravity more than 1.025	Urine special instructions
Coproporphyrin (screen)	Negative	Random or 24-hour specimen
Creatine	Male: up to 40 mg/24 hr Female: up to 80 mg/24 hr	24-hour urine
Creatinine	Male: 1–2 g/24 hr Female: 0.8–1.8 g/24 hr	24-hour urine
Cystine (screen)	Negative	Random specimen
Glucose (quantitative)	Negative	24-hour specimen
Hemosiderin	Negative	Random specimen
Indican (qualitative)	Negative	Random specimen
Ketones	Negative	Random specimen
Melanin	Negative	Random specimen
Myoglobin	None present	Random specimen
Osmolality	50–1200 mOsm/kg urine H_2O	Random specimen
pH	4.8–7.8	Random specimen
Phosphorus	Up to 1 g/24 hr	24-hr specimen
Porphobilinogen	Negative	24-hr specimen
Porphyrins (screening)	No fluorescence	Random specimen
Potassium	25–100 mEq/24 hr	24-hr specimen
Protein (quantitative)	Up to 100 mg/24 hr	24-hr specimen
Protein (qualitative)	Negative	Random specimen
Seminal fructose	Fructose normally present	Special instructions
Serotonin	Negative	24-hr specimen
Sodium	130–260 mEq/24 hr	24-hr specimen
Specific gravity	1.002–1.030	Random specimen
Sperm count	Greater than 20 million/ml Motility 60% at ½ hr to 3 hr, majority grade 3	Special instructions
Sulfonamides	Negative	Random specimen
Three glass test	Same as routine urinalysis	Special instructions
Uric acid	200–800 mg/24 hr	24-hr specimen
Urobilinogen (qualitative)	Urobilistix 0.1–1.0 Ehrlich unit	Random specimen
Urobilinogen (semi-quantitative)	0.1–1.0 Ehrlich unit/2 hr	2-hr specimen, afternoon collection.
Uroporphyrin	Negative	Random or 24-hr specimen

ANTIMICROBIAL DRUG DOSAGE*

	ADULTS		CHILDREN		USUAL INTERVAL
	ORAL Daily Dosage	PARENTERAL Daily Dosage	ORAL Daily Dosage	PARENTERAL Daily Dosage	Between Doses
Amikacin		15 mg/kg		15 mg/kg	q8-12h
Amoxicillin	0.75-1.5 Gm		20-40 mg/kg		q8h
Amphotericin B		0.25-0.6 mg/kg[2]		0.25-1 mg/kg[2]	
Ampicillin	2-4 Gm	2-12 Gm	50-100 mg/kg	100-200 mg/kg[5]	q6-8h[5]
Azlocillin		8-18 Gm		200-300 mg/kg[6]	q4-6h
Bacampicillin	800-1600 mg		25-50 mg/kg		q12h
Carbenicillin	4-8 tablets[7]	30-40 Gm[8]	50-65 mg/kg	100-600 mg/kg	q6h[9]
Cefaclor	0.75-1.5 Gm		20-40 mg/kg		q8h
Cefadroxil	2 Gm		30 mg/kg		q12-24h
Cefamandole		1.5-12 Gm		50-150 mg/kg	q4-8h
Cefazolin		1-6 Gm		25-100 mg/kg	q6-8h
Cefoperazone		2-12 Gm		100-150 mg/kg	q6-8h
Cefotaxime		2-12 Gm		100-200 mg/kg	q4-6h
Cefoxitin		3-12 Gm		80-160 mg/kg	q4-8h
Ceftizoxime		2-12 Gm			q8-12h

* From The Medical Letter: *Handbook of Antimicrobial Therapy*, revised edition, 1984, pp. 40-47.

1. Or refer to the nomogram in FA Sarubbi, Jr, and JH Hall, Ann Intern Med, 89:612, 1978.
2. Given intravenously once a day, over a period of two to six hours. Begin with test dose and increase slowly. Dosage should be adjusted according to susceptibility of organism and serum concentration of drug. In fungal meningitis intrathecal administration may be necessary, in a dose of 0.1 mg initially, increased gradually to 0.5 mg every 48-72 hours, depending on the condition of the patient. Pediatric intrathecal doses should be one-third to one-half the adult dose.

USUAL MAXIMUM DOSE/DAY	NEWBORN (Parenteral) Up to 1 Week Dosage and Interval	1-4 Weeks Dosage and Interval	DOSAGE INTERVAL For Creatinine Clearance (ml/min) 80-50	50-10	<10
1.5 Gm	15 mg/kg/day q12h	15-22.5 mg/kg/day q8-12h	12h[1]	24-36h[1]	36-48h[1]
3 Gm	Not recommended	Not recommended	8h	12h	12-24h
1 mg/kg[3]	0.1-1 mg/kg/day[2]	0.1-1 mg/kg/day[2]	Change not required[4]		
12 Gm	50-100 mg/kg/day q12h	100-200 mg/kg/day q8h	8h	8h	12h
24 Gm			4-6h	8h	12h
1600 mg			12h	12h	24h
40 Gm	200-300 mg/kg/day q8h	400 mg/kg/day q6h	4-6h[10]	2-3 Gm q6h[10]	2 Gm q12h[10]
4 Gm			Change not required		
2 Gm			12-24h	24h	36h
12 Gm		50-150 mg/kg/day q4-8h	1-2 Gm q6h[10]	1-2 Gm q8h[10]	0.5-1 Gm q12h[10]
6 Gm	30 mg/kg/day q12h	30-60 mg/kg/day q8-12h	8h	0.5-1 Gm q8-12h[10]	0.5-1 Gm q24h[10]
12 Gm			Change not required		
12 Gm	100 mg/kg/day q12h	150 mg/kg/day q8h	4-6h	6-12h	12h
12 Gm			1-2 Gm q8h[10]	1-2 Gm q12h[10]	0.5-1 Gm q12-24h[10]
12 Gm			0.5-1.5 Gm q8h[10]	0.25-1 Gm q12h[10]	0.25-1 Gm q24-48h[10]

3. Or up to 1.2 mg/kg given every other day.
4. Amphotericin B is potentially nephrotoxic; temporary interruption of therapy may be required when the serum creatinine exceeds 3 mg/dl.
5. For meningitis in children caused by ampicillin-sensitive *H. influenzae* type b, Medical Letter consultants recommend up to 400 mg/kg/day. Meningitis should be treated q4h.
6. Up to 450 mg/kg/day in patients with cystic fibrosis.
7. Tablets contain 382 mg of indanyl sodium carbenicillin.
8. For septicemia or other severe infections; 4-8 grams/day is usually sufficient for urinary tract infections.

ANTIMICROBIAL DRUG DOSAGE (continued)

	ADULTS		CHILDREN		USUAL INTERVAL
	ORAL Daily Dosage	PARENTERAL Daily Dosage	ORAL Daily Dosage	PARENTERAL Daily Dosage	Between Doses
Cefuroxime		2.25-9 Gm		50-100 mg/kg[11]	q8h
Cephalexin	1-4 Gm		25-50 mg/kg		q6h
Cephalothin		2-12 Gm		75-125 mg/kg	q4-6h
Cephapirin		2-12 Gm		40-80 mg/kg	q4-6h
Cephradine	1-4 Gm	2-8 Gm	25-50 mg/kg	50-100 mg/kg	q6h[9]
Chloramphenicol	50-100 mg/kg	50-100 mg/kg[12]	50-100 mg/kg	50-100 mg/kg[12]	q6h
Cinoxacin	1 Gm				q6-12h
Clindamycin	0.6-1.8 Gm	0.6-3.6 Gm	10-25 mg/kg	10-40 mg/kg	q6h
Cloxacillin	2-4 Gm		50-100 mg/kg		q6h
Colistimethate		2.5-5 mg/kg		2.5-5 mg/kg	q8h
Cyclacillin	1-2 Gm		50-100 mg/kg		q6h
Dicloxacillin	1-2 Gm		12.5-25 mg/kg		q6h
Erythromycin	1-2 Gm	1-4 Gm IV[14]	30-50 mg/kg	15-50 mg/kg IV[14]	q6h
Flucytosine	50-150 mg/kg		50-150 mg/kg		q6h

9. Parenteral doses can be given q4-6h.
10. Parenteral dose for adults.
11. Up to 200-240 mg/kg/day, divided every 6 to 8 hours, for bacterial meningitis.
12. Intravenous administration; chloramphenicol is not effective when given intramuscularly. Dosage should be adjusted according to serum concentrations.
13. Initial dosage. Subsequent dosage must be based on determination of serum concentrations. For premature infants throughout the first month of life, initial dosage is 25 mg/kg/day.
14. By continuous drip or slow intermittent infusion.
15. If treatment is essential, begin with 15-25 mg/kg q24h and adjust daily dose to maintain the plasma concentration between 50 and 75 mcg/ml.
16. In some cases of meningitis some consultants also give gentamicin intrathecally in single daily doses of up to 5 mg for adults and 1 or 2 mg for infants until CSF cultures are negative.

USUAL MAXIMUM DOSE/DAY	NEWBORN (Parenteral) Up to 1 Week Dosage and Interval	1-4 Weeks Dosage and Interval	DOSAGE INTERVAL For Creatinine Clearance (ml/min) 80-50	50-10	<10
9 Gm			8h	8-12h	24h
4 Gm	Not recommended	Not recommended	6h	8-12h	24-48h
12 Gm	40 mg/kg/day q12h	60 mg/kg/day q8h	6h	8h	12h
12 Gm			6h	8h	12h
8 Gm	Not recommended	Not recommended	6h	8h	12-72h
4 Gm	25 mg/kg/day[13] q24h	25-50 mg/kg/day[13] q12-24h	Change not required		
1 Gm			0.25 Gm q8h	0.25 Gm q12-24h	Not recommended
4.8 Gm	Unknown	Unknown	Change not required		
4 Gm	Not recommended	Not recommended	Change not required		
5 mg/kg	Not recommended	Not recommended	Not recommended		
2 Gm			6h	12-24h	24h
4 Gm	Not recommended	Not recommended	Change not required		
4 Gm	Not recommended	Not recommended	Change not required		
150 mg/kg	Not recommended	Not recommended	6h	12-24h	Not recommended[15]

17. Infants 2000 grams or less should get 7.5 mg/kg q12h; those more than 2000 grams should get 10 mg/kg q12h.
18. Less than 20 kg: 50 mg. Twenty to 40 kg: 100 mg. More than 40 kg: 200 mg.
19. Usually given with an acidifying agent.
20. Dosage for anaerobic bacterial infections. First dose should be 15 mg/kg loading dose. Dosage should be reduced with severe hepatic disease.
21. The manufacturer recommends an initial test dose of 200 mg.
22. The manufacturer recommends monitoring bleeding time in patients receiving more than 4 grams per day for more than three days and also recommends that all patients receiving the drug be given 10 mg of vitamin K per week prophylactically.
23. For gram-negative meningitis in children, the manufacturer recommends an initial loading dose of 100 mg/kg.

ANTIMICROBIAL DRUG DOSAGE (continued)

	ADULTS		CHILDREN		USUAL INTERVAL
	ORAL Daily Dosage	PARENTERAL Daily Dosage	ORAL Daily Dosage	PARENTERAL Daily Dosage	Between Doses
Gentamicin	Not recommended	3-5 mg/kg[16]	Not recommended	3-7.5 mg/kg[16]	q8h
Griseofulvin					
Microsize	0.5-1 Gm		11 mg/kg		q24h
Ultramicrosize	0.33-0.66 Gm		7.25 mg/kg		q24h
Kanamycin		15 mg/kg		15-20 mg/kg	q8-12h
Ketoconazole	200-400 mg		50-200 mg/kg[18]	q24h	
Methenamine hippurate[19]	2 Gm		25-50 mg/kg		q12h
Methenamine mandelate[19]	4 Gm		50-75 mg/kg		q6h
Methicillin		4-12 Gm		100-200 mg/kg	q4-6h
Metronidazole[20]	30 mg/kg	30 mg/kg	30 mg/kg	30 mg/kg	q6h
Mezlocillin		6-18 Gm		300 mg/kg	q4-6h
Miconazole[21]		200-3600 mg		20-40 mg/kg	q8h
Moxalactam[22]		2-12 Gm		150-200 mg/kg[23]	q8h
Nafcillin	2-4 Gm	2-9 Gm	50-100 mg/kg	100-200 mg/kg	q6h[9]

24. One mg is equal to 1600 units.
25. The interval between parenteral doses can be as short as 2 hours for intial intravenous treatment of meningococcemia, or as long as 12 hours between intramuscular doses of penicillin G procaine.
26. Patients with severe renal insufficiency should be given no more than one-third to one-half the maximum daily dosage, i.e., instead of giving 24 million units per day, 10 million units could be given. Patients on lower doses usually tolerate full dosage even with severe renal insufficiency.
27. By continuous IV infusion. Although not recommended, the intramuscular dose for adults is 2.5-3 mg/kg/day divided into 4 to 6 equal doses.
28. Sulfisoxazole or trisulfapyrimidines.
29. Parenteral doses can be given q6-8h.
30. Tetracycline or oxytetracycline. The oral dose of methacycline or demeclocycline for adults is 600 mg daily in two to four divided doses. The oral dose of doxycycline for adults is 100 mg once or twice a day. The oral dose of minocycline for adults is 100 mg twice a day. The parenteral dose of doxycycline or minocycline is 100-200 mg/day, in one or two doses.

USUAL MAXIMUM DOSE/DAY	NEWBORN (parenteral) Up to 1 Week Dosage and Interval	1-4 Weeks Dosage and Interval	DOSAGE INTERVAL For creatinine Clearance (ml/min) 80-50	50-10	<10
5 mg/kg	5 mg/kg/day[16] q12h	7.5 mg/kg/day[16] q8h	8-12h[1]	12-24h[1]	24-48h[1]
			Change not required		
			Change not required		
1.5 Gm	15-20 mg/kg/day q12h[17]	15-20 mg/kg/day q8-12h	24h[1]	24-72h[1]	72-96h[1]
1 Gm			Change not required		
4 Gm	Not recommended	Not recommended	12h	Not recommended	Not recommended
4 Gm	Not recommended	Not recommended	6h	Not recommended	Not recommended
12 Gm	50-75 mg/kg/day q8-12h	100-150 mg/kg/day q6-8h	6h	8h	12h
4 Gm	15 mg/kg once, then 7.5 mg/kg q12h	15 mg/kg once, then 7.5 mg/kg q12h	Change not required		
24 Gm	150-225 mg/kg/day q8-12h	225-300 mg/kg/day q6-8h	4-6h	6-8h	8-12h
3600 mg			Change not required		
12 Gm	100 mg/kg/day[23] q12h	150 mg/kg/d[23] q8h	0.5-3 Gm q8h[10]	0.25-2 Gm q8-12h[10]	0.25 Gm q12h to 1 Gm q24h[10]
12 Gm	40 mg/kg/day q12h	60-80 mg/kg/day q6-8h	Change not required		

31. For oral administration. Parenteral doses are given q6-12h.
32. Doxycycline can be administered in the usual dosage in patients with renal insufficiency, but is not recommended for infections of the urinary tract in such patients.
33. Infants 2000 grams or less should get 75 mg/kg q12h in the first week, and 75 mg/kg q8h when they are one to four weeks old; those more than 2000 gm should get 75 mg/kg q8h in the first week, and 100 mg/kg q8h when they are one to four weeks old.
34. Each tablet contains 80 mg trimethoprim and 400 mg sulfamethoxazole. Double-strength tablets are also available; the usual dosage of these is 1 tablet q12h. Suspensions contain 40 mg trimethoprim and 200 mg sulfamethoxazole per 5 ml. Parenteral dosage ranges from 8-20 mg/kg/day trimethoprim and 40-100 mg/kg/day sulfamethoxazole.
35. The usual maximum daily dose is 4 tablets orally or 1200 mg trimethoprim - 6000 mg sulfamethoxazole intravenously.

ANTIMICROBIAL DRUG DOSAGE (continued)

	ADULTS		CHILDREN		USUAL INTERVAL
	ORAL Daily Dosage	PARENTERAL Daily Dosage	ORAL Daily Dosage	PARENTERAL Daily Dosage	Between Doses
Nalidixic acid	4 Gm		Not recommended		q6h
Netilmicin		4-6.5 mg/kg		5.5-8 mg/kg	q8h
Nitrofurantoin	200-400 mg	Not recommended	5-7 mg/kg	Not recommended	q6h
Oxacillin	2-4 Gm	2-12 Gm	50-100 mg/kg	100-200 mg/kg	q6h[9]
Penicillin G[24]	1-2 Gm	1.2-24 million U	25-50 mg/kg	100,000-250,000 U/kg	q6h[25]
Penicillin V[24]	1-2 Gm		25-50 mg/kg		q6h
Piperacillin		12-24 Gm		200-300 mg/kg	q4-6h
Polymyxin B		1.5-2.5 mg/kg[27]		1.5-2.5 mg/kg[27]	q6h
Rifampin	0.6 Gm		10-20 mg/kg		q12-24h
Spectinomycin		2 Gm once		40 mg/kg once	
Streptomycin		1-2 Gm		20-30 mg/kg	q12h
Sulfonamides[28]	2-4 Gm	100 mg/kg	150 mg/kg	100 mg/kg	q6h[29]
Tetracyclines[30]	1-2 Gm	0.75-1 Gm IV	25-50 mg/kg	10-20 mg/kg IV	q6h[31]
Ticarcillin		200-300 mg/kg		200-300 mg/kg	q4-6h
Tobramycin		3-5 mg/kg		6-7.5 mg/kg	q8h
Trimethoprim	200 mg		4 mg/kg		q12h
Trimethoprim-sulfamethoxazole	4 tablets[34]	8-20 mg/kg[34] (trimethoprim)	8-20 mg/kg[34] (trimethoprim)	8-20 mg/kg[34] (trimethoprim)	q6-12h
Vancomycin	0.5-2 Gm[36]	2 Gm IV	50 mg/kg[36]	40 mg/kg IV[37,38]	q6-12h

36. Only for treatment of pseudomembranous colitis.
37. Sixty mg/kg/day may be needed for staphylococcal central-nervous-system infections (UB Schaad et al, J Pediatr, 96:119, 1980).

USUAL MAXIMUM DOSE/DAY	NEWBORN (Parenteral) Up to 1 Week Dosage and Interval	1-4 Weeks Dosage and Interval	DOSAGE INTERVAL For Creatinine (ml/min) 80-50	50-10	<10
4 Gm	Not recommended	Not recommended	6h	6h	Not recommended
6.5 mg/kg	5 mg/kg/day q12h	7.5 mg/kg/day q8h	8-12h	12-24h	24-48h
400 mg	Not recommended	Not recommended	6h	Not recommended	Not recommended
12 Gm	50-75 mg/kg/day q8-12h	100-150 mg/kg/day q6-8h	Change not required		
24 million units	50,000-150,000 U/kg/day q8-12h	75,000-250,000 U/kg/day q6-8h	Change not required		See note 26
4 Gm	Not recommended	Not recommended	6h	8h	12h
24 Gm			4-6h	6-12h	12h
2.5 mg/kg	Not recommended	Not recommended	Not recommended		
0.6 Gm			Change not required		
4 Gm	Not recommended	Not recommended	No change	Not recommended	Not recommended
2 Gm	Not recommended	Not recommended	24h	24-72h	72-96h
8 Gm	Not recommended	Not recommended	6-8h	8-12h	12-24h
2 Gm	Not recommended	Not recommended	Not recommended[32]		
24-30 Gm	150-225 mg/kg/day q8-12h[33]	225-300 mg/kg/day q8h[33]	4-6h	2-3 Gm q6-8h[10]	2 Gm q12h[10]
5 mg/kg	4 mg/kg/day q12h	6 mg/kg/day q8h	8-12h[1]	12-24h[1]	24-48h[1]
200 mg			12h	18-24h	24-48h
See note 35	Not recommended	Not recommended	12h	18h	24h
2 Gm	30 mg/kg/day[38] q12h	30-45 mg/kg/day[38] q8h	1 Gm q24-72h[10,39]	1 Gm q3-7d[10,39]	1 Gm q5-10d[10,39]

38. Peak serum concentrations should be monitored.
39. Alternatively, see nomogram in RC Moellering, Jr, et al, Ann Intern Med, 94:343, 1981.

IDENTIFICATION OF POTENTIAL HAZARDOUS MATERIAL IN CARGO*

A. Internal Identification from Shipping Papers (Most Positive Method)

- A sample shipping paper is shown below (formats vary; NA number may be used instead of UN).

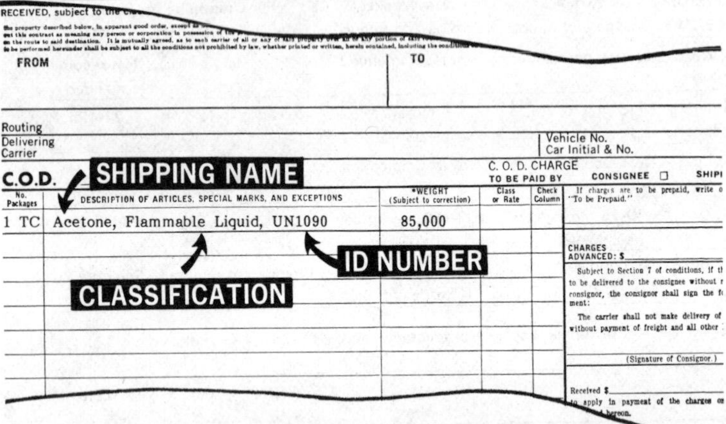

RECEIVED, subject to the ...

FROM | TO

Routing
Delivering Carrier | Vehicle No. Car Initial & No.

C.O.D. | C. O. D. CHARGE TO BE PAID BY CONSIGNEE ☐ SHIP...

No. Packages	DESCRIPTION OF ARTICLES, SPECIAL MARKS, AND EXCEPTIONS	*WEIGHT (Subject to correction)	Class or Rate	Check Column
1 TC	Acetone, Flammable Liquid, UN1090	85,000		

If charges are to be prepaid, write ... "To be Prepaid."

CHARGES ADVANCED: $

Subject to Section 7 of conditions, if ... to be delivered to the consignee without ... consignor, the consignor shall sign the ... ment:

The carrier shall not make delivery of ... without payment of freight and all other ...

(Signature of Consignor.)

Received $ ... to apply in payment of the charges on ... hereon.

- Shipping papers are commonly required to be (a) in the cab of the motor vehicle; (b) in the possession of a train crew member; (c) in a holder on the bridge of a vessel; or (d) in the possession of an aircraft pilot.

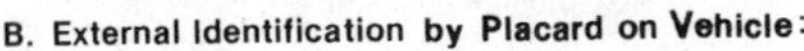

B. External Identification by Placard on Vehicle:

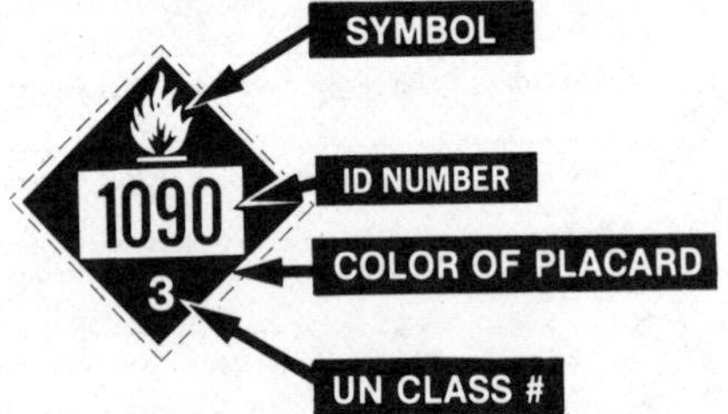

- Emergency Service Vehicles carry Dept. of Transportation (DOT) *EMERGENCY RESPONSE GUIDEBOOK* (DOT-P 5800.2), which gives guides to emergency action to be taken by fire-fighters, police and other emergency services, and gives specific identification of substances by ID Number.
- The above information can also be obtained by calling CHEMTREC TOLL FREE PHONE NUMBER (1-800-424-9300).

  Note: Outside the continental United States or in the District of Columbia, call instead: 202-483-7616.

C. General Recommendations When Approaching Scene of an Accident Involving Any Cargo

- Move and keep people away from accident scene.
- Do not walk on or touch any spilled material.
- Avoid inhalation of all gases, fumes and smoke, even if no hazardous materials are involved.
- Do not assume that gases or vapors are harmless because of lack of smell.
- If more than ① person is involved in an emergency response action, it is very important that an on-the-scene leader be designated (predesignation during emergency action preplanning is strongly recommended) and that you know who is in charge of handling.

* Based on information from *Hazardous Materials: 1980 Emergency Response Guidebook*. U. S. Department of Transportation (DOT), Research and Special Programs Administration/Materials Transportation Bureau, 1980.

FURTHER EXTERNAL IDENTIFICATION AIDS FOR POTENTIAL HAZARDOUS MATERIALS IN VEHICLES

UN CLASS #	UN CLASS NAME	COLOR	SYMBOL
1	Explosives/Blasting agents	Orange	
2	Gases Red: flammable Green: nonflammable	Red or green	
3	Flammable and combustible materials	Red	
4	Flammable solids	Red and white	
5	Oxidizers and organic peroxides	Yellow	
6	Poisons (white diamond/ black letters)	White and black	
7	Radioactive materials	Yellow and white	
8	Corrosives (black diamond/ white letters)	Black and white	
•	Substances that should *not* be treated with water	Blue	

EMERGENCY COMMUNICATIONS

INTERNATIONAL MORSE CODE

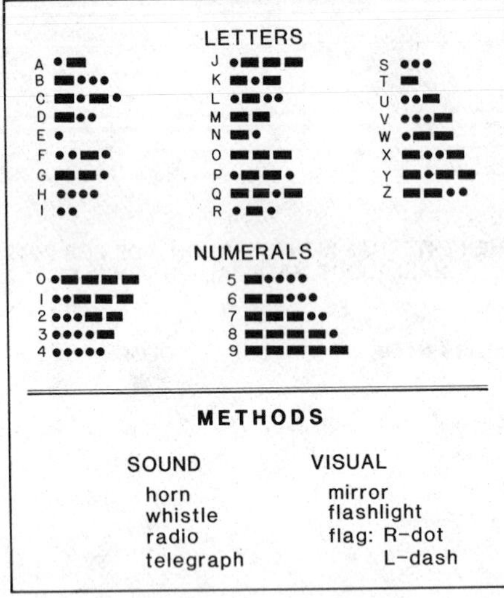

OFFICIAL CB RADIOTELEPHONE 10 CODE

10- 1 **Receiving Poorly**
10- 2 **Receiving Well**
10- 3 **Stop Transmitting**
10- 4 **OK, Message Received**
10- 5 **Relay Message**
10- 6 **Busy, Stand By**
10- 7 **Out Of Service, Leaving Air**
10- 8 **In Service, Subject To Call**
10- 9 **Repeat Message**
10-10 **Transmission Completed, Standing By**
10-11 **Talking Too Rapidly**
10-12 **Visitors Present**
10-13 **Advise Weather/Road Conditions**
10-16 **Make Pickup At** ______
10-17 **Urgent Business**
10-18 **Anything For Us?**
10-19 **Nothing For You, Return To Base**
10-20 **My Location Is** ______
10-21 **Call By Telephone**
10-22 **Report In Person To** ______
10-23 **Stand By**
10-24 **Completed Last Assignment**
10-25 **Can You Contact** ______?
10-26 **Disregard Last Information**
10-27 **I Am Moving To Channel** ______
10-28 **Identify Your Station**
10-29 **Time Is Up For Contact**
10-30 **Does Not Conform To FCC Rules**
10-32 **I Will Give You A Radio Check**
10-33 **EMERGENCY TRAFFIC AT THIS STATION**
10-34 **Trouble At This Station, Help Needed**
10-35 **Confidential Information**
10-36 **Correct Time Is** ______
10-37 **Wrecker Needed At** ______
10-38 **Ambulance Needed At** ______
10-39 **Your Message Delivered**
10-41 **Please Tune To Channel** ______
10-42 **Traffic Accident At** ______
10-43 **Traffic Tieup At** ______
10-44 **I Have A Message For You (Or** ______ **)**
10-45 **All Units Within Range Please Report**
10-50 **Break Channel** ______
10-60 **What Is Next Message Number?**
10-62 **Unable To Copy, Use Phone**
10-63 **Net Directed To** ______
10-64 **Net Clear**
10-65 **Awaiting Your Next Message/Assignment**
10-67 **All Units Comply**
10-70 **Fire At** ______
10-71 **Proceed With Transmission in Sequence**
10-73 **Speed Trap At** ______
10-75 **You Are Causing Interference**
10-77 **Negative Contact**
10-84 **My Telephone Number Is** ______
10-85 **My Address Is** ______
10-91 **Talk Closer To Mike**
10-92 **Your Transmitter Is Out Of Adjustment**
10-93 **Check My Frequency On This Channel**
10-99 **Mission Completed, All Units Secure**
10-200 **Police Needed At** ______

Note: Any 10-Code signal may be reversed by stating it as a question. For example, 10-20? would mean "What Is Your Location?" or 10-36? "What Is The Correct Time?"

LAND TO AIR SIGNALS (USAF) *

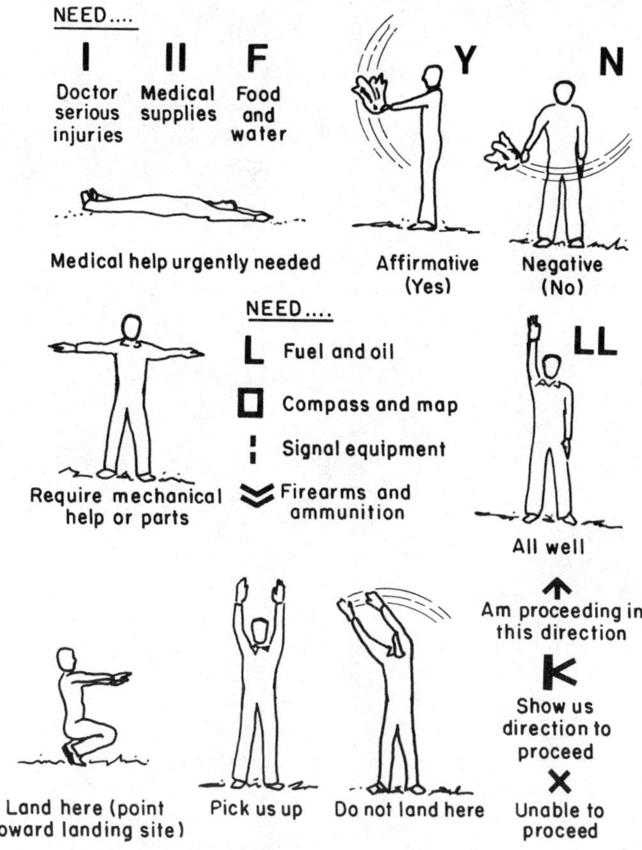

* Dark black letters and pattern signals (positioned above or to the right of the human figure) have comparable meaning to the associated human figure signal. These letters and patterns may be formed by trampling snow, digging trenches in soil or sand, or making mounds of any available material to make the pattern detectable from the air. Patterns must be large enough to be seen from the air — long limbs of pattern should be 15 to 18 feet; short limbs, 10 to 12 feet; all should be 3 feet in width. Figures, smoke signals and flashing reflectors serve as general signals.

Index

Note: Page numbers in *italics* indicate illustrations; those followed by (t) indicate tables.

Abalone poisoning, 530
Abandonment, of patient, 727–729
Abasin poisoning, 476
Abbreviations, commonly used, 759–768
Abdomen, injuries of, 678–680
  classification of, 6(t)–7(t)
  muscles of, *408*
  regions of, *143*
Abdominal pain, 141–148
  conditions associated with, 142(t)–143(t)
  diagnosis of, 141–148, 144(t)–146(t)
  in acute cholecystitis, 145(t)
  in acute pancreatitis, 145(t)
  in aortic aneurysm dissection, 146(t)
  in appendicitis, 145(t)
  in ectopic pregnancy, 436–437
  in hemorrhage, 144(t)
  in incarcerated hernia, 145(t)
  in infection, 145(t)
  in inflammation, 144(t), 145(t)
  in intussusception, 145(t)
  in obstruction, 145(t)
  in peptic ulcer, 144(t)
  in perforation, 144(t)
  in poisoning, 147(t)
  in pregnancy, 434
  in superior mesenteric artery thrombosis, 146(t)
  in surgical vs. nonsurgical abdomen, 141
  in ureteral stone, 146(t)
  in volvulus, 145(t)
  laboratory tests for, 147(t)
  management of, 148
  of vascular origin, 146(t)
  patient history in, 145
  patient instructions in, 141
  physical examination in, 146–147
  radiologic and visual tests in, 147–148
  types of, 140
Abdominal thrust, 38–40, *39*
Abdominal wall, congenital defects of, 458
Abortion, defined, 730
  self-inflicted, vaginal burns from, 188
  spontaneous, 434–435
  therapeutic, for rape victim, 97
Abrasions, 680. See also *Wound(s)*.
  of cornea, 282
  of hand, 339
  of penis, 320
Abruptio placentae, 442(t)
Abrus precatorius poisoning, 474
Abscess, 148–153
  alveolar, 149
  anorectal, 149
  Bartholin's glands, 150
  brain, 150
  breast, 150
  cold, 150
  collar-button, 150–151
  dental, 149
  epidural, 151
  gas, 151
  ischioanal, 151
  nasal septum, 151
  palmar space, 151
  perianal, 151
  perineal, 152
  perinephric, 326
  perirenal, 326
  peritonsillar, 152
  periurethral, 152
  pilonidal, 152–153
  pulmonary, 153
  retroperitoneal, 153
  retropharyngeal, 153
  stitch, 153
  subdiaphragmatic, 153
  suburethral, 153
  tendon sheath, 338
  tubo-ovarian, 330–331
Absinthe poisoning, 474, 566
Acacia poisoning, 474
Acetaldehyde poisoning, 474
Acetaminophen, 85
  poisoning from, 474, *475*
    N-acetylcysteine for, 471(t), *475*
  toxicologic values for, 777(t)
Acetanilid poisoning, 474
Acetarsone poisoning, 474
Acetazolamide, for mountain sickness, 160
Acetic acid poisoning, 476, 477
Acetic anhydride poisoning, 477
Acetoarsenite poisoning, 476
Acetohexamide poisoning, 476
Acetone, poisoning from, 476
  toxicologic values for, 777(t)
Acetonitrile poisoning, 476
Acetophenetidin poisoning, 476
N-Acetyl procainamide, toxicologic values for, 779(t)

Acetylarsen poisoning, 518
Acetylcarbromal poisoning, 476
Acetylcholine chloride poisoning, 476
N-Acetylcysteine, for acetaminophen poisoning, 471(t), *475*
Acetylene poisoning, 476
Acetylsalicylic acid, and Reye's syndrome, 252
  for pain, 85
  ingestion test for, 134
  poisoning from, 466(t), 477, 488, 591–593
Achalasia, 306
Achilles tendon rupture, 406(t)
Acid(s). See also specific acids.
  burns from, 185, 477
    of eye, 187
    of fingernail, 543
  poisoning from, 477
Acidosis, in blood transfusions, 118
  management of, 79–83
  metabolic, 361–364, 362(t)–363(t)
  respiratory, 362(t)
Aconite poisoning, 477, 530
Acquired immune deficiency syndrome, 233–236
Acridine poisoning, 477, 522–523
Acrolein poisoning, 477
Acromioclavicular separations, 386, 387(t)
Acrylaldehyde poisoning, 477
Acrylonitrile poisoning, 477
ACTH poisoning, 511
ACTHAR poisoning, 511
Activated charcoal, for poisons, 467–468
Acupressure, 91
Acupuncture, 91
Acute brain syndrome, 623–624
Acute mountain sickness, 160
Acute necrotizing ulcerative gingivitis, 702–703
Acute respiratory distress syndrome, 627–630
  and blood transfusion, 118
Acute situational reaction, 618
Adalin poisoning, 502
Addiction, 58–61
  defined, 58–59
  narcotic, 59–61
  tests for, 133–134
Addisonian crisis, 273
Adenitis, mesenteric, 313
Adhesions, conjunctival, 285
  intestinal, 303
Adhesives. See also *Glue*.
  cyanoacrylate, skin welding by, 666
Adrenal cortical hyperfunction, 274
Adrenal cortical insufficiency, acute, 273
Adrenal disorders, 273–274
Adrenal hyperplasia, congenital, 454
Adrenalin, as psychomimetic, 537
  poisoning by, 524
Advanced cardiac life support, 30(t), 31(t), 35
Aerosinusitis, 414
  in divers, 167(t)
Aerosols, as hallucinogens, 539(t)
Aerotitis, 269
Agranulocytosis, 360
Agrostemma githago poisoning, 478, 530
AIDS, 233–236
Air embolism, arterial, 720
  in blood transfusions, 118
  in dialysis, 324(t)
  in divers, 162, 164(t)
  venous, 722
Air travel, and otitis media, 269
  restrictions on, 163–168
Airway, esophageal gastric tube, 41, *41*
  esophageal obturator, 41, *41*
  nasopharyngeal, 40
  oropharyngeal, 40
Airway maintenance, 38–45
  abdominal thrust for, 38–40, 39, *39*
  back blows for, 38–40, *39*
  chest thrusts for, 38–40, *39*
  cricothyrotomy in, 44, *45*
  endotracheal intubation for, 42–43, *43*
  esophageal gastric tube airway in, 41, *41*
  esophageal obturator airway in, 41, *41*
  head tilt with neck or chin lift for, 38
  in head injuries, 346
  in spinal cord injuries, 427
  jaw lift for, 38
  nasopharyngeal airway in, 40
  nasotracheal intubation in, 42
  oropharyngeal airway in, 40
  tracheostomy in, 44–45
Airway obstruction, by foreign object, 297–298
  complete, signs of, 34(t)
  congenital, 453
  in asthma, 631–632
  in cancer patients, 448(t)
  in croup, 634–634
  in epiglottitis, 635
  localization of, 34(t), 295
  management of, 38–45. See also *Airway maintenance*.
Akee poisoning, 478
Alcohol(s), and Antabuse, 521–522
  higher, poisoning from, 478
  isopropyl, poisoning from, 525
  methyl, poisoning from, 555–556
  poisoning from, 478, 525
  rubbing, poisoning from, 590, 613
  wood, poisoning from, 555–556
Alcohol intoxication, blood alcohol levels in, 131(t), 132
  blood analysis in, 130–131, 131(t)
    permit for, 734, 735
  breath analysis in, 130
  clinical examination in, 132–133
  excitement states in, 279
  headache and, 207
  history and habits in, 132
  modifying factors in, 132–133
  tests for, 130–133

Alcohol intoxication (*Continued*)
 tests for, permits for, 734, 735
Alcohol withdrawal, neonatal, 457
Alcoholic encephalitis, 232, 433
Alcoholic neuritis, 420
Aldehyde poisoning, 478
Aldrin poisoning, 478
Aldrite poisoning, 478
Alfalfa poisoning, 478
Alimentary tract, poison removal from, 462
Alkali(es). See also specific alkalies.
 burns from, 185
  of eye, 187
 poisoning from, 478
Akaloid poisoning, 479, 491
Alkalosis, management of, 79–83
 metabolic, 363(t), 365, 366(t)
 respiratory, 363(t)
Alkron poisoning, 572
Alkyl mercury compound poisoning, 479
Alkyl sodium sulfate poisoning, 479
Allergic contact dermatitis, 566, 660, 664, 665(t)
Allergic reactions, 154–156
 anaphylactoid, 155–156
 angioedema in, 155
 emergency kit for, 154
 in blood transfusion, 118
 serum, 155–156
 to antisera, 155–156
 to antitoxins, 155–156
 to cosmetics, 512
  and eyelid edema, 283
 to drugs, 154–156
 to food, headaches in, 210
 to insect bites and stings, 154–156, 690–691
 to local anesthetics, 483–484
 to mercury diuretics, 554
 to nylon, 566
Allethrin poisoning, 479
Allguard poisoning, 613
Allium sativum poisoning, 479
Allyl cinerin poisoning, 479
Allyl dibromide poisoning, 479
Aloin poisoning, 479
Alpha rays, effects of, 16
Altitude sickness, 160
Aluminum acetate poisoning, 479
Aluminum ammonium sulfate poisoning, 479
Aluminum chloride poisoning, 479
Aluminum poisoning, 479
Aluminum salt poisoning, 479
Alveolar abscess, 149
Amanita poisoning, 561–562
Amantadine hydrochloride poisoning, 537
Amberjack poisoning, 531
Amenorrhea, 328
American nightshade poisoning, 582
American plum poisoning, 480
American woodbine poisoning, 573
Amidopyrine poisoning, 480
Amidryl poisoning, 521
Amines, mixed, injury from, 590
Aminoazotoluene poisoning, 594
Aminophenazone poisoning, 480
Aminophylline, dosage and administration of, 52(t)–53(t)
 poisoning from, 480
 toxicologic values for, 779(t)
2-Aminopyridine poisoning, 480
Aminopyrine poisoning, 480
2-Aminothiazole poisoning, 480
Amitril poisoning, 608
Amitriptyline poisoning, 608
Amizol poisoning, 480
Ammonia, for resuscitations, 52(t)–53(t)
 poisoning from, 480–481
Ammoniated mercury poisoning, 481
Ammonium chloride poisoning, 481
Ammonium picrate poisoning, 481
Ammonium sulfite poisoning, 481
Amnionitis, 435–436
Amniotic membranes, dressings from, 184–185
 premature rupture of, 445
Amobarbital sodium, dosage and administration of, 52(t)–53(t)
 toxicologic values for, 777(t)
Amoebic dysentery, 239, 314(t)–315(t)
Amphedroxyn poisoning, 556
Amphetamines, abuse of, 539(t)
 dependence on, 482
 poisoning from, 481–482, 556
Ampicillin sodium, dosage and administration of, 52(t)–53(t)
Ampicillin trihydrate, dosage and administration of, 52(t)–53(t)
Amputated parts, permit for disposal of, 736
 reattachment of, 672–674, 691
Amygdalin poisoning, 482
Amyl acetate poisoning, 482
Amyl alcohol poisoning, 482
Amyl nitrate, as cyanide antidote, 469(t)
 dosage and administration of, 52(t)–53(t)
 poisoning from, 482
Amytal, toxicologic values for, 777(t)
Anal fissures, 308
Analgesia. See also *Pain*.
 in head injuries, 347
Analgesics, narcotic, 83–84. See also *Narcotics*.
 non-narcotic, 84–86
  nonprescription, 85
  prescription, 85
  usage of, 85
 topical, 86–87
Anaphylactic shock, 154–155, 690–691
Anasadol poisoning, 591
Anatomical gifts, permits for, 747–748
Anemia, aplastic, 360
 hemolytic, 358
 profound, air travel and, 168
 sickle cell, 360, 361

Anesthesia, general, and prolonged postoperative coma, 229–231
  carbon dioxide retention in, 231
Anesthetics, and malignant hyperthermia, 711–712
  general, drug potentiation of, 230–231
  inhalation, 90–91
    poisoning from, 483
  intravenous, poisoning from, 483
  local, 87–90, *88*, *89*
    poisoning from, 483–484
Aneurysm, aortic, dissecting, 715–719
Angel dust, 575, *576*, 577(t)
Angel's trumpet poisoning, 484
Angina, Ludwig's, 702
  Prinzmetal, 191
  Vincent's, 702–703
Angina pectoris, 190–191
Angioedema, 155
  of eye, 282
Angiography, digital subtraction, 140
Anhydrous calcium sulfate poisoning, 582
Anhydrous hydrazine poisoning, 589
Aniline poisoning, 484
Ankle, dislocations of, 403
  fractures of, 402–403
  ligaments of, *401*
  nerve blocks for, *89*
  splinting of, 375(t)
  sprain of, 402
Anorectal abscess, 149
Anorectal emergency conditions, 308–309
Anorectal polyps, 313
Anoxia, in divers, 164(t)
Ant bites, 169
Ant paste poisoning, 484
Ant powder poisoning, 485
Ant stings, 693
Antabuse poisoning, 521–522
Anthrax, 236
Antibiotics, and neuromuscular weakness, 422
  poisoning from, 485
Anticholinergics, physostigmine salicylate for, 471(t)
  poisoning from, 466(t)
Anticholinesterases, atropine as antidote for, 469(t)
Anticoagulants, hemorrhage and, 359–360
  protamine sulfate for, 470(t)
  vitamin K for, 470(t)
  poisoning from, 485
Antidepressants, for pain, 85
  tricyclic, physostigmine salicylate for, 471(t)
    poisoning from, 466(t), 608
Antidotes, for poison, 468, 469(t)–471(t)
Antifebrin poisoning, 474
Antifreeze poisoning, 526
  ethanol for, 469(t)
Antihistamine poisoning, 485
Antimicrobial drugs, dosage of, 782(t)–789(t)
  selection of, 262(t)–264(t)
Antimony, food contamination with, 531
  poisoning from, 485
    dimercaprol for, 470(t)
Antimony oxide poisoning, 554
Antiperspirant poisoning, 515
Antipyrine poisoning, 480
Antisera, allergy to, 155–156
Antitoxins, allergy to, 155–156
Antu poisoning, 485
Anxiety states, 278–281. See also *Excitement states*.
Aortic aneurysm, dissecting, 715–719
  abdominal pain in, 146(t)
Aortic rupture, 216–217
Apgar score, 450
Apiol, oil of, toxicity of, 566
Aplastic anemia, 360
Apnea, neonatal, 456
Apomorphine hydrochloride poisoning, 463, 485–486
Appendicitis, 309–310
  pain in, 145(t)
Apple(s), bitter, poisoning from, 511
  seeds from, poisoning from, 486
Apricot pit poisoning, 486
Aralen diphosphate poisoning, 506–507
Arbor vitae poisoning, 486
Arbovirus infections, 236–237
Arecoline poisoning, 486
Arenavirus infections, 236–237
Argemone oil poisoning, 486
Arm, anatomy of, *411*
  immobilization of, 20, 23
  injuries of, classification of, 6(t)–7(t)
    crushing, 681
  muscles of, *410*
  peripheral nerve injuries of, 425–427
Arnica poisoning, 486
Arochlor poisoning, 573
Arrhythmias. See *Cardiac arrhythmias*.
Arsenic, food contamination with, 531
  poisoning from, 486–487
    dimercaprol for, 470(t)
    from color pigments, 487
Arsenic trioxide poisoning, 487
Arsenic trisulfide poisoning, 487
Arseniuretted hydrogens, poisoning from, 487
Arsine poisoning, 487
Artane poisoning, 487
Arterial blood gas values, 780(t)
Arterial embolism, 719, 720
Arterial injuries, 712–713
Arterial thrombosis, 721
Arteritis, temporal, 713
Arthritis, aseptic, 404
  gouty, 366
  of cervical spine, and headache, 207
  septic, 404–405
Arthrocentesis, 104
Artificial blood, 119, 747

Artificial ventilation. See *Resuscitation; Ventilation.*
Arum spp., poisoning from, 487
Arylam poisoning, 501
Asarum europaeum poisoning, 487
Asbestos poisoning, 487
Asphalt burns, 185
  of eye, 187
Asphyxiation, 157–159
Asimina triloba poisoning, 488
Aspidum poisoning, 488
Aspiration, meconium, 452
  pericardial sac, 110–112
  peritoneal, 112
Aspiration pneumonia, 638
Aspirin, and Reye's syndrome, 252
  for pain, 85
  ingestion test for, 134
  poisoning from, 466(t), 477, 488, 591–593
  toxicologic values for, 776(t), 779(t)
Asthma, 631–634
  remedies for, poisoning from, 488
Ata poisoning, 480
Atabrine, toxicity of, 587
Ativan poisoning, 493
Atrial fibrillation, 191, *192*
Atrial flutter, 191, *192*
Atrial tachycardia, *193*
  paroxysmal, 191
Atrioventricular block, *192*, 196
  third-degree, *192*, *194*, 199
Atropine, as antidote, 469(t)
  dosage and administration of, 52(t)–53(t)
  in CPR, 30(t)
  indications for, 84
  intratracheal injection of, 108–109
  poisoning from, 488–489
    physostigmine salicylate for, 471(t)
Aureomycin poisoning, 507
Auripigment poisoning, 487
Authorization, for emergency care, 734–750. See also *Permit(s).*
Autopsies, 67
Autotransfusions, 119
Autumn crocus poisoning, 489
Avantine poisoning, 547
Aventyl poisoning, 566, 608
Avulsed parts, disposal of, permit for, 736
Avulsion, incomplete, of nail, 340, *341*
  of ear, 700
  repair of, 672–674, 691
Azalea poisoning, 489
Azo dye poisoning, 522–523
Azodrin poisoning, 567–568
Azulfidine, toxicity of, 599

Baby powder poisoning, 489
Bacilli, antimicrobial drugs for, 262(t)–263(t)
Bacitracin poisoning, 489
Back. See also *Spinal cord; Spine; Vertebra(e).*
  crushing injuries of, 681
  ligaments of, *386*
  muscles of, *409*
  sprains of, 382–383
  strains of, 382–383
Bacterial endocarditis, acute, 191–193
Bacterial infections, with mass victims, 12
Bacterial meningitis, 247–248
Bacterial pneumonia, 637–638
BAL, for heavy metal poisoning, 489
  poisoning from, 489
Balanitis, 326
Banana oil poisoning, 482
Banana peel scrapings, 537
Bandage(s), *670*. See also *Dressings.*
  triangular, *373*
Bandaging, 104–105
Baneberry poisoning, 489
Banthine poisoning, 556
Barbenyl poisoning, 575
Barbiturates, 538(t)
  anesthetic potentiation by, 231
  poisoning from, 489–490
  toxicologic values for, 777(t)
Barium poisoning, 490
Barotrauma, 159–168
  and air travel, 163–168
  in divers, 159–163, 164(t)–167(t)
Barracuda, bites of, 169–170
  poisoning from ingestion of, 491, 531
Bartholin's gland abscess, 150
Basal skull fracture, 349
  bleeding from ear in, 270
  otorrhea in, 272
Baseball finger, 335, 342, 394
Bat bites, 170
Battered child syndrome, 458–459
Battered female syndrome, 328–329
Battered male syndrome, 329
Batteries, disc, ingestion of, 299–300
Battle's sign, 349
Baytex poisoning, 567–568
Bead tree poisoning, 552
Bean poisoning
  broad, 527
  calabar, 499
  castor, 503
  djenkol, 522
  fava, 527
  horse, 527
  jequirty, 547
  lima, 549
  Mexican jumping, 558
  precatory, 584
  stinging, 561
  Windsor, 527
Bedbug bites, 170
Bee stings, 154–156, 691–692
Beech creosote poisoning, 512
Beechnut poisoning, 491

Beef tapeworms, 314(t)–315(t)
Bell's palsy, 420
Belladonna poisoning, 491
  physostigmine salicylate for, 471(t)
Benadryl poisoning, 521
Bends, 161–162, 164(t)
Benne poisoning, 594
Bennett's fracture, 393
Benzahex poisoning, 492
Benzanthrone poisoning, 491
Benzedrine poisoning, 481–482
Benzene poisoning, 491–492
Benzethonium chloride poisoning, 492
Benzidine dye poisoning, 522–523
Benzidine poisoning, 493
Benzidine test, for blood, 133
Benzodiazepine poisoning, 493
Benzylchloride poisoning, 493
Beriberi, cerebral, coma in, 232
Beryllium poisoning, 493–494
Beryllium oxide poisoning, 554
Beta rays, effects of, 16
Betel nut poisoning, 486
Bhang. See *Marijuana*.
BHC poisoning, 492
Bichloride of mercury poisoning, 494
Bidrin poisoning, 567–568
Bilberry poisoning, 610
Bile duct injuries, 681–683
Biofeedback, analgesic, 91
Biologic warfare, 12
Bird of paradise poisoning, 494
Birth. See also *Delivery; Labor; Pregnancy.*
  live, defined, 729
  premature, defined, 729
Birth control pills, toxicity of, 494
Birth trauma, 456
Bishydroxycoumarin, and hemorrhage, 359–360
Bismuth poisoning, 494
Bismuth subnitrate poisoning, 494
Bismuth subsalicylate poisoning, 494–495
Bites, 169–176
  ant, 169
  barracuda, 169–170, 491, 531
  bat, 170
  bedbug, 170
  black widow spider, 170, 176
  brown spider, 170, 176
  camel, 171
  cat, 171
  chigger, 171
  dog, 171
  eel, 171
  flea, 171–172
  fly, 172
  Gila monster, 172
  horse, 172
  human, 172
  insect, 172
    allergic reactions to, 154–156
Bites *(Continued)*
  insect, of eyelid, 289
  kissing bug, 172
  llama, 172
  louse, 172
  mite, 172
  mosquito, 172
  octopus, 173
  rabies treatment for, 169
  rat, 173
  rattlesnake, 173–176
  shark, 173
  snake, 173–176
  spider, 170–171, 176
  tick, 175(t), 176
  treatment of, 169
Bitter almonds, oil of, poisoning from, 495
Bitter apple poisoning, 511
Bittersweet poisoning, 597
Bitumen burns, 185
Blaasoportoby poisoning, 530, 602–603
Black cherry poisoning, 491, 504
Black eye, 288–289
  in anterior fossa fracture, 349
Black laurel poisoning, 495
Black ulna poisoning, 531
Black varnish tree, dermatitis from, 665(t)
Black widow spider bites, 170, 176
Bladder, catheterization of, 105–106
  injuries of, 319
Bladen poisoning, 567–568
Bladex poisoning, 567–568
Blast injuries, mass, 12
    nuclear, 13
Bleach poisoning, 495
Bleaching powder poisoning, 544–545
Bleeding. See *Hemorrhage*.
Bleeding heart poisoning, 495
Blepharitis, 282
Blighia sapida poisoning, 495
Blightox poisoning, 522
Blindness. See also *Vision loss*.
  hysterical, 620
Blisters, 657
Blistex poisoning, 522
Blood, in stool, 304–306, *305*
  tests for presence of, 133
Blood clotting. See *Clotting*.
Blood flukes, 314(t)–315(t)
Blood gases, arterial, normal values for, 780(t)
Blood pressure cuff, as tourniquet, 354
Blood sausage poisoning, 530
Blood substitutes, 119, 747
Blood tests, for alcohol, 130–131, 131(t)
  normal values for, 773(t)
    permit for, 734, 735
Blood transfusions, 118–119
  autotransfusion, 119
  blood substitutes for, 119, 747
  refusal of, form for, 747
Blood vessels. See also *Arteries; Veins; Venous*.

Blood vessels (*Continued*)
  foreign bodies in, 301
  lacerated, repair of, *676*
Bloodroot poisoning, 495
Blowfish poisoning, 530, 602–603
Blow-out fracture, of orbit, 290
Blue bottle stings, 694
Blue lupin poisoning, 511
Blue mold dust poisoning, 522
Blue rocket poisoning, 477
Blue velvet, 609
Blueberry leaf poisoning, 495
Blueweed poisoning, 495
Bluing, laundry, poisoning from, 495
Body positioning, in emergencies, *26*
Body surface area, estimation of, for burns, 178, *180*, 180(t), 181(t)
  West nomogram for, *74*
Boils, 148–149. See also *Abscess*.
Bombings, 12
  nuclear, 12–13, *13*
    flash burns from, 187
Borate poisoning, 495–496
Boric acid poisoning, 495–496
Borneol poisoning, 500
Boron poisoning, 495–496
Boron oxide poisoning, 496
Botete poisoning, 530, 602–603
Botulism, 237, 496
  vs. tick paralysis, 175(t)
Boutonniere deformity, 335, 342
Bovine tetanus antitoxin, 137
Boxer's fracture, 393
Boxwood poisoning, 496
Boyle's law, 159
Bradycardia, 193–196
Brain, abscess of, 150
  concussion of, 348
    excitement states in, 279
    headache in, 210
  edema of, 346–347
    high altitude, 161
  injuries of. See *Head injuries*.
  tumors of, headache in, 207
Brain death, 417
  signs of, 63–64
Brass chills, 554
Breakbone fever, 238
Bream poisoning, 530, 531
Breast abscess, 150
Breath analysis, in alcohol intoxication, 130
Breech delivery, 438–439
Bretylium tosylate, dosage and administration of, 52(t)–53(t)
  in CPR, 30(t)
Bright's disease, 326
Brill-Zinsser disease, 252, 254(t), 259
Brionia poisoning, 496
British anti-lewisite, for heavy metal poisoning, 489
  poisoning from, 489
Broad bean poisoning, 527
Bromadal poisoning, 502
Bromate poisoning, 497
Bromides, anesthetic potentiation by, 231
  poisoning from, 497
Bromine poisoning, 497–498
Bromoform poisoning, 498
Brompton's solution, 84
Bronchial foreign bodies, 297–298
Bronchiolitis, 634
Bronchitis, 634
Bronchospasm, 631–634
Broom top poisoning, 498
Brown spider bites, 170, 176
Brucellosis, 259
Brucine poisoning, 498
Bubonic plague, 249
Buckeye poisoning, 498
Buckthorn poisoning, 498
Buerger's disease, 721
Bullet wounds, 680
  in mass casualties, 13–14
  of chest, 219
Bullous myringitis, 270
Bundle branch block, *195*
Buphanine poisoning, 498
Bupivacaine hydrochloride, contraindications to, 90
Burbot poisoning, 531
Burns, 177–190
  acid, 185, 477, 543
    of eye, 187
    of fingernail, 543
  age and physical condition in, 179
  agents causing, 179
  alkali, 185, 478
    of eye, 187
  amniotic membrane dressings for, 184–185
  asphalt, 185
    of eye, 187
  bitumen, 185
  body surface area of, *74*, 178, *180*, 180(t), 181(t)
  caustic, 185, 186, 478
    of eye, 187
    of vagina, 188
  cement, 186
  classification of, 179–182
  chemical, 186
  concrete, 186
  depth of, 178, *182*
  dressings for, 184–185
  electrical, 186
  escharotomy in, 184
  evaluation of, 178–182, *180*, 180(t), 181(t)
  flash, 187
  fluid administration in, 183–184, 183(t)
  friction, 187
  gasoline, 187
  hydrofluoric acid, 543
  location of, 178–179
  lye, 551

Burns (*Continued*)
  magnesium, 188
  major, 179–182
  management of, 182–185
    at scene, 177
    during transport, 177
  metal, of ear, 186
    of eye, 187
  minor, 179
  moderate, 179
  napalm, 188
  of conjunctiva, 286
  of cornea, 287
  of ear, 186
  of esophagus, 187, 478, 551
  of eye, 187
  of eyelid, 288
  of mouth, 188, 478, 551
  of mucous membranes, 188, 478, 551
  of respiratory tract, 158, 188
  of scalp, 189
  of vagina, 188
  pavement, 188–189
  phosphorus, 188–189
  pitch, 185
  prevention of, 178
  radiation, 189
    solar, 189
    therapeutic, 139
    x-ray, 190
  requiring special management, 185–190
  rocket fuel, 589–590
  rule of nines for, 180(t)
  slag, of ear, 186
    of eye, 187
  slight, 179
  sun, 189
  tar, 185
    of eye, 187
  tear gas, 190
  time elapsed since, 179
  titanium tetrachloride, 190
  ultraviolet lamp, 286–287
  war gas, 14, 190, 612–613
  x-ray, 190
Bursitis, 405
  of hip, 407
Bushmaster bites, 173–176
Butabarbital, toxicologic values for, 777(t)
Butalbital, toxicologic values for, 777(t)
Butamben picrate poisoning, 498
Butane poisoning, 498
Butanol poisoning, 498
Butazolidin poisoning, 579
Butesin picrate poisoning, 498
Butisol, toxicologic values for, 777(t)
Buttercup poisoning, 588
Butterfly bandage, *670*
n-Butyl alcohol poisoning, 498
n-Butyraldoxime poisoning, 499
Caddis fly stings, 692–693
Cadmium, food contamination with, 531
  poisoning from, 499
    CaEDTA for, 470(t)
Cadmium oxide poisoning, 554
Café coronary, 38–40, *39*
Caffeine poisoning, 499
Caffeine-withdrawal headache, 207
Caine preparations, for nerve blocks, 87–90, *88, 89*
  poisoning from, 483–484
  topical, 86
Caisson disease, 161–162, 164(t)
Cajeput oil, poisoning, 566
Calabar bean poisoning, 499
Caladium poisoning, 487, 499
Calcium, serum, deficiency, 369
    in children, 454
  excessive, 366–367
  normal values for, 775(t)
Calcium arsenate poisoning, 500
Calcium arsenite poisoning, 500
Calcium chloride, dosage and administration of, 52(t)–53(t)
  in CPR, 30(t)
Calcium disodium edetate poisoning, 526
Calcium disodium ethylenediaminetetra-acetate, as antidote, 470(t)
Calcium gluconate, dosage and administration of, 52(t)–53(t)
Calculi, gallbladder, 32, 145(t), 310
  urinary, 327–328
California fern poisoning, 511
Calla lily poisoning, 500
Calomel poisoning, 500
Caltha palustris poisoning, 500
Cambogia poisoning, 500
Camel bites, 171
Camellia poisoning, 500
Camphor poisoning, 500
Camphorated oil poisoning, 500
Cancer patients, emergencies in, 447, 448(t)–449(t)
Candidiasis, vaginal, 332(t)
Cannabis sativa. See *Marijuana*.
Cannulation, venous, 119–129
    femoral vein, 120(t), 123, *123*
    internal jugular vein, 120(t), 123–128, *124, 125*
    pediatric, equipment for, 127(t)
    peripheral vein, 120–122, 120(t), *121*
    sites for, 120(t)
    subclavian vein, 120(t), 123–129, *129*
Cantharides poisoning, 500
Cantril bites, 173–176
Capillary blanching test, in shock, 649(t)
Capillary leak syndrome, 627
Capsine poisoning, 520
Carbamate pesticide poisoning, 500
Carbamazepine, toxicologic values for, 777(t)

p-Carbamylaminophenylarsenic acid poisoning, 500
Carbarsone poisoning, 500
Carbaryl poisoning, 501
Carbazoate poisoning, 481
Carbinol poisoning, 555–556
Carbolic acid poisoning, 578
Carbon dioxide, poisoning from, 501
  in divers, 164(t)
  retention of, in general anesthesia, 231
Carbon disulfide poisoning, 501
Carbon monoxide poisoning, 501–502
  and smoke inhalation, 158–159
  in divers, 164(t)
Carbon tetrachloride poisoning, 502
Carbonic poisoning, 477
Carbonic acid anhydride poisoning, 501
Carbonic acid gas poisoning, 501
Carbonyl chloride poisoning, 580
Carbromal poisoning, 502
Carbuncles, 150
Cardiac arrest, at birth, 451
  causes of, 35
  management of, 32(t)–33(t). See also *Resuscitation.*
  warning signs of, 35–36
Cardiac arrhythmias, agonal, 37
  in dialysis patients, 324(t)
  pacemaker for, 110, *111*
    failure of, 201–202
  syncope of, 432
  ventricular, without pulse, 37
Cardiac compression, closed chest external, 48, 49(t)
  open chest internal, 50
Cardiac dysrhythmias, cardioversion for, 50–51, *50*
  defibrillation for, 51
Cardiac emergencies, 190–206
  electrocardiogram in, *192–195*
  encephalopathy in, 199–200
  in hypertensive crisis, 199–200
Cardiac injuries, 217
Cardiac pacemakers, 110, *111*
  failure of, 201–202
Cardiac resuscitation. See *Resuscitation.*
Cardiac tamponade, 202
  as oncologic emergency, 449(t)
  pericardial sac aspiration in, 110–112
  pericardial sac effusion for, 110–112
Cardiogenic shock, 647. See also *Shock.*
  signs and symptoms of, 650(t)
  treatment of, 651(t)
Cardiopulmonary resuscitation. See *Resuscitation.*
Cardiovascular disease, air travel in, 163–168
  in children, 453
  structural, 453
Cardiovascular system, poison removal from, 467
Cardioversion, 50–51, *50*
Cargo, identification of potential hazardous material in, 790–791
Caricella, 237
Carolina jasmine poisoning, 535
Carotid sinus syncope, 432
Carpal dislocations, 392
Carpal scaphoid fractures, 392
Cashew nut oil, dermatitis from, 502, 665(t)
Cassia oil poisoning, 509
Cast(s). See also *Splinting.*
  patient instructions for, 376
  types of, 376
Castor bean extract poisoning, 503
Castor bean poisoning, 503
Castrix poisoning, 503
Cat bites, 171
Cat scratch fever, 171
Catapres poisoning, 509
Caterpillar stings, 692–693, 694
Cathartics, for poisoning, 467
Catheter, runaway, 301
  Swan-Ganz, 116
Catheterization, bladder, 105
  central venous, 106
  nasal, 109–110
Catheterization setup, 77
Cauliflower ear, 270
Causalgia, 421
Caustic burns, 185, 186, 478
  of eye, 187
  of vagina, 188
Cavallas poisoning, 531
CB code, 792
Cedar, red, poisoning from, 486
  white, poisoning from, 552
Cedar oil poisoning, 503
Cellulitis, of hand, 339
  of orbit, 284–285
  synergistic necrotizing, 689–691, 689(t)
  treatment of, 149, 249
Cement burns, 186
Centigrade-Fahrenheit temperature conversion, 772
Central retinal artery occlusion, differential diagnosis of, 293(t)
Central retinal vein occlusion, differential diagnosis of, 293(t)
Central venous pressure, 106
Centripetal compressive wrapping, 726, *726*
Cephalgia, 207–215. See also *Headache(s).*
  Horton's, 211
Cerebellar hemorrhage, 714–715
Cerebral beriberi, coma in, 232
Cerebral edema, control of, 346–347
  high altitude, 161
Cerebral emboli, 719
  and prolonged postoperative coma, 231
Cerebral hypoxia, and prolonged postoperative coma, 231
Cerebral thombosis, and prolonged postoperative coma, 231

Cerebrocardiopulmonary resuscitation, 37. See also *Resuscitation.*
Cerebrospinal fluid, collection of, 114–116
headache in, 213–214
normal values for, 115(t), 780(t)
Cerebrovascular accident. See *Stroke.*
Cerebrovascular disorders, and prolonged postoperative comas, 231
Certificate, birth, 729–730
death, 730
Cerumen, 270
and hearing loss, 270, 271
Cervical spine. See also *Neck.*
dislocations of, 381
fractures of, 381
immobilization of, 20, 23, 374(t)
Cesarean section, 438
after maternal death, 439
Cevadine poisoning, 611
Chain saw injuries, 684
Chalazion, 282
Chancre, hard, 237
soft, 237
syphilitic, 253
Chancroid, 237
Charcoal, for poison adsorption, 467–468
Charcoal hemoperfusion, in poisoning, 467
Chelidonne poisoning, 503
Chem Hex poisoning, 492
Chemical(s), mind-effecting, 536–539
Chemical burns, 186
Chemical-induced dermatoses, 661
Chemical pneumonitis, beryllium-induced, 494
Chemical warfare, 14
Chemistry values, normal, 775(t)–776(t)
Chemopodium poisoning, 503
Cherry poisoning, 504
black, 491, 504
finger, 527
Jerusalem, 547
wild, 498
Chest, flail, 218
injuries of, 216–222
aortic rupture in, 216–217
bullet, 219
cardiac trauma in, 217
classification of, 6(t)–7(t)
compression, 219
contusion, 219
crushing, 219, 681
diaphragmatic injury in, 218
excitement states in, 279
hemopericardium in, 219
initial considerations in, 216
intercostal nerve block for, *221*, 222
penetrating/perforating, 219
pneumothorax in, 220–221, *220*
special emergency procedures for, 222
stab, 219
subcutaneous emphysema in, 221
tracheobronchial rupture in, 221
Chest (*Continued*)
injuries of, treatment priorities in, 216
muscles of, *408*
Chest thrust, 38–40, *39*
Chickenpox, 237
differential diagnosis of, 260(t)–261(t)
Chigger bites, 171
Chilblain, 704–706
Child(ren), abuse of, 458–459
cardiovascular diseases in, 453
digoxin dosage in, 198(t)
drug dosages in, 73, 73(t), *74*
emergencies in, 450–460
endocrine and metabolic disorders in, 453–455
venous cannulation in, equipment for, 127(t). See also *Venous cannulation.*
Chile saltpeter poisoning, 591
China oil poisoning, 574
Chinaberry poisoning, 552
Chinawood oil poisoning, 609
Chloral hydrate poisoning, 504
Chloramine T poisoning, 504
Chloramphenicol poisoning, 504
Chlorate poisoning, 504
Chlordane poisoning, 504
Chlordiazepoxide, poisoning from, 493, 504
toxicologic values for, 777(t)
Chlorinated lime poisoning, 544–545
Chlorinated prophylene propane poisoning, 514
Chlorine poisoning, 505
Chlormethane poisoning, 557
Chloroacetophenone poisoning, 505
Chlorobenzalmalononitrile poisoning, 505
Chlorobenzene poisoning, 505
Chlorodinitrobenzene poisoning, 505–506
Chloroform poisoning, 483, 506
Chloromycetin poisoning, 504
Chloronaphthalene poisoning, 506
Chloronitrobenzene poisoning, 506
Chlorophenothane poisoning, 515
Chloropicrin poisoning, 506, 607
Chloroquine phosphate poisoning, 506–507
Chlorothiazide poisoning, 507
Chlorpheniramine poisoning, 507, 585
Chlorpromazine hydrochloride, poisoning from, 507
with narcotics, 84
Chlortetracycline hydrochloride poisoning, 507
Chlorthion poisoning, 567–568
Chlor-trimeton, toxicity of, 585
Choanal atresia, 453
Chokecherry poisoning, 507
Chokes, in decompression sickness, 162, 164(t)
Choking, 38–40, *39*
Cholecystitis, 32, 310
acute, pain in, 145(t)
Cholinergic poisoning, 466(t)
Choroid, injuries of, 286
Choroiditis, 282

Christmas rose poisoning, 540
Chromate poisoning, 507–508
Chromic acid poisoning, 507–508
Chronic obstructive pulmonary disease, coma in, 228
Chrysarobin poisoning, 508
Cicuta virosa poisoning, 508
Cigar poisoning, 508
Cigarette poisoning, 508
Ciguatera, 530
Ciliary body injuries, 286
Cimetidine poisoning, 508
Cinchonine poisoning, 509
Cineol poisoning, 509
Cinnamon oil poisoning, 509
Ciodrin poisoning, 567–568
Citrate intoxication, and blood transfusion, 118
Citrate acid poisoning, 509
Claviceps purpurea poisoning, 530
Clavicle, fractures of, 385
  splinting of, 374(t)
Clam poisoning, 530
Cleaning compound poisoning, 509
Cleaning fluids, as hallucinogens, 539(t)
  poisoning from, 509
Climbing lily poisoning, 535
Clinoril poisoning, 600
Clonidine poisoning, 509
Clorox poisoning, 544–545
Closed chest external heart compression, 48, 49(t)
Clostridial myonecrosis, 688–691, 689(t)
Clotting, disorders of, 355–358, 356(t)–357(t). See also *Coagulopathy.*
  normal values for, 774(t)
Clotting factor deficiencies, 359
Cluster headaches, 211
Coagulation. See *Clotting.*
Coagulopathy, 355–358, 356(t)–357(t)
  and blood transfusions, 118
  consumption, 355–358, 356(t)
  disseminated intravascular, 355–358, 356(t)
Coal oil poisoning, 548
Coal tar dye poisoning, 522–523
Coal tar naphtha poisoning, 563
Cobalt poisoning, 510
  CaEDTA for, 470(t)
Cobalt oxide poisoning, 554
Cobra bites, 173–176
Cocaine, 539(t)
  in speedballs, 597
  poisoning from, 510
Cocci, antimicrobial drugs for, 263(t)
Coccidioidomycosis, 249
Coccyx, fractures of, 385
Coco de mono nut poisoning, 610
Codeine, abuse of, 538(t)
  dosage and administration of, 52(t)–53(t)
  indications for, 84
  poisoning from, 510
Coelenterate stings, 695
Colchicine poisoning, 510–511
Cold, common, 237–238
Cold abscess, 150
Cold exposure, 706–708. See also *Hypothermia.*
Cold injury, focal, 704–706
Colitis, ulcerative, 313–314
Collar-button abscess, 150–151
Colle's fracture, 391–392
  reversed, 391–392
Colocynth poisoning, 511
Colon. See also *Intestine(s).*
  injuries of, 683
Colonial spirit poisoning, 555–556
Color pigment poisoning, 487
Columbia spirit poisoning, 555–556
Columbine poisoning, 511
Coma, 222–232
  causes of, common, 222, 417
    rare, 229
  diabetic, 223
    differential diagnosis of, 227(t)
    vs. insulin shock, 227(t)
  Glasgow Scale for, 226(t)
  hepatic, 228
  hyperosmolar nonketotic, 228–229
  hysterical, 620
  in acute infectious diseases, 222
  in chronic obstructive pulmonary disease, 228
  in electrical shock, 226–227
  in emphysema, 228
  in meningitis, 222
  in Wernicke's encephalopathy, 232
  management of, 224(t)–225(t)
  myxedema, 277–278
  prolonged postoperative, 229–232
  psychogenic, 232
  uremic, 229
Commitment, involuntary psychiatric, 622–623. See also *Psychiatric emergencies.*
Common cold, 237–238
Communicable diseases, 232–265. See also *Infections.*
  clean techniques for, 232–233
  control techniques for, 232–233
  prophylaxis for, 233
  symptom control in, 233
  treatment of, 233
Compartment syndromes, 405, 406(t)
Compound 42 poisoning, 613
Compound 497 poisoning, 517
Compound 1068 poisoning, 504
Compound 1080 poisoning, 528–529
Compressed air sickness, 161–162, 164(t)
Compression injuries, of arteries, 713
  of chest, 219
Compressive centripetal wrapping, 726, *726*
Computerized tomography, 140

Concrete burns, 186
Concussion, brain, 348
  excitement states in, 279
  headache in, 210
Condylar fractures, 389
Condyloma acuminatum, 238
Cone shell stings, 693
Congestive heart failure, 196–197
Coniine poisoning, 511
Conjunctiva, adhesions of, 285
  burns of, 286
  foreign bodies of, 286
  hemorrhage in, in divers, 164(t)
  injuries of, 286–287
Conjunctivitis, 282
  differential diagnosis of, 292(t)
Consciousness, altered, 222–232. See also *Coma*.
  causes of, 222
  evaluation of, in head injuries, 343, 345(t)
  loss of. See also *Coma; Syncope*.
    episodic, differential diagnosis of, 430(t)–431(t)
Consent, 739–743
  for minors, 738(t), 739, 740
  free choice, defined, 739
  informed, defined, 739
Consent forms, 734–750. See also *Permit(s)*.
Consumption coagulopathy, 355–358
Contact dermatitis, 556, 660. See also *Allergic reactions*.
  urushiol, 664, 665(t)
Contact lens, irrigating, 286
  removal of, 291
Contusions, 376–377, 681. See also *Wound(s)*.
  of artery, 713
  of chest, 219
  of finger, 340
  of hand, 339–340
  of heart, 217
  of kidney, 318
  of nose, 414
  of penis, 320
Conversion hysteria, 620–621
Convulsions, 266–269. See also *Seizures*.
Copper poisoning, 511
    CaEDTA for, 470(t)
Copper oxide poisoning, 554
Copperhead bites, 173–176
Coprinus atramentarius poisoning, 530
Co-ral poisoning, 567–568
Coral snake bites, 173–176
Coral stings, 693
Corn campion poisoning, 478
Corn cockle poisoning, 478
Corn lily poisoning, 611
Corn rose poisoning, 478
Cornea, abrasions of, 282
  burns of, 287
  examination of, 281
  foreign bodies of, 287–288, 288
  injuries of, 287–288
Cornea (*Continued*)
  penetrating wounds of, 288
  staining of, 281, 287
  superficial wounds of, 288
  ulcers of, after foreign body removal, 288
    differential diagnosis of, 292(t)
Coroner's cases, 65, 66(t)
  autopsy in, 67
Corozate poisoning, 522
Corpse, disposal of, 68
Corticosteroids, anesthetic potentiation by, 230
Corticotropin poisoning, 511
Cortisone poisoning, 512
Coryza, 237–238
Cosmetics, allergic reaction to, 512
    and eyelid edema, 283
Cottonmouth bites, 173–176
Coumachlor poisoning, 613
Coumadin poisoning, 613
Court testimony, 754–755
Cow cabbage poisoning, 541
Cow parsnip poisoning, 541
Cowbane poisoning, 508
Cowhage poisoning, 561
Cow-itch poisoning, 561
Cowslip poisoning, 500
Coxsackievirus infections, 240
Coyotillo poisoning, 498
Crab eye poisoning, 547
Cramps, heat, 708–709, 710(t)
  menstrual, 329
Cranial arteritis, 713
Cranial injuries. See *Head injuries*.
Cranial nerves, evaluation of, in head injuries, 343
Craniotomy burr hole sites, *351*
Crank poisoning, 481–482
Crayon poisoning, 512
Creosote poisoning, 512
Crepe paper poisoning, 571
Crib death, 459–460
Cricothyrotomy, 44, *45*
Criminal evidence, at emergency scene, 2
Croton oil poisoning, 512
Croup, 634–635
Crowfoot poisoning, 588
Crude thyroid extract poisoning, 606
Crushing injuries, 681
  of chest, 219, 681
Cryotherapy sprays, topical, 86
Cryptitis, anorectal, 308
Cryptococcosis, 249
Culdocentesis, 106–107
Curare poisoning, 512
Cushing's syndrome, 274
Cyanide poisoning, 513
  antidotes for, 469(t)
Cyanoacrylate adhesives, skin bonding with, 666
Cyclamen poisoning, 514
Cycrimine hydrochloride poisoning, 514

Cyst, ovarian, rupture of, 331
torsion of pedicle of, 333
Cystisine poisoning, 514
Cystitis, 322–323
Cytomegalovirus infection, 238

D-14 poisoning, 522
Dacryocystitis, 283
Daffodil poisoning, 563
Dakin's solution, 544–545
Dalmane poisoning, 493, 529
Dalton's law, 160
Dandy fever, 238
Daphne poisoning, 514
Darnel poisoning, 550
Darvon poisoning, 585
Datura stramonium poisoning, 514
DD compound poisoning, 514
DDD poisoning, 514, 602
DDT poisoning, 515
Dead on arrival cases, 65
Deadly nightshade poisoning, 491
Deafness. See *Hearing loss*.
Death, brain, 417
signs of, 63–64
certification of, 64, 730
conclusive signs of, 63
definition of, 61–62
presumptive signs of, 62–63
time of, criteria for, 61–62
Death camas poisoning, 615
Death cases, autopsies in, 67
coroner's, 65, 66(t)
dead on arrival, 65
disposal of remains in, 68
medical examiner's, 65, 66(t)
notification of kin in, 65–67
organ donation in, 68
permit for, 736, 747–748
religious rites in, 68, 69(t)–72(t)
Death certificates, 64, 730
Death fish, 530, 602–603
Deathmore poisoning, 613
Debridement, of wounds, 668
of hand, 336, *337*
Decaborane poisoning, 589
Decompression sickness, 161–162, 164(t)
Decon poisoning, 613
Deferoxamine, for iron salts, 471(t)
Defibrillation, 51
Degloving injuries, 686–687
Deglutition, muscles of, disorders of, 425
Dehydration. See *Fluid; Fluid replacement*.
Delirium, 618–619
Delirium tremens, 279, 525
Delivery, breech, 438–439
emergency, 436–438, *440–441*
fetal injury in, 456
home, 433–434
obstetric cord prolapse and rupture in, 436
Delivery *(Continued)*
uterine inversion after, 436
Delnay poisoning, 567–568
Delphinium poisoning, 515
Delta-Cortef poisoning, 584
Deltasone poisoning, 584
Deltra poisoning, 584
Demerol poisoning, 553
Demeton poisoning, 515, 567–568
Dendrite, 284
Dengue, 238
Dengue-like fevers, 236–237
Dental. See *Tooth*.
Deodorant poisoning, 515
Deodorizer poisoning, 515
Depakene, toxicologic values for, 779(t)
Depilatory poisoning, 515
Depressants, 538(t)–539(t)
Depression, 619–620
De Quervain's disease, 342
Dermatitis, allergic, 556, 660. See also *Allergic reactions*.
beryllium, 493
Dermatologic disorders, 657–666
Dermatomes, *426*, *428*
Derris poisoning, 515
Desipramine poisoning, 608
Desoxyephedrine hydrochloride poisoning, 556
Desoxyn poisoning, 556
Detergent poisoning, 516, 595
Dexamethasone, dosage and administration of, 52(t)–53(t)
Dexedrine poisoning, 481–482
Dextroamphetamine sulfate poisoning, 516
Dextrolevomethadone hydrochloride, 539(t)
Dextrose, dosage and administration of, 52(t)–53(t)
for insulin shock, 470(t)
Devil's apple poisoning, 514
Diabetes insipidus, 275–276
Diabetes mellitus, coma in, 223
differential diagnosis of, 227(t)
vs. insulin shock, 227(t)
ketoacidosis in, treatment of, 223–226
Diacetylmorphine poisoning, 541
Diagnostic procedures, consent form for, 736
equipment for, 75(t)
Dialysis, in poisoning, 467
peritoneal, 112–113
renal, emergencies in, 323, 324(t)–325(t)
Dialkylphosphate poisoning, 567–568
Diaminodiphenyl poisoning, 493
Diaphragm, injuries of, 218
rupture of, 218
Diaphragmatic hernia, 306–307
neonatal, 452
Diarrhea, 311(t), 312
Diazepam, dosage and administration of, 52(t)–53(t)
intratracheal injection of, 108–109
poisoning from, 493, 516
toxicologic values for, 777(t)

Diazepam (*Continued*)
  with fentanyl, 84
Diazinon poisoning, 567–568
Diazomethane poisoning, 516
Dibenzoxapine poisoning, 505
Diborane poisoning, 496, 589
Dibrom poisoning, 567–568
Dibucaine, topical, 86
Dicaphthon poisoning, 567–568
Dichapetalum cymosum poisoning, 596
Dichapetalum toxicarium poisoning, 516
Dichloren poisoning, 566
Dichlorobenzene poisoning, 516
Dichlorodifluoromethane poisoning, 516
Dichlorodiphenyltrichlorethane poisoning, 515
Dichloroethane poisoning, 516
Dichloroethylether poisoning, 516
Dichlorohydrin poisoning, 516
Dichloronitroethane poisoning, 525
Dichlorophene poisoning, 517
2,4-Dichlorophenoxyacetic acid poisoning, 517
Dicoumarin poisoning, 517
Dicumarol poisoning, 517
Dieffenbachia poisoning, 487, 517
Dieldrin poisoning, 517
Diethylamine poisoning, 518
Diethyl-betachlorethylamine poisoning, 518
Diethylene ester poisoning, 518
Diethylene glycol poisoning, 518, 526
Diethylstilbestrol, for pregnancy prevention, in rape victim, 97
  poisoning from, 518
Diflunisal, 85
Digit. See *Finger(s); Toe(s).*
Digital nerve blocks, 90
Digital subtraction angiography, 140
Digitalis poisoning, 197–199, 198(t), 518–519
Digitalis purpurea, 518–519
Digoxin, dosage and administration of, 52(t)–53(t)
    in children, 198(t)
  poisoning from, 196–199
  toxicologic values for, 777(t)
Dilantin, poisoning from, 579–580
  toxicologic values for, 779(t)
Dilaudid poisoning, 519
Dimenhydrinate poisoning, 519
Dimercaprol, as antidote, 470(t), 489
  poisoning from, 489
Dimetane poisoning, 519
Dimethoate poisoning, 567–568
Dimethyl lysergic acid, 538(t)
Dimethyl phthalate poisoning, 519
Dimethyl sulfoxide, poisoning from, 520
  topical, 87
Dimethylcarbinol poisoning, 547
Dimethylhydrazine, unsymmetrical, poisoning from, 590
Dimethylketone poisoning, 476
Dimethyltryptamine, 537, 538(t)
Dinitrobenzene poisoning, 520
Dinitrocresol poisoning, 520
Dinitrophenol poisoning, 520
Dinitrotoluene poisoning, 520–521
Dioxane poisoning, 521
Dioxin poisoning, 521
Diphenhydramine, dosage and administration of, 52(t)–53(t)
  poisoning from, 521
Diphenoxylate poisoning, 521
  nalaxone for, 469(t)
Diphenylhydantoin poisoning, 579–580
Diphtheria, 238–239
Dipterix poisoning, 567–568
Disasters. See also *Mass civilian casualties; Triage.*
  guidelines for, 17–19
  individual preparedness for, 18–19
  individual responsibility to community in, 19
  potable water for, 19
Disc batteries, ingestion of, 299–300
Disclosure permit, 734
Diseases, communicable, 232–265. See also *Communicable diseases.*
  psychosomatic, 624–625
  reportable, 100–102, 751–752
Disk, herniated, 383–384
Dislocation, of ankle, 403
  of cervical spine, 381
    skull traction for, 114
    splinting of, 20, 23, 374(t)
  of fingers, 395
  of hip, 397
  of humerus, 386–387
  of knee, splinting of, 375(t)
  of lunate, 392
  of patella, 399, 400(t)
  of penis, 320
  of shoulder, 386–387
  of tarsus, 403
  of toe, 395, 404
  of wrist, 392
  perilunar, 392
  splinting of, 376. See also *Splinting.*
  sternoclavicular, 385
  temporomandibular, 381
  treatment of, 379–380
  with mass casualties, 14
Disseminated intravascular clotting, 355–358, 356(t)
Disulfiram poisoning, 521–522
Di-Syston poisoning, 567–568
Dithane poisoning, 522
Dithicarbamate poisoning, 522
Dithiopropanol, as antidote, 489
Diuretics, mercury, poisoning from, 554
  thiazide, poisoning from, 604
Diuril poisoning, 507
Diverticular disease, 312
Divers, air travel by, 168
Diving hazards, 162–163, 164(t)–167(t)
Divinyl ether poisoning, 483
Djenkol bean poisoning, 522

DMSO, poisoning from, 520
  topical, 87
DMT, 537, 538(t)
Doctor. See *Physician.*
Dog bites, 171
Dog parsley poisoning, 514
Doll's eye maneuver, 344, 345(t)
Dolophine, 539(t)
  poisoning from, 555
Donovanosis, 241
Dopamine, in CPR, 30(t)
Doppler test, 133
Doriden, poisoning from, 535
  toxicologic values for, 778(t)
Dormiral poisoning, 575
Douches, burns from, 188
Dowklor poisoning, 504
Doxepin, for pain, 85
Dramamine poisoning, 519
Dressings, amniotic membrane, 184–185
  for burns, 184–185
  for hand injuries, 338
Dromoran poisoning, 556
Drowning, 157–158
  as diving hazard, 165(t)
Drugs. See also generic names of specific drugs.
  abuse of, 59–61, 536–540
  addiction to, 59–61. See also *Narcotics.*
  allergic reactions to, 154–156, 661
  and excitement states, 279
  antimicrobial, selection of, 262(t)–264(t)
  controlled, 93–95
    classification of, 94
    prescription of, 95(t)
  depressant, 538(t)–539(t)
  dose conversions for, 772(t)
  dosage of, in children, 73, 73(t), *74*
  emergency, commonly used, 52(t)–55(t)
  hallucinogenic, 536–539
  in pregnancy, 436
  intraglossal injection of, 108
  intratracheal injection of, 108–109
  lethal or toxic blood levels of, 472
  monitoring of, 777(t)–779(t)
  narcotic. See *Narcotics.*
  normal values for, 777(t)–779(t)
  prescription, controlled, 94, 95(t)
    restrictions on, 93–95
  psychomimetic, 536–539
  specimen requirements for, 777(t)–779(t)
  stimulant, 539(t)
  toxicologic values for, 777(t)–779(t)
  withdrawal from, neonatal, 457
Drug addiction, 59–61
  tests for, 133–134
Drug dependence, 58
Drug habituation, 58
Drug-induced toxic epidermal necrosis, 659, 661
Drunkenness. See *Alcohol intoxication.*
Dulcamara poisoning, 597
Dumb cane poisoning, 487, 517
Dutchman's breeches poisoning, 495
Dwarf bay poisoning, 514
Dwarf tapeworms, 314(t)–315(t)
Dye, aniline, 484
  azo, 522
  benzidine, 522
  coal tar, 522
Dye poisoning, 522–523
  acridine, 522
  hair, 536
  phthalein, 523
  shoe, 523, 594
  triphenyl, 523
Dying patients, termination of care for; permit for, 749–750
  triage and, 7(t). See also *Triage.*
Dymelor poisoning, 476
Dysentery, 239, 314(t)–315(t)
Dysmenorrhea, 329
Dysrhythmias, cardioversion for, 50, *50*
  defibrillation for, 51

E605 poisoning, 572
Ear, avulsion of, 700
  bleeding from, 270
  burns of, 186
  cauliflower, 270
  cerumen in, 270, 271
  contusions of, 270
  disorders of, 269–273
  examination of, 269
  foreign bodies in, 296
  hematoma of, 270
  infections of, 270, 271–272. See also *Otitis.*
  swimmer's, 272
Ear squeeze, in divers, 165(t)
Earache, 271
  headache and, 215
Eardrum, burns of, 186
  rupture of, in divers, 165(t)
Earthquakes, 17–19. See also *Mass civilian casualties; Natural disasters; Triage.*
Earwax, 270, 271
Ecchymosis, of eyelid, 288–289
    in anterior fossa fracture, 349
Echovirus infections, 240
Eclampsia, 444
Ectopic pregnancy, 436–437
Ectropion, 283
Eczema, 661
  varicose, 724
EDB poisoning, 526
Edema, cerebral, control of, 346–347
    high altitude, 161
  digital, compressive centripetal wrapping for, 726, *726*
  of eyelid, 283

Edema (*Continued*)
pulmonary 627–630
acute, 203
high altitude, 161
in dialysis patients, 325(t)
EDTA, toxicity of, 526
Eel, bites of, 171
poisoning from ingestion of, 530, 531
El perrito stings, 694
Elavil poisoning, 608
Elbow, fractures of, 389
nursemaid's, 390
pitcher's, 389
splinting of, 375(t)
Electrical burns, 186
Electrical shock, 226–227
Electrocardiography, in cardiac emergencies, *192–195*
portable unit for, 76
Electrolyte balance, basic elements in, 80(t)
daily requirements for, 81
maintenance of, 79–83
Electrolyte imbalance, in cancer patients, 449(t)
Electrolyte replacement, for mass casualties, 82–83
solutions for, 82
Electromechanical disassociation, 37, 199
Elephant's ear poisoning, 487, 517
Elephant's scratchwort poisoning, 561
Elgetol poisoning, 520
Embolism, 719–720
air, arterial, 720
in blood transfusions, 118
in dialysis patients, 324(t)
in divers, 162, 164(t)
venous, 722
arterial, 719, 720
cerebral, 719
and prolonged postoperative coma, 231
fat, and prolonged postoperative coma, 231
in cancer patients, 449(t)
in dialysis patients, 324(t)
peripheral artery, 719
pulmonary, 639–640
saddle, 639
Emergency bag, contents of, 74–79
precautions for, 79
Emergency care, consent to, 739–743. See also *Consent; Permit(s).*
defined, 727
for minors, consent for, 738(t), 739, 740
for service personnel and dependents, 753
follow-up after guidelines for, 728–729
legal duty to supply, 728
permits and authorizations for, 734–750. See also *Permit(s).*
physician's responsibilities in, 752–753
priority classification for, for individual, 5
for mass casualties, 5–8. See also *Mass civilian casualties; Triage.*
refusal to supply, 728
Emergency care (*Continued*)
standards of care in, 733
Emergency case log, 730–731
Emergency case records, 730–732
Emergency communications, 792–793
Emergency kit, for allergic reactions, 154
Emergency medical supplies, 74–79
precautions for, 79
Emergency medicine, achievements in, 56–58
defined, 727
education in, 57–58
organizational achievements in, 56–57
technical improvements in, 57
Emergency problem analysis, 1–4
Emergency scene, analysis of, 1–2
history-taking at, 2
life support measures at, 3–4. See also *Life support.*
physical examination at, quick initial, 2–3
systematic, 3–4
quarantine of, 1
triage at, 5–9. See also *Triage.*
Emergency services, defined, 727
Emergency water sterilizers, poisoning from, 544–545
Emetics, 54(t)–55(t), 463
Emetine poisoning, 523
Emotional hyperventilation, 280
Emotional problems, 615–627. See also *Psychiatric emergencies.*
Emphysema, coma in, 228
in divers, 165(t)
of eyelids, 283
subcutaneous, 221
Empty bladder syndrome, 318
Encephalitis, alcoholic, 232, 433
viral, 236–237, 239–240
Encephalopathy, and hypertensive crisis, 199–200
Wernicke's, 232, 433
Endep poisoning, 608
Endocarditis, acute bacterial, 191–193
Endocrine disorders, in children, 453–455
Endocrine emergencies, 273–278
Endophthalmitis, 284–285
Endotracheal injections, 108–109
Endotracheal intubation, 42–43, *43*. See also *Airway maintenance.*
Endrin poisoning, 523
Enema, in poisoning, 467
English ivy poisoning, 523
English yew poisoning, 601
Enterovirus infections, 240
Entropion, 283
Eosin poisoning, 523
Ephedrine poisoning, 524
Epicondylitis, 407
Epidemic, management principles for, 12
Epidemic parotitis, 248–249
Epidemic pleurodynia, 240, 249–250
Epididymitis, 323
Epidural abscess, 151

Epidural hemorrhage, 350
Epiglottitis, 635–636
Epileptic seizures, 266–269. See also *Seizures*.
Epinephrine hydrochloride, dosage and administration of, 52(t)–53(t)
  as psychomimetic, 537
  for anaphylactic shock, 154
  in CPR, 30(t)
  intratracheal injection of, 108–109
  poisoning from, 524
  with lidocaine, contraindications to, 90
Epiphyseal injuries, 379
Epistaxis, 414–416, *415*
  in divers, 165(t)
EPN poisoning, 524, 567–568
Epoxy resin poisoning, 524
Epsom salts poisoning, 551
Equanil, poisoning from, 553
  toxicologic values for, 778(t)
Equine tetanus antitoxin, 137
Ergot poisoning, 524
Erysipelas, 658
Erythema multiforme, 661
Erythrityl tetranitrate poisoning, 525
Erythroblastosis fetalis, severe, 452
Escharotomy, 184
Eserine poisoning, 581
Esophageal gastric tube airway, 41, *41*
Esophageal obturator airway, 41, *41*
Esophagitis, reflux, 308
Esophagus, burns of, 187, 478, 551
  foreign bodies in, 298–299
  perforation of, 303
  varices of, 316
Essence of vinegar poisoning, 476
Essential oil poisoning, 566. See also *Oil(s)*.
Estimulex poisoning, 556
Estrogens, conjugated, for pregnancy prevention, in rape victim, 97
Ethanol, for ethylene glycol poisoning, 469(t)
  for methanol poisoning, 469(t)
  poisoning from, 525
  toxicologic values for, 777(t)
Ethchlorvynol, poisoning from, 525
  toxicologic values for, 777(t)
Ether poisoning, 483
Ethide poisoning, 525
Ethine poisoning, 477
Ethoheptazine, 85
Ethosuximide, toxicologic values for, 777(t)
Ethyl alcohol, for pain, 86
  poisoning from, 525
Ethyl chloride poisoning, 483, 525
  topical spray, 86
Ethyl gasoline poisoning, 526–527
Ethyl nitrate poisoning, 589
Ethylene poisoning, 483
Ethylene chlorohydrin poisoning, 526
Ethylene dibromide poisoning, 526
Ethylene glycol poisoning, 526
  ethanol for, 469(t)
Ethylene oxide poisoning, 526
Ethylene trichloride poisoning, 607
Ethylenediamine tetra-acetic acid poisoning, 526
Etrafon poisoning, 608
Eucalyptol poisoning, 527
Euonymin poisoning, 527
Evidence, criminal, at emergency scene, 2
Exanthems, common, differential diagnosis of, 260(t)–261(t)
Excitement states, 278–281
  and brain concussion, 348
  common causes of, 278
  control measures for, 278–279
  drug-induced, 279
  hyperventilation in, 280
  in alcoholism, 279
  in chest and pulmonary conditions, 279
  in head injuries, 279–280
  in thyrotoxicosis, 281
  manic, 281
  phobic, 281
Expert witness, 754–755
Explosions, mass injuries from, 12
Extensor pollicis longus, examination of, 335
External ear squeeze, in divers, 165(t)
Extracranial headache, 209(t). See also *Headache(s)*.
Extradural hemorrhage, 350
Extreme unction, 69(t)–72(t)
Extremities. See also *Arm; Leg*.
  immobilization of, 20, 23
  injuries of, classification of, 6(t)–7(t)
Eye, angioedema of, 282
  black, 288–289
    in anterior fossa fracture, 349
  burns of, 187
  disorders of, 281–294
    nontraumatic, 282–285
    traumatic, 285–291
      contact lens removal in, 291
      vision loss in, differential diagnosis of, 294(t)
    treatment of, general principles of, 281–282
  examination of, 281
    in head injuries, 343, 345(t)
  foreign bodies in, 296
  herpetic infections of, 284
  lacrimator gases in, 612–613
  mustard gas in, 612–613
  penetrating injury of, and sympathetic ophthalmia, 291
  red, differential diagnosis of, 292(t)
Eye patch, 287
Eye strain, 210
Eyelashes, inversion of, 285
Eyelid, burns of, 288
  ecchymosis of, 288–289
    in anterior fossa fracture, 349
  edema of, 283

Eyelid *(Continued)*
emphysema of, 283
eversion of, 283
injuries of, 288–289
insect bites of, 289
inversion of, 283
lacerations of, 289

Facial nerve, laceration of, 699
paralysis of, 420
Factor VIII deficiency, 359
Factor IX deficiency, 359
Fahrenheit-centigrade conversion table, 772
Fainting. See *Syncope*.
False grape poisoning, 573
False hellebore poisoning, 611
False morel poisoning, 531, 540
Familial periodic paralysis, 425
Fancy leaf caladium poisoning, 487, 499
Fasciitis, necrotizing, 688–691, 689(t)
Fat embolism, and prolonged postoperative coma, 231
Fava bean poisoning, 527
Favism, 527
Febrile illnesses. See *Fever(s)*.
Feces, blood in, 304–306, *305*
impacted, 302–303
Feet. See *Foot*.
Felons, 151
Femoral head and neck fractures, 397
Femoral hernia, 306
Femoral shaft fractures, 397
Femoral vein cannulation, 120(t), 123, *123*
Fenfluramine hydrochloride poisoning, 527
Fenoprofen, 85
Fentanyl, indications for, 84
Fenthion poisoning, 567–568
Ferbam poisoning, 522
Fer-de-lance bites, 173–176
Fern, male, poisoning from, 488
Ferrous salts. See *Iron salts*.
Fetal circulation, persistence of, 453
Fetus, effects of drugs on, 436
maturity of, estimation of, 439–441
Fever(s), breakbone, 238
dandy, 238
dengue-like, 236–237
headache and, 210
hemorrhagic, 236–237
in dialysis patients, 324(t)
metal fume, 554
Monday morning, 554
nonspecific, treatment of, 234(t)
parrot, 250
polymer flume, 583
Q, 255(t)
rat bite, 173
requiring treatment, signs and symptoms of, 235(t)
Rocky Mountain spotted, 176, 252, 255(t)

Fever(s) *(Continued)*
scarlet, 252
treatment of, 234(t)
typhoid, 259
typhus, 252, 254(t)–255(t), 259
undulating, 259
yellow, 265
Fiberoptiscopy, 140
Fibrillation. See also *Cardiac arrhythmias*.
atrial, 191, *192*
ventricular, 36–37, *193*
defibrillation for, 51
prophylaxis for, 206
Fibrinogen coagulation test, 133
Fibrinolytic disorders, 355–358, 356(t)–357(t)
Fibromyositis headache, 213
Fibula, fractures of, 402
splinting of, 375(t)
Filariasis, 240
Finger(s), abscess of, 151, 152
baseball, 335, 342, 394
compressive centripetal wrapping of, 726, *726*
contusions of, 340
dislocations of, 395
fractures of, 393–395
splinting of, 338, 340, 375(t)
infections of, 338
injuries of. See also *Hand, injuries of*.
mallet, 335, 342, 394
nerve injuries of, 335, 341
ring removal from, 114, 333
splinting of, 375(t)
tendon injuries of, 336, 342
repair of, 677
Finger cherry poisoning, 527
Fingernail, abscess of, 152
acid burns of, 543
hematoma of, 339
incomplete avulsion of, 340, *341*
Fingernail bed, laceration of, 340, *340*
Fingernail polish poisoning, 563
Fingernail polish remover poisoning, 563
Fire ant stings, 693
Fire bombs, mass injuries from, 12
Fire bush poisoning, 586
Fire extinguisher poisoning, 527–528
Fire thorn poisoning, 586
Fires, evacuation principles in, 178
Fireworks poisoning, 528
Fish poisoning, 531, 602–603
Fish tapeworms, 314(t)–315(t)
Fishhook removal, 681, *682*
Fissures, anal, 308
Fistula, tracheoesophageal, congenital, 458
Flail chest, 218
Flash burns, 187
of eye, 286–287
Flavin poisoning, 522–523
Flea bites, 171–172
Flexor digitorum profundus, examination of, 335

Flexor digitorum superficialis, examination of, 335
Flexor tendons, injuries of, 336, 341–342
examination in, 335
repair of, *677*
Flexor tenosynovitis, suppurative, 338
Fluid, daily requirements for, 81
output of, daily, 82
estimation of, 82
Fluid loss, estimation of, 80
Fluid replacement, 79–83
in burn patients, 183–184, 183(t)
in mass casualties, 82–83
solutions for, 82
Flukes, 314(t)–315(t)
Fluorescein poisoning, 523
Fluorescein staining, corneal, 281, 287
Fluoride poisoning, 528
Fluorine poisoning, 589
Fluoroacetate poisoning, 528–529
Fluoroscopy, 139
Flurazepam, dosage and administration of, 52(t)–53(t)
poisoning from, 493, 529
Flutter valve, for tension pneumothorax, 220, *220*
Fly bites, 172
Flying, restrictions on, 163–168
Foley catheter, for nasal packing, 109–110
Follow-up care, guidelines for, 728–729
Food, allergic reactions to, 154–156
headache in, 210
oral burns from, 188
poisoning from, 529–533
Foot, disorders of, 403–404
immersion, 704–706
ligaments of, *401*
nerve blocks for, *89*
splinting of, 375(t)
trench, 704–706
Forced expiratory volume, test of, 135
Foreign bodies, 295–301
general considerations in, 295
in airway, 297–298
localization of, 34(t), 295
removal of, 38–40, *39*
in bronchi, 297–298
in circulation, 301
in conjunctiva, 286
in cornea, 287–288, *288*
in ear, 296
in esophagus, 298–299
in eye, 296
in intestine, 300
in larynx, 297–298
in musculoskeletal system, 300–301
in nose, 296
in sclera, 290
in stomach, 299–300
in throat, 297
in trachea, 297–298
Foreign bodies (*Continued*)
in vagina, 301
removal of, 295–296
from airway, 38–40, *39*
x-rays of, 295
Formaldehyde poisoning, 533
Formalin poisoning, 533
Formic acid poisoning, 533
Foundry worker's ague, 583
Fournier's gangrene, of scrotum, 321
Four-o'clock poisoning, 533
Fowler position, modified, *26*
Fowler's solution poisoning, 486–487
Foxglove poisoning, 518–519
Fracture(s), Bennett's, 393
blood loss estimation for, 379
boxer's, 393
carpal scaphoid, 392
Colle's, 391–392
reversed, 391–392
condylar, 389
greenstick, *380*, 381
immobilization of, 20, *23*, 373–376, 374(t)–375(t), See also *Splinting*.
in mass casualties, 14
maxillofacial, 699
of ankle, 402–403
of cervical spine, 381
splinting, 20, *23*, 374(t)
of clavicle, 385
of coccyx, 385
of elbow, 389
of epiphysis, 379, *380*
of femoral head and neck, 397
of femoral shaft, 397
of fibula, 402
of finger, 393–395
splinting of, 338, 340
of hip, 397
of humerus, 388–389
of jaw, 381, 699, *701*
air travel and, 168
of malleolus, 403
of metacarpal, 393
of metatarsus, 404
splinting of, 338
of navicular, 392
of nose, 416
of orbit, 290, 699, *700*
of os calcis, 403
of patella, 402
of pelvis, 395–397
of penis, 320
of radius, 390–391
distal, 391–392
of head, 390
of ribs, 218–219, 385
intercostal nerve block for, 218, *221*, 222
of scapula, 386
of skull, anterior fossa, 349
basal, 349
bleeding from ear in, 270

Fracture(s) *(Continued)*
of skull, depressed, 348
compound, 349
linear, without depression, 348
middle fossa, 349
otorrhea in, 272
posterior fossa, 350
of sternum, 218, 385
of tarsus, 404
of testis, 318–320
of thumb, 393
of tibia, 402
of toe, 404
of tooth, 696–699, 698(t)
of ulna, 390–392
of vertebrae, 381, 384–385
cervical, 381
thoracic, 219
of wrist, 392
Smith's, 391–392
splinting of, 20, 23, 373–376, 374(t)–375(t)
sternoclavicular, 385
stress, 406(t)
supplies for, 77
supracondylar, 389
treatment of, 379–380
types of, *380*
Free choice consent, 739. See also *Consent*.
French chalk poisoning, 600
Freon poisoning, 516, 533
Friar's cowl poisoning, 477
Friction burns, 187
Frostbite, 704–706
Frostnip, 704–706
Fuel, rocket, injury from, 589–590
Fuel oil burns, 187
Fugu poisoning, 531, 602–603
Fumarin poisoning, 613
Fumigants, soil, 596
Fungal infections, 249
antimicrobial drugs for, 263(t)
Fungicide poisoning, 531
Furacin poisoning, 565
Furniture polish poisoning, 534
Furosemide, dosage and administration of, 52(t)–53(t)

Gadolinium chloride poisoning, 534
Galactosemia, 455
Galerina venenata poisoning, 534
Gallbladder, injuries of, 681–683
perforation of, 303–304
Gallstones, 32, 310
pain in, 145(t)
Gamboge poisoning, 500
Gamekeeper's thumb, 342
Gamma rays, effects of, 16
Gammexane poisoning, 492
Gangrene, Fournier's, of scrotum, 321
gas, 688
Gangrene *(Continued)*
progressive synergistic, 688–691, 689(t)
Gantanol poisoning, 599
Gantrisin poisoning, 599
Gardenal poisoning, 575
Gardening products, poisoning from, 473
Garlic poisoning, 479
Gas(es), nerve, 14
poisonous, mass casualties from, 14
war, 14, 612–613
burns from, 190
Gas abscess, 151
Gas gangrene, 688
Gasoline burns, 187
Gasoline poisoning, 526–527, 534–535, 613
Gastric hemorrhage, aspirin-induced, 488
Gastric lavage, 107, 467
setup for, 77
Gastric suction, in poisoning, 467
Gastritis, aspirin-induced, 488
Gastrocnemius tear, 406(t)
Gastroenteritis, 311(t), 312
Gastrointestinal tract, bleeding in, 304–306, *305*
test for, 133
emergencies involving, 301–317
neonatal, 307
vascular, 316
infections of, 302
parasitic, 313, 314(t)–315(t)
inflammation of, 302
injuries of, 683
obstruction of, 302
poison removal from, 462
Gastroschisis, 458
Gelsemium poisoning, 535
General anesthesia, 90–91. See also *Anesthetics*.
General Information about Surgery form, 742–743
Genital herpes, 242
Genital wart, 238
Genitourinary conditions, 319–328
traumatic, 319–322
Gentamicin, toxicologic values for, 778(t)
Gentian violet poisoning, 522–523
German measles, 252
differential diagnosis of, 260(t)–261(t)
Giardia, 314(t)–315(t)
Gila monster bites, 172
Gingilli poisoning, 594
Gingivitis, acute necrotizing ulcerative, 702–703
Ginkgo tree, dermatitis from, 665(t)
Glasgow Coma Scale, 226(t)
Glaucoma, 283–284
and headache, 210
differential diagnosis of, 292(t), 293(t)
Globus, 620–621
Gloriosa poisoning, 535
Glucide poisoning, 590
Glue, as hallucinogen, 539(t)

Glue *(Continued)*
poisoning from, 582
skin welding by, 666
Glutamic acid poisoning, 535
Glutethimide, poisoning from, 535–536
toxicologic values for, 778(t)
Goiter, congenital, 453
Gold, dimercaprol for, 470(t)
Gold salts poisoning, 536
Golden celandine poisoning, 503
Golden chain poisoning, 548
Golden ragwort poisoning, 594
Gonorrhea, 240–241
postexposure prophylaxis for, 256
Good Samaritan laws, 728, 733
Gout, 366
Gram stain, 107–108
Granulocytopenia, 360
Granuloma inguinale, 241
Grape hyacinth poisoning, 563
Grease gun injuries, 683
Green hellebore poisoning, 611
Greenstick fracture, *380*, 381
Groupers poisoning, 531
Gruthion poisoning, 567–568
Guaiacol poisoning, 536
Gum arabic poisoning, 474
Gunshot wounds, 680
in mass casualties, 13–14
of chest, 219
Gymnothorax flavimarginatus poisoning, 536
Gynecologic conditions, 328–333

Haff disease, 531
Hair dye poisoning, 536
Hair remover poisoning, 515
Hair spray poisoning, 536
Hallucinogens, 536–539
Halon poisoning, 516
Halothane poisoning, 483
Halowax poisoning, 506
Hamstring tears, 398
Hand, abscess of, 150–151
cellulitis of, 339
collar-button abscess of, 150–151
hematoma of, 339–340
incision sites in, *337*
infections of, 338
injuries of, 333–342
abrasion, 339
analgesics for, 339
anesthesia in, 335
antibiotics for, 338, 339
closure of, 336–338
contusion, 339–340
debridement of, 336, *337*
dressings for, 338
final preoperative cleaning of, 335–336
follow-up care of, 339
grease gun, 683

Hand *(Continued)*
injuries of, history-taking in, 334
initial general measures in, 333–336
laceration, 340
motor function testing in, 334
nerve, 334, 341
nerve blocks for, *88*
nerve examination in, 334
paint gun, 683
postoperative care of, 338–339
preliminary cleaning of, 333–334
puncture, 341
ring removal in, 114, 333
splinting of, 338–339, 375(t)
staple gun, 685
tear gas gun, 505, 686
tendon, 336, 341–342
repair of, *677*
tendon examination in, 335
tourniquet for, 335
x-rays for, 334
Hand, foot, and mouth disease, 240
Hangover headache, 207
Hard chancre, 237
Hashish, 538(t)
Hayweed poisoning, 541
Hazardous materials, identification of, 790–791
Head injuries, 343–353. See also specific types; e.g., *Skull fractures*.
airway maintenance in, 346
bleeding from ears in, 270
cerebral edema in, 346–347
classification of, 6(t)–7(t)
differential diagnosis of, 347
emergency care of, axioms for, 352–353, 353(t)
while awaiting transport, 24
excitement states in, 279–280
general considerations in, 343
helmet management and removal in, 25
initial neurologic examination in, 343–344, 345(t)
level of, localization of, 344, 345(t)
lumbar puncture in, 353
pain control in, 347
patient instructions for, 353(t)
sedation in, 346
shock in, 346
Head tilt with neck or chin lift, 38
Headache(s), 207–215
alcohol excess, 207
algorithm for, *208*
caffeine-withdrawal, 207
causes of, *208*, 209(t)
concussion, 210
cluster, 211
earache and, 215
extracranial, 209(t)
eye strain, 210
febrile, 210
food allergy, 210

Headache(s) *(Continued)*
glaucoma, 210
hangover, 207
herpetic, 210–211
histamine, 211
hunger, 211
hypertensive, 211
hypoglycemic, 211
hypotensive, 212
in altitude sickness, 160
in arthritis of cervical spine, 207
in brain tumors, 207
in hyperviscosity conditions, 211
in increased intracranial pressure, 212
in poisoning, 215
inflammatory, 209(t)
meningeal irritation, 212
migraine, 212–213
vision loss in, 294(t)
mixed, 209(t)
muscle contraction, 209(t)
myofibrositis, 213
orthostatic, 212
psychogenic, 213, 214
remedies for, poisoning from, 540
sinus, 213
spinal puncture, 213–214
sunlight, 214
tension, 213, 214
toothache and, 215
toxic, 215
traction, 209(t)
treatment of, algorithm for, *208*
uremic, 215
vascular, 209(t)
vasopressor, 215
Hearing loss, and cerumen, 270, 271
in aerotitis, 269
rapid onset, 271
Hearing tests, 269
Heart. see also *Cardiac.*
injuries of, 217
Heart attack. See *Cardiac arrest.*
Heart block, *192*, 196
complete, *192*, *194*, 199
pacemaker for, 110, *111*
failure of, 201–202
Heart failure, congestive, 196–197
Heartburn, 308
Heat, warm moist, for pain, 87
Heat cramps, 708–709, 710(t)
Heat exhaustion, 709, 710(t)
Heat prostration, 709, 710(t)
Heat stress disorders, 708–712, 710(t)
differential diagnosis of, 710(t)
iatrogenic, 711–712
Heather poisoning, 540
Heatstroke, 709–711, 710(t)
Heavy metal poisoning, BAL for, 489
food-borne, 489
Hedeoma poisoning, 573
Heimlich maneuver, 38–40, *39*
Hellebore poisoning, 611
Helleborein poisoning, 540
Helmets, removal of, 25
Helvella poisoning, 531, 540
Hematologic values, normal, 773(t)
Hematoma, extradural, 350
of ear, 270
of hand, 339–340
of nose, 416
subungual, 339
Hematoma block, 90
Hematuria, post-traumatic, 318, *319*
Hemlock, poison, poisoning from, 511, 583
water, poisoning from, 508
Hemodialysis, 112–113
emergencies in, 323, 324(t)–325(t)
in poisoning, 467
Hemolytic anemia, 358
Hemolytic reactions, in blood transfusion, 118
Hemolytic streptococcal infections, 241
Hemoperfusion, charcoal, in poisoning, 467
Hemopericardium, 219
Hemophilia, 359
Hemoptysis, in divers, 165(t)
massive, 641
Hemorrhage, 353–361
abdominal, pain in, 144(t)
after tonsillectomy, 701–702
after tooth extraction, 700–701
after varicose vein ligation, 724
and anticoagulant therapy, 359–360
protamine sulfate for, 470(t)
vitamin K for, 470(t)
cerebellar, 714–715
chemical control of, 354–355
conjunctival, in divers, 164(t)
control of, 353–355
epidural, 350
esophageal, in Mallory-Weiss syndrome, 316
extradural, 350
from ear, 270
from nose, 414–416, 415
in divers, 165(t)
from peptic ulcer, 304–306
from rectum, 304–306, 309
gastric, aspirin-induced, 488
gastrointestinal, 304–306, *305*
test for, 133
general measures for, 355
in arterial injuries, 712–713
in cancer patients, 449(t)
in clotting disorders, 356(t)–357(t), 359
in dialysis patients, 324(t)
in fibrinolytic disorders, 355–358, 356(t)–357(t)
in fractures, blood loss estimation for, 379
in hypoprothrombinemia, 359
in platelet disorders, 356(t)–357(t), 361
in polycythemia, 360
in pregnancy, antepartum, 442, 442(t)
ectopic, 436

Hemorrhage (*Continued*)
in pregnancy, first trimester, 441–442
in spontaneous abortion, 434–435
in sickle cell crisis, 360–361
intracerebral, 714
intracranial, 350–351, 714–715
mechanical control of, 353–354
medical control of, 354–355
postcircumcision, 321
postoperative, 355
postpartum, 442–443
pulmonary, 641
spontaneous, 355
subarachnoid, 715
subdural, 715
vascular, guide to, 356(t)–357(t)
vitreous, differential diagnosis of, 294(t)
Hemorrhagic fevers, 236–237
Hemorrhoids, 308–309
bleeding, 306
Hemostasis, 353–355
Hemp, Indian. See *Marijuana*.
Henbane poisoning, 544
Henry's law, 160
Henware poisoning, 491
Heparin, and hemorrhage, 359–360
dosage and administration of, 52(t)–53(t)
poisoning from, 540
protamine sulfate for, 470(t)
Hepatic coma, 228
Hepatitis, viral, 242, 243(t), *244*
Heptachlor poisoning, 540
Heracleum lanatum poisoning, 541
Hernias, 306–307
diaphragmatic, neonatal, 452
incarcerated, pain in, 145(t)
Herniated disk, 383–384
Herniated nucleus pulposus, 383–384
Heroin, 538(t)
overdose of, 541
with cocaine, in speedball, 597
Herpangina, 240
Herpes, genital differential diagnosis of, 332(t)
ocular, 284
Herpes simplex, 242
Herpes simplex keratitis, 284
Herpes zoster, 421
Herpes zoster ophthalmicus, 284
Herpetic headache, 210–211
HETP poisoning, 567, 568
Hexamethylenetetramine poisoning, 541
Hexylresorcinol poisoning, 542
Hiatal hernia, 308
Hiccups, 636
High altitude cerebral edema, 161
High altitude pulmonary edema, 161
High altitude sickness, 160
High-impulse CPR, 37
Hip, bursitis of, 405, 407
dislocations of, 397
disorders of, nontraumatic, 407
fractures of, 397
Hip (*Continued*)
splinting of, 375(t)
Hip pointers, 395
Hippomane mancinella poisoning, 542
Histadyl hydrochloride poisoning, 507
Histamine headache, 211
Histamine poisoning, 542
Histoplasmosis, 249
History-taking, at emergency scene, 2
Hives, 664–666
Holly poisoning, 542
Homatropine poisoning, 542
Homeless patients, 626
Homicidal threats, 620
Honey poisoning, 531, 542
Hookworms, 314(t)–315(t)
Hordeolum, 285
Hornet stings, 695
Horse bean poisoning, 527
Horse bites, 172
Horseradish poisoning, 511
Horton's cephalgia, 211
Household cleaners, poisoning from, 509
Household products, poisoning from, 473
Human bites, 172
Human tetanus–immune globulin, 136
Humerus, dislocations of, 386–387
fractures of, 388–389
splinting of, 374(t)
Hunger headaches, 211
Hurricanes, 17–19. See also *Mass civilian casualties; Triage*.
Hyacinth poisoning, 542
Hydrazine, anhydrous, poisoning from, 589
Hydeltra poisoning, 584
Hydrocarbon poisoning, 542
Hydrocele, 323–326
Hydrochloric acid poisoning, 477
Hydrofluoric acid poisoning, 543
Hydrogen, liquid, burns from, 589
Hydrogen peroxide poisoning, 590
Hydrogen selenide poisoning, 544
Hydrogen sulfide poisoning, 544
Hydromorphone hydrochloride, 84
poisoning from, 519
Hydrophobia, 250–251
Hydroquinone poisoning, 544
HydroThinner intoxication, 604
Hydroxyzine, with meperidine, 84
Hymenoptera stings, 154–155, 691–692
Hyoscyamus poisoning, 544
Hyperaldosteronism, 274
Hyperammonemia, 455
Hyperbaric oxygen therapy, 163
Hyperbilirubinemia, 454–455
Hypercalcemia, 366–367
in cancer patients, 449(t)
Hyperemesis gravidarum, 443
Hyperesthesia, hysterical, 621
Hyperglycemia, in diabetes mellitus, 223–226, 227(t). See also *Diabetic coma*.

Hyperinsulinism, 223, 274, 466(t)
  dextrose for, 470(t)
  vs. diabetic coma, 227(t)
Hyperkalemia, 367
  in cancer patients, 449(t)
  in dialysis patients, 324(t)
Hypermagnesemia, 368
Hypernatremia, 368–369
Hyperosmolar nonketotic coma, 228–229
Hyperoxia, in divers, 166(t)
Hyperparathyroidism, acute, 275
Hyperpituitarism, 276
Hyperpotassemia, 367
Hypersensitivity reactions, 154–156
Hypertension, and headache, 211
  in pregnancy, 443–444
  pulmonary, with persistence of fetal circulation, 453
Hypertensive crisis, and encephalopathy, 199–200
  cardiac emergencies in, 199–200
  in pheochromocytoma, 273–274
Hyperthermia, malignant, iatrogenic, 711–712
Hyperthyroidism, 276–277
Hyperuricemia, in cancer patients, 499(t)
Hyperventilation, 280
  diagnosis of, 430(t)–431(t)
Hyperviscosity conditions, headaches in, 211
Hypervitaminoses, 611–612
Hypnosis, 91–92
Hypnotics, poisoning from, 466(t)
Hypocalcemia, 369
  in children, 454
Hypocarbia, in divers, 165(t)
Hypochlorite poisoning, 544–545
Hypoglycemia, 369
  diabetic. See *Insulin shock*.
  in children, 453–454
Hypoglycemic headache, 211
Hypokalemia, 370
  in cancer patients, 449(t)
  in dialysis patients, 325(t)
Hypomagnesemia, 370
Hyponatremia, in cancer patients, 449(t)
Hypoparathyroidism, 275
Hypopharynx, foreign object in, 38–40, *39*, 298–299. See also *Foreign bodies*.
Hypopituitarism, 275–276
Hypoprothrombinemia, 359
Hypotension, and chlorpromazine hydrochloride, 507
  in dialysis patients, 325(t)
  orthostatic, syncope in, 432
Hypotensive headaches, 212
Hypothermia, and prolonged postoperative coma, 232
  core, 706–708
  in blood transfusion, 119
  in dialysis patients, 325(t)
  in divers, 166(t)
Hypothyroidism, 277–278
Hypovolemic shock, 647. See also *Shock*.
  neonatal, 451
  signs and symptoms of, 650(t)
    treatment of, 651(t)
Hypoxia, and prolonged, postoperative coma, 231
  in air travel, 168
  in divers, 164(t)
Hysteria, 620–621
  differential diagnosis of, 430(t)–431(t)
Hysterical paralysis, 425, 621

Ibuprofen, 85
Ice packs, 86–87
Ichthyosarcotoxism, 531
Identification, by caregiver, at emergency scene, 1
Iliac crest injuries, 395
Ileus, paralytic, 303
Ilex aquifolium poisoning, 542
Imipramine poisoning, 608
Immersion foot, 704–706
Immunization, tetanus, 135–137
    for hand injuries, 334
Impetigo contagiosum, 658
Increased intracranial pressure, headaches in, 212
Indelible ink poisoning, 545
Indelible pencil poisoning, 545
Inderal poisoning, 585–586
Indian hemp. See *Marijuana*.
Indian marking nut, dermatitis from, 665(t)
Indian poke poisoning, 545
Indian tobacco poisoning, 550
Indigo poisoning, 545
Industrial hernia, 307
Industrial injuries, 755–757
Infant botulism, 237, 496
  vs. thick paralysis, 175(t)
Infantile paralysis, 240, 250
Infections. See also *Communicable diseases*.
  antimicrobial drugs for, 262(t)–264(t)
  arbovirus, 236–237
  arenavirus, 236–237
  coxsackievirus, 240
  cytomegalovirus, 238
  dengue, 238
  echovirus, 240
  enterovirus, 240
  excitement states in, 280
  fungal, 249
    antimicrobial drugs for, 263(t)
  gastrointestinal, 302
    parasitic, 313, 314(t)–315(t)
  hemolytic streptococcal, 241
  herpes simplex, 242
    genital, 332(t)
    in mass casualties, 12
    ocular, 284
  mycotic, 249

Infections *(Continued)*
mycotic, antimicrobial drugs for, 263(t)
neonatal, 455–456
of ear, 270, 271–272
of hand, 338
of scrotum, anaerobic, 321
of soft tissue, 688–691, 689(t)
of vagina, 331(t), 332(t), 333
of wounds, 674, 688–691
parasitic, 313, 314(t)–315(t)
poliovirus, 240, 250
requiring treatment, signs and symptoms of, 235(t)
respiratory, viral, 237–238
treatment of, 234(t)
rickettsial, 252, 254(t)–255(t)
antimicrobial drugs for, 264(t)
staphylococcal, of skin, 658
streptococcal, of skin, 658
hemolytic, 241
soft tissue, 688–691, 689(t)
Infectious diseases. See *Communicable diseases*.
Infectious mononucleosis, 242–244
differential diagnosis of, 260(t)–261(t)
Inflammatory headache, 209(t). See also *Headache*.
Influenza, 245
Information, release of, 750–752
Informed consent, defined, 739. See also *Consent*.
Inguinal hernia, 306–307
Inhalation anesthetics, 90–91
poisoning from, 483
Injection, intraglossal, 108
intratracheal, 108–109
Injuries. See also *Wound(s)* and specific types.
critical, defined, 7(t)
mass, 9–19. See also *Mass civilian casualties; Triage*.
minor, defined, 6(t)
moderate, defined, 6(t)
most severe, defined, 7(t)
multiple, classification of, 6(t)–7(t)
severe, defined, 6(t)
Ink, indelible, poisoning from, 545
Ink eradicator poisoning, 545
Inkberry poisoning, 582
Inky cap poisoning, 530, 545
Insect bites, 172
allergic reaction to, 154–156, 690–691
of eyelid, 289
Insect stings. See *Sting(s)*.
Insecticides, organophosphate, poisoning from, 567–569
Insomnia, 621–622
Insulin poisoning, 545
Insulin shock, 223, 274, 466(t)
dextrose for, 470(t)
vs. diabetic coma, 227(t)
Insurance, malpractice, 733
Intercostal nerve block, 221, 222
Intermittent abdominal compression, with CPR, 37
International Morse code, 782
Interstitial pneumonia, 245
Intervertebral disk, herniated, 383–384
Intestinal flukes, 314(t)–315(t)
Intestinal round worms, 314(t)–315(t)
Intestinal parasites, 313, 314(t)–315(t)
Intestine(s). See also *Colon; Gastrointestinal tract*.
adhesions of, 303
foreign bodies in, 300
injuries of, 683
intussusception in, 302
obstruction of, 302–303
congenital, 458
perforation of, 303–304
congenital, 458
Intocostrin poisoning, 512
Intracerebral hemorrhage, 714
Intracranial disease, vision loss in, 293(t)
Intracranial hemorrhage, 350–351, 714–715
Intracranial pressure, increased, headache in, 212
Intraglossal injections, 108
Intraocular pressure tonometry, 108
Intraperitoneal perforation, 303–304
Intratracheal injections, 108–109
Intravenous anesthetics, poisoning from, 483
Intravenous starter set, 74
Intubation. See also *Airway maintenance*.
endotracheal, 42–43, *43*
nasotracheal, 42
Intussusception, 302
pain in, 145(t)
Inversine poisoning, 552
Iodate poisoning, 545
Iodide poisoning, 545
Iodine poisoning, 545
Iodoform poisoning, 546
Ionizing radiation. See *Radiation*.
Ipecac, fluid of, 463, 546
syrup of, 463
dosage and administration of, 54(t)–55(t)
Iridocyclitis, 284
differential diagnosis of, 292(t)
Iris, injuries of, 290
Iris poisoning, 546
Iritis, 284
differential diagnosis of, 292(t)
Iron oxide poisoning, 546
Iron salts poisoning, 546
deferoxamine for, 471(t)
Ischioanal abscess, 151
I-sedrin poisoning, 524
Isocyanate poisoning, 590
Isodrin poisoning, 517
Isolan poisoning, 567–568
Isoniazid poisoning, 546–547
Isophen poisoning, 556
Isopropyl alcohol poisoning, 525, 547

Isoproterenol, dosage and administration of, 54(t)–55(t)
in CPR, 30(t)
poisoning from, 547
toxicologic values for, 778(t)
Isotope production facility accidents, 14–16, 15(t), 17(t)
Isotron poisoning, 516
Isuprel poisoning, 547
Itai-itai disease, 499
Italian asp stings, 694
Itch, washermans', 665(t)
Itching. See *Pruritus*.
Ivray poisoning, 550
Ivy, English, poisoning from, 523

Jack-in-the-pulpit poisoning, 547
Jake poisoning, 609
Jamestown weed poisoning, 514
Japanese lacquer tree, dermatitis from, 665(t)
Jatropha nut oil poisoning, 547
Jaw, dislocations of, 381
fractures of, 381, 699, *701*
air travel and, 168
splinting of, 374(t)
Jaw lift, 38
Jehovah's witnesses, transfusion refusal form for, 747
Jellyfish stings, 695
Jequirty bean poisoning, 547
Jerusalem cherry poisoning, 547, 597
Jet bead tree poisoning, 589
Jimsonweed poisoning, 488, 491, 514
Joints, of finger, contusions of, 340
of hand, infection of, 338
Jonquil poisoning, 563
Jugfish poisoning, 531, 602–603
Jugular vein, internal, venous cannulation of, 120(t), 123–128, *124*, *125*
Jute poisoning, 548

Kawasaki's disease, 245–246
vs. toxic shock syndrome, 258
Keratitis, 294
differential diagnosis of, 292(t)
herpetic, 284
Kerosene, burns from, 187
poisoning from, 548
Ketamine poisoning, 483, 537, 575
Ketoacidosis, diabetic treatment of, 223–226
vs. hyperinsulinism, 227(t)
Kidney, injuries of, 318
Kissing bug bites, 172
Kiszka poisoning, 531
Knee, disorders of, 398–402, 400(t)
fractures of, 399–402, 400(t)
ligaments of, *401*
Knee (*Continued*)
splinting of, 375(t)
Knife wounds, 685
of chest, 219
Knockout drops, 504
Korlan poisoning, 567–568
Krait bites, 173–176

Labarraque's solution, 544–545
Labor. See also *Delivery*.
cord prolapse and rupture in, 446
length of, 437
precipitate, emergency delivery in, 436–438, 440–441
premature, 444–445
true, signs of, 437
Laburnum poisoning, 548
Lacerations, follow-up care of, 678, 679(t)
of arteries, 713
of bladder, 318
of conjunctiva, 287
of eyelid, 289
of facial nerve, 699
of hand, 340
nerves of, 336, 341
of nail bed, 340, *340*
of nose, 416
of parotid duct, 699
of penis, 320
of scalp, 351–352
of tendons, 377–378, 378(t), 677
repair of, 669–674, *670–675*
Lachman test, 399
Lacquer tree, dermatitis from, 665(t)
Lacrimator war gases, 612–613
Lactic acid poisoning, 477, 548
Land to air signals, 793
Lanoxin, toxicologic values for, 777(t)
Lantana poisoning, 548
Lapis lazuli poisoning, 610
Large intestine, injuries of, 683. See also *Intestine(s)*.
Larkspur poisoning, 515
Larval stings, 693
Laryngeal atresia, 453
Laryngeal foreign bodies, 297–298
Laryngeal obstruction, subglottic, 634–635
Laryngitis, 637
subglottic, 635–636
Laryngotracheobronchitis, 634–635
Last rites, 69(t)–72(t)
Lathyrism, 531
Laudanum poisoning, 560
Laundry bleach poisoning, 495
Laundry bluing poisoning, 495
Laundry detergent poisoning, 595
Laurel poisoning, 495, 548
Lavage, gastric, 107
equipment for, 77
Lawn mower injuries, 684

Lead, food contamination with, 531
poisoning from, 531
CaEDTA for, 470(t)
dimercaprol for, 470(t)
Lead arsenate poisoning, 548
Lead oxide poisoning, 554
Lead salts poisoning, 548–549
Left bundle branch block, *195*. See also *Cardiac arrhythmias*.
Leg, anatomy of, *413*
immobilization of, 20, *23*, 375(t), 376
injuries of, classification of, 6(t)–7(t)
crushing, 681
soft tissue, 406(t)
muscles of, *412*
peripheral nerve injuries of, 425–427
Legionnaire's disease, 246
Lemon grass oil poisoning, 549
Length, U.S.-metric conversion table for, 771(t)
Leprosy, 246
Lethane poisoning, 549
Lewisite, 613
Liability cases, 732
Librium, poisoning from, 493, 504
toxicologic values for, 777(t)
Lice, 659–660
Lidocaine, dosage and administration of, 54(t)–55(t)
for local/regional anesthesia, 87–90, *88*, *89*
in CPR, 30(t)
intratracheal injection of, 108–109
topical, 86
Life lines, 109
Life support, advanced cardiac, 30(t), 31(t), 35
at emergency scene, 3–4
basic, 27, *28*, 31(t). See also *Resuscitation*.
decision tree for, *29*
termination of, permit for, 749–750
Life support unit, 35
Ligaments, injuries of, management of, 378(t)
of ankle, *401*
of back, *386*
of foot, *401*
of knee, *401*
injuries of, 398–399, 400(t)
of lower extremity, *401*
of neck, *382*
of pelvis, *396*
of ribs, *386*
of shoulder and upper extremity, *388*
Lighter fluid poisoning, 549
Ligustrum vulgare poisoning, 584
Lilacin poisoning, 602
Lily, calla, poisoning from, 500
climbing, poisoning from, 535
corn, poisoning from, 611
Lily of the valley poisoning, 549
Lima bean poisoning, 549
Limbitrol poisoning, 608
Lime poisoning, 549
chlorinated, 544–545
Lindane poisoning, 492, 549
Lip, suturing of, *671*
Lipstick poisoning, 549
Liquid measures, equivalent, 771(t)
Lithium carbonate poisoning, 550
toxicologic values for, 777(t), 778(t)
Live birth, defined, 729
Liver, injuries of, 683–684
Llama bites, 172
Lobelia poisoning, 550
Local anesthetics, 87–90, *88*, *89*. See also *Caine preparations*.
poisoning from, 483–484
Lockjaw, 256–257
Locoweed poisoning, 484
Locust poisoning, 495, 550
Lolium temulentum poisoning, 550
Lomotil poisoning, 550
Long board, for immobilization, *23*
Lorazepam poisoning, 493
Lorchel poisoning, 531, 540
Louse bites, 172
LSD, 538(t)
Lubricating oil poisoning, 566
Ludwig's angina, 702
Lumbar puncture, 114–116
headache and, 213–214
in head injuries, 353
Lumbar spine, dislocations of, 384
Luminal poisoning, 575
Lunate, dislocation of, 392
Lung. See also *Pulmonary*.
abscess of, 153
burns of, 158, 188
disorders of, 630–642
smoke inhalation in, 158–159
Lupine poisoning, 550
Lye poisoning, 551
Lymphangitis, 725
Lymphatic system emergencies, 725–726
Lymphogranuloma venereum, 246
Lymphopathia venereum, 246

Macassar oil, 591
Mace, 505
Magnesium, burns from, 188
poisoning from, 551
serum, deficient, 370
excessive, 368
toxicologic values for, 778(t)
Magnesium oxide poisoning, 554
Magnesium sulfate poisoning, 551
Magnolia poisoning, 551
Mahimahi poisoning, 531, 603
Maidenhair tree, dermatitis from, 665(t)
Malaria, 246–247
Malathion poisoning, 551
Male fern poisoning, 488

Malignant hyperthermia, iatrogenic, 711–712
Malignant pustule, 236
Malleolar fractures, 403
Mallet finger, 335, 342, 394
Mallory-Weiss syndrome, 316
Malpractice, 732–734
insurance for, 733
statute of limitations on, 733
Mancellier poisoning, 542
Mandelamine poisoning, 541
Mandible, fractures of, 381, 699
air travel in, 168
splinting of, 374(t)
Mandrake poisoning, 552
Maneb poisoning, 522
Manganese oxide poisoning, 554
Manganese poisoning, 551
Mango, dermatitis from, 665(t)
poisoning from, 552
Manic-depressive psychosis, 624
Manic states, 280. See also *Excitement states.*
Manzanillo poisoning, 542
Maple syrup urine disease, 455
Marcozole poisoning, 556
Marijuana, 538(t), 552
Marine animals, poisoning from ingestion of, 522, 602–603
stings of, 693
Marsh marigold poisoning, 500
Masks, ventilatory, 46, 47, *47*
Mass Casualty Incident, defined, 5
Mass civilian casualties, 9–19
communication in, 10(t)
contamination abatement in, 10(t)
emergency treatment areas for, 11(t)
evaluation and care in, 10(t)–11(t)
fluid and electrolyte replacement for, 82–83
hospital admission for, 11(t)
medical emergencies in, 14
morgue for, 11(t)
public relations for, 11(t)
security for, 11(t)
supplies and personnel for, 10(t)
surgical area for, 11(t)
sustenance for, 11(t)
teamwork in, 11(t)
transport in, 10(t), 20–27
triage for. See *Triage.*
victim tagging in, 5–8, 11(t)
MAST, 113–114
air travel and, 168
Masterwort poisoning, 541
Mastitis, 329
Mastoiditis, 271
Mastopathy, 329
Match poisoning, 552
Match test, of ventilatory capacity, 135
Maxilla, fractures of, 381, 699, *701*
air travel in, 168
Maxillofacial fractures, 699
Mayapple poisoning, 552
Meadow saffron poisoning, 489, 510–511
Measles, 247
differential diagnosis of, 260(t)–261(t)
Measurements, U.S.-metric equivalent, 770(t)–772(t)
Mecamylamine poisoning, 552
Meconium aspiration, 452
Median nerve, examination of, 334
Medical examiner's cases, 65, 66(t)
Medical information, release of, permit for, 734
Medicine, storage of, in catastrophe, 14
Medicolegal evidence, at emergency scene, 2
Melia azedarach poisoning, 552
Melitoxin poisoning, 517
Meniere's disease, 417–418
Meningeal irritation, headache in, 212
Meningitis, bacterial, 247–248
coma in, 222
neonatal, 456
spinal puncture in, 114–116
Meningococcemia, 248
Meningoencephalitis, 236–237, 239–240
Meningomyelocele, 457
Meniscus tear, 398–399, 400(t)
Menorrhagia, 329
Menstrual period, absence of, 328
abnormally profuse, 329
bleeding between, 329–330
painful, 329
Mental illness, 615–627. See also *Psychiatric emergencies.*
Mental institution, treatment in, 616
involuntary, 622–623
Mentally incompetent adults, consent for, 745
Meperidine, dosage and administration of, 54(t)–55(t)
indications for, 84
poisoning from, 553
Meprobamate poisoning, 553
toxicologic values for, 778(t)
Merbromin poisoning, 553–554
Mercaptan poisoning, 553
Mercocresol poisoning, 553–554
Mercresin poisoning, 553–554
Mercurochrome poisoning, 553–554
Mercurophylline poisoning, 554
Mercurous chloride poisoning, 500
Mercury, ammoniated, poisoning from, 481
bichloride of, poisoning from, 494
poisoning from, 553
dimercaprol for, 470(t)
penicillamine for, 470(t)
Mercury antiseptics, poisoning from, 553–554
Mercury diuretics, poisoning from, 554
Mercury oxycyanide poisoning, 554
Mercuzanthin poisoning, 554
Mersalyl poisoning, 554
Merthiolate poisoning, 553–554
Mescal poisoning, 554
Mescaline, 538(t), 554
Mesenteric adenitis, 313

Mesenteric vascular occlusion, 316
Metabolic acidosis, 361–364, 362(t)–363(t)
 in blood transfusions, 118
 management of, 79–83
Metabolic alkalosis, 363(t), 365, 366(t)
 management of, 79–83
Metabolic disorders, 361–372
Metabolic resuscitation, at birth, 451
Metacarpal fractures, 393
Metacide poisoning, 567–568
Metal burns, of ear, 186
 of eye, 187
Metal fume fever, 554
Metal poisoning, BAL for, 489
 food-borne, 531
Metaldehyde poisoning, 555
Metatarsal fractures, 404
Methadone, abuse of, 539(t)
 poisoning from, 555
Methamphetamines, abuse of, 539(t)
 dependence on, 482
 poisoning from, 481–482, 556
 with Percodan, 597
Methanol, poisoning from, 555–556
  ethanol for, 469(t)
 toxicologic values for, 778(t)
Methantheline bromide poisoning, 556
Methaqualone poisoning, 556
Methedrine. See *Methamphetamine(s).*
Methemoglobinemia, 472
Methenamine poisoning, 541, 556
Methimazole poisoning, 556
Methol poisoning, 552
Methorphinan hydrobromide poisoning, 556
Methoxamine, dosage and administration of, 54(t)–55(t)
Methoxychlor poisoning, 557
Methoxyphenol poisoning, 536
Methyl acetate poisoning, 557
Methyl alcohol poisoning, 555–556
Methyl bromide poisoning, 557
Methyl cellosolve poisoning, 557
Methyl chloride poisoning, 557
Methyl ethyl ketone poisoning, 558
Methyl formate poisoning, 558
Methyl hydrate poisoning, 555–556
Methyl iodide poisoning, 558
Methyl salicylate, poisoning from, 558, 591–593
 topical, 87
Methyl violet poisoning, 558
Methylcyanide poisoning, 476
Methylene blue poisoning, 523, 557
Methylene dichloride poisoning, 557
Methylergonovine, dosage and administration of, 54(t)–55(t)
Methylmalonic acidemia, 455
Methylmorphine poisoning, 510
Methylprednisolone sodium succinate, dosage and administration of, 54(t)–55(t)
Methylrosaniline chloride poisoning, 558
Methyprylon, toxicologic values for, 778(t)
Methysergide maleate poisoning, 558
Meticortelone poisoning, 584
Meticorten poisoning, 584
Metric-U.S. equivalent measurements, 770(t)–772(t)
Metrorrhagia, 329–330, 330(t)
Metubine iodide poisoning, 512
Mexican jumping bean poisoning, 558
Mickey Finn, 512, 559
Migraine headaches, 212–213
 vision loss in, 294(t)
Military anti-shock trousers, 113–114
 air travel in, 168
Military personnel and dependents, emergency care of, 753
Milk sickness, 531
Milkweed poisoning, 559
Miltown poisoning, 553
Mimosa poisoning, 559
Mind-affecting chemicals. See *Hallucinogens.*
Mineral oil poisoning, 566
Minors, emergency care of, permits for, 738(t), 739, 740
  who may sign, 745
Mipafox poisoning, 567–568
Miscarriage, 434–435
Mistletoe poisoning, 559
Mites, 172, 659–660
Mittelschmerz, 330
Mock orange poisoning, 478
Model airplane glue, as hallucinogen, 539(t)
 poisoning from, 582
Modified Fowler position, *26*
Modified Sims position, *26*
Modified Trendelenburg position, *26*
Molluscum contagiosum, 248
Monday morning fever, 554
Moniliasis, vaginal, 332(t)
Monkshood poisoning, 477, 559
Monoamine oxidase inhibitors, anesthetic potentiation by, 231
Monochlorobenzene poisoning, 505
Mononucleosis, infectious, 242–244
  differential diagnosis of, 260(t)–261(t)
Monosodium L-glutamate poisoning, 559
Monteggia's fracture, 391
Moonflower poisoning, 484
Moonseed poisoning, 559
Morbus strangulatorius, 702
Morel poisoning, 531, 540
Morgue, for mass civilian casualties, 11(t)
Morning glory seeds, as hallucinogen, 537, 560
Morphine, abuse of, 539(t)
 dosage and administration of, 54(t)–55(t)
 indications for, 84
 poisoning from, 560
Morse code, 792
Mosquito bites, 172

Moth repellent poisoning, 561
Mother of pearl poisoning, 560
Motion sickness, 418
Motor function, evaluation of, 424(t)
  in head injuries, 343–344, 345(t)
Mountain laurel poisoning, 561
Mountain sickness, 160
Mountain tobacco poisoning, 486
Mousebane poisoning, 477
Mouth, burns of, 188, 478, 551
  trench, 702–703
Mower injuries, 684
Mucocutaneous lymph node syndrome, 245–246
Mucous membrane, burns of, 188, 478, 551
  disorders of, 657–666
  poison removal from, 462
Multiple injuries, classification of, 6(t)–7(t)
Mumps, 248–249
Murder, threats of, 620
Muriatic acid poisoning, 477
Murine typhus, 252, 254(t), 259
Mucuna pruriens poisoning, 561
Muscarine poisoning, 561
Muscle contraction headache, 209(t). See also *Headache(s)*.
Muscle relaxant poisoning, 561
Muscle strength, evaluation of, 424(t)
Muscle weakness, evaluation of, 424(t)
Muscles, disorders of, acute, 423(t)
  injuries of, management of, 378(t)
  of deglutition, disorders of, 425
  of lower extremity, *412*
  of respiration, disorders of, 425
  of trunk, *408–409*
  of upper extremity, *410*
Musculoskeletal disorders, 372–413
  analgesia in, 372
  diagnosis of, 372–373
  follow-up evaluation in, 373–376
  general considerations in, 372–376
  initial immobilization for, 373, 374(t)–376(t)
  transport in, 372. See also *Transport*.
  treatment of, 373
  x-rays in, 372–373
Musculoskeletal foreign bodies, 300–301
Mushroom(s), hallucinogenic, 538(t)
  poisoning from, 561–562
Mushroom miasma, 562
Musquash root poisoning, 508
Mussel poisoning, 562
Mustard gas, 612–613
Mustargen poisoning, 566
Mustine poisoning, 566
Myasthenia gravis, 418–420
  neonatal, 457
Mycotic infections, 249
  antimicrobial drugs for, 263(t)
Myocardial infarction, *194*, 200–201
  pacemaker for, 110, *111*
    failure of, 201–202
Myofasciitis, headache in, 213
Myofibrositis, headache in, 213
Myonecrosis, clostridial, 688–691, 689(t)
Myopathy, acute, 423(t)
Myositis, streptococcal, 689–691, 689(t)
Myringitis, bullous, 270
Myristicin poisoning, 562
Mysoline, toxicologic values for, 779(t)
Mytilotoxism, 531–532
Myxedema coma, 277–278

Nabam poisoning, 522
Nail. See *Fingernail*.
Nail polish poisoning, 563
Nail polish remover poisoning, 563
Naked lady poisoning, 489
Naloxone, as antidote, 469(t)
  dosage and administration of, 54(t)–55(t)
  intratracheal injection of, 108–109
Naloxone hydrochloride test, 133–134
Napalm burns, 188
Naphazoline hydrochloride poisoning, 585
Naphtha poisoning, 563
Naphthalene poisoning, 563
Naphthalin poisoning, 563
Naphthol poisoning, 563
Naphthylamine poisoning, 563
α-Naphthylthiourea poisoning, 485
Naproxen, 85
Naproxen sodium, 85
Narcan test, 133–134
Narcissus poisoning, 563
Narcotics, addiction to, 59–61
    tests for, 133–134
  administration of, 84
  choice of, 84
  contraindications to, 83–84
  dosage of, 84
  indications for, 83
  opium derivative, test for, 134
  poisoning by, 466(t), 563
    nalaxone for, 469(t)
  prescription requirements for, 95
  sensitivity to, in myxedema, 277–278
  types of, 59
Narcylene poisoning, 477
Nasal septum, abscess of, 151
  injuries of, 416
Nasopharyngeal airway, 40
Nasotracheal intubation, 42
Natural Death Act, 64, 749–750
Natural disasters, 17–19. See also *Mass civilian casualties; Triage*.
  guidelines for, 17–18
  individual preparedness for, 18–19
  individual responsibility to community in, 19
  potable water in, 19
Nausea and vomiting, in pregnancy, 443
Navicular, fractures of, 392

Near-drowning, 157–158
Neck. See also *Cervical spine.*
  dislocation of, 381
  fracture of, 381
  ligaments of, *382*
  penetrating wounds of, 684
  splinting of, 374(t)
  strain of, 381–382, 422
  whiplash injuries of, 381–382, 422
Necrotizing fasciitis, 688–691, 689(t)
Needle, contaminated, puncture by, algorithm for, *244*
Negligence, 732. See also *Malpractice.*
Nembutal, toxicologic values for, 778(t)
Neonate, alcohol withdrawal in, 457
  Apgar score of, 450
  baptism of, 70(t)–71(t)
  birth certificate for, 729–730
  birth injuries of, 456
  death certificate for, 730
  emergency conditions of, 450–453
  gastrointestinal emergencies in, 307
  resuscitation of, 451
Neostigmine bromide poisoning, 563–564
Nephritis, 326
Nerve(s), distribution of, *428*
  facial, laceration of, 699
  lacerated, repair of, 677
  of hand, examination of, 334
    injuries of, 334, 341
  peripheral, of extremities, injuries of, 425–427
Nerve block(s), 87–90, *88*, *89*. See also *Anesthetics, local.*
  intercostal, *221*, 222
Nerve gases, 14, 564
Neuralgia, 420
Neuritis, 420
  cervical, in whiplash injuries, 381–382, 422
  optic, differential diagnosis of, 294(t)
  peripheral, in pregnancy, 421
  retrobulbar, 421
    differential diagnosis of, 294(t)
Neurologic deficit, reversible ischemic, 722
Neurologic disorders, 416–433
  general considerations in, 416–417
  in children, 456–457
  in divers, 166(t)
Neurosis, signs of, 617(t). See also *Psychiatric emergencies.*
Neutrons, 16
Niacin poisoning, 564
Nickel poisoning, 564
  CaEDTA for, 470(t)
  dimercaprol for, 470(t)
Nickel carbonyl poisoning, 564
Nickel oxide poisoning, 554
Nicotine poisoning, 508, 564
Nicotinic acid poisoning, 564
Nifos poisoning, 602
Night blooming cereus poisoning, 564
Nightshade, American, poisoning from, 582
  deadly, poisoning from, 491
  poisoning from, 597
Niran poisoning, 572
Nitrate poisoning, 565
Nitric acid poisoning, 477, 565
Nitric oxide poisoning, 565
Nitrite poisoning, 565
Nitrobenzene poisoning, 565
Nitrochlorobenzene poisoning, 565
Nitrochloroform poisoning, 506
Nitrofurazone poisoning, 565
Nitrogen poisoning, 566
Nitrogen mustard poisoning, 566
Nitrogen oxide poisoning, 569–570
Nitrogen tetraoxide poisoning, 590
Nitroglycerine, dosage and administration of, 54(t)–55(t)
  poisoning from, 590
Nitroprusside poisoning, 566
Nitrous oxide, 90–91
  poisoning from, 483
Nodal paroxysmal tachycardia, *192*, 201
Noludar, toxicologic values for, 778(t)
Nongonococcal urethritis, 249
Non-soap cleaner poisoning, 595
Norisodrine poisoning, 547
Normal values, table of, 773–781
Norpramin poisoning, 608
Nortriptyline poisoning, 566, 608
Nose, conditions of, 414–416
  contusions of, 414
  foreign bodies in, 296
  fractures of, 416
  hematomas of, 416
  lacerations of, 416
  landmarks in, *415*
  packing of, 109–110
Nosebleed, 414–416, *415*
  in divers, 165(t)
Notification of kin, 65–67
Nuclear bombs, 12–13, *13*
  flash burns from, 187
Nuclear magnetic resonance, 140
Nuclear power plant accidents, 14–16, 15(t), 17(t)
Nursemaid's elbow, 390
Nutmeg poisoning, 562
Nuts, cashew, dermatitis from, 502, 665(t)
  coco de mono, poisoning from, 610
  Indian marking, dermatitis from, 665(t)
  jatropha, poisoning from, 547
  tung, poisoning from, 609
  Venezuela, poisoning from, 610
Nux vomica, 598–599
Nyctal poisoning, 502
Nylon, allergy to, 566

Oakleaf poison ivy, 665(t)
Obesity cures, poisoning from, 566

Obstetric emergencies, 433–446
  general considerations in, 433–434
  supplies for, 77
Obstruction, intestinal, 303
Occupational hernia, 307
Occupational injuries, 755–757
Octa-Klor poisoning, 504
Octalox poisoning, 517
Octopus bites, 173
Oculocephalic test, 344, 345(t)
Oculovestibular test, 344, 345(t)
Oil(s), argemone, poisoning from, 486
  banana, poisoning from, 482
  beechnut, poisoning from, 491
  cajeput, poisoning from, 566
  camphorated, poisoning from, 500
  cashew nut, dermatitis from, 502, 665(t)
  castor, poisoning from, 503
  cedar, poisoning from, 503
  China, poisoning from, 574
  chinawood, poisoning from, 609
  cinnamon, poisoning from, 509
  coal, poisoning from, 548
  croton, poisoning from, 512
  essential, poisoning from, 566
  eucalyptus, poisoning from, 527
  fuel, burns from, 187
    poisoning from, 548
  gingilli, poisoning from, 594
  Hell, poisoning from, 547
  jatropha nut, poisoning from, 547
  laurel, poisoning from, 495, 548
  lemon grass, poisoning from, 549
  linseed, poisoning from, 550
  lubricating, poisoning from, 566
  Macassar, poisoning from, 591
  mineral, poisoning from, 566
  nutmeg flower, poisoning from, 562
  of absinthe, poisoning from, 474, 566
  of almond, poisoning from, 565
  of apiol, poisoning from, 609
  of bitter almonds, poisoning from, 495
  of cassia, poisoning from, 509
  of mirbane, poisoning from, 565
  of nutmeg, poisoning from, 562
  of pennyroyal, poisoning from, 573
  of rosemary, poisoning from, 590
  of saffron, poisoning from, 590–591
  of sage, poisoning from, 591
  of sassafras, poisoning from, 591
  of sweet birch, poisoning from, 558
  of tansy, poisoning from, 600
  of turpentine, poisoning from, 609
  of vitriol, poisoning from, 477
  of wintergreen, poisoning from, 558
  of wormseed, poisoning from, 503
  olive, adulteration of, 547
  pear, poisoning from, 482
  pine, poisoning from, 581
  teaberry, poisoning from, 558
  tung, poisoning from, 609
Oil(s) *(Continued)*
  Turkey red, poisoning from, 547
Oleander poisoning, 566–567
OMPA poisoning, 567–568
Omphalocele, 458
Oncologic emergencies, 447, 448(t)–449(t)
Operative and treatment permit, 743–744. See also *Permit(s)*.
Ophthalmia, sympathetic, 291
Opium derivatives test, 134
Opium poisoning, 567
Optic neuritis, differential diagnosis of, 294(t)
Orbital cellulitis, 284–285
Orbital fractures, 290, 699, *700*
Orchitis, 318–320
Organ donation, 68
  permit for, 736, 747–748
  uniform donor card for, 747–748
Organic brain syndrome, 623–624
  acute, 417
Organic phosphate poisoning, 532
Organophosphate poisoning, 567–569
  atropine for, 469(t)
Ornithosis, 250
Oropharyngeal airway, 40
Oropharynx, foreign bodies in, 298–299
Orthodichlorobenzene poisoning, 569
Orthopedic disorders. See *Musculoskeletal disorders*.
Orthopedic supplies, 77
Orthostatic headaches, 212
Orthostatic hypotension, syncope in, 432
Os calcis fractures, 403
Osgood-Schlatter disease, 402
Osmium tetroxide poisoning, 569
Ostochondral separation, 217
Otitis externa, 271–272
  in divers, 166(t)
Otitis media, 272
  and barometric change, 269
  and mastoiditis, 271
  in divers, 166(t)
Otorrhea, 272–273
Ouabain poisoning, 569
Ovarian cyst, rupture of, 331
  torsion of pedicle of, 333
Ovulatory pain, 330
Oxalic acid poisoning, 569
Oxazepam poisoning, 493
Oxides of nitrogen poisoning, 569–570
Oxygen, liquid, 590
  poisoning from, 570
    in divers, 166(t)
Oxygen therapy, hyperbaric, 163
Oxyphenbutazone, poisoning from, 579
Oxyquinolone derivative poisoning, 570–571
Oxytocin poisoning, 583
Oxyuriasis, 314(t)–315(t), 664
Oyster poisoning, 532
Ozone poisoning, 571

Pacemaker, 110, *111*
  failure of, 201–202
Pagitane poisoning, 514
Pain, abdominal. See *Abdominal pain.*
  acupressure for, 91
  acupuncture for, 91
  antidepressants for, 85
  biofeedback for, 91
  ethyl alcohol for, 86
  hypnosis for, 91–92
  in ear, 271
  in head injuries, 347
  in poisoning, 472
  in tooth, 696
  local anesthetics for, 87–90, *88, 89*
  management of, 83–93
    by narcotics, 83–84
    medical, 83–91
    nonmedical, 91–93
  menstrual, 329
  ovulatory, 330
  phenothiazines for, 85
  referred, 141
  regional anesthetics for, 87–90, *88, 89*
  religion and prayer for, 91
  somatic, 140
  topical agents for, 86–87
  transcutaneous nerve stimulators for, 91
  L-tryptophan for, 86
  visceral, 140
Paint gun injuries, 683
Paint poisoning, 571
Paint remover poisoning, 571
Paint thinner poisoning, 604
Palmar space abscess, 151
Pamaquine naphthoate poisoning, 571
Pamelor poisoning, 566
Pancreatic disorders, 274
Pancreatic injuries, 684
Pancreatitis, 313
  acute, pain in, 145(t)
Panda sign, 349
Panic state, 620–621. See also *Excitement states.*
Panmyelotoxicosis, 532
Panophthalmitis, 284–285
  differential diagnosis of, 292(t)
Pansy poisoning, 571
Pantopon poisoning, 571
Paper product poisoning, 571
Paracetamol poisoning, 474, *475*
  N-acetylcysteine for, 471(t), *475*
Parachlorometacresol poisoning, 572
Parachlorometaxylenol poisoning, 572
Paradichlorobenzene poisoning, 572
Paradoxical respiration, in chest injuries, 218
Paraldehyde poisoning, 572
Paralysis, acute, 422–425
    differential diagnosis of, 423(t)
  facial nerve, 420
  familial periodic, 425
Paralysis (*Continued*)
  hysterical, 425, 621
  in spinal cord injuries, 427–429
  noncentral neuropathic, causes of, 425
  of central nervous system origin, causes of, 425
  tick, 175(t), 176
Paralytic ileus, 303
Paranoia, 624. See also *Psychiatric emergencies.*
Paraphimosis, 326
Paraphos poisoning, 572
Paraquat poisoning, 572
Parasitic infections, 313
  antimicrobial drugs for, 264(t)
Parathion poisoning, 532, 567–568, 572
Parathyroid disorders, 275
Parathyroid intoxication, acute, 275
Paregoric poisoning, 572
Paresis, acute, 422–425
Paresthesias, 661–662
  hysterical, 425, 621
Paris green poisoning, 573
Paronychia, 152
Parotid duct, laceration of, 699
Parotitis, 704
  epidemic, 248–249
Paroxon poisoning, 567–568
Paroxysmal tachycardia, nodal, *192,* 201. See also *Cardiac arrhythmias.*
Parrot fever, 250
Parthenocissus quinquefolia poisoning, 573
Patella, dislocations of, 399, 400(t)
  fractures of, 402
  rupture of, 398–399, 400(t)
Patient history, analysis of, at emergency scene, 2
Pavement burns, 188–189
Pawpaw poisoning, 488
PCB poisoning, 573
PCP poisoning, 575, *576,* 577(t)
Peach pit poisoning, 573
Pear oil poisoning, 482
Pediatric emergencies, 450–460
Pediculosis, 659–660
Pelletierine poisoning, 573
Pelvic inflammatory disease, 330–331
Pelvis, fractures of, 395–397
  ligaments of, *396*
  splinting of, 375(t)
Pencils, indelible, poisoning from, 545
Penetrating wounds, 684
  in mass casualties, 13–14
  of chest, 219
  of cornea, 288
  of eye, and sympathetic ophthalmia, 291
  of iris, 290
  of heart, 217
  of neck, 684
Penicillamine, for mercury poisoning, 470(t)
Penis, injuries of, 320
    zipper, 687

Pennyroyal poisoning, 573
Pentaborane, 590
Pentazocine hydrochloride, 85
  poisoning from, 573
  naloxone for, 469(t)
Pentazocine lactate, 85
Pentobarbital, toxicologic values for, 778(t)
Pentothal sodium poisoning, 573–574
Pentylenetetrazole poisoning, 574
Peptic ulcer, bleeding from, 304–306
  pain in, 144(t)
Pepto-Bismol, 54(t)–55(t)
Perch poisoning, 532
Perchlorates, 590
Percodan, 597
Perforating wounds, 685. See also *Penetrating wounds*.
  of chest, 219
Perforation, intraperitoneal, 303–304
  of bladder, 318
  of esophagus, 303
Perfume poisoning, 515, 574
Perianal abscess, 151
Periapical abscess, 149
Pericardial effusion, 202
Pericardial sac aspiration, 110–112
Pericardial tamponade, in cancer patients, 449(t)
Pericarditis, *194*, 202–203
  in dialysis patients, 325(t)
Pericoronitis, 149
Perilunar dislocations, 392
Perineal abscess, 152
Perinephric abscess, 326
Periodontal abscess, 149
Peripheral arteries, embolism of, 719
  thrombosis of, 721
Peripheral facial nerve paralysis, 420
Peripheral nerve. See *Nerve(s)*.
Peripheral neuritis, in pregnancy, 421
Peripheral vein cannulation, 120–122, 120(t), *121*
Perirenal abscess, 326
Peritoneal aspiration, 112
Peritoneal dialysis, 112–113
  in poisoning, 467
Peritonsillar abscess, 152
Periurethral abscess, 152
Permit(s), 734–750
  for blood alcohol test, 734, 735
  for diagnostic procedures, 736
  for disposal of severed or amputated parts, 736
  for emergency care, 734–750
  for immediate treatment, 737
  for information disclosure, 734
  for mentally incompetent adults, 745
  for minors, who may sign, 745
  for organ donor, 736, 747–748
  for photographs, 745–746
  for surgery, treatment without, 736–737
Permit(s) *(Continued)*
  for termination of life support, 749–750
  for therapeutic procedures, 736
  requirements for, 737–739
  telegraph, 746
  telephone, 746
  valid, types of, 746
  verbal, 746
  written, 746
Pernio, 704–706
Persian insect powder poisoning, 586
Pertussis, 265
Peru balsam poisoning, 574
Pesticide poisoning, 574–575
    carbamate, 400
  food-borne, 529
    organophosphate, 567–569
Petroleum distillate poisoning, 575
Petroleum naphtha poisoning, 563
Phalanges. See *Finger(s)*; *Toe(s)*.
Phallodine poisoning, 532
Pharyngitis, 703
Phemerol poisoning, 492
Phenacetin poisoning, 476
Phencyclidine, abuse of, 538(t)
  poisoning from, 575, *576*, 577(t)
Phenobarbital, poisoning from, 575
  toxicologic values for, 778(t)
Phenol, poisoning from, 477, 578
  topical, 86
Phenolphthalein poisoning, 578
Phenoltetrachlorphthalein poisoning, 523
Phenosulfonphthalein poisoning, 523
Phenothiazines, anesthetic potentiation by, 231
  extrapyramidal reactions to, 280–281
  for pain, 85
  poisoning from, 578–579
Phenyl mercuric acetate poisoning, 582
Phenyl salicylate poisoning, 579
Phenylbutazone poisoning, 579
Phenylhydrazine poisoning, 579
Phenytoin, dosage and administration of, 54(t)–55(t)
  poisoning from, 579–580
  toxicologic values for, 779(t)
Pheochromocytoma, 273–274
Philodendron poisoning, 487, 580
Phimosis, 326
Phlebothrombosis, 722–723
Phobias, 281. See also *Psychiatric emergencies*.
Phosdrin poisoning, 567–568
Phosgene poisoning, 580
Phosphamidon poisoning, 567–568
Phosphine poisoning, 580
Phosphoretted hydrogen poisoning, 580
Phosphoric acid poisoning, 580
Phosphorus, burns from, 188–189
  poisoning from, 580–581
Photographs, permit for, 745–746
Photophthalmia, 286–287

Phthalein dye poisoning, 523
Phycomycosis, 249
Physic nut tree poisoning, 547
Physical examination, quick initial, 2–3
systematic, 3–4
Physician, as witness, 754–755
Physician-patient relationship, establishment of, 727–728
Physostigmine salicylate, as antidote, 471(t)
poisoning from, 581
atropine for, 469(t)
Phytolacca poisoning, 582
Picric acid poisoning, 581
Picrotoxin poisoning, 581
Pieris japonica poisoning, 549
Pigeonberry poisoning, 582
Pigments, arsenic, poisoning from, 487
Piles, 308–309, 306
Pilocarpine, poisoning, 581
Pilonidal abscess, 152–153
Pine oil poisoning, 581
Pinks poisoning, 582
Pinworms, 314(t)–315(t), 644
Pit viper bites, 173–176
Pitch burns, 185
Pitcher's elbow, 389
Pituitary disorders, 275–276
Pituitary extracts, posterior, poisoning from, 583
Pituitary hypersecretion, 276
Pituitary insufficiency, 275–276
Pival poisoning, 613
Placenta previa, 442(t)
Placidyl, poisoning from, 525
toxicologic values for, 777(t)
Plague, 249
Plantaris tendon rupture, 406(t)
Plasmapheresis, in poisoning, 467
Plaster of paris poisoning, 582
Plastic glue, abuse of, 539(t)
poisoning from, 582
Plastic poisoning, 582
Plastic surgery techniques, *670–675*
Platelet disorders, 356(t)–357(t), 361
Pleural effusion, 637
Pleuritis, 637
Pleurisy, 637
Pleurodynia, epidemic, 240, 249–250
Plum, American, poisoning from, 480
Plumbism, 548–549
PMA poisoning, 582
Pneumatic trousers, 113–114
air travel in, 168
Pneumonia, 637–638
aspiration, 638
bacterial, 638
congenital, 455–456
interstitial, 245
viral, 245, 638
Pneumonic plague, 249
Pneumonitis, chemical, beryllium-induced, 494
Pneumothorax, 638–639
in divers, 167(t)
in neonate, 452–453
spontaneous, 638–639
tension, 220, *220*
therapeutic, 639
traumatic, 220–221
Poison(s). See also specific poisons.
adsorption of, 467–468
antidotes for, 468, 469(t)–471(t)
classification of, 460–461
defined, 460
precipitation of, 468
radiopaque, 461
removal of, after hypodermic administration, 462
from alimentary tract, 462
from circulation, 467
from gastrointestinal tract, 462
from mucous membranes, 462
from skin, 462
from wounds, 462
unknown, identification of, 464(t)–465(t)
Poison hemlock, 511, 583
Poison ivy, 583, 662–663, 665(t)
Poison kit, 77–78
Poison oak, 583, 662–663, 665(t)
Poison ryegrass, 550
Poison sumac, 583, 662–663, 665(t)
Poisoning, 460–615
abdominal pain in, 147(t)
cathartics for, 467
charcoal hemoperfusion in, 467
emergency kit for, 77–78
emetics for, 463
enema in, 467
gastric lavage in, 467
gastric suction in, 467
gastrointestinal bleeding in, 306
headaches in, 215
legal considerations in, 462
peritoneal hemodialysis in, 467
plasmapheresis in, 467
removal from further external toxin exposure in, 462
removal from further internal toxin exposure in, 462–467
reporting of, 462
self-induced, 462
syrup of ipecac for, 54(t)–55(t), 463
treatment of, general considerations in, 462
initial axioms for, 460–461
supportive, 468–472
urine pH adjustment in, 467
vomiting in, contraindications to, 463
Poinsettia poisoning, 582
Poisonous gases, mass casualties with, 14
Pokeweed poisoning, 582
Poliomyelitis, 250

Poliovirus infections, 240, 250
Polish, fingernail, poisoning from, 563
  furniture, poisoning from, 534
  shoe, poisoning from, 594
  silver, poisoning from, 595
Polish kiszka poisoning, 530
Polychlorinated biphenyl poisoning, 573
Polycythemia, 360
  headache in, 211
Polymer fume fever, 583
Polyps, anorectal, 313
Pomegranate poisoning, 583
Pondimin poisoning, 527
Poppy poisoning, 583
Pork tapeworms, 314(t)–315(t)
Porphyria, acute intermittent, 371
Portuguese man-of-war stings, 694
Possum bug stings, 694
Postcircumcision bleeding, 321
Posterior pituitary extract poisoning, 583
Pot. See *Marijuana*.
Potable water, 19
  sterilizers for, poisoning from, 544–545
Potassium, daily requirements for, 81
  deficiency of, 370
  excessive, 367–368
  normal values for, 776(t)
Potassium chlorate poisoning, 504, 583
Potassium ion poisoning, 583
Potassium oxylate poisoning, 583
Potassium permanganate, poisoning from, 584
  vaginal burns from, 188
Potassium nitrate poisoning, 593
Potato poisoning, 532, 584, 597
Prayer, as analgesic, 91
Precatory bean poisoning, 584
Precordial thump, 48, *49*
Prednisolone, poisoning, 584
Prednisone poisoning, 584
Preeclampsia, 443–444
Pregnancy, abdominal pain in, 434
  chest thrust in, *39*, 40
  delivery in, breech, 438–439
    cesarean section, 438
      after maternal death, 439
    difficult vaginal, 438–439
    emergency nonhospital, 437–439, *440–441*
  drugs in, 436
  ectopic, 436–437
  fetal maturity estimation in, 439–441
  hemorrhage in, antepartum, 442, 442(t)
    first trimester, 441–442
    in ectopic pregnancy, 436
    in spontaneous abortion, 434–435
    postpartum, 442–443
  hyperemesis gravidarum in, 443
  hypertension in, 443–444
  premature labor in, 444–445
  premature membrane rupture in, 445
  peripheral neuritis during, 421
  prevention of, in rape victim, 97
Pregnancy (*Continued*)
  syncope in, 445–446
  therapeutic and diagnostic precautions in, 328
  umbilical cord prolapse and rupture in, 446
  uterine inversion in, 446
  vena cava syndrome in, 446
Premature birth, defined, 729
Prestone poisoning, 526
Priapism, 326–327
Prickly poppy poisoning, 486
Primidone, poisoning from, 584
  toxicologic values for, 779(t)
Primrose poisoning, 584
Primula poisoning, 584
Privet poisoning, 584
Privine poisoning, 585
Procainamide, dosage and administration of, 54(t)–55(t)
  in CPR, 30(t)
  poisoning from, 585
  toxicologic values for, 779(t)
Prochlorperazine, dosage and administration of, 54(t)–55(t)
Proctitis, 309
Progressive synergistic gangrene, 688–691, 689(t)
Prolan poisoning, 585
Pronestyl, poisoning from, 585
  toxicologic values for, 779(t)
Proparacaine, dosage and administration of, 54(t)–55(t)
Propanone poisoning, 476
Prophenpyridamine poisoning, 585
Propoxyphenes, 85
  poisoning from, 585
    naloxone for, 469(t)
Propranolol, dosage and administration of, 54(t)–55(t)
  poisoning from, 585–586
Prostatitis, 327
Prostigmine poisoning, 563–564
Protamine sulfate, for heparin overdose, 470(t)
Protriptyline poisoning, 608
Pruritus, 662
  due to varicose eczema, 724
Pruritus ani, 663
Pruritus vulvae, 664
Psilocybin, as hallucinogen, 538(t)
  poisoning from, 561–562
Psittacosis, 250
Psychiatric emergencies, 615–627
  acute situational reaction as, 618
  delirium as, 618–619
  depression as, 619–620
  drug therapy for, 625
  evaluation in, 616, 617(t)
  homicidal threats as, 620
  hospitalization in, 616
    involuntary, 622–623
  hysteria as, 620
  in runaways and chronically homeless, 626

Psychiatric emergencies (*Continued*)
insomnia as, 621–622
involuntary treatment of, 622–623
manic depression as, 624
neuroses as, 617(t), 621
paranoia as, 624
psychophysiologic illness as, 624–625
psychoses as, 617(t), 623–624
schizophrenia as, 624
suicidal ideation as, 619–620
violent behavior as 626–627
Psychogenic coma, 232
Psychogenic headaches, 213, 214
Psychomimetic drugs, 536–539
Psychophysiologic illness, 624–625
Psychoses. See also *Psychiatric emergencies.*
manic-depressive, 624
paranoic, 624
signs of, 617(t), 623
subacute, 623–624
types of, 623–624
Psychosomatic illness, 624–625
Psychotherapeutic drugs, usage guidelines for, 625
Pterygium, 285
Puffer poisoning, 532, 602–603
Pulmonary. See also *Lung; Respiratory.*
Pulmonary abscess, 153
Pulmonary artery embolism, 639–640
Pulmonary conditions, excitement states in, 279
Pulmonary disease, chronic obstructive, coma in, 228
Pulmonary edema, 627–630
acute, 203
high altitude, 161
in dialysis patients, 325(t)
Pulmonary hemorrhage, 641
Pulmonary hypertension, with persistence of fetal circulation, 453
Pulmonary irritant war gases, 612–613
Puncture wounds, 684
of hand, 341
Punicine poisoning, 573
Puss caterpillar stings, 694
Pyelonephritis, 327
Pyracantha poisoning, 586
Pyramidon poisoning, 480
Pyrethrum poisoning, 586
Pyribenzamine poisoning, 609
Pyridine poisoning, 586
Pyrocatechol poisoning, 586
Pyrogallic acid poisoning, 586–587
Pyrogallol poisoning, 586–587
Pyrogenic reactions, in blood transfusion, 119
Pyrolan poisoning, 587

Q fever, 255(t)
Quaalude poisoning, 556
Quadriceps muscle, rupture of, 400(t)
tear of, 398
Quarantine, of emergency area, 1
Quaternary ammonium salts poisoning, 587
Quinacrine hydrochloride poisoning, 587
Quinidine, poisoning from, 587
toxicologic values for, 779(t)
Quinine poisoning, 587
Quinsy, 152

Rabies, 250–251
immunization for, 251
treatment for, indications for, 169
Racephedrine poisoning, 524
Radial nerve, examination of, 334
Radiation, burns from, 189–190
dose-effect relationship for, 17(t)
effects of, 16, 17(t)
injuries from, mass, 14–16, 15(t), 17(t)
magnitude of, 16
protection from, 15(t)
Radiation exposure team, 16
Radioactive isotope production facility accidents, 14–16, 15(t), 17(t)
Radiography. See *X-rays.*
Radiology. See *X-rays.*
Radionuclide imaging, 140
Radiotelephone 10 code, 792
Radius, distal, fractures of, 391–392
head of, fractures of, 390
subluxation of, 390
shaft of, fractures of, 390–391
splinting of, 375(t)
Ragwort poisoning, 588
Ranunculus scleratus poisoning, 588
Rape, 96–99
definition of, 96
laboratory and evidence kit for, 99
medicolegal documentation in, 98–99
physical examination in, 96
permit for, 739, 741
physical injuries in, treatment of, 96
pregnancy prevention in, 97
psychologic damage in, prevention and treatment of, 96–97
seminal fluid test in, 134–135
venereal disease prevention and treatment in, 97
Rat bites, 173
Rat killer poisoning, 588
Ratsbane poisoning, 516
Rattlesnake bites, 173–176
Rauwolfia alkaloid poisoning, 588
Raynaud's phenomenon, 725
Rectal sphincter tone, evaulation of, in head injuries, 344
Rectum, abscess of, 149
bleeding from, 304–306, 309
polyps of, 313
prolapse of, 307–308

Rectum (*Continued*)
strictures of, 309
Red cedar poisoning, 486
Red sage poisoning, 548
Red snapper poisoning, 531, 532
Red squill poisoning, 588
Referred pain, 141
Reflex(es), evaluation of, in head injuries, 344
Reflex neurovascular syndrome, 421, 725
Reflux esophagitis, 308
Refrigerating agent poisoning, 588
Release from responsibility form, 731, *731*
Release of information, 750–752
Religious rites, in death and dying cases, 68, 69(t)–72(t)
Renal calculi, 327–328
Renal dialysis emergencies, 323, 324(t)–325(t)
Rengas tree, dermatitis from, 665(t)
Reportable diseases and conditions, 100–102, 751–752
child abuse as, 459
epilepsy as, *268*, 269
poisoning as, 462
unusual occurrences as, 731–732
Reserpine poisoning, 588
Resorcinol poisoning, 588
Respiration, paradoxical, in chest injuries, 218–219
Respiratory acidosis, 362(t)
Respiratory alkalosis, 363(t), 365
Respiratory arrest, in divers, 167(t)
Respiratory burns, 158, 188
Respiratory disorders, 630–642
clinical evaluation in, 630
laboratory tests in, 630–631
pediatric, 457–458
Respiratory distress, and foreign bodies, 297–298
evaluation of, 31(t)
Respiratory distress syndrome, 457, 627–630
and blood transfusion, 118
Respiratory failure, acute, 631
Respiratory infections, viral, 237–238, 637–638
treatment of, 234(t)
Respiratory muscles, disorders of, 425
Resuscitation, abdominal thrust in, 38–40, *39*
advanced cardiac life support in, 30(t), 31(t), 35
airway clearance in, 38–40, *39*
airway maintenance in, 38–45
at birth, 450–451
back blows in, 38–40, *39*
cardiac compression in, closed chest external, 48, 49(t)
open chest internal, 50
cardioversion in, 50–51, *50*
cerebrocardiopulmonary, 37
chest thrust in, 38–40, *39*
cricothyrotomy in, 44, *45*
drugs for, 52(t)–55(t)
endotracheal intubation in, 42–43, *43*
Resuscitation (*Continued*)
esophageal gastric tube airway in, 41, *41*
esophageal obturator airway in, 41, *41*
foreign object removal in, 38–40, *39*
further research in, 37
high-impulse, 37
in electrical shock, 226–227
intermittent abdominal compression in, 37
life support decision tree for, *29*
life support phase of, 27, *28*
life support unit in, 35
nasopharyngeal airway in, 40
nasotracheal intubation in, 42
oropharyngeal airway in, 40
precordial thump in, 48, *49*
successful, after cardiac arrest, 36
techniques of, 38–55
termination of, 37, 61–64
tracheostomy in, 44–45
ventilation in, 46–47, *47*. See also *Ventilation*.
Retinal artery occlusion, differential diagnosis of, 293(t)
Retinal detachment, differential diagnosis of, 294(t)
Retinal injuries, 290
Retinal vein occlusion, differential diagnosis of, 293(t)
Retrobulbar neuritis, 421
differential diagnosis of, 294(t)
Retroperitoneal abscess, 153
Retropharyngeal abscess, 153
Reversible ischemic neurologic deficit, 722
Reye's syndrome, 252
Rhinorrhea, 641
Rhinovirus, 237–238
Rhodanate poisoning, 604–605
Rhododendron poisoning, 589
Rhodotypos kerroides poisoning, 589
Rhubarb poisoning, 532, 589
Ribs, fractures of, 218–219, 385
intercostal nerve block for, 218, *221*, 222
splinting of, 374(t)
ligaments of, *386*
Ricin poisoning, 589
Ricinus communis poisoning, 503
Rickettsial infections, 252, 254(t)–255(t)
antimicrobial drugs for, 264(t)
Rickettsial pox, 255(t)
Right bundle branch block, *195*. See also *Cardiac arrhythmias*.
Ring, removal of, 114, 333
Rinne hearing test, 269
Roach poisoning, 532
Roach paste poisoning, 589
Rocket fuels, injuries from, 589–590
Rocky Mountain spotted fever, 176, 252, 255(t)
Rodenticide poisoning, 588
Roentgenography. See *X-rays*.
Ronnel poisoning, 567–568
Rope burns, 187

Rosary pea poisoning, 584
Rosemary oil poisoning, 590
Rotenone poisoning, 590
Roundworms, 314(t)–315(t)
Rubella, 252
differential diagnosis of, 260(t)–261(t)
Rubeola, 247
differential diagnosis of, 260(t)–261(t)
Rubbing alcohol poisoning, 590, 613
Rule of nines, for burns, 180(t)
Rumex acetosa poisoning, 590
Runaways, 626
Rupture, of Achilles tendon, 406(t)
of amniotic membranes, premature, 445
of aorta, 216–217
of diaphragm, 218
of kidney, 318
of ovarian cyst, 331
of patella, 398–399, 400(t)
of plantaris tendon, 406(t)
of quadriceps muscle, 400(t)
of umbilical cord, 436
tracheobronchial, 221
ventricular, 190
Russian fly poisoning, 500

Saccharin poisoning, 590
Saccharinol poisoning, 590
Sacral vertebrae, 385
Saddle embolus, 639
Saffron poisoning, 590–591
Safrole poisoning, 591
Sage poisoning, 591
St. Anthony's fire, 658
Sal ammoniac poisoning, 481
Salicylanilide poisoning, 591
Salicylates. See also *Aspirin*.
poisoning by, 466(t), 591–593
ingestion test in, 134
toxicologic values for, 776(t), 779(t)
Salicylazosulfapyridine poisoning, 599
Salol poisoning, 579
Salpingitis, acute, 330–331
Salt, daily requirement for, 81
poisoning from,, 591, 596
Saltpeter poisoning, 591
Salygran poisoning, 554
Samarium chloride poisoning, 593
Santonin poisoning, 503
Saponin poisoning, 593
Sausage cyanosis, 532
Scabies, 659–660
Scalded skin syndrome, 658–659
Scalp, burns of, 189
lacerations of, 351–352
Scapula, fractures of, 386
splinting of, 374(t)
Scarlatina, 252
differential diagnosis of, 260(t)–261(t)
Scarlet fever, 252
differential diagnosis of, 260(t)–261(t)
Scarlet red poisoning, 594
Schizophrenia, 624. See also *Psychiatric emergencies*.
Schraden poisoning, 567–568
Sciatica, 421–422
Scleral injuries, 290
Scleritis, 285
Scoke poisoning, 582
Scopolamine poisoning, 594
physostigmine for, 471(t)
Scoporius poisoning, 498
Scorpion stings, 694
Scotch broom poisoning, 498
Scotchguard poisoning, 613
Scrotum, anaerobic infection of, 321
Fournier's gangrene of, 321
injuries of, 318, 321–322
Scrub typhus, 255(t), 259
SCUBA diving, 162–163, 164(t)–167(t)
Sea anemone stings, 694
Sea bass poisoning, 531, 532
Sea nettle stings, 694
Sea onion poisoning, 597
Sea snake bites, 173–176
Sea urchin stings, 695
Secobarbital, toxicologic values for, 779(t)
Seconal, toxicologic values for, 770(t)
Sedation, in head injuries, 346
Sedatives, anesthetic potentiation by, 231
poisoning by, 466(t)
Seizures, 266–269
age group factors in, 266
causes of, 266
differential diagnosis of, 430(t)–431(t)
epileptic, further evaluation of, 268
further management of, 268–269
initial treatment of, 267
reporting of, 268, 269
further evaluation of, 268
further management of, 268–269
grand mal, treatment of, 267
in dialysis patients, 325(t)
in poisoning, 468–472
neonatal, 456
reporting of, *268*, 269
types of, 266
Selenium poisoning, 594
Senecio poisoning, 532, 594
Seminal fluid test, in rape, 134–135
Sensory evaluation, in head injuries, 344
Sepsis, neonatal, 456
Septic abortion, 435
Septic arthritis, 404–405
Septic shock, 647. See also *Shock*.
signs and symptoms of, 650(t)
treatment of, 651(t)
Septra poisoning, 599
Serax poisoning, 493
Serpasil poisoning, 588

Service personnel and dependents, emergency care of, 753
Serum desensitization, 102–103
Serum disease, 155–156
Serum sensitivity, 102–103
Serum shock, 156. See also *Shock*.
Sesame oil poisoning, 594
SEVIN poisoning, 501
Sexual assault, 96–99. See also *Rape*.
 examination in, permit for, 739, 741(t)
Shark bites, 173
Sheep dip poisoning, 594
Shellac poisoning, 594
Shellfish poisoning, 532
Shin splints, 406(t)
Shirlan poisoning, 591
Shock, 642–656
 anaphylactic, 154–155, 690–691
 cardiogenic, 647
  signs and symptoms of, 650(t)
  treatment of, 651(t)
 cellular metabolism in, monitoring of, 647(t)
 defined, 642–643
 electrical, 226–227
 hypovolemic, 647(t)
  in neonate, 451
  signs and symptoms of, 650(t)
  treatment of, 651(t)
 in head injuries, 346
 in toxic shock syndrome, 257–258
 insulin, 223, 274, 466(t)
  dextrose for, 470(t)
  vs. diabetic coma, 227(t)
 organ perfusion in, monitoring of, 647(t)
 patient history in, 643–647
 pneumatic trousers for, 113–114
  in air travel, 168
 rapid physical review for, 646(t)
 septic, 647
  signs and symptoms of, 650(t)
  treatment of, 651(t)
 serum, 156
 severity of, physiologic evaluation of, 643, 647(t), 648(t)–649(t)
 signs and symptoms of, 643, 650(t)
 treatment of, 650–656, 651(t)
  initial general measures in, 644(t)–645(t)
 types of, 643–647
Shoe cleaner poisoning, 594
Shoe dye poisoning, 523, 594
Shoe polish poisoning, 594
Shoeguard poisoning, 613
Short board, for immobilization, 23
Shoulder, anatomy of, *388*
 dislocations of, 386–387
 splinting of, 374
Shoulder separations, 386, 387(t)
Sickle cell crisis, 360–361
Sierra fish poisoning, 531
Signals, emergency communication, 792
  land to air, 793
Silver compound poisoning, 595
Silver polish poisoning, 595
Silver salt poisoning, 595
Sims position, modified, *26*
Single photon envasion computerized tomography, 140
Singultus, 636
Sinox poisoning, 520
Sinus arrest, 196. See also *Cardiac arrhythmias*.
Sinus bradycardia, 193–196. See also *Cardiac arrhythmias*.
Sinus headaches, 213
Sinus squeeze, 414
 in divers, 167(t)
Sinus tachycardia, *192*, 203. See also *Cardiac arrhythmias*.
Sinusitis, 641–642
 in divers, 167(t)
662 poisoning, 492
Skin, disorders of, 657–666. See also *Dermatitis*.
 contagious and communicable, 657–660
 foreign bodies in, 300–301
 poison removal from, 462
 welded, 666
Skin diving hazards, 162–163, 164(t)–167(t)
Skull fractures, anterior fossa, 349
 basal, 349
  bleeding from ear in, 270
  otorrhea in, 272
 depressed, 348
  compound, 349
 linear, without depression, 348
 middle fossa, 349
 posterior fossa, 350
Skull traction, 114
Skunk cabbage poisoning, 611
Slag burns, of ear, 186
 of eye, 187
Small intestine, injuries of, 683. See also *Intestine(s)*.
Smallpox, 252
 differential diagnosis of, 260(t)–261(t)
Smelter shakes, 554
Smith's fracture, 391–392
Smoke inhalation, 158–159
Smoke irritant war gases, 612–613
Snail bait poisoning, 595
Snake bites, 173–176
Snorkeling, hazards of, 162–163, 164(t)–167(t)
Snowdrop poisoning, 598
Snuff, 595
Soap poisoning, 595
Soapberry poisoning, 478
Sodium, deficiency of, 370–371
 excessive, 368
Sodium arsenate poisoning, 596
Sodium arsenite poisoning, 596
Sodium bicarbonate, dosage and administration of, 54(t)–55(t)

Sodium bicarbonate (*Continued*)
in CPR, 30(t)
Sodium chloride, daily requirements for, 81
poisoning from, 591, 596
Sodium cyanide poisoning, 596
Sodium fluoroacetate poisoning, 596
Sodium hydroxide poisoning, 596
Sodium ion poisoning, 596
Sodium nitrite, as cyanide antidote, 469(t)
poisoning from, 596
Sodium sulfite poisoning, 596
Sodium thiosulfate, as cyanide antidote, 469(t)
Sodomy, forced, 99
Soft chancre, 237
Soft tissue avulsion, repair of, 672–674
Soft tissue injuries, 667–691. See also *Wound(s)*.
cleaning of, 668
debridement of, 668–669
examination of, 668
management of, initial, 667–669
Soil fumigant poisoning, 596
Solanine poisoning, 532, 597
Somatic pain, 140
Sominex poisoning, 597
Somnifacients, prescription warnings for, 95
Somonal poisoning, 575
Sorrel poisoning, 590
Spanish bayonet poisoning, 597
Spanish fly poisoning, 500
Specimen collection setup, 78
Speed. See *Amphetamines*.
Speedballs, 597
Spider bites, black widow, 170, 176
brown spider, 170, 176
tarantula, 176
Spider lily poisoning, 597
Spinal cord compression, nontraumatic, 429
traumatic, 427–429
Spinal cord injuries, traction in, 114
Spinal puncture, 114–116
headache in, 213–214
in head injuries, 353
Spine. See also *Back; Vertebra(e)*.
cervical. See also *Neck*.
arthritis of, headache in, 207
dislocations of, 381
fractures of, 381
splinting of, 374(t)
dislocations of, 384
fractures of, 219, 381, 384–385
immobilization of, 20, 23, 374(t)
injuries of, with cord compression, 427–429
Spirits of camphor poisoning, 500
Spirochetes, antimicrobial drugs for, 264(t)
Spleen, injuries of, 685
perforation of, 303–304
Splinters, 300–301
Splinting, 20, 23, 373–376, 374(t)–375(t)
of cervical spine, 20, 23, 374(t)
of finger, 340
of hand, 338
Splinting (*Continued*)
patient instructions for, 376
types of, 373, 374(t)–375(t)
Spotted cowbane poisoning, 508
Spouse abuse, 328–329
Sprains, 376–377, 377(t)
in catastrophes, 14
of ankle, 402
of back, 382–383
Spurred rye poisoning, 524
Squamous cell cervical intraepithelial neoplasia, 260
Squaw mint poisoning, 573
Squaw weed poisoning, 594
Squill poisoning, 597
Squirrel poisons, 597
Stab wounds, 685
of chest, 219
Staggerbush poisoning, 598
Staining, corneal, 281, 287
Stannic salt poisoning, 598
Stannous salt poisoning, 598
Staphylococcal infections, of skin, 658
Staple gun injuries, 685
Star anise poisoning, 598
Star of Bethlehem poisoning, 598
Statutes of limitations, on malpractice, 733
Stenosing tenovaginitis, 342
Steri-Strips, *670*
Sternoclavicular dislocations, 385
Sternoclavicular fractures, 385
Sternum, fracture of, 218, 385
Steroids, anesthetic potentiation by, 230
Stevens-Johnson syndrome, 661
Stillbirth, defined, 730
Stimulants, 539(t)
poisoning by, 466(t)
Sting(s), 691–695. See also *Bites*.
ant, 169
bee, 154, 691–692
blue bottle, 694
caddis fly, 692
caterpillar, 692–693, 694
cone shell, 693
coral, 693
fire ant, 693
hornet, 695
insect, allergic reaction to, 154–155, 690–691
jellyfish, 695
larval, 693
marine animal, 693
Portuguese man-of-war, 694
puss caterpillar, 694
sea anemone, 694–695
sea nettle, 694–695
sea urchin, 695
scorpion, 694
stingaree, 695
stingray, 695
yellow jacket, 695
wasp, 695

Stingaree stings, 695
Stinging bean poisoning, 561
Stingray stings, 695
Stinkweed poisoning, 514
Stitch abscess, 153
Stoddard solvent poisoning, 598
Stokes-Adams syndrome, 203
Stomach. See also *Gastric.*
  foreign bodies in, 299–300
  perforation of, 303–304
Stomatitis, ulcerative fetid, 702–703
Stool, blood in, 304–306, *305*
  impacted, 302–303
Straddling injuries, 318, 321–322
Strains, 376–377
  in catastrophes, 14
  of back, 382–383
  of neck, 381–382, 422
Stramonium, 598
Strelitzia poisoning, 494
Strength, evaluation of, 424(t)
Streptococcal infections, hemolytic, 241
  of skin, 658
Streptococcal myositis, 688–691, 689(t)
Streptodornase poisoning, 598
Streptokinase poisoning, 598
Stress fractures, 406(t)
Stroke, causes of, differential diagnosis of, 716(t)
  prevention of, 718(t)
  treatment of, 717(t), 718(t)
Strychnine, 598–599
STP poisoning, 539
Stud gun injuries, 685
Stye, 285
Subarachnoid hemorrhage, 715
Subarachnoid puncture, 114–116
Subclavian vein cannulation, 120(t), 123–129, *129*
Subcutaneous emphysema, 221
Subdiaphragmatic abscess, 153
Subdural hemorrhage, 350–351, 715
Subluxation, of radial head, 390
Subpoenas, 753–754
Subrogation cases, 732
Subungual hematoma, 339
Suburethral abscess, 153
Sudden infant death syndrome, 459–460
Suicidal ideation, 619–620
Suicide and suicide attempts, 103–104
  vs. self-poisoning, 462
Suladyne poisoning, 599
Sulfadiazine poisoning, 599
Sulfamethizole poisoning, 599
Sulfamethoxazole poisoning, 599
Sulfisoxazole poisoning, 599
Sulfocyanate poisoning, 604–605
Sulfonamide poisoning, 599
Sulfotepp poisoning, 567–568
Sulfur chloride poisoning, 599
Sulfur dioxide poisoning, 600
Sulfur poisoning, 599
Sulfuric acid poisoning, 477, 600
Sulfuryl chloride poisoning, 600
Sulindac poisoning, 600
Sunburn, 189, 664
Sunlight headache, 214
Sunstroke, 712
Suntan creams and lotions, poisoning from, 600
Superglue, skin bonding with, 666
Superior mesenteric artery thrombosis, abdominal pain in, 146(t)
Superior vena cava syndrome, in cancer patients, 449(t)
Suppurative flexor tenosynovitis, 338
Supracondylar fractures, 389
Supraventricular tachycardia, *192, 193,* 204–205. See also *Cardiac arrhythmias.*
  nodal paroxysmal, *192,* 201
Surgery, consent to, 739–743
  permit for, 743–744
  refusal to be informed of, 743
Surgical setup, 78
Suture abscess, 153
Suturing, 669–674, *661–665*
Swan-Ganz catheter, 116
Sweet pea poisoning, 600
Swimmer's ear, 272
Symblepharon, 285
Symbols, commonly used, 769
Symmetrel poisoning, 537
Sympathetic ophthalmia, 291
Syncope, 620, 720–721
  carotid sinus, 432
  causes of, 432
  differential diagnosis of, 430(t)–431(t)
  in pregnancy, 445–446
  vasopressor, 620
    differential diagnosis of, 430(t)–431(t)
Syndrox poisoning, 556
Synergistic necrotizing cellulitis, 688–691, 689(t)
Syntho-San poisoning, 492
Synthroid poisoning, 606
Syphilis, 253–256
  hard chancre in, 237
  postexposure prophylaxis for, 256
  soft chancre in, 237
Syrup of ipecac, 463
  dosage and administration of, 54(t)–55(t)
Systox poisoning, 515, 567–568

T_3 poisoning, 606
T_4 poisoning, 606
Tachycardia. See also *Cardiac arrhythmias.*
  atrial, *193*
  nodal paroxysmal, *192,* 201
  sinus, *192,* 203

Tachycardia (*Continued*)
supraventricular, *192, 193,* 204–205
ventricular, *193,* 205–206
prophylaxis for, 206
vs. supraventricular tachycardia with aberrant ventricular conduction, 205
without pulse, 37
Tagamet poisoning, 508
Talc poisoning, 600
Talwin poisoning, 573
Tanacetum vulgare poisoning, 600
Tandearil poisoning, 579
Tannic acid poisoning, 600–601
Tannin poisoning, 600–601
Tansy poisoning, 600
Tapazole poisoning, 556
Tapeworms, 314(t)–315(t)
Tar burns, 185
of eye, 187
Tar poisoning, 601
Tar camphor poisoning, 563
Tarantula bites, 176
Tares poisoning, 550
Tarsus, dislocations of, 403
fractures of, 404
Tartaric acid, 601
Taxus baccata poisoning, 601
TCA poisoning, 601
TCDD poisoning, 601
TCE poisoning, 601
TDE poisoning, 601
Teaberry oil poisoning, 558
Tear gas burns, 190
Tear gas gun and pen injuries, 505, 686
Teel poisoning, 594
Teething powder poisoning, 601
Teflon poisoning, 601
Tegretol, toxicologic values for, 777(t)
Tellurium poisoning, 602
Temperature conversion table, 772
Temperature variation emergencies, 704–712
Temporal arteritis, 713
Temporomandibular dislocations, 381
Temporomandibular joint syndrome, 702
Tempra. See *Acetaminophen.*
Tendinitis, acute, 378
Tendon(s), Achilles, rupture of, 406(t)
injuries of, 377–378, 378(t)
of hand, examination of, 335
lacerated, repair of, 677
plantaris, rupture of, 406(t)
Tendon sheath abscess, 338
Tenosynovitis, flexor, suppurative, 338
Tenovaginitis, stenosing, 342
Tension headaches, 213, 214
Tension pneumothorax, 220, *220*
TEPP poisoning, 567–568, 602
Terpin hydrate poisoning, 602
Terpineol poisoning, 602
Test(s), 130–135
alcohol intoxication, 130–133
blood. See *Blood tests.*
Test(s) (*Continued*)
Doppler, 133
fibrinogen coagulation, 133
for knee disorders, 398–399, 400(t)
for presence of blood, 133
hearing, 269
Lachman, 399
naloxone hydrochloride, 133–134
narcotic addiction, 133–134
oculocephalic, 344, 345(t)
oculovestibular, 344, 345(t)
opium derivative, 134
Rinne, 269
salicylate ingestion, 134
seminal fluid, 134–135
tilt, 649(t)
tuning fork, 269
ventilation, 135
vision, 281
Weber, 269
wrinkle, 334
Testimony, court, 754–755
Testis, fracture of, 318–320
torsion of, 321
Tetanus, 256–257
Tetanus immune globulin, dosage and administration of, 54(t)–55(t)
Tetanus immunization, 135–137
for hand injuries, 334
Tetany, 371–372
Tetrachlorethane poisoning, 601
Tetrachlorodiphenylethane poisoning, 514, 601, 602
Tetrachloroethylene poisoning, 602
Tetraethyl lead poisoning, 602
Tetraethylpropyrophosphate poisoning, 602
Tetrafluoroethylene poisoning, 602
Tetrahydronaphthalene poisoning, 602
Tetralin poisoning, 602
Tetramethyl disulfide poisoning, 605
Tetramethylthiuram disulfide poisoning, 602
Tetraodon poisoning, 532
Tetraodontiae poisoning, 602–603
Tetrin poisoning, 567–568, 602
Thallium poisoning, 603
Theobromine poisoning, 603
Theophylline, poisoning from, 603
toxicologic values for, 779(t)
Therapeutic procedures, consent forms for, 736
Thermometer conversion chart, 772(t)
Thiamine hydrochloride poisoning, 604
Thiazide diuretics poisoning, 604
Thimerosal poisoning, 553–554
Thimet poisoning, 567–568
Thiocyanate poisoning, 604–605
Thioglycolate poisoning, 605
Thionyl chloride poisoning, 605
Thiophos poisoning, 572
Thioridazine, for pain, 85
Thiosulfil poisoning, 599

Thiouracil poisoning, 605
Thiram poisoning, 605
Thomas slag, 605
Thoracentesis, 116, *116*
Thoracic spine. See *Spine.*
Thoracostomy, 116–118, *117*
Thoracotomy, closed, 216
Thorax. See *Chest.*
Thorazine poisoning, 507
Thorium oxide poisoning, 605
Thorn apple poisoning, 514
Threadworms, 314(t)–315(t)
Threshold limit value (TLV), 473
Throat, burns of, 188
  foreign bodies in, 297
Thromboangiitis obliterans, 721
Thrombocytopenia, 356(t)–357(t), 361
Thrombophlebitis, 723
  postinjection, 724
Thrombosis, 721
  cerebral, and prolonged postoperative coma, 231
  superior mesenteric artery, abdominal pain in, 146(t)
Thuja poisoning, 486
Thumb. See also *Finger(s); Hand.*
  fractures of, 393
  gamekeeper's, 342
Thymol poisoning, 605–606
Thyroid, radioactive uptake by, treatment for, 15
Thyroid disorders, 276–278
Thyroid extract poisoning, 606
Thyroid storm, 276–277
Thyrotoxicosis, 276–277
  congenital, 454
Tibia, fractures of, 402
  splinting of, 375(t)
Tibial tubercle fragmentation, 402
Tic douloureux, 422
Tick bites, 175(t), 176
Tick paralysis, 175(t), 176
Tick typhus, 255(t), 259
Tilt test, in shock, 649(t)
Tin poisoning, 606
  food-borne, 531
Tincture of opium poisoning, 560
Tinnitus, 273
Titanium tetrachloride, burns from, 190
  poisoning from, 606
TLV (threshold limit value), 473
TNT poisoning, 608
Toadfish poisoning, 532, 602–603
Toadstool poisoning, 606
Tobacco poisoning, 606
Toe(s), dislocation of, 395, 404
  fracture of, 393–395, 404
  splinting of, 375(t)
Toenail. See *Fingernail.*
Tofranil poisoning, 608
Toluene, as hallucinogen, 539(t)
  poisoning from, 491–492, 606
Toluidine poisoning, 606
Tomarin poisoning, 613
Tomato poisoning, 532, 597
Tomography, computerized, 140
Tongue, retroflexion of, 297
Tonometry, intraocular pressure, 108
Tonsillectomy, bleeding after, 701–702
Tonsillitis, 152, 703
Tooth, abscess of, 149
  extraction of, bleeding and pain after, 700–701
  fracture of, 696–699, 698(t)
  injury of, magnitude of, *697*
  luxation of, 696–699, 698(t)
  painful, 215, 696
Tooth powder poisoning, 607
Toothache, 696
  headache and, 215
Toothpaste poisoning, 607
Tourniquet, 354, 667–668
  for hand injuries, 335
Toxaphene poisoning, 607
Toxic epidermal necrosis, 658–659, 661
  vs. toxic shock syndrome, 258
Toxic shock syndrome, 257–258
Toxicologic values, 777(t)–779(t)
Trachea, foreign object in, 38–40, *39*, 297–298
Tracheobronchial injuries, 686
Tracheobronchial rupture, 221
Tracheoesophageal atresia, 458
Tracheoesophageal fistula, 458
Tracheostomy, 44–45
Trachoma, 258, 285
Traction, skull, 114
Traction headache, 209(t)
Transcutaneous nerve stimulators, 91
Transfer of care, 27
Transfusions. See *Blood transfusions.*
Transient ischemic attacks, 721–722
Transient situational disorders, 618
Transport, of injured, 20–27
    body positioning in, *26*
    by one person, *21*
    by two people, 22
    by three or more people, 22
Transverse processes, spinal, fractures of, 384
Traumatic pneumothorax, 220–221
Tremetol poisoning, 607
Trench foot, 704–706
Trench mouth, 702–703
Trendelenburg position, modified, *26*
Trephination, for intracranial hemorrhage, 350, 351, *351*
Triage, 5–9. See also *Mass civilian casualties.*
  for mass civilian casualties, 10(t)
  judgement evaluation in, 8–9
  multiple injury classification in, 6(t)–7(t)
  victim tagging for, 5–8, 11(t)
Triage team, 10(t)
Trialkylthiophosphate poisoning, 607

Triangular bandage, *373*
Triavil poisoning, 608
Tribromethane poisoning, 498
Trichiasis, 285
Trichlorfon poisoning, 567–568
Trichloroacetic acid poisoning, 477, 601
Trichlorobenzene poisoning, 607
Trichloroethylene poisoning, 483, 607
Trichloromethane poisoning, 506
Trichloronitromethane poisoning, 506, 607
2,4,5-Trichlorophenoxy acetic acid poisoning, 607–608
Trichomonas vaginalis, 332(t)
Tricresol poisoning, 608
Tricyclic antidepressants, poisoning from, 466(t), 608
physostigmine salicylate for, 471(t)
Trigeminal neuralgia, 422
Trigger fish poisoning, 531
Trihexyphenidyl poisoning, 487
Trilene poisoning, 607
Trinitrobenzene poisoning, 608
Trinitrotoluene poisoning, 608
Tri-*o*-cresyl phosphate poisoning, 609
Triorthocresyl phosphate poisoning, 609
Tripelennamine hydrochloride poisoning, 609
Triphenyl dye poisoning, 523
Trithion poisoning, 567–568
L-Tryptophan, for pain, 86
TTD poisoning, 521–522
Tuberculosis, 258–259
d-Tubocurarine chloride poisoning, 512
Tubo-ovarian abscess, 330–331
Tulip poisoning, 609
Tullidora poisoning, 498
Tumors, brain, headache in, 207
Tung oil poisoning, 609
Tuning fork tests, 269
Turpentine poisoning, 609
2-4-D poisoning, 609
Tylenol. See *Acetaminophen*.
Typhoid fever, 259
Typhus, 252, 254(t), 255(t), 259

UDMH, 590
Ulcer, beryllium, 493
corneal, after foreign body removal, 288
differential diagnosis of, 292(t)
peptic, bleeding from, 304–306
pain in, 144(t)
varicose, 724
Ulcerative colitis, 313–314
Ulcerative fetid stomatitis, 702–703
Ulna, fractures of, 390–392
splinting of, 375(t)
Ulnar nerve, examination of, 334
Ultramarine poisoning, 610
Ultrasonography, 140
Ultraviolet lamp burn, 286–287
Umbilical cord prolapse and rupture, 446
Uncal syndrome, 344–346
Unconsciousness. See also *Coma; Syncope*.
episodic, differential diagnosis of, 430(t)–431(t)
Undulant fever, 259
Uniform Anatomical Gift Act, 68
Uniform donor card, 747–748
Unsymmetrical dimethylhydrazine poisoning, 590
Unusual occurrence reports, 731–732
Upper extremity. See *Arm*.
Uradal poisoning, 502
Uranium dioxide poisoning, 610
Uremia, coma in, 229
headache in, 215
Ureteral stone, 327
abdominal pain in, 146(t)
Urethra, injuries of, 321–322
Urethral catheterization, 106
Urethritis, 328
nongonococcal, 249
Urgency evaluation, 5–9
Urinary retention, 327
Urine, blood in, tests for, 133
normal values for, 780(t)–781(t)
pH adjustment of, in poisoning, 467
Urised poisoning, 556
Urticaria, 664–666
Urushiol contact dermatitis, 664, 665(t)
Uterus, inversion of, postpartum, 446
rupture of, 442(t)
Uveitis, 284
differential diagnosis of, 292(t)

Vabrocid poisoning, 565
Vaccinium uliginosum poisoning, 610
Vagina, burns of, 188
foreign bodies in, 301
injuries of, 322
Vaginitis, 331(t), 332(t), 333
Valium poisoning, 493, 516
toxicologic values for, 771(t)
Valproic acid, toxicologic values for, 779(t)
Vanadium pentoxide poisoning, 610
Vapam poisoning, 610
Varicella, 237
differential diagnosis of, 260(t)–261(t)
Varices, esophageal, 316
Varicose ulcer, 724
Varicose veins, 723–724
Varidase poisoning, 598
Varnish poisoning, 610
Varnish remover poisoning, 610
Variola, 251
differential diagnosis of, 260(t)–261(t)
Vascular disorders, 712–726
abdominal pain, 146(t)

Vascular emergencies, in cancer patients, 449(t)
Vascular headache, 209(t)
Vascular occlusion, mesenteric, 316
Vasopressin, toxicity of, 583
Vasopressor headache, 215
Vasopressor syncope, 620
  differential diagnosis of, 430(t)–431(t)
Vasopressor syndrome, 720–721
Vasopressors, intraglossal injection of, 108
Veins, varicose, 723–724
Vena cava syndrome, 446
Venereal diseases, 259–261. See also specific types.
  in rape victim, 97
Venereal wart, 238
Venerupin poisoning, 532
Venezuela nut poisoning, 610
Venous air embolism, 722
Venous cannulation, 119–129
  femoral vein, 120(t), 123, *123*
  internal jugular vein, 120(t), 123–128, *124*, *125*
  pediatric, equipment for, 127(t)
  peripheral vein, 120–122, 120(t), *121*
  sites for, 120(t)
  subclavian vein, 120(t), 123–129, *129*
Venous system, foreign bodies in, 301
Ventilation, expired air, 46–47, *47*
  manual, 47
  mechanical, 47
Ventilation test, 135
Ventilators, mechanical, 47
Ventox poisoning, 477
Ventral hernia, 307
Ventricular asystole, 36
Ventricular fibrillation, 36–37, *193*. See also *Cardiac arrhythmias*.
  defibrillation for, 51
  prophylaxis for, 206
Ventricular hypertrophy, left, *195*
Ventricular rupture, acute, 190
Ventricular tachycardia, *193*, 205–206. See also *Cardiac arrhythmias*.
  prophylaxis of, for, 206
  vs. supraventricular tachycardia with aberrant ventricular conduction, 205
  without pulse, 37
Verapamil, dosage and administration of, 54(t)–55(t)
Veratrine poisoning, 611
Veratrum californicum poisoning, 611
Veratrum viride poisoning, 611
Verruca acuminata, 238
Verruca vulgaris, 238
Versene poisoning, 526
Vertebra(e). See also *Back; Spine*.
  dislocations of, 381, 384
  fractures of, 219, 381, 384–385
  transverse processes of, fractures of, 384
Vertigo, 432–433
  in Meniere's disease, 418
  in motion sickness, 418
Vincent's angina, 702–703
Vinegar, essence of, poisoning from, 476
Vinyl chloride poisoning, 611
Violet poisoning, 611
Viosterol poisoning, 611–612
Viper's bugloss poisoning, 495
Viral encephalitis, 236–237
Viral infections. See *Infection(s)*.
Viral hepatitis, 242, 243(t), *244*
Viral pneumonia, 245, 638
Virginia creeper poisoning, 573
Visceral pain, 140
Vision loss, hysterical, 294(t)
  in retrobulbar neuritis, 421
  malingering, 294(t)
  sudden, differential diagnosis of, 293(t)–294(t)
Vision tests, 281
Vitamin A poisoning, 532, 612
Vitamin B deficiency, coma in, 232
Vitamin B_{12} hydrochloride poisoning, 604
Vitamin C poisoning, 476, 477
Vitamin D poisoning, 611–612
Vitamin K, for dicumarol overdose, 470(t)
Vitamin K_1 poisoning, 612
Vitreous hemorrhage, differential diagnosis of, 294(t)
Vitriol, oil of, poisoning from, 477
Vivactil poisoning, 608
Volcanic eruptions, 17–19. See also *Mass civilian casualties; Natural disasters; Triage*.
Volume, U.S.-metric conversion table for, 770(t)
Volvulus, 316
  pain in, 145(t)
Vomiting, 317
  induction of, 463
    syrup of ipecac for, 54(t)–55(t), 463
Vulva, injuries of, 322
Vulvovaginitis, 331(t), 332(t), 333

War gases, 14, 612–613
  burns from, 190
Warfarin, and hemorrhage, 359–360
  poisoning from, 613
Warficide poisoning, 613
Wart, genital, 238
  venereal, 238
Wartime injuries, management of, 9–19. See also *Mass civilian casualties; Triage*.
Washerman's itch, 665(t)
Wasp stings, 695
Water. See also *Fluid*.
  daily requirements for, 81
  potable, 19
Water glass poisoning, 613

Water hemlock poisoning, 508
Water moccasin bites, 173–176
Water sterilizers, emergency, poisoning from, 544–545
Waterfront cocktails, 613
Waterproofing agent poisoning, 613
Weber hearing test, 269
Weight, U.S.-metric conversion table for, 770(t)–771(t)
Welded skin, 666
Welder's flash, 286–287
Wernicke's encephalopathy, 232, 433
West nomogram, for body surface area, *74*
Whiplash injuries, 381–382, 422
Whipworms, 314(t)–315(t)
White cedar poisoning, 552
White hellebore poisoning, 611
Whitelow, 151
Whooping cough, 265
Whortleberry, poisoning, 610
Wife, battered, 328–329
Wild black cherry poisoning, 504
Wild cherry poisoning, 498
Wild pepper poisoning, 514
Wild sage poisoning, 548
Wild tobacco poisoning, 613
Wild wood vine poisoning, 573
Wind chill table, *705*
Windshield glass injuries, 686
Windsor bean poisoning, 527
Wisteria poisoning, 614
Witness, physician as, 754–755
Wolfsbane poisoning, 477, 486
Wood alcohol poisoning, 555–556
Wood creosote poisoning, 512
Wood naphtha poisoning, 555–556
Wood poisoning, 614
Wood spirit poisoning, 555–556
Wool sorters' disease, 236
Wooly shig stings, 694
Wooly worm stings, 694
Worker's compensation, 755–757
Wormseed poisoning, 503
Wormwood poisoning, 474
Wound(s). See also *Injuries* and specific types.
  abrasion, 680
  bullet, 680
    in mass causalties, 13–14
    of chest, 219
  cleaning of, 668
  closure of, 669–674, *670–675*
  contusion, 681
  crushing, 681
  debridement of, 668
    in hand injuries, 336, *337*
  degloving, 686–687
  dressings for, 677–678
  examination of, 668
  fishook, 681, *682*
  follow-up care of, 678, *679*
  gas abscess of, 151
Wound(s) *(Continued)*
  gas formation in, 688, 689(t)
  grease gun, 683
  infection of, 674, 688–691
  laceration, 667–674, *670–677*
  paint gun, 683
  penetrating, 684
    in mass casualties, 13–14
  perforating, 685
  poison removal from, 462
  postoperative care of, 677–678
  puncture, 684
  stab, 685
  staple gun, 685
  stitch abscess of, 153
  stud gun, 685
  tear gas pen and gun, 686
  tetanus-prone, 135–136
  windshield glass, 686
  with severed parts, repair of, 672–674, 691
  wringer-type, 686–687
  zipper, 687
Wrapping, centripetal compressive, 726, *726*
  for ring removal, 114
Wringer-type injuries, 686–687
Wrinkle test, 334
Wrist, dislocations of, 392
  fractures of, 392
  nerve blocks for, *88*
  splinting of, 375(t)

Xylene poisoning, 491–492, 614
Xylol poisoning, 491–492
X-rays, 137–140
  alternatives to, 140
  burns from, 139, 190
  fluoroscopic, 139
  for foreign object localization, 295
  gonad protection from, 139
  in abdominal pain, 147–148
  in poisoning, 461
  indications for, 137–138
  interpretation of, 138–139
  ordering views for, 138, 138(t)
  ownership of, 139
  specialized studies in, 140
  transferral of, 139

Yage, 539
Yaupon poisoning, 614
Yellow cedar poisoning, 486
Yellow fever, 265
Yellow jacket stings, 695
Yellow jasmine poisoning, 535
Yew poisoning, 601, 614
Yucca poisoning, 597

Z-plasty, 674
Zarontin, normal and toxic levels of, 777(t)
Zeneb poisoning, 522
Zerlate poisoning, 522, 614
Zinc chills, 554
Zinc chloride poisoning, 614
Zinc cyanide poisoning, 614
Zinc dimethyldithiocarbamate poisoning, 614
Zinc oxide poisoning, by ingestion, 615
  by inhalation, 554
Zinc phosphate poisoning, 615
Zinc poisoning, food-borne, 532
Zinc stearate poisoning, 615
Zinc sulfate poisoning, 615
Zipper injuries, 687
Ziram poisoning, 522, 614
Zygadenus venenosus poisoning, 615

Emergency Telephone Numbers

	Area Code	Number
Ambulance		
Air Ambulance		
Fire Department		
Police Department		
Sheriff's Office		
Highway Patrol		
Mobile Emergency Unit		
Central Disaster Number (if not 911)		
Burn Center		
Rape Center		
Mental Crisis Center		
Alcohol Detoxification Center		
Dental Emergency (24-hour)		
Local Body Organ Bank†		
*National Body Organ Bank†	800	24-DONOR
Medical-Surgical Supply		
Pharmacy		
Hospitals		
Misc.		

*Indicates 24-hour telephone information service. Dial 1 before all of these numbers.
†See also *8–13, Organ Donation*.